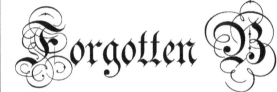

ISBN 978-1-5278-7514-2
PIBN 10916214

1 MONTH OF
FREE
READING

at
www.ForgottenBooks.com

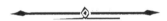

By purchasing this book you are eligible for one month membership to ForgottenBooks.com, giving you unlimited access to our entire collection of over 1,000,000 titles via our web site and mobile apps.

To claim your free month visit: www.forgottenbooks.com/free916214

English
Français
Deutsche
Italiano
Español
Português

www.forgottenbooks.com

Mythology Photography **Fiction**
Fishing Christianity **Art** Cooking
Essays Buddhism Freemasonry
Medicine **Biology** Music **Ancient
Egypt** Evolution Carpentry Physics
Dance Geology **Mathematics** Fitness
Shakespeare **Folklore** Yoga Marketing
Confidence Immortality Biographies
Poetry **Psychology** Witchcraft
Electronics Chemistry History **Law**
Accounting **Philosophy** Anthropology
Alchemy Drama Quantum Mechanics
Atheism Sexual Health **Ancient History**
Entrepreneurship Languages Sport
Paleontology Needlework Islam
Metaphysics Investment Archaeology
Parenting Statistics Criminology
Motivational

CONTENTS OF VOLUME IV.

DISEASES OF THE GENITO-URINARY SYSTEM.

[1] Though properly belonging in Vol. V., with Diseases of the Nervous System, this section has been placed here for convenience.

CONTRIBUTORS TO VOLUME IV.

BAER, B. F., M. D.,
> Professor of Obstetrics and Gynæcology in the Philadelphia Polyclinic and College for Graduates in Medicine, and Dean of the Faculty; Obstetrician to Maternity Hospital; President of the Obstetrical Society of Philadelphia, etc.

BYFORD, WILLIAM H., M. D.,
> Professor of Gynæcology in the Rush Medical College, Chicago.

DELAFIELD, FRANCIS, M. D.,
> Professor of Pathology and Practical Medicine in the College of Physicians and Surgeons, New York.

DUDLEY, EDWARD C., A. B., M. D.,
> Professor of Gynæcology in the Chicago Medical College, Chicago.

DUHRING, LOUIS A., M. D.,
> Professor of Skin Diseases in the University of Pennsylvania, Philadelphia.

EDES, ROBERT T., M. D.,
> Jackson Professor of Clinical Medicine in Harvard University, Boston, Mass.

ENGELMANN, GEORGE J., M. D. (Berlin),
> Professor of Obstetrics and Gynæcology in the St. Louis Polyclinic and Post-Graduate School of Medicine.

GOODELL, WILLIAM, M. D.,
> Professor of Clinical Gynæcology in the University of Pennsylvania, Philadelphia.

GROSS, SAMUEL W., A. M., M. D.,
> Professor of the Principles of Surgery and of Clinical Surgery in the Jefferson Medical College of Philadelphia.

JACOBI, MARY PUTNAM, M. D.,
> Professor of Materia Medica and Therapeutics in the Women's Medical College, New York, and Professor of Diseases of Children at the New York Post-Graduate School.

JAGGARD, W. W., A. M., M. D.,
> Professor of Obstetrics in the Chicago Medical College, Medical Department Northwestern University; Obstetrician to Mercy Hospital, Chicago.

JENKS. EDWARD W.. M.D.. LL.D.. Detroit, Michigan,

Formerly Professor of Medical and Surgical Diseases of Women and Clinical Gynæcology in the Chicago Medical College, and in the Post-Graduate Medical School of New York.

KEYES, EDWARD L., A.M., M.D..

Professor of Genito-Urinary Surgery and Syphilis in the Bellevue Hospital Medical College, New York; Surgeon to Bellevue Hospital; Consulting Surgeon to the Charity Hospital.

NORRIS. WILLIAM F., A.M., M.D.,

Clinical Professor of Ophthalmology in the University of Pennsylvania, Surgeon to Wills Ophthalmic Hospital, Philadelphia.

REEVE, J. C., M.D., Dayton, Ohio,

Formerly Professor of Materia Medica and Therapeutics in the Medical College of Ohio.

SKENE. ALEXANDER J. C., M.D.,

Professor of Gynæcology in the Long Island College Hospital, Brooklyn, and in the Post-Graduate Medical School of New York.

STELWAGON, HENRY W., M.D.,

Physician to the Philadelphia Dispensary for Skin Diseases; Chief of the Skin Dispensary of the Hospital of the University of Pennsylvania, Philadelphia.

STRAWBRIDGE, GEORGE, M.D.,

Clinical Professor of Otology in the University of Pennsylvania, Philadelphia.

THOMAS, T. GAILLARD, M.D.,

Clinical Professor of Diseases of Women in the College of Physicians and Surgeons, New York; Surgeon to the New York State Woman's Hospital.

TYSON, JAMES, A.M., M.D.,

Professor of General Pathology and Morbid Anatomy in the University of Pennsylvania; Physician to the Philadelphia Hospital, Philadelphia.

WILSON, JAMES C., A.M., M.D.,

Physician to the Philadelphia Hospital, and to the Hospital of the Jefferson College; President of the Pathological Society of Philadelphia.

ILLUSTRATIONS.

ILLUSTRATIONS.

DISEASES OF THE GENITO-URINARY SYSTEM.

DISEASES OF THE KIDNEYS, INCLUDING THE PELVIS OF THE KIDNEYS.

By ROBERT T. EDES, M. D.

Anomalies of Shape, Size, Number, and Position.

THE kidneys are two glandular organs, of a concavo-convex shape so characteristic as to be frequently used as a term of comparison, situated on each side of the vertebral column, with the longer diameters nearly parallel thereto, but slightly convergent toward the upper extremity, and extending from about the upper border of the eleventh rib on the left side and the middle of the corresponding rib on the right to the second or third lumbar vertebra. Hence they are somewhat less than half covered by the last two ribs.

The upper extremity is a little the wider and the thinner, and by this peculiarity and a recollection of the position of the vessels (from the front, vein, artery, ureter) the two kidneys may be assigned to their proper sides after removal from the body.

They are behind, and at their upper extremities nearly in contact with, the peritoneum, resting, with their more or less voluminous envelope of adipose tissue, upon the great muscles of the loins. The fat which in the normal condition surrounds the kidneys varies, as might be supposed, within wide limits, and is by no means devoid of importance, since its deficiency is undoubtedly a predisposing cause for some of the displacements hereafter to be described. In this fatty mass may also be situated perinephritic abscesses, and into it spread with considerable facility morbid growths originating in the kidney itself.

At the middle of the inner borders of the kidneys are situated the hiluses into which enter veins, arteries, ureters, nerves, and lymphatics, united by connective tissue and forming a sort of pedicle.

The normal weight of each kidney is to be expressed by a rough average as from four and a quarter avoirdupois ounces, or one hundred and twenty grammes, on the one hand, to seven ounces, or two hundred grammes, on the other; but since a deficiency in the size of one is not unfrequently compensated by an increase in the other, it would be safer to give the weight of the pair as from two hundred and forty to four hundred grammes, the lesser number representing those organs which are not only small but anæmic, and the larger those which are either distinctly hypertrophied or much congested: many diseased kidneys will also be found within these limits.

The size of the kidney is in a general way proportioned to the size of the body: the proportion is stated as 1 to about 240. A disproportionate change in the size of both kidneys without any change in structure is a true hypertrophy, and may be met with in persons whose habits as regards the ingestion of fluids (especially such as are freely secreted by the kidneys—for instance, beer or other forms of dilute alcohol) tend toward excess, or where a disease like diabetes throws a large amount of diuretic material into the circulation.

The deep position of the kidneys makes them usually inaccessible to physical exploration to any practical extent. In stout persons they are so entirely covered by their own immediate envelope of fat, by the adipose tissue of the mesentery, and by the thick abdominal walls as to be completely indistinguishable. In thinner persons deep palpation with both hands may enable us to say that there is a diminished resistance to pressure, as in the case of movable kidney, or that there is or is not any decided enlargement. Slighter changes in size cannot be accurately determined, although Bartels[1] states that he was once enabled to detect a considerable enlargement in a case of parenchymatous nephritis by double palpation. In moderately thin persons the lower end of the kidney can be more or less distinctly felt.

A position upon the hands and knees (not the gynecological semi-prone position), allowing the whole abdomen to gravitate directly away from the backbone, is said to afford, by the varying concavity of the lumbar region on the two sides, information as to the absence of either kidney from its usual place. When the kidney, however, is displaced, and when it comes decidedly forward from increase in its own size or from the pressure of a tumor behind it, it may very often become extremely accessible.

Percussion gives even less information than palpation, since the dulness of the lumbar muscles extends laterally beyond that of the kidneys, and is of itself so complete as to offer no change from the addition or subtraction of the resistance of the underlying organ.[2]

The most marked anomaly in the shape of the kidneys when both are present, and the only one which possesses a clinical interest, is that known as the horseshoe kidney, being a more or less complete fusion of the organs of each side in front of the vertebral column and the great vessels. This fusion is usually at the lower end, but may be in the middle or at the upper end. Sometimes there is a portion lying directly in front of the vertebral column so large and thick as to appear almost like a middle lobe or a third kidney. In a few rare instances this portion has formed a pulsating enlargement mistaken for an aortic aneurism or other abdominal tumor. In others compression of the great vessels has given rise to phlebitis, or the abnormal position of the ureters has obstructed the passage of the urine, with the results, as regards the secondary affection of the kidneys, to be described below.

[1] Ziemssen, vol. xv.

[2] It is probable that Simon's method of thrusting the hand into the rectum and large intestine might be made available by a person with a small hand and arm for diagnosis in doubtful cases where the value of the information to be obtained would be sufficient to compensate for the risk of serious injury.

The removal of the kidneys may be accomplished through the rectum—and has been effected many times by myself and assistants—in cases where a complete autopsy is refused. The manœuvre is not very difficult through a large and especially a female pelvis, but under other circumstances may be somewhat fatiguing. Considerable post-mortem information in regard to other organs may be obtained in the same way.

These instances are, however, among the curiosities of medicine, and no rule for their diagnosis can be laid down. A horseshoe kidney is usually discovered only after death, and with no special frequency in cases of renal disease.

Variations in the number of the kidneys possess this point of practical interest, that diseases affecting a single organ are more dangerous than if another exists which can take upon itself extra duty. Apparent absence of one kidney may be due to atrophy, attended with very small size of the renal vessels; in which case a small mass of connective tissue is found at the upper end of the ureter, which is usually illy developed. The other kidney is usually hypertrophied.

The kidney may fail to be developed. In this case there are no vessels corresponding to the renal artery and vein, and the ureter is stated to be invariably absent, but the writer has seen a specimen where the left ureter terminated superiorly in a rounded cul-de-sac, no kidney or supra-renal capsule being present. The other kidney was of rather large size in proportion to the size of the patient, but of the usual form. This defect is apt to be associated with some anomaly of the genital organs.

Another condition, apparently similar, but really due to a fusion of the two embryonic kidneys, is sometimes found. In this the single organ, situated upon one side, is irregular in form and in the number and origin of its vessels. There are usually two ureters, arising one above or beside the other, and directed to their proper positions in the floor of the bladder. A single ureter arising from a single kidney has been seen to empty upon the opposite side of the bladder.

Supernumerary kidneys have been noted. In one case an extra pair, situated below the others, were intensely inflamed, while the normal organs were not so.

A position of one kidney has been noticed considerably higher than normal, so as to push the spleen from its place. A more common anomaly, however, is the situation of one kidney at a point much below the usual, most commonly at the brim of the pelvis. When this happens the kidney itself is usually more or less distorted in form, and receives its blood-supply from several small arteries which enter it at irregular points, forming as it were several small hiluses. They may originate from the aorta or from one or both iliacs. The ureter is correspondingly short. This position is of some importance, since a pelvic tumor is formed which has in one instance proved an obstacle in child-birth, while in another the misplaced kidney itself underwent an acute nephritis from the pressure of the fœtal head. The kidney tumor has in a few instances been felt in this position during life, but its nature has not been diagnosticated.

Floating Kidney.

The most clinically important change in the position of the kidney is not a permanent one, but varies from time to time with the posture of the patient and the altered conditions of pressure—externally by dress or apparatus, or internally by the other abdominal organs. It is known as floating or wandering kidney. In this affection the kidney ceases to be firmly imbedded in the fat usually found in the lumbar region, constituting a support and packing for these organs as well as for the suprarenal capsules, and is allowed more or less liberty of movement, which is restrained by a pedicle consisting of the ureter, vessels, and nerves, with more or less connective tissue. As it passes downward and forward it comes into more intimate relations with the peritoneum, which usually covers only the anterior surface, often with an intervening layer of fat, so that it may even gain a sort of special investment or meso-nephron.

The extent of the excursions of which the tumor thus formed is capable must naturally vary considerably. Sometimes the organ can be pushed or make its own way forward so as to come into contact with the anterior abdominal wall on the same side, and not much lower than the normal position, or it may pass considerably downward, and thus be confounded with tumors arising from the pelvis.

This affection is much more frequent among women than in men, and the right kidney is more frequently movable than the left: both, however, are sometimes dislocated. It is observed in a much larger proportion of cases in the laboring classes than in those whose work is less severe and carried on in less constrained attitudes. Judging from the relative amount of the literature of the subject, it would appear to be much less frequently observed in this country than among the lower classes of Germany, where so large a proportion of the severest outdoor labor is carried on by women.

Various causes are assigned for this displacement. It is stated to be usually congenital, but is not described as found post-mortem in children with at all the frequency that it occurs in adults; and it is certainly possible in adults to fix in many cases the beginning of the disease with a reasonable degree of certainty. That a certain amount of predisposition, or peculiarly favorable position of the kidney, or an unusual laxity of connective tissue, exists in a certain number of cases is undoubtedly true.

The next most important factor is undoubtedly a laxity of the abdominal walls, affording a less firm and unyielding support to the contained viscera, and a deficiency, usually an acquired one, of the fat surrounding the kidney, which enables it in the normal condition to be supported by the layer of peritoneum passing across its front from the spinal column to the flank. This is seen in a certain set of cases where the trouble dates from an acute disease or a rapid emaciation. The well-known influence of repeated pregnancies is undoubtedly exerted in this way.

Another set, especially those exceptional cases which occur in strongly-built and not thin persons, are referable to severe shocks received in gymnastic exercises, hard riding, or falls from a horse.

One of the most frequent causes, and one which accounts for the fact of the affection being most prevalent among the working classes, is the use of a tight strap or cord to support the garments. Corsets, which exercise a more even pressure over a larger surface, do not have this effect. The right kidney, from the position of its superior extremity in front of the liver and its slightly higher place in the abdomen, appears to be more influenced by this pressure than the left. The movements of respiration, especially when reinforced by the forced inspiration and compression of the abdominal viscera accompanying violent exertion, appear to assist in the dislodgment · already favored by the pressure of the girdle.

According to Müller Warnek,[1] who has laid especial stress on this method of causation, a slighter degree of displacement is possible in this way without or preceding the full development of wandering kidney. A pressure is exercised upon the descending duodenum with which the right kidney is brought into intimate relations behind, and bound down by, the peritoneum; which leads, as Bartels supposes, to a hindrance in the passage of food from the stomach, and consequent dyspeptic phenomena. In these cases, when the kidney has become a more freely movable one and has dropped farther down in the abdominal cavity, the pressure on the duodenum ceases, the consequent symptoms disappear, and give place to the dragging sensations and severe colicky attacks which are apt to characterize an older case.

SYMPTOMATOLOGY.—There is great variety in the kind and amount of effect which the movable kidney exercises on the general organism and the local effects it produces. Neither the local nor the general symptoms are necessarily proportionate in severity to the amount of the displacement.

It may be said in advance that, contrary to what might be expected, the symptoms are not usually connected with any disturbance in the urinary function, and, although exceptions are not unknown, the rule is for a displaced kidney to be an otherwise healthy one. Cystitis and uterine affections have been observed in this connection, but it is doubtful if any relation other than coincidence or a mutual dependence upon impaired general nutrition and overwork exists between them. The partial stoppages which might be supposed to arise from the twisting of the ureters are not frequently observed.

Hysteria and hypochondriasis have been frequently attributed to this lesion, and might undoubtedly find their exciting cause in anxiety about a tumor of unknown character and origin; but there seems no good reason to connect them in any other relation of causation. It is undoubtedly true that many pains and discomforts exist in these cases which are neither satisfactorily explained nor gotten rid of by being called hysterical. These abdominal pains, especially of a dragging character, and also the sensation as of something falling or moving about in the abdomen, particularly when the patient assumes the upright posture or makes unusual exertions, are very naturally connected with the existence of the actual condition which is likely to give rise to them. Müller Warnek has recorded the frequent coincidence of flatulent dyspepsia and dilatation of the stomach depending on retention, and its consequent fermentation, in connection with the movable kidney and its supposed pressure on the duodenum. It is not probable, however, that all the symptoms are to be explained so simply, but it is quite as likely that the dragging and tension of the pedicle may have a remoter effect through the renal and sympathetic nerves.

Severer attacks occasionally occur with violent colic and inflammatory symptoms, the tumor formed by the misplaced organ becoming exceedingly sensitive to pressure. These have been attributed to some incar-

[1] *Berl. klin. Woch.*, 1877, 38.

ceration, but there is no evidence that this accident occurs, and it has not been found after death. They are probably due to a localized peritonitis of the investment of the kidney, or perhaps to simple neuralgia. Icterus and hepatitis, consequent upon a circumscribed peritonitis set up by the pressure of the movable kidney upon the liver, have been observed.

Death is not one of the usual results of this affection but a recent surgical writer (Keppler[1]) has called attention to cases where long-continued dyspeptic symptoms, with constant pain and the chagrin and melancholy due to inability to work, have been followed by death from exhaustion, and nothing except a movable kidney has been found at the autopsy.

There can be no doubt that in many cases the symptoms are more severe than might be supposed from the ordinary descriptions, and are very unfairly characterized as hysterical. On the other hand, many cases are attended with but the mildest form of the symptoms just described, and the patients, ignorant of any tumor either from its discomfort or from having felt it, live in health and comfort for many years.

DIAGNOSIS.—The diagnosis of this condition, if the physician keeps in mind the possibility of its occurrence, is usually not difficult. In many cases a tumor has been felt by the patient which when called to the attention of the physician is recognized by its shape. In some cases in thin persons the form of the kidney, even to its hilus with the strongly-beating artery, can be made out. It glides easily from between the fingers, and can be moved more or less remotely from its normal position, to which, however, it returns without difficulty, especially when the patient assumes the recumbent position. The excursions are of course limited to a certain length of radius, of which the origin of the renal vessels is the centre, and seldom go much beyond the median line toward the side opposite to that on which the movable organ belongs.

The usual statement of text-books, that a depression or lessened resistance is to be felt in the loins of the side from which the kidney is absent, and a diminution of the normal dulness, which returns again when the organ is replaced, rests, as regards the majority of cases, rather upon theoretical considerations than on actual observation. The thickness of the lumbar muscles, upon which the kidney rests, is such that the dulness on percussion is not capable of much change. In most persons the outer limit of dulness in this region is not that of the outer edge of the kidney, but of the extensor dorsi communis. Palpation and percussion therefore in the renal region are not likely to be of much value in diagnosis, although an occasional case appears to justify the ordinary statement. The hand-and-knee position described above would be more likely than any other to show an existing depression.

Palpation for the purpose of finding the tumor, if it be not at once evident, or for examining it after it is found, should be bimanual, one hand being placed in the space between the ribs and the crest of the ilium of the supine patient and pressed strongly upward, while the surface rather than the points of the fingers of the other hand should be carried and pressed with some firmness into the relaxed abdominal parietes. In this way the kidney may be caught between the two hands and examined more or less completely according to the thickness of the abdominal walls. Sometimes the kidney can be partly grasped between the fin-

[1] *Arch. für Klin. Chirurg.*, 1879.

ger and thumb of one hand. In this way the size, shape, and sensitiveness of the tumor can be determined, as well as its position and movability.

A movable kidney may of course present some difficulties of diagnosis from other abdominal tumors. The liver is sometimes, though very rarely, movable, and never to the same extent as a wandering kidney, and as it is pushed downward discloses its much greater bulk. The base of the gall-bladder may occasionally be quite movable, but its excursions are of a more limited radius, being of course executed only by the base and not the whole organ.

The spleen, when it descends so as to be distinctly felt below the ribs, is much less movable, and if it descends deeply without great enlargement, its absence from its proper place is demonstrable by percussion. The splenic tumor is also larger, firmer, and more closely applied to the abdominal walls than the floating kidney. The left kidney, it should be remembered, is less frequently movable than the right.

A small ovarian tumor might be mistaken for a movable kidney low down in the abdomen, or vice versâ. The latter error has actually been committed, and has led to an attempted removal of the supposed cyst. The more easy movability of the kidney upward and of the ovary downward or laterally, as well as the shape, and in many cases the result of a vaginal examination, should be sufficient to make the distinction, which, if an exact diagnosis be absolutely necessary, may be confirmed by aspiratory puncture.

A malignant omental tumor might at the first examination present points of difficulty in diagnosis, but even if it were single and counterfeited with considerable accuracy the shape of the kidney, neither of these conditions would be likely to continue for any length of time.

TREATMENT.—The treatment usually suggested for this affection is based partly on the fact that many cases are hysterical, and also on that other more important one, that very little can be done to restrain the vagaries of the offending organ.

A correct diagnosis, it has been frequently remarked, is often sufficient to relieve the patient's mind, and secondarily her body, and may be all that is necessary in cases where the symptoms are all psychical and have arisen from the discovery of a tumor of unknown nature.

As a relief from the more serious annoyances the avoidance of certain disturbing causes may be of value, and such will consist in a proper regulation of the bowels and consequent avoidance of straining, and the choice of an occupation as little laborious and involving as little work in the upright posture as possible. No tight, narrow girdle should be worn about the upper part of the abdomen.

On the other hand, the use of a tight bandage over the whole abdomen is usually recommended, and seems to be useful in a small proportion of cases. It can of course act only by rendering the whole abdomen a little more tightly packed, and cannot exercise much restraint on any special portion of its contents. Pads of various shapes worn under the bandage may bring a little more local pressure to bear. One shaped like a carpenter's square, with an ascending branch to check the lateral movements, and a horizontal one to prevent the descent of the tumor, has been proposed. A truss with pads adapted to the loins and a front pad over the kidney has also been used.

It is impossible to read the history of many cases of this affection without becoming convinced that while the majority need but the mental assurance of the harmlessness of the tumor to restore their mental equilibrium, and others find their troubles bearable or capable of relief by mechanical appliances, no inconsiderable number are incapacitated from labor and the enjoyment of life by the necessity for great care in their movements, or suffer from severe symptoms, as pain and dyspepsia, which demand a more active treatment.

·This has been afforded by operative surgery in two ways. Of these the most obvious is removal of the offending organ. It has now been clearly shown, by the number of nephrectomies that have been performed, that one healthy kidney is sufficient to support the function of urinary elimination ; and if one kidney can be clearly shown to be healthy, the other can be safely removed. Such an operation undoubtedly adds to a patient's risks, since any subsequent renal affection is likely to prove fatal ; but it has been now done a considerable number of times for the relief of the affection in question, and with good results. R. P. Harris[1] has collected 16 cases with 10 recoveries, the organ removed in 3 out of the 6 fatal cases being diseased. Only 2 of these operations were by the lumbar incision, both being saved. They have since been reported.

The operation has usually been done by the abdominal incision, which offers the advantages of greater accessibility of the pedicle for the purpose of ligating the arteries, and also greater ease in getting at the kidney itself, since it has often formed a partly separate pouch in the peritoneum, from which it would not be so easy to dislodge it by the lumbar incision. The latter operation is, as just stated, by no means impracticable nor specially dangerous. Of course it is desirable to avoid for some time after the operation anything which, like the use of diuretics or the excessive secretion of water, will throw any increased work upon the remaining kidney until it has had time to accommodate itself to them.

A singular case of attempted excision of a tumor supposed to be a wandering kidney, which could not be found after the incision was made, is recorded.[2] In this case the symptoms, which, as well as the physical signs, had pointed distinctly to a movable kidney, disappeared after the operation. The author compares this case to another, in which great relief was experienced from a pretended operation for the removal of normal ovaries.

The other operation consists in the fixation of the movable organ. In one case a curved needle bearing a strong tape ligature was passed into the abdominal muscles, through the kidney, and out again. The ligature remained for some time, giving a certain amount of relief from the distressing symptoms, but maintaining a constant discharge until it came away without having accomplished any permanent benefit. The kidney was afterward removed by a lumbar incision, and a deep cicatrix found running longitudinally along the otherwise healthy organ.[3]

In other cases[4] a dissection has been made until the kidney was reached, which was then, with its adipose capsule, stitched firmly into

[1] Am. Journ. Med. Sci., July, 1882.   [2] Hygeia, 11, 12, 1880, Svensson.
[3] A. W. Smyth, New Orleans Med. and Surg. Journal, Aug., 1879.
[4] Hahn, "Fixation of Movable Kidney," Am. Journ. of Med. Sci., April, 1882, from Cbl. für Chirurgie, 1881.

the wound. In one of these cases the kidney became somewhat loosened again, but it is possible that the risk of this accident might be avoided by some modification in the operative procedure. If this operation can be made a successful one, and generally accepted, of which as yet the paucity of cases hardly permits us to judge, it is manifestly far preferable to removal, since it leaves in its place an organ usually perfectly capable of performing its functions.

Polyuria; Diabetes Insipidus.

Polyuria is the name of a symptom the presence of which may be easily ascertained beyond a doubt, but which is notwithstanding occasionally overlooked. Its existence is to be determined by measuring the urine. In extreme cases this may be unnecessary, but slighter forms may easily escape notice if this is not done. The quantity of urine normally secreted varies considerably, owing to many causes, of which the principal are—the quantity of fluid ingested, not necessarily in the form of beverages, but of food more or less succulent; the activity of the other secretions, especially those of the skin and the intestines, and the presence of substances which increase the rapidity of its flow through the kidney or stimulate the glandular cells; and, to a certain extent also, individual peculiarities.

The quantity of water furnished by the kidneys depends largely upon the excess of pressure in the vessels, and especially in the Malpighian coils, over that in the interior of the tubes, and is consequently influenced by the general blood-tension.

The second factor of importance is the calibre of the renal vessels, especially the arterioles; and the third, the freedom of exit of the formed secretion from the uriniferous tubes. A certain amount of back pressure, so far from diminishing the amount of urine, seems to increase it, as shown in some of the cases of surgical polyuria, where the normal amount is considerably exceeded, while the renal parenchyma is being gradually destroyed.

The arterioles of the kidney being, like all other arterioles in the body, under the control of the nervous system through the vaso-motor nerves, it is easy to see how the various affections of this controlling element may act upon the secretion of urine; neither is it possible to deny (although by far the most important factor in the rapidity of the urinary secretion has been shown to be the blood-pressure) that the nervous system may have a direct effect upon the secreting renal parenchyma.

The normal quantity of urine for an adult of medium height and weight and ordinary habits as regards the ingestion of liquids may be stated as fifty fluidounces, or a liter and a half, which is of course to be considered as only a very rough approximation. One liter on the one hand, and two liters on the other, can hardly be considered pathological limits, unless the increase or decrease takes place under circumstances which ought to produce the opposite effect.

Frequency of micturition, especially if nocturnal, is often considered almost a proof of polyuria, but can at most only justify a presumption of it, which is to be confirmed or not by exact measurement. Any existing polyuria is likely to be greater during the night. Frequency of micturition may mean polyuria, or, on the contrary, may coexist with a considerably diminished total amount of urine; in which case it means only increased irritability of the bladder, and is then a purely nervous symptom; assuming, of course, the absence of inflammatory trouble. The rapidity with which the secretion accumulates in the bladder has a certain influence in determining the need for micturition; that is, a bladder containing five ounces of urine which has been gradually accumulating for some hours retains it with greater ease than if the same amount had been rapidly secreted, as, for instance, after a full meal with an abundant supply of fluids.

Polyuria is often, or always if persistent, an important symptom, and the suggestions made by it can easily be added to and confirmed by a more minute examination of the urine. Thus we may have the following combinations indicating important diseases:

Polyuria, moderate, with diminished specific gravity, albumen usually in small amount, and some casts; in chronic interstitial nephritis.

Polyuria, with pus and mucus and débris from the urinary passages, usually turbid and often alkaline and offensive; in irritation of the kidneys depending on lesions of the deeper urinary passages, prostate, or bladder (surgical polyuria);

Polyuria, with increase of urea (azoturia);

Polyuria, with increase of phosphates (phosphaturia);

Polyuria, with increased specific gravity and sugar; in diabetes mellitus;

Polyuria, with decreased specific gravity and diminished or normal solids; in diabetes insipidus.

These conditions have many points of mutual contact and resemblance, but the affection which is the subject of the present essay is diabetes insipidus—i. e. that form of polyuria which is accompanied by no abnormal constituents except occasionally inosite, a very little sugar, or a very small amount of albumen. In the cases where these constituents might lead to difficulties in the way of diagnosis the absence of other symptoms of the disease likely to be mistaken will suffice to mark off the affection as entirely distinct.

The normal elements may be decreased, normal, or increased. The disease thus defined includes not only diabetes insipidus, but many cases of so-called phosphaturia and azoturia, which, if not exactly coinciding, have many points in common.

In some cases which, from the character of the urine as well as from the other symptoms, should evidently be classed as diabetes insipidus, the quantity of urine, although somewhat increased, is not very excessive, reaching perhaps two liters, but in the great majority is discharged in much larger quantity. In a case which came under the observation of the writer by the kindness of H. E. Marion the amount of urine gradually rose from two or three gallons to five or six and seven, and on one occasion the patient, a girl of fifteen, after some unusual excitement is supposed to have passed eight gallons in the course of twenty-four hours. Of this eleven quarts was by actual measurement, and passed in the presence of her mother in the course of the afternoon.

The urine in these cases is, as would naturally be supposed, of a very pale color and of low specific gravity, which from 1005 to 1010, representing the usual range, may in extreme cases fall to or even below 1001 as measured by the ordinary urinometer. I have seen no case recorded where the specific gravity of such a urine has been determined by instruments of greater delicacy. Its odor is comparatively faint, but it is somewhat prone to decomposition. The solid constituents are often somewhat increased in the twenty-four hours, especially the urea, which may be present in double the usual amount. This is probably the result of an increased metamorphosis from the passage of so large an amount of water through the tissues.

It is not always true, however, that the solids are increased, and the difference in the amount of destructive metamorphosis taking place in different cases is probably closely connected with the clinical differences which may be observed in regard to the amount of wasting and affection of the general health. The phosphates are frequently increased, as found by Dickenson and Teissier; and such an increase has probably about the same meaning as the increase in urea. In other cases, however, they take part in the general diminution of solids, as in the case of Marion just alluded to, where they were reported as absent, which undoubtedly means simply present in so small amount as to escape the usual clinical tests.

Among the concomitant symptoms the most necessarily and closely connected with the increased discharge of fluid is its increased ingestion, so that the disease has been called polydipsia instead of polyuria, it being assumed that the thirst is the initial and important symptom upon which the diuresis naturally depends. It has been observed in many cases, however, that the quantity of water drunk is very much below that which is passed. In the case last spoken of the water ingested in the form of drink was but a small fraction of the quantity of the urine, so that the patient drank but two or three pints while passing many gallons. In cases where the beginning of the disease has been carefully observed patients have distinctly stated that the increased discharge began before they felt increased thirst. This of course takes no account of the quantity of water contained in solid or semi-solid food. Polyphagia is occasionally seen, as in the oft-quoted case of Trousseau, the terror of restaurant-keepers. So intense is the craving for water that in several instances where attempts have been made to limit its amount the unfortunate patient has drained the chamber-pot. Emaciation is probably connected with increased metamorphosis, as indicated by the increased secretion of urea and phosphates. Dryness of the skin has been frequently noted, and has been said to mark the distinction between polyuria and polydipsia, in the former the skin being dry, and in the latter moist. In one case, however, where copious perspirations were noted, the patient stated positively that the polyuria began a number of days before increased thirst was experienced. In another very extreme case, attended, however, with no wasting, night-sweats occurred. Pruritus has been mentioned as affording another point in the resemblance which undoubtedly exists between the severer cases of this disease and diabetes mellitus. Dyspeptic symptoms have been noted in some cases, and œdema may take place, as in many wasting diseases.

The nervous symptoms are perhaps the most important in the severer cases. In some which have been examined post-mortem distinct nervous lesions have been found, such as the remains of tubercular meningitis, tumors involving the cerebellum, and softening of the floor of the fourth ventricle; in others the patients are known to have been syphilitic.

Severe headache is a symptom of some importance, occurring in a considerable number, but not the majority, of cases. Atrophy of the optic nerve was present in two reported cases, to which the writer can add a third where failing vision, headache, and emaciation were the principal and earliest phenomena, while at a later period the atrophy was demonstrable by the ophthalmoscope. The polyuria in this case, though marked, was not excessive, and the patient, a young man, after remaining for some years in a condition of chronic invalidism, died. Chronic interstitial nephritis had of course been suspected and sought for, but no evidence of it found beyond the symptoms already stated; neither were there any more definite cerebral symptoms.

Finally, it should be stated that a great many cases of this kind have no marked symptoms at all except the essential one, and so long as they are supplied with a sufficient amount of fluid live in comfort with their single inconvenience.

The diabète phosphatique of Teissier[1] should be cited in this connection. In only a small proportion of his cases where an excess of phosphates was noted was the quantity of the urine also increased, and in these the symptoms seem as appropriate to the polyuria as to the phosphaturia. It is worthy of note, however, that one series of his cases is connected with disease of the nervous system; another alternates or coexists, as does also diabetes insipidus, with diabetes mellitus; and his fourth class closely resembles, with the exception of the increase of phosphates (if this can be looked upon, after what has been said above of the increase of solid urinary constituents, as an exception at all), the affection last named—*i. e.* diabetes mellitus. In fact, many of these cases of Teissier read like what would have evidently been called, without a quantitative analysis, simply polyuria or diabetes insipidus.

According to Teissier, the presence of an excess of phosphates in the blood is sufficient to determine a polyuria. It is possible that in many cases where a polyuria accompanies phthisis, as noted in many of his cases, the symptom may be really due to actual organic (perhaps amyloid) disease of the kidney.

The COURSE AND TERMINATION naturally vary greatly with its etiology and the diseases with which it is associated. In some cases where nutrition is but little affected, and no attempt is made to check the natural appetite for water, the disease may go on for years with no essential change or impairment of the general health, as in the remarkable one quoted by Dickenson, where a French infant had at the age of three impoverished her family by her demand for water, which seems to have been an expensive luxury, and at a later period kept her husband—to whom, however, she bore eleven children—in a constant state of impecuniosity by the same depraved appetite. At the age of forty she drank in the presence of a scientific commission within ten hours fourteen quarts of water, of which she returned through her kidneys ten to their astonished gaze.

---

[1] *Du Diabète phosphatique*, par L. S. Teissier, Paris, 1877.

When polyuria is merely a symptom of cerebral inflammation, of central tumor, of syphilis, or of phthisis, the course and prognosis will of course be that of the primary disease. It occasionally comes on during pregnancy, and in one such case it is stated to have ceased two days after delivery, and in another the secretion, uninfluenced by parturition, resumed its normal quantity when lactation was fully established.

· It is very rare, if indeed it ever happens, for life to be terminated by diabetes insipidus unaccompanied by any other disease, although from its association with many and severe affections, both of the nervous system and of the kidneys, it must of course not unfrequently happen that a patient dies in, though not on account of, the polyuric state. It is strange to observe, however, as has been often before remarked, how thin a shell of renal structure will suffice to carry on not only the usual, but an excessive, flow of water.

The ORIGIN of diabetes insipidus has been found in several conditions. Greater disposition toward it exists in early life, although it is by no means confined to youth. After middle life polyuria is likely to awaken the suspicion either of chronic interstitial nephritis or of prostatic disease, or other affection of the urinary passages setting up a sympathetic irritation of the kidney. It has been found to originate during convalescence from acute diseases, with perhaps preference for meningitis. Syphilis has its share of cases, as in most other organic nervous diseases. Shocks of various kinds, including fright, sudden or prolonged immersion in cold water, the rapid ingestion of large quantities either of water or of alcoholic fluids, are undoubted potent factors. In this respect, again, we may see the resemblance between diabetes without sugar and true or saccharine diabetes. It is favored by the hysterical diathesis. A very interesting case of severe hysteria with hemianæsthesia and hemiplegia and other marked symptoms varied for a time between almost complete anuria and the most profuse discharge of over two hundred ounces per diem.

A most interesting group of cases has been recorded by Weil,[1] where out of a family of 91, 28 were polyuric. The head of the family, a polyuric, lived to the age of eighty-three, while his descendants were robust, many of them attaining a good old age. There were no anomalies of the circulation, and the persons affected were not alcoholics. Their only complaint was of a troublesome thirst, and they declined treatment.

The PATHOLOGY of diabetes insipidus, so far as is positively known, may be gathered from the previous account of its etiology and symptoms. It is evidently of nervous origin in the great majority if not all cases. It is often connected with distinct lesions of the nervous system, and attended with other nervous symptoms. In some cases it occurs in connection with a well-marked hysterical diathesis. The copious flow of pale urine as a sequel to the hysterical paroxysm is well known, and the same thing often attends a severe nervous headache in either sex. It is probable that the polyuria attending lesions of the urinary passages is a reflex nervous phenomenon, since it may be present when there is no suspicion of organic renal disease.

Guyon[2] states that surgical polyuria occurs under three conditions—

[1] *Cbl. für die Med. Wiss.*, 1884, p. 263, from *Virch. Arch.*, xcv.
[2] *Leçons cliniques sur les Maladies des Voies urinaires*, Paris, 1881.

painful excitation of the sensibility of the deeper portion of the urethra or the vesical mucous membrane; repeated attempts to urinate during the night; retention of urine more or less complete, but especially when there is distension of the bladder. Of the first cause he gives an instance in the case of a young man who had a polyuria whenever a bougie was passed beyond a urethral stricture.

Where, however, polyuria, especially chronic, is due to habitual over-distension, it is in the highest degree probable that it is at least partly due to structural alteration of the kidney. The well-known experiment of Bernard, by which an increased flow of urine was induced by a puncture of the floor of the fourth ventricle, and those of Eckhard on section of the splanchnic nerves, show how it is possible for nervous affections to influence the secretion of urine, though the path or paths of the influence are by no means completely made out.

One of the most noticeable points in the pathology of the more excessive cases of polyuria is the disproportion which often exists between the amount of fluid ingested and the amount discharged, the latter often exceeding the former several times. The source of the excess of water has not been satisfactorily determined, but it is evident from a careful experiment of Watson, repeated by Dickenson, that the body has under some circumstances the power of appropriating water from the atmosphere instead of discharging aqueous vapor through the lungs and skin as usual. In the experiments referred to persons affected with extreme polyuria were weighed immediately after passing water, and again after as long an interval as they were able to restrain their thirst, of course being also without food and under observation, when it was found that the weight had been increased by a number of ounces. In Dickenson's case, weighing thirty pounds more or less, where the amount of urine excreted daily was from seven to nine liters, the gain in weight at several observations was as follows: in three hours, $15\frac{1}{2}$ oz.; in five hours twenty minutes, $19\frac{3}{4}$ oz.; in three and a half hours, $3\frac{3}{4}$ oz.

The DIAGNOSIS of this affection rests, in the first place, upon the determination of a permanent increase in the quantity of urine passed considerably above the normal, and, as has been already remarked, may require a measurement of the daily amount—a procedure which it is well to make a matter of routine in any cases where urinary trouble may be present. The increase being found, if it be very great it will only remain to determine whether sugar be present, which will be indicated by the specific gravity and the appropriate chemical tests. Traces of sugar are sometimes found in cases of polyuria which do not present the characteristics of saccharine diabetes, and can hardly be considered to materially affect the character of the disease.

A specific gravity decidedly above normal, with an excessive quantity of urine, is not likely to belong to anything but diabetes mellitus, though the chemical tests should never be neglected. If, however, the polyuria be only moderate, it becomes necessary to exclude surgical affections of the urinary passages, especially an enlarged prostate, often attended with retention and distended bladder. Pyelitis and hydro-nephrosis may also give rise to the same condition of over-activity of the kidneys. The appropriate surgical examinations with the sound may be necessary, but the presence of pus, bacteria, and the epithelium of the urinary passages in the surgical urine, as well as its frequent alkalinity, may direct a very strong suspicion before the sound is used. The age of the patient also will be of considerable weight in this connection.

A point of real difficulty of diagnosis, and great importance for treatment and prognosis, is the distinction between simple polyuria not excessive, but attended by constitutional symptoms, such as impaired nutrition, dyspepsia, and severe headache, from chronic interstitial nephritis, which often makes its appearance with similar symptoms. Mistakes between these two affections have undoubtedly occurred, and can in many cases hardly be avoided except by reserving the diagnosis for a time. The similarity is rendered still more deceptive by the undoubted occurrence of a trace of albumen or a hyaline cast or two in cases of nervous disturbance, without justifying a diagnosis of progressive renal disease. High arterial tension also is likely to be found in both conditions. Nothing but repeated and careful examinations of the urine and of the circulation, especially at times when the nervous symptoms are less marked, and often a considerable amount of time, can fix the diagnosis.

Hypertrophy of the heart, and even slight dropsy, will undoubtedly be extremely decisive symptoms, but are not likely to occur until after a time when the doubt no longer exists. In other cases it may be highly important to carefully exclude organic cerebral disease before making a diagnosis of simple polyuria.

It is hardly appropriate to speak of a diagnosis from azoturia or phosphaturia, since these conditions are extremely likely to exist coincidently with typical polyuria and to make a part of the same disease. It is of much importance, however, to ascertain their presence with reference to the probable effect of the disease on the nutrition.

In regard to the TREATMENT, it may be remarked, to begin with, that restriction of water, although naturally diminishing somewhat the discharge of urine, does not cure the disease, but, on the contrary, in many cases augments not only the discomfort of the patient, but tends to the dryness of the skin, dyspeptic and nervous disturbances, and emaciation. Patients may recover flesh, strength, and spirits on being allowed to drink ad libitum, even although the inconvenience of excessive urination be thereby somewhat increased. Sufficient food and drink should therefore be allowed, although a patient may be ordered to observe such moderation as will not put his powers of endurance to too severe a test.

Of the drugs proposed, nearly all have offered some prospect of success, and have been accordingly reckoned almost specifics. Opium has in some cases been found as useful in these cases as in diabetes mellitus, and probably, as in that disease, by diminishing the sensitiveness of the nervous system. Valerian and valerianate of zinc, recommended by Trousseau and apparently successful in his hands, have reckoned both failures and successes in the hands of others. Nitric acid, in the dose of from 1 to 5 drachms per diem of the dilute in a large quantity of water, is said to have been highly efficacious in one series of cases.[1] It is given until aching of the jaws and teeth, with some gingivitis, denoting its constitutional action, is produced. It was more successful than any other drug in Marion's case, although the specific symptoms were not produced, the patient being now in good health or free from

[1] Kennedy, *Practitioner*, vol. xx. p. 95.

her trouble. Atropia from its general action in diminishing secretion has been tried, and with occasional alleged success, but with many more failures. Pilocarpine from its action on the skin might be of value in those cases where the skin is very dry, but has no very general applicability.

The drug most frequently employed, and which can claim a larger proportion of successes than any other, is ergot in full doses, half a drachm or a drachm (2 to 4 cubic centimeters of the fluid extract) several times per diem. Its method of action is undoubtedly in the contracting effect which it exercises on the renal arterioles. In many cases it has decidedly diminished the amount of urine, and in some a permanent cure seems to have resulted.

In estimating the value of drugs in certain cases of this affection its not infrequent neurotic origin should be borne in mind, as well as the very capricious effect of supposed remedies in the hysterical diathesis. Unfortunately, many cases remain rebellious to all drugs, and can only be rendered as little uncomfortable as possible.

What has been said of treatment applies only to the well-marked cases of diabetes insipidus. Polyuria, as a symptom of other diseases or of surgical affections, is hardly likely to call for treatment other than that of the disease upon which it depends.

Albuminuria.

Albuminuria signifies a condition in which albumen appears in the urine, and has by some writers been made of equal significance with nephritis or Bright's disease. It is hardly necessary to say that this coincidence is far from being an exact one, and that the symptom may exist without Bright's disease, and also Bright's disease without the symptom. For our present purposes albuminuria will be taken to mean those conditions in which albumen may be found in the urine without the existence of decided diffuse nephritis. As a symptom, and a highly important one, of Bright's disease it will be considered elsewhere.

Albumen is secreted in the kidneys chiefly in the Malpighian capsules, where, if at all abundant, it may be easily demonstrated after death by hardening the kidneys by boiling. This coagulates the albumen in situ, where it may be shown by sections prepared in the usual method. It has been supposed that albumen is normally secreted in the capsules of the healthy kidney, and afterward absorbed by the epithelium lower down; but this view can easily be shown to be erroneous by subjecting a kidney which has not secreted albuminous urine to the process just described, which shows no coagulated albumen in the place where it ought to be most abundant.

The albumen found in the urine is chiefly that which forms the most important portion of the blood-serum, although other albuminoid bodies have from time to time made their appearance and have some diagnostic importance. Semmola[1] states that the albumen appearing in the urine in true Bright's disease differs from that found with the cardiac or amyloid kidney. The distinction can, according to him, be shown in

[1] *Archives de Physiologie*, 2d Serie, tome ix., and 3d Serie, tome iv.

the appearance of the precipitate to a practised observer, and also by a more rapid diffusibility through animal membranes. He admits, however, that he has in vain sought for any distinct and clear chemical test by which the difference can be recognized.

Fibrin may occur in inflammatory conditions in the form of coagulated masses, and hence cannot affect the question of the presence of albumen. Casein has not been detected with certainty. Various albuminoid bodies, called albuminose, paralbumen, metalbumen, and serum-globulin, are occasionally met with in renal disease, and may give rise to some confusion during an analysis. They are at present, however, more suitable for chemical than for clinical study.

A variety of albumen is said to occur in osteomalacia which is not coagulated by heat alone nor by heat and nitric acid. This has been called Bence Jones's albumen, but has been seen by others. Peptone has been found in urine, but usually in such specimens as have been or which afterward become albuminous. Its exact signification when alone cannot be more exactly stated, as it has appeared in a variety of diseases, though not in perfect health.

Finally, a protein body, a ferment called nephrozymase, may be thrown down from every urine by an excess of alcohol.

Hæmoglobin gives a dark-red color to the urine, which on boiling forms a brown coagulum floating on the surface.

Hæmoglobinuria may be produced in animals by the intravenous injection of large quantities of water, causing a dissolution of the corpuscles, but the degree of hydræmia necessary to produce this condition is much in excess of any met with in diseases of the human being.

Human hæmoglobinuria may be the result of various pathological conditions, among which may be mentioned some infectious diseases, jaundice, burns, and the effects of many poisons, as well as the transfusion of sheep's blood.

Intermittent hæmoglobinuria, which is attended with fever, is usually the result of cold acting upon predisposed persons. The color of the urine and of the coagulum, together with the absence of red corpuscles under the microscope, will distinguish urine of this character from others which are also coagulable by heat.

Several methods are in use for the detection of albumen. Of these, boiling is perhaps the oldest and most generally employed, and if conducted with due care is a very delicate and useful test. The urine to be tested should be clear and slightly acid, when on boiling the albumen, if present, will be precipitated in whitish flocculi, more or less abundant according to the amount, or, if the quantity is very small, as a turbidity. The flocculi soon settle to the bottom of the tube when it cools, and the thickness of the deposit formed gives an approximation to a quantitative estimate. It is to the proportionate thickness of this deposit that the terms 30 or 50 per cent. of albumen are commonly but incorrectly applied. If the quantity is very small, it may not be distinctly perceptible until after cooling.

If alkaline or very slightly acid urine is boiled, a deposit of phosphates will be thrown down which closely resembles that from albumen, while, on the other hand, the albumen remains undissolved unless in large amount. These deposits of phosphates differ a little in appearance from an albuminous one, but in order to be accurate acetic or nitric acid should be added, drop by drop, to the hot urine, when the phosphates will be redissolved and the albumen, if present, precipitated. It is better, however, to add the acid cautiously to the point of slight acidity before boiling. A recent work[1] gives the following directions for this reaction, which is then "absolutely conclusive and surpassed in delicacy by no other:" "The urine is first made distinctly acid with some drops of acetic acid, and then about one-sixth of its volume of a concentrated solution of chloride of sodium or sulphate of sodium or magnesium added. If the urine contains albumen, a precipitate of coarser or finer flakes appears on boiling." This reaction may be used as a quantitative test by diluting and acidifying, if necessary, a known quantity of urine, washing the precipitate on a weighed filter, drying, and weighing the whole.

An exceedingly delicate and convenient test is that by nitric acid. The acid is placed in the bottom of a conical wine-glass, and the urine, filtered if necessary, allowed to flow on top of it from a pipette, so as to disturb the plane of junction of the two fluids as little as possible, and leave a distinct line of demarcation. At this plane of union, if albumen be present, will be formed an opaque white line varying in thickness according to the amount of albumen, so that after some practice and with care an approximate estimate of the percentage may be made. A deposit of urates may sometimes be formed a little above the plane of union, but it may be distinguished by its position, by its less distinct limitation on the upper surface, and also by its disappearance on warming. In a very concentrated urine and in cold weather this error may be conveniently avoided by previous warming of the urine and of the reagent. The same remark applies to the brine test.

A crystalline precipitate of nitrate of urea may give rise to error if the urine be very concentrated or the experiment conducted in the cold. This may be distinguished by its disappearance on warming or by the microscope. The action of the nitric acid on the coloring matter of the urine, forming a dark band at the point of junction, may obscure the reaction, but with care will not give rise to mistakes.

Another test recently introduced, which presents some advantages over the nitric acid, and is certainly quite as delicate, consists in a saturated solution of common salt in water acidulated with about 5 per cent. of the dilute hydrochloric acid of the *Pharmacopœia*. This solution should be used exactly in the manner described for nitric acid. There is no change of color at the line of junction, and no precipitate takes place there except albumen or peptone, or resins when they have been administered. The opaque line of precipitate may, if the amount of albumen present be small, require a short time to form, so that in cases of doubt it is well to allow the test-glass to stand for a few minutes. It will, however, show very distinctly in any cases in which nitric acid shows any precipitate. The line does not, however, increase in thickness and density in proportion to the amount of albumen so exactly as that produced by nitric acid, so that the brine test is not so useful for approximately quantitative use as the nitric acid, although fully as delicate. If it be desired to distinguish peptone from albumen, it may be done by a comparison of this test

[1] *Die Lehre vom Harn*, Salkowski und Leube.

with the nitric acid, which does not throw down peptone. If a deposit occur, which may consist of resin, the addition of more urine will dissolve it if resin, while albumen will not be affected.

Picric acid is a delicate and often a convenient test. The dry acid may be dissolved in the urine, or a saturated solution used into which the urine may be slowly dropped, each drop making a slight whitish cloud as it slowly falls through the yellow solution.

The iodo-hydrargyrate of potassium is perhaps the most delicate test of all: Potassii iodidi, 3.32 gm.; Hydrarg. bichlor., 1.35 gm.; Acidi acetici, 20 c.c.; Aq. destill. q. s. ut fiat 100 c.c.—Tanret's test. It may be used in the same way as the nitric acid or brine, or simply inter-mixed. Its only disadvantage is that it throws down alkaloids, but as this will not happen unless the alkaloid be taken in large quantity— as might happen, for instance, in the case of quinine—the chances of error from this source are not very great if this peculiarity be borne in mind.

Ferrocyanide of potassium in an acid solution has recently been pro-posed as a convenient test. It may be made up into pellets with citric acid or used in the same combination in the form of papers.

The phenic-acid test is prepared as follows:

Ac. phenic. glacial. (95 per cent.),   ℥ij;
Ac. acet. puri.,   ℥vij;
M.   Add liq. potassæ,   ℥ij–℥vj.
Millard.

This is said to be very delicate, but the writer has no experience with it.

Tungstate of sodium is another recent addition to the list, which it is evident is already long enough for practical purposes.

Several of the tests mentioned have recently been prepared in the form of papers saturated with known quantities of the reagent and dried. They may be carried in the pocket-book and applied at the bedside, if desired, in a test-tube small enough to be very conveniently carried in the vest pocket. The iodo-hydrargyrate is perhaps the most useful. It is the most delicate, and a plan has been proposed for making with it a quan-titative estimate of considerable accuracy by means of a standard solu-tion or piece of gray glass adjusted by such a solution, with which the precipitate produced can be compared as to its opacity.

Exact quantitative examinations for albumen may be made by several processes, but that by boiling, if carried out with the precautions described in works on chemistry, is as accurate as any, and probably the best adapted to the needs of the practitioner if he should wish for such results.

For clinical purposes, however, it will rarely if ever be found useful to determine the amount of albumen more accurately than can be done by the various approximations mentioned above.

When even the smallest trace of albumen is discoverable by any of these methods, the question of the integrity of the kidneys at once arises —a question which a few years ago would have been considered as settled in the unfavorable sense by the same occurrence.

It is necessary to distinguish, first of all, between an essential and an accidental albuminuria, the first referring to that condition where the albumen is secreted with the urine and forms an essential part of it, and the other to the accidental admixture from the presence of pus or blood, which may have made its appearance at any point below the secreting tubes. When hemorrhage takes place from the kidney, albumen is of course present in the urine, but its signification under these circumstances is entirely different from that which it bears when unaccompanied by the corpuscular elements of the blood.

No means at present exist for determining whether a small amount of albumen present in the urine is more than enough to be accounted for by the pus or blood known to exist by the presence of its corpuscular elements or of its coloring matter. An approximate estimate may be made by one familiar with such examinations, but no rule can yet be laid down. Such a rule might be approximately established by a succession of counts with the hæmocytometer of the corpuscles found in albuminous urine of known percentage, or estimates of hæmoglobin by color tests.

The exact conditions of the kidney or of the blood which may cause the appearance in the urine of albumen without blood or pus—that is, of true albuminuria—have been the subject of much experiment and argument, which it would be impossible to reproduce, even in outline, within the limits of this article; and this is the less to be regretted since they have as yet led to no practical or generally accepted conclusion. A few of the more important facts bearing on the question may, however, be stated here. ·

Albumen other than serum-albumen, when introduced into the circulation either by injection into the veins subcutaneously, or if in very large quantity by the mouth, is rapidly excreted by the kidneys. This albumen also, if collected from the urine of the first animal and injected into the vein of a second, again comes through the kidneys. The albumen, however, which is obtained from the urine of an ordinary case of albuminuria —that is, serum-albumen—does not behave in this way, but is not excreted through healthy kidneys. These facts seem to show that the appearance of albumen in the urine in ordinary cases of renal disease is not to be attributed to any change in its quality approximating it to egg-albumen, for instance, but is due to the condition of the kidneys.

Disturbances of the renal circulation, especially those giving rise to venous stasis, are very likely to cause albuminuria; a temporary ligature of the renal vein causes albumen to appear in the urine after its removal, and ligature of the ureter has the same effect.

The albuminuria succeeding the collapse of Asiatic cholera or yellow fever seems to have a somewhat similar origin, being the result of re-establishment of the circulation after extreme anæmia of the kidney. Clinical facts in general seem to point to simple disturbance of the circulation and to alterations in the kidneys themselves as the usual causes of albuminuria, though in many cases the lesion seems to be a slight and temporary one.

Some other conditions under which such disturbances and alterations may arise, exclusive of Bright's disease, are the following:

Munn[1] found albumen in small quantities in 11 per cent. of cases. presenting themselves for life insurance, supposing themselves healthy and having no lesions of heart or lungs. It is not stated whether casts were found in these cases or not, and their value as representing healthy

[1] *New York Medical Record,* xv. 297.

persons cannot, it is obvious, be correctly estimated until some time has elapsed. It is well known that renal lesions may be exceedingly slow in their progress, and it is by no means improbable that a part of these cases may have been really in the early stages of a chronic form of Bright's disease. Albumen has been found in the urine of boys and adolescents, as well as in that of healthy soldiers, tested immediately after rising : in most of these cases the amount was extremely small. Certain conditions, moreover, may greatly increase the proportion of cases in these same classes in which albumen is present. Thus, fatiguing exercise will bring it on in some persons, and the urine of a body of soldiers if examined late in the day after severe drill shows a much larger proportion of albuminurics than if examined after rising. The urine of the pedestrian Weston is said to have contained not only albumen, but casts. It is certainly not true that fatiguing exercise will cause albuminuria in everybody, and it is not claimed, even by those who report these and similar cases, that they prove albumen to be a normal constituent. Some of the cases are distinctly described as delicate without being actually ill. Cases have been reported where cold bathing has been followed by temporary albuminuria. Here it is in the highest degree probable that a disturbance in the circulation is produced by contraction of the cutaneous arterioles ; and it is possible that we may find in this increased sensitiveness of certain persons an explanation of the occurrence of acute dropsy as a sequel to scarlatina or as the result of exposure in only a small proportion of the cases where the exposure takes place. It is hardly necessary to admit, on the basis of these observations, that albumen is a constituent of healthy urine, although this may be shown at some future day by still more delicate tests, but simply that the renal circulation may in certain sensitive persons be sufficiently influenced by slight and transient causes to permit albumen to pass into the urine. It is the almost unanimous conclusion of practical writers, taking fully into the account these recently-ascertained facts of albuminuria in alleged health, that the presence of albumen in the urine in sufficient quantity to be detected by any of the ordinary tests is a decidedly serious symptom.

The influence of many well-recognized pathological states in bringing about venous stasis, and that delay of the blood in the renal—and more especially the Malpighian—vessels which seems the most essential factor in the secretion of albumen, is well known, and its recognition is of much importance in diagnosis and prognosis, since the unfavorable signification of albuminuria in certain cases is liable to be overrated, and a diagnosis of chronic renal disease made to depend upon symptoms which really belong to some other affection. How far alteration in the capillaries and epithelium is in each case concerned in the production of albuminuria it is often impossible to say, since any alteration in these elements which can be observed after death is almost certain to be complicated with lesions which can disturb the local circulation.

Cardiac obstructive disease is very likely to be accompanied by albuminuria, and the state of the kidneys by which this condition is brought about is undoubtedly venous congestion. The urine in a case of this kind is usually scanty, of high specific gravity, high colored, often with a deposit of urates, while the albumen appears in small quantity. A few hyaline casts are not infrequently seen, and do not materially increase the gravity of the prognosis so far as renal disease is concerned. The kidney which furnishes this urine is usually a little harder and a little denser than normal, but with a nearly normal microscopic structure, exhibiting but little more than capillaries well filled with blood, and in the interior of some of the tubes casts similar to those found in the urine during life.

Doubt may occasionally arise as to the diagnosis between a congested kidney consequent upon valvular disease of the heart and an interstitial nephritis with hypertrophy of the heart. In the latter case, however, the urine, although containing albumen, is usually much more copious and of low specific gravity. Diminished power of the heart without valvular lesion may have as a consequence albuminuria which disappears if the heart recovers its vigor.

In many of the cases in which albumen appears in the urine temporarily it is not easy to say whether an actual nephritis may not be present, though not sufficiently severe to give rise to other symptoms.

In almost any febrile disease of sufficient intensity albumen is often found, and when such a case terminates fatally without renal symptoms, the condition of the kidneys, consisting in more or less granular degeneration of the epithelium, is often spoken of as parenchymatous nephritis. If it is correctly called so, it is certainly very different from the idiopathic form, whether acute or chronic, since it is very rare for typhoid fever, for example, either to present the symptoms of acute nephritis during life or to terminate in chronic Bright's disease. In scarlatina, and rarely in other fevers, a distinct nephritis is present, but a degeneration of structure sufficient to produce albuminuria is in many instances a result merely of a high temperature.

Many applications to the skin produce albuminuria, but in almost all, if not all, of these an actual nephritis has been found to exist. The same is true of poisoning with strong acids, phosphorus, and arsenic.

A very important form of albuminuria is that found during pregnancy, more frequent with a first child or with twin pregnancy, and often associated with other symptoms of nephritis. It is probable, however, that in many instances it is a result of impeded abdominal circulation, although it is very rarely that the gravid uterus can press directly on the renal veins. In the severer cases a well-marked parenchymatous nephritis exists; but it should be distinctly borne in mind that if every instance of albuminuria in pregnancy is due to nephritis, it is certainly a form of the disease which may lead neither to severe symptoms nor to chronic disease. On the other hand, the appearance of albumen in the urine of a pregnant woman, though not necessarily calling for active interference of any kind, should always be a danger-signal, and put the physician on the lookout for other indications of actual renal disease.

In many nervous affections albumen may be found in the urine. It can be produced, as was shown long ago by Bernard, by a puncture in the floor of the fourth ventricle near to the point where a similar puncture gives rise to diabetes. Lesion of the cerebral peduncles, section, destruction, or irritation of the spinal cord, and irritation of the renal nerves are also causes of this symptom. It is by no means difficult to account for this phenomenon by the changes which take place in the renal circulation under influence of the vaso-motor nerves which originate or pass through the peduncles, pons, and spinal cord, although it is highly probable that similar results might follow irritation transmitted from a distance. These facts are not without practical importance, for they give rise to very considerable chances of error in diagnosis; as, for instance, where a patient suffering from severe headache, with possibly gastric symptoms, is found to have albumen and casts in his urine, which is also copious and of low specific gravity. It might not be easy to decide that such a case was not one of interstitial nephritis with symptoms far from unusual, and yet it might perfectly well be a cerebral tumor. The diagnosis would demand a thorough search for other symptoms, such as double optic neuritis on the one hand, as indicating cerebral disease and cardiac hypertrophy, with high arterial tension on the other, as connected with nephritis. A careful consideration of the order of their occurrence is also desirable.

After an epileptic attack albumen may appear in the urine for a short time, disappearing within a few hours. This occurrence might lead to an erroneous diagnosis of uræmic convulsions if the examination happened to be made shortly after a fit and not repeated at a later period. Transitory mania may perhaps be placed in the same category.

Chronic mental disease, like general paralysis of the insane, is frequently accompanied by albuminuria, and even temporary mental disturbance in a sensitive person has been known to excite the symptom.

In narcotic poisoning both by alcohol and by opium a similar state of things sometimes occurs. With alcohol, however, distinction is to be made between chronic cases, where a suspicion of parenchymatous nephritis may be fairly entertained, and acute alcoholism or delirium tremens, where the albumen appears and disappears within a few days. In a patient profoundly under the influence of opium the urine may contain not only albumen, but casts, and the diagnosis of uræmic coma is very likely to be made if nothing is known about the history—an error which might be of great consequence, as tending to discourage the efficient treatment necessary in opium-poisoning or causing the waste of time on inefficient measures.

It is obvious from what has been said that the diagnosis of albuminuria as a symptom is sufficiently simple with a little care in chemical manipulation, but that its significance is not so easy to determine in every case, since it is found in so many cases unconnected with chronic or progressive renal disease, and on the other hand may be absent while serious nephritis is going on.

Albuminuria, as defined at the beginning of this article—that is, occurring in the absence of chronic and serious renal disease—is only to be diagnosticated by the exclusion of such diseases, by careful consideration of all the symptoms present, such as changes in the quantity and specific gravity of the urine, in the force, rhythm, and size of the heart, and of the arterial tension, as well as the relation of the amount of albumen to the amount of urine and character of the sediment as indicating one or the other form of nephritis. Thus a very small amount of albumen with a highly concentrated urine is not likely to be met with in the usual forms of nephritis, but is often found in connection with valvular disease of the heart.

Treatment is but rarely directed to this symptom, since, when albumen is present in but small quantity, as usually happens, it is of little or no consequence except as an important element in diagnosis, while the few cases in which the amount is large enough to constitute a serious drain upon the system are almost exclusively cases of actual Bright's disease, and hence do not come under this head. The administration of astringents, especially tannic and gallic acids, has been found to diminish the quantity of albumen in the urine.

(A copious bibliography of this subject will be found in an article by Ellis in the *Boston Medical and Surgical Journal,* vol. i., 1880.)

Renal Colic; Renal Calculus.

Renal colic is the appellation of a group of symptoms caused, in by far the greater proportion of cases, by the passage of a renal calculus through the ureter, or sometimes merely its engagement in the upper extremity and impaction or subsequent falling back. Other foreign bodies large enough to cause distension and obstruction, such as clots of fibrin or portions of hydatid cysts, may give rise to the same phenomena. Most physicians, however, have seen cases where the same set of symptoms have not been followed either by the discharge of the stone per urethram or by evidence of its continued sojourn anywhere in the urinary organs. They may occur in persons of a neuralgic tendency in connection with the uric or oxalic diathesis. The conclusiveness of such cases, as proving the possibility of a purely neuralgic or spasmodic attack, must of course depend upon the carefulness and intelligence of the patient and the opportunities of the physician for observation extending over years. As it is admitted, however, that these symptoms may occur without the demonstrated presence of a calculus, it would be perhaps better nomenclature to apply the term renal colic to painful and spasmodic affections of the kidney and ureter, however caused, and to describe the passage of a calculus or other obstruction under its own name.

Calculi of various kinds, sizes, and shapes may be found in the pelvis of the kidney. They are most frequently composed of uric acid, which may exist alone or with layers of phosphates superimposed. They are usually in concentric layers, more or less irregular in shape, and of a reddish-brown color of various shades. Soft concretions of urates are occasionally noted. Oxalate of lime is the material of many small calculi, and may be the nucleus of a larger one or occur in alternate layers with uric acid. These stones are of a dark grayish-brown and are exceedingly rough and irritating. Among the most frequent constituents of renal calculi are to be found phosphates, either of lime or the triple salt of ammonia and magnesia. They may form layers with other material, or constitute alone the largest and most curiously shaped of all the renal calculi. Their surface may be smooth and almost polished, or roughened, eroded, and almost crystalline in texture.

Cystine rarely forms a renal calculus, and xanthic oxide still more rarely. Masses of fibrin resulting from renal hemorrhage are described. They are said to be of the consistency of wax, tough and elastic. Coagula of the ordinary form may also give rise to the same set of symptoms.

On one occasion the writer saw the dilated pelvis of the kidney filled with hundreds of spherical brownish soft masses from the size of a mustard-seed to that of a pea, easily crushed in the fingers, burning with the smell of albumen, and leaving but a small amount of ash.

The size of renal calculi may vary from almost microscopic grains, which then usually take the collective name of sand or gravel, and are most commonly composed of uric acid, up to masses of some ounces in weight, completely filling a dilated pelvis.

It is doubtful in what way renal calculi originate, their constituents being always present in the urine, but rarely crystallizing out. The uric-acid infarction of new-born children can hardly be considered as accounting for any large number of cases, although it might be the basis of calculi in young children. The uric and phosphatic deposits some-times found in the tubes of the more mature kidney may possibly, when dislodged, be a point upon which additional quantities of the same sub-stances are deposited, but anything which delays in the pelvis or in some of its calices a concentrated urine, especially if much mucus be present, may be regarded as favoring the agglomeration of deposits. A previous pyelitis is perhaps the usual cause of phosphatic deposits. Small uric-acid calculi may sometimes be found in considerable numbers in the sul-cus surrounding some of the papillæ, and of a size which could hardly afford any marked symptoms in passing down the ureter. These, if any inflammation were to arise, would form a mass with pus or mucus which might serve as a nucleus for a phosphatic calculus. These suppositions are, however, rather theoretical and fragmentary, and do not cover all the cases. Constitutional predisposition has been much discussed, though not a great deal is known about it. A gouty tendency, however, undoubtedly favors the production of uric-acid calculi.

A small renal calculus, when formed, may be the beginning of several quite different sets of phenomena. Of these, the simplest and most favor-able event is its descent through the ureter into the bladder, with its sub-sequent expulsion with the jet of urine from the urethra. If the calculus be small and smooth, the passage through the ureter may be attended with little or no uneasiness, but if it is large enough to fill or distend the tube, and especially if the stone be irregular and rough, its descent gives rise to excessively severe symptoms. These are pain in the back at the level of the kidney, in the side and groin corresponding to the ureter affected, sometimes shooting down the thigh; with retraction of the testicle; usually no fever, but much general depression; feeble pulse, coldness and paleness of the surface, fainting, and vomiting. The begin-ning of the attack is usually sudden, corresponding to the entrance of the calculus into the ureter, and the pain continues without intermission, though with some remissions, until its discharge into the bladder. The pain is usually of the severest, and is described as cutting or tearing in character. It is probable that an attack may sometimes end by the cal-culus, which has become engaged in the ureter, falling back into the pelvis instead of advancing through the ureter. In this case the pain ceases for the time, to be perhaps subsequently renewed, or, if the stone grow larger, so that it cannot re-enter the ureter, giving place to the symptoms due to irritation of the pelvis.

The urine is usually diminished in amount until the arrival of the calculus at the bladder, when the fluid that has been retained is suddenly discharged with the stone. Constant attempts to pass water during the passage downward of the calculus are the consequence of sympathetic irritation of the bladder, and not of accumulation of urine therein. The urine is likely to be bloody, but is not necessarily so. The smoothness or roughness of the surface of the stone is of much importance as determining the presence of this symptom.

The DIAGNOSIS of renal colic is usually not difficult, but it may not always be readily distinguished from hepatic or intestinal colic. The suddenness of the attack and intensity of the pain, its location in the side and downward to the groin, will in most cases make the condition very characteristic.

From hepatic colic or the passage of a gall-stone the situation of the pain, which is in the latter affection naturally somewhat farther forward, the tenderness on pressure in the same region, and often the whitish color of the stools or the presence of jaundice, as well as the history of former attacks, will usually make the distinction a matter of a high degree of probability.

Intestinal colic is usually referred to the middle of the abdomen, is accompanied by constipation, while the movements of the intestines and of flatus are often distinctly perceived by the sensation of the patient or the ears of the bystanders, and on the whole the attack is less severe and the pain less intense.

As has already been stated, it is probable that symptoms closely resembling if not identical with those of the passage of a calculus may occur when the substantial cause of them does not make its appearance ; and although many of these may perhaps be accounted for by the ill-success of the search or by the calculus having ceased to pursue its downward course and having become quiescent in the kidney, yet it is well for the practitioner to be prepared for an occasional disappointment in obtaining tangible proof of the nature of the attack. Time may be required to decide whether an attack is due to calculus, or is simply one of the spasmodic or neuralgic paroxysms mentioned above.

If after careful watching no stone makes its appearance, and on the other hand the pain does not continue and no pus gives evidence of pyelitis, it is highly probable that no stone is or has been present.

A true neuralgia of the kidney may undoubtedly exist. Lumbago and lumbar neuralgia may simulate renal colic, but are almost always much less severe, the pain less sharp and more dull and aching, aggravated by movement, while the sympathetic phenomena, especially those connected with the urinary apparatus, are wanting.

The diagnosis of the character of the calculus can sometimes be made with a reasonable degree of probability. If crystals of uric acid or of oxalate of lime have been or are present in considerable quantity, it is highly probable that a possible stone may consist of those substances. These crystals, however, are of little value in proving the presence of a stone.

The important diagnosis of the occlusion of a ureter by a calculus, and at the same time that of the soundness of the opposite kidney, may be made with great certainty if the urine, which has previously been purulent, bloody, or containing renal epithelium or casts, suddenly becomes clear coincidently with the occurrence of symptoms of the impaction of a stone.

It is not of course necessary that in every case of impaction the flow of urine from the affected side should be entirely stopped, since the calculus may be of such a shape as to permit the passage of urine past it.

The PROGNOSIS in this affection is extremely favorable, so far as the recovery from the individual attack is concerned, since if the stone is small enough to enter the ureter it will probably be successful in forcing its way through sooner or later. It is of course possible that this pain, like any other of excessive severity, might cause death, but such an occurrence must be extremely rare.

Perforation of the ureter may occur, with consequent peritonitis. A permanent plugging of the ureter from failure of the calculus to pass will give rise to changes in the kidney to be subsequently described.

In cases where only a single kidney exists, and this becomes obstructed, the symptoms of suppression of the urine may come on, including death by coma if the obstruction is not relieved. Ten days is the limit assigned by Ebstein beyond which recovery is not to be expected, but he mentions a case in which it took place after thirteen days of anuria. It must be remembered that a painful obstruction, or in fact any severe shock to one kidney, may produce a very great diminution in the amount of urine even when the other is sound. This is undoubtedly the result of nervous sympathy.

One attack of renal colic renders another very probable, either immediately or after months or years. Several hundred small calculi may follow each other in rapid succession, or, on the other hand, a single one may leave the patient in peace for a long time. Much depends on the character of the calculus, the diathesis and habits of the patient, and upon the treatment.

The subsequent history of the renal calculus belongs to surgery. After it has reached the bladder and failed to be discharged, it increases in size and is removed by lithotomy or lithotrity. The urethra, however, will usually permit to pass any stone which has come through the ureter. The patient who has just experienced relief from renal colic should be instructed to pass his water into a vessel which can be examined, and if the calculus do not soon make its appearance he should void the urine when stooping forward or even lying on his face, so as to bring the stone to the orifice of the urethra. It may catch in the urethra and demand surgical interference.

The TREATMENT of the paroxysm consists chiefly in relieving the pain, which may be partly done by the hot bath or hot applications. Opium, or preferably morphine subcutaneously, is likely to be called for in large doses. Attention has been called to the danger of morphine in sufficient dose to relieve severe pain in cases where, as in renal colic, the pain is likely to be suddenly terminated by the natural progress of the affection, thus destroying the physiological antagonism which exists between pain and morphine, and allowing the drug to exercise its full power to an extent which may be over-narcotic. The use of atropine with the morphine will mitigate to some extent its danger, without interfering with its analgesic effects.

In the milder cases ether and chloroform may be of value given by the mouth, while in excessively severe ones anæsthetics by inhalation may be called for, and their use continued for hours. This course also is not without its inconveniences. The writer has seen a case where a somewhat prolonged maniacal attack, with delusions lasting several days, came on after the long-continued use of chloroform to relieve the pain incident to the passage of a multitude of small uric-acid calculi.

The use of diluents has been suggested as hastening the passage, but there is no reason to doubt that the pressure upon the calculus is always sufficient to move it forward as rapidly as its shape and size will permit. The relaxation of the spasmodically contracted ureter is of much more importance than an excessive vis-a-tergo applied to the calculus.

The treatment of the incipient calculus in the kidney or of the condition which gives rise to it must naturally vary according to its chemical constitution, which can only be certainly determined after its discharge, but as to which an approximate opinion can be formed from a knowledge of the tendencies and diseases of the patient and from an examination of the urine.

The use of a largely-diluted solution of citrate of lithia or of acetate, citrate, or tartrate of potassium will probably prevent the deposition of uric-acid sand, and might even dissolve a small calculus, although the proofs of this having actually been done are not conclusive. If the urine be largely diluted the risk of the formation of a calculus of another kind —i. e. phosphatic—is not great. Simple water would be of great value in many cases, both as dissolving uric acid and as promoting the metamorphosis of tissue, upon some abnormality of which the accumulation of uric acid is supposed to depend. The benzoate of lithia, by the destructive action which Garrod has shown benzoic acid or its derivative hippuric acid to have upon uric acid and the solvent action of the lithia, may be of value. The phosphatic deposit, on the other hand, although beneficially influenced by a sufficient supply of water, is not so amenable to chemical influence as the other form, because it is much easier to render the urine alkaline than acid when any irritation of the urinary passages is present.

The vegetable acids, however, pass into the urine, and may render it acid if in sufficient quantity. Benzoic acid becomes hippuric acid, and can be used to make the urine more acid, as it causes very little gastric irritation even in considerable doses. Boric acid also passes into the urine, and acidifies as well as disinfects it, and might perhaps be used to promote the solution of a phosphatic stone, though the writer is unaware of any instance in which this has actually been done. It does much toward diminishing suppuration in the urinary passages, upon which phosphatic urine largely depends.

The conditions which lead to the deposit of oxalate of lime are not sufficiently well known to make the prophylaxis of this calculus easy by any chemical means, except by dilution of the urine and by a general tonic regimen with abundant exercise.

Although it is not usual for a calculus to be arrested in the ureter after having once fairly entered, this sometimes occurs, and the result is stoppage of the flow of urine upon that side, dilatation of the ureter, followed in turn by dilatation of the pelvis, and finally atrophy of the renal substance. This does not happen suddenly, however. The urinary passages do not rapidly dilate to any considerable extent, and their increase in calibre under pressure from within has been considered a growth rather than a distension. This condition will be treated under the head of Hydro-nephrosis.

Calculous Pyelitis.

When a calculus remains in the pelvis of the kidney without completely obstructing the flow of urine, it usually increases in size, while the resulting irritation may be the cause of fresh deposits either upon the surface of the original calculus or in the form of new concretions. In this way immense deposits of urinary salts may be formed. Thus, in a case given in detail in the second series of *Boston City Hospital Reports* there was found upon the one side a calculus which when perfectly clean and dry weighed 204 grammes, filling the whole dilated pelvis and sending prolongations into the calices, so that its shape was compared to that of a hippopotamus. The resemblance was made more complete by the wrinkling and roughness of the exterior. In the other kidney were several hundred calculi, from the size (and shape) of a large almond down to that of white mustard-seed. The latter were composed of two apparently distinct substances—one a reddish-brown, looking like uric acid, and the other of the color and polish of white marble ; both, however, were phosphates.

The amount of local disturbance produced in the pelvis of the kidney by the presence of a foreign body seems to depend somewhat upon the character of its surface. Rough and uneven calculi, such as oxalate of lime, are apt to produce inflammation much more rapidly than smooth and polished ones, but it is seldom that any calculus remains without some pyelitis. At first only a loss of polish of the mucous membrane, with a little increase of mucus, may be observed, to which succeed roughening and suppuration with occasional fibrinous deposit. The pelvis, more or less dilated, may then contain a quantity of muco-purulent urine, with perhaps some blood, in which are concealed the stones which have given rise to this condition, and often phosphatic deposits not converted into calculi.

Pyelitis is divided by some foreign writers into catarrhal and diphtheritic—a distinction rather of degree than of kind. The mucous membrane of the pelvis may, like other mucous membranes rarely, and like serous membranes often, throw out a fibrinous exudation which takes the form of false membrane. This indicates intensity of inflammation, but has no necessary connection with diphtheria. A true diphtheritic pyelitis, that is, connected with the general disease known as diphtheria, is of course a conceivable lesion, but certainly not a common one.

The renal symptoms—especially true albuminuria, so common and of such grave import in this disease—are due to lesions of the secreting substance, and not of the pelvis. It is important, but not always easy, to decide whether there is more albumen present than is to be accounted for by the pus. The pyelitis may be acute or chronic, being character-i.ed by the intensity of the attack and the rapidity with which the symptoms subside. The prospect of a given attack being acute is decided largely by the supposed cause : a small calculus passing into the ureter undoubtedly gives rise in most instances to a localized pyelitis, which subsides after the cause of irritation has disappeared. An inflammation from a larger one remaining is naturally of slower development, but may be more acute while the calculus remains rough and irritating, and partially subside when it becomes covered with a smoother coating of phosphates. The mucous membrane, however, is not likely to regain a completely healthy condition.

The mucous membrane in severe pyelitis may be deeply eroded, and even perforated, so that the contents of the pelvis escape and give rise to abscess in the perinephritic or prevertebral cellular tissue, which may be discharged through the loins with resulting cure, or the establishment of a fistula, from which issues pus and at times calculi. Among the rarer results of perforation may be mentioned gastro-nephric and duodeno-nephric fistulæ. These might be diagnosticated by the presence of food and other intestinal contents in the urine, provided that the ureter were still pervious. Vomiting of calculi and urine has been reported by the older writers.

The writer is indebted to J. R. Chadwick for references to two modern cases—one where such a fistula was diagnosticated during life ;[1] and another where a gastro-nephric fistula was found after death.[2] In the latter case a diagnosis would have been impossible, as the kidney was disorganized and the ureter occluded. The extent to which the renal secreting substance suffers in calculous pyelitis varies considerably, and is very probably connected with the amount of pressure exercised either by the calculus itself when it attains a large size or by the urine in cases of obstruction. It is rare for either pyelitis or hydro-nephrosis to exist entirely independently.

The changes which take place are those of atrophy. Interstitial suppurative nephritis seems to follow this form of pyelitis much less frequently than that which is due to extension upward of disease in the lower urinary passages.

Corresponding to the pressure of solid or fluid, the papillæ are eroded and the straight tubes shortened. In the cortical substance, which soon becomes diminished in thickness, the interstitial tissue is hypertrophied, dense, and hard, while the tubes become smaller or in time disappear. The Malpighian bodies are changed to dense masses of connective tissue, but are still plainly recognizable, irregularly crowded together instead of being arranged as usual in more or less symmetrical double rows. The cortex of the kidney may thus become but little more than a mere skin stretched over a large stone, with perhaps here and there a piece of renal structure recognizable and in a comparatively normal condition.

The extremer grades of hydro-nephrosis do not seem to be met with in this form of atrophy, but the pelvis is considerably dilated, while its internal capacity is also added to by the atrophy of the renal substance. The interior of the cyst thus formed usually retains distinct traces of its original division into infundibula, and may be, as already stated, almost filled by the calculus. Kidneys undergoing this process of degeneration

[1] *Giornale di Anat. e Fis. path.*, iii. p. 370.　　　[2] Marquezy, *Thèse de Paris*, 1856.

often furnish up to a short time before death a normal, or even more than normal, amount of urine, and one is often astonished to find how little disturbance of elimination has been caused in cases where the true kidney-structure seems to the naked eye to have been almost entirely destroyed.

The DIAGNOSIS of a calculus remaining in the pelvis of the kidney depends chiefly on the determination of hæmaturia and pyelitis for which no other cause can be found, and upon the presence of pain in one loin. It is naturally greatly assisted by the presence or history of renal colic. An aching pain in the loins, more or less permanent, is a frequent but not invariable symptom. It may be such as to prevent the patient from standing upright, and cause him to assume an habitually stooping posture in standing or walking. A careful examination of the urine in conjunction with this symptom, especially if an unusually abnormal condition has been preceded by an exacerbation of the pain, may make the diagnosis almost certain. In the beginning of a case occasional not severe hæmaturia, with some increase of mucus or a little pus, may be all that can lead to the suspicion of calculus as the cause of pain. At a later period an increase of these symptoms, with a considerable quantity of the peculiar irregular epithelium lining the pelvis, may be observed. The latter constituent, however, can hardly be looked upon as entirely conclusive of pyelitis, since the lower urinary passages may give rise to cells of about the same form and size, and the irregularity is likely to be increased beyond recognition by the presence of inflammation. They may also undergo change of form in the urine. The presence of transparent or other casts denotes the irritation of the renal parenchyma.

The point of chief difficulty in the diagnosis of pyelitis is the determination of the origin of the pus, whether from the kidney or the bladder. Cystitis may be only partly excluded by the absence of dysuria. A point of considerable weight is the reaction of the urine, that from the kidneys being usually acid, while that from the bladder, when cystitis of much severity exists, is alkaline or rapidly becomes so. The pus coming from the kidneys is more intimately mixed with the often profuse urine than when formed in the bladder. The whole of it does not in the former case completely subside, but remains in sufficient quantity to form a turbid or opalescent mixture—the polyuric trouble of Felix Guyon, according to whom this condition in an acid urine is strongly indicative of renal as distinguished from vesical lesion. In cystitis the pus subsides in more or less distinct masses, but if the urine is alkaline, or when it becomes so, is altered to a ropy consistency usually spoken of as muco-purulent.

The procedure recommended by Thompson may be resorted to in order to determine whether the urine comes from the kidneys loaded with cellular detritus, or whether the addition is made in the bladder. This consists in washing out thoroughly the bladder with several successive quantities of water through a single catheter, until the water comes away clear and the bladder has contracted itself around the instrument, when the urine from the kidneys will for a time come through direct and comparatively uncontaminated.

In cases where the urine is alkaline in the kidney, which may happen, distinctions founded on the reaction cannot be of value, and the same may be said of cases where cystitis is known to exist, but where there is in addition a possibility of a renal calculus. In these some such mechanical procedure as that just described must be resorted to.

The presence of a calculus as a cause of pyelitis cannot always be demonstrated, but may be more or less strongly suspected according to the conclusiveness with which any other cause can be excluded, by the definiteness and character of the local pain, the history of renal colic, the presence of uric-acid crystals in the urine, and perhaps in some cases the results of palpation. The exploring-needle may be used, and may of course, if reaching the calculus and giving a characteristic grating feeling and sound, give absolutely positive results; but a failure to strike a stone could hardly be regarded as proof positive of its absence.

The diagnosis of renal calculus from lumbago or neuralgia should rest, in case the pain is severe enough or long-continued enough to really cause the question to arise, upon an examination of the urine.

A very important point in diagnosis, especially when the question of operative procedure arises, is that of the soundness of the other kidney. Accidental circumstances will sometimes permit this to be determined; as, for instance, when one ureter is suddenly blocked by a calculus, and at the same time the urine, which has previously been found purulent, bloody, and containing renal cells and casts, becomes clear and normal until the obstruction is removed and the abnormal ingredients reappear. Cases of exstrophied bladder, where of course it is possible easily to separate the urine of the two kidneys, may be, from their rarity, practically left out of the account. Various proposals for obtaining the separate urine of the two kidneys have been made. A small catheter has been passed into the female ureter through the dilated urethra. In the female also a finger in the vagina may succeed in temporarily blocking one ureter, while the secretion of the other alone is filling the bladder, a catheter with a bent portion at the end being used for making counter-pressure from the inside. It would probably remain doubtful in most cases how successful this manœuvre had been in completely stopping the flow of urine, although experiments upon the dead body have been made by Polk,[1] who proposes the method, with entire success. The male bladder offers greater difficulties, which are at present insurmountable. A point opposite the lower end of the ureter can, it is true, be reached with some difficulty in the rectum, and it is possible that a catheter might be so adjusted as to make counter-pressure to the finger in this position, but there could be no certainty that the occlusion was complete.

The whole hand in the rectum, after Simon's method, would enable the object to be accomplished with more certainty, but this procedure has risks of its own. A staff with flattened extremity, as suggested by Weir,[2] may more conveniently, though with somewhat less certainty, be used for pressing from within the rectum on the ureter where it passes over the brim of the pelvis. A compressorium consisting of an empty and folded bag, to be introduced into the bladder and there expanded by the introduction of metallic mercury, has been described and used, with the result of partly checking the flow of urine.[3] The proposition to pinch up the extremity of one ureter in the bladder by means of the lithotrite is still

[1] *New York Med. Journ.*, Feb. 17, 1883.   [2] *Ibid.*, Dec. 27, 1884.
[4] See Weir's article, just quoted.

more open to the objection of great uncertainty, and would, to say the least, demand very special skill to obtain even a chance of success.

None of these procedures have as yet been put to practical use, and it is doubtful whether any of them, unless we except perhaps the use of a staff in the rectum, would be justified for purely diagnostic purposes, considering the great risks involved. For the present, at least, the possibility of separating the secretion of one kidney from that of the other must be looked upon as depending chiefly upon accident, and in case of contemplated operation it is not possible to assure one's self of the integrity of the other kidney before the abdomen is opened. In many cases after opening the abdomen both kidneys may be examined before deciding upon further steps. Lawson Tait considers an exploratory incision distinctly indicated whenever abdominal disease not malignant threatens the life of the patient. The soundness of the other kidney, however, may be considered highly probable if in spite of demonstrated extensive disease of one kidney a sufficient quantity of urine with a normal amount of urea and salts continues to be formed.

The SYMPTOMS arising from a large calculus producing destruction of the renal substance, when both kidneys are affected or one is insufficient to supplement the partial or total loss of the other, may closely resemble those of diffuse nephritis, either interstitial or parenchymatous, or perhaps it would be more correct to say that these forms of nephritis are the symptoms of such a change. Thus we may have polyuria, albumen, and casts, dyspnœa, dropsy, and uræmia. The enormous calculus described above as resembling a hippopotamus had given rise to no marked symptoms until palpitation, dyspnœa, and œdema were complained of; the heart was hypertrophied.

The TREATMENT of calculi remaining in the kidney is, so far as medical means are concerned, that which has been already described, and, to say the least, is not a high degree of efficiency. Rest, diuretics, and solvents of the kind already spoken of, and narcotics, may afford relief, and in the case of quite small calculi, such as sometimes remain in the kidney even when not too large to pass through the ureter, solution is possible; but there is even less reason to suppose that large calculi can be dissolved in the kidney than that the tendency to their formation can be counteracted.

Surgery, however, offers in some cases complete relief. Two operations have been undertaken for this purpose, of which the surgical details are here inappropriate, but the indications for which may very properly be discussed from a medical point of view. These are nephrotomy or nephro-lithotomy, the removal of the stone through an incision in the pelvis or secreting substance of the kidney; and nephrectomy, or the removal of the whole gland with its contents. It is obvious that the indications for these two operations are quite different, although cases are likely to arise where it will be well to change the plan from the former to the latter during the operation.

When a sinus exists from the inflamed and perforated pelvis, or an abscess connected with the kidney has been recently opened, it may be dilated or enlarged by incision sufficiently to allow the passage of an exploring finger and forceps. The large arterial and venous branches which surround the pelvis make it safer to trust rather to dilatation or tearing to get through to its interior than to incision, which must, if necessary, be practised with great care. Experience has shown that an incision can be made through the renal substance without great danger, the hemorrhage being chiefly venous. This incision has been made in several cases, and where the secreting portion is much atrophied is obviously of still less consequence than in the healthy kidney. After the removal of the calculus, drainage may be established for a time until the pelvis has resumed its normal condition or the purulent discharge has diminished.

If no sinus exists, but a diagnosis has been clearly made, or even if symptoms of sufficient severity exist to justify a strong suspicion and decisive treatment, an incision may be made along the edge of the erector spinæ or the great mass of muscle attached to the spinal column and passing through the quadratus lumborum. An incision outside of the quadratus lumborum will come upon the kidney, but too far outside to make a direct access to the pelvis practicable. If it be known, however, that the cut must be made through the kidney itself, then the primary incision through the skin may be made in the exterior line, and will be less deep. Measuring along the last rib two inches from its extremity, and then at right angles an inch and a half downward and inward, will indicate a point at which a puncture will reach the renal pelvis. This may be made the central point of an incision, though it is often necessary to utilize the whole space from the last rib to the crest of the ilium. After reaching and exploring the kidney with the finger, the incision may be carried cautiously through the pelvis and enlarged by dilatation or tearing.

In order to feel the calculus it may be necessary to have counter-pressure made from the front of the abdomen in order to lift or fix the kidney, and a case has been mentioned where the finger, having failed to reach a calculus behind, was carried around and in front of the kidney with success. If the calculus is too large or too irregular to be removed whole, it may be broken and extracted piecemeal.

This lumbar method is undoubtedly to be preferred when it is known that a simple nephrotomy will be sufficient or when the more or less diseased kidney is to be treated as a cyst or abscess by drainage. It is open to the objection that if it be found desirable to change the operation into an nephrectomy, it is not quite so easy to remove a large mass in this way as by laparotomy, and the pedicle is much less accessible. The objection is not sufficient, however, to contraindicate it in many cases, for additional room can be obtained by resection of the last rib. So far as the writer is aware, laparotomy has never been performed for the simple removal of a calculus.

Nephrectomy, or removal of the kidney, may be required for various conditions, among which is to be reckoned a renal calculus with pyelitis of sufficient severity to threaten life or give rise to constant suffering; but as it is often indicated for other reasons, its consideration will be deferred.

Pyelitis may be excited by the presence of other foreign bodies, among which are coagula and parasites. An acute pyelitis may accompany an acute nephritis. Occasionally also an idiopathic pyelitis is said to be met with, but it must be difficult in such a case to exclude the presence of some irritant which has escaped observation.

Secondary Pyelitis.

Pyelitis is most frequently excited by the propagation of an inflammatory process upward from the bladder, and hence it is, with its resulting effects upon the renal structure, one of the most important complications of chronic cystitis and of surgical affections in the lower urinary passages. Anatomically, a pyelitis of this character differs but little from that of local origin described above, except that the contents of the inflamed cavity do not include deposits of urinary salts unless such have been formed secondarily. It is, however, more likely to be severe, and especially to affect the true renal substance more rapidly and more seriously, and consequently to be attended with constitutional symptoms in an acute form.

Two factors are of especial importance in determining the rate of development and severity of pyelitis supervening on affections of the urinary passages: First, the amount of obstruction which exists to the exit of the urine; and, secondly, the character of the cystitis as regards decomposition of the urine. It is obvious that whatever sends urine back into the ureters, or, what is the same thing, prevents its passage downward, will by keeping it longer in contact with the mucous membrane intensify whatever morbid action such an irritant would have, and of course a putrid or ammoniacal urine will induce inflammatory action, while a normal secretion might remain for a long time innocuous. Hence it is that we may have hydro-nephrosis and pyelitis entirely distinct from each other, but are very likely to have both combined in most cases.

It is especially in surgical affections of the urinary passages, involving, as many of them do, considerable obstruction with a more or less intense cystitis, that we meet with the combination of the two conditions. Such are enlarged prostate with its usual obstruction and frequent chronically-distended bladder, with ammoniacal, purulent, and decomposing urine, or stricture with frequent over-contraction of the bladder, forcing the urine backward as well as forward. In diseases of the female generative organs we are more likely to have the hydro-nephrosis and pyelitis as separate affections, since the compression which so frequently arises in cases of cancer or of pelvic inflammation is likely to be above the bladder, thus preventing the regurgitation of urine as well as its passage downward.

Two conditions of the renal substance seem to result from pyelitis of this kind: one, a chronic nephritis already described, with increased formation of connective tissue, atrophy of the tubes and the Malpighian bodies (the latter, however, remaining recognizable, although crowded together), and a general, and at times extreme, shrinking of the whole organ. The other is more acute, and consists in the formation of abscesses of small size, which in the medullary portion are somewhat elongated and arranged parallel to the tubes, and in the cortical portion preserve a less degree of regularity, though still having some reference to the columnar arrangement of the masses of convoluted tubes. The intervening structure is usually in a marked condition of parenchymatous degeneration. This is the so-called surgical kidney.

Whether the one or the other of these processes shall take place probably depends chiefly on the infectiousness of the cystitis or of the urine contained in the bladder and backing up into the kidneys, although it is not necessary that any degree of dilatation should be present for this condition to arise. Sometimes also the surgical kidney may be found when the original cystitis is not at all severe.

The DIAGNOSIS of a pyelitis supervening on a cystitis is not always easy, but may frequently be inferred, and it is possible that by careful treatment of the cystitis it may be reduced to a very low grade of severity, while the pyelitis still remains, which will permit the diagnosis to be somewhat more conclusive.

If the urine comes acid, but pus-laden, from the kidney, it will soon assume the contrary reaction in the bladder, and the pus will be changed by the ammonia into so-called muco-pus; the cells supposed to be characteristic of the pelvis of the kidney will, like the pus-cells, be so altered by the same causes, and so intermixed with similar cells from the bladder, that the distinction will be difficult or impossible. The presence of a few hyaline casts is very likely to be noticed, and indicates irritation, or perhaps a more decided implication, of the renal substance. Nothing, however, can be inferred from failure to find them. Hæmaturia is not so necessary an accompaniment of this form of pyelitis as of that arising from a mechanical irritant in the kidney. If, however, the urine does not become rapidly altered in the bladder, or if by any of the processes mentioned above the kidney urine can be obtained in a condition of comparative purity, the microscopic indications become more precise.

A dull pain and tenderness in the loins and along the course of the ureters is a symptom of value, though by no mean conclusive, and should lead to a suspicion of pyelitis. A polyuria of short duration may be a purely nervous symptom, but a persistent flow of pale urine, which fails to settle clear, and of which the turbidity is caused by pus, is due in great probability to renal disease, and if it could be shown to come in this condition from the kidney would almost certainly denote pyelitis.

The rational SYMPTOMS are of the greatest value as determining the extent and severity of the disease, although it may be impossible to distribute them with absolute exactness between the various organs involved —that is, bladder, pelvis, and renal substance.

The occurrence of a single chill, or even of several, with rapid subsidence of the fever, is not conclusive, since the ordinary urinary fever supervening on surgical operations, even so slight as passing the catheter, is not necessarily connected with renal disease.

A long-continued fever, not especially intense and of a more or less distinctly intermittent type, especially if becoming at some definite period decidedly more intense, is likely to mean the invasion of a new tract of mucous membrane, such as that of the renal pelves or even of the kidney-substance itself. Continued or remittent urinary fever is of very grave import. With this fever will appear the dry red tongue and the distressing anorexia, nausea, and vomiting, with either constipation or diarrhœa.

The TREATMENT of this form of pyelitis, so far as it differs from that of the calculous variety, depends largely upon that of the causative cystitis, though not entirely, since if it has once assumed the chronic condition it does not necessarily subside even if the cystitis be cured. The essentials of treatment may be said to be drainage from below and washing from below and from above. The measures for carrying the first of these indications are those which are also required for the causative cystitis, and, being chiefly surgical, a minute description of them does not come within the scope of this article. They may be simply catheterization, dilatation, divulsion or section of a stricture of the urethra, drainage of the bladder through the rectum or through the perineum.

It is not out of place, however, even in a strictly medical essay, to point out the extreme importance, not only in the way of treatment, but of prophylaxis, of securing a free exit for the urine. Even that small degree of obstruction or hindrance which leads a person to habitually put a little extra strain upon the bladder in order to expel its contents, especially if it be allowed occasionally to become dilated, may gradually lead to dilatation of the ureters, and thus make an easy passage upward for inflammatory and decomposed urine if such should afterward be formed as a consequence of cystitis by retention. The washing of the bladder from the urethra may be done with a great variety of antiseptics and acids: nitric acid in the proportion of 1 per mille may be used to change the reaction of the urine. Carbolic acid should be carefully used, from the danger of its absorption in poisonous amounts. Boric acid is a safe and quite efficient antiseptic.

Washing from above, which is evidently that which alone can directly affect the renal pelvis, must be done with such drugs as can be safely given internally, so that carbolic acid cannot be of much use in this way. Salicylic acid loses a part, but not all, of its antiseptic properties in its passage through the blood and kidneys. Boric acid passes readily into the urine, alters its reaction, and seems to have some antiseptic action. It is unirritating in the stomach, and may be given in doses of 30 centigrammes or 5 grains to the extent of 1 or 2 grammes per diem. Benzoic acid and the benzoate of sodium, ammonium, or lithium have been found to be of value in cystitis, and as they can only reach the bladder by previously passing over the pelvic mucous membrane, they should also have a good effect here. It is obvious that constitutional symptoms arising from cystitis and its consequent nephritis may demand the most attention, and should evidently be of a decidedly supporting character, the details of which have no special reference to the disease, but to the general condition. Quinine may be called for as an antipyretic.

The question of removal of a kidney for pyo-nephrosis is less likely to arise in this form than the other, since from its causation it is much more likely to be bilateral; but if under any peculiarity of anatomical arrangement, such as greater dilatation of the one ureter, it should be found that one kidney was nearly healthy while the other was in a state of pyelitis, and purulent inflammation was giving rise to serious constitutional disturbance, such an operation might be undertaken.

The operation of nephrectomy, or removal of the kidney, may be required for various lesions, most of which include more or less pyelitis, and it may be considered once for all in this place. It has now been practised more than one hundred times. A table including 100 cases is given by R. P. Harris in the *American Journal of the Medical Sciences* for July, 1882, and many have been recorded since.[1] It can, of course, hardly be expected that the removal of one of a pair of vital organs, under circumstances where it is often the case that the other is not

[1] Weir, *New York Med. Journ.*, Dec. 27, 1884.

completely capable of carrying on the additional work, should present the same favorable array of statistics as ovariotomy; but it gives no small number of recoveries in cases which without it would undoubtedly have proved fatal, and it must be considered as having a legitimate and well-defined place among the major operations.

There are two distinct methods, besides, of course, all the minor differences of detail called for in the individual case. The kidney may be reached from the loin by an incision along the outer edge of the erector spinæ, as already described for nephrotomy. It is to be enucleated from its capsule of fat by the fingers, and a ligature or ligatures passed around the pedicle consisting of the veins, arteries, and ureter. The kidney is then cut off, possibly leaving a little renal substance if the pedicle be short and accessible with difficulty. The wound is left partly open for drainage. This method has the advantage of avoiding the peritoneum and the handling of other abdominal organs. Its disadvantages are, in some cases, the want of room, and when undertaken for the relief of floating kidney the difficulty of finding the organ, which is likely to be at the end of a pouch formed of peritoneum. In cases of calculous pyelitis, where it may be at the beginning of the operation uncertain whether merely an incision for the removal of a stone or a total removal of a kidney of normal size may be necessary, this line of approach presents decided advantages.

The other method is by abdominal incision or laparotomy, which is usually made through the linea alba, though in a number of cases the outer edge of the rectus abdominis on the side corresponding to the organ to be removed has been taken as the guide. The steps of the operation are similar to those of ovariotomy where the pedicle is tied and returned to the abdominal cavity. This operation may be one of choice, from the greater ease with which the pedicle can be reached and the possibility of increasing the length of the incision in case of necessity for the removal of a very large tumor. In one case a crucial incision was made. When the kidney to be removed is a wandering one, and especially when a kidney has become fixed in an anomalous position, this is by far the easiest, and sometimes the only practicable, method.

Antiseptic precautions are of course to be used.

Hydro-nephrosis.

Obstruction to the discharge of urine from the body naturally produces special disorders in the secreting and discharging organs. If the obstruction exist below the neck of the bladder, as in stricture of the urethra or enlarged prostate, then the bladder is the organ primarily affected, and it may become distended, sacculated, its muscular coat hypertrophied, its mucous membrane affected with catarrhal inflammation, and its contents changed from the normal by the addition of mucus, of pus, of bacteria, or a deposit of earthy phosphates from the ammoniacal reaction produced by decomposition of the urea.

The effects of distension of the bladder will sooner or later make themselves felt in the upper urinary passages, and will then give rise to the same dilatation of the ureters and the renal pelvis as occurs when the obstruction is higher up. As regards the rapidity with which such changes progress, much depends upon the degree of obstruction as well as upon the amount of urine secreted. It probably, however, never takes place suddenly.

In a case which came under the observation of the writer a partial paralysis of the bladder, probably existing from infancy, had in the course of three or four years, during which large quantities of light urine were passed, given rise to dilatation of the ureters, slight dilatation of the pelvis of the kidneys, atrophy of the parenchyma, and hypertrophy of the left ventricle.

Obstructions in the course of the ureters may exist at their opening into the bladder, which may be contracted by chronic cystitis; at a point immediately above this from compression by morbid growths, especially of the uterus, one of the most common causes of hydro-nephrosis, or even from retroflexion of the uterus when pregnant; at any point in its course by a twisting or sharp angle, as in movable kidney, although this is a much rarer accident than might be supposed; or at the brim of the pelvis, where it may be bound down by old peritoneal adhesions, and at its junction with the renal pelvis, which may be formed in such a manner as to constitute a valve, so that the urine escapes slowly or with great difficulty; or where it may be blocked by a calculus or other deposit in the cavity of the pelvis.

Obstructions by a twist or angle or by a valvular opening may, it is obvious, be temporary or intermittent in their action, and probably some arrangement of this kind was present in the cases which have been reported of relief of hydro-nephrosis by gentle massage of the abdomen.

Above the point of obstruction the ureter and pelvis are found dilated and the walls somewhat thinned. The kidney and its pelvis form a more or less irregular rounded pouch, with the tense cylindrical tube of the ureter attached to it below. The kidney itself becomes in various degrees atrophied. In some cases it retains nearly all its secreting structure, and is merely spread out upon the surface of the sac; in others, while the pelvis is but little dilated, the true kidney substance atrophies almost completely, and becomes a mere shell enclosing a cavity continuous with the pelvis and broken up by fibrous septa into subordinate cavities representing the original calices. A partial hydro-nephrosis is sometimes observed affecting only the calices.

Whether the one or the other of these conditions shall result depends, as has already been remarked, upon the completeness and suddenness of the obstruction. If the ureter of a rabbit is ligatured, the second condition—that is, atrophy of the kidney with but little dilatation—is observed. The pressure of urine soon puts a stop to further secretion, and there is no time for a slow and gradual dilatation of the pelvis and ureter. When, as is much more frequently the case in the human subject, the obstruction is more gradual or incomplete, the back pressure is for a long time insufficient to completely stop the passage of fluid through the renal capillaries, so that the pelvis and ureter, though allowing their contents to pass out only under a considerable vis-a-tergo, have time to accommodate themselves to the change, and dilate gradually, attaining sometimes enormous dimensions. The size of a hydro-nephrotic sac varies greatly: 60 liters of contents is certainly a very extreme case.

The sac is usually white and glistening, thinner at some places than at others, and lined with a smooth, pale, and atrophied mucous membrane. The muscular layer has degenerated, and perhaps partly disappeared. The liquid contained in the sac, supposing no inflammatory products to have been mingled therewith, is at first nearly identical with urine, and always contains urea. Afterward its character changes from the absorption of the urinary salts and the secretion of mucus. The contents may be dark-colored from hemorrhage or somewhat gelatinous. At a later period again they become serous and may contain cholesterin.

The description just given, as well as that of the symptoms, applies to simple hydro-nephrosis. When the sac has become inflamed we have the very common combination with pyelitis, and the affection is called pyo-nephrosis. The progress of a case of hydro-nephrosis may be in rare cases to recovery by spontaneous re-establishment of the permeability of the ureter. In others it persists a long time without giving rise to trouble. If inflammation supervene, it is obvious that fever, either simply irritative or of pyæmic character, may be a severe or even a fatal concomitant, or that in this condition a perforation may take place. When the tumor is large it may from its bulk alone produce disturbance of the circulation, dyspnœa, palpitation, and œdema of the lower limbs.

As regards the influence of this lesion on the secretion of urine, everything must depend on the amount of renal atrophy. A single kidney may undoubtedly be completely atrophied by this as by any other lesion without producing serious symptoms, since, as has been repeatedly demonstrated, the other is sufficient to carry on the work under ordinary circumstances ; but if, as very frequently happens, both kidneys are involved, there must come a time when the renal substance no longer suffices, and the usual results of suppression of urine follow. It is possible, however, for extensive changes to take place in both kidneys before symptoms of insufficient secretion arise.

Hydro-nephrosis, in the entire absence of inflammatory symptoms and in the presence of conditions likely to cause it known to exist in the lower urinary passages, may be rather suspected than diagnosticated until the appearance of a tumor. Some dull pain in the loins without irradiations in any direction may exist, but so common a symptom can have but little weight in diagnosis. For an early recognition of swelling in suspected cases where nothing can be felt anteriorly, it has been recommended that the patient be placed upon the hands and knees, when the flank upon the affected side, instead of falling slightly forward and leaving a shallow depression outside of the erector spinæ, will remain full or protuberant. When an enlargement evidently connected with the kidney makes its appearance after obstruction to the passage of urine is known to exist, the diagnosis may often be very simple ; but if the tumor be the first phenomenon observed, as may easily happen when the obstruction is situated high up or even at the commencement of the ureter, it may require to be distinguished from several other kinds of tumor occupying the lumbar region, or, since hydro-nephrosis of a movable or misplaced kidney sometimes takes place, from tumors of the abdomen in general. From solid malignant tumors of the kidney the feeling of comparative elasticity and fluctuation will in most cases distinguish it, though an encephaloid kidney may be so soft as to render the second of these points of comparatively little value. Absence of hæmaturia and of the cancerous cachexia, though not conclusive, would have much weight.

A hydatid cyst might counterfeit a hydro-nephrosis, but instances of this affection having its primary seat in the kidney are of extreme rarity. An ordinary cystic kidney is most likely to be connected with chronic diffuse interstitial nephritis, which will have made itself manifest by the usual symptoms, and is moreover unlikely to attain the dimensions of a large or even moderate hydro-nephrosis. In a thin person the ureter might, if felt dilated through the abdominal walls, clear up the diagnosis. Extreme cases of cystic kidney with comparatively little nephritis may, however, present great similarity and cause difficulty in diagnosis.

From most other tumors of the abdominal cavity those of the kidney present the important distinction that they are situated behind the peritoneum, and consequently behind the intestines, so that the surface of a renal tumor is likely to be crossed by a more or less extensive area of percussion resonance, representing usually the large intestine. This criterion is, however, not absolute, since a renal tumor may push the colon completely to one side, or, on the other hand, tumors not connected · with the kidney may allow the intestine to come between themselves and the abdominal wall.

An ovarian cyst is more manifestly attached to the pelvis, and its history will disclose the fact of its having arisen from below. A gravid uterus should also, when small, be manifestly connected with the pelvis, and when larger be accompanied by the usual symptoms of pregnancy. The same may be said of extra-uterine pregnancy, which may be mentioned as among the conditions possibly giving rise to difficulties in diagnosis.

The most efficient aid to diagnosis, when it is of importance that such should be accurately made, is the aspirator-needle, which will procure a fluid more or less characteristic of the tumor into which it is thrust. In hydro-nephrosis the contents are a somewhat dilute urine, with perhaps mucus; in a solid tumor, blood, with pieces of tissue recognizable by the microscope; in a cystic tumor, fluid which is perhaps somewhat urinous, but much more changed than in simple hydro-nephrosis, and perhaps containing solid-looking bodies with concentric and radiating striation; in hydatid cysts, hooks and fragments of scolices; in ovarian cysts, the various contents, fluid and semi-fluid, but not urinous, generally found therein.

With all these means, however, cases will occasionally arise in which expert diagnosticians may be lead astray, and the difficulties become considerably greater when the dilated pelvis is that of a displaced or unusually-placed kidney. Such cases have been subjected to operation under the impression that an ovarian cyst was present.

The medical TREATMENT of hydro-nephrosis is nil. In many cases nothing is demanded by the immediate necessities of the case, and atrophy, if it be probable that only one kidney is involved, may be allowed to take place without interference. It is possible that in some instances manipulation of the tumor might relieve the obstruction and allow the tumor to subside when a slight twist or angle in the ureter is the cause. The fact of an occasional spontaneous subsidence of such a tumor shows that something of this kind has taken place.

The surgical treatment of affections of the lower urinary passages, as both a prophylactic and therapeutic measure, has already been spoken of under the head of Pyelitis. It would, however, be only in a minority of cases of pure hydro-nephrosis that the seat of obstruction could be efficiently reached by surgery.

Puncture and aspiration of the sac may very properly be resorted to, and may prove of value—in the first place, as a more or less temporary relief; and secondly, as a means of re-establishing the flow through the natural passages by the relief of pressure and consequent opening of the valvular fold, which has occasionally been observed at the junction of the ureter with the pelvis.

In a case where the obstruction is known to be irremediable, and where the hydro-nephrosis, if existing only on one side, is likely to increase, it is not desirable to make the puncture too early or to repeat it too frequently, since by allowing the pressure to increase the atrophy of the kidney will be more rapidly accomplished, and the need of frequently emptying the sac will not arise so often in the future. On the other hand, if there is a prospect of a restoration, if both kidneys are affected, or if the kidney not involved in the hydro-nephrosis is known to be seriously impaired in function, and it is desirable to preserve the secreting structure as long as possible, the punctures should be so arranged as to keep the pressure at its minimum. This must, however, be regarded as a temporary expedient. The puncture may be made either from the back or front, though in most cases the latter position, if the puncture be made with a small clean needle, would be the more convenient, and equally safe notwithstanding its traversing the peritoneum.

A hydro-nephrosis may be treated either by removal or by drainage. Both of these methods have been resorted to, and are to be employed according to the circumstances of the individual case. A pyo-nephrosis naturally demands interference more peremptorily and more promptly than a simple hydro-nephrosis, because it exposes the patient to the dangers not only of its pressure and of its tendency to destruction of the renal substance, but to those more urgent ones of purulent infection or of perforation and perinephritic abscess. Removal is to be undertaken by the ordinary rules of laparotomy. Drainage has been arranged in cases where removal was impossible or unadvisable by stitching the edges of an opened sac to the external wound. It is possible that the choice between the two operations can be made only after the primary incisions and explorations have advanced sufficiently to enable the extent of adhesions and the amount of healthy renal substance to be approximately determined.

Staples of Dubuque states, on the basis of 71 cases collected by him, that "63 per cent. of patients operated on are cured by lumbar nephrectomy, 68 per cent. by open methods in general, and up to date 100 per cent. by either lumbar incision and drainage or the creation of a fistula."

Malignant Growths.

As pathological rarities only, and having but little clinical interest, may be mentioned, as occurring in the kidneys, fibroma, lipoma, myxoma, anginoma, and adenoma. Malignant growths originating in or involving the kidneys, sarcoma or carcinoma, are, however, more frequent and more important.

Sarcoma, primitive or secondary, of the kidney is a somewhat rare occurrence, but most frequent in children. The whole kidney may be transformed into a mass occupying its place and somewhat resembling it in form, but many times exceeding it in bulk and weight. Such a tumor may largely distend the abdominal cavity and compress its contents. Upon section we often find a substance varying greatly in consistence, from almost fibrous hardness to cavities filled with grumous material broken down by fatty degeneration and often colored by hemorrhage. In the interior may be found remains of the pyramids and cortical substance occupying their usual relative positions, but as it were distended, these portions being surrounded by a much thicker layer of purely abnormal neoplasm, probably connected with the capsule and its surrounding fat. In other cases all traces of normal form and structure may have disappeared. The microscopic structure of such a growth presents no peculiarity except so far as the arrangement of cells in the normal gland may be followed to a certain extent in the less-altered portions of the tumor. Besides this total destruction of the kidney, it is not uncommon to find nodules involving a part of one or both the organs, and more or less distinctly marked off from the healthy portion.

The origin of sarcomata involving the kidneys may be the subperitoneal cellular tissue or the neighboring organs. As a primary disease sarcoma of the kidneys is very rare.

True cancer or carcinoma of the kidney is not a common disease, and is said to have been found 12 times in 447 cases of cancer of various organs. It may be primary or secondary, and a description of the gross appearances would be essentially the same as that of the sarcoma. The tumor does not, however, usually attain so large a size, and the amount of degeneration of neighboring organs and of ulceration is greater. Calculi are often found in cancerous kidneys.

The SYMPTOMS produced by either sarcoma or carcinoma may be none at all for a time. Dull pains in the loins or referred to the hypochondrium—which, however, from their indefiniteness can have but little diagnostic importance—are among the early phenomena. Pains like nephritic colic may appear. The urine usually shows little of importance. There may be sympathetic disturbance of micturition, but unless hemorrhage occurs there is not likely to be anything in the urine discoverable by the microscope to fix the nature of the trouble. Fragments of cancer-structure in the very rare cases in which they are said to have been found would of course be conclusive, but evidence based on the alleged discovery of cancer-cells in the urine must be received with the utmost caution, recollecting the great variety of shapes and sizes assumed by the epithelium of the urinary passages. Hæmaturia is a symptom occurring in only a portion of the cases, its appearance in a given case evidently depending on the way in which the tumor invades the kidney and increases in size. If growing in such a way as to compress the ureter at an early stage before any erosion of the mucous membrane has taken place, blood, even if set free in the pelvis, cannot reach the bladder. If hæmaturia is present before any tumor can be felt, it has only a subordinate value, but if occurring after the discovery of such a tumor, the combination is of the highest significance. At a later period all the symptoms of compression of other abdominal viscera arise—anorexia, vomiting, jaundice, œdema, ascites, emaciation, and death.

When a tumor has become evident, it is to be diagnosticated from cystic disease and from hydro-nephrosis, with which it agrees in position and possibly in form. From the former of these its hardness and rapid growth, the invasion of other organs, and the cachexia will serve to distinguish it. Hæmaturia is not present in cystic disease. From hydronephrosis or pyo-nephrosis the diagnosis has already been stated. On the right side it might not in every case be easy to distinguish a morbid growth of the kidney from one affecting the liver, and a similar difficulty might arise on the other side with the spleen. The diagnosis is to be made by a careful location of the tumor by palpation and percussion and the absence of symptoms likely to occur in connection with affections of the organs named. In children psoas abscess and degeneration of the lumbar lymphatic glands should also be considered.

A sarcoma of the kidney has been mistaken and punctured for an empyema. A sarcoma behind the kidney, pushing it forward, is very difficult to distinguish from a similar growth affecting the organ itself, especially as it is likely to give rise to signs of renal irritation discoverable by the microscope. A slight pyelitis, distinguished by pus and the absence of any cellular elements to indicate an origin at a lower point, has been observed in such a case.

The results of exploratory puncture have been before alluded to. If a piece can be brought away large enough to be examined microscopically, it may settle the diagnosis, not only as to a malignant growth, but also as to its kind.

The distinction between carcinoma and sarcoma cannot always be made during life, nor indeed, without a microscopical examination, after death. It is of importance chiefly with reference to prognosis after operation for removal of the organ. A more rapid growth, a greater tendency to invade other organs, and a more marked cachexia would speak in favor of carcinoma, while a tumor gradually attaining a very large size, and not spreading beyond the kidney and its immediate envelopes, is more likely to be a sarcoma.

There is no TREATMENT known to be of value in cancer or sarcoma of the kidney, except so far as it may diminish pain or regulate the secretions. Surgically, removal of the diseased organ is the only expedient to be thought of. Although nephrectomy has been shown to be a perfectly practicable operation, and one that is usually well borne when the other kidney is sound, it has not proved very successful with malignant growths, even as a temporary expedient. This is partly at least to be accounted for by the difficulties lying in the way of diagnosis in the earlier stages, and the reluctance with which so serious an operation would naturally be resorted to until hopes based either on the uncertainties of diagnosis or mistaken reliance on medical treatment have been given up. Cases, however, have been reported where patients have recovered from the operation, and the disease has not returned for some months. When an operation has been resorted to, the tumor has usually become too large to be extracted through the loin, and laparotomy has been the course pursued. According to Billroth,[1] out of 33 operations for tumors of the kidney, 13 have been cured.

Cysts.

Three kinds of cysts are met with in the kidney besides those connected with the growth of parasites.

Kidneys congenitally affected with cystic degeneration contain a large number of sacs lined with a vascular membrane, among the partitions of which are found the remains of secreting structure. Both kidneys are equally affected, and are enlarged and more or less lobulated. They are occasionally so large as to constitute an obstacle to labor, and various operative procedures, even evisceration, have been required to accomplish the delivery of the fœtus affected. The cysts are filled with fluid of various degrees of darkness of color from almost perfect limpidity to almost black. The fluid in the smaller cysts, at least, contains some of the urinary solids. The slighter degrees of this affection do not render a child necessarily non-viable, but with the larger some accident is likely to happen.

The formation of these cysts has been referred to an intra-uterine chronic nephritis, but another theory accounts for them by a vice of development. The fact that when the lesion is unilateral, as sometimes happens, there is apt to be a deficiency of some other part of the genito-urinary apparatus on the same side, and that several infants with cystic degeneration have been born of the same mother, speaks strongly in favor of the latter theory.

Serous cysts of later origin do not usually attain so large a size, or rather the kidney does not, on account of their smaller number. They are lined with a thinner membrane, and their contents are nearly clear, but coagulable, comprising uric acid, carbonate of lime, and cholesterin. Occasionally a single cyst attains considerable dimensions and produces by its pressure atrophy of part of the kidney. These cysts are supposed to arise in consequence of the blocking of a tube.

The third class of cysts closely resemble the first in appearance and in form, and contain more or less serous or gelatinous fluid, with albumen, blood-corpuscles, and pus, as well as the peculiar colloid bodies previously mentioned. They undoubtedly arise from the distension of tubes and of Malpighian bodies. These cysts are usually associated with chronic interstitial nephritis, and in fact they are rarely absent in cases of this kind, although the extreme degree—that is, where the cysts assume the most prominent position while the contracting nephritis falls into the background—are less common. In these latter cases the organ may be almost transformed into a mass of rounded bodies somewhat resembling a bunch of grapes.

The SYMPTOMS of the first two of these conditions—that is, of the cysts which are not connected with an active nephritis and attract attention simply as tumors—depend on the pressure they exert; and a diagnosis is to be made by a knowledge of their history and by the rules already given. The symptoms and diagnosis of the third variety are involved in those of chronic interstitial nephritis.

[1] *Mittheil. der Aerzte in Nieder Oesterreich*, Bd. x. p. 161 et seq.

There is no reason to suppose that any drug has any therapeutic action on such kidneys, so far as the cysts are concerned. It should always be remembered that a kidney may contain a large number of cysts, and yet scattered portions of secreting substance enough be left to carry on the function indefinitely.

It might under some circumstances be justifiable to remove a cystic kidney on account of the pressure exercised on other organs, but as the cysts do not increase rapidly in size, punctures several times repeated, so as to empty a number of them, would in most cases prove as effectual an operation, and, what is of greater importance, would not involve the loss of any portion, even if small, of secreting structure which may be left.

Tuberculosis.

The tubercles which are found in the kidney in cases of general miliary tuberculosis have usually no clinical interest, since the kidney is not, even in children, one of the points where tubercular localization is most intense, and renal tubercles are consequently but little advanced when death takes place from the extension of the disease in other organs. They present no symptoms which are perceptible among the much graver ones attending the progress of the disease elsewhere.

In the disease known as tubercle of the kidney, caseous nephritis, or nephro-phthisis, masses of caseous material are deposited in the renal parenchyma which may soften, break down, and communicate with each other and with the calices and pelvis. In some cases it is probable that the disease originates in or immediately underneath the mucous membrane of the urinary passages. This process of breaking down continues much in the same way as that of a phthisical lung, until the kidney becomes little more than a hardened, irregular, knobby shell enclosing a ragged, ulcerated cavity with thickened, pus-secreting walls and filled with pus, more or less blood, and débris of kidney-structure and tubercle. In such portions of renal substance as may remain it is not unusual to find miliary tubercle. If obstruction of the ureter exists, a pyo-nephrosis may exist in addition. Rupture into the peritoneal cavity or into the intestine has occurred.

It is probable that in this affection are included two processes, differing in pathology and etiology and to some extent in clinical history. It is probable that true tubercle may originate in the kidney as a result of either tubercle or cheesy inflammation elsewhere, as in the lungs, bodies of the vertebræ, or scrofulous glands. In this case there are no marked symptoms until the process of softening and breaking down has reached the mucous membrane of the pelvis. Besides this, renal phthisis sometimes succeeds, as a more local invasion, to tubercle or cheesy inflammation of the urinary passages, and in this case the symptoms appear simply as aggravations of those already present and depending upon ureteritis and pyelitis. Renal phthisis is seldom if ever an independent disease. It is often associated, besides the affections already named as standing in etiological relationship with it, with cheesy inflammation of the testicle, vesiculæ seminales, and much less frequently of the ovaries and Fallopian tubes.

The DIAGNOSIS of tubercle in the kidney before it has reached the pelvis is probably impossible. Pain in the back or slight albuminuria, as has been already stated, is of no diagnostic value except as pointing to some renal irritation, as to the cause of which it tells nothing. In the presence of tubercle elsewhere it might be regarded as suspicious.

After cavities have become connected with the pelvis or have extended from it, the symptoms become more marked. In the urine are to be found pus, some blood, epithelium of the urinary passages and often of the kidneys, in many cases in the form of casts; and it is claimed that masses of caseous matter as large perhaps as the head of a pin may be found, which will of course make the diagnosis almost a matter of certainty. If the urine containing such a deposit is acid, it is almost certain that the lesion is mainly in the kidney and that the bladder is but slightly if at all affected. It is also stated that the bacillus of tubercle has been found. The presence of this parasite will not only testify as to the presence of the clinical condition known as phthisis of the kidney, but will also make it sure that the affection depends upon tubercle in the strictest pathological sense, and will influence the prognosis accordingly. Inoculation of purulent sediment from the urine of a patient suffering from tuberculosis of the urinary passages has produced tubercle in the iris of the rabbit. This procedure has been suggested as a means of diagnosis as to the character of a chronic catarrh of these passages before the appearance of tubercle elsewhere.[1]

If pyelitis have already been present, the change in the appearance of the urine will be less characteristic, but there may be a marked aggravation of symptoms when the contents of softened masses are added to the secretions of the mucous surface. There is likely to be much fluctuation in the quantity of débris present from day to day. Urinary fever of the hectic or subcontinued type, with anorexia, nausea, dry tongue, and diarrhœa, is present. In some cases the enlarged and irregular kidney may be felt.

The PROGNOSIS of this condition is in the highest degree unfavorable, although the finding of cicatrices in kidneys where symptoms of renal phthisis have been present suggests that it is possible for caseous masses in these organs, as well as in the lungs, to undergo absorption and healing.

The TREATMENT must be, in the first place, constitutional by tonics and reconstituents, and local by the use of such antiseptics as are eliminated through the kidney, as boric or benzoic acid or the benzoates. But little, however, is to be expected from it.

Parasites.

The most important parasite which is known to inhabit the kidney is the immature tapeworm of the dog, or Tænia echinococcus. It is decidedly rare in this country to meet with this affection in any part of the body, and as the kidney is not one of the organs most likely to be chosen as its habitat, the condition is not one which comes often under the observation of physicians.

[1] Ebstein, *Centralblatt für die Med. Wiss.*, 1882, p. 918, from *Deutsch. Arch. f. klin. Med.*, xxxi. S. 63.

It is hardly necessary to describe here the structure or contents of the hydatid cyst which forms the home of the parasite, nor its etiology, since these topics belong to general pathology, and the cyst is the same in whatever organ it may be seated. When it affects the kidney, it is usually the left—more frequently that of a man between thirty and forty years of age.

A hydatid cyst may be situated upon any part of the kidney. If small, it may never make its presence known. A larger one may give rise to those vague pains in the back found with so many diseases of the kidney and characteristic of none of them. A cyst may open in any direction, but is more likely to empty into the pelvis of the kidney. When this happens, the smaller cysts or pieces of the larger ones often enter the ureter and give rise to renal colic, and possibly, later, to a pyelitis. Other points of discharge are the intestines, the lungs, or the abdominal walls.

After a hydatid cyst has reached a certain size its presence may be recognized by palpation, but the diagnosis between it and other tumors of the kidney must be very difficult unless characteristic fragments make their appearance in the urine at the same time that the tumor diminishes in size, or unless they can be obtained by puncture. The hydatid thrill, if it can be obtained, will be an important factor in diagnosis.

The TREATMENT of this affection in the kidney presents no special points of difference from that of similar cysts in the liver; with this important exception, that besides punctures with large and small trocars, incisions, electrolysis, etc., the resource of complete extirpation still remains. Cures have been obtained by repeated punctures and subsequent suppuration, and by partial removal through the abdominal walls and subsequent drainage.

Among the parasites of the kidney it is customary to mention the Strongylus gigas, which is a worm somewhat resembling the ascaris and inhabiting the pelvis. It is not very infrequent among the Carnivora, but since only seven cases have been described in the human subject since the seventeenth century, and only a part of these are admitted as genuine by certain authors, its diagnosis, prognosis, and treatment must depend more upon theory than upon experience. The diagnosis is to be made, if at all, on the basis of a pyelitis and the discovery of the eggs of the parasite in the urine.

The Distoma hæmatobium is a parasite found chiefly in the blood-vessels, and especially those of the portal system. It is occasionally, however, met with in the veins of the kidney and also in the urinary passages. Its eggs pass into the pelvis and ureters, and there begin their development, which, however, is soon arrested, as they rapidly perish in the urine.

These parasites appear to produce either by a direct action or by the occlusion of vessels, ulceration, and hemorrhages from the urinary mucous membrane, including that of the bladder. These effects are supposed to be due to the blocking of the smaller vessels by the worms themselves. An adherent deposit consisting of masses of distoma eggs and grains of uric acid sometimes forms in grayish-yellow patches within the ureter, and gives rise to stricture, with dilatation and hydro-nephrosis above. This parasite has been considered the cause of the endemic hæmaturia of hot countries, but as cases of this affection have been carefully examined for the distoma with negative results, it must be considered as only one among several causes. Strongyli are said to have been found in some of the cases.

Nothing is known of an appropriate TREATMENT for the distoma. An abundant flow of urine might perhaps carry off more rapidly such individuals as have found their way into the urinary passages, and, considering the character of the deposit described above as causing stoppage of the ureter, treatment directed against the uric-acid diathesis might diminish the risk of this particular form of trouble.

Diseases of the Ureters.

Absence of the ureter may take place when one kidney is congenitally absent, though this is not an absolute rule, since the ureter may terminate above in a rounded sac. When a single kidney exists, consisting of the fusion of two, there are usually two ureters opening in the usual position. In one instance, in which only one kidney and one ureter were present, the ureter opened into the bladder on the side opposite to that upon which the kidney was situated.

Not very infrequently two ureters exist in connection with a normal kidney, remaining separate for the whole or a part of their course to the bladder. This condition is merely a sort of exaggeration of the separation between the two branches of the renal pelvis.

A few instances have been noted where a ureter or a fistula connected therewith has opened outside of the bladder at a point near the urethra. This malformation gave rise to symptoms of incontinence of urine, and in one case was remedied by operation.

Abnormal openings of the ureter into the uterus and vagina as the results of pelvic inflammations, and upon the external surface as the result of wounds, have occurred. They are more or less amenable to surgical treatment, and belong to the domain of surgery and gynecology rather than to medicine.

Occlusion of the ureter has already been spoken of in connection with the hydro-nephrosis and pyelitis to which it gives rise. This occlusion results from pressure exerted either at the vesical orifice from cystitis; a little higher up from malignant disease connected with the uterus or a fibroma surrounding the ureter; from contracting adhesions resulting from pelvic inflammation; or from sharp flexions of the tube itself, perhaps also from valvular folds of the mucous membrane. Sometimes its obliteration seems to be the result of old inflammation of the mucous membrane of the ureter itself in connection with that of the renal pelvis. In the latter case the occlusion may be complete at several points, while at others a collection of dry, cheesy, or putty-like material occupies the cavity of the ureter as well as the pelvis of the atrophied kidney.

Cancer is not known primarily to invade the ureter.

Tubercle is not infrequently found in the form of small granulations in cases of general tuberculosis, and it is possible that this deposit may be among the earlier ones; hence a chronic catarrh of the urinary passages without some known cause should be looked upon with suspicion, and the development of phthisis as far as possible guarded against.   The presence of these small tubercles in the ureter, if none are present or no ulceration exists in the kidney, are of little or no local importance.

Inflammation of the ureter often exists in connection with cystitis and pyelitis, and in fact constitutes the means by which the higher urinary passages become gradually involved in the diseases below.

The DIAGNOSIS of this condition as a distinct disease is hardly possible, and is besides unnecessary, as the treatment to be directed thereto would be included in that called for by the more extensive and obvious inflammation of the kidney and bladder.

DISEASES OF THE PARENCHYMA OF THE KIDNEYS, AND PERINEPHRITIS.

By FRANCIS DELAFIELD, M. D.

CHRONIC CONGESTION OF THE KIDNEY.

SYNONYMS.—Passive congestion; Cyanotic induration.

It is now generally recognized that we must separate from the other forms of kidney disease the condition of chronic congestion. Since Traube first called attention to the causation and characters of this lesion, all authors have recognized its special character, although there are still minor differences of opinion concerning it.

ETIOLOGY.—Chronic congestion of the kidney may be produced by any mechanical cause which interferes with the escape of the blood from the renal veins. Thrombi of the veins, tumors pressing on the veins, emphysema of the lungs, hydro-pneumothorax, pericarditis,—all may produce this lesion. As to how often it is produced by the pregnant uterus is still a question. But the most common cause of all is organic disease of the heart. Practically, the lesion comes under consideration as a complication of heart disease, of aneurism of the arch of the aorta, and of emphysema of the lungs.

LESIONS.—If the congestion has not existed for a long time, we find the kidneys increased in size and their weight great in proportion to their size. They are of an unnatural hardness—a hardness which can be imitated by injecting the blood-vessels of a normal kidney with water. The capsules are not adherent, the surfaces of the kidneys are smooth. Both the cortical and pyramidal portions are congested, and this congestion gives the entire organs a peculiar reddish, livid color. No lesions are found in the Malpighian bodies, tubes, stroma, or blood-vessels, except that the epithelium of the convoluted tubes may be a little swollen.

If the congestion has lasted for a longer time, the kidneys may continue to be large or they may be somewhat reduced in size; the weight remains out of proportion to the size. There are the same unnatural color and consistence. The capsules are now often slightly adherent and the surfaces of the kidneys finely nodular. In the cortex there may be patches of new connective tissue enclosing atrophied tubules, or there may be a more diffuse growth of connective tissue separating the tubes from each other. In the convoluted tubules the epithelial cells may be swollen and finely granular, or very much swollen and coarsely granular, so as to nearly fill the tubes, or flattened so that the cavities of the tubes are unnaturally large. The tubes may also contain cast-matter and detached and broken epithelial cells. The capsules of the Malpighian bodies may be a little thickened and the capsular endothelium swollen. In the pyramids the epithelium of the straight tubes may be granular and detached, and there is often cast-matter in the looped tubes. It is difficult to tell whether there is any real change in the veins of the kidney.

As a result of the same interference with the venous circulation, similar changes are found in other parts of the body—in the lungs, liver, spleen, stomach, small intestine, and pia mater. In all these organs there is, first, simply a venous congestion, then after a time structural changes are added. Formation of new connective tissue and of new functional cells of the particular organ, degeneration of these cells, dilatation and tortuousness of the small veins and capillaries, are regularly present. The kidney lesion, therefore, is only one of a number of lesions, all dependent on a common mechanical cause.

SYMPTOMS.—Of the persons who die with chronic congestion of the kidney, a large number present marked symptoms during life, but it is difficult to determine how largely these symptoms are due to the congestion of the kidney.

A congestion of the kidney of only a few days' duration does not seem usually to give rise to any symptoms. Even if such a congestion is prolonged to two or three weeks, as we see in some cases of hydropneumothorax from perforation of the lung, there may be no renal symptoms and no changes in the urine. On the other hand, it is extremely rare for organic heart disease or emphysema of the lungs to prove fatal without some disease of the kidneys.

The question is still further complicated by the fact that both in cardiac disease and emphysema there may be either chronic congestion of the kidney or chronic diffuse nephritis with the same symptoms.

After excluding the cases of cardiac hypertrophy secondary to kidney disease and the cardiac diseases with complications, I find in my casebooks 137 cases in which the patients died simply from heart disease, changes in the viscera due to the disturbance of the venous circulation, and kidney disease. Of these cases, 84 presented the lesions of chronic diffuse nephritis; 53 were in the state of chronic congestion. Of the cases of chronic diffuse nephritis, 27 were large white kidneys, 29 atrophied kidneys, 28 could not be classed as either large white or atrophied. In these cases there existed during life certain regular symptoms. There were changes in the urine, dropsy, headache, delirium, convulsions, coma, dyspnœa, vomiting, cough, hæmoptysis, loss of flesh and strength.

As regards the quantity of the urine, there was a very great variety until shortly before the patient's death ; then the urine was usually diminished in amount, sometimes suppressed. A very marked decrease in the amount of urine was more constant in the cases of chronic diffuse nephritis than in those of chronic congestion. But in several cases both of chronic diffuse nephritis and of chronic congestion the patients passed from thirty to forty ounces of urine up to the time of their deaths.

Albumen and casts were often present—nearly always with the large white kidneys, not nearly as constantly with atrophied kidneys or with the cases of chronic congestion. In cases of chronic congestion the albumen was usually in small amount and often not accompanied with casts.

The specific gravity of the urine was apt to be low with chronic diffuse nephritis and high with chronic congestion, but there were many exceptions to this rule. With large white kidneys, atrophied kidneys, simple diffuse nephritis, and chronic congestion the specific gravity might be either normal, high, or low up to the time of death.

Transudation of the serum into the subcutaneous connective tissue and the serous cavities was a very constant symptom. It was a little more constant, and perhaps usually reached a greater degree, in the cases of chronic diffuse nephritis than in those of chronic congestion.

Headache, delirium, convulsions, and coma occurred in a moderate number of all the cases.

Dyspnœa was a very frequent symptom in all the cases.

Vomiting was also present in many cases.

Cough, with mucus or muco-purulent sputa, sometimes with hæmoptysis, was a very common symptom.

Many of the patients lost flesh and strength and became anæmic.

COURSE OF THE DISEASE.—There is a great deal of similarity in the histories of patients who suffer from the combination of cardiac and renal disease. There is first the history of the heart disease. A patient goes on for a number of years, sometimes apparently perfectly well and unconscious that his heart is diseased, sometimes more or less troubled with cough, cardiac dyspnœa, and palpitation. But after a longer or shorter time there is a marked change for the worse. Either gradually or rapidly the cough becomes worse, the dyspnœa greater, the functions of the stomach are disturbed, the patient loses flesh and strength, dropsy is developed, and finally cerebral symptoms. Some die suddenly, some with exhaustion, some with dropsy, some with dyspnœa, some comatose. It is always possible for the patient to recover from the first attack of this kind, sometimes even from a second, but eventually there comes an attack which proves fatal.

The most striking cases are those in which cardiac disease exists for many years without giving any symptoms, and then the symptoms are developed rapidly. Such persons, although they have organic disease of the heart, may seem to enjoy perfect health. They may even be able to take long walks, climb mountains, or perform laborious work. On some day they suddenly become sick. Sometimes the exciting cause of the attack is a pleurisy or a pericarditis, sometimes there is no apparent cause. The first symptom is usually dyspnœa, and this is not an ordinary cardiac dyspnœa. It is a very distressing and constant dyspnœa, which does not allow the patients to lie down. They pass days and nights sitting in a chair, fatigued, ready to sleep, but kept awake by the constant dyspnœa. Some of these patients will die at the end of a few days; others live longer and develop dropsy, anæmia, and cerebral symptoms.

When the chronic congestion of the kidneys is secondary to emphysema of the lungs, the course of affairs is much the same. The patient goes on for a number of years with the ordinary symptoms of emphysema, and then gradually or suddenly becomes worse. Dyspnœa, dropsy, anæmia, cerebral symptoms make their appearance, and the case terminates in the same way as the cardiac cases.

DURATION.—How long congestion of the kidneys may exist without producing symptoms it is hard to say. Certainly it may exist for a number of days without any apparent disturbance of the functions of the kidney. Whether it may exist for a time, give symptoms, and then disappear, is uncertain; the rule seems to be that the lesion, when once well established, persists up to the death of the patient.

TREATMENT.—It must be acknowledged that we can hardly hope for a cure of the lesion of the kidneys, and that even alleviation of the symptoms is not always possible. The mechanical cause of the obstruction to the venous circulation cannot be removed, and it is not only the functions of the kidneys that are disturbed, but those of the lungs, liver, spleen, stomach, and small intestine. Still, we can do something. The iodide of potassium, convallaria, caffeine, and digitalis may be of service in equalizing and strengthening the heart's action, and at the same time act as diuretics. Inhalations of the nitrite of amyl dilate the arteries and capillaries, and so unload the veins. Opium is the great remedy for the dyspnœa, although it must be given with caution. Inhalations of ether may render the patient's last days more comfortable.

BRIGHT'S DISEASE OF THE KIDNEYS.

AFTER considering separately the condition of chronic congestion of the kidney, we find that there are a group of kidney diseases characterized by certain rational symptoms, changes in the urine, and alterations in the structure of the kidneys which are popularly known by the name of Bright's disease.

Various attempts have been made to classify these cases.

1. All the kidney lesions have been supposed to correspond to the stages of an inflammatory process—a stage of congestion, a second stage of exudation, and a third stage of contraction.

2. The disease has been divided, according to its clinical symptoms, simply into acute and chronic Bright's disease.

3. The gross appearances have been taken as a standard, and the cases are classed as examples of large white kidney, atrophied kidney, waxy kidney, etc.

4. The kidneys have been compared to mucous membranes, and authors speak of catarrhal and croupous nephritis.

5. The disease has been classified, according to the particular part of the kidney affected, into parenchymatous, tubular, glomerular, interstitial, and diffuse nephritis.

With our present knowledge of the subject it seems to me most convenient to speak of acute and chronic parenchymatous nephritis and acute and chronic diffuse nephritis. I include under the head of parenchymatous nephritis all those kidneys in which the lesions are strictly confined to the epithelial cells lining the tubules and the capsules of the glomeruli; under the head of diffuse nephritis, those kidneys in which the lesions involve the tubes, stroma, glomeruli, and arteries; under the head of interstitial nephritis, those kidneys in which the essential morbid changes are in the stroma.

This classification seems to me to be theoretically correct, but yet I must admit that from a clinical standpoint nearly all the cases may be conveniently arranged into the two classes of acute and chronic Bright's disease.

GENERAL SYMPTOMS OF BRIGHT'S DISEASE.—There are a certain number of symptoms common to all the varieties of Bright's disease, and it is convenient to consider them before going on to the special description of each of these varieties. These symptoms are—

Changes in the Urine.—Healthy adults usually secrete during the twenty-four hours from 40 to 50 ounces of urine of a light-yellow color, of acid reaction, of a specific gravity of 1015 to 1025, and holding in solution a number of excrementitious substances. Small amounts of albumen and of sugar seem to be, in some persons, physiological ingredients of the urine.

In most cases of Bright's disease the quantity of the urine at some time in the course of the disease deviates from the normal standard. Either the urine is increased in amount or diminished or suppressed, and in the course of the same case the urine may be at one time increased, at another diminished.

We find in healthy persons that the quantity of urine varies with the amount of fluids that are imbibed and with the condition of the skin and the bowels—that nervous influences and certain drugs will increase or diminish the amount of urine. Physiologists teach us that the amount of urine excreted varies with the degree of the blood-pressure in the renal arteries or with the rapidity with which the blood circulates through these arteries.

The urine may be very much increased or diminished in amount as the result of various morbid conditions. Scanty urine or suppression of urine is observed in the course of acute parenchymatous and acute diffuse nephritis and in the early stages of the development of the large white kidney. During the course of any case of chronic Bright's disease there are usually periods during which the urine is scanty or suppressed, especially toward the close of the disease. The kidney lesions which complicate scarlet fever, yellow fever, and cholera are often attended with suppression of urine. Any diseases accompanied by a well-marked rise of temperature are apt to be associated with a diminution in the amount of urine. Injuries to the urethra, even very slight ones, may be followed by complete suppression of urine, without any changes in the kidneys except congestion.

Marked diminution in the amount of urine occurring in the course of acute and chronic Bright's disease is usually associated with the development of cerebral symptoms—headache, restlessness, delirium, muscular twitchings, convulsions, stupor, and coma. Such a change in the amount of the urine usually lasts only a few days and may terminate fatally, or the quantity of urine will increase and the patient get better. There are, however, cases in which the suppression of urine lasts for several days without the development of uræmic symptoms. Whitelaw[1] relates a

[1] *Lancet*, September, 1877.

case of suppression of urine lasting for twenty-five days in a boy eight years old. The suppression began twelve weeks after an attack of scarlatina. There were no uræmic symptoms, and the child recovered completely.

The suppression of urine due to injuries of the urethra gives rise to symptoms of great prostration—rigors, vomiting, and collapse—rather than to uræmic symptoms.

Suppression of urine is also produced by occlusion of the ureters by calculi, new growths, etc. It is a curious fact that in these cases the patients continue to live for a number of days (9 to 11, Roberts), and no uræmic symptoms are developed until a few hours before death.

The most marked examples of persistent increase in the quantity of urine are afforded by cases of diabetes mellitus and diabetes insipidus. But a daily excretion of from 70 to 100 ounces is common enough with atrophied kidneys, with large white kidneys, and with waxy kidneys.

It is exceedingly difficult to form any rational idea of the causes of the variations in the amount of urine in the course of the same case, and in different cases with similar kidney lesions. Various explanations have been attempted, ascribing these changes to the hypertrophy of the left ventricle of the heart, to changes in blood-pressure, to lesions of the arteries, to changes in the composition of the blood, to lesions in particular portions of the kidneys. But any one who tries to apply these explanations to any number of actual cases will find many difficulties.

The most evident causes of diminution in the amount of urine seem to be an abnormal condition of the circulation of the blood and either congestion or structural changes of the kidneys.

The specific gravity of the urine varies from day to day and from hour to hour in the same person, having a regular relation to the quantity of urine passed. But a long-continued deviation from the normal specific gravity is usually an evidence of disease. The highest specific gravities obtain with saccharine diabetes. Abnormally high specific gravities also often occur in the urine of patients with a high temperature, with chronic congestion of the kidneys, and in some cases of acute and chronic parenchymatous nephritis.

Low specific gravities are the rule in diabetes insipidus and with acute and chronic diffuse nephritis. In chronic diffuse nephritis the specific gravity remains low even if the quantity of urine passed is very small. When there is almost suppression of urine from occlusion of the ureters the urine that is passed is of low specific gravity.

These changes in specific gravity correspond of course to the amount of solid matter in solution in the urine, and may depend upon a change in the relative proportion of the fluid and solid constituents of the urine, or upon an absolute increase or decrease of the solid portions.

Any change in the absolute amount of solid matter excreted in the urine must depend upon changes in the composition of the blood, or in the circulation of the blood through the kidneys, or in the structure of the kidneys themselves. All these three conditions seem to exist in Bright's disease, and either together or separately may diminish the daily excretion of solid matter.

It is not necessary here to enumerate the different solid constituents of the urine. A change in the amount of many of them merely indicates disorders of the digestive process. Urea seems to be the most important of the excretory substances, and its quantity is regularly diminished both in acute and chronic Bright's disease.

Blood is found in the urine in a considerable number of cases of Bright's disease. If it is present in large quantities, the urine will be of a reddish color; if in smaller quantities, of a smoky color; and if in still smaller quantities, the color will not be changed. Blood is found regularly with acute diffuse nephritis, with the more severe cases of acute parenchymatous nephritis, with the exacerbations of chronic diffuse nephritis, and with suppurative nephritis. The blood seems to. be derived from the tufts of vessels in the Malpighian bodies.

Albumen in the urine is a very common symptom of renal disease, but it is not confined to such cases. It is also found without any structural lesions of the kidneys.

1. There are some individuals whose urine, for many years, will contain small quantities of albumen, and yet their general health is good and they never develop any renal symptoms. In some of these cases the urine is always somewhat diminished in quantity, and in some there is also a little sugar in the urine.

2. In a large number of perfectly healthy persons small amounts of albumen will appear as a temporary condition after muscular exercise, sea-bathing, eating certain kinds of food, etc.

3. Albumen may be present in considerable amount for weeks or months in the urine of young persons, and then disappear altogether. The general health may continue good or be somewhat depreciated. After a time the albumen disappears and the patients have no further trouble.

4. General convulsions, concussion of the brain, and transfusion of blood often produce a temporary albuminuria.

Some observers believe that albumen is always present in the urine, but in such small amounts as to elude the ordinary tests.

Both physiological and pathological albuminuria is most constant and abundant after eating.

The albumen is not all of the same character. Most of it is serum-albumen, but with it is a smaller amount of globulin and sometimes of peptones. As yet the serum-albumen seems to be of the principal practical importance.

Pathological albuminuria is most constant and the albumen is most abundant with acute and chronic parenchymatous nephritis, with acute diffuse nephritis, and with the large white variety of chronic diffuse nephritis. It is least constant and least abundant with the atrophic variety of chronic diffuse nephritis, with some waxy kidneys, with interstitial nephritis, and with chronic congestion of the kidney. A variety of explanations have been given to account for the production of albumen by diseased kidneys, but none of them are very satisfactory.

The albuminuria has been ascribed to disease of the epithelium of the Malpighian bodies; to increase of the blood-pressure within the renal arteries, either with or without disease of the arterial walls; to slowing of the blood-current in the arteries; to diminution of the blood-pressure in the arteries; to congestion of the renal veins; to changes in the composition of the blood; to changes in the epithelium of the renal tubules.

For practical purposes it is to be remembered that large amounts of albumen regularly indicate structural changes in the kidneys; that small amounts of albumen are found without any kidney lesions, with chronic congestion of the kidney, and with chronic diffuse nephritis; that chronic diffuse nephritis may exist without albuminuria for a long time.

In many cases of kidney disease we find in the urine bodies of cylindrical shape called casts. The same bodies are also found within the tubules of diseased kidneys. Concerning the nature and origin of these bodies we are still ignorant. We only know that they are formed within the kidney tubules and are carried thence into the urine. With the exception of the blood-casts, which are composed simply of a number of blood-globules pressed together, all casts seem to be formed of a peculiar homogeneous hyaline substance to which other elements may be added. Hyaline casts are composed entirely of such material. Waxy casts are formed of the same substance, which becomes denser. Epithelial casts are made by the adhesion of epithelial cells to the surface of hyaline casts. Nucleated, granular, and fatty casts are hyaline casts with the fragments of degenerated epithelium incorporated in them.

Occasionally hyaline casts are found in the urine of healthy persons. They also occur as a temporary condition after severe muscular exertion, with typhlitis, with renal calculi, and with jaundice. Most frequently, however, they are associated with structural disease of the kidneys. Usually they are found in albuminous urine, and in proportion to the amount of albumen, but we may find casts without albumen and albumen without casts.

With chronic congestion of the kidney the casts are hyaline and few in number. With acute parenchymatous nephritis there are hyaline, granular, nucleated, and epithelial casts. With chronic parenchymatous nephritis there are hyaline, granular, and nucleated casts. With acute diffuse nephritis there are blood, epithelial, hyaline, granular, nucleated, and fatty casts. With chronic diffuse nephritis there are hyaline, waxy, granular, fatty, nucleated, and epithelial casts.

An accumulation of serum in the subcutaneous connective tissue, in the serous cavities, and in the lungs is one of the regular symptoms of Bright's disease. It usually appears first in the feet or in the face. Such dropsy is said to be due to a low specific gravity of the blood-serum; to the loss of albumen; to the scanty elimination of urine; to hydræmia plethora; or to changes in the walls of the blood-vessels.

The functions of the stomach are often disordered, either with or without the existence of chronic gastritis. Loss of appetite, nausea and vomiting, oppression after eating, etc. continue and grow worse throughout the disease. Vomiting is also a frequent concomitant of the so-called uræmic attacks.

Diarrhœa often occurs with dropsy and a scanty excretion of urine, and may then be of service to the patient, but it sometimes becomes very profuse, rebellious to treatment, and is of positive injury.

Dyspnœa associated with Bright's disease seems to occur in several different ways. It may be of mechanical origin from œdema of the lungs or from hydrothorax. It may be a purely nervous phenomenon, ɹr it may depend upon a complicating heart lesion. The nervous dyspnœa seems to be allied to the uræmic vomiting and cerebral symptoms; it is often most distressing.

In the course of chronic Bright's disease disturbances of vision occur dependent on three different conditions: (1) There may be a loss of vision, usually temporary, without any discoverable lesion of the eye. (2) There may be simple neuro-retinitis. (3) There may be the characteristic nephritic retinitis with hemorrhages and fatty degeneration of the retina. These two forms of retinitis are often the first symptoms of renal disease.

Neuralgic pains, most frequently referred to some part of the head or face, but also to other parts of the body, are prominent symptoms in some cases.

The Blood.—Both in acute and chronic Bright's disease the patients often become markedly anæmic and pale. This change in the color of the patient corresponds to an alteration of the composition of the blood with the details of which we are not as yet fully acquainted. The blood seems to be thinner and more watery.

Cerebral Symptoms.—Headache, drowsiness, stupor, sleeplessness, delirium, coma, muscular twitchings, and general convulsions are of frequent occurrence. The headache and drowsiness may continue during the course of the disease for many months. The stupor, sleeplessness, delirium, coma, muscular twitchings, and general convulsions are apt to occur in attacks which last for several days, and then pass away or terminate in the death of the patient. With such cerebral symptoms are often associated dyspnœa, vomiting, increased temperature, and diminution in the excretion of urine. The entire group of symptoms is commouly known by the name of uræmia.

It is a matter of great practical importance to determine the cause of these cerebral symptoms, for otherwise there can be no rational treatment of them. It is evident that such cerebral symptoms must depend upon anatomical changes in the brain or its membranes, or upon a change in the composition of the blood which circulates through the brain, or upon the quantity of blood supplied to the brain.

It is to be remembered that such cerebral symptoms occur most frequently with the atrophic form of chronic diffuse nephritis; that they are often the first symptom of renal disease; that the same person may have several such attacks, with no cerebral symptoms during the interval; that the urine is usually, but not always, diminished during the attack, and becomes more abundant when the attack ceases; that such attacks also occur with the chronic congestion of the kidney due to cardiac disease, in pregnant women without kidney disease, and with diseased arteries and high arterial tension without kidney disease.

Anatomical changes in the brain or its membranes do exist in a considerable number of cases of chronic Bright's disease. Chronic meningitis with thickening of the pia mater and an increase of serum is quite common; anæmia and œdema of the brain-tissue are often seen. But there are a great many cases with cerebral symptoms without such lesions, and with such lesions without cerebral symptoms.

The composition of the blood is undoubtedly changed in most of the cases with cerebral symptoms. It is natural to look for such changes as are due to perversion of the excretory function of the kidneys, and to ascribe the cerebral symptoms to the poisoning of the blood by urea, by urea transformed into carbonate of ammonia, or by the other excretory matters which should be eliminated by the urine.   Moreover, it has been demonstrated that there is a very marked increase in the amount of urea contained in the blood in such cases.   On the other hand, we find that suppression of urine with accumulation of urea in the blood may exist for a long time without cerebral symptoms if the suppression is due to obstruction of the ureters; that with chronic congestion of the kidney, puerperal convulsions, and diseased arteries urea is excreted in fair amount, although cerebral symptoms exist; and that even in cases of cerebral symptoms with chronic diffuse nephritis there may be no increase of urea in the blood.

In most of the cases with cerebral symptoms, however, there are other changes in the composition of the blood, concerning the exact nature of which we are still ignorant.   In most cases of chronic Bright's disease the patients become pale and the blood is thin and watery ; and this is also often the case with chronic congestion of the kidney and with diseased arteries.   In pregnancy the quantity of blood is said to be increased : in cholera a considerable part of the fluid portions of the blood is lost.

Changes in the amount of blood in the brain may be due to lesions of the cerebral arteries or to contraction of these arteries ; to changes in the arteries in other parts of the body ; to organic disease or functional disorder of the heart ; or to a change in the whole amount of blood contained in the body.

It seems to me probable that the so-called uræmic symptoms are most frequently due to disturbances of the circulation of blood.   Such disturbances of the circulation produce in the brain cerebral symptoms; in the lungs, dyspnœa ; in the stomach, vomiting ; in the kidneys, suppression of urine.

With the atrophic form of chronic diffuse nephritis we have all the conditions necessary for an irregular circulation—hypertrophy of the left ventricle, diseased arteries, and hydræmic plethora.   In the other cases with cerebral symptoms there are also conditions present capable of interfering with the circulation.

Acute Parenchymatous Nephritis.

PATHOLOGICAL ANATOMY.—The lesions of acute parenchymatous nephritis vary with the intensity of the inflammatory process.

(1) Mild Cases.—The kidneys are of normal size and weight.   The capsules are not adherent, the surface of the kidney is smooth, the cortex is of normal color or rather pale.   The epithelial cells lining the convoluted tubes are swollen and granular.

(2) More Severe Cases.—The kidneys are increased in size.   The cortex is thick and whitish, with white striæ extending in to the bases of the pyramids.   The epithelium of both the convoluted and straight tubes and of the Malpighian bodies is swollen and granular.   There is cast matter in the tubes.

(3) The Most Severe Cases.—The increase in the size of the kidneys is still more marked. The epithelium of most of the tubes is not only swollen and granular, but is also in many tubes detached from their walls. A great deal of cast-matter, and sometimes blood, is found in the tubes. There are no changes in the stroma or in the blood-vessels of the kidneys.

ETIOLOGY.—Acute parenchymatous nephritis occurs both as a primary and secondary lesion. The idiopathic cases occur without assignable cause or after exposure to cold, and are not very common. The secondary cases are seen very frequently. They complicate a variety of other diseases. With pneumonia, typhus fever, and typhoid fever the nephritis is usually of mild type. With yellow fever and acute atrophy of the liver the nephritis is very severe. With scarlatina, diphtheria, pyæmia, peritonitis, phosphorus- and arsenic-poisoning the severity of the nephritis varies with the different cases.

SYMPTOMS.—(1) The Idiopathic Cases.—The urine is diminished in quantity and may be suppressed ; its specific gravity continues nearly normal ; it contains albumen, usually in large amounts, sometimes blood : in some cases very few casts are seen, in others there are large numbers of hyaline, granular, and nucleated casts.

As regards the other symptoms, it is convenient to divide the idiopathic cases into three classes. In the first class dropsy and anæmia are the most marked symptoms ; with these there are loss of appetite and a depreciation in the general condition of the patient. In the second class cerebral symptoms are more prominent. There will be delirium, convulsions, stupor, coma, and with these persistent vomiting, dyspnœa, and great prostration, but no dropsy. The third class suffer from the symptoms of both the other classes. Dropsy, anæmia, loss of appetite, cerebral symptoms, vomiting, dyspnœa, and prostration are all present.

(2) The Secondary Cases.—The condition of the urine varies with the intensity of the nephritis. In the mild cases the urine is unchanged. In the more severe cases we find the urine diminished in quantity, containing albumen in varying amount, sometimes blood. Hyaline and granular casts are often present, but are not very numerous. Dropsy does not usually occur except with the parenchymatous nephritis of scarlatina. Nausea and vomiting are not infrequent, but it is often difficult to tell whether they are due to the primary disease or to the nephritis. Cerebral symptoms — convulsions, delirium, stupor, and coma — occur with the more severe cases.

DURATION.—(1) The Primary Cases.—The class of cases characterized by cerebral symptoms are of short duration. The bad cases die at the end of a few days, the milder cases recover within a few weeks. The class of cases characterized by dropsy last longer, often for several months.

(2) The Secondary Cases.—The renal symptoms continue during the course of the primary disease, and may disappear with the termination of this disease. But if the nephritis is severe the renal symptoms may continue for months after the primary disease has run its course. Albumen and casts are especially apt to persist for a long time. Such a persistence of the nephritis is especially apt to occur with scarlatina and diphtheria.

PROGNOSIS.—(1) The Primary Cases.—The cases characterized by both dropsy and cerebral symptoms usually end fatally. The cases characterized by cerebral symptoms alone are also very apt to die. The cases characterized by dropsy and anæmia often get well, but the albumen and casts may persist for a long time, and the patient may have several attacks of such a nephritis.

(2) The Secondary Cases.—Here the prognosis varies with the intensity of the nephritis. The more severe forms of the inflammation may add very much to the danger of the primary disease or may persist for a long time afterward.

TREATMENT.—(1) The Primary Cases.—In the cases characterized by dropsy the first indication is to get rid of the dropsy, and this is to be done by the methodical use of diuretics, cathartics, and diaphoretics. It will be found, however, that there is a great difference in the different cases as regards the precise time when these remedies will take effect and the dropsy decrease. Usually it is the best plan during the first few weeks of the disease to keep the patient confined to bed or to the house, and on a milk diet. From time to time efforts should be made to reduce the dropsy, but if these efforts produce no effect they should be discontinued and then tried again. In addition to the dropsy the condition of the stomach and the anæmia require treatment. For the stomach the milk diet is perhaps the most efficacious treatment. For the anæmia iron given by the mouth, combined with daily inhalations of oxygen gas, is of very great service. It is very important in these cases to guard against relapses. If possible, the patients should not return to their ordinary pursuits for a year after their apparent recovery, but should spend that time in travelling and improving their health in every possible way.

In the cases characterized by cerebral symptoms it must be confessed that treatment is not very efficacious. Diuretics have no effect, cathartics seem to do no good. Systematic sweating, the use of pilocarpine in small doses twice a day, inhalations of nitrite of amyl, the administration of chloral hydrate, caffeine, digitalis, and convallaria, and the use of fluid food in small doses, are indicated.

(2) The Secondary Cases.—While the primary disease, to which the nephritis is secondary, is running its course there is little to be done for renal symptons. If, however, these symptoms persist after the termination of the primary disease, then the main indication is to improve the general health in every possible way.

Chronic Parenchymatous Nephritis.

A good deal of confusion is connected with this name, for the reason that many authors include in this one class all the large white kidneys except the waxy ones, and such kidneys present a variety of lesions. There are, however, a moderate number of cases in which the morbid changes are confined to the epithelium of the tubes and to the Malpighian bodies. All the kidneys, no matter what their gross appearance may be, which present changes in the stroma and blood-vessels, as well as in the tubes, belong properly to the class of chronic diffuse nephritis. I confine the name of chronic parenchymatous nephritis, therefore, to those kidneys in which the inflammatory process runs a chronic course and is confined to the epithelium of the tubes and the Malpighian bodies.

LESIONS.—The kidneys are regularly increased in size, often weighing sixteen or twenty ounces. The capsules are not adherent, the surface of the kidney is smooth. The cortex of the kidney is thick and white, with white striæ running into the bases of the pyramids; the pyramids are large and red. The epithelium of most of the tubes and of the Malpighian capsules is swollen, granular, and detached. Cast-matter is present in the tubes. There may be an increase in the number of the small cells which cover the tufts of vessels in the Malpighian bodies.

ETIOLOGY.—This form of nephritis is not very common. It may follow acute parenchymatous nephritis and chronic congestion of the kidney; it is one of the complications of chronic pulmonary phthisis, and it occurs as an idiopathic disease.

SYMPTOMS.—There is a good deal of variety in the different cases as to the quantity and specific gravity of the urine. Usually the quantity is somewhat diminished, and the specific gravity is between 1020 and 1030.

Albumen is regularly present in considerable quantity, but it may be scanty, and may even disappear altogether for a time. Hyaline and granular casts are usually present, but in small numbers.

Dropsy is a regular symptom, and often goes on to general anasarca, although the degree of the œdema varies from week to week. Occasionally a case will run its course without any dropsy.

The functions of the stomach are disturbed, and the patients suffer from loss of appetite, nausea, and vomiting.

Muscular twitchings, convulsions, stupor, and coma only occur in the very severe cases.

Dyspnœa is often produced by the dropsy, sometimes is simply a nervous phenomenon.

Bronchitis with cough and expectoration may be a complication.

DURATION.—The course of the disease is slow; it lasts for months and years. The cases vary a good deal in the number and severity of the symptoms. Some cases run their course with nothing but the changes in the urine, loss of appetite, and a moderate degree of anæmia. In other cases the dropsy is the most prominent symptom, and in still others the cerebral symptoms predominate. There may be intervals of weeks and months during which all the symptoms, except the changes in the urine, disappear and then come on again.

PROGNOSIS.—The prognosis of chronic parenchymatous nephritis is not good, but still it is not so bad as that of chronic diffuse nephritis: some of the cases recover and never have any further indications of kidney disease.

TREATMENT.—The main indications for treatment are to improve the digestion, remove the dropsy, and restore the blood to a natural condition. It is usually necessary for the patient to give up his ordinary business and if possible to pass the winter months in a warmer climate.

Acute Diffuse Nephritis.

This form of nephritis has been described under a variety of names. It has been called acute Bright's disease, acute desquamative nephritis, acute tubular nephritis, croupous nephritis, acute albuminuria, the first stage of chronic Bright's disease, acute parenchymatous nephritis, glomerulo-nephritis, and acute interstitial nephritis.

MORBID ANATOMY.—The kidneys are increased in size, the capsules are not adherent, the surfaces are smooth. There may be an intense congestion of the entire kidney, including its pelvis, or the cortex is of an opaque white color mottled with red spots, and the pyramids are red. The tissue of the kidney is usually moist and succulent. In the tubes the epithelial cells are swollen, granular, and detached. Cast-matter and blood are found in many of the tubes. In the Malpighian bodies the cells which line the capsules are increased in size and number, sometimes to such an extent as to compress the tuft of vessels. The stroma of the kidney is infiltrated with serum, pus-cells, and blood.

ETIOLOGY.—Most of the cases of acute diffuse nephritis occur after exposure to cold or as a complication of scarlatina.

SYMPTOMS.—(1) The Idiopathic Cases.—Of these we may distinguish two sets of cases. In the first set of cases the invasion of the disease is acute. A person who has previously been usually in good health, after exposure to cold and wet will be suddenly attacked with rigors, a febrile movement, and pain in the back. There will be frequent and painful micturition, the urine being only passed a few drops at a time, or it is completely suppressed.

The urine is bloody or of a brownish smoky color. It is of low specific gravity. It contains a very large amount of albumen, numerous hyaline, granular, epithelial, and blood casts and renal epithelium, and sometimes pus-cells. Later in the disease fatty casts are also present.

The patient soon develops dropsy, the extent of which varies in the different cases. Sometimes it involves only the face, sometimes the hands and feet, or there may be general subcutaneous œdema, serum in the serous cavities, œdema of the lungs and of the glottis. The patients lose their appetite; often there are nausea and vomiting. As a rule, there are cerebral symptoms—headache, drowsiness, stupor, delirium, muscular twitchings, convulsions, and coma. In the milder cases there will be only headache and periods of drowsiness, alternating with periods of irritability. In the severe cases there will be dyspnœa, delirium, repeated convulsions, and coma.

These are the regular symptoms of the disease—symptoms varying in their number and development with the intensity of the nephritis. In the worst cases the cerebral symptoms are developed early and the patients die at the end of a few days. In other cases the symptoms continue for months, and at the end of that time terminate either in the death or recovery of the patient. Albumen and casts in the urine may persist long after all other symptoms have disappeared. In other cases the disease runs a very mild course; the patients are not at any time seriously ill, and they recover completely at the end of two or three weeks. In still other cases the acute inflammation is succeeded by chronic diffuse nephritis. Relapses and repeated attacks of the disease occur in some persons.

The course of the disease may be modified by complicating inflammations. Pericarditis, pleurisy, peritonitis, pneumonia, cystitis, and inflammations of the joints and muscles are not uncommon.

PROGNOSIS.—In the larger number of cases the prognosis is good. The milder cases recover after two or three weeks; more severe cases last for several months. The bad cases die at the end of a few days with cerebral symptoms, or all the symptoms continue and the patient dies at the end of several months, or they pass on to the lesions and symptoms of chronic diffuse nephritis, or they die from some complicating inflammation.

TREATMENT.—In the mild cases but little treatment is required. The patients should be kept in bed, should have a fluid diet, the bowels should be moved, and the restlessness should be quieted by the bromides, chloral hydrate, or opium. If the dropsy is a marked feature, more active purgatives are to be employed, hot-water or hot-air baths are to be used, and jaborandi may be of service. When the urine is very scanty, wet or dry cups over the region of the kidneys and hot fomentation over the same region are of much service. For the more marked cerebral symptoms treatment is not very satisfactory. As the patients get better iron and tonics are usually indicated. Great care must be used to prevent relapses. All exposure to cold must be avoided; the patient is to be kept in the house or sent to a warm climate for some time after he is apparently well. So long as albumen and casts persist in the urine the patients must not be considered well, although they may present no renal symptoms.

(2) In the second set of cases the invasion of the disease is not acute, and the symptoms may at first be so slight that the patient will hardly notice them. Usually the first symptoms are referable to the stomach. The patients lose their appetite, are troubled with nausea, and vomit occasionally. There may be a moderate amount of pain in the back, general languor, and indisposition for mental or physical work. Then they notice a change in the urine; they pass much less than before. The urine remains of its ordinary color or is a little smoky; its specific gravity is less; it contains a good deal of albumen, sometimes a little blood, and large numbers of hyaline, granular, and epithelial casts.

Dropsy makes its appearance at first in the face or feet; it may remain confined to these regions or extend to the rest of the body and become a general dropsy. The cerebral symptoms are slight—headache, irritability, drowsiness. The blood becomes thin and watery and the patients unnaturally pale. There may be dyspnœa either dropsical or nervous. The symptoms continue for weeks or months.

PROGNOSIS.—These cases, as a rule, do well, and recover at the end of a few weeks or months. But in some the symptoms continue and the patients go on to have chronic diffuse nephritis.

TREATMENT.—In the mild cases it is only necessary to keep the patients in the house, put them on a milk diet, keep the bowels open, and after a time give them iron. If the dropsy is more marked, we must try to get rid of it by cathartics, sweating, and diuretics. If the anæmia is marked, inhalations of oxygen must be combined with the administration of iron.   In these cases also it is important to guard against relapses.

The Acute Diffuse Nephritis of Scarlatina.

Most cases of scarlatina are complicated either by acute parenchymatous or diffuse nephritis.   Some confusion has arisen from the attempt to describe scarlatinal nephritis as if it was one disease, while really there are two anatomical forms of nephritis which occur as complications of scarlatina.   When we try to fix the time during the course of scarlatina when the kidney lesions are developed, we meet with the same difficulty —that statistics have been compiled on the supposition that there is only one form of scarlatinal nephritis.   If we take all the cases together, we find that kidney symptoms may be developed from the very first day of scarlet fever to the end of the ninth week—that the largest number of cases develop symptoms on the fourteenth day, the next largest on the twenty-first day, and next to this on the seventh day (Tripe).   It seems probable that parenchymatous nephritis belongs to the first weeks of the disease, diffuse nephritis to the later weeks.

SYMPTOMS.—The urine is diminished in amount, and may be suppressed.   Its specific gravity is low, its color is bloody or smoky; it contains blood, large amounts of albumen, and numerous hyaline, granular, and epithelial casts.

The patients lose their appetites, and suffer from nausea and occasional vomiting.   There is a febrile movement, usually not very severe, pain in the back and limbs.   They become unnaturally peevish and irritable and complain of headache, the irritability alternating with drowsiness.   In the more severe cases delirium, convulsions, and coma are developed.   The color of the patients is changed, the skin and mucous membranes becoming pale.   Dropsy is developed—sometimes only a little puffiness of the face, hands, or feet, sometimes general anasarca.   Synovitis and muscular rheumatism are frequent complications, while pericarditis, pleurisy, and pneumonia occur less often.

The disease runs its course within a moderate length of time, although the changes in the urine often persist long after all the other symptoms have disappeared.   The ordinary cases recover after from one to three weeks; the very bad cases die at the end of a few days.   In a few cases the symptoms continue and the patient develops chronic diffuse nephritis.

PROGNOSIS.—The prognosis is quite good.   The larger number of the cases recover completely.   In the more severe cases, however, the patients may die with cerebral symptoms, or all the symptoms will continue and the patient die after several weeks.

TREATMENT.—The indications for treatment are the same as in the idiopathic form of acute diffuse nephritis.

Chronic Diffuse Nephritis.

This is the most common and the most important form of kidney disease.   It has been described under a variety of names—chronic Bright's disease, croupous, catarrhal, interstitial, tubal, and parenchymatous nephritis; fatty, granular, atrophied, cirrhotic, and large white kidney.

Although all patients with chronic diffuse nephritis suffer from essentially the same symptoms, yet there is a good deal of difference as to the way in which these symptoms are developed and as to the predominance of some symptoms over others. Although the minute lesions of the kidneys are essentially the same in all cases, yet the gross appearance varies a good deal. There is, therefore, a practical convenience in distinguishing certain varieties of chronic diffuse nephritis. Of late years, however, the tendency to do this has been carried very far, especially as regards the atrophic form of chronic diffuse nephritis. Writers speak as if there were only two forms of chronic diffuse nephritis—the large white kidneys and the atrophied kidneys—and as if each of these had a distinct clinical history. More than this, the changes in the blood-vessels and in the circulation which so often complicate chronic Bright's disease have attracted so much attention that the arterial changes have been regarded as the most important part of the disease, so that we even hear of Bright's disease without any lesion of the kidneys. It is also customary to describe separately those kidneys of which the arteries have undergone waxy infiltrations.

I do not think that either the lesions or the symptoms are such as to justify such views. After separating the true cases of chronic parenchymatous nephritis—cases in which only the epithelium of the tubes and of the Malpighian capsules is changed—all the other kidneys of chronic Bright's disease present essentially the same lesions and give rise to the same symptoms.

We can indeed often tell during the life of the patient whether he has large white or atrophied or waxy kidneys, but in many cases such a diagnosis is impossible.

MORBID ANATOMY.—There is good deal of variety in the gross appearances and size of the kidneys. Most numerous are the so-called atrophied kidneys. These kidneys are usually diminished in weight, the kidneys weighing together three or four ounces, but often they weigh up to ten or twelve ounces. The capsules are adherent, and when they are stripped off portions of the kidney-tissue adhere to them. After stripping off the capsules the surface of the kidney is left finely or coarsely nodular. The cortex is thinned and of a red or grayish mottled color; the pyramids are small or of normal size, sometimes studded with small white concretions of urate of soda. There are often small cysts both in the cortex and pyramids.

Next in frequency come the so-called large white kidneys. Of these a certain number are not examples of chronic diffuse nephritis at all, but of acute or chronic parenchymatous nephritis. Of the large white kidneys which belong to chronic diffuse nephritis we can distinguish three varieties—the simple large white, the waxy large white, and the large white of cardiac disease.

The gross appearance of the kidneys is very much the same whether they are or are not the seat of waxy infiltrations. They are increased in size, weighing together from sixteen to twenty ounces. The capsules are not adherent; the surfaces of the kidneys are smooth and pale, often mottled by large stellate veins. The cortex is thickened, of white or white mottled with red, or yellow or grayish color. In the very waxy kidneys the gray or white color has a semi-translucent appearance. The pyramids are large and red, contrasting with the cortex. We find some kidneys of the same color and general appearance as large white kidneys, but with atrophied cortex and adherent capsules.

The large white kidneys due to cardiac disease are increased in size and weight. The capsules are not adherent, the surfaces are smooth. The cortex is thickened and of a peculiar pinkish-white color; the cortical striæ may still be visible. The pyramids are of a somewhat darker red than the cortex. The whole coloring is entirely different from that of chronic congestion of the kidneys, and the texture, although firm, is not of the stony hardness of that lesion.

Besides the atrophied and the large white kidneys, there are a large number of kidneys which are not diminished in weight and which do not resemble either the large white or the atrophied kidneys. These kidneys weigh together from nine to twenty ounces. The capsules are sometimes adherent, sometimes not. The surface of the cortex may look like that of a normal kidney or be finely or coarsely nodular. The cortex is of normal thickness or thickened; it is of a variety of colors. Sometimes it is not to be distinguished from a normal kidney, or it may be gray or gray mottled with yellow or red or white, or of a diffuse red color. The pyramids are of natural size or large, of red or pale color. I do not know a good name for these kidneys, but their appearance differs altogether from that of the large white or atrophied kidneys.

Still another class may be made of those kidneys which pass from the condition of chronic congestion into that of chronic diffuse nephritis. These kidneys retain the color and the hardness of chronic congestion, but the capsules are adherent, the surfaces finely nodular, and the cortex irregular.

Minute Lesions.—Nearly all the component parts of the kidneys undergo morbid changes. In the tubes the epithelial cells undergo marked changes, especially in the cortex. The epithelial cells are swollen, finely or coarsely granular, or fatty or completely disintegrated, or the seat of hyaline degeneration. They may be detached from the walls of the tubes, or sometimes they are in place, but flattened. The tubes may contain cast-matter, blood, pus-cells, small polygonal cells. The calibre of the tubes is often changed. The tubes may be dilated either in the form of cylindrical or sacculated dilatations; the latter often form cysts of considerable size. Such dilatations regularly affect groups of tubes, as if they were due to obstruction of the large tubes in the pyramids. In other cases the tubes are denuded of epithelium, become smaller, fall together, and look like connective tissue. The membranous wall of the tubules may be thickened or it may undergo waxy degeneration.

The Malpighian bodies are changed. Their capsules may be thickened, contracted, or dilated. The flat cells which line the capsules are increased in size, sometimes in number. The capillary tuft may be dilated or its walls may be thickened; it may be completely obliterated and changed into a ball of fibrous tissue, or it may be the seat of waxy infiltration. Often the Malpighian bodies are much closer together than they are in a normal kidney.

In the stroma, especially in the cortex, there is a new growth of connective tissue. This new connective tissue is in patches of varying size, surrounds Malpighian bodies and blood-vessels, and may be continuous with the capsule of the kidneys.

The arteries are frequently changed. There is a general thickening of all their coats, usually a simple sclerotic thickening.

All these changes, when they have once begun in the kidneys, have a natural tendency to go on and become more and more marked. There is much difference in different kidneys in the predominance of one or more of these changes over others. In one kidney the changes in the tubes will be most marked, in another those in the Malpighian bodies, in another those in the stroma. But there seems no good reason for believing that these changes are developed successively—that there is first a lesion of the stroma, then a lesion of the tubes, or first a lesion of the tubes, and then of the stroma. The earliest examples of chronic diffuse nephritis, obtained from persons dying accidentally of other diseases, show that the lesions are diffuse at the very outset.

In the atrophied kidneys the new connective tissue is in patches. In the earliest stages of the lesion these patches are confined to the region close to the capsule; later in the disease the whole thickness of the cortex is involved. The tubes embraced within these areas of new connective tissue are atrophied and collapsed. The rest of the cortex-tubes exhibit marked degenerative changes in the epithelium, and often cast-matter. Dilatation of the tubes is very common. The Malpighian bodies are usually much altered—the capsules thickened, the tufts atrophied. Occasionally there is waxy degeneration of the Malpighian tufts. There are some atrophied kidneys in which the changes in the stroma are very slight.

In the large white kidneys there is much variety. In some of them one is surprised to find how slight the minute lesions are. In others the principal changes are in the epithelium of the tubes, so that it may be difficult to tell whether they are examples of parenchymatous or of diffuse nephritis. In many others there is a very marked production of new connective tissue either in patches or diffuse. The large white kidneys which are waxy differ from the others only in the addition of the waxy degeneration of the Malpighian tufts and arteries to the other lesions. I have no knowledge of any kidneys in which waxy degeneration exists without the presence of the regular lesions of diffuse nephritis.

In the large white kidneys of cardiac disease the large thickened arteries are a prominent feature.

ETIOLOGY.—Chronic diffuse nephritis is more common in males than in females. It is said to occur at nearly all ages; the maximum liability is in persons between the ages of forty-five and fifty-five years. The disease prevails principally in temperate climates; in New York it is of very common occurrence. Persons who are habitually intemperate, who have constitutional syphilis, who suffer from privation, are very liable to the disease. There is a disposition in certain families to the development of the disease. Not that it is, strictly speaking, hereditary, but there will be a number of examples of it in the same family. A number of brothers and sisters or of more distant relatives in the same family will at different times suffer from the disease. There seems also to be some sort of relationship between chronic diffuse nephritis and pulmonary phthisis. Not only does nephritis complicate phthisis, but in the same family some members have phthisis, others nephritis.

Acute diffuse nephritis and chronic congestion of the kidney may be followed by chronic diffuse nephritis.

Heart disease, emphysema, phthisis, cirrhosis of the liver, chronic inflammation of the bones and joints, gout, rheumatism, and chronic arteritis, are often complicated by the disease.

SYMPTOMS.—It is sometimes impossible to tell which of the varieties of chronic nephritis exists in a given patient, but in other cases the diagnosis can be made. If, however, we correct our clinical diagnosis by post-mortem observations, we find that we may be mistaken about even the (apparently) most characteristic cases. There is more difference in the earlier stages of these cases than in the later ones. In hospitals, where the patients come to die, all the cases of chronic diffuse nephritis are a good deal alike.

The atrophied kidneys present us with a very great variety of clinical histories. It is impossible to describe all the different ways in which the disease may begin and run its course, but we may enumerate some of them :

1. Persons may have atrophied kidneys for a number of years without any renal symptoms; they die from accident or from some other disease, and at the autopsy the kidneys are found to be far advanced in disease.

2. The disease of the kidneys exists, but it gives no symptoms until the patient suffers from some severe accident or is attacked by some acute disease, and then the renal symptoms are suddenly developed.

3. The patient will very slowly lose flesh and strength, the appetite will be capricious, either mental or bodily exertion is an effort, but there are no positive symptoms, except that the urine is of rather low specific gravity, and in the evening urine there will be occasionally a trace of albumen. In this condition these patients may continue for years. They may improve very much under treatment, and finally die from some other disease without ever developing any renal symptoms. Other cases, however, do after a time develop all the characteristic symptoms.

4. For several months the patients do not feel well: the appetite is lost, there is nausea and occasional vomiting, they become pale and anæmic, do not sleep well at night, are irritable and easily worried, are troubled with headache. The urine continues normal or is of low specific gravity or contains a little albumen. Then they suddenly become worse and the regular symptoms are developed.

5. In other cases headache or sleeplessness or dyspnoea or loss of vision may precede all the other symptoms by several weeks.

6. Severe neuralgic pains in different parts of the body, coming on in attacks and very rebellious to treatment, may precede the other symptoms for months.

7. The very first symptoms may be an attack of convulsions. The patient may have been apparently in good health, and while sitting quietly in a room or lying in bed will be seized with a general convulsion. In some of these cases the convulsions are repeated; between them the patient remains partly or completely unconscious, and dies in

a few days. In other cases one or two convulsions are followed by the development of the other symptoms of the disease.

8. With valvular disease of the heart and atrophied kidneys we may get the same combination of symptoms which I have described in the section on chronic congestion of the kidneys.

9. The patient may first notice that he is passing too much urine. This urine is of low specific gravity, and occasionally contains a little albumen and hyaline casts. Then the health begins to fail: there are dyspeptic symptoms, headache, occasional œdema of the legs. From time to time the patient becomes worse; the urine is diminished in quantity, the headache is more marked; he cannot sleep, he has dyspnœa, he vomits, the muscles of the face twitch, or there may be general convulsions or delirium or partial or complete coma. Such attacks may last for days or weeks, and then either terminate fatally, or the patient gets better and may be able to return to his ordinary business for a time. In this way the same patient may suffer from a number of such attacks.

10. In some cases dropsy is a prominent feature from the very first and goes on to general anasarca.

The following history would answer for many of the cases of atrophied kidneys: A woman, thirty-eight years old, was in good health, fat and robust, until January, 1873. Then she caught cold; her feet became œdematous; she had headache, pain in the back, vomiting; her eyesight was impaired; her urine was increased in amount and passed more frequently. She continued in this condition and losing flesh and strength until June, 1873, when she came into the hospital. At that time the urine was diminished to eighteen ounces in twenty-four hours; it contained a considerable amount of albumen and hyaline and granular casts. Her color was still good. There was moderate œdema of the feet. After this the urine increased in amount to eighty ounces daily—specific gravity 1002, albumen diminished. The dropsy disappeared, and the patient left the hospital feeling very well on September 29, 1873. In December, 1873, she returned to the hospital with nausea and vomiting, dyspnœa, cough, no dropsy; urine 80 to 100 ounces daily. She had become feeble and anæmic, and there was well-marked hypertrophy of the left ventricle of the heart. She again improved, and was discharged after two weeks. In March, 1874, she returned. The urine was now scanty, and she was troubled with vomiting, dyspnœa, cough, sleeplessness, slight convulsive movements of the voluntary muscles, no dropsy. By the end of April she was again feeling well, and left the hospital. In June, 1874, she returned with all the old symptoms and œdema of the legs. On July 20 she had two general convulsions. After this she again improved for a time, but in September all the symptoms returned, and she was delirious a good deal of the time. Urine 40 to 50 ounces daily, specific gravity 1005, moderate amount of albumen, no casts. By the end of September she again was sleepless, had several slight convulsions, and died October 2. The kidneys were a typical picture of the red atrophied kidneys with thickened arteries.

We may say in general that with the atrophied kidneys the so-called uræmic symptoms—headache, sleeplessness, delirium, convulsions, coma, dyspnœa—are very apt to occur, and that early in the disease. The urine is regularly increased in amount and of low specific gravity, except during the uræmic attacks, when it is diminished ; but the uræmic attacks may come on while the patient is passing 30 to 40 ounces of urine of a specific gravity of 1020. Albumen is regularly present only in small amounts, and not constantly, but exceptionally there will be a good deal. Casts are hyaline, not constant, but exceptionally in considerable numbers. Dropsy may be absent throughout the disease, or a little œdema of the face and legs may come and go, or there may be marked general anasarca. Not unfrequently during the uræmic attacks the temperature runs up to 99° to 100°. Hypertrophy of the left ventricle of the heart is a frequent complication, but I have not found it in as large a proportion of cases in New York as it is described by English and German writers.

The duration of the disease is very uncertain. In fact, we seldom know what its real duration is, for the reason that there is no necessary relation between the development of the kidney lesions and the appearance of the symptoms. After the appearance of the kidney symptoms some of the patients die in a few days ; others go on for months and years with either constant or intermittent symptoms.

The Large White Kidney.—These cases are more readily recognized than the cases of atrophied kidneys, for the reason that dropsy is more constant and occurs earlier in the disease, and that albumen is regularly present in the urine.

In many of the cases œdema of the face or feet is the first symptom. Often the patients will tell you that it is the only symptom, and that they would feel perfectly well if they could only get rid of the swelling. Closer questioning, however, will usually show that the functions of the stomach are disturbed, that there is occasional headache, that the eyesight is impaired, and that the patient has been passing less urine.

In some cases impairment of vision is the first symptom that attracts the attention of the patient. In some cases disturbances of digestion, or neuralgic pains, or gradual loss of health and strength, or a diminished amount of urine, will be the first symptoms, and may last for weeks before other symptoms are developed. Or the patient may be attacked suddenly as if with acute diffuse nephritis. The urine will contain blood and numerous casts ; the dropsy and the other symptoms are rapidly developed. In some of the cases complicated with cardiac disease the history will be that of heart disease rather than that of kidney disease.

When the disease is fairly established the dropsy is always a prominent symptom, often very distressing to the patient. In some patients when once developed it continues to increase steadily up to the time of their death ; in others the dropsy comes and goes, sometimes disappearing altogether for weeks and months.

The functions of the stomach are usually disturbed, the patients lose appetite, have nausea and vomiting, oppression after eating, etc. But some persons retain a good appetite for a long time, even though they vomit occasionally. Diarrhœa is often developed ; sometimes only enough to carry off part of the dropsy, sometimes profuse, persistent, and uncontrollable. The blood becomes thin and watery, and the skin, the mucous membranes, and the sclerotic assume an unnatural white appearance. The patients lose both mental and bodily vigor, and become less and less fit to carry on their ordinary occupations.

Of the uræmic symptoms, headache and dyspnœa occur at any time in the course of the disease, but convulsions, delirium, and coma belong to its later stages.

The urine is regularly first diminished and afterward increased, but the quantity often varies very much from day to day. The specific gravity is regularly low, albumen is constant and in large amount; casts are usually present in considerable numbers, especially during the exacerbations of the disease, when hyaline, granular, and epithelial casts are found, but in other cases hardly any casts can be found. Blood is sometimes present in the urine during the exacerbations of the nephritis.

The disease varies much in its course and duration. Some cases progress steadily, getting worse from day to day, and die at the end of a few months from the time at which the first symptoms appeared. Other persons go on living for years, the symptoms improving or disappearing for weeks or months, and then coming again. Finally, the patients die—some in an exacerbation of the disease with bloody urine and acute symptoms; some with excessive dropsy; some with delirium, convulsions, and coma; some suddenly; some with complicating disease.

The following histories may serve to illustrate the course of the disease

A male, thirty years old, of intemperate habits, for one year before his death noticed that his urine was sometimes scanty and high-colored, sometimes abundant and pale, and that his eyesight became impaired. For four months there was occasional nausea and vomiting. For six weeks there was occasional headache, dyspnœa, and œdema of the feet, the urine more scanty. For nine days before death he passed from one to four ounces of urine daily, specific gravity 1014, albumen 50 per cent., numerous hyaline, granular, and epithelial casts. The man was now feeble and anæmic, had headache, was drowsy, vomited occasionally, had twitching of muscles of face; continued drowsy, but with his mental faculties quite clear, so that he was able to transact some business an hour before he died. Death was sudden while lying quietly in bed. The kidneys weighed twenty ounces, surfaces smooth, cortex thick and white, pyramids large and red. The Malpighian bodies showed a marked increase in the size and number of the capsule cells; the cortex-tubes were dilated; in some the epithelium was flattened, in others swollen, granular, and detached; in the pyramid-tubes the epithelium was swollen and detached; there was cast-matter in some of the tubes, both in the cortex and pyramids; there was a very extensive new growth of new connective tissue in the cortex, partly diffuse, partly in patches.

A male, forty-one years old, six years before his death caught cold while bathing, and suffered with dropsy, a febrile movement, prostration, scanty urine which contained albumen, blood, and numerous casts. After a few weeks all the symptoms disappeared and he returned to his business. He continued to enjoy good health for about eighteen months; then in the winter the urine became scanty and contained blood, albumen, and numerous casts. General anasarca was rapidly developed. The dropsy lasted for six months, and then disappeared, but the urine from that time always contained varying amounts of albumen and casts. For nearly two years after this time the man continued to feel well, was actively engaged in business, had no dropsy, but the urine still contained

casts and albumen. Then the dropsy returned again, and was very considerable. But the appetite and digestion continued good, there was no
headache, the patient was intelligent and cheerful. The dropsy, a moderate diarrhœa, and the change in the urine were the only symptoms.
In two months the dropsy had again disappeared and the patient returned
to his work. After this time, however, the patient was never as well : a
little œdema of the legs was present much of the time; he became gradually more and more anæmic and feeble, and finally died with marked
dropsy and anæmia about six years from the time of the first appearance
of kidney symptoms.

The Large White Kidneys with Waxy Infiltration.—It is well known
that in certain persons a peculiar morbid change takes place in the
viscera. The walls of the blood-vessels and some of the glandular
cells become infiltrated with a peculiar translucent substance. This
morbid change is commonly known by the name of waxy or amyloid
infiltration. It is known that such an infiltration occurs regularly in
persons who have chronic inflammations of the bones and joints, constitutional syphilis, and pulmonary phthisis. It is also known that this
new substance is colored in a special way by iodine and some of the aniline colors. Beyond this we have no real knowledge of what the substance is or how it is produced.

In other parts of the body the waxy infiltration can hardly be said to
produce any local symptoms. If one has a waxy liver or spleen, these
organs may give the physical evidences of their enlargement, but that
is all. We look upon such patients as suffering from some general
changes concerning the nature of which we are ignorant, but not as
suffering simply from disease of the liver or spleen.

It seems at first sight natural to think of waxy kidneys in the same
way—not as examples of kidney disease, but as parts of a general morbid
condition. This view has been adopted by most authors. They describe
the waxy kidneys as something different from the other forms of nephritis. But really this is an error. In the vast majority of cases the waxy
kidneys are simply a variety of chronic diffuse nephritis. It is possible
(Cohnheim) to have waxy infiltration of the Malpighian bodies without
other lesion of the kidney, but this is a rare exception. The rule is that
we find the ordinary lesions of chronic diffuse nephritis ; and, more than
this, we often find the nephritic lesions very much farther advanced than
the waxy infiltration. The association of the lesions is not at all such as
to give the idea that the waxy infiltration is produced first and the other
lesions afterward. It is also not uncommon to find waxy infiltration of
the Malpighian tufts without similar changes in any other part of the
body.

The type of the nephritis varies in different cases. Most of the kidneys resemble the large white kidneys, some the atrophied, some those
which are neither large white nor atrophied. The clinical history varies
in the same way, and is that of a large white or atrophied kidney, as the
case may be. The only difference is that in some patients (not in the
majority) there is a very large amount of urine passed of low specific
gravity.

As a matter of fact, in most cases of waxy kidneys we simply make
the diagnosis of chronic diffuse nephritis, and if we add to this that of

waxy infiltration it is because the patients have had syphilis or bone or joint disease. Even in this way we are often enough deceived, as in the following case :

A woman, twenty-six years old, came into the hospital on January 25, 1876. She had contracted syphilis five years before. For two years she had suffered from dyspnœa and frontal headache. For seven months there was occasional œdema of the face and feet. At the time of her admission to the hospital she was very pale and anæmic; the urine was of a specific gravity of 1008, abundant, and contained no albumen or casts. The liver was very large and smooth. It was supposed that she had waxy liver and kidneys. She grew steadily weaker, continued to have a little œdema, vomited occasionally, developed the physical signs of bronchitis, with a temperature of 104° Fahr., and died on April 3, 1876. At the autopsy the aortic valves were found thin and insufficient. There was muco-pus in both the large and small bronchi, with irregular spots of red hepatization in the lung. The liver and spleen were large and waxy. The kidneys weighed together four ounces, and presented the ordinary lesions of atrophied kidneys, with only commencing waxy infiltrations of a few of the Malpighian tufts.

The Large White Kidney of Heart Disease.—This variety of chronic diffuse nephritis seems to be secondary to organic disease of the heart, and, less frequently, to emphysema of the lungs. The urine is diminished in amount, sometimes suppressed ; it is dark-colored, the specific gravity varies between 1010 and 1030 ; albumen is absent altogether or present in small amount ; hyaline and granular casts may be present, but are not constant. Dropsy may be absent or moderate or excessive. Cerebral symptoms—vomiting, cough, dyspnœa, anæmia—are usually present. Some of the patients die suddenly, some with dropsy, some with urgent dyspnœa.

The examples of chronic diffuse nephritis which are neither atrophied kidneys nor large white kidneys are numerous. Some of them give the clinical history of the large white kidneys, some that of the atrophied kidneys, some do not correspond to that of either ; but they all exhibit some of the characteristic symptoms of chronic nephritis—changes in the urine, dyspnœa, vomiting, cerebral symptoms, dropsy, anæmia.

The following histories will show the course of the disease in some of these cases :

Case 1.—A male, forty years old, came into hospital on October 9, 1881. The patient was a beer-drinker, but denied rheumatism and syphilis. He said that he had been perfectly well until fourteen months before ; then he had an attack of lobar pneumonia which confined him to the house for four weeks. Since that time he has never felt as well and has had occasional dyspnœa. Nine months ago the dyspnœa became so troublesome that he had to give up work, and he also began to suffer from severe headaches. Three weeks ago the urine became scanty and dropsy appeared in the legs and scrotum. When admitted to the hospital the patient was large and fat. There was dropsy of the legs and of the scrotum, marked dyspnœa, sibillant râles over both lungs; 10 ounces of urine in twenty-four hours, specific gravity 1023, albumen 10 per cent.; hyaline and epithelial casts. The urine on Oct. 12 was 13 ounces ; on Oct. 14, 42 ounces ; on Oct. 18, 54 ounces. On this last day he had several convulsions, became comatose, and died October 19. At the autopsy the pia mater was thickened and there was an increase of serum beneath it. The heart weighed fourteen ounces, the aortic and mitral valves were a little thickened, the walls of the ventricles were unnaturally hard. In the lungs there were a few old hard miliary tubercles. The kidneys weighed sixteen ounces, surfaces smooth, capsules not adherent, cortex and pyramids of red color, urates in the pyramids. The cortex-tubes showed marked changes in their epithelium, but the Malpighian bodies, stroma, and arteries were nearly normal.

Case 2.—A female, forty-five years old, was admitted to the hospital December 5, 1881. Denied rheumatism, syphilis, and intemperance. She had considered herself strong and well until two months before. Then she had a sudden attack of dyspnœa, dizziness, faintness, and cardiac palpitation. After this she was never well, complained of pain about the heart, headache, attacks of dyspnœa, dropsy of the face, hands, and feet. The urine was scanty and dark-colored. She is now emaciated and anæmic, has moderate œdema of the legs, complains of dyspnœa, headache, and nausea. The heart's action is feeble and irregular, and there is a presystolic murmur. On December 19 she vomited blood. On January 2 she had a chill, followed by a temperature of 102°. On January 5 she became drowsy, then had twitchings of the muscles of the face; became semi-comatose, and died January 11. While she was in the hospital the urine varied in amount from 1 to 6 ounces daily; it contained a very large amount of albumen and a few hyaline casts. After death the pia mater looked sodden and finely granular. The walls of its arteries were a little thickened, and there were little clumps of endothelial cells on its outer surface. The mitral valve of the heart was thickened and stenosed. The kidneys were of medium size, their capsules slightly adherent, their surfaces finely nodular, the cortex of normal thickness, red mottled with yellow spots. There was an extensive growth of diffuse connective tissue separating the tubes both in the cortex and pyramids. The tubes were large and contained much cast-matter. Most of the Malpighian bodies were normal.

COMPLICATIONS.—The most frequent complication of chronic diffuse nephritis is disease of the heart. We find cardiac lesions and renal lesions associated in three different ways:

1. Valvular lesions or dilatation of the ventricles produce chronic congestion of the kidney, with its changes into parenchymatous or diffuse nephritis or the large white kidney of cardiac disease.

2. Chronic diffuse nephritis is followed by the development of hypertrophy of the left ventricle. This may occur with all the varieties of chronic diffuse nephritis, but is most common with the atrophied kidneys.

3. Valvular lesions and chronic nephritis occur in the same persons, but neither can be said to depend upon the other.

The arteries are often diseased, the aorta and the arteries throughout the body. There may be a simple sclerosis and thickening of the wall of an artery, or endarteritis deformans, or obliterating arteritis.

Cerebral apoplexy may occur with all the varieties of chronic diffuse nephritis, but much more frequently with atrophied kidneys.

Thickening of the pia mater, with increase of serum beneath it, is often seen.

Dilatation of the lateral ventricles of the brain sometimes occurs, and may give rise to cerebral symptoms.

Pericarditis is seen more frequently with the atrophied kidneys.

Pneumonia is especially apt to be fatal when it occurs in persons already suffering from chronic diffuse nephritis.

Emphysema and chronic bronchitis are often associated with the atrophied kidneys.

Phthisis is found with all the varieties of chronic nephritis.

Peritonitis occurs in a few cases as a complicating inflammation.

Cirrhosis of the liver is found quite frequently.

PROGNOSIS.—In every case of chronic diffuse nephritis the natural course of the morbid changes in the kidney tissue is to become more marked and involve more and more of the kidney. The effect upon the general health of the patient is not in any exact relation to the degree of the kidney lesion. These two facts render the prognosis of chronic diffuse nephritis very uncertain. The disease is always a very serious one, and terminates regularly in destroying life, but the length of time that will elapse before this fatal termination, and the precise way in which death will take place, are difficult to determine beforehand.

TREATMENT.—There seems no good reason for believing that we can directly influence the development of the lesions in the kidneys. It is possible that such a development may be indirectly delayed by improving the general health of the patient.

There is good reason to believe that some of the symptoms which occur regularly in patients who have chronic diffuse nephritis are dependent not upon the nephritis, but upon other causes. We may therefore look for indications for treatment in three different directions:

1. To delay the development of the disease by improving the general health of the patient.

2. To treat those symptoms which are not produced by the kidney disease.

3. To treat those symptoms which are produced by the kidney lesions.

To fulfil the first indication the most potent influences that we have are the giving up of business and of vicious habits and causing the patient to live year after year in the most suitable climates. Generally speaking, warm climates are to be preferred, but the individual disposition of each patient must always be consulted.

Of less efficacy, but still of importance, are the improvement of the digestion by means of drugs and the feeding of the patient.

In every patient suffering from chronic diffuse nephritis there are a number of symptoms which seem to depend directly upon other conditions, and not upon the kidney lesions; for if these conditions are removed the symptoms disappear, although the kidney lesions continue. To this category of symptoms seem to belong the headache, delirium, stupor, coma, and convulsions, the nervous dyspnœa, the vomiting in part, the dropsy in part, the diminution of urine in part. All these symptoms are due to disturbances of the circulation, and the disturbances of the circulation are produced by a number of causes which may act separately or together. Changes in the valves and walls of the heart, in the force and regularity of the heart's contraction, in the walls and size of the arteries and capillaries, and in the volume and composition of the blood, each, separately or associated, may interfere with the proper circulation of the blood, and this interference usually takes the form of too much blood in the veins and too little blood in the arteries.

Anatomical changes in the valves of the heart, in its walls, and in the walls of the arteries and capillaries cannot be influenced by any means at our command. The force and regularity of the contractions of the heart can, however, be very decidedly modified by drugs. Opium in moderate doses makes the heart's action slower and stronger; iodide of potassium makes the heart's action more regular; convallaria makes the heart's action slower and stronger; digitalis increases the force of the heart's action, but at the same time contracts the arterioles; aconite and veratrum viride make the heart's action slower and more feeble.

The size of the arteries and capillaries can also be altered by drugs. Nitrite of amyl and nitro-glycerin relax and dilate the whole arterial and capillary system; chloral hydrate dilates the arterioles (Fothergill).

The volume of the blood can be diminished by bloodletting and by eliminating the plasma of the blood indirectly by sweating, purging, or diuresis.

The symptoms which can be ascribed directly to the presence of the kidney disease are—(1) The changes in the composition of the blood. We have still very little exact knowledge of what these changes are, but we may say generally that there is an increase in the relative quantity of the watery constituents of the blood and of the excrementitious products which should be eliminated by the kidneys. (2) The changes in the quantity of urine probably depend partly on the changes in the circulation, partly on the composition of the blood, and partly upon the structural changes in the kidneys. The albumen and casts seem to be directly due to the kidney lesion. (3) The changes in the nutrition of the patient, the disturbances of digestion, and some of the headaches, all seem to belong directly to the kidney disease.

Now let us try to apply these principles to the practical treatment of the different symptoms.

The Urine.—As regards the presence of albumen and casts, it is doubtful whether we are able to do anything, although it is customary to give the tr. ferri chloridi and the bichloride of mercury in order to diminish the excretion of albumen. As regards the quantity of urine, we must distinguish whether the patient is in the ordinary course of the disease, whether he is having an uræmic attack, or whether he is having an acute exacerbation of the nephritis with congestion of the kidney and blood in the urine. Under the circumstances last mentioned the indications are to apply wet or dry cups over the lumbar region, to use hot fomentations to the back or hot-air baths, to open the bowels freely, to put the patient on a milk diet, and, if the heart's action is too strong, to give aconite in small doses.

If during the ordinary course of the disease the urine is constantly diminished, diuretics are often of good service, although the cases differ as to the particular drugs which answer best. The preparations of digitalis, the diuretic pill of digitalis, squills, and bichloride of mercury, the iodide and acetate of potash, and jaborandi in small doses, are the most reliable agents of this class. Sometimes the frequent use of milk or of water in small quantities (half an ounce or an ounce every half hour) will answer the purpose. There can never be any use in continuing the employment of diuretics in these cases if after a fair trial they do not increase the flow of urine.

During the progress of uræmic attacks diuretics do not act, and the same is often the case with cathartics and diaphoretics. The urine is only to be increased by the same means which are indicated for the relief of the whole uræmic condition, and of these we will speak later.

The dropsy in many cases will vary in amount, and even disappear at times without any treatment. It is regularly most marked with the large white kidneys and with those kidneys which are neither large white nor atrophied, especially when there is complicating heart disease and the patient is anæmic. Generally speaking, it is best to keep dropsical patients in bed most of the day. We attempt to get rid of the œdema by the skin, the bowels, and the kidneys, to regulate the heart's action, and to improve the condition of the blood. Hot-air baths or hot-water baths repeated every day, the milder hydragogue cathartics, and the different diuretics may all be used with advantage. If the dropsy is excessive, it may be necessary to tap the peritoneal or pleural cavities or to puncture the skin of the legs and scrotum. Sometimes bandaging the legs so as to exert moderate pressure seems to assist in getting rid of dropsy. To regulate the heart's action we find that digitalis, convallaria, and the iodide of potash are often of service. To improve the condition of the blood the systematic use of iron and oxygen is indicated. The most hopeless cases are those in which there is complicating heart disease and those in which the dropsy steadily increases, although the patient is passing from 60 to 100 ounces of urine daily.

Disturbances of the stomach are of different kinds and dependent upon different conditions. There may be simply loss of appetite or discomfort after eating, or nausea, flatulence, and vomiting; and these symptoms will be associated with chronic catarrhal gastritis or with a stomach that is anatomically normal. Sometimes, although there is occasional nausea and vomiting, the appetite continues good, or as part of an uræmic attack there will be constant vomiting.

The habitual dyspeptic disturbances are to be treated like other cases of gastric dyspepsia. A regulated diet, the vegetable bitters, the mineral acids, or the alkalies are sometimes of service. The repeated and persistent vomiting of uræmic attacks is a most distressing symptom and one often very difficult to control. The patients must be fed with small quantities of fluid food or of prepared meat. The most efficient remedies are those addressed to the condition of the circulation. Hypodermic injections of morphia, enemata of chloral hydrate, inhalations of nitrite of amyl, convallaria in small doses by the mouth, are all of service.

The anæmia from which the patients suffer is to be combated by the systematic use of iron and oxygen. Any efficient preparation of iron will answer, but it must often be given in considerable doses. Sometimes the bichloride of mercury in small doses answers better than iron. The oxygen should be inhaled for from five to thirty minutes twice a day.

The so-called uræmic attacks, although they have a general similarity, yet vary in their manifestations in different cases. In some cases the patient develops an unnatural restlessness and anxiety, an inability to sleep, now and then a sudden twitch of one of the facial muscles, and headache. Or a patient whose color is still good will only complain of pain in the epigastrium and moderate dyspnœa, and yet will be in bed and evidently seriously ill. Or a patient who has been troubled with dyspeptic symptoms and gradual loss of strength suddenly develops vomiting, intense headache, sleeplessness, a single convulsion followed by facial paralysis. A man with a previous history of chronic Bright's disease becomes persistently anæmic and dropsical ; he has constant dyspnœa, cannot lie down, cannot sleep, and yet looks drowsy and stupid ; is mildly delirious and has very little intelligence ; then gradually becomes unconscious, then comatose, and so dies. Or there are first attacks of dyspnœa, either spasmodic or from exertion, but which are temporary and can be relieved. Then the dyspnœa becomes more constant and severe ; the patient cannot lie down at all, all remedies become less and less efficacious, and the dyspnœa only ends with the life of the sufferer. In other cases a patient will suddenly become unconscious, although not comatose ; he will lie flat in bed, the skin livid and bathed in perspiration, the respiration labored and rapid, with coarse râles all over the lungs, the heart's action rapid and feeble, the temperature perhaps a little elevated ; or sudden and profound coma or noisy delirium or repeated convulsions may be the prominent features.

There is hardly a limit to the variety of the precise manner in which all these symptoms—restlessness, sleeplessness, headache, vomiting, delirium, convulsions, and coma—may present themselves. It is to be remembered that although all these symptoms are always dangerous, and often fatal, yet patients may pass through a number of such attacks before the fatal one arrives.

To relieve these attacks the most effectual remedies are opium, chloral hydrate, nitrite of amyl, convallaria, digitalis, caffeine, bloodletting, purging, sweating, and cathartics.

Opium is a very valuable remedy, but great judgment is required in selecting the preparation and the dose for each case. The old doctrine that opium is a dangerous drug for patients suffering from Bright's disease is perfectly true, but it is equally true that it is also a valuable remedy. Generally speaking, the more marked the uræmic attack the larger the dose of opium that will be borne. It is always well to try to obtain a free movement from the bowels, although this is not always possible.

In the milder cases the fluid extract of convallaria in ten-minim doses will often diminish the frequency of the heart's action, increase the production of urine, and improve the general condition of the patient.

In the earlier stages of dyspnœa five-grain doses of the iodide of potash with a little opium will sometimes keep the patient comfortable for months. For the severe attacks of dyspnœa dry cups over the chest and inhalations of oxygen are of service. In the worst and most uncontrollable dyspnœa it seems justifiable to keep the patient under the influence of ether or chloroform.

SUPPURATIVE NEPHRITIS AND PYELO-NEPHRITIS.

SUPPURATIVE inflammation of the tissue of the kidney and of its pelvis and calices occurs under several different conditions: It is the result of injuries; it is due to emboli; it occurs without discoverable causes; it is secondary to cystitis, the cystitis being due to strictures of the urethra, to stone in the bladder, to paraplegia, to operations on the urethra, bladder, and uterus, to gonorrhœa, to enlarged prostate.

Chronic suppurative pyelo-nephritis is often caused by the presence of calculi in the pelvis of the kidney.

1. Suppurative Nephritis from Injury.—Gunshot wounds, incised or punctured wounds, falls, blows, and kicks are the ordinary traumatic causes. If the injury is a very severe one, it causes the death of the patient in a short time; if it is less severe, suppurative inflammation may be developed.

The inflammatory process may be diffuse, so that the whole of one or both kidneys is converted into a soft mass composed of pus, blood, and broken-down tissue, or it is circumscribed, and one or more abscesses are found in the kidney which may communicate with the pelvis.

SYMPTOMS.—Rigors mark the beginning of the suppuration, and are often repeated through its course. A febrile movement is developed which is apt to assume the hectic character with sweatings. There is often vomiting. There may be very severe pain, referred to the region of the inflamed kidneys. The urine is diminished or suppressed; it contains blood alone or blood and pus.

In the bad cases the patients pass into the typhoid condition, become delirious, and die comatose or with a very rapid or febrile pulse. Or the disease is protracted, the patients become more and more emaciated, and finally die exhausted.

In other cases the symptoms abate, the urine returns to its natural condition, and the patients recover.

TREATMENT.—The management of these cases is rather surgical than medical. The external wound is to be treated antiseptically, and the general condition of the patient to be looked after in the ordinary way.

Such traumatic abscesses are of infrequent occurrence. I have no personal knowledge of them.

2. Abscesses produced by Emboli.—In ordinary endocarditis with vegetations on the valves it often happens that fragments of the vegetations become fixed in the branches of the renal arteries. When this is the case infarctions are produced, usually of the white variety.

With malignant endocarditis, with surgical pyæmia, and with the curious cases called idiopathic pyæmia, small emboli seem to find their way into the smallest branches of the renal artery. They do not produce infarctions, but small abscesses. In these cases the kidneys are increased in size and dotted with little white points surrounded by a red zone. These little white points are formed by an infiltration of pus-cells between the tubes, and in the larger foci by a breaking down of the kidney-tissue. Colonies of micrococci are sometimes, but not always, found in the Malpighian tufts, the veins, and the abscesses.

SYMPTOMS.—These embolic abscesses can hardly be said to have any clinical history. Whatever symptoms may belong to them are lost in those of the general disease from which the patient is suffering.

3. Idiopathic Abscesses.—Occasionally cases of abscesses of one of the kidneys are met with. They last a long time, and when the patient dies both the kidney tissue and the pelvis are involved to such an extent as to render the anatomical diagnosis difficult. The greater part of the kidney-tissue is destroyed and replaced by sacs full of pus; the pelvis is dilated and its walls thickened. The surrounding connective tissue is thickened; perforations and sinuses may extend into the surrounding connective tissue, into the large intestine, and through the diaphragm into the lung.

SYMPTOMS.—At first these cases are apt to be very obscure. An irregular febrile movement accompanied with rigors comes and goes, lasting for shorter or longer periods. The patients lose appetite, vomit occasionally, and become emaciated and anæmic. With this there may be pain over the region of one of the kidneys.

After a time a tumor may make its appearance in the position of one kidney—a tumor which can be felt through the anterior abdominal wall. If the abscess communicates with the pelvis of the kidney and the ureter remains pervious, pus and fragments of kidney-tissue are discharged with the urine. The pus is usually discharged at intervals, and at such times the size of the tumor diminishes. In other cases the pus burrows in other directions—into the retro-peritoneal connective tissue, the peritoneal cavity, the colon, or through the diaphragm into the lung. These cases are apt to run a protracted course and terminate fatally.

TREATMENT.—The only plan of treatment likely to cure the patient is a surgical one—either to extirpate the diseased kidney, or to cut down on the abscess and treat it on the antiseptic plan like any deep abscess.

4. Suppurative Pyelo-Nephritis with Cystitis.—Lesions.—Usually both kidneys are affected. They are increased in size, and both the kidneys and their pelvis are congested. The mucous membrane of the pelvis is thickened and coated with pus or patches of fibrin. Scattered through the kidneys are abscesses and purulent foci of different sizes. The smallest foci are not visible to the naked eye, but with the microscope we find collections of pus-globules between the tubes, with swelling and degeueration of the epithelium within the tubes. The larger purulent foci look like white streaks or wedges running parallel to the tubes and surrounded by zones of congestion. The larger abscesses replace considerable portions of the kidney.

The ureters in some cases are inflamed, their walls thickened, their inner surface coated with pus or fibrin. The bladder presents regularly the lesions of acute or chronic cystitis.

ETIOLOGY.—For the production of this form of nephritis inflammation of the bladder seems to be necessary. How the inflammatory process is transmitted from the bladder to the kidneys is still uncertain, but it seems probable that it is effected by bacteria. The cases of cystitis in which a suppurative nephritis is likely to be developed are those due to strictures of the urethra, stone in the bladder, operations on the urethra, bladder, and uterus, paraplegia, gonorrhœa, and enlarged prostate.

SYMPTOMS.—When the nephritis occurs with cystitis due to stone in the bladder, strictures, or operations on the genito-urinary tract, the symptoms are much the same. The patient has first the symptoms belonging to the cystitis, then he is attacked with rigors, followed by a febrile movement. The rigors are often repeated; the febrile movement is very irregular and often accompanied by profuse sweating. There is a rapid change in the general condition of the patient. He becomes much prostrated and emaciated from day to day. The face is drawn and anxious, the tongue dry and brown, the pulse rapid and feeble, and delirium is developed, and the patient finally dies in a condition resembling that of typhoid fever or of pyæmia. The urine is diminished in amount; it may be suppressed. It contains blood, pus, and mucus. The pus and mucus belong to the cystitis; the blood seems to be derived both from the kidneys and the bladder.

Cases of suppurative nephritis complicating gonorrhœa are fortunately not common, but several of them have been observed. Murchison [1] describes two cases, in both of which the cerebral symptoms were very marked—delirium, convulsions, and coma. I have seen one such case. The patient was a prostitute who came into the hospital with a specific vaginitis. After a few days she developed symptoms of an acute cystitis; then after a few more days she was attacked with rigors and a febrile movement, passed rapidly into the typhoid condition, and died. At the autopsy there were found acute cystitis, pyelitis, and numerous small abscesses in both kidneys.

When suppurative nephritis complicates the cystitis due to enlarged prostate, the clinical symptoms are somewhat different. The patients are usually men over fifty. They have generally suffered from the symptoms of enlarged prostate—retention of urine, either constant or intermittent, and more or less cystitis, with pus and mucus in the urine in varying amount. Sometimes, however, no such history is obtained; the patients assert that they have had no previous bladder trouble. The first symptom is diminution in the amount of urine passed and the appearance of blood. The quantity of urine is only a few ounces or it is completely suppressed. The blood is present in considerable amount; often the patients seem to pass pure blood instead of urine. The patients rapidly become prostrated and very anxious. There are usually no rigors, and there may be no febrile movement. After this the prostration becomes more marked, the pulse is rapid and feeble, the skin cold and bathed in perspiration, and the patients die in collapse at the end of a few days.

PROGNOSIS.—Suppurative nephritis secondary to cystitis is a very fatal disease; so far as I know, all the cases die.

TREATMENT.—The treatment for these cases is altogether a preventive one directed to the cystitis. In the cases of paraplegia, stone in the bladder, stricture, and enlarged prostate constant care must be used to prevent the accumulation of urine in the bladder and the development of cystitis.

In all cases of operation on the genito-urinary tract the supervention of cystitis is to be guarded against.

[1] *Lancet,* 1875, p. 80.

PERINEPHRITIS.

The loose connective tissue which is situated around and beneath the kidney may become the seat of suppurative inflammation, and in this way abscesses of considerable size are formed.

LESIONS.—The connective tissue behind the kidney seems to be the usual point of origin of the inflammatory process, and it is here that the pus first collects. After the abscess has reached a certain size the suppuration seems to have a natural tendency to spread and the pus burrows in different directions—backward through the muscles; downward along the iliac fossa, even as far as the perineum and scrotum or vagina; forward into the peritoneal cavity, the colon, or the bladder; upward through the diaphragm. The kidney is either compressed by the abscess or its tissue also becomes involved in the suppurative process. The soft parts around the abscess become thickened.

ETIOLOGY.—Perinephritis is either secondary or primary. The secondary cases are due to extension of· the inflammation from abscesses in the vicinity, such as are formed with caries of the spine, pelvic cellulitis, puerperal parametritis, perityphlitis, suppuration of the kidneys, and pyelo-nephritis. The primary cases occur after exposure to cold, after contusions over the lumbar region, great muscular exertion, and without discoverable cause. The lesion is said to complicate typhus and typhoid fever and smallpox. The disease occurs both in children and adults, most of the cases reported having been between the ages of twenty and forty years.

SYMPTOMS.—The disease begins regularly with pain and tenderness referred to the lumbar region on one side between the lower border of the ribs and the crest of the ilium, sometimes to a point above or below this. At about the same time are developed repeated rigors, a febrile movement with evening exacerbations, sweating, loss of appetite, vomiting, and prostration. These are all the symptoms for from one to two weeks. Then the skin over the lumbar region on one side becomes red and œdematous; the corresponding thigh is kept flexed and rigid, for any movement of it gives pain. Then the lumbar region becomes more and more swollen until fluctuation can be made out, and finally the abscess breaks through the skin. If such cases are left to run their course the abscess may reach a very large size. If the pus does not extend backward, but in some other direction, the symptoms are more obscure, for the local symptoms of an abscess in the back are absent.

If the abscess ruptures into the peritoneal cavity, the symptoms of acute general peritonitis are suddenly developed. If it perforates into the colon or bladder, the pus is discharged with the feces or the urine. If the perforation is through the diaphragm, there will be empyema, or the lung becomes adherent and pus is coughed up from the bronchi. As soon as the abscess is opened and the pus escapes the acute constitutional symptoms subside.

Trousseau believes that the inflammatory process sometimes stops short of the production of pus. In such cases of course there are no evidences of the formation of an abscess.

The disease may terminate in different ways:

1. The inflammation may terminate in resolution (Trousseau).

2. The abscess is opened by operation or spontaneously and the patient recovers.

3. Although the abscess is opened either by the surgeon or spontaneously, the suppurative process continues and the patient dies exhausted, usually with waxy viscera.

4. Perforation into the peritoneum, the pleura, or the lung causes death.

TREATMENT.—The main point in treatment is to discover the abscess and to open it. The longer the suppurative process goes on and the larger the abscess, so much the worse is the prognosis.· It is proper to explore with the aspirator after the disease has lasted for a few days, even if no fluctuation can be made out. The abscess is to be opened and treated on antiseptic principles.

HÆMATURIA AND HÆMOGLOBINURIA OR HÆMATINURIA.

By JAMES TYSON, A. M., M. D.

THE above terms are applied, the first to a condition of urine in which, of the constituents of blood, red discs at least are present; the second to that in which, while no corpuscles are found, blood coloring matter is abundant. Each of these conditions has been repeatedly observed as a distinct state at the moment when urine is passed; but it is also to be remembered that a true hæmaturia may, in the course of a few hours, become a hæmatinuria or hæmoglobinuria, by solution or disintegration of the red blood-discs. So far as I know, this subsequent solution and conversion can take place only in an alkaline urine; but as any urine through decomposition may become alkaline, it is evident that any hæmaturia may, in the course of time, become a hæmoglobinuria—a fact sometimes overlooked. I have, for example, known urine to be sent from Southern parts of the United States which, when shipped, contained blood-corpuscles, but which, when received in Philadelphia, contained no blood-discs, only large amounts of blood coloring matter. Especially does this occur in warm weather, when urine decomposes quickly. Such a hæmoglobinuria might be characterized as secondary. Doubtless, too, a more rapid solution is contributed to in some instances by the state of the blood-discs themselves, which are at times disintegrated before or at the moment they leave the blood-vessels, at others are intact, and at others, still, may be just ready to fall to pieces. In the hæmoglobinuria, where the blood-corpuscles have been secondarily dissolved and disintegrated, their remnants may be found in the shape of dark-brown or red granules, which form a sediment of varying bulk.

The immediate cause of this dissolved state of the blood-discs, where not due to the solvent action of an alkaline urine, appears to be the difference in degree of the cachexia which is at the bottom of the renal hemorrhagic tendency.

The term hæmaturia is applied to blood in the urine from whatever part of the urinary passages it may come, whether the bladder, ureters, kidney, or even urethra; whereas the blood in primary hæmoglobinuria always comes directly from the kidney.

In this paper I shall confine myself to the consideration of renal hæmaturia and hæmoglobinuria in the strict sense of the term; nor will I include such renal hæmaturia as constantly occurs in the first stage of acute Bright's disease.

Emphasizing again that all primary hæmoglobinurias are renal, it is

104

important to be able to say of a given hæmaturia whether it is renal or not. Even coarse methods are often sufficient to settle the question. Blood from the kidney, so far as my experience goes, is never discharged in the shape of clots, at least large enough to be recognized as such by the naked eye. More frequently coagula of blood are passed when hemorrhage takes place into the pelvis of the kidney. These coagula generally cause severe pain in their descent, and by this symptom are distinguished from coagula from the lower part of the ureter and bladder.

The smoky hue, which is characteristic of the presence of small quantities of blood in an acid urine, affords presumptive evidence that the blood is renal in its origin, because the conditions which are associated with blood from other parts of the genito-urinary tract are very apt to be associated with an alkaline urine, to which blood imparts a bright-red hue. This is, however, not invariable, as smoke-hued urine may be due to admixture of blood from the bladder and parts of the genito-urinary tract other than the kidney.

The microscope affords valuable assistance in determining the source of blood in the urine. In addition to blood-discs or their molecular débris, tube-casts made up of cemented blood-discs or their débris are very constantly, although not invariably, found in such urine. This evidence is conclusive, and, although sometimes wanting, the invariable absence of clots from blood descended from the kidney, together with the absence of irritation of the bladder, makes it usually quite easy to recognize a renal hæmaturia.

It is scarcely necessary to say that all urine containing blood or hæmoglobin contains albumen, the quantity varying with that of these substances present. Any further deviations from the normal composition of the urine are, in the main, due to admixture of other constituents of blood.

Causes which give rise to Hæmaturia and Hæmoglobinuria.

Hæmaturia is due to a variety of causes, which may be local or general. Local hæmaturia is caused by wounds, blows upon the kidney, or falls in which the kidney receives the force of the blow, as in striking the edge of a fence in falling; from cancer of the kidney, impacted calculus, parasites, embolism, acute Bright's disease; also poisoning from carbolic acid, cantharides, and mustard. General causes of hæmaturia are malaria, purpura, scurvy, blood-dyscrasias due to continued and eruptive fevers, especially typhus fever and smallpox, septicæmia and pyæmia, and cholera. Finally, it must be admitted that there is a hemorrhagic diathesis manifested by hæmaturia and hæmoglobinuria.* Primary hæmoglobinuria may be produced by any of the general causes just named, or by the prolonged inhalation of arseniuretted hydrogen and carbonic acid, and the introduction of numerous substances into the blood, as iodine, arsenic, etc.

While a rupture of the blood-vessels of the kidney may be supposed to be at the bottom of a certain proportion of cases of hæmaturia, it is by no means a necessary condition of their occurrence, as it is well known that in inflammations there may be extravasations of blood without rupture of ·

the blood-vessels. There is implied, however, in all these conditions an alteration of the vessel-walls which permits such transudation. Indeed, Ponfick[1] goes so far as to say that even transudations of hæmoglobin through the blood-vessels of the kidney are impossible without the presence of serious diffuse nephritis. There is every reason to believe, however, that simple alterations of the blood are of themselves sufficient to cause such transudations. Take, for instance, the extravasations in purpura, which are not confined to the vessels of the kidney. It is impossible to conceive inflammatory conditions so general as would have to be presupposed in this disease.

Hæmaturia from Local Causes.

It is unnecessary to consider in detail the local causes of hæmaturia. It is evident how injuries and blows upon the kidney, and impacted calculus may produce hemorrhage. The history of nephritic colic or of gravel in urine, along with blood, would suggest the latter cause. Nor is it necessary to detail the phenomena of hemorrhagic infarction which succeeds embolism and is the direct cause of hemorrhage into the tubules of the kidney. Hæmaturia is by no means a constant symptom in sarcoma and cancer of the kidney. A small amount of blood in the urine is a constant symptom in acute nephritis, where it is due to a rupture of the blood-vessels of the Malpighian tuft. It is accompanied by blood-casts and other symptoms of acute Bright's disease. Carbolic acid, cantharides, oil of mustard, and similar substances produce hæmaturia by causing congestion and inflammation of the kidney.

The parasites which may cause hemorrhage in the substance of the kidney are the Bilharzia hæmatobia, the Filaria sanguinis hominis, the Strongylus gigas, and possibly common intestinal worms which may reach the kidney through fistulous openings. The first is a thread-like worm three or four lines in length, which was discovered by Bilharz, and infests the small vessels of the mucous and submucous tissue of the veins of the intestinal tract, the pelvis of the kidney, ureter, bladder, and more rarely of the kidney itself. It is very frequent in Egypt, where Griesinger found it 117 times in 363 autopsies; also in South Africa (Cape of Good Hope), where it gives rise to an endemic hæmaturia. It has been studied by Bilharz, John Harley, and William Roberts.

The Filaria sanguinis hominis is a long, narrow microscopic worm, not wider than a red blood-disc, and one seventy-fifth of an inch long, which infests the blood. Hemorrhages result from its accumulation in the vessels, causing rupture. The cases which have been studied occurred mostly in India, China, and Australia.

The Strongylus gigas is a large worm, resembling the ordinary lumbricoid, but larger, the male being from ten to twelve inches long and one-fourth of an inch wide, while the female is sometimes more than a yard in length. It infests the kidneys and urinary passages of certain lower animals (the dog, wolf, horse, ox, etc.), but rarely those of man.

---

[1] "Ueber die Gemeingefährlichkeit der essbaren Morchel," *Virchow's Archiv,* Bd. lxxxviii. S. 47.

Malarial Hæmaturia and Hæmoglobinuria.

SYNONYMS.—Intermittent hæmaturia; Paroxysmal hæmaturia; Malarial yellow fever; Swamp yellow fever; Paroxysmal congestive hepatic hæmaturia (Harley).

Perhaps the most important form of hæmaturia and hæmoglobinuria resulting from general causes is that due to malarial poisoning. I prefer the term malarial to intermittent or paroxysmal, not only because it more precisely indicates the cause of the condition, but also because the contion itself is by no means always intermittent, sometimes continuing without interruption until checked by appropriate treatment; and I have known it to continue uninterruptedly for a year, in spite of all treatment.

The first complete report of an undoubted instance of this affection appears to have been published by Dressler in 1854,[1] although incomplete and uncertain cases were reported prior to this date—one as early as 1832 by Elliotson.[2] G. Troup Maxwell of Ocala, Florida, writes me, in 1883, that he first observed cases in Florida thirty years ago, and published an article on the disease in the *Oglethorpe Medical Journal*, Savannah, Ga., July, 1860. George Harley[3] early contributed to our accurate knowledge of the subject in 1865, and since then numerous papers and reports of cases have appeared in English and American journals, the southern part of the United States being a fertile scene of the affection, while it is by no means rare in the Middle States.

Two degrees of the disease are met with—a milder form, in which other symptoms as well as the hæmaturia are less pronounced, and of which instances occur in the Middle States as well as the South and West of the United States. Of this kind seem to be the cases studied by Harley and other English physicians. In addition to this, there is a second, more malignant, form, attended by great prostration, vomiting, and yellowness of the skin, along with copious discharges of bloody urine. Instances of the latter are numerous in the Southern States of this country, where they have recently been studied with much care; also in the East and West Indies and in tropical countries generally. In neither degree of the disease is it necessary that the red corpuscles of the blood should be present. They may be represented by their coloring matters alone, when the condition is called a hæmoglobinuria or a hæmaturia.

The Milder Form.—The subjects, in my experience of eight cases. have been, with one exception, men, and I believe the experience of others included more men than women. They are generally able to recall a history of exposure to malaria, and often of distinct attacks of malarial fever, intermittent or remittent. The hæmaturia appears suddenly, and when paroxysmal may occur daily or on alternate days or a couple of times a week, or even at longer intervals. When the attacks occur at longer intervals, say of ten days or two weeks, if the disease is left alone the interval is apt to gradually diminish until the passage of bloody urine becomes daily. The urine in the morn-

---

[1] "Ein Fall von intermittirender Albuminurie und Chromaturie," *Virchow's Archiv*, Bd. vi. S. 264, 1854.
[2] "Clinical Lecture on Diseases of the Heart, with Ague (and Hæmaturia)," *London Lancet*, 1832, p. 500.
[3] "Intermittent Hæmaturia," *Medico-Chirurg. Trans. London*, 1865.

ing may be perfectly clear, and at two o'clock is evidently bloody. It continues so through one or two acts of micturition, and then becomes clear again; or it may be bloody on rising and clear up by noon. Sometimes the bloody urine is preceded or accompanied by a sense of weariness and chilly feeling, or sometimes simply by cold hands and feet or by cold knees, or by pallor and blueness of the face, or by accelerated pulse, or by no other symptoms whatever. There is sometimes a sense of fulness in the region of the kidney and sacrum. The attacks are often induced by exposure to cold.

Harley states that in one of the two cases which he reported there was a slight jaundice, and in the second a "sallowness which appeared to be due to a disturbance of the hepatic functions," but in none of the cases which I have met was this symptom present. In the more malignant form occurring in the tropics and the Southern States of America, jaundice is a constant symptom.

While a majority of cases of malarial hæmaturia are intermittent, many are continuous, and of my eight cases only three were distinctly intermittent. One of these cases I published in a clinical lecture in the *Philadelphia Medical Times* as far back as September 1, 1871.

Negroes are not exempt from this milder form of the disease, as they seem to be from the more malignant form of the South. While writing this paper I was consulted by a negro thirty-one years old who had a true malarial hæmoglobinuria, which yielded promptly to the treatment by quinine. But this was the only negro out of seven cases.

The duration of the disease is very various, and if neglected may be indefinite. Stephen Mackenzie[1] reports a case which lasted twenty-three years.

PHYSICAL AND CHEMICAL CHARACTERS OF THE URINE.—The urine is usually acid in reaction when passed, sometimes neutral, rarely alkaline, and ranges in specific gravity from 1010 to 1028. It is always albuminous, and always tinged by blood coloring matters, the depth of color varying from the trifling degree known as smoke-hued to a dark-red or claret color. Sometimes it is even darker, and is often compared to porter, though this degree of coloration is more characteristic of the malignant form. The urine deposits a dark, reddish-brown sediment, generally copious, but varies in quantity with the degree of coloration of the urine. This sediment is made up chiefly of red blood-discs or the granular débris resulting from their disintegration.

Casts of the uriniferous tubules are also often present. They are usually made up of aggregated red blood-discs or the granular matter referred to; but they may also be hyaline or hyaline with a moderate amount of granular matter attached. Granular urates also at times contribute to the sediment and also adhere to the casts. Renal and vesical epithelium may occur. Crystals of oxalate of lime and of uric acid are sometimes present, while blood-crystals have been found by Gull[2] and Grainger Stewart, and a hæmatin crystal once by Strong.[3]

That red blood-discs are at times exceedingly scarce, and even totally absent at the very moment when urine is passed, is a well-recognized fact; while that the coloring matter present is still that of the blood.

[1] "On Paroxysmal Hæmoglobinuria, *London Lancet*, vol. i., 1884, p. 156.
[2] *Guy's Hosp. Reports*, 1866, p. 381.   [3] *British Med. Journ.*, 1878, vol. ii. p. 103.

even though no corpuscles are present, is easy of demonstration by the production of Teichmann's hæmin crystals,[1] by spectrum analysis, or by the guaiacum test.

In the matter of the presence or absence of blood-discs, it is to be remembered that these may be present at the moment the urine is passed, but disappear by subsequent solution if the urine happens to be alkaline or becomes so secondarily. It is an interesting fact, too, that colorless blood-corpuscles are often present intact, even when red discs are absent. While I have frequently examined urine sent me from the South in which the coloring matter of the blood and no corpuscles were present, only one of the cases coming under my own observations furnished urine of this character. The proportion of urea varies, and bears no evident relation to the condition itself.

PATHOLOGY AND MORBID ANATOMY.—The pathology of malarial hæmaturia consists, as yet, chiefly of theoretical deductions. We can only conclude that the malarial poison acts upon the blood and blood-vessels, impairing the integrity of both. This goes so far occasionally as to produce an actual destruction of blood-discs, and always so alters the capillaries that they permit the transudation of blood-elements ordinarily retained.

The morbid anatomy is scarcely more precisely defined. Ponfick[2] goes so far as to say that the exudation of hæmoglobulin is not possible without the concurrence of marked diffuse nephritis. Recently Lebedeff[3] has sought to investigate the more minute alterations of the kidney in hæmoglobin exudation, but without very definite results. These, however, on the whole, seem to confirm Ponfick's view as to the presence of an inflammatory process, as also do those of Litten[4] and Lassar.[5]

DIAGNOSIS.—The diagnosis of this condition is not usually difficult. We have first to determine whether the hemorrhagic discharge is from the kidney rather than the bladder or ureters. The former is the case when tube-casts are found. But tube-casts are not always present even when the hemorrhage is from the kidneys. The absence of clots and of vesical irritation, and of pain in the course of the ureters, is characteristic of blood from the kidneys. Finally, all hæmoglobinurias are renal.

It being certain that the blood comes from the kidney, we have to distinguish it from that due to cancer, to calculus-irritation, and to cachexias, as purpura and scurvy ; or to grave forms of infectious disease, septicæmia, pyæmia, etc. ; or, finally, to poisonous substances introduced into the blood, such as arsenic, iodine, arseniuretted hydrogen, carbonic acid and carbonic oxide gas, and even certain species of edible fungi.

The diagnosis is greatly aided if it is found we have to do with a

---

[1] Place a drop of the sediment upon a glass slide and allow it to dry. Mix thoroughly with a few particles of common salt and cover with a thin glass cover, under which allow two or three drops of glacial acetic acid to pass. Carefully warm the slide for a few seconds over a spirit-lamp, and when most of the acetic acid is evaporated, examine by the microscope. Hæmin crystals will be seen to crystallize out as the mixture cools.

[2] "Ueber die Gemeingefährlichkeit der essbaren Morchel," *Virchow's Archiv*, Bd. lxxxviii. S. 476, 1882.

[3] "Zur Kenntniss der feineren Veränderungen der Nieren bei der Hämoglobinausscheidung," *Virchow's Archiv*, Bd. xci. S. 267, Feb., 1883.

[4] "Verhandl. des Vereins für innere Medicin," *Deut. Med. Wochenschr.*, No. 52, Dec. 20, 1883.

[5] *Ibid.*, No. 1, Jan. 3, 1884.

hæmoglobinuria rather than a hæmaturia. For although the former condition is produced by toxic and septic agencies of another kind, the attending symptoms, when it is thus produced, are so characteristic that it is not likely that error can be made.

To aid in distinguishing it from cancer we have the history of malarial exposure, and often that of other forms of malarial disease; and, notwithstanding the seeming drain upon the system, none of the cases I have ever seen present the profound anæmia of cancer. The bloody discharge in cancer of the kidney is always a true hæmaturia; there are always blood-discs in the urine. There is often pain in the region of the kidney in cancer, but never in malarial hæmaturia.

In calculous disease there is almost always pain before or during the hæmaturic attack, and characteristic crystalline sediments often appear in the urine.

The disease, being comparatively rare in this latitude, is sometimes overlooked on this account. Of the 8 cases which I have noted during sixteen years, 5 originated in Pennsylvania, 1 in New Jersey, 1 in Delaware, and 1 in North Carolina.

TREATMENT.—The treatment is distinctly that of malarial disease, and I have seldom seen more brilliant and satisfactory results than have followed the use of quinine in a case accurately determined, although such success is not invariable; and I have known the disease to resist for a long time the most thorough and judicious use of anti-malarial remedies. Usually, however, I take hold of a case of this kind with considerable confidence. When there are distinct remissions my practice has been to administer 16 to 20 grains of sulphate of quinia in the usual manner of anticipation of the paroxysm in intermittent fever—from 3 to 5 grains every hour until the required amount is taken; the whole amount may be taken in two doses, or even in one dose. Where there is no distinct remission I more usually direct 3 to 5 grains every three hours, until the hemorrhage ceases or decided cinchonism is produced.

The advantage well known to accrue in malarial disease from the combination of mercurials with quinine applies to hemorrhagic malaria as well, although I usually reserve the mercurial until I have ascertained whether the simple quinine treatment answers the purpose. If the usual method fails, I give 8 or 10 grains of calomel in the evening, followed by a saline in the morning, before reinstituting the quinine treatment. In the case of the colored man alluded to who had malarial hæmoglobinuria 36 grains of quinine failed to break the attack; but the same quantity, given after 10 grains of calomel had acted, succeeded.

Where these means failed I have not found the other methods of treatment commonly resorted to in obstinate malarial disease to be any more efficient. I allude to the treatment by arsenic or by iron and arsenic. Indeed, in the only two cases in which, after failure with the quinine treatment, iron and arsenic were used at my suggestion, they failed absolutely. In the one case, under the care of James L. Tyson, this treatment was carried out most faithfully. After four weeks' treatment with quinine without effect, Fowler's solution was given, at first in 5-drop doses three times daily, subsequently increased to 10 and 15, along with 20- and 30-drop doses of tincture of the chloride of iron, until œdema of the eyelids occurred, when the arsenic was discontinued, but the iron continued. In two or three days the arsenic was recommenced in 3- and 4-drop doses for three or four weeks longer without effect. Fluid extract of ergot in 20-drop doses was then substituted for the iron, alternating with the arsenic for two weeks longer, when some slight favorable change was apparent, but it was temporary. Repeatedly throughout the treatment the patient complained of weariness and backache, cold feet and knees, headache and acceleration of pulse, and a feeling of utter wretchedness; and then again he would feel quite comfortable for a day or two, but with little or no change in the urine, except occasionally in the morning, when it would sometimes be quite light-hned, but after breakfast would again assume its bloody character. A sojourn at the seaside for two weeks was without effect.

It will appear from the above that ergot, which has been found useful in some forms of hæmaturia, is of little service here, as is attested by two other cases in which I tried it faithfully. At the same time, it is a remedy which should be tried in case of failure with others.

The usual astringents, mineral and vegetable, of known efficacy in the treatment of hemorrhagic conditions, should be used alone or in conjunction with the specific anti-malarial treatment after the latter has been found of itself insufficient. To this class of remedies belong the mineral acids, persulphate of iron, acetate of lead, alum, gallic acid, catechu, kino, the astringent natural mineral waters, etc.

Rest is certainly an important adjuvant in the treatment of this form of malarial disease. I have known a recurrence to take place after a long drive.

It is claimed for many natural mineral waters that hemorrhage from the kidneys is one of the affections cured by their use. Chalybeate and alum springs might be expected to be of advantage by the local action of these astringents in their transit through the kidneys, and they frequently are. The following case illustrates their efficiency: The patient was a lawyer who consulted me in June, 1881, at the suggestion of W. W. Covington of North Carolina. He had frequently had chills, and a congestive chill in 1873. Three months before I saw him he began to pass bloody urine. He had no other symptoms, except a soreness and weakness in the neighborhood of the sacrum, extending into the outer part of the left thigh. The urine passed for me at the time of his visit was dark reddish-brown in color, acid in reaction, had a specific gravity of 1028, highly albuminous, and deposited a sediment of almost tarry consistence, which was made up almost entirely of blood-corpuscles. There were no tube-casts. He had been a dyspeptic since seventeen years of age, and medicines disagreed with him; but he was treated faithfully with quinine, iron, arsenic, ergot, benzoate of lime, all without the slightest effect. At the end of about a year from the time he consulted me he heard of the Jackson Spring, located in Moore county, North Carolina, fifteen miles distant from Manly Station on the Raleigh and Augusta Railroad. He went there, and remained one week. He stated that for the first two or three days the water acted decidedly on his kidneys, and he voided a number of clots of blood. On the third day all traces of blood disappeared, and it recurred but once since, on a very cold day in November last, but again disappeared after a day or two in the house. Unfortunately, no precise analysis of this water seems to have been made, but from what my friend writes it evidently contains iron and sulphur, and magnesia is also said to be present. It is promptly diuretic. Since this occurred I have used the water of alum springs in other instances with advantage.[1]

The following are some of the chalybeate and alum springs the waters of which may be expected to be of service in hæmaturia: Orchard Acid Springs, New York; Rockbridge Alum Springs, Pulaski Alum Springs, Bath Alum Springs, Stribling Springs, and Bedford Alum Springs, all in Virginia. In all of these waters iron and alum are both present, accompanied, in many instances, by free sulphuric acid, by which their efficiency is increased. In one of my cases the hemorrhage disappeared temporarily under the use of the water from the Bedford Springs, Penna., but again returned. These waters contain a little iron, but no alum. Subsequently, the same patient was promptly relieved by quinine, which had not been previously tried.

But the cases most promptly relieved by the alum waters are the non-malarial cases depending, upon hemorrhagic diathesis without other local disease. A remarkable instance of this kind was related to me by letter by J. Macpherson Scott of Hagerstown, Md. After enormous doses of quinine had been used under the supposition that it was malarial, it was promptly and totally cured.

Malignant Malarial Hæmaturia.

The second more serious form of this disease, as it occurs in the tropics and the southern part of the United States, is characterized by such increased intensity of all the symptoms that it may be well called malignant. Singularly, however, the disease has seemed to be much more prevalent during the last fifteen years. My attention was first called to it in September, 1868, when I received specimens of urine and the history of some cases from R. D. Webb of Livingston, Ala., who wrote also that it was not known in that part of his State prior to 1863 or 1864.

In this, as in the milder form, there is a distinct but more invariable history of malarial exposure, and the attack often begins as an ordinary case of chills and fever, there being often one or two paroxysms before the hæmaturia appears. At other times the hemorrhage ushers in the disease suddenly. The urine is often black and almost tarry in consistence, and passed in unusually large quantities—it is said as much as a pint every fifteen or twenty minutes until a couple of quarts have been passed, or one or two gallons in the course of twelve hours. But after twenty-four hours the quantity diminishes. Epistaxis sometimes occurs, but is not often profuse. Distressing nausea, and vomiting of bilious and even black matter, like that of black vomit, also occur. Intense jaundice rapidly supervenes—said to come on sometimes in the course of an hour, often in from two to six hours. The tongue is brown and dry. The bowels are at times constipated, and at others loose. Although the patient may be feverish at first, with a temperature of 104° to 106°, and the skin dry, the pulse rapidly becomes small and feeble until it is

[1] See the report of a case treated successfully by Rockbridge alum-water by Radcliffe, *Med. News*, Jan. 12, 1884.

scarcely perceptible. Drowsiness and coma sometimes intervene, and at others the mind is clear until the moment of death, which frequently supervenes within twenty-four or sixty hours; or the symptoms may subside, to be repeated again the next day if not prevented by treatment. If recovery takes place, which it sometimes does, and lately more frequently, convalescence is slow and tedious, the patient remaining for weeks in an enfeebled and anæmic state.

In this form, especially, of the disease it often happens that the coloring matter and the débris of blood-discs only are found in the urine, very few and often no entire ones being discernible: in other words, we have a true hæmoglobinuria or hæmatinuria. The urine is of course albuminous. A specimen recently received from North Carolina and analyzed by Wormley contained no corpuscles, but revealed the spectroscopic band characteristic of hæmoglobin. It contained $2\frac{1}{2}$ per cent. of urea. The specific gravity of the urine ranges between 1010 and 1020, being lower when it is copious.

As to the jaundice, it is evidently a hæmatogenetic, and not a hepatogenetic, form with which we have to deal. It is due, not to the retention of bile, but to the disintegration of blood-corpuscles and the solution of their coloring matter, which diffuses through the tissues and stains them yellow or yellowish-green. This form too, apparently, is more frequent in males, and negroes appear to be exempt. This is not the case with the milder form, for it will be remembered that one of my patients was a negro.

Autopsies reveal the same intense yellow coloration of internal organs —lungs, liver, spleen, stomach, kidneys—anæmia rather than congestion, while the blood is dark-hued and is indisposed to coagulate. The spleen is often enlarged.

The TREATMENT for the breaking of the paroxysm is pre-eminently quinine or quinine with mercurials, and although this does not always succeed, there seems to be no other remedy. The quinine may be given hypodermically. The nausea has been controlled by morphia and lime-water, by carbolic acid, and by creasote. In addition, restorative measures are necessary, including the free use of stimulants. Turpentine has been used in large doses ($f\overline{3}j$), it is said with advantage, in Alabama.

CHYLURIA.

By JAMES TYSON, A. M., M. D.

THE term chyluria is applied to a condition of urine in which the secretion is admixed with fat in a minute state of subdivision, whence the urine acquires a milky or chylous appearance. The proportion of fat varies greatly between such as gives a mere opalescence to the secretion and that which makes it absolutely indistinguishable, in appearance, from milk, while even the characteristic odor and taste of urine are often wanting. The further resemblance of such urines to milk is found in the fact that, on standing, a cream-like substance rises to the surface. On the other hand, a spontaneous coagulation into a jelly-like substance containing fibrin proves an unmistakable relation to blood.

The chemical composition of such a urine, having a specific gravity of 1013 and neutral in reaction, is given by Beale,[1] as follows:

Water	947.4
Solid matter	52.6
Urea 7.73	
Albumen 13.00	
Uric acid 0.00	
Extractive matter with uric acid 11.66	
Fat insoluble in hot and cold alcohol, but soluble in ether . . 9.20 ⎫	
Fat insoluble in cold alcohol . . . . 2.70 ⎬ 13.90	
Fat soluble in cold alcohol . . . . 2.00 ⎭	
Alkaline sulphates and chlorides 1.65	
Alkaline phosphates . . . . ⎫ 4.66	
Earthy phosphates . . . . ⎭	

Such urines are of course albuminous, as will have been seen from the table. They therefore coagulate when boiled or on the addition of an acid. They also exhibit a tendency to spontaneous coagulation more or less complete, which is apt to be followed by later disintegration of the clot. The proportion of solids is larger than in ordinary urines.

Microscopically, the urine is found to contain, in addition to its usual elements, immense numbers of molecular particles easily soluble in ether, and therefore fatty in their composition. It may be rendered perfectly clear by the addition of ether, and again approximately milky after evaporating the ether and shaking the residue; but now the microscope shows the oil in the shape of oil-drops and not molecules. Oil-drops are also sometimes sparsely present in the fresh fluid, but the fatty particle is commonly molecular. Indeed, the molecules are commonly so small that an

[1] *Urinary and Renal Derangements and Calculous Disorders*, Philada., 1885, p. 73.

aggregated mass of them appears like a delicate cloud under the microscope, rather than a collection of individual particles. Blood-corpuscles may also be present, sometimes in sufficient quantity to produce a distinct pink coloration, but no unusual proportion of leucocytes is common. The pink tinge, and even an almost bloody appearance, is very apt to precede the chyluria. This bloody character sometimes gradually increases until the chyluria has become a hæmaturia, so that we have sometimes a chyluria spoken of as a first stage of hæmaturia. Tube-casts do not occur. Chyluria is seldom constant, and a specimen of urine passed a couple of hours after one white as milk may be, again, perfectly clear and in all respects natural. Thus, a second specimen, passed by the same patient as that of which the analysis is given above, was almost clear. It had a specific gravity of 1010 and a slightly acid reaction, and contained a mere trace of deposit, consisting of a little epithelium, a few cells larger than lymph-corpuscles, and a few small cells, probably minute fungi. Not the slightest precipitate was produced by the application of heat or addition of nitric acid. The following is Beale's analysis :

Water	978.8
Solid matter	21.2
Urea	6.95
Albumen	0.00
Uric acid	.15
Extractive matters with uric acid	7.31
Fat insoluble in hot and cold alcohol, but soluble in ether	
Fat insoluble in cold alcohol	.00
Fat soluble in cold alcohol	
Alkaline sulphates and chlorides	5.34
Alkaline phosphates	1.45
Earthy phosphates	.15

DISTRIBUTION OF THE DISEASE.—By far the largest majority of instances of the disease originate in tropical and subtropical climates. Thus, India, China, and South America—and in South America, Brazil, and Guiana—are countries in which it is common. It is said to be rarer on the coast of South America than in the interior ; yet it is especially partial to insular countries, and most of the cases observed in this country originate in the West Indies—in Barbadoes and Cuba, in Bermuda and the island of Trinidad. Many cases occur in Bahia, Guadeloupe, Madagasear, the Isle of Bourbon, and Mauritius. Indeed, the first important study of the subject was based on cases observed in the latter island by Chapotin.[1] In Africa both Egypt and the Cape of Good Hope are favorite localities, and in Australia, Brisbane has furnished many cases.

At the same time, cases do originate in temperate climates, and although the disease is rare in Europe and North America, Dickinson has collected five cases from his own practice or that of others, which undoubtedly originated in England. I know of but one case of certain North American origin, that of a woman reported by McConnell to the Medico-Chirurgical Society of Montreal, April 27, 1883. She was thirty-three years old, a native of the province of Ontario, and had had the disease eleven years. At the time of her death, which appears to have been from tubercular phthisis, there were cavities in the apices of both lungs.

[1] Thèse, *Topographie médicale de l'Ile de France.* 1812.

SUBJECTS ATTACKED.—There seems no election as to nativity, natives and foreigners being indiscriminately attacked in the countries in which it occurs. There is some difference of opinion as to whether the disease is more frequent in males or females; which is a reason for believing that it occurs with nearly equal frequency in both.

It is more common in middle life, but Prout reports an instance in a child eighteen months old, and Rayer one in a woman at seventy-eight years. She had had it, however, since she was twenty-five, or about fifty-three years. Dickinson was consulted with regard to a boy of five, and mentions a case fatal at twelve. Roberts says: "Chylous urine prevails mostly in youth and middle age."[1] Of 30 cases collected by him, 3 were under twenty; 7 between twenty and thirty; 11 between thirty and forty; 6 between forty and fifty ; and 3 over fifty.

The subjects of the disease are apt to be pale and relaxed as to their tissues, but while this may be a possible result of the disease, it can hardly be regarded as a predisposing cause.

PATHOLOGY AND ETIOLOGY.—The precise mode in which chyluria is brought about is unknown. It is to be inferred, in view of our existing knowledge, that there has been produced, in some way, in each instance a communication between the urinary and chyliferous systems, although exactly where such communication is has as yet only been guessed at. It may be in the kidney itself, or its pelvis, or the ureter, or in the bladder. Cases originating in the tropics have been found associated with elephantiasis, but this is not very frequent. Dilatation of cutaneous lymphatics, producing cutaneous papules and vesicles and a discharge of lymph from them, has also been noted coincident with chyluria.

Prout,[2] among the earlier writers on this subject, and more recently Bence Jones,[3] Waters, Bouchardat, Robin, Bernard, and Egel, did not consider a positive lesion necessary, but ascribed the condition to a vice of nutrition and blood-making, accompanied by a slight consequent textural alteration in the blood-vessels of the kidney, through which the elements of the chyle transuded. Waters[4] says that "the main pathological feature of the complaint is a relaxed condition of the capillaries of the kidney," which permits the transudation.

The results of examination of the blood, in cases of chylous urine, by Bence Jones, Rayer, and Crevaux, who found in certain instances an excess of fat, have been quoted in support of these views, but these examinations seem to have been microscopical and not chemical, and the results have not been confirmed by recent observers. Such views were also upheld on theoretical grounds by Bouchardat,[5] based on the greater commonness of the disease in warm climates. He reasoned that when the heat-producing elements, whether absorbed from food or produced by metamorphoses of other proximate principles, are in excess, and an elevated external temperature does not favor their consumption, their elimination is attempted by certain organs, notably the liver and kidneys. The effort by the kidneys seems, however, to be attended by a structural change in the blood-vessels, as the result of which blood is

[1] *Urinary and Renal Diseases,* 4th ed., Philada., 1885, p. 344.
[2] *Stomach and Renal Diseases,* 4th ed., London, 1843.
[3] *Lectures on Pathology and Therapeutics,* 1868, p. 256.
[4] *Med.-Chir. Trans.,* vol. xiv. p. 221, 1862. [5] *Ann. de Thérapeutique,* 1862.

eliminated with fat, especially at the beginning of the disease. Later the blood disappears, but the albumen remains some time longer, disappearing finally with the fat.

Bernard and Robin also compared the blood of such cases to that of geese artificially fattened, being that condition of blood which is normal after digestion but transient. Egel also held similar views, ascribing the imperfect elaboration to the effect of hot climates.

Gubler[1] first suggested that chylous urine was due to a passage of chyle directly into the urinary passages, and that this was immediately preceded by a dilatation of the renal lymphatics similar to that known to occur on the surface of the body and attended by the local flow alluded to.

·Vandyke Carter,[2] of Bombay, suggested that the communication was between the lacteals and lymphatics of the lumbar region and those of the kidney. Those who have seen the semi-diagrammatic drawing of a dissection of the lymphatics as seen from behind, in the remarkable case of Stephen Mackenzie,[3] cannot fail to be impressed with the probability of such communication.

That a chylous urine is the direct result of a discharge of chyle into the urinary passages at some point between the kidney and the neck of the bladder, is further rendered likely by the experience of W. H. Mastin of Mobile, Alabama, with a case of chylous hydrocele: W. H. W., a native of Alabama, aged twenty-two, presented himself with a hydrocele. Mastin tapped the sac and drew off a white milk-like fluid, which was sent to me for examination. It was perfectly white and nudistinguishable by the eye from milk. Upon microscopical and chemical examination, I found it presented all the physical and chemical characters of chyle. Six months later, the sac having refilled, Mastin evacuated eight ounces more of the same fluid—some of which was again sent to me—and then laid open the sac freely. Examining the cavity carefully, he found it smooth, polished, and pearly white, but at its upper portion, just where it began to be reflected over the testis, was a small, round, granular-looking mass about the size of an ordinary English pea. This he sliced off with a pair of scissors, and at once recognized the patulous mouths of three or four small vessels which did not bleed. These he dissected back for a short distance, and found that they passed into the connective tissue around the upper border of the testis. He then passed a ligature around the mass and brought the ends of the ligature to the outside, excised all the front wall of the tunica, and closed the sac. The patient recovered, and there was no return of the hydrocele. Although it is to be regretted that the patulous vessels were not watched for a few minutes, I do not think there can be any reasonable doubt that there was here a lymphatic varix, and that the chylous fluid in the tunica was the result of leakage through its walls. Since the patient had had gonorrhœa, Busey,[4] in his remarks on this case, suggests that the obstruction to the onward movement of the lymph, and the cause, therefore, of the dilatation and rupture, was inflammation attacking a single gland or an area of lymphatics.

[1] *Gazette médicale de Paris*, 1858, p. 646.   [2] *Med.-Chir. Trans.*, vol. xlv., 1862.
[3] *Trans. Path. Soc. of London*, vol. xxxiii. p. 394, 1882.
[4] *Occlusion and Dilatation of Lymph-Channels*, by Samuel C. Busey: A series of papers reprinted for private distribution from the *New Orleans Medical and Surgical Journal*, from Nov., 1876, to March 1878.

If it be acknowledged, then, that in chyluria some direct communication must exist between the lymphatic and urinary systems, how is this communication brought about? Various causes have been supposed at different times to be responsible for this condition, among them traumatism in its various modes of occurrence, such as being thrown from a horse. Mental shock has also been held responsible. So, also, syphilis and hereditary tendency. But most cases still remained unaccounted for when, on August 4, 1866, Wücherer first detected in the chylous urine of a woman in the Misericordia Hospital at Bahia an unknown worm. In 1872 it was announced that Timothy R. Lewis had found in the blood, and also in the urine, of a person suffering with chyluria in Calcutta, a delicate thread-like worm about $\frac{1}{70}$ of an inch long and $\frac{1}{3500}$ of an inch wide. This observation was confirmed by Palmer and Charles. Lewis named it Filaria sanguinis hominis. Since then the filaria has been found in the blood and urine of many cases. Lewis found six in a single drop of blood from the ear, and estimated 700,000 as approximately correct for the whole body. But Mackenzie calculated that there were in the blood of his patient from 36,000,000 to 40,000,000 embryo filariæ. These minute nematodes, discovered by Wücherer and Lewis, proved to be, as was indeed early suspected, the larvæ of a larger filaria which was discovered by Bancroft of Brisbane, Queensland, Australia, in December, 1876, first in a lymphatic abscess in the arm, and afterward in the fluid of hydrocele of persons infested with the smaller worm. The parent worm is about the thickness of a human hair and three or four inches long. It was named, by Cobbold, Filaria Bancrofti. Lewis himself found, in August following, a male and female of the parent worm, in a scrotum infiltrated with chylous fluid, in a case of elephantiasis. The female contained ova with embryos precisely like those found in the blood and urine. The worms are viviparous, but abortions seem frequent, ova being frequently discharged unhatched.

It has been rendered highly probable, by the researches, first, of Manson in China, and later of Lewis in India and Sonsino in Egypt, that the filaria in its fully-developed form is introduced into the stomach and intestines of man with water. Thence it makes its way into the blood and lacteal system, where it reproduces the embryo filariæ. These embryonic or larval filariæ are taken from the human blood by a mosquito, in the body of which it undergoes further development, after which the perfect Filaria Bancrofti is deposited in water, through which it again reaches the stomach of man, and thus the disease is perpetuated.

One of the most singular features in the history of the filaria is its nocturnal habit. It is found in the blood only at night, unless, as Mackenzie has shown, night be converted into day—that is, if the hours of sleeping and waking be reversed. In Mackenzie's case the worms appeared about seven o'clock in the evening, increased up to midnight, and disappeared by eight or nine o'clock in the morning. What becomes of them at the time when they are undiscoverable in the blood is as yet unknown.

Acknowledging filariæ to be the essential cause of chyluria, the precise method in which they operate to cause the obstruction, dilatation, and rupture of the lymphaties is a matter of speculation. The embryo filariæ are so lithe and small that they move among the corpuscles apparently without harming them, but the ova in which the embryos lie coiled up, and which are often discharged unhatched, are large enough to cause obstruction in the smaller lymphatics and lymph-passages of the lymphatic glands, and thus cause the phenomena of chyluria, as well as of the other diseases of the lymphatic system with which it is often associated, or which may occur independently of it, such as elephantiasis, cutaneous lymph-vesicles with their chylous and lymphous discharges, lymph scrotum, chylous hydrocele, and other diseases of the lymphatics. Indeed, the total number of affections other than chyluria which are found associated with filariæ exceed those of chyluria. Among the diseases with which it is said to be associated is erysipelas.

It is evident, therefore, that notwithstanding the fact that the discovery of the Filaria sanguinis hominis has shed a flood of light upon the subjcet of chyluria, the fact must not be overlooked that not a few cases of the disease have occurred in which the most careful search has failed to find this parasite in the blood. Careful examinations, during waking and sleeping hours, have been made without result, so that we cannot deny altogether the possibility of the disease occurring independent of filariæ as the cause. It is common, therefore, to speak of parasitic and non-parasitic chyluria.

On the other hand, the filaria embryo is often found in the blood of persons apparently in perfect health. Manson tells us that out of every ten Chinamen taken at random, at Amoy, the blood of one will contain filariæ.

MORBID ANATOMY.—There can hardly be said to be any morbid anatomy of chyluria, unless we regard the lymphatic lesions which sometimes accompany it as a part of the disease. Again and again do we read the reports of autopsies at which the kidneys were found normal, and where lesions have been noted they were such as are found due to other causes, and the coincidence was accidental.

SYMPTOMATOLOGY.—Apart from the characteristic urine of the condition, there are no symptoms which can be regarded as in any way peculiar to the disease. The mode of onset is usually sudden, and yet many patients experience no symptoms whatever, and would be quite unaware that they were afflicted in any way, were they not aware of the fact that they are passing lactescent urine. Since the discharge is, however, a drain of very valuable nutrient and force-producing material, most patients sooner or later gradually grow weaker; and this symptom of weakness becomes sometimes very marked, so that they fall into a condition of extreme debility, even to fainting on exertion.

Another symptom sufficiently frequent to deserve mention is pain in lumbar region, sometimes very severe, sometimes on one side, at others on both.

Painful micturition, due to obstruction, is also a symptom traceable directly to the condition of the urine. The disposition of chylous urine to coagulate has already been alluded to. The coagulation taking place in the bladder, it is the clot which sometimes obstructs the urethra and makes urination difficult or impossible. Plugs of coagulum are ejected, sometimes with considerable force, after prolonged straining, and with this comes relief to the symptoms, which may be reproduced through the operation of the same cause.

Other symptoms which are occasionally present may have an accidental relation to the affection, while they may be due to it. Such are headache, nausea, and other gastric symptoms.

Mention has been made, too, of the concurrence of superficial lymphatic leakage, especially on the lower part of the abdomen, the thighs, and the legs. Such leakage is often from little vesicular elevations which are evidently dilated lymphatic vessels. The presence of such leakage should suggest the examination of urine for lesser degrees of chyluria. In like manner, the urine should be examined in case of elephantiasis, lymph-scrotum, and chylous hydrocele, with which also chyluria is sometimes associated.

The effect of intercurrent febrile states, whether symptomatic of local inflammation, as of the lungs, or whether the result of the idiopathic fevers, has often a singular effect on chyluria in causing its disappearance for a time. It would seem that states of high vascular tension, however induced, tend to make it cease.

While chyluria has made its appearance, for the first time, in a number of cases during pregnancy, this condition in other instances has caused it to disappear, especially toward the later months ; whence it would seem that the pressure of the rising womb has a favorable effect.

The DIAGNOSIS of chyluria consists in the recognition of the chylous state of the urine. This, ordinarily very easily recognized, might be taken in its slight degrees for phosphatic or uratic or purulent conditions of the urine, and vice versâ. The disappearance of the first on the addition of acids, of the second on the application of heat or alkalies, will resolve any doubt, while the microscope will detect the pus-corpuscles in the last. None of the reagents named will dissolve the fatty molecules of a chyluria, while ether will cause the fluid to clear up completely.

The PROGNOSIS is usually favorable. Very rarely is an attack fatal, and when such is the case it is from exhaustion—from the drain to which the system.is subject. Tubercular phthisis is therefore a not infrequent immediate cause of death.

TREATMENT.—On the supposition that filariæ are the essential cause of the disease, the rational indication would be first to destroy them by the introduction into the blood of some parasiticide ; and, second, to repair the lesion of communication between the lymphatic .system and the urinary passages. As yet no agent is known which would not be as fatal to the host as to the filaria, if used in sufficient quantity to destroy the latter ; nor has it ever been possible to find the point of communication between the two systems, although treatment has been directed to producing closure of such communication, and with some show of success. Thus, in a case under his care Dickinson of London injected into the empty bladder twelve ounces of a solution of perchloride of iron, containing at first two drachms of the tincture to the whole quantity, gradually increased to four drachms. The solution was retained in the bladder for from eight to twelve minutes with little or no inconvenience. The operation was repeated almost daily for twelve days. The effect was always to check the milky flow and to substitute a clear urine. But after the operation had been repeated a certain number of times there was a decided rise of temperature, with headache, nausea, lumbar pain, hæmaturia, and albuminuria which continued a short time after the hæmaturia ceased. Singularly, too, with the subsidence of these symptoms, the chyluria remained absent for some time. The injections were resumed on its return, and each time were followed by relief. In the course of their use, however, the strength of the solution was increased to an ounce of the perchloride to twelve ounces of water, and the strongest solutions were retained in the bladder for as much as an hour, the weaker longer. Ultimately, however, the use of the injections became so painful that they had to be discontinued.

Another measure, employed by Bence Jones, was abdominal pressure by means of a belt. This also, in his experience, relieved the lumbar pain. In his case, which was about eight years under observation, Dickinson applied the pressure by a sort of tourniquet about an inch below the umbilicus. This lessened, though it did not stop, the pulsation in the femoral arteries. It also was successful at first, the chylosity lessening, and finally ceasing, but on the removal of the belt the chylous character gradually returned, and in sixteen hours was as bad as before. Repeated trials were followed by the same transient effect, but no cure. Under this treatment, however, combined with a liberal diet and rest, the patient gained many pounds in weight, and was able to leave the hospital and resume her occupation as dressmaker, the pursuit of which, and the absence of the favorable conditions of hospital-life, as invariably caused a return of the symptom and its resulting debility, which again caused her to seek admission.

Rest, therefore, and an abundance of good nourishing food, tend at least to counteract the exhausting effects of the disease, and even to cause the discharge to cease. Tonics, and especially chalybeates, are indicated for the former purpose.

As the relaxing effects of warm climates and warm weather seem to predispose to the condition and to aggravate it, removal to cooler latitudes and places is indicated.

Astringents, internally administered, naturally suggested themselves at an early date, and were used by Prout, Priestley, and Bence Jones. The latter especially thought gallic acid useful. He reports a case in which the disease did not return after its long-continued use. Goodwin of Norwich, England, also reports a case in which the chyluria was controlled by the gallic acid, but returned in four or five days after the remedy was discontinued. It again disappeared on resuming the drug, and the patient could at any time render the urine nearly normal in appearance by taking it. The case was lost sight of before it could be regarded as cured. Waters also reports a case which apparently recovered completely after nine weeks' treatment by gallic acid. He gave at first 30 grains a day, which were gradually increased to 135 a day, and then gradually reduced.

Other astringents which have been used are tannic acid, matico, or acetate of lead, nitrate of silver, the mineral acids.

Mangrove was successfully used in a case related by Bunyan of British Guiana. It was used in the shape of a decoction at the suggestion of a negress, an ounce being taken four times a day. In seven days the patient was so much relieved that the remedy was discontinued for two days, but the symptoms returned. They again disappeared when the drug was resumed, and two subsequent attacks were immediately cut short by the remedy. Roberts suggests that it may act as a parasiticide, aud suggests larger and sustained doses of the iodide of potassium for the same purpose.

Retention of urine, when present, should be treated like the same symptoms under other circumstances, by catheterization, washing out the bladder with tepid water, warm fomentations, and similar measures. It has even been suggested to wash out the bladder with ether under these circumstances.

As it seems impossible for the embryo filariæ to develop in the human body into the fully-developed Filaria Bancrofti, it is evident that with the death of the latter, which must occur sooner or later, the production of embryos must cease, while those previously produced must sooner or later also die, and in this way a spontaneous cure take place—just as a person infested with trichinous disease will ultimately recover if the introduction of the trichinæ cease and he is able to survive the irritation caused by the presence of the parasite in his muscles. In this manner we may account for the spontaneous disappearance of the disease in so many instances where all treatment has proved unavailing.

DISEASES OF THE BLADDER.

By EDWARD L. KEYES, M. D.

Inflammation.

THE bladder is a patient organ, and rather slow to resent injuries from within or without. It never inflames on account of such general causes as the influence of cold, anæmia, cachexia, or a depressed state of the general system. Any of these causes may act as adjuvants, but alone they are not effective. Thus a chilling of the legs, inoperative upon an individual with a healthy bladder, is a prime factor in exciting inflammation in the bladder of an old man with an enlarged prostate ; while the simple passage of a sound upon an individual suffering from anæmia might provoke a cystitis which the same traumatic cause would not have produced upon a patient in a thoroughly healthy condition.

Yet inflammation of the bladder is very common. It is sometimes a malady, more often a symptom produced by some other malady (stricture, prostatic enlargement, stone), and only to be overcome by detecting and removing its cause. The causes of inflammation of the bladder therefore include nearly all the maladies to which the bladder is liable.

The varieties of cystitis take name from that tissue of the viscus which is involved, and from the modality of the inflammation.

We have—

1. Cystitis mucosa
   - Acute
     - suppurative ;
     - diphtheritic ;
     - gangrenous.
   - Chronic
     - catarrhal ;
     - membranous.

2. Interstitial cystitis, where the muscular coat of the bladder is involved.

3. Peri-cystitis, para-cystitis, where the peritoneal surface or surrounding structures are inflamed.

This short section upon a surgical subject, only being granted a few pages in a medical work, cannot include a description of all these conditions, or more than a general outline of acute and chronic catarrhal cystitis. Suffice it to say for the other varieties that interstitial cystitis depends upon mucous cystitis or peri-cystitis, and is an inflammation of the muscular coat of the bladder, sometimes culminating in abscess, sometimes in concentric hypertrophy—*i. e.* contracture of the bladder. Peri-cystitis and para-cystitis occur in connection with peritonitis and pelvic cellulitis, and the peripheral inflammation may extend inward and involve the muscular and later the mucous coat.

All these conditions are grave only in proportion to the intensity of the malady causing them and to which they are subordinate.

Gangrenous cystitis occurs after injury, and occasionally in profound septicæmic conditions (puerperal) or after intense cantharidal poisoning. It is fatal.

True diphtheria of the bladder occasionally, but very rarely, accompanies general diphtheritic conditions, and is a very grave malady. Membranous cystitis is less grave, may be partial or complete. I have a fibrinous east of a female bladder which was extruded through the meatus. This malady occurs sometimes as a late complication of advanced chronic cystitis mucosa in the male. Recovery is quite possible.

Cystitis mucosa is a common disorder, constantly encountered by the physician as well as the surgeon. The irritable bladder, sometimes called cystitis, demands description here, as it may go on to become subacute or even acute cystitis of the vesical neck.

Irritability of the bladder is a neurotic and not an inflammatory condition, although it may lead to the latter state and terminate in it. The bladder is said to be irritable when the calls to urinate are too frequent, generally with little or no pain. As a rule, the urine is clear, containing no pus or a quantity entirely disproportionate to the frequency of the call to urinate.

In true irritability of the bladder the patient sleeps all night, although he may have have to empty his bladder every hour or two by day. There is sometimes a sense of weight, heat, or throbbing, more or less intense, in the perineum; the desire to urinate is normal but imperious; the satisfaction after the act is complete, and no pain accompanies its performance.

This condition of things is generally either neurotic directly, or indirectly (reflex). In children it may be caused by a tight prepuce, especially if irritated by retained smegma, by teething, by the existence of intestinal worms; and it may accompany chorea. It gets well by lapse of time or is cured by removal of the cause. In the adult it is most common in young men and recent widowers, and is often an expression of sexual distress due to sexual stimulation without relief, to sexual excess, or to improper sexual hygiene. The irritation of acrid urine will also cause it, as well as such peripheral troubles as a narrow meatus urinarius, a tight prepuce, urethral stricture, moderately enlarged prostate, kidney irritation (stone in the kidney, etc.). It appears in old men, sometimes, apparently, as a forerunner of organic prostatic changes.

Such stimulation as a glass of wine or beer, pleasant company, absorbing occupation, may cause it to disappear temporarily. It is habitually better in dry, clear weather, and worse in damp seasons when the wind is east. Worry, anxiety, fatigue, depression of spirits, and similar causes aggravate the condition. It is better for the first twenty-four hours after sexual intercourse, and worse than it was before during the next following twenty-four hours.

The SYMPTOMS of pure irritability are simply a frequent desire to urinate during the waking hours, the act not being attended by pain and the urine being reasonably clear.

The PATHOLOGY of this affection is not definitely known. It seems to be an essential neurosis involving the sensitive nerves of the deep urethra and neck of the bladder, attended, if long continued, by surface congestion of the deep urethra and neck of the bladder, and ultimately the phenomena of inflammation; for the very mechanical act of allowing the bladder incessantly to empty itself too often, and to squeeze its own neck, will, in many cases, after a time, lead to traumatic inflammation of mild type.

TREATMENT.—Marriage is a very effective treatment of pure vesical irritability when there is a sexual element in the case.

If any peripheral or local cause exists (stricture, contracted meatus, dense acid urine), its removal will effect a cure. Alkaline diluents, notably the citrate of potassium in gr. v–xxx doses, administered midway between meals, copaiba, or cubebs in moderate doses, often gives relief. Tonics, the tincture of the chloride of iron, and arsenical preparations are often of great value. The tincture of hyoscyamus in ℳx–lx doses may be combined advantageously with any of these remedies.

One of the most efficient of all methods of treatment is the use of the conical steel sound, as large as the urethra will admit without violence. The sound should be warmed, lubricated, and gently carried into the bladder at intervals of two to four days. The daily passage of the sound is objectionable, even if it gives relief at first, for it is liable to kindle a slow inflammation in a urethra unaccustomed to its use. When a sound is inserted it should not be left an instant in the bladder, but should be gently withdrawn as soon as it has been fully inserted. If left in the urethra, it does no good, and may act upon the cut-off group of muscles in the membranous urethra, causing them to contract spasmodically, as in the physiological performance of the coup-de-piston after urination. Such contraction bruises the sensitive mucous membrane of the urethra against the hard sound, and does mechanical damage.

The sound acts in three ways: It (1) mechanically distends the irritable contracted cut-off muscle and seems to quiet its contractile tendency. It (2) squeezes all the blood from the passively congested vessels of the irritated mucous membrane, thus ensuring a new supply of blood to the part and an improved circulation in the reaction which follows the irritation. It (3) mechanically, by contact, blunts the sensibility of the terminal sensitive nerves in the mucous membrane of the deep urethra. In this way the sound acts, and its effects generally last several days, often a week. Its good effect is also instantaneous. The slight feeling of weight and discomfort in the perineum which the patient has before its use is gone instantly, and replaced by a feeling of comfort. When this immediate sense of relief is not experienced, it is doubtful whether such a case will yield to the simple treatment by sounding.

It is a mistake to suppose that any ointments smeared upon a sound do good in this condition. - Mercurial, belladonna, and other ointments are used, but they are all and entirely rubbed off the sound before it reaches the deep urethra, and their good effect probably resides solely in the imagination of the physician and the credulity of the patient. Ointments are undoubtedly of service in some obstinate cases, notably strong tannic-acid mixtures, and sometimes iodoform, but these cannot be carried to the deep urethra by being rubbed upon a sound. The cupped sound may be used to effect this very neatly, the little cups on the sides of the curve of the sound being filled with the ointment which it is proposed to carry down and apply to the affected spot. A few drops of a mild nitrate-of-silver injection also give decided good results in some cases. The solution should vary between two and ten grains in the ounce of water, and may be accurately applied by means of a Bigelow or an Ultzmann syringe, a few drops being thrown into the membranous urethra. After the application, which should be made only when the patient has a full bladder, urination will wash out the canal and good effects may be looked for—not immediately, as after sounding, but after the irritation produced by the stimulating application has subsided.

Acute Cystitis.

Acute cystitis sometimes involves only the neck of the bladder; in other cases the whole mucous lining of the bladder is included in the morbid process.

The causes of acute cystitis may be grouped under six heads:

1. Traumatic.—Under this head may be ranged all injuries from with-out, with or without fracture of the pelvic bones—wounds, rupture of the bladder, the pressure of the child's head during labor; injuries from within, as during the use of instruments, by stone, or pedunculated tumor. The list may be increased by such chemical traumatisms as those produced by ammoniacal urine in cases of atony or paralysis, by excessively acid urine in neurotic conditions of the neck of the bladder. Such chemical causes, it will be observed, commonly act in conjunction with another cause. Irritating injections without any co-operative cause are capable of lighting up acute cystitis.

2. Extension of neighboring inflammation—gonorrhœal cystitis and that attending prostatic inflammation, pelvic abscess, pelvic cellulitis, peritonitis from neoplasms growing at the vesical neck, tubercle, cancer, etc.

3. Medicinal—from cantharides, sometimes cubebs or turpentine.

4. Specific—in diphtheritic, puerperal, septicæmic conditions.

5. The influence of cold when chronic inflammation already exists.

6. Neurotic—actual, from extreme and long-continued neuralgia of the vesical neck; reflex, from irritation at a distance, tight meatus, stricture, inflammation of the seminal vesicles, kidney irritations.

SYMPTOMS.—The symptoms of acute cystitis are (1) frequent painful urination by night as well as by day, the pain being greatest at the close of, and immediately after, the act, and the pain persisting more or less between the acts, radiating from the perineum; (2) moderate fever, some-times announced by chill; (3) commonly great despondency and a depression of spirits totally disproportionate to the degree and significance of the local inflammation; (4) the urine invariably is milky, with pus: it may at first be acid and of normal odor; it is often tinged with blood, especially toward the end of the act of urination. In extreme cases the urine may contain membranous or sloughy shreds or gangrenous gases. The urine eventually becomes alkaline, and finally deposits lumps of pus and abundant triple phosphate crystals.

Complications occurring with the cystitis yield appropriate symptoms.

Such possible complications are congestion and engorgement of the prostate, possibly going on to abscess; epididymitis, orchitis, inflammation of the seminal vesicles, inflammation running up the ureters, pyelitis, surgical kidney; abscess in the walls of the bladder or in the connective tissue about the same; very rarely peritonitis or suppurative phlebitis in the veins about the neck of the bladder.

The pathological changes produced by acute cystitis are similar to analogous changes upon the other mucous membranes: patches of more or less brilliant uniform or punctate redness, perhaps surrounding small ecchymotic areas; a softened, swollen mucous membrane; enlarged follicles near the neck of the bladder, perhaps ulcerated spots; possibly false or true diphtheritic exudations (such exudations have been especially noted in cantharidal cystitis); possibly interstitial abscess of the bladder-wall, or even suppurative phlebitis in the veins about the prostate and neck of the bladder, as observed by Walsham[1] in a case of cystitis due to over-distension. This last complication is happily exceptionally rare.

The PROGNOSIS varies with the cause of the cystitis, and as the latter often cannot be entirely removed, the acute cystitis may only be moderated so as to be made to assume the chronic form. When the cause can be entirely removed, acute cystitis gets well and leaves the bladder absolutely sound.

TREATMENT.—Acute cystitis from whatever cause requires a uniform general line of treatment. Anodynes are essential both for the patient's comfort and to prevent the constant straining to empty the bladder to which the unremitting, painful desire to urinate impels him. Hyoscyamus is a favorite in the form of tincture in $\mathfrak{m}$xx–ʒj doses, or any of the opiates by the mouth, or in suppository preferably combined with extract of belladonna in small dose. Sometimes quarter- or half-grain suppositories of extract of belladonna alone at intervals of six to eight hours keep the tenesmus more in check than anything else, but belladonna used too freely may bring on retention by causing spasm of the cut-off muscles. Camphor is useful, especially in strangury from cantharides. Rest in bed is essential in most cases, preferably with the hips raised. Heat in some form, as a hot poultice, fomentation, spongio-piline, hot-water rubber bottle, etc. over the hypogastrium preceded by a mustard plaster, gives great comfort. Hot-water hip-baths of short duration and frequently repeated are of service in most cases.

Alkalies are valuable, especially in the beginning of an attack—liq. potassæ $\mathfrak{m}$v–xx doses, citrate of potassium gr. x–xx, combined with an anodyne or some demulcent drink.

Infusions and extracts of corn-silk, dog-grass root, buchu, pareira brava, uva ursi, etc. are of some assistance, but generally not so comforting as some of the bland diuretic waters—Bethesda, Mountain Valley, Poland, Glenn, Vichy, Wildungen, Buffalo Lithia. Distilled water or rain-water, especially if taken warm, is a good diluent diuretic. On the advent of acute cystitis all instrumentation upon the bladder should, if practicable, be postponed, all stimulating drugs (cantharides, turpentine, cubebs, alcohol) stopped, and stimulating foods avoided. Asparagus, coffee, salt, pepper, mustard, acids, and a highly nitrogenized diet are not allowable. The rectum should be kept empty and complications treated as they arise.

---

[1] *London Lancet*, May 10, 1879, p. 665.

Chronic Cystitis (Catarrh of the Bladder).

Catarrh of the bladder is chronic inflammation of the mucous membrane of the urinary reservoir, with more or less thickening of the walls of the bladder. This malady, so apt to persist for years, is probably more commonly encountered by the physician than acute cystitis. Acute cystitis, however, frequently complicates the chronic malady by occasional outbursts of acute symptoms. Thus an attack of the stone is acute calculous cystitis interrupting the course of chronic vesical inflammation due to stone. Catarrh of the bladder may follow acute cystitis, or it may commence insidiously as a subacute disorder, and be catarrh, in the popular sense, from the first.

The causes of catarrh of the bladder are never single. It always takes two causes to produce true catarrh of the bladder—one mechanical, and one chemical. After a traumatism inflicted on a healthy bladder, with proper care the patient recovers entirely. If, however, he insists upon keeping up and about, continues to drink liquor, and does not avoid straining at urination, the membrane about the neck of the bladder, irritated by the ammonia from the decomposing urine, secretes an excess of viscid mucus, the pus becomes gelatinized by the ammonia, the constant straining leads to hypertrophy of the muscular coat, the nerves lose their acute sensitiveness, and the milder persistent malady, chronic catarrh, is set up, to continue perhaps for an indefinite period.

Infiltrations of the bladder-walls with tubercle or cancer, urinary calculus, and, notably, enlarged prostate, stricture of the urethra, tumors of the bladder, hernia of the bladder, exstrophy, over-distension of the bladder from stricture, spasm of the urethra, coma, paralysis, or other cause, may be the traumatic element, while the liberated ammonia from the alkaline decomposing urine furnishes the chemical element; and the two causes, if continued, occasion and maintain the condition known as chronic catarrh of the bladder. In coma or the delirium of typhoid fever or paraplegia or hemiplegia (sometimes) the bladder becomes over-distended and atonied, perhaps paralyzed. Here the use of the catheter appropriately, with great gentleness, may relieve the patient without even the intervention of acute cystitis; while, on the other hand, acute cystitis may come on and be cured, or, if ammoniacal urine be allowed to accumulate and the bladder be not washed out so long as it is unable to entirely expel its contents, chronic cystitis, catarrh, results. I have known several cases of partial paraplegia and other disorders in which the patient could void no drop of urine except through a catheter, where there never had been any chronic catarrh, no stringy mucus, hardly a pus-corpuscle, through long years of the disability, owing to intelligence in the attention to emptying and washing out the bladder instituted by the physician having first charge of the case.

As prominent among the causes of chronic catarrh in a purely medical aspect it may be well to insist upon the ease with which this condition is sometimes brought about by the physician himself. A man with a weakened bladder may carry a pint or much more clear urine in his bladder constantly during many years as a residual deposit which his weakened bladder cannot throw off. Excess over the fixed residuum produces a desire to urinate, and the patient, mainly by voluntary contraction of the

abdominal walls, voids that excess. If now the physician finds this globular accumulation in the patient's belly, and in his zeal to do all that is
possible forgets his caution, he may throw the patient first into an acute
cystitis (if haply he escapes collapse), and then into chronic vesical catarrh
—an affair perhaps of a lifetime. Surgeons have noticed, and especially
Sir Henry Thompson has pointed out, that a dirty catheter may poison
the urine and bring about a cystitis which otherwise might have been
avoided; and observers from all time have noticed that the sudden entire
evacuation of the contents of a bladder long accustomed to over-distension is in itself a grave cause of serious inflammatory disturbance to the
mucous membrane of the bladder. Recently much attention has been
called to this condition and its possible fatal termination by Sir Andrew
Clarke, under the name of catheter fever.

The deductions from a knowledge of these facts are obvious: they
are—(1) always to thoroughly cleanse, and then to disinfect, a catheter on
each occasion before its use; and (2) never to empty entirely at a first
sitting a bladder which has been long habituated to over-distension; and
when, finally, the bladder is emptied, always irrigate it with a disinfecting solution (borax) after each emptying.

SYMPTOMS.—Chronic cystitis varies in grade, and its symptoms vary
with the grade of the inflammatory process. There is probably no pain
more intense than that endured by a man with severe general cystitis in
its last stages, when the unceasing tenesmus wrings groans from his lips,
the sweat from his body, doubles his frame in agony, and converts his
facial expression into a distorted tragedy. The sight is pitiable and never
to be forgotten. On the other hand, a man may continue about and at
his work with a patient flabby bladder containing constantly more or less
stringy mucus and ammoniacal urine, suffering little or no pain or tenesmus, and perhaps having no subjective symptoms except a slight sense of
weight in his lower belly and a rather frequent desire to urinate.

Between these limits the symptoms range, but in a general way it may
be said that the symptoms of chronic vesical catarrh are these: frequent
calls to urinate, attended by more or less pain, especially toward and after
the termination of the act. The sense of satisfaction normally felt after
urination is generally absent. Motion, particularly jolting as in rough
riding, causes pain. This pain is referred to the lower part of the belly,
to the perineum, to the end of the penis, the urethra, the anus. The
straining after urination may be absent or of the most intense character,
leading to prolapse of the rectum and causing excruciating torture. The
urine always contains pus scattered through it, and generally also more or
less pus in that semi-solid condition known as stringy mucus. Stringy mucus
is pus gelatinized by the ammonia of the decomposing urine. These clots
of muco-pus contain gritty crystals of the ammonio-magnesian phosphate.
More or less blood is to be found in the urine, especially during acute
paroxysms. Pure blood sometimes follows the urine after each act of
urination. Bacteria abound in the fluid, which varies in odor greatly in
different cases, not always strictly in accordance with the severity of the
actual inflammatory process. Thus, the urine may be simply sweetish
in its odor, ammoniacal, flat, and stale, or be possessed of a putrid, sickening sweetness of indescribably nauseating power. Again, it may be
rankly rotten. The bottom of the chamber in some cases becomes cov-

ered with a thick coating of the viscid muco-pus, which strings out and reluctantly follows the fluid when the vessel is inverted. Sometimes the urine contains shreds of false membrane or putrid masses of sloughy tissue.

PATHOLOGY.—In chronic cystitis the mucous membrane of the bladder undergoes gradual thickening, loses its pink salmon tint, and becomes gray in color. The thickening extends to the submucous layer, and more or less to the muscular walls as well. In cases of prolonged chronic cystitis attending atony of the bladder, notably with hypertrophied prostate, the cavity of the organ is large, its walls seemingly thinned and flabby, its internal coat roughened by the crossing of bundles of muscular fibres or perhaps perfectly smooth. In other conditions (concentric hypertrophy), where there has been a serious obstacle to the free outflow of urine without any atony of the muscular coat (stricture of the urethra, some cases of stone and of enlarged prostate), the walls of the bladder may be enormously thickened to the extent of an inch or more, the inside surface rough, perhaps ulcerated.

The thickening of the muscular bands within the bladder often causes them to stand out in bold relief, like the muscular bundles in the heart-cavity. These prominent bundles enclose spaces of various sizes and shapes, and from the bottoms of these spaces sometimes the mucous membrane protrudes between the muscular bands and forms pouches of varying size (sacculated bladder). These pouches consist of mucous membrane alone covered with peritoneum, and may become the seat of encysted stone.

If there has been a subacute grade of the surface inflammation before death, there may be livid spots on the mucous surface of the bladder, punctate or larger ecchymoses, reddened areas from which the epithelium is more or less detached, ulcers with or without sloughs or diphtheritic covering, perhaps perforations of the bladder and infiltration of urine, enlarged mucous follicles, granulations, fungosities, etc. Heterologous deposits, tumor, cancerous and tubercular ulcers, cysts, stone, complete the possibilities of what may be encountered in the bladder at an autopsy upon a patient with chronic cystitis.

The chronic like the acute varieties of cystitis may involve the whole of the inside of the bladder or only a portion of it.

The PROGNOSIS, like that of acute cystitis, varies mainly with the cause. If the latter can be entirely removed (stone), the bladder gets perfectly well. Not so, however, unless all the causes are removed. Thus, a phosphatic stone may grow in a bladder as a result of enlarged prostate and chronic cystitis. The presence of the stone excites the chronic cystitis, and subjects the patient to a crisis of acute cystitis from time to time. The removal of such a stone will by no means cure the chronic cystitis; its removal is only one step in the treatment of the cystitis.

As far as life is concerned, the prognosis of chronic cystitis is good. A patient may live many years with chronic cystitis, particularly if he treats his bladder properly. Although, as generally encountered, chronic cystitis is not curable, few maladies yield results to treatment more gratifying to the physician and the patient than the one under consideration.

The legitimate ultimate termination of chronic cystitis is by chronic inflammation of the ureter and pelvis of the kidney on both sides, interstitial kidney changes, and finally death by suppression. Generally, this end may be almost indefinitely postponed by well-directed efforts of palliative treatment.

TREATMENT.—The acute outbursts of inflammatory disturbance occurring during the course of chronic cystitis require the same means for their relief as those already indicated when considering the treatment of acute cystitis—all the prohibition of stimulants, the use of bland mineral waters, demulcent decoctions, infusions, and alkaline draughts. The anodynes, the rest, the heat, the hip-bath, are all indicated here for the acuter symptoms, just as they are in the acute malady, but very much more can be done both in a prophylactic and in a curative way. A milk diet, even an exclusive milk diet, is an element of great value in cases of chronic cystitis. I have two patients, both old men, now under observation, one of whom recovered entirely from cystitis with complete atony, necessitating the constant use of the catheter, by means of an exclusive milk diet. He takes one gallon of milk a day, and nothing else, and lives among his fellow-men at his work and amusements in entire contentment. He has remained absolutely well on this diet during many years. The other patient could not take milk after fair trial, but gradually emerged from the very jaws of death, due to prolonged chronic cystitis and double pyelitis, by the free use of koumiss, which his wife daily prepared for him. Vichy and milk in equal parts, taken cold, is another form of using the milk diet, and the more modern peptonized milk another.

Light white and red wines, or even a little gin or old brandy, are of decided advantage in the majority of enfeebled old men with chronic cystitis. The patient should be clothed with the utmost care. The feet and legs should be clad in wool unless in the very hottest season, and flannel should constantly encase the belly and loins. Nothing is more detrimental to chronic cystitis than chilling the legs.

Another word is necessary in favor of the internal use of alkaline remedies. Even where the urine is alkaline, ammoniacal, putrid, if the stomach will take an alkaline medicine kindly the effect is generally beneficial, for the urine, especially in old men who are prone to these maladies, is quite certain to be acid at the fountain-head. And even if the urine is immediately altered by chronic pyelitis through ammoniacal decomposition before it enters the ureter, yet it will generally irritate the pelvis of the kidney and the ureter and the bladder less if it be secreted in a bland alkaline state than if it be discharged into the irritated area full of uric acid.

Turpentine, copaiba, cubebs, and the muriate of iron are of service in selected cases, but ordinary astringents seem to possess little or no value. Benzoic acid, in ten-grain doses in capsules, sometimes improves the ammoniacal condition of the urine, but the stomach often rejects it. Boracic acid, which has of late been much talked about, in five- to ten-grain doses in water, three or four times a day, is of value occasionally. Quinine is serviceable where the nerve-force is failing. I have been unable to procure any very decided advantage from the use of salicylic acid or the salicylate of sodium by the mouth.

The most important general surgical principle in connection with chrouic vesical catarrh is that which concerns emptying the bladder thoroughly and ensuring its cleanliness. In many, perhaps most, conditions of chronic inflammation of the bladder from atony, paralysis, obstruction, or other cause the bladder fails to empty itself entirely. There remains, therefore, a fixed residuum always in the bladder; and although this is diluted and partly evacuated at each act of urination, yet some of the pus, the bacteria, the ammoniacal ferment, remains constantly in the bladder ready to contaminate each new portion of urine as it descends from the kidneys. This must be disposed of, and the bladder washed out, if a permanently satisfactory treatment is to be instituted.

The soft-rubber catheter is to be preferred where it will pass, otherwise the woven silk or the French Mercier instrument, and the bladder should receive attention at least once in the twenty-four hours, and oftener if required. The last drops of urine should be drawn off and the bladder washed with water at about 100° F., in which is dissolved some borax— a heaping teaspoonful to the pint—or other substance capable of disinfecting the contents or mildly stimulating the circulation of the bladder.

Carbolic acid has not yielded good results in my hands. A host of remedies have been employed, but it is doubtful whether anything can do more good than the water mechanically, borax as a disinfectant, dilute nitric acid, ℥i–x to the pint, as a stimulant, or, in some cases, nitrate of silver, gr. ½–x to the ounce, used with caution. The injections should be practised through the catheter which withdraws the urine, and repeated according to their effect. For cleansing purposes an injection of simple warm water may be used at each introduction of the catheter. A fountain syringe with two-way stopcock is the most convenient instrument to use for the purpose of simply washing the bladder, because the wash may be repeated indefinitely until it returns clear, without readjusting the nozzle in the catheter.

Very extreme, long-protracted cases of chronic vesical catarrh justify the performance of lateral cystotomy for their relief, or the modification quite recently proposed by Thompson[1]—a median perineal incision involving only the membranous urethra, through which a large soft-rubber catheter is passed and tied in for a few days or longer.

Neurosis of the Bladder.

The most common vesical neurosis is neuralgia of the neck of the bladder, with or without the accompaniment of irritability of the bladder, spasmodic stricture, or vesical spasm. Irritability of the bladder has been already considered at the beginning of the section on Cystitis. The other neurotic conditions are always more or less interwoven with each other, and they may each and all of them complicate inflammatory states of the deep urethra, prostate, and vesical neck.

The CAUSES of this set of affections are most varied, and range from irregular sexual hygiene (the most common of all) through inflammatory local conditions, peripheral irritations (the most obstinate of which is

[1] *Brit. Med. Journ.,* Dec. 9, 1882, p. 1131.

chronic inflammation of the seminal vesicles, with or without true spermatorrhœa), up to organic changes in the spinal cord and brain.

The PROGNOSIS in neurotic states varies with the cause. Some cases are easily controlled; others absolutely defy all and every treatment of which I have any knowledge.

The TREATMENT involves a removal, if possible, of the cause. Local measures which have been found most effective in subduing the deep urethral irritation are—(1) the gentle passage of a soft bougie or conical steel sound into the bladder at intervals of one to seven days. The instrument should be removed at once. Sometimes it is necessary to cut a narrow meatus or a stricture in the pendulous urethra in order that a sound of large-enough size may be employed to put the sensitive deep urethra sufficiently on the stretch. (2) The application to the deep urethra and prostatic sinus of pastes of tannin or iodoform with the cupped sound or other apparatus, or the injection of the deep urethra with strong solutions of tannin or mild solutions (gr. i–x to ʒj) of nitrate of silver. (3) In the most extreme cases, those furnishing all the symptoms of stone, even cystotomy is justifiable. It nearly always furnishes a temporary, sometimes permanent, relief.

Medical measures include all the bland diluent mineral waters, alkaline and tonic remedies, already considered in discussing Irritability of the Bladder.

Atony and Paralysis.

Atony of the bladder is more or less lack of expulsive force, due to failure in power of the muscles of the bladder, the nerves remaining sound. Paralysis is the same condition perhaps more pronounced, but due to central origin. A patient may be unable to pass water in more than a dribbling stream, but if he has true organic stricture or spasm of the deep urethra, the muscular coat of his bladder may perhaps not be to blame for his imperfect urination. The question of atony may be decided in such a case by introducing a catheter of any size that will pass. If there is atony, the stream flows sluggishly from the mouth of the catheter, and toward the end is influenced by the breathing of the patient. If there is no atony, the stream rushes through the catheter, and maintains its force until the last drop flows away. In paralysis and extreme atony the influence of the descent of the diaphragm during inspiration is noticed during the whole course of the flow of the sluggish stream through the catheter.

The CAUSES of atony are over-distension of the bladder, voluntary (by persistently neglecting the call to urinate), involuntary retention (from fever, coma, stricture, large prostate), and a certain intrinsic, sometimes inherited, tendency to weakness on the part of the bladder, noticed by some people during their entire lives.

Atony is most common, often a part of their malady, in old men with enlarged prostate. Paralysis of the bladder accompanies certain organic changes due to injury or disease in the spinal cord or brain. Both in atony and in paralysis the bladder may be constantly distended to a certain extent, perhaps to its utmost limit, as a passive sac, and the excess of urine over this uniform residuum may dribble away involuntarily (false incontinence), or may be expelled in small portions by repeated acts of urination performed in the ordinary way or by the aid of great straining and assistance from the voluntary contractions of the muscular walls of the abdomen. No condition of incontinence of urine can be considered proved until demonstrated by the passage of a catheter. Both atony and paralysis may get well under proper treatment in favorable cases. Many cases are incurable, but the discomfort they tend to cause may be almost entirely counteracted.

TREATMENT.—Under all circumstances where the bladder cannot empty itself, the catheter should be used, and the bladder should be washed out, kept clean, and disinfected. All the suggestions laid down for catheterization and vesical injection in the section on Chronic Cystitis are applicable here and need not be repeated. It is particularly necessary to disinfect the catheter on each occasion before it is introduced. This is best effected by washing the catheter outside and inside with a 5 per cent. solution of carbolic acid in water, and finally washing it outside with clean water, before its introduction. If the bladder is over-distended, it should not, as a rule, be entirely emptied at the first introduction of the catheter, for fear of possible collapse, or, what is more to be dreaded, setting up acute cystitis by suddenly taking off all the internal pressure from the vessels in the walls of the weakened bladder, to which pressure the circulation has become accustomed. If, therefore, the bladder is emptied inadvertently, it is better to inject a few ounces of warm water containing borax in solution (a teaspoonful to the pint), and leave it in until the next catheterization. The quantity left in may be reduced at each sitting. By careful attention to these means most cases of over-distension due to atony or paralysis may be relieved without the intervention of cystitis, or with so little that it does not become a serious factor in the case.

The medical treatment of these cases is less important than the mechanical. Under the latter alone and improvement in general health curable cases often get well. Milk diet is of service, and iron and tonics of considerable value in proper cases. Electricity has not yielded satisfactory results in my hands, and I have not derived the advantage from ergot which is often claimed for it. In cases of atony I think I have seen good results sometimes follow the use of strychnine internally in pretty full doses. The same remedy under the skin acts more promptly and more effectively if it is to do any good at all. In true paralysis of central origin the cure of the bladder depends upon relief of the original disease and local treatment to the bladder.

Hysterical women sometimes feign paralysis in order apparently to secure the sympathy and personal attention of the physician. The application of the actual cautery above the pubes, and entrusting a female nurse with the function of catheterization, is generally effective treatment in these cases.

Hemorrhage from the Bladder.

After all sorts of wounds and injuries to the bladder, and in cases of rupture of the viscus, blood is found in the urine. In certain medical conditions, in scurvy, hemorrhagic eruptive diseases, cases of vicarious menstruation, it has been noticed. In strangury due to cantharides, or in any condition of acute or chronic cystitis with considerable spasm of the bladder, the urine contains more or less blood. Especially is this true if ulceration exist at or near the neck of the bladder, as in tubercular or cancerous cystitis.

In cases of stone in the bladder one of the cardinal symptoms is vesical hæmaturia, while in villous growth often the only symptom of the malady is repeated attacks of more or less profuse bleeding from the bladder coming on unexpectedly, without obvious exciting cause, and showing no regularity in the length of the intervals between the hemorrhages or the intensity or duration of the latter. Outbursts of unexpected hemorrhage are not uncommon in connection with some cases of enlarged prostate and chronic cystitis, while these outbursts are the rule, sooner or later, in most cases of true cancer of the bladder.

The DIAGNOSIS is often very important—that is, in a given case to decide whether the blood comes from the bladder or from the kidney. This may usually be ascertained by a very simple manœuvre, especially when the flow of blood is not excessive : a silver catheter of short curve is introduced and the urine drawn off, the bladder gently washed several times without moving the catheter, and the shade of red in the wash noted. Now, the bladder being slightly distended with warm water, the point of the catheter is moved somewhat roughly in all directions and made to touch different portions of the wall of the bladder. The water is now allowed to escape, and its deepened color will decide that the hemorrhage has a vesical origin, for manipulations of a silver catheter in a healthy bladder will not occasion a flow of blood. In doubtful cases on two occasions I succeeded in locating the point whence the blood escaped as follows : In one I passed a soft catheter, and washed the bladder until the wash escaped nearly clean; I then withdrew the catheter until the point reached the membranous urethra (the bladder having been left full of clean water), and immediately passed the instrument again and withdrew the contents of the bladder, which were now brilliantly colored, thus locating the bleeding point in the prostatic sinus. In the other case, that of a young man with moderate stricture, whose urine was nearly solid with blood, I noticed that no blood escaped by the meatus between the acts of urination ; therefore the bleeding point was posterior to the membranous urethra. Was it in the prostate, the bladder, or the kidney? To decide this I passed a soft catheter and washed the bladder until the wash flowed clear. I then injected some warm water, withdrew the catheter, and caused the patient to empty the bladder. The flow was brilliant with blood. In both these cases I effected a cure by one application of solid nitrate of silver through the urethra to the prostatic sinus.

The TREATMENT of vesical hæmaturia is the treatment of the cause, which, if possible, must be ascertained. For the symptom itself the internal use of iron, turpentine, opium, gallic and tannic acids, are of service. I have not derived any advantage from ergot. Locally, rest in bed, ice over the region of the bladder, and avoidance of straining at urination are generally all that is necessary. I have had good results from injecting the bladder with a solution of alum, gr. i–ij to ʒj of warm water, and cures have been effected by injecting nitrate of silver in solution. It is not well to inject iron in solution, since this substance makes a hard clot, and a soft clot is preferable. When the bladder fills up with a solid clot of blood, the best treatment, according to my experience, is to administer opium freely and diluent drinks. The urine slowly dissolves the clot, which has already arrested the hemorrhage, in most cases by its pressure, and the blood flows away as a dark coffee-ground material, sometimes nearly black. If the catheter is used, the clot broken up or dissolved with pepsin or other substance, and washed or pumped out, a new clot is apt to form at once; and although this treatment is based on high authority, and is often practised successfully, it is a question whether the patient would not in many cases do as well, or better, by being let alone, soothed by opium, until the urine dissolves the clot and nature relieves him.

New Growths in the Bladder.

These belong strictly to the province of surgery, but they fall also under the notice of the physician. Tubercular disease may involve the whole mucous surface or only the neck of the bladder; cancer may infiltrate its walls or grow out as a solid tumor in the vesical cavity; fibrous, sarcomatous, and myomatous new formations, polypi, and cysts, simple and hydatid, have been encountered; villous growths, both benign and cancerous, may occur. These morbid deposits give rise either to recurrent hemorrhage or to varying grades of chronic cystitis. The diagnosis is often difficult, the treatment generally palliative. Much has been done of late in an operative way for the relief of tumors of the bladder, and some brilliant results have been secured by operations through the perineum as well as above the pubes. A tumor of moderate size may be detected by the searcher within the bladder, and often may be grasped in a lithotrite and measured. Such a tumor can generally be plainly felt by conjoined palpation in a thin subject, one hand pressed firmly down behind the pubes and two fingers of the other hand passed into the rectum. Recently, Sir Henry Thompson has advocated vesical exploration for purposes of diagnosis through a median incision in the perineum, as for median lithotomy, and has practised it a number of times with a large measure of success. I have made the same exploration several times, and have encountered and successfully removed one tumor. The expedient is worth bearing in mind for use in any obscure cases. It is probably less objectionable and more likely to yield valuable information than the exploration by introducing the whole hand into the rectum (Simon's method).

SEMINAL INCONTINENCE.

By SAMUEL W. GROSS, A. M., M. D.

DEFINITION.—By the term seminal incontinence, which is synonymous with involuntary or abnormal seminal emissions, pollutions, and spermatorrhœa, is meant the involuntary discharge of semen beyond the limits of health. Although usually described as a distinct disease, it is symptomatic of, and, as a rule, primarily dependent upon, weakness or exhaustion, along with exaggerated irritability, excitability, impressibility, or mobility of the centres which preside over erection and ejaculation. Hence it should be regarded as a motor neurosis, and not as a functional disorder of the testes.

CLASSIFICATION.—Involuntary seminal losses embrace three conditions, which constitute as many varieties of the affection, and which may exist separately, or pass into one another, or be combined. These varieties are, first, nocturnal losses or pollutions, which occur during sleep, and are generally attended with an erection, erotic dream, and pleasurable sensation; secondly, diurnal pollutions, which take place when the patient is awake, are excited by trivial mechanical or psychical causes, and are associated with imperfect erection and diminished sensation; and, thirdly, spermorrhagia, or spermatorrhœa, in the strict acceptation of that term, which is characterized by a constant escape of a slight amount of seminal fluid, without the orgasm, pleasurable sensation, or impure thoughts, or during micturition and defecation.

1. Nocturnal Pollutions.—By far the most common of the varieties of seminal incontinence is the first, or that in which the emissions occur during sleep under the influence of an erotic dream, and which may, therefore, be regarded as an exaggeration of the normal or physiological condition. In health, provided the subject leads a continent life, the number of emissions varies greatly, and as they are merely reflex signs of distension of the seminal passages, they are not pathological nor are they attended with ill effects. The knowledge of this fact is of great practical importance, as it frequently enables the physician to assure his patient that the emissions are not abnormal, thereby relieving his mind of a great weight. It is, of course, to be remembered that the frequency of nocturnal pollutions depends upon age, climate, habits, temperament, constitution, diet, and predisposition, and that young men who suffered during childhood from nocturnal incontinence of urine are particularly obnoxious to them. Their frequency also varies greatly in the same person, and it is scarcely possible to determine what constitutes the standard

of health merely by the intervals of their repetition, since a number which would be normal in one person would be abnormal in another. In men, however, who possess sound nervous systems and who do not trouble themselves with sexual matters an emission every fortnight is a sign of excellent health ; and even if they should occur at intervals of several days, they are not inconsistent with temporary good health. The latter statement is well exemplified by a case which came under my observation in 1882. A druggist, twenty-seven years of age, had had for six years from three to five emissions a week, and occasionally two during a single night, attended with erections and voluptuous dreams, without the slightest evidence of impairment of his health. In all such cases, however, as well as in those in which the emissions have occurred at longer intervals for a number of years, it only requires a little longer time for general symptoms to manifest themselves.

Nocturnal pollutions are to be regarded as pathological when they occur in married or single men who indulge in regular intercourse ; when they are followed by backache, headache, enfeeblement of the functional powers of the brain, mental depression, and bodily or mental lassitude ; when they take place without erections or dreams ; when they accompany or follow acute or chronic diseases ; when they coexist with diurnal pollutions or spermorrhagia ; and, finally, when they are complicated by one of the varieties of impotence, which may be the only indication that the emissions are abnormal or one of the effects of impairment of the functions of the genital nervous centres. The associated symptoms of myelasthenia and cerebrasthenia vary very much in degree in men of apparently the same amount of vigor and tolerance, and in whom the pollutions occur with equal frequency, or they may even be absent altogether.

2. Diurnal Pollutions.—Ejaculation of semen during the day is fortunately of comparatively infrequent occurrence, since it indicates a more serious condition than do losses of seminal fluid occurring when the patient is asleep, the genital organs and the centres which preside over them being highly impressible or in a state of irritable weakness. In what may be regarded as the lesser form of the affection the ejaculation is due to slight peripheral irritation, induced, for example, by friction of the clothing, crossing of the legs repeated several times, horseback exercise, driving over rough streets, riding in railway-cars, or even shaving, combing the hair, or shampooing the head ; while in the more aggravated variety an emission is induced by psychical irritation, such as reading libidinous books, the sight of indecent pictures, dwelling upon sexual ideas, or the mere sight of a female. In the former of these varieties there is a fair erection, but the sensibility is blunted ; in the latter the erection is flabby or the penis is flaccid and there is little if any pleasure.

3. Spermorrhagia.—In the third phase of the affection, which is still more uncommon than the second variety, there is a continuous passive loss of semen, without erection or sensation—a condition which depends upon paralysis and dilatation of the orifices of the ejaculatory ducts, and which is most conspicuous during the acts of micturition and defecation. The existence of spermatorrhœa, in the restricted sense of the term, is denied by some authors, but I have myself met with it in five instances, and typical cases have been recorded by other modern writers.

CLINICAL HISTORY.—Seminal incontinence usually supervenes upon the interruption of sexual intercourse, especially when the subject has been accustomed to excessive venereal indulgence, or, as more frequently happens, upon the abandonment of the habit of masturbation. Any one of these varieties may exist separately, but they gradually pass into each other, and are variously intermixed in the advanced grade of the affection. In the mild type there is increased frequency in the occurrence of nocturnal pollutions, ejaculation taking place at intervals of several days or for two or three nights in succession, when there is a respite for a week or ten days. The emissions are associated with disturbances of the nervous system, referable to the brain or spinal cord or to the cerebro-spinal axis, of which mental lassitude and muscular debility are the most common signs. When, as the result of the increase in the irritability of the ejaculatory centre and of the progressive weakness or exhaustion of the entire nervous system, the case goes on from bad to worse, it usually pursues the following course: Abnormal frequency of the nocturnal pollutions is associated with pain in the back, headache, muscular fatigue, and incapacity for sustained mental effort. With the increase in the number of the emissions erection becomes imperfect, ejaculation on coition is frequently precipitate, and the patient complains of dulness of perception, impairment of memory, mental dejection, a dull pain in the occipital region, weakness of vision, vertigo, palpitation of the heart, trembling and numbness of the limbs, shortness of the breath, flatulence, constipation, and other signs of gastric derangement. Diurnal pollutions are now superadded, and intercourse is impracticable, either from failure of erection or from premature ejaculation. The general symptoms, too, are more serious. The patient constantly broods over his condition, assumes that he has permanently lost his virility, and the mental anxiety and dejection verge upon or merge into a condition of sexual hypochondrism. The gait is unsteady; the hands and feet are habitually cold; he is subject to wandering neuralgic and rheumatoid pains; passes restless nights; loses flesh and color; shuns society; imagines that every one recognizes his condition, and fears to look one in the face; and is utterly incapacitated for mental or physical exertion. With the still further increase of the irritable weakness of the genitalia and nervous centres the semen flows continuously out of the urethra, and its discharge is augmented during defecation and micturition. Finally, the man becomes a confirmed hypochondriac, and should he have inherited a tendency to insanity, epilepsy, ataxia, or other nervous disorders, he may lapse into one of these conditions.

In the early stage of seminal incontinence, when the nocturnal pollutions overstep the natural limits, the ejaculated fluid is unchanged. When, however, the pollutions are more frequent and diurnal discharges coexist, the semen is watery and scanty; the spermatozoids are smaller, comparatively few in number, and their movements are liable to be abolished in less than an hour, while spermatic crystals form more rapidly and more abundantly than in health. In the worst cases, or those characterized by diurnal and nocturnal pollutions and by the presence of semen in the urine, the spermatozoids are either entirely absent, or, if they are present, they are motionless, stunted, or variously deformed. In these advanced cases the ejaculated fluid, which consists principally of the secretions of the seminal vesicles and the prostate, frequently undergoes fatty degencration, as indicated by granular epithelium, by molecular detritus, and even by oil-globules in the protoplasm of the altered zoosperms. The entire absence of spermatozoids, constituting the condition known as azoospermatorrhœa, is of infrequent occurrence.

An examination of the genital organs discloses elongation of the prepuce in nearly one-fourth of all cases; a rigid and pointed penis in one-tenth; relaxation of the scrotum in about one-eighth; irritable testes in 1 example out of every 25; varicocele in 1 case out of every 50; coldness of the genitalia in 1 case out of every 17; a feeling of heat in 1 case out of every 33; and irritability of the bladder in 1 case out of every 25. It will, moreover, be found that seminal incontinence is complicated by feebleness of erection, with precipitate ejaculation on coition, in 22 per cent. of all cases; by the occurrence of ejaculation on attempting intercourse, before penetration, simultaneously with erection, or even before erection, in 16 per cent.; and with total impotence in 5 per cent. of all cases. Prostatorrhœa is also a not infrequent complication, while urethral strictures and hyperæsthesia are nearly always present.

ETIOLOGY AND PATHOGENY.—Seminal incontinence is not a separate entity, but one of many symptoms of general or local disorders, or of both combined. In the majority of instances it must be looked upon as a neurosis, diurnal and nocturnal pollutions representing a motor neurosis with spasm of the seminal vesicles, and spermorrhagia indicating a motor neurosis with dilatation and paresis of the orifices of the ejaculatory ducts. In all of the varieties there is increased susceptibility of the cerebral and spinal genital centres to factors which in healthy persons are not productive of ill effects.

Like other nervous disorders, involuntary seminal emissions sometimes manifest themselves in several members of the same family through several generations, being the result of inherited predisposition. In this class of cases the subjects are of a nervous, excitable, or irritable temperament, somewhat anæmic, and possibly suffered during infancy from nocturnal enuresis. Among the predisposing causes the most common is indulgence in erotic fancies, which terminates in increased reflex impressibility of the centres which preside over the genital organs.

The affection is, however, usually acquired, being met with particularly in single subjects toward the termination of the second decade and between the second and third decades. Of these cases, at least nine-tenths can be traced to masturbation, while the remainder will be found to have had gonorrhœa or to have masturbated, suffered from gonorrhœa, or indulged their sexual propensities in various ways. Seminal incontinence is not common as the result of sexual coition, and it is highly probable that when married men are affected the sexual excess is engrafted upon a previously vicious habit. From a practical point of view, it is of the first importance to be aware of the fact that one or more strictures of the urethra will be found in 80 per cent. of all cases, and that decided hyperæsthesia of the prostatic portion of the urethra is present in 94 per cent. of all instances.

The rational explanation of morbid seminal emissions seems to be as follows: Under the influence of erotic ideas, masturbation, sexual excesses, or unsatisfied sexual excitement produced by dallying with women, exaggerated irritability of the genital organs is induced, and is followed by subacute or chronic inflammation and abnormal sensibility of the urethra, particularly of its prostatic division, which terminate, in cases characterized by diurnal pollutions and spermorrhagia, in relaxation and dilatation of the orifices of the ejaculatory ducts. As the natural result of the constant excitability of the terminal filaments of the nerves distributed to the prostatic urethra, these nerves are alive to the slightest impressions, act as peripheral sources of irritation, and induce permanent increased mobility or irritability of the cerebral and spinal genital centres, through which the motor nerves of the ejaculatory apparatus are thrown into action, and an emission ensues.

Seminal incontinence is an occasional accompaniment of injuries of the spine, and it is also met with during the progress of or convalescence from acute and chronic diseases which are marked by disturbances or exhaustion of the central nervous system. Thus, it may be symptomatic of phthisis, variola, typhus, progressive muscular atrophy, and incipient bulbar paralysis, ataxia, and paraplegia; while the habitual use of opium and chronic alcoholism predispose to its occurrence.

Of the local causes referable to the genitalia, by far the most important and most frequent are hyperæsthesia and inflammation of the prostatic portion of the urethra, which are generally induced by masturbation. These lesions constitute the primary source of the trouble in the large majority of cases, and tend not only to excite reflex pollutions, but to maintain the disorder by keeping the mind occupied with sexual matters. Other common local causes are found in congenital narrowing of the meatus, organic stricture of the urethra, a redundant prepuce, balanitis, and the accumulation of smegma. Among the more infrequent etiological factors may be mentioned herpes of the prepuce, congenital shortness of the frenum, spasmodic stricture, polypus of the deep urethra, spermatocystitis, and epididymitis.

Among the remaining exciting causes of pollutions are diseases of the anus and rectum, as hemorrhoids, morbid growths, ascarides, fissures, ulcers, pruritus, and painful eruptions. The nerves of the rectum and anus being derived from the same region as those of the genitalia, it is not surprising that the ejaculatory centre should respond to an impulse transmitted from them. In habitual constipation straining at stool may also excite an emission through the consentaneous action of the muscles of the abdomen, rectum, and seminal vesicles; but this is only observed when the orifices of the ejaculatory ducts are paralyzed and patulous.

ANATOMICAL CHARACTERS.—There are no records of the morbid appearances which appertain to seminal incontinence in its early stage, but that the hyperæsthesia of the prostatic urethra depends upon chronic or subacute inflammation is rendered certain by the concomitant symptoms, by exploration with the sound, aided by the finger in the rectum, and by the results of treatment. In the advanced stage, post-mortem inspection has disclosed stricture of the urethra, injection of the mucous membrane of the deep portion of the urethra, dilatation and excoriation of the orifices of the ejaculatory ducts, and suppuration of the prostate and the seminal vesicles. The changes which occur in the nervous centres are unknown.

DIAGNOSIS.—The microscope affords the only positive mode of determining whether the fluid which is discharged from the urethra during pollutions, or constantly moistens that canal in spermorrhagia, or is expelled at stool or with the urine, or is brought away by the bulb of the explorer, is seminal in its character. Should spermatozoids be detected, there can be no doubt as to its true nature, but their absence is not an evidence that the case is not one of spermatic incontinence, since in the condition known as azoospermatorrhœa the exhausted sexual apparatus furnishes a thin, transparent, watery fluid which may be entirely devoid of fertilizing elements, and contains cylinder epithelial cells, epithelium which has undergone fatty or colloid degeneration, a few lymph-corpuscles, an abundance of fatty detritus, and a few small shining bodies which are the remains of the badly-evolved spermatozoids. Under these circumstances, the history of the case, the fact that the subject is or was a masturbator, and the associated nervous symptoms are aids in forming a diagnosis; and this is especially true of cases in which a fluid is expressed at stool, and which in the majority of instances is the altered secretion of the prostate. Under the microscope the thin, more or less milky prostatic fluid will be found to contain cylinder epithelium, numberless colorless and refracting granules of lecithin, and minute yellowish concentric amyloid concretions; and, after it has slowly dried upon the slide, crystals of phosphate of magnesium or of ammonio-magnesian phosphate will make their appearance.

Should a microscopical examination be impracticable, we may assume that the discharge which occurs during defecation in the subjects of too frequent nocturnal pollutions is an evidence of coexisting prostatorrhœa; while we may frame the rule that the flocculent sediment contained in the urine and the discharge at stool of persons suffering from both nocturnal and diurnal pollutions, and a slight continued discharge from the urethra represents semen. In the last event we may moreover assume, especially if the patient be impotent, that the orifices of the ejaculatory ducts are relaxed.

PROGNOSIS.—Nocturnal emissions are very amenable to treatment, particularly when they are kept up by appreciable local lesions, the only cases which are, as a rule, rebellious being those in which the pollutions are associated with chronic inflammation of the seminal vesicles. In expressing an opinion in a given case the physician should, however, be influenced by the severity of the signs of nervous exhaustion. If the general symptoms point to involvement of the cord alone, the prognosis is far better than when signs of cerebrasthenia are present; but the outlook is bad if, in addition to cerebral and spinal exhaustion, the patient is a sexual hypochondriac. Nocturnal pollutions occurring during the progress of acute or chronic general disorders are also, as a rule, readily checked. The prognosis in the same class of cases is, moreover, far better when the usual local lesion—namely, morbid sensibility of the prostatic urethra—has been induced by gonorrhœa rather than by masturbation; and it is also more favorable when the pollutions occur in mature years from sexual excesses than when they are due early in life to masturbation.

Even when the emissions occur during the day from trivial psychical or mechanical causes, ample experience has convinced me that the prognosis is far better than many writers would lead one to believe. These cases are, however, less tractable than those of nocturnal pollutions, but they finally recover with the exercise of a little patience. The worst outlook is when the emissions are passive, or occur without the orgasm, or during urination and defecation. In this class of cases not only are the ordinary remedies applicable to the other varieties demanded, but measures will have to be resorted to to overcome the paralyzed and dilated orifices of the ejaculatory ducts. Although the prognosis is not as favorable, I have never seen an example of spermorrhagia that did not finally yield to treatment.

TREATMENT.—Certain hygienic and moral rules must be observed in the management of all the varieties of seminal incontinence. The diet should be plain, nutritious, and digestible; the evening meal should be light and dry; and spirits and malt liquors, as well as stimulating articles of food, should be eschewed. As the morning fulness of the bladder is very liable to produce an erection, that organ should be thoroughly emptied on retiring; and as pollutions usually occur toward morning, the patient should set an alarm-clock one hour before the time at which he has generally observed that the emissions take place, in order that he may be awakened to relieve the bladder of its contents. He should also sleep upon a hair mattress without much covering. Everything calculated to induce a flow of blood to the genitalia, such as horseback exercise, driving over rough roads, and railway travelling, should be interdicted. Masturbation and sexual intercourse must be abandoned, and the subject should be informed that the enforced rest of the organs will possibly result in temporary increased frequency of the pollutions. Chaste associations should be cultivated, and erotic thoughts and desires be banished. To attain this end the mind and body should be kept pleasantly occupied by gymnastic exercises and the study of any subject which the patient may fancy. If, however, he be not in full health, or if there are commencing or marked signs of spinal or cerebral exhaustion, mental and physical exercise should be taken in moderation.

In the treatment of involuntary seminal emissions a thorough examination should be made of the genital and associated organs, with the view of detecting and getting rid of any reflex or eccentric lesions or causes which predispose to, or even excite and maintain, them in impressible subjects. If the patient has a redundant prepuce, it should be removed; if the meatus be contracted, it should be enlarged; while balanitis, herpes, hemorrhoids, rectal fissure or ulcer, or pruritus should be treated in the usual way. In not a few mild cases, particularly those dependent upon phimosis, a contracted meatus, or a stricture just behind the orifice, it will be found that operative interference is quite sufficient to bring about relief. Habitual constipation, which is met with in about one-third of all instances, demands particular attention, either by enemata of temperate water or a pill composed of one-tenth of a grain each of aloin and extract of belladonna, administered every eight hours.

In the section on the etiology and pathogeny of seminal incontinence attention is called to the fact that hyperæsthesia of the prostatic urethra is nearly always present. While it is undoubtedly true that the genital nervous centres may be highly impressible without the intervention of hyperæmia, inflammation, and abnormal sensibility of the prostatic urethra, it is none the less true that those lesions are the most constant and most important of all the causes which excite and maintain the disorder, especially in masturbators, in whom, moreover, strictures may be looked for in about eight-tenths of all cases. As a rule, the coarctations will be formed just behind the meatus, but others may be present posteriorly. Be this as it may, a knowledge of their existence is of the first importance, as they aggravate the morbid condition of the prostatic urethra and serve to keep up a peripheral source of spinal neurasthenia.

For the detection of a stricture the exploratory or acorn-headed soft bougie should be resorted to, as it is the only instrument with which coarctations of large calibre and granular patches can be accurately defined, and with which abnormal discharges can be withdrawn for minute examination. One being selected which fills the meatus, it is warmed and well oiled, and inserted as far as the bladder. Should its introduction be arrested, smaller sizes are successively employed until one will pass without difficulty. On its withdrawal the abrupt shoulder of the bulb coming in contact with the posterior face of the stricture imparts to the touch a sensation as if it had jumped over a band, while a granular patch conveys the impression of a limited roughness of the canal. Hyperæsthesia of the urethra is readily determined by the nickel-plated steel bougie, and its existence should never be based upon the passage of the soft explorer alone, as the latter is productive of far more pain than the former. In conducting these examinations a contracted meatus or a stricture just behind the orifice should first be divided, in order that the instruments for exploration may correspond to the normal calibre of the urethra. Unless this point receives attention the examination will be likely to prove valueless. Should one or more strictures be present, the case must be referred to a surgeon.

From the preceding considerations it follows that the treatment, whether it be local or general, must at the outset be of a calming and sedative nature, the end in view in the great majority of instances being to overcome the exaggerated irritability of the genital nervous centres and the abnormal sensibility of the deep urethra. By the indiscriminate employment of strychnia, cantharides, phosphorus, and cold ablutions great harm is done, and the management of involuntary seminal emissions is brought into disrepute.

Of the local remedies to overcome the hyperæsthesia of the prostatic urethra, there is not one entitled to so much confidence as the nickel-plated conical steel bougie, passed at intervals of four days, and at once withdrawn for the first few insertions, after which, with the decrease of the sensibility, the intervals should be shortened, and it should be retained longer, until it is inserted every forty-eight hours and permitted to remain in the canal for a few minutes. The size of the first instrument is to be gauged by that of the meatus if it be normal, and if it be found necessary during the course of the treatment the orifice should be enlarged, in order that bougies of progressively increasing sizes may be introduced until they correspond to the full calibre or distensibility of the urethra, as indicated by the urethrameter. Unless these precautions be observed the measure will not bring about the desired result.

As a rule, the bougie will meet the indication, but in exceptional instances a small, circumscribed area of tenderness remains, which comprises the sinus pocularis, and which proves rebellious to instrumentation. Under these circumstances it becomes necessary to apply a drop or two of a solution of nitrate of silver to the spot, which is best done with a small syringe attached to a perforated bulbous explorer. The ordinary forms of porte-caustique charged with the fused nitrate are objectionable, as the remedy does not come in contact with the orifices of the ejaculatory ducts contained within the sinus pocularis, and its application cannot be properly controlled. From an ample experience I can confidently recommend the use of a thirty-grain solution, repeated every four days. Provided the patient be kept in bed for a few hours, the pain and desire to urinate will not last more than thirty minutes. When the affection proves to be more than ordinarily obstinate, flying blisters, made by pencilling cantharidial collodion first on the one side of the perineal raphé, and, after the surface has healed, on the opposite side, will prove serviceable.

In addition to these measures great assistance will be derived on retiring from the hot sitz-bath, or from a sponge or cloth dipped in water at a temperature of at least 105° F. and applied to the perineum and lower part of the spine. Cold applications are to be studiously avoided.

Of the general remedies, not a single one is comparable to bromide of potassium, which not only diminishes the reflex excitability of the cord and suspends sexual desires and the power of erection, but corrects the acidity of the urine and exerts an anæsthetic effect upon the mucous membrane of the urethra. I am in the habit of administering from three to four scruples of the salt at bedtime, and if I find that it sets up signs of bromism I diminish it for a time, and afterward promote its excretion by the kidneys by combining with it about fifteen grains of bitartrate of potassium. Should the patient be anæmic, the dose should be reduced to one drachm, and three grains of quinine along with twenty-five drops of the tincture of the chloride of iron should be ordered every eight hours. When, on the other hand, the patient is robust and plethoric or in full health, I frequently add to the bromide ten drops of veratrum viride or tincture of gelsemium, or administer the bromide in half an ounce of the infusion of digitalis.

Another remedy which diminishes the reflex mobility of the genitospinal centre, at the same time that it reduces the secretion of the seminal fluid, is the sulphate of atropia. Given in the average dose of the one-sixtieth of a grain on retiring, so that the patient may sleep through its disagreeable action, it will be found to be an invaluable addition to the treatment.

When the bromide of potassium and atropia do not agree with the patient, I substitute the monobromide of camphor and extract of belladonna in the proportion of ten grains of the former to one-third of a grain of the latter. In the remaining anaphrodisiacs, such as lupulin, camphor, and conium, I have not the slightest confidence.

Under the plan of treatment thus outlined the majority of cases of nocturnal and diurnal pollutions recover ; but if the spinal genital centre still remains too impressible, galvanization with the anode to the lumbar region and the cathode to the perineum will prove highly serviceable. When the condition is one of spermorrhagia, after the hyperæsthetic symptoms have subsided the relaxed and paralyzed orifices of the ejaculatory ducts may be restored to their normal condition by the continuous current, the negative reophore being placed in the rectum and the positive on the perineum or the lumbar vertebræ. Should galvanization fail, the induced current may be passed through a negative catheter electrode in the prostatic urethra to the anode resting on the perineum or spine; but this mode of application requires great caution, and a feeble power should be employed at the commencement. For this reason the rectal is preferable to the urethral reophore. In the absence of electrical apparatus the tonicity of the muscles of the ejaculatory ducts may be greatly improved, and even restored, by the use of the cooling sound, by the application of a thirty-grain solution of nitrate of silver, and by cold sitz-baths. In these cases half a drachm of the fluid extract of ergot after each meal, or fifteen drops of a mixture composed of six drachms of the tincture of the chloride of iron and two drachms of the tincture of cantharides, will also prove valuable. The operations of castration and excision of portions of the vas deferens need only be mentioned to be condemned.

To sum up the results of my experience in the management of seminal incontinence, I may add that the steel bougie, bromide of potassium, and atropia are especially adapted to cases of nocturnal and diurnal pollutions, and that after the hyperæsthesia has been relieved electricity, ergot, and strychnia are the most reliable agents in spermorrhagia. The end having been accomplished, moderation in sexual intercourse should be enjoined if the patient is married; continence in thought and action should be observed if he remains single; and matrimony should be advised if his circumstances and inclination warrant it. Marriage should not, however, be encouraged if the emissions are not arrested, as I have met with several cases in which the patient was rendered miserable by this act, from the fact that he deemed his case beyond all hope, as the emissions still continued.

DISPLACEMENTS OF THE UTERUS.

By E. C. DUDLEY, A. B., M. D.

THE title of this article is not to be taken in a restricted sense, inasmuch as the uterus is anatomically so connected with adjacent organs that the displacements of the uterus cannot be intelligently considered or satisfactorily presented without at the same time incidentally taking into account the displacements, causative, resultant, or concurrent, of the ovaries, Fallopian tubes, rectum, vagina, and bladder.

Normal Location and Position of the Uterus.[1]

In the works on anatomy and gynecology which we are accustomed to consult the uterus is represented as having a straight or nearly straight canal—as lying about midway between the symphysis pubis and the hollow of the sacrum, its axis corresponding to that of the pelvic inlet. They generally agree that its position is one of slight, and only slight, anteversion; some admit that slight anteflexion may not be injurious, but most would pronounce the organ anteverted or anteflexed to a degree that would endanger health if by conjoined manipulations its anterior wall could be felt through the anterior wall of the vagina. The classical idea of the normal position of the uterus presupposes a distended bladder and rectum occupying the anterior and the posterior thirds of the pelvic cavity. Such an arrangement would leave for the uterus only the intermediate space, and would constitute a condition seldom or never realized in health.

Suppose a straight line coincident with the vesico-vaginal wall (Fig. 1) to be continued through the cervix to the sacrum. This line represents approximately the antero-posterior diameter of the pelvis. The length of the vesico-vaginal wall is two and a half inches, and, supposing the cervix to be just midway between the symphysis and the sacrum, the distance from its posterior wall to the sacrum must also be two and a half inches. Add to the sum of these two parts of this antero-posterior diameter one inch for the cervix, and the antero-posterior diameter of the pelvis becomes six inches instead of the normal four and one-third; which proves that the cervix must normally be much nearer to the hollow of

---

[1] The importance of a distinction between location and position will become apparent hereafter: by the former is meant the situation of the organ regardless of its attitude, by the latter is meant the attitude alone. To change an object from one place to another is to change its location; to turn it over or bend it upon itself is to change its position

the sacrum than to the symphysis. Since the length of the vesico-vaginal wall plus the diameter of the cervix measures three and one-half inches, it follows that the distance from the posterior wall of the cervix to the hollow of the sacrum must be the difference between four and one-third and three and one-half inches, or five-sixths of an inch.

Again, suppose the uterus (Fig. 1) to be carried bodily upward and backward, its axis remaining the same, until the cervix reach its normal

Fig. 1.

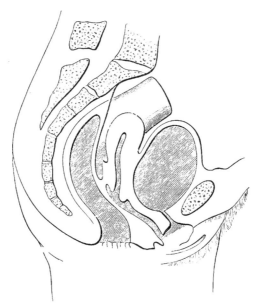

The Classical Representation of the Pelvic Organs.

position near the hollow of the sacrum; then would the body of the uterus impinge upon the bony sacrum. It is therefore clear that the anteversion must be the normal position, because the uterus and sacrum would otherwise occupy the same space.

Fig. 2 represents, according to Schultze,[1] the location and position of the virgin uterus and its surroundings, the bladder, rectum, and vagina being empty and collapsed. The angle of about 90° which the cervix forms with the vagina measures the forward inclination of the cervix, but is subject to slight variations in consequence of the physiological

[1] *Archiv für Gynäkologie*, 1875, Band viii. p. 134, and *Lageveranderungen der Gebarmutter*, Berlin, 1881.

Ely Van de Warker makes a full and critical study of the normal movements of the unimpregnated uterus in the *N. Y. Medical Journal*, xxi. p. 337, and of the normal position and movements of the unimpregnated uterus in the *American Journal of Obstetrics*, xi. p. 314. His conclusions substantially agree with those of Schultze.

Frank P. Foster (*American Journal of Obstetrics*, xiii. p. 30) presents a valuable paper giving a résumé of the literature, with original observations, in which he takes exceptions in part to the views of Schultze.

movements of the uterus. The body is furthermore bent forward upon the cervix, so that its anterior surface rests upon the empty bladder. The angle of the normal anteflexion, according to careful measurements by Schultze, is about 48°; Fritsch says that 90° is the physiological limit. This question will be further considered under the subject of pathological anteflexions.

Normal Movements of the Uterus.

Strictly, the uterus can have no absolutely normal position or location, because it has a certain normal range of movements which depend to some extent upon respiration, intra-abdominal forces, and locomotion, but more

FIG. 2.

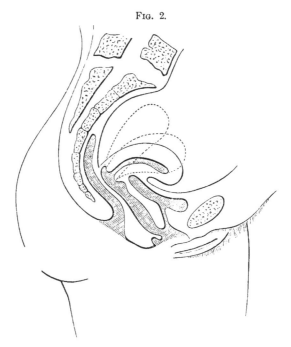

The Correct Representation of the Pelvic Organs.

especially upon the varying quantity of material in the rectum and bladder. Its normal position, then, varies within the limits of its normal movements. If the body of the uterus rest upon the bladder, it must rise as the bladder becomes distended, and, conversely, if the urine be drawn through a catheter while the woman is lying on her back, the uterus, notwithstanding the opposing influence of its own weight, immediately follows the receding wall of the bladder and returns through an angle of 45°, or possibly even 90°, to its accustomed position. The dotted lines in Fig. 2 indicate the degree of version and flexion consequent upon the varying quantity of fluid in the bladder.

The full rectum forces the uterus in the opposite direction, toward the symphysis, and thereby counteracts the influence of the bladder. This anterior movement is, however, somewhat limited, and is confined to the cervical portion, except when the body has been forced back into close proximity with the rectum by the over-distended bladder.

Normal Supports of the Uterus.

The uterus is maintained in its normal position and location by the following agents:

a. The uterine ligaments;
b. The pelvic floor.[1]

a. Physiologically, these ligaments are relaxed; the state of tension would be pathological; they do not fix the uterus; they only tend to limit its movements to their normal range. Backward displacement of the body is resisted by the round ligaments, backward displacement of the cervix by the utero-vesical ligaments and by the vesico-vaginal wall. Forward and downward displacements are resisted by the utero-sacral ligaments, and excessive lateral motion by the broad ligaments. This restraining power is doubtless greater in the utero-sacral than in any of the other ligaments.

b. The pelvic floor, which is the chief support of the uterus, is divided into two segments, the pubic and the sacral. The pubic segment[2] is composed of bladder, urethra, anterior vaginal wall, and bladder peritoneum. It is attached in front to the symphysis pubis and laterally to the anterior bony walls of the pelvis. The sacral segment[3] is composed of rectum, perineum, posterior vaginal wall, and strong tendinous and muscular tissue. It is attached to the coccyx, to the sacrum, and to the posterior wall of the bony pelvis.

Permeating the pelvic floor in all directions, entering into the composition of its single parts, binding them together, and sending its processes to the bony pelvis, is the pelvic connective tissue, upon the integrity of which depends the integrity of the pelvic floor as a uterine support. Its pernicious influence as a pathological factor will be considered hereafter. The old idea that the uterus is supported by the vaginal walls or by the perineum or by the uterine ligaments is obsolete; they are important parts of the pubic and sacral segments, and as such contribute their share, but the pelvic floor as a whole supports the uterus. The various uterine supports are to a great extent the seat of motor influence. They consequently not only resist excessive movement, but also serve to return the organ from its physiological migrations.

DEFINITION AND NOMENCLATURE OF DISPLACEMENTS.—In the foregoing pages the normal location, position, movements, and supports of the uterus have been defined. Those conditions are pathological which induce changes to positions or locations beyond the defined limits, or which so fix the organ that its normal movements are prevented. The displacements are divided into mal-locations and malpositions.

The mal-locations in which the entire uterus occupies a place outside

[1] For a description of the female pelvic floor see Hart's *Atlas.*
[2] Hart and Barbour's *Manual of Gynecology.*   [3] *Ibid.*

its normal limits are as follows : ascent, retro-location, ante-location, lateral location, descent.

The malpositions are determined by excessive change in the inclination of the uterine axis. They are further divided into flexions, in which the organ is bent upon itself in an abnormal degree, manner, or direction ; and versions, in which the axis of the unflexed uterus inclines in an abnormal degree or direction. The malpositions are retroversion, retroflexion, lateral version, lateral flexion, anteversion, anteflexion.

SYMPTOMS AND DIAGNOSIS IN GENERAL.—Each variety of displacement may be indicated by its own group of symptoms and physical signs. These will be presented in the study of the special lesions. To avoid repetition, those symptoms and signs which pertain to no special displacement, but which belong to all alike, will be mentioned at once. They may arise either from the displacement itself or from its possible complications, of which the following are examples : Metritis, ovaritis, salpingitis, atresia and stenosis, cystitis, vesical catarrh, rectitis, rectal catarrh, periuterine cellulitis and peritonitis, uterine catarrh, tumors, cicatrices, etc.

Uterine displacement may be a cause or an effect of associated complications, or together with them it may be a concurrent result of some common cause, or it may have had primarily no pathological connection with them. The symptoms of displacement refer to the pelvic organs or to the nervous system. Among the symptoms which refer to the pelvic organs are—difficulty in walking and standing; pelvic pain, more or less constant; dysmenorrhœa, menorrhagia, sterility, frequent abortion, constipation, painful or difficult defecation, dysuria, polyuria, tenesmus, etc. Among the symptoms which refer to the nervous system are—neuralgia in various parts, paralysis, hysteria, nervous dyspepsia, anæmia, chlorosis, spinal irritation, etc.

The final diagnosis must always depend upon direct examination of the uterus itself. The first division of the above group of symptoms is not likely to escape notice as indicative of displacement, but the nervous symptoms are constantly disregarded or treated without reference to their possible pelvic origin. The frequent dependence of these nervous phenomena upon displacement is proved by their persistence in many cases after ordinary treatment, by their prompt disappearance upon permanent replacement and retention of the uterus by mechanical means, and by their equally prompt recurrence upon removal of the support. The presence, therefore, of the second division of the group or any part thereof, even though the first be absent, will justify, may even necessitate, a careful investigation into the state of the pelvic organs.

That examination which results only in giving the name to a special variety of displacement, and does not include the complicating lesions, would not furnish a sufficient guide to the therapeutic indications, and is therefore inadequate. The successful treatment, for instance, of an anteflexion dependent upon inflammation of the utero-sacral ligaments must include the removal of the inflammation.

An important prerequisite to examination is the absence of material in the rectum and bladder. The full rectum distorts the vaginal walls, deprives the examiner of the space necessary for the introduction of the speculum, and throws the uterus out of its accustomed position. Much more troublesome is the presence of even a small quantity of urine in the bladder, because it causes the patient to render the abdominal muscles tense when the hand is placed over the lower portion of the abdomen for bimanual palpation, and makes it impossible to engage the uterus between the hand and the examining finger. The distended bladder by pushing the uterus upward and backward makes bimanual palpation almost use-less. It is not surprising that conflicting opinions are common, when one day the patient is examined with rectum and bladder full, another day empty; one day in the dorsal, another in Sims's or the knee-chest posi-tion; one day with the cylindrical or bivalve speculum, another day with Sims's or Simon's.

For digital examination the dorsal position is preferred : the patient should be drawn close to the edge of a bed, or preferably a table, the thighs being flexed, the feet about fifteen inches apart, and the knees widely separated. The examiner should stand facing the patient, never at the side. The index finger of the left[1] hand, lubricated with vaseline or oil, then slowly advances over the perineum into the vagina, noting the condition of the perineum, the presence or absence of cicatrices or of sub-involution of the vagina or perineum, the capacity of the vagina, the con-dition, size, and direction of the cervix, its distance from the sacrum and vulva, its mobility or fixation. Now, for the first time, the right hand is pressed well down behind the pubes, and the uterus is engaged between it and the examining finger. (See Figs. 16 and 17.) In this way the examiner may determine more accurately the position, location, and size of the entire organ ; may detect the possible presence of complicating tumors, both inflammatory and non-inflammatory ; may also note, if possible, the location and condition of the ovaries, which, especially in the posterior displacements, are liable to be prolapsed and excessively sensitive, and to constitute, therefore, a most intractable complication. The index finger sweeps around the cervix in search of tender places which may be the result of former cellulitis or the expression of some neurosis. Above all, the digital examination requires a light, gentle, delicate touch.

In exploring the uterine cavity to learn its position the fine silver-wire probe of Emmet—not the sound—should be used. The uterus, if freely movable, is liable to be thrown out of its accustomed position by the heavier, unyielding sound. The sound also causes much more pain and exposes the patient to great danger of cellulitis. The frequent lighting and relighting of pelvic inflammation by injudicious slight manipulations of the uterus doubtless led Emmet to the utterance of a prophecy which ought to become classical : "A great advance in the treatment of the diseases of women will be made whenever practitioners become so im-pressed with the significance of cellulitis as to apprehend its existence in every case. The successful operator in this branch of surgery will always be on the lookout for the existence of cellulitis, and take measures to guard against its occurrence."

When the probe or the sound is used without the speculum, the patient

---

[1] The left-hand method of examination is incomparably superior to the right. The palmar surface of the index finger is more easily directed toward the left side of the pelvis, which is especially subject to disease. Its tactile sense is more acute and more easily educated. The stronger right hand should be free to palpate the surface of the abdomen in conjoined manipulation.

should be on the back and the index finger of the left hand should be used as a guide. The bivalve and cylindrical specula are almost useless in explorations of the interior of the uterus. The exploration is most effectually and gently made with Sims's speculum, the patient being in the left latero-prone position. In some cases the probe cannot be passed by any other method.

Ascent of the Uterus.

This mal-location may result from traction above or from pressure below. The organ may be drawn upward and backward by shortening of the utero-sacral ligaments, which results from inflammation and which usually induces a troublesome form of anteflexion. The enlarged pregnant uterus sometimes becomes attached by adhesive inflammation to a portion of the peritoneum in one of the higher zones of the pelvis or in the abdomen, and the organ may consequently remain fixed in its elevated position after involution. A tumor connected with the uterus or its appendages which has grown too large to be retained in the pelvis may, upon rising into the abdomen, drag the uterus with it. Pressure below may come from excessive distension of the rectum or bladder, or from a large accumulation of menstrual fluid in the vagina, or from a tumor originating in any portion of the pelvis below the level of the uterus. In diagnosis, prognosis, and treatment this displacement is wholly subordinate to the more significant lesions of which it is only the incidental result.

Retro-location of the Uterus.

The uterus may be forced back into a post-normal location by the presence of a tumor in front or by the distended bladder, or it may be drawn back and fixed by peritoneal adhesions. Retro-location is liable to induce vesical irritation by putting the vesico-vaginal wall on the stretch and thereby dragging on the neck of the bladder. This intractable symptom is sometimes relieved by Emmet's buttonhole operation of urethrotomy, for an account of which see section on Anteflexion. This operation would obviously be applicable also for the relief of the same symptom when caused by ascent of the uterus.

Ante-location of the Uterus.

The causes of this displacement are similar to those which produce retro-location; they are—distension of the rectum, post-uterine hæmatocele, post-uterine tumors, and peritoneal adhesions. Ante-location often causes vesical irritation, consequent upon the invasion by the uterus of that space which belongs to the bladder.

Lateral Locations of the Uterus.

The entire uterus is often displaced to the right or the left by a tumor or by an inflammatory exudate. The latter occurs as a product of cellulitis, usually in the left broad ligament, and crowds the organ toward the opposite side of the pelvis. After resolution the ligament, shortened by inflammatory contraction, draws the uterus to the affected side and fixes it there. Lateral displacement from this cause often accompanies laceration of the cervix, the cellulitis having occurred on the side corresponding to the laceration.

Descent or Prolapse of the Uterus.

The nature of this displacement is clearly indicated by its name. It is convenient to distinguish three degrees of descent: In the first the organ is displaced downward and forward until sufficient space has been gained between the cervix and the sacrum to permit the body to turn back into extreme retroversion; in the second the cervix descends to the vulva; in the third the uterus protrudes partially or wholly through the vulva, constituting a condition sometimes called procidentia.

ETIOLOGY AND CLINICAL HISTORY.—Descent may be the result of any or all of the following causes: I. Pressure from above; II. Weakening of the supports; III. Increased weight of the uterus; IV. Traction from below. Either of the above conditions being the primary cause, the others singly or combined may result.

I. Pressure from above may depend upon the presence of a pelvic or abdominal tumor, ascites, fecal accumulations, tight or heavy clothing, etc.

II. The uterine supports may be weakened and relaxed in consequence of subinvolution, senile atrophy, abnormally large pelvis, increased weight of the uterus, pressure from above, traction from below, etc.

III. Increased weight of the uterus may be caused by congestion, subinvolution, hypertrophy, hyperplasia, pregnancy, fluid in the endometrium, uterine tumors, etc.

IV. Traction from below may be due to vaginal cicatrices, abnormally short vagina, falling of the pelvic floor, etc.

Obviously, descent of the vesico- and recto-vaginal walls, or, more comprehensively, the sacral and pubic segments of the pelvic floor, involves also concurrent descent of the uterus. Descent of the vagina, therefore, must be studied in connection with the descent of the uterus. Excessive descent of the vaginal walls usually originates with parturition.

In labor the anterior wall of the vagina is so depressed, stretched, and shortened by the advancing head that during and after the second stage the anterior lip of the cervix may be seen behind the urethra. If the puerperium progress favorably, with prompt involution of the uterus, vagina, perineum, and peritoneum, the relaxation of the vesico-vaginal wall and of the utero-sacral supports disappears and the uterus resumes its normal multiparous location and position.[1] But if the enlarged uterus remain in the long axis of the vagina, with its fundus incarcerated in the hollow of the sacrum between the utero-sacral ligaments, and with its sacral supports so stretched that they cannot recover their contractile power, and with involution of all the pelvic organs arrested, the descent

[1] The anteflexion of the multiparous uterus is less than that of the virgin.

may not only persist, but may even progress with constantly increasing cystocele to the third degree of prolapse. The downward influence of the above conditions may be materially increased by rupture of the perineum, and consequent prolapse of the recto-vaginal wall into a pouch called rectocele.

In the great majority of cases of complete prolapse the posterior vaginal wall in its descent is peeled off from the rectum, leaving the

Fig. 3.

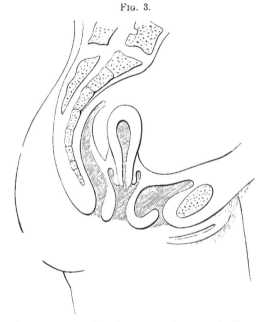

First Degree of Prolapse of the Post-partum Uterus. The posterior vaginal wall has been changed from its normal forward direction to a vertical direction by perineal rupture and anterior displacement of the cervix; the vesico-vaginal wall descends in cystocele, becomes hypertrophied, and drags the heavy uterus after it. The descending uterus carries with it a reduplication of the vaginal walls.

latter in its normal position. In rare instances the lower portion of the rectum is also found to have extruded in extreme rectocele, making a pouch below and in front of the anus, where fecal matter may accumulate and remain in hard scybalæ.

Obviously, complete prolapse of the uterus is only an incident to the prolapse of the pelvic floor. The whole mechanism is in all respects analogous to that of hernia. The extruded mass drags after it a peritoneal sac, which, hernia-like, contains small intestine. This sac forces its way to the pelvic outlet and extrudes through the vulva, having the inverted vagina for its covering.

In descent of the first degree the location of the uterus is either changed to a lower level, the position remaining normal, or, as is more common, the cervix having moved nearer to the symphysis and the organ turns back into retroversion. In a given case suppose the vaginal walls from some cause to have become relaxed and to have settled to a lower level in the pelvis.   As an associated fact the uterus to which these walls are attached must then also occupy a place correspondingly nearer to the vulva—*i. e.* the location of the uterus has changed, so that space enough intervenes between it and the hollow of the sacrum for the former to turn back into the position of retroversion or retroflexion. If, on the contrary, the descending uterus still maintains its normal ante-version and anteflexion, it must occupy space which belongs to the blad-der.   The vesical irritation consequent upon this mal-location has gen-erally been ascribed to the anteversion and anteflexion, which are therefore oftentimes wrongly pronounced pathological.   The prompt relief which follows permanent replacement of the organ in the normal location, even though in so doing its anteposition be exaggerated, proves that the symp-toms depend upon the mal-location, not upon the anteposition.   The im-portance of a clear distinction, therefore, between location and position becomes apparent.   Vesical irritation, moreover, is sometimes caused by the dragging of the uterus upon the neck of the bladder.   This traction occurs not only in ascent, but also when the organ descends below a certain level.

In the foregoing paragraphs traction due to the falling pelvic floor has been discussed as a cause of descent.   The impairment of the uterine supports may, however, be such that instead of falling and dragging the

FIG. 4.

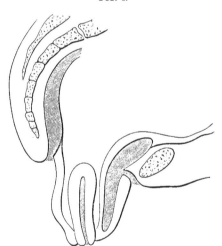

Showing Extreme Descent of the Uterus and of the Pelvic Floor, and the Hernial Character of the Lesion.

uterus after them, they simply permit it to descend along the vaginal canal by the force of its own weight, and to carry with it the reduplicated vaginal walls.   This influence is generally enforced by the increased weight of the diseased organ.   The vagina more readily becomes a track for the descending uterus when from any cause the normal forward direc-tion of the vaginal canal changes toward the vertical: this change may occur either as the result of a forward displacement of its upper extremity, involving anteposition of the cervix, or of a retro-displacement of its lower extremity in consequence of rupture or subinvolution of the perineum. (See Fig. 3.) Descent in the track of the vagina is obviously combined with some degree of retroversion, because the axes of the uterus and vagina then correspond.

The PATHOLOGICAL ANATOMY may involve all the displaced organs. The circulation throughout the pelvis is impeded by traction upon the vessels, and the entire pelvic contents therefore become the subject of venous congestion, with consequences disastrous to local innervation and nutrition.

The ovaries may suffer concurrent displacement, with resulting inflammatory and cystic enlargement. The peritoneum which enters into the formation of the uterine ligaments and of the pelvic floor is dragged along with the uterus.

The vagina is hypertrophied and swollen. Its mucous membrane becomes the seat of acute vaginitis and chronic catarrh. In the third degree of descent the exposed vagina, no longer lubricated by the normal secretions of the uterus, becomes dry, parchment-like, œdematous, eroded, and ulcerated. Sometimes the cul-de-sac of Douglas is distended by downward pressure of the intestines, by a small tumor, or by ascitic fluid, and a consequent hernial sac may protrude into the vagina through some portion of the posterior vaginal fornix. The anterior fornix is subject to a similar accident. These conditions are designated enterocele vaginalis, anterior and posterior.

The rectum and bladder are subject to inflammation and chronic catarrh, and the bladder especially to concurrent descent. The uterus may be enlarged from any one or all of a variety of causes—congestion, subinvolution, hypertrophy, and hyperplasia. Its cervix is often the seat of extreme erosion or so-called ulceration. The endometrium, in order to relieve the organ of its surplus blood, gives forth an excessive secretion of mucus, which upon being increased in quantity becomes vitiated in quality. This is termed uterine catarrh. The enlargement of the uterus often pertains more to the cervix than to the body, especially in prolapse of the second and third degrees. An explanation of this may be found in Figs. 5 and 6.

Apparent elongation and disproportionate circular enlargement of the cervix are conditions which almost every standard author wrongly calls hypertrophic elongation and circular hypertrophy. The question of elongation is easily settled by placing the patient in the knee-chest position. Then the uterus by its own weight falls toward the diaphragm, the vagina unfolds, and the apparent uterovaginal attachment $X'Z'$ (Figs. 5 and 6) disappears, disclosing the actual attachment, XZ. Further, the point of the sound, passed into the bladder while the

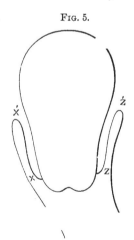

FIG. 5.

Descent of the Virgin Uterus into the Vaginal Canal, showing the Reduplicated Vaginal Walls. The utero-vaginal attachment, points X and Z, appears to be at X' and Z'. The apparent increase of length in the vaginal portion of the cervix due to the reduplication is measured by the distance from X and Z to X' and Z'.

cervix is exposed by Sims's speculum, may be placed against the anterior wall of the cervix at Z, which would be impossible if the attachment were at Z'.

The comparatively small amount of hypertrophy in disproportionate circular enlargement is proved by the operation of trachelorraphy or by bringing the points a and b (Fig. 6) together with uterine tenacula, the organ being exposed by Sims's speculum. Then the out-rolled intracervical mucous tissues are rolled back, the proper diameter of the cervix is restored, and a laceration on one or both sides, extending past the vaginal attachment, becomes apparent.

FIG. 6.

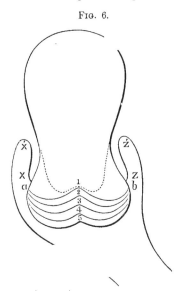

Descent of the Uterus, showing Excessive Circular Enlargement of the Lacerated Cervix, consequent upon Reduplication of the Vaginal Walls and Out-rolling of Intracervical Tissues. The divided fragments of the os externum are at a and b. The curved lines forming the angles 1, 2, 3, 4, and 5 indicate the gradual process of the eversion. The angle of the laceration at point 1 has been forced down by the swelling and out-rolling of the mucous and submucous tissues of the cervix to point 5. The apparent os externum is at point 5. The utero-vaginal attachment X and Z seems to be at X' and Z'. The vaginal portion of the cervix therefore appears much larger and longer than it actually is.

Hypertrophy or hyperplasia usually causes a nearly symmetrical enlargement of the entire organ. At any rate, those cases in which the reduplication of the vaginal walls does not almost entirely explain the great elongation so called, or in which great disproportionate circular enlargement has not been caused by laceration of the cervix, are the rare exceptions. The great merit of having secured general assent to the foregoing proposition, and of having given to the subject a new and right direction, must be accorded to Emmet. The cervix now is seldom amputated except for malignant disease.

Congestion of the uterus consequent upon obstruction in the stretched and displaced veins is often so extreme as to induce a state analogous to erection. Measurements by the probe just before and a few minutes after replacement generally show an appreciable decrease in the length of the uterine canal. If the prolapse has been of the third degree, the difference may amount to one or even two inches. It is important not to confound the enlargement of congestion with increase in the solid constituents of the organ.

SYMPTOMS AND COURSE.—A dragging sensation and pelvic and abdominal pain are generally present. Rectocele and cystocele and rectal and vesical catarrh often cause painful and severe functional disturbances of the rectum and bladder. In descent of the third degree excoriations of the exposed vagina and cervix sometimes cause extreme suffering. The course is ordinarily chronic, but attacks of acute vaginitis and pelvic peritonitis are not uncommon. The peritonitis sometimes effects a spontaneous cure by peritoneal adhesions which fasten the uterus in an elevated position and hold it permanently. The symptoms of descent may be so severe as to necessitate absolute rest in bed. In other cases they are often attended with very little discomfort.

DIAGNOSIS is by inspection, palpation, and exploration. The prolapsed uterus may be distinguished from cystocele, rectocele, inverted uterus, and fibroid tumor by the presence of the os externum. The sound may be passed through the urethra into the cystocele, and the finger through the anus into the rectocele. The length of the uterus may be determined by the sound, the size, shape, position, extent of descent, and difficulty of replacement by conjoined manipulation.

PROPHYLAXIS.—This requires such measures during labor as may be necessary to prevent long and powerful pressure upon the pelvic floor. After labor any injury to the perineum should be promptly repaired. The vagina should be kept clean by irrigations. The urine, if necessary, should be regularly drawn and the bowels moved daily without straining. If conditions be present likely to induce subinvolution—such, for example, as pelvic inflammation or laceration of the cervix—they should receive treatment at the proper time. Undue relaxation of the pelvic floor necessitates a more prolonged rest in bed, the use of astringent douches, and the application of a pessary when the patient resumes the upright position.

TREATMENT.—The first indication is replacement, which in the first and second degree of descent is not difficult unless the uterus be held down by cicatrices or by a tumor. Complicating pelvic cellulitis and peritonitis may render replacement dangerous or impossible, and may for a time contraindicate all direct treatment. Replacement of the organs from the third degree of prolapse is accomplished in the inverse order of their descent: first, the posterior vaginal wall, then the uterus, and last the anterior vaginal wall. Not infrequently the completely prolapsed uterus and pelvic floor, hernia-like, become strangulated. Then taxis will usually suffice if supplemented by hot applications, elastic pressure, anodynes, and the knee-chest position. Should these fail anæsthesia may be required.

Undue pressure from above should if possible be removed. The clothing should be loose, and the weight of the skirts supported from the shoulders either by straps or preferably by buttoning them upon a waist made for the purpose. This waist is a good substitute for the corset, which under all circumstances and in all its forms is injurious. Increased uterine weight from subinvolution or congestion is to be overcome by appropriate means. Enlargement of the uterus when due to hypertrophy or hyperplasia is generally incurable. Amputation of the cervix for what was formerly considered circular hypertrophy and hypertrophic elongation is now seldom or never required for the purpose of decreasing uterine weight. Amputation except for malignant disease has given place to the operation of trachelorrhaphy. Tumors exerting pressure above or traction below should if possible be removed. Regulation of the bowels and general tonics are usually necessary. The knee-chest position assumed several times a day causes the uterus to gravitate toward the diaphragm, and thereby gives temporary rest to the overburdened supports. While in this position the patient should separate the labia, so that the air may rush in and the vagina become expanded. The measures enumerated above, together with rigid care of the diet and of such other hygienic requirements as the individual case may demand, are essential as adjuvants to the more special treatment which almost every case requires.

In exceptional cases of sudden descent, even to the third degree, replacement alone is sometimes followed by permanent relief; but if the descent has been gradual it always recurs immediately after replacement. Measures are therefore required for the maintenance of the uterus in its normal location and position. This indication is fulfilled by pessaries and by operations.

Pessaries.—The function of the pessary is not only to maintain the uterus on the health level in its normal location, but also, if possible, in its normal position, which requires the cervix to be about one inch from the sacrum. The cervix being thus placed, the organ cannot turn back into retroversion, because in so doing the fundus would encounter the sacrum. The direction of least resistance would then be forward into the normal anterior position. The application of the pessary is then based upon the general proposition that if the cervix be normally placed the body of the uterus will in the absence of complications take care of itself. Since the vagina at its upper extremity is attached to the cervix, displacement of the latter is clearly impossible if the upper extremity of the vagina be sustained in its normal location. The pessary restores and maintains the relations of the relaxed vaginal walls by crowding the posterior vaginal cul-de-sac backward into the hollow of the sacrum. It thereby also holds the attached cervix within a proper distance of the sacrum. The Hodge pessary or some modifications thereof fulfils this purpose in ordinary cases more satisfactorily than any other.

The curves of the pessary demand careful attention in its application. When the uterus is below the normal level, the broad ligaments are necessarily rendered more tense than natural, and the blood-vessels, more especially the veins, which are looped one upon the other, and which traverse these ligaments to and from the uterus, are made to collapse. This causes venous congestion and consequent increase in weight of the uterus—a condition favorable to malposition, uterine catarrh, and pathological changes in structure. A pessary which will raise the uterus to the health level clearly fulfils an indication. A pessary which raises it above the health level renders the broad ligaments tense and reproduces a condition which it was designed to relieve. Maintenance of the uterus upon the health level depends largely upon the curves of the pessary.

FIG. 7.

FIG. 8.

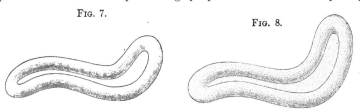

The Emmet Curves.　　　　　The Albert Smith Curves.

The accompanying cuts illustrate the shape and curve of the Hodge pessary as modified by Emmet and Albert Smith. Fig. 7 represents the curve of Emmet, and Fig. 8 that of Albert Smith. For convenience let us characterize that curve which rests in the posterior vaginal cul-de-sac as the uterine curve, and that which occupies that part of the vagina adjacent to the pubis the pubic curve. The acuteness and length of the uterine curve determine the height to which the pessary will lift the uterus. The longer and more acute the curve, the higher the uterus will be lifted, and vice versâ. The smaller curve of the Emmet modification will answer the average indication more nearly than the sharper curve of the Albert Smith modification, which may lift the uterus too high. The pubic should generally be proportioned to the uterine curve; that is, the greater the uterine, the greater the pubic curve. A pessary properly adjusted in all other respects may, by pressure upon the urethra and neck of the bladder, create vesical tenesmus and urethral irritation. This calls for increase in the pubic curve. The pubic curve may, however, be so great that the lower part of the pessary occupies the centre of the vulva, where it may create irritation. For this condition lessening of the pubic curve is the remedy. The pessary should not be so wide as to distend the vagina. Its length should be measured by the distance from the lower extremity of the symphysis pubis to the posterior vaginal cul-de-sac, less the thickness of the finger. If properly adjusted it should sustain the pelvic floor in its normal relations and the uterus in stable equilibrium.

The uterus in the first and second degrees of descent is usually either retroverted or retroflexed. The reader is therefore referred to the remarks on the application of pessaries in the treatment of these displacements.

In advance prolapse dependent upon extensive injuries to the perineum and other parts of the pelvic floor, and usually associated with extreme subinvolution of all the pelvic organs, the axis of the vagina is often changed from its forward oblique to the vertical direction. (See Fig. 3.) The downward traction of the prolapsing cystocele and rectocele upon the fornix of the vagina may then be so great that the pessary is inadequate to maintain in place the upper extremity of the vagina. The cervix then moves forward, the corpus turns back, and the whole uterus easily descends in a vertical direction along the prolapsing walls of the vagina to the second or third degree of prolapse. In this condition pessaries which disappear within the vagina are liable to be forced out with the prolapsing pelvic floor, or if retained seldom maintain the uterus in position. In such cases the various cup pessaries which are supplied with external attachments and abdominal belts are often used, but they are inadequate, because they either so fix the uterus as to prevent its normal movements, or they hold it in such unstable equilibrium that it may assume any one of the various malpositions, anterior, posterior, or lateral; and they are open to the further serious objection of constantly reminding the patient of their presence. As an expedient the uterus may sometimes be held within the pelvis by means of a large Albert Smith pessary with extreme uterine and pubic curves. The rational treatment, however, requires first an operation on the anterior vaginal wall to restore the fornix of the vagina to its normal place in the hollow of the sacrum, and with it the attached cervix; and second, an operation at the vaginal outlet to bring the posterior wall in contact with the anterior, and thereby to restore the lower extremity of the vagina to its normal place under the pubis.

ANTERIOR ELYTRORRHAPHY.—Numerous operations on the vaginal

walls have been devised for the purpose of narrowing the vagina, and thus preventing descent along the vaginal canal, but they are temporary in their results, because, as long as the direction of the vagina remains vertical, its walls again become dilated by the prolapsing uterus and the former condition is re-established. The operation to be effective is performed as follows: A Sims's speculum of long blade, perforated at its extreme end, to which the cervix has been attached by a piece of silver wire, passing through the perforation and the posterior lip, is introduced, the patient being in Sims's position. The cervix is thereby drawn by the point of the speculum far back into the hollow of the sacrum. The author finds this preferable to the method described by Emmet, who has the cervix held back by a sponge probang in the hand of an assistant. The space in the anterior part of the pelvis is now so increased that the uterus readily falls forward into decided anteversion. While the uterus is thus held in position by its attachment to the blade of the speculum, the operator with two uterine tenacula finds in the loose vaginal tissue on either side of the cervix two points which can be brought together in front of the cervix. Then at each of the two lateral points a surface is denuded with the curved scissors about one-half

FIG. 10.

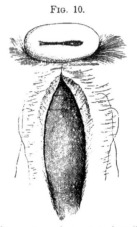

FIG. 9.

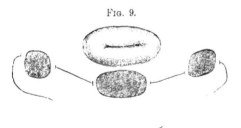

The First Suture before Twisting in Emmet's Operation for Procidentia (Emmet).   Folds on the Anterior Vaginal Wall formed after Twisting the First Suture (Emmet).

inch square, and in front of the cervix a surface an inch long by half an inch wide across the anterior vaginal wall close to the uterine attachment. A No. 26 silver-wire suture is then passed, as shown in Fig. 9, and twisted as shown in Fig. 10, so as to secure the lateral denuded surfaces in contact with the larger surface in front of the cervix.

Inasmuch as the operation often fails at the point of the first suture, the author has usually introduced two or three of this kind instead of one. Two longitudinal folds are now formed on the anterior vaginal wall, which serve as guides for denuding and turning in the remaining redundant tissue by a line of sutures, which should extend forward along the centre of the vesico-vaginal wall until the folds are lost in the vaginal surface near the neck of the bladder. Sometimes the redundant tissue about the urethra cannot be disposed of by turning it in from side to side. Then it is desirable to make a crescentic denudation across the lower portion of the vagina, its concavity being on the uterine side, and to unite the margins below to those above by means of a curved line of sutures. The completed operation is shown in Fig. 11.

The after-treatment requires the self-retaining Sims's sigmoid catheter in the urethra for a week or frequent catheterization, absolute rest in bed, hot-water vaginal douches, regulation of the bowels, and the removal of

Fig. 11.

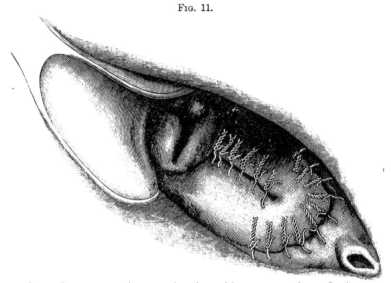

Emmet's Operation for Procidentia and Urethrocele completed. Sims's Speculum, Left Latero-prone Position (Emmet).

the sutures on the twelfth day. After the completion of the operation the cervix is maintained near the hollow of the sacrum, and the organ remains normally anteverted and anteflexed, making an acute angle with the vesico-vaginal wall, which has now been restored to its normal direction and length. Unfortunately, it is not unusual to abandon the patient after this operation, in the vain hope that the uterus and anterior vaginal wall will maintain their normal relations without the support of the perineum and posterior vaginal wall. This is a great mistake, because the cystocele and procidentia almost always completely reappear within a few months. Anterior elytrorrhaphy, therefore, is simply one of the steps in the treatment.

PERINEORRHAPHY.—This is the name usually applied to the repair of the ruptured perineum, but the scope of the operation has been extended to include also the surgical treatment of rectocele and relaxation of the posterior vaginal wall. The most scientific operation yet devised is the one proposed by Emmet,[1] which is performed as follows: The patient being etherized and in the lithotomy position, the operator seizes with a tenaculum the crest of the rectocele or posterior vaginal wall at a point which can be drawn forward without undue traction—point *a*. With another tenaculum the lowest caruncle or vestige of the hymen (point *b*),

[1] *Trans. Am. Gynæcological Society*, 1883; *Principles and Practice of Gynecology*, 3d ed.

and with another the posterior commissure of the vulva (point c), are
hooked up. The triangle included between these points defines one-half
of the surface to be denuded. The three tenacula are now placed in the
hands of assistants, the sides of the triangle are made tense by traction,
and the included surface denuded. The tenaculum at *c* is then removed,
and the middle point of the line *a b* is caught and drawn toward the
interior of the vagina in the direction of the vaginal sulcus on that side,
and the sutures are introduced, as in Fig. 13. The same thing is then
repeated on the other side, and the sutures are all tightened, forming a
line of union running back into each sulcus, as shown in Fig. 14.

The essential part of the operation inside the vagina almost always
succeeds, but the external part of the rupture at the posterior commissure

FIG. 12.

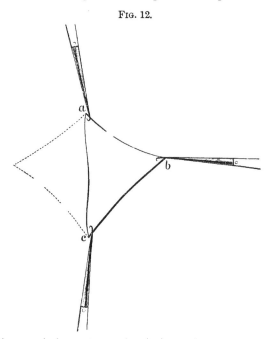

a is at the crest of the rectocele; *b* at the caruncle just within the labium; and *c* at the posterior commissure. The cut represents that half of the surface to be denuded which is on the operator's right.
The dotted lines represent the other half, on the left.

often fails to unite; furthermore, the operation as described by Emmet does
not overcome the patulous condition of the introitus vaginæ in case of great
relaxation of the vagina. The author has sought to obviate the first of
these difficulties by the use of deep silver sutures instead of the superficial
ones described by Emmet. They should be introduced before tightening
the vaginal sutures, and should be passed far around in the posterior
vaginal wall, their points of entrance and exit being the same as for the
three lower unsecured superficial external sutures in Fig. 14. The second
difficulty may be overcome by further denuding a triangular surface
in the vaginal sulcus on each side, the base of the triangle corresponding

to the line *a b*, Fig. 12, and its apex being in the vaginal sulcus at a distance corresponding to the degree of relaxation. This increases the length of the lines of union running into the sulci represented by *d b* and *e f*, Fig. 14. In the vaginal portion of the wound silk or catgut is preferable to silver, the latter being difficult to remove.

Fig. 13.   Fig. 14.

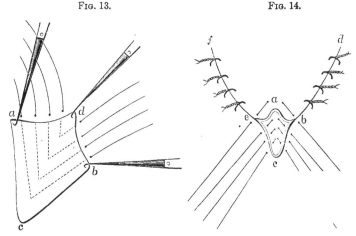

Fig. 13. The Sutures in Place. When secured they will unite *a d* with *b d*, and lift the perineum up in contact with the anterior vaginal wall.

Fig. 14 All the Vaginal Sutures Twisted. One suture, including the crest of the rectocele and the labium majus on either side, and three superficial external sutures, are yet to be secured   The lines *a d* and *d b*, Fig 13, have been brought into coincidence by means of the sutures, and now form the line of union *d b*. The tissues between the lines *a c* and *c b*, Fig. 13, have been so lifted up and are so held under the line of union *d b* that the line *c b*, Fig. 13, has been reduced to *c b*, Fig. 14, which makes the external portion of the wound insignificant in extent.

Emmet is entitled to great credit for having given to the profession an operation which brings the posterior vaginal walls up against the anterior more perfectly than any other, and which, being mostly inside of the vagina, is therefore followed by very little of the pain during convalescence which formerly rendered perineorrhaphy one of the most trying operations in gynecology. The operation furthermore has demonstrated the former teachings relative to the direction of perineal rupture[1] and the tissues involved to be incorrect, or at least inadequate.

Retroversion.

Retroversion is that position of the uterus in which the fundus is posterior to the axis of the pelvic inlet. If the cervix be in its normal place near the sacrum, retroversion is scarcely possible, because it is prevented by the proximity of the over-arching sacrum. (See Fig. 2.) The first degree of prolapse must therefore precede any considerable backward turning of the uterus. When the cervix has been displaced downward

[1] At the meeting of the American Medical Association in June, 1883, the author presented a paper describing the transverse laceration of the perineum and its operative treatment, which was published with illustrations in the transactions by the journal of the Association, Dec. 22, 1883. This communication referred only to the recent rupture and the immediate operation.

and forward so far that its distance from the sacrum is equal to or greater than the length of the uterus, retroversion to any extent becomes possible. (See Figs. 3 and 16.)

ETIOLOGY AND HISTORY.—From the above it follows that the causes of commencing retroversion must be identical with the causes of the first degree of prolapse. After the puerperium the relaxation of the supports and the weight of the organ may persist, and spontaneous replacement may be prevented by the pressure and weight of the intestines upon the anterior surface. Every act of defecation forces the cervix forward and downward, and the uterus, being in the axis of the vagina, and having therefore little support below, must depend upon the subinvoluted peritoneal suspensory ligaments and pelvic fascia, which are inadequate. This condition is very often induced by abortions, with resulting increased weight and relaxation of the vaginal walls. Local peritonitis and cellulitis may permanently fix the corpus in its retroverted position by cicatricial bands and adhesions.

SYMPTOMS AND COURSE.—The displacement and its complications usually cause bearing-down sensations, a feeling of heaviness in the pelvis, exhaustion upon walking and standing, especially the latter, and constipation. After the puerperium the extreme engorgement of the pelvic organs often produces uterine hemorrhage, which should not be confounded with the returning menstruation. Especially after abortion the hemorrhage often persists for a long time unless cured by treatment. Gradual or sudden replacement may occur spontaneously, or the causes may continue active, and even be enforced by cystocele and rectocele. The displacement may also be complicated by disease and displacement of the ovaries. Organic disease of the uterine walls may induce a superadded retroflexion. The heavy organ may descend along the relaxed subinvoluted vaginal walls even to complete procidentia.

DIAGNOSIS AND PROGNOSIS.—The symptoms outlined in the preceding paragraph indicate the probability of displacement, but the diagnosis depends upon direct examination of the uterus. Conjoined manipulation and the probe will usually show the retroverted organ with the cervix displaced toward the pubes and with the corpus in the hollow of the sacrum. The introduction of the probe is contraindicated by cellulitis and peritonitis. In certain cases of anteflexion, as represented in Fig. 23, the cervix is bent forward in the vaginal axis as in retroversion. The condition is in reality one of retroversion of the cervix with high anteflexion of the corpus, which may usually be detected by careful conjoined examination. The prognosis with treatment is generally favorable both for speedy relief and ultimate recovery.

TREATMENT.—As in descent, the treatment consists in removing cellulitis, peritonitis, and other complications, in the use of pessaries, and in operations on the anterior and posterior vaginal walls if needed. Inasmuch as the treatment corresponds to that of retroflexion, it will be presented under that subject.

Retroflexion.

ETIOLOGY AND PATHOLOGY.—Retroflexion is that displacement in which the organ is bent backward upon itself. It usually results from, and is associated with, retroversion, but for convenience the double displacement will be termed retroflexion. It may be caused by the great weight of the corpus, the soft flexible state of the uterine walls during and after involution, intra-abdominal forces, downward' pressure during defecation, tight clothing, and not commonly by the obstetric bandage.

The ovaries, unless fixed elsewhere by adhesions, are displaced with, and held down on either side of, the corpus, sometimes enlarged from inflammation, often adherent, and always extremely sensitive. Chronic metritis, cellulitis, and peritonitis, with adhesions more or less firm, are usually present, and not infrequently as the result of gonorrhœa, abortion, or injudicious treatment. Peritoneal adhesions between the corpus

FIG. 15.

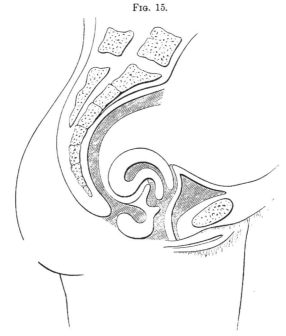

Extreme Retroflexion, with Hypertrophy of the Corpus, which impinges upon the rectum and compresses the recto-vaginal wall.

and the cul-de-sac of Douglas sometimes make replacement impossible. In rare cases the displacement is congenital.

SYMPTOMS AND COURSE.—Among the most pronounced symptoms are profuse uterine catarrh, menstrual disorders, sterility, abortion, weakness, pain in the back, painful defecation, rectal tenesmus, the symptoms of pelvic inflammation, neurasthenia, and other nervous symptoms. The uterine catarrh is due to an effort on the part of the engorged pelvic organs to relieve themselves by an exaggerated secretion of mucus from the uterus, which upon being increased in quantity becomes vitiated in quality, and therefore pathological. Menorrhagia and abortion may also result from congestion. Dysmenorrhœa and sterility result from the general anæmic condition and from the inflammatory complications, and from the obstruction in the uterine canal or in the blood-vessels at the angle of flexure. (See Pathology of Anteflexion.) The rectal symptoms are caused by the pressure of the corpus uteri upon the rectum, which gives the sensation to the patient of an overloaded bowel.

Should pregnancy occur, the rapid growth of the uterus may induce spontaneous reposition at about the fourth month, when the fundus rises out of the pelvis, but if the corpus be incarcerated under the sacral promontory from adhesions or from any other cause, the uterus will, unless manually replaced, relieve itself by abortion.

Abdominal pains, nervous dyspepsia, and neuralgia in distant parts of the body are often present; indeed, the nervous symptoms may be of the most exaggerated character, and may comprise all that is implied by the word hysteria in its most comprehensive signification.

DIAGNOSIS.—Digital touch discloses the cervix low in the pelvis, and the fundus uteri is felt through the posterior vaginal wall in the cul-de-sac of Douglas. Conjoined manipulation with the index finger of the left hand, first in the vagina and then in the rectum, and the right hand over the hypogastric region, will show the size, form, consistency, and location of the uterus, the degree of the flexure, and the difficulty of replacement. An inflammatory exudate or hæmatocele, posterior to the uterus, or a fibroid in the posterior uterine wall, may be mistaken for the retroflexed corpus. The probe will always verify the diagnosis, but if there be great tenderness with fixation in the cul-de-sac of Douglas, treatment should be directed against the inflamed condition, and the final diagnosis made by repeated examinations or after the disappearance of the inflammation. Great and lasting injury is often done in the attempt to complete the diagnosis at the first examination. The presence of a fibroid in the posterior uterine wall with post-uterine inflammation is a serious complication both in diagnosis and treatment. If the rectum be overloaded with fecal matter, the diagnosis should be deferred. The displacement is distinguished from the presence of an ovary or small ovarian tumor in the pouch of Douglas by careful bimanual examination and by the probe.

TREATMENT OF RETROVERSION AND RETROFLEXION.—The objects of treatment are replacement and retention of the uterus. The obstacles to replacement are cellulitis, peritonitis, and fixation of the uterus, and these complications often require weeks, and in severe cases months, of treatment preparatory to replacement. Some of the general therapeutic suggestions under the subject of descent are also applicable to the retropositions. Rest, massage, careful regulation of the bowels, feeding, and general tonics are essential. For the inflammation small blisters over the inguinal regions frequently repeated, and the daily application of the cotton and glycerin plug to the cervix, and dry cupping over the sacrum, are most efficacious. The glycerin may be combined with alum, tannin, chloral hydrate, or iodoform. Thymoline in small quantities partially destroys the disagreeable iodoform odor. The most useful and essential topical application is the hot-water vaginal douche, but its use will be followed by failure and disappointment if it be applied in the ordinary way. The following is quoted from a paper by the author which was published in the *Chicago Medical Gazette,* Jan. 1, 1880:

" *Ordinary Method of Application.*	" *Proper Method of Application.*
" I. Ordinarily, the douche is applied with the patient in the sitting posture, so that the injected water cannot fill the vagina and bathe the cervix uteri, but, on the contrary, returns along the tube of the syringe as fast as it flows in.	" I. It should invariably be given with the patient lying on the back, with the shoulders low, the knees drawn up, and the hips elevated on a bed-pan, so that the outlet of the vagina may be above every other part of it. Then the vagina will be kept continually overflowing while the douche is being given.
" II. The patient is seldom impressed with the importance of regularity in its administration.	" II. It should be given at least twice every day, morning and evening, and generally the length of each application should not be less than twenty minutes.
" III. The temperature is ordinarily not specified or heeded.	" III. The temperature should be as high as the patient can endure without distress. It may be increased from day to day, from 100° or 105° to 115° or 120° Fahr.
" IV. Ordinarily, the patient abandons its use after a short time."	" IV. Its use, in the majority of cases, should be continued for months at least, and sometimes for two or three years. Perseverance is of prime importance."

" A satisfactory substitute for the bed-pan may be made as follows: Place two chairs at the side of an ordinary bed with space enough between them to admit a bucket; place a large pillow at the extreme side of the bed nearest the chairs; spread an ordinary rubber sheet over the pillow, so that one end of the sheet may fall into the bucket below in the form of a trough. The douche may then be given with the patient's hips drawn well out over the edge of the bed and resting on the pillow, and with one foot on each chair; the water will then find its way along the rubber trough into the bucket below." The Davidson syringe, which has an interrupted current, is preferable to any of the fountain syringes.

As the tenderness disappears the cotton plugs may be increased in quantity, and thereby made to serve as temporary support for the uterus until a more permanent pessary can be substituted. The sluggish circulation in the pelvis and torpid condition of the bowels may be much relieved by the daily application of the wet pack. A small flannel sheet folded lengthwise to the width of two feet, dipped in very hot water, and dried by passing it through a wringer, is wound about the hips and covered by another dry one. At the end of a half hour, during which time the patient maintains the recumbent position, the sheets are removed. When the tenderness has been sufficiently reduced, gentle attempts at replacement may be made every day or two by conjoined manipulation. The patient's tolerance of manipulation may thus be observed and the way prepared for complete replacement and permanent retention after the subsidence of the inflammation.

In retroversion and retroflexion always replace the uterus before adjusting the pessary, otherwise the instrument will press upon the sensitive uterus, when one of three unfortunate results must occur: (1) The pessary may not be tolerated on account of pain; (2) the pessary may be forced down by pressure from above so near to the vulva that it will fail to do the least good; (3) the uterus, finding it impossible to hold its position against the pessary, instead of taking its proper position will often be bent over it in exaggerated retroflexion, with the cervix between the pessary and the pubes and the body between the pessary and the sacrum, or the whole organ may slip off to one side of the instrument into a malposition more serious than the one for which relief is sought. The safest and most effective method of replacement is by conjoined manipulation, as represented in Figs. 16 and 17. The dotted lines in the former indicate the gradual elevation of the corpus out of the hollow of the sacrum to the pelvic brim, where it may be anteverted by the fingers of the right hand pressed well down behind its posterior wall. During the process of anteversion the index finger of the left hand in the anterior fornix of the vagina presses the cervix back to its place in the hollow of the sacrum, as in Fig. 17. Efficient reposition of the uterus is very often impossible without anæsthesia.

FIG. 16.

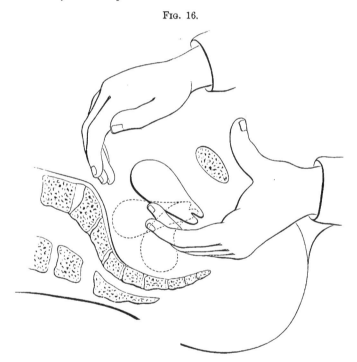

Commencing Reposition of the Retroverted or Retroflexed Uterus by Conjoined Manipulation (modified from Schultze).

The replacement is not usually accomplished by drawing the fundus forward and pushing the cervix back directly in the median line. In most cases the fundus sweeps around the arc of a circle on the left side of the pelvis, and the cervix on the right. This is owing to the greater frequency of cellulitis on the left side, and consequent shortening of the left broad ligament. After replacement the organ is to be held in position by a suitable pessary.

Bimanual replacement has two great advantages over the more familiar methods of the sound or repositor: first, it is more effective and more permanent; second, the lever action of the sound or repositor, by which the operator may unwittingly use an undue and dangerous amount of force, is avoided in the use of the hands, through which the operation is not only constantly under his control, but also within his appreciation.

FIG. 17.

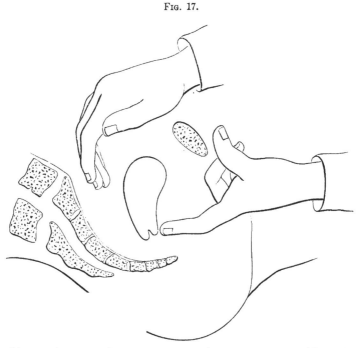

Completed Reposition of the Retroverted or Retroflexed Uterus by Conjoined Manipulation (modified from Schultze).

Inasmuch as the pessary fulfils its indications by sustaining the pelvic floor, and thereby holding the cervix in the hollow of the sacrum, the same general principles, and in fact the same pessaries, which are applicable to prolapse apply also to retroversion and retroflexion. Indeed, the first step in the genesis of the retro-positions has been shown to be prolapse. The student is therefore referred to the general remarks on the adjustment of pessaries for prolapse.

The operations of elytrorraphy and perineorraphy, especially the latter, already described in the treatment of descent, are often of the utmost importance in the treatment of the posterior displacements, and should therefore be carefully studied in this connection.

In the adjustment of the pessary it is desirable, if possible, to avoid direct pressure upon any part of the uterus. Pessaries designed to prop up the body of the uterus by pressure upon the posterior wall to correct the posterior malpositions, and upon the anterior wall to correct the anterior malpositions, are very liable to induce metritis and perimetritis, and are therefore generally unsafe. In certain cases, however, the vaginal walls, especially the posterior, may be so relaxed from subinvolution and other causes that the instrument, though very long, fails to maintain the cervix in its normal place. Under such conditions a pessary may be required to act directly upon the uterus. The Schultze's sleigh pessary represented in Fig. 19 fulfils this indication. Schultze's figure-of-eight pessary, or a long Albert Smith pessary with its uterine curve made so extreme as to bring the upper part of the instrument in front of the cervix instead of behind, answers the same purpose.

Fig. 18.

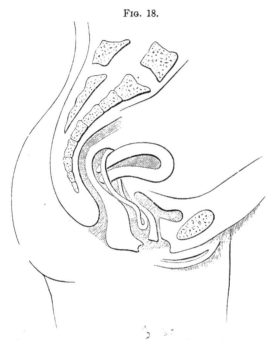

Showing the Pelvic Organs sustained by the Emmet Pessary after reposition of the prolapsed, retroverted or retroflexed uterus.

Thomas's retroflexion pessary, with its bulbous upper extremity, is a long, narrow instrument of extreme uterine curve. It lifts the uterus very high, and is specially applicable in cases of great relaxation of the pelvic floor and of complicating prolapse of the ovaries (Fig. 21). The bulbous portion is sometimes made of soft rubber.

A properly-adjusted pessary gives to the patient no consciousness of its presence. If the instrument cause pain it should be removed and search made for the tender places; it should then, if possible, be remoulded into such shape that it will not exert pressure upon them. Often a slight indentation at some point will enable the patient to wear it with comfort.

Sometimes when the corpus has been firmly bound back by peritoneal adhesions they may be broken up by very forcible conjoined manipulation under ether, but the operation is dangerous, and should therefore be undertaken only by an expert operator. In place of this operation Lawson Tait has proposed to open the abdomen, break the adhesions, and stitch the fundus uteri to the abdominal wound. This operation in the hands of such an operator as Tait is probably not more dangerous than breaking up firm adhesions by forcible conjoined manipulation.

In certain cases in which replacement is impracticable or impossible on account of inflammation or adhesions a soft rubber ring may be inserted, and will often give decided relief by lifting the uterus and pelvic floor nearer to the health level. In the treatment of all displacements coition

FIG. 19.

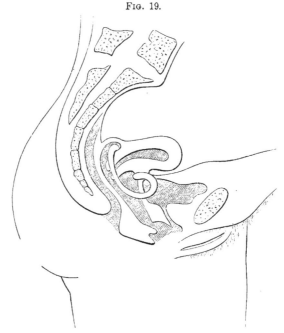

Schultze's Sleigh Pessary in place, as adjusted for prolapse, retroversion, or retroflexion with great relaxation of the vaginal walls (after Schultze).

should be forbidden or permitted only with great moderation, and the pessary should be kept clean by copious daily applications of the vaginal douche. Every three or four weeks the instrument should be removed and the pelvic organs carefully examined.

It should be urged that no man can safely apply the pessary until he has fully appreciated its indications and contraindications. Few practitioners possess naturally the mechanical skill necessary to its proper adjustment. Of this thousands of unfortunate women bear witness. Its dangers in inefficient hands are in striking contrast with its usefulness when judiciously employed.

Many cases of displacement, both anterior and posterior, are so complicated by prolapsed and adherent ovaries, by advanced disease of the ovaries and Fallopian tubes, and by peritoneal adhesions, that not only replacement, but even palliation, is impossible; then, as a final resort, the activity of the pelvic organs, both physiologically and pathologically. may be put at rest by the removal of the ovaries and Fallopian tubes.

William Alexander of Liverpool has devised an ingenious operation of shortening the round ligaments for the radical cure of descent and

Fig. 20.

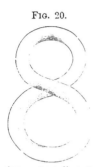

Front View of Schultze's Figure-of
Eight Pessary. The upper opening is intended to hold the cervix.
This pessary has the uterine and
pubic curves, as in Figs. 7 and 8.

Fig. 21.

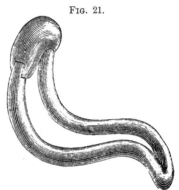

Thomas's Retroflexion Pessary.

of the posterior displacements. He reports twenty-two cases of the operation in his own practice and several more in the practice of other surgeons, with almost uniform success in completely curing the displacements. The operation, although new, gives promise of a brilliant and successful future.

Lateral Versions and Flexions.

The lateral malpositions which often complicate retroversion and retroflexion are usually the result of inflammation in a broad ligament or in the uterus itself, or in both. Their treatment is that of the causa·tive inflammation, and follows the general principles which have been laid down for the treatment of other versions and flexions.

Pathological Anteversion.

Sometimes the physiological angle of flexure becomes obliterated in consequence of chronic metritis, resulting in permanent straightening of the uterus, and the cervix becomes elevated and fixed above, or the corpus depressed and fixed below, the normal level. This constitutes pathologi·cal anteversion (Fig. 22).

ETIOLOGY.—The exaggerated anteversion of early pregnancy is phys-iological, the exaggerated anteversion of the uterus in chronic metritis is pathological. Elevation of the cervix and depression of the corpus may be induced by peritoneal adhesions. Increased weight from a mural fibroid may also depress the corpus.

The SYMPTOMS are due to the pelvic inflammations already mentioned and other complications. The increased weight of the uterus, which is usually hypertrophied from metritis, generally causes a dragging sensation, especially if the organ be also prolapsed. The enlarged corpus occupying the territory of the bladder often induces persistent vesical irritation or even cystitis. Menorrhagia, when present, is the result of the metritis or a fibroid rather than of the displacement per se.

DIAGNOSIS AND PROGNOSIS.—The displacement is recognized by digital touch, which discloses the anterior wall of the uterus parallel to the anterior wall of the vagina, with the fundus close to the symphysis and the cervix elevated. Conjoined examination will show the size, shape,

FIG. 22.

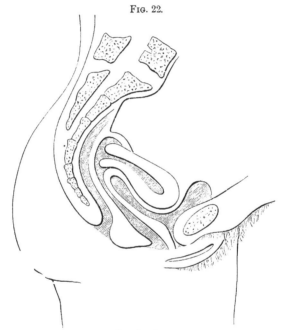

Pathological Anteversion.

hardness, and degree of fixation. Exaggerated anteversion of the healthy uterus is not necessarily pathological in its results. This is illustrated by the anteversion of early pregnancy. The prognosis is therefore good if the causes can be removed.

TREATMENT.—Inasmuch as exaggerated anteversion is the position taken by the uterus in chronic metritis, it follows that the treatment is often that of chronic metritis. For the treatment of metritis, perimetritis, fibroids, menorrhagia, etc. the reader is referred to the special literature of those subjects. Irritable bladder, which is often a mechanical result of the displacement and enlargement, may sometimes be relieved by means of an Albert Smith or Hodge pessary, which lifts the organ to a higher level away from the bladder. In thus elevating the uterus the anteversion may be rather increased than diminished, which proves that the symptoms were dependent not upon the anteposition, but rather upon descent and antelocation. Should the parts be too sensitive to tolerate the hard-rubber pessary or a flexible rubber ring, the daily application of medicated pledgets of cotton will give support to the uterus and decrease the tenderness until the more permanent instrument can be worn. The numerous anteversion pessaries designed to elevate the corpus by direct pressure on the anterior wall of the uterus generally irritate the organ, and thereby aggravate the inflammatory complications. They are therefore to be used with extreme caution.

Pathological Anteflexion.

DEFINITION.—The normal forward bending of the corpus upon the cervix uteri when the bladder is empty makes an angle of which the approximate physiological limits are between 45° and 90° : the flexure would generally be pathological if less than 45° or more than 90°. Furthermore, if the flexure, whether it be normal or abnormal in extent,

FIG. 23.

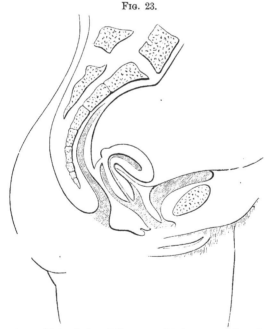

Congenital Anteflexion. Both cervix and body are flexed forward.

does not disappear upon filling the bladder, but remains constant under all conditions, the rigidity makes the flexure pathological. Anteflexion is therefore pathological if the mobility at the angle of flexure is increased or diminished or absent.

ETIOLOGY AND PATHOLOGY.—Anteflexion may be congenital or acquired. By congenital is meant not defective fœtal development, but failure of the immature child uterus to develop at puberty, a failure which usually pertains alike to the uterus, Fallopian tubes, ovaries, and vagina. In congenital anteflexion the uterus is bent upon itself almost double, the body and cervix both pointing in the direction of the pelvic outlet, with the cervix somewhat elongated and situated in the long axis of the vagina. (See Fig. 23.)

Acquired anteflexion may be simply an exaggeration of the normal flexure, due either to increased weight of the corpus from the presence

FIG. 24.

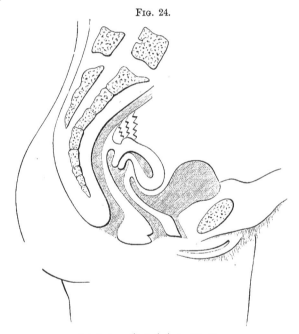

Anteflexion with Post-uterine Fixation

of the uterine fibroid near the fundus or to unequal growth of the uterine walls or to unequal involution. A very frequent cause of anteflexion is thickening of the posterior wall of the uterus from the products of inflammation, and a corresponding atrophy of the anterior wall from prolonged pressure at the angle of flexure. Post-uterine cellulitis and peritonitis involving the utero-sacral ligaments is a frequent and dis-couraging complication. Sometimes the inflamed ligaments contract and drag the anteflexed uterus upward and backward, where it may be permanently fixed by peritoneal adhesions. (See Fig. 24.)

A constriction of the uterine canal at the point of flexure may, by confining the secretions above, produce inflammation in the body of the uterus, Fallopian tubes, and ovaries analogous to the cystitis, ureteritis, pyelitis, and nephritis which follow stricture of the male urethra. The peri-uterine inflammations, having the relation either of cause or effect of the flexure, often bind the pelvic organs together in a mass of exu· date, with resulting failure of nutrition, nerve-irritation, and constant pain, which sometimes render the patient's life miserable and useless.

SYMPTOMS AND COURSE.—The numerous symptoms due to the inflammatory and other complications should not be confounded with those of the displacement. The symptoms of anteflexion are polyuria and dysuria, dysmenorrhœa and sterility.

The vesical symptoms are produced either by the rigidity of the uterine tissue at the angle of flexure, which prevents the body from rising out of the way of the filling bladder, or by the inflammatory shortening of the utero-sacral ligaments, which, by drawing the uterus upward and backward, put the vesico-vaginal wall on the stretch, thereby causing traction upon the neck of the bladder.

The dysmenorrhœa may depend upon the presence of constriction of the uterine canal at the angle of flexure. This causes the blood to accumulate and to coagulate in the body of the uterus, from which it is expelled at intervals by uterine contractions simulating labor-pains. The pain when due to this cause is therefore always very severe just before the passage of a clot. Furthermore, the dysmenorrhœa may be caused by obstruction in the veins at the angle of flexure, which causes intense venous congestion of the entire body of the uterus; pain is then due to the pressure of the swollen vessels upon the nerve-filaments and to a consequent irritable condition of the muscular tissue of the uterus. Sometimes upon the establishment of the flow the uterine canal becomes temporarily straightened; this removes the cause of the vascular obstruction, and together with the flow gives relief.

Sterility is very commonly associated with anteflexion. The fact that dilatation and incision of the constricted canal have frequently been followed by conception has been accepted as proof that the sterility is due to the constrictive obstruction. This mechanical theory is questioned by many, who say that the dilatation cures sterility by straightening the uterus and thereby removing the venous obstruction and the consequent congestion.

DIAGNOSIS.—The educated touch which distinguishes the normal version, flexion, and movements of the uterus will appreciate the anatomical differences between pathological and normal anteflexion. The degree of flexure, the mobility or rigidity, and the size, shape, location, and consistency of the uterus may be ascertained by conjoined manipulation. The presence of post-uterine cellulitis is recognized by the pain caused in dragging the uterus slightly forward and by increased thickness and tenderness in the region of the utero-sacral ligaments, which may be felt by vaginal or rectal touch. Anteflexion is distinguished from a fibroid in the anterior wall of the uterus by the probe. When the diagnosis of anteflexion is obscured by the presence of cellulitis, it is usually better to wait for absorption of the exudate than to subject the patient to needless danger from the probe. Should it be necessary to pass the probe, the danger is decreased by gentle manipulation, which is facilitated by Sims's speculum and the latero-prone position. The common error of mistaking the normal version and flexion of a prolapsed uterus for pathological version and flexion has been exposed in a previous paragraph. (See Etiology and Clinical History of Descent.)

TREATMENT.—If complicating cellulitis or peritonitis exist, in the relation of either cause or effect to the flexure, its removal becomes the prime indication, because unless removed it is a positive contraindication to the more direct treatment of the malposition itself. Chronic metritis, hyperplasia, hypertrophy, and irremovable tumors sometimes render cure impossible. Improvement of the general health, treatment of complications, and palliation then become the only resources.

The direct treatment of pathological anteflexion has for its object the straightening of the uterine canal, which is usually accomplished either by division of the cervix or by dilatation. But before considering the treatment more specifically, it should be remembered that surgical treatment of anteflexion in cases of dysmenorrhœa and sterility is only justifiable when the anteflexion is pathological. To say that most women who suffer from dysmenorrhœa and sterility have anteflexion is only saying that in the majority of such cases the uterus is in its normal position.

The Marion-Sims operation of dividing the cervix is open to two objections: first, its results are apt to be only temporary, in consequence of rapid contraction upon healing of the wound; second, it has frequently been followed by death. Dilatation by means of tents is also transient in its results, and dangerous to life. Both Sims's operation and dilatation by tents have given frequent and serious warnings in the shape of pelvic inflammations, which, if not destructive to life, have been almost as disastrous in their influence upon health.

The following, with some modifiations, is an abstract of a valuable contribution[1] by Goodell of Philadelphia, in which he gives positive endorsement to rapid dilatation as proposed by Ellinger and others. The instruments recommended are two Ellinger dilators, which are preferred on account of the parallel action of their blades. The dilatation is commenced with the smaller instrument and completed with the larger, which has powerful blades that do not spring or feather. The light instrument needs only a ratchet in the handle, but the stronger one has a screw which forces the handles together and the blades apart. To prevent injury to the fundus when the instrument is open, the length of the blades is limited to two inches. The larger instrument has a dilating power of one and a half inches, and has a graduated arc in the handles which indicates the divergence of the blades. Goodell's modification of Ellinger's dilators is provided with serrated blades, to prevent them from slipping out of the canal during the process of dilatation.

For dysmenorrhœa or sterility due to flexion or stenosis the method of operation is as follows: A suppository containing a grain of the aqueous extract of opium is introduced into the rectum, the patient etherized, and the uterus exposed by Sims's speculum. The cervix is held by a tenaculum, and the smaller dilator is introduced as far as it will go. Upon gently stretching open that portion of the uterine canal which it occupies, the stricture above so yields that when the blades are closed they will pass higher. By repeating this manœuvre a cervical canal is tunnelled out which before would not admit the finest probe. Should the os

[1] *American Journal of Obstetrics*, 1884, p. 1179.

externum or cervical canal be too small to admit the instrument, a pair of pointed scissors may be substituted, and by the same opening and closing motions the canal may be prepared for the introduction of the smaller dilator. As soon as the cavity of the uterus has been entered the handles are brought together. This dilator is then withdrawn, the larger one introduced, and its handles slowly screwed together. If the flexure be very marked, the larger instrument after being withdrawn should be introduced with its curve in the opposite direction to that of the flexure, and the final dilatation made with the dilator in this position. But in reversing the curve the operator should take care not to rotate the organ upon its own axis, and not to mistake a twist thus made for a reversal of the flexure; the ether is then withheld, and the instrument allowed to remain in place until the patient begins to flinch, when it is removed. The best time for the dilatation is midway between the monthly periods. In the majority of cases the dilatation should be carried to about one and a quarter inches. The infantile uterus which has failed to develop at puberty has thin, unyielding walls, and should therefore not be dilated more than three-fourths of an inch or an inch. In using the larger instrument it is usually necessary to have the assistant make decided counter-traction with the vulsella forceps to prevent the blades of the dilator from slipping out. The cervix is sometimes lacerated, but not sufficiently to produce unpleasant results.

Goodell's statistics include one hundred and fifty operations of full dilatation under ether, with no fatal result and without serious inflammatory disturbance. As precautions against cellulitis, peritonitis, and metritis the patient should be fortified for the operation with moderate doses of opium and full doses of quinine, and for two or three days after the dilatation this should be continued and supplemented by the application of an ice-bladder over the abdomen.

After forcible dilatation under ether the cervical canal rarely returns to its previously angular or contracted condition. The cervix shortens and widens, and the plasma thrown out thickens and stiffens the uterine walls. In a small minority of cases the operation must be repeated. Dysmenorrhœa or sterility, if dependent solely upon the flexure, is cured by the dilatation. The comparative safety of forcible dilatation in the hands of a skilful and experienced gynecologist may be contrasted with its great danger when undertaken by an operator unacquainted with the special requirements of uterine surgery. Peri-uterine inflammation is a positive contraindication to the operation.

Post-uterine inflammation, which has drawn the anteflexed or anteverted uterus upward and backward by the contraction of the uterosacral ligaments, often produces traction upon the vesico-vaginal wall and neck of the bladder, with a constant desire to micturate. For the relief of this intractable symptom, which sometimes goes on to cystitis, Emmet has proposed a most satisfactory remedy known as his buttonhole operation of urethrotomy.[1] He makes a longitudinal opening about five-eighths of an inch long through the urethro-vaginal wall, between the meatus and the neck of the bladder, without cutting through either. To prevent the opening from healing together, the margins of the mucous membrane of the urethra are united with fine catgut sutures to the mar-

[1] Emmet's *Principles and Practice of Gynecology*, 3d ed., pp. 275 and 761.

gins of the mucous membrane of the vagina. According to Emmet, the operation relieves irritation due to traction on the neck of the bladder by freeing the pelvic fascia at the fixed point where it converges to its pubic attachment. The operation is equally applicable for the relief of this symptom when due to inflammation in any other part of the pelvis. The same result may be secured, but less satisfactorily, by forcible dilatation of the urethra.

From personal experience the author can testify to the gratifying effects of this operation. Vesical irritation caused by post-uterine inflammation and consequent contraction of the utero-sacral ligaments is often wrongly attributed to the mechanical pressure of the anteflexed fundus uteri upon the bladder, which is manifestly impossible, if the contracted utero-sacral supports hold the entire uterus back away from the bladder.

The various anteflexion and anteversion pessaries which have been devised for the purpose of propping up the corpus are almost useless. Their false reputation depends upon the relief which they frequently give to complicating prolapse, the symptoms of which have been wrongly attributed to anteflexion or anteversion. The same pessaries therefore may be applied as in descent. (See Etiology and Clinical History of Descent.) Intra-uterine stem pessaries designed to straighten the flexed uterus are sometimes effective, and always dangerous.

DISORDERS OF THE UTERINE FUNCTIONS.

By J. C. REEVE, M. D.

MENSTRUATION with its disorders is the only subject to be considered under this head. In its monthly recurrence it is most intimately conneeted with, and dependent upon, ovulation, each menstrual discharge being the sign and evidence of the maturation and expulsion of one ovum or more. This proposition is denied by some, but the evidence adduced against it, while sufficient to show that the two processes may be dissociated, and may sometimes occur independently, is not strong enough to invalidate the truth of the general statement.

Menstruation may be entirely absent, the flow may be excessive, or it may be accompanied by severe pain; and these derangements have been designated from time immemorial as amenorrhœa, menorrhagia, and dysmenorrhœa. The time is long past, however, when these affections could be treated as distinct diseases. Each of them may be caused by influences so various—and, above all, may depend upon pathological conditions so different, and even dissimilar—that the name applied to each is indefinite, and, like the term dropsy, only incites inquiry as to some abnormal condition of which the deranged flow is the symptom. A due appreciation of this fact is of prime importance, because treatment cannot be instituted with expectation of success until the particular form of each derangement has been distinguished.

The great majority of cases of uterine derangement depend upon changes of structure. Those considered purely functional are largely in the minority, and would be still less in number with a more intimate knowledge of pathology or with greater skill in examination. No argument is needed, therefore, to show that a direct and thorough examination of the organs concerned is essential to rational treatment of this class of affections. There are obvious difficulties in the way of such an investigation, different from and far greater than attend the investigation of the diseases of any other organ of the body. With tact and proper demeanor, however, these difficulties can be generally overcome, but in any other than trifling cases, and especially in those continuing for any considerable time, the practitioner will do injustice to himself as well as to his patient if he do not insist upon this indispensable investigation.

A due appreciation of the influence of uterine disorders and diseases upon other and remote parts of the body is necessary to a correct estimate of their importance, and often of great practical value in treatment. Through the sympathetic nervous system pathological conditions of the uterus modify the processes of organic life, and by direct or reflex action affect the cerebro-spinal system in its centre or at any point of its terminal ramifications. That the stomach responds readily to uterine excitations is shown in pregnancy, and uterine disease often causes disorders of the digestive organs the origin of which may not be suspected. Eructations, vomiting, and the various forms of indigestion are not uncommon. The bowels are irregular in action, constipation alternating with diarrhœa, and flatulent distension may occur even to a degree demanding special treatment. Failure of general nutrition and impoverished blood are the consequences of this disturbed digestion; without good blood there is no sound innervation, and the nervous system is soon in such a condition as to respond unduly to even insignificant impressions. Normal menstruation is marked by a nervous erethism which shows itself by irritability, fits of despondency, and exhibitions of temper. There are therefore abundant reasons why nervous diseases should be very frequently seen as a remote effect of uterine disorders.

A very large proportion of these reflex diseases first occur at the period of puberty, many present striking exacerbations at every menstrual period, and some are so closely associated with this function as to be cured only by remedies addressed to it. Headache, neuralgia, hysteria in its varied forms, chorea, catalepsy, epilepsy, and even mania, have been repeatedly shown to have their origin in the sexual organs. The reproach often directed at gynecologists, of a disposition to magnify their specialty, falls pointless before such important facts; and since it is not uncommon for diseases of organs in close proximity to the uterus, as those of the urethra, bladder, and rectum, to be mistaken for or confounded with diseases of the uterus itself, there is abundant warrant for urging the closest scrutiny as to a possible uterine origin of remote diseases, especially those of a nervous character.

Amenorrhœa.

The term amenorrhœa signifies the absence of menstruation. It occurs in two different forms: First, those cases in which menstruation has never occurred—emansio mensium; second, those in which it has disappeared after having been established—suppressio mensium.

The following pathological schedule may assist in the study of the subject. It need scarcely be said that it is not presented as correct in every particular, nor with the idea that the dividing-lines between physiological and pathological conditions can be always determined, but as a convenient guide to follow in the study of the subject:

A. Amenorrhœa (absent menstruation) from

 a, anatomical conditions: want of development of organs, atresia of passages;

 b, physiological influences: delayed puberty, idiopathic;

 c, pathological causes: constitutional diseases, disease of the sexual organs, the cachexiæ.

B. Amenorrhœa (secondary or suppressed menstruation):

 a, anatomo-pathological: atresia of passages, atrophy of organs;

 b, physiological: pregnancy, nursing, premature change of life;

 c, pathological: besides those given above—A–c—are psychical influences and exposure or taking cold during menstruation.

Absence or want of due development of some of the sexual organs is not of very infrequent occurrence. The ovaries are very rarely found wanting ; they are more often checked in development and present the characteristics of early life. This condition may be the cause of delayed, irregular, or scanty menstruation, making a more or less near approach to amenorrhœa. Absence of the uterus is often combined with absence or with an undeveloped condition of the vagina, but this canal may be perfect and no change of the external organs be present to indicate that the uterus is wanting. It may also exist in a rudimentary form, and may be found corresponding in size and shape to the uterus of any period of early life.

Absence of the ovaries not only causes amenorrhœa, but checks the progress of the bodily development and prevents the sexual changes of puberty. When the ovaries are wanting there is almost always absence of the Fallopian tubes, uterus, and vagina. The symptomatology of absence of the uterus is not generally striking, the lack of menstruation being the principal sign ; exceptionally, however, it is otherwise. In some cases where the ovaries are present and the uterus wanting, the most aggravated affections of the nervous system show themselves.

Congenital atresia of the genital canal may occur in any part of its course. Imperforate hymen is the most frequent as it is the least dangerous form, being more than twice as common as atresia of the vagina and three times as frequent as that of the cervix uteri. The vagina may be extremely small in calibre, closed in part or the whole of its course, or only a fibrous cord indicate where it should be. The uterus may be closed at the internal or external os; the latter is the more frequent. An occlusion at one point does not preclude the existence of other closures higher up. The effect of a closed canal with a recurring secretion above is evident, and gives rise to a well-marked class of cases. The organs above become distended, and the distension increases until an opening is made by art or the retained fluid bursts a passage for escape. This may occur outwardly with immediate relief and cure, or into the peritoneal cavity, causing speedy death. The time at which the uterus may be expected to give way under such distension cannot be stated, as the power of resistance of the organ differs and the amount of secretion each month may vary widely. Scanzoni in one case evacuated eight pounds of blood, the result of seven months' accumulation, and found the uterine wall as thin as paper. Bernutz states that the average time before interference is necessary is three or four years, and gives a case first operated upon in the tenth year of its course.

Menstrual retention is not at first indicated by pronounced symptoms. Suspicion of the nature of the case may be first excited by the severity of those symptoms which at every period announce the approach of menstruation and known as the menstrual molimen. As distension increases these become extreme, with rectal and vesical tenesmus and severe uterine colic. The nervous system sympathizes, as with all menstrual derangements, and there may be rigor, fainting, or even convulsions.

Whenever a patient presents such symptoms an examination should be insisted upon. It will generally reveal a smooth, soft, and fluctuating tumor, projecting externally if the case be one of imperforate hymen, or higher up if the vagina be occluded. If the uterus has become distended, there will be a round, smooth, elastic tumor above the pubes. Diagnosis will be·more or less difficult according to the seat of the obstruction. Cases of imperforate hymen may be readily diagnosed by sight, if touch and the history are not sufficient. When the occlusion is deeper, the patient should be placed under the influence of an anæsthetic. By one finger in the rectum and the thumb in the vagina, and a sound in the bladder, the seat and extent of the obstruction may be determined. Should it be necessary, the urethra may be dilated and a finger passed into the bladder in order to make a diagnosis. Rectal exploration is of great assistance in discovering the uterine enlargement and its character. Scanzoni calls attention to the difference in the cervix when the atresia is at the internal or external os. In the latter case the cervix will be obliterated; in the former, it will be unchanged. With a perfect vagina and a cervix of this character retention may be taken for an early pregnancy, especially as it is not uncommon for sympathetic mammary symptoms and gastric troubles to be present. Time will demonstrate the nature of the case if a diagnosis cannot be made at once.

The age at which the menstrual flow is established varies greatly. The average age of puberty in this country, as appears from Emmet's tables made up of 2330 cases, is 14.23 years, and these are believed to be the only American statistics. A close correspondence may be noted between this and the statistics of the four largest cities of France, which give 14.26 as the average. But that it is not unusual for the appearance of menstruation to be delayed is shown by the fact that of the above 2330 cases, 288 only menstruated at sixteen years and 254 more between that age and twenty-three. The circumstances which may influence, within physiological limits, the appearance of menstruation should be considered in connection with cases of this kind. Climate and social position are the principal ones. The epoch of puberty descends in the scale of age in proportion to the average height of the temperature of various countries, and vice versâ. Social position and city life show a marked effect in hastening puberty as compared with the simpler manners and plainer life of rural populations. It amounts to an average of something over a year, and is explained by the influence of enervating and luxurious habits, of light reading and the drama, the chief subject of both being the grand passion, but especially of a freer intercourse between, and the co-education of, the sexes, and the greater extent to which music is cultivated and enjoyed.

· Among pathological conditions giving rise to amenorrhœa it would seem that disease of the ovaries should occupy the first rank in frequency and importance. The reverse is the truth. The ovaries are rarely inflamed, and when so amenorrhœa is not always the result. They are frequently the seat of cystic degeneration, producing tumors of large size, yet so long as but a small portion of one of the organs remains unaffected Graäfian vesicles may still be furnished and menstruation continue. It is by the influence of remote pathological conditions that the menstrual flow is most frequently restrained, and especially by those general affections known as cachexiæ, all of which exhibit marked depression and low grade of vital power and activity, if not more pronounced pathological processes. Chlorosis, the relations of which to menstruation are intimate, and which seems to be sometimes the offspring of amenorrhœa, exerts a marked retarding influence, amounting to an average of one year and a half. The scrofulous cachexia is still more potent: Scanzoni states that of 31 well-marked cases, in 19 menstruation did not occur until the twenty-first year.

Amenorrhœa which is the result of pulmonary tubercular disease comes frequently under observation. It may occur at a very early period of the disease, before there is any great amount of deposit in the lungs, when it is rather the expression of want of vital force than of the exhausting effect of the disease. Under these circumstances it is only to the laity a subject of serious consideration; to the physician it is but a symptom.

The suppression as well as the absence of menstruation may be caused by atresia of the passages, this form differing from the congenital only etiologically, and in the fact that the flow has been once established. The acquired atresiæ are mostly the result of violent inflammations or traumatic influences. The vulva and vagina, or either, may be closed from sloughing after difficult labors or gangrene following the septic fevers. Occlusion of the cervix uteri may follow labor or amputation of the part, but a far more frequent cause is the application of severe caustics, happily less frequent now than formerly. Lawson Tait says he has never met with atresia of this part from any other cause.

The mode of diagnosis has already been given, and in regard to symptomatology there is only to be noted the statement of Bernutz, that there is far greater intolerance of retention from acquired than from congenital atresia.

Atrophy of the uterus is a normal process after the menopause, but it sometimes occurs much earlier in life, and then causes scanty and irregular menstruation or amenorrhœa. Attention was first called to this condition by Simpson as a process sometimes following parturition under the name of super-involution. Several labors in rapid succession have been stated to be a cause, but Simpson and Courty both give a case after a single birth. Uterine atrophy may also result from the pressure of tumors, and it has been observed in paraplegias the result of defective innervation.

The deranged menstruation is the one prominent symptom of this condition, and a diagnosis is to be made by exploration. The cervix is found small and the body light when lifted on the finger. Bimanual examination and the introduction of the sound will reveal the true condition of the organ. The latter process should be cautiously conducted on account of a frequent change of texture in the uterine walls which allows the instrument to pass through them with the use of but very little force.

Amenorrhœa is physiological during nursing and pregnancy. The former needs no attention, the latter only in regard to diagnosis. A sudden cessation of menstruation, the patient presenting all the appearances of good health, should immediately excite suspicion as to the nature of the cause. It needs but little experience to distinguish and manage these cases in the lower social ranks. The case is different, however, in a family of good position, with an anxious mother urgent for active measures, where no suspicions will be tolerated and the imputation of possible pregnancy be warmly resented. Time is here the sure ally of the physician, and an examination should be deferred until such a period has been reached that pregnancy can be positively negatived or determined.

The influence of acute diseases in suppressing menstruation is not marked. During convalescence from them the flow frequently ceases from general debility. All chronic diseases depressing and exhausting in nature cause suppression, as albuminuria, cirrhosis, and cancer. Tuberculosis is as fruitful in interrupting the return as in preventing the appearance of the flow, and suppression from this cause is very frequent. Under impaired nutrition and depressed powers vital force is engaged wholly in maintaining existence; there is none for any function relating to the propagation of the species. In this class the disappearance is gradual; the flow becomes scanty and irregular in recurrence, and finally ceases. This form of amenorrhœa differs in no material point from the similar class already considered; it is but a symptom of disease of some vital organ or of some general abnormal condition.

Suppression from psychical influences is not at all uncommon. Fright, grief, bad news, sudden or prolonged anxiety, frequently cause this disturbance of function. The mental impression need not be very profound. Amenorrhœa is a common event with girls who go away from home to boarding-school. In these cases it is not probable that there is any pathological condition of the sexual organs; a change in their innervation is a phrase which will best serve to explain the origin of the derangement or to express our ignorance. The diagnosis of this form may be a matter of deep interest when it occurs directly after marriage, as it not infrequently does, and gives ground for the belief that pregnancy has occurred. Still more important is it when the suppression follows illicit intercourse, the fear of pregnancy then exerting a powerful emotional influence. Some cases are on record, and the writer has met with two: in both the function resumed its course after a time without remedies.

Exposure to storm, getting the feet wet, and the sudden application of cold to the genitals frequently cause suppression. All the conditions, however, are not well understood. The bathing- and fishing-women of Europe are said to ply their vocation without reference to menstruation, and to suffer no inconvenience. In these cases the increased flow of blood to the pelvic organs oversteps the narrow line which separates physiological from pathological congestion, and may even pass on to inflammation.

The SYMPTOMS are well marked—at first, local, as severe backache, increased heat and pressure in the pelvic region, discomfort passing on to pain, even uterine colic. If the impression be severe enough to affect the general system, there will be febrile action more or less intense, and various nervous symptoms, spasmodic or convulsive.

The therapeutics of amenorrhœa must be directed in accordance with the conditions which cause it. But the strictly scientific method cannot be followed at the outset. This method presupposes a direct examination of the organs as the first step. For obvious reasons this must be deferred until special symptoms show its necessity. For treatment the cases may be classified, in some instances according to the schedule, but more frequently according to the cause or leading features, and very generally without reference to whether there is absence merely or suppression of the function.

In amenorrhœa from atresia the measures of relief will be purely surgical; the treatment, therefore, does not fall within the scope of this article.

The physician is frequently consulted in cases where menstruation has occurred once or twice, perhaps at long intervals, and not appearing regularly the fears of friends are excited. This is the normal course of establishment in a large proportion of cases. Time and assurance and regimen are alone needed, provided there is no evidence of deteriorated health. Absence of the function alone does not demand treatment—a fact which should be kept steadily in mind.

In a still larger class of cases the amenorrhœa depends upon, and is the direct result of, some pronounced cachectic condition, as chlorosis, scrofula, or a more or less active tubercular disease of the lungs. The treatment of this class resolves itself into that of the disease causing the derangement, and the reader is referred to the articles on the corresponding subjects.

The cases requiring more direct consideration therapeutically are those closely allied to the preceding, in which delay in appearance depends upon want of development of the body or general feebleness of constitution, or those in which absence follows and continues unduly after some severe disease. In all these cases the treatment is to be indirect rather than direct. The absent function is to be restored by improving nutrition, by increasing bodily vigor, and by using every means to establish the general health on a firm basis. Measures for this purpose should be addressed to every particular of the habits, occupation, and surroundings of the patient. They do not differ from those of a general tonic course, but in some particulars a special influence may be exerted upon the function at fault. The clothing should be warm, especially about the pelvis and lower extremities, due care of the feet being impressed in proportion to the universal neglect shown by girls and women in regard to these important parts of the person. The diet should be of plain, wholesome, substantial food, and in many cases one of the lighter wines may be added to the principal meal of the day with decided advantage. Gymnastics may be prescribed, but outdoor life should be urged, with horseback riding as the very best mode of exercise for promoting the flow. A change of air and scene exerts a well-known and powerful influence in improving nutrition and modifying vital actions. It should be rather from the city to the country for these cases. Special advantages may be derived from a residence at the seaside on account of the beneficial effects of surf-bathing. A scientifically-conducted hydropathic establishment is very desirable for its regular hours, well-ordered diet, and treatment by baths and douches. Or a watering-place may be preferred where a chalybeate water may exert a special influence in addition to those of moderate indulgence in the gayety and amusement of such a place.

Inquiry as to school-life and educational work should never be omitted. The general mode of education of girls is faulty in the extreme. No attention is paid to the great change of puberty, which amounts to a revolution in the economy, and instead of aiding the vital forces drawn upon for effecting this change, they are still further depressed by sedentary life in close rooms or strongly urged in another direction. No two leading organs of the body can be pushed in development at the same time with impunity. There is no exception here: either the brain and nervous system or the sexual organs will suffer. In this direction is often found a potent cause of all the forms of uterine derangement—a fact which cannot have escaped the observation of every physician. The writer has always urged an entire break in the school-life of girls of at least one year's duration at the time when signs of puberty begin to manifest themselves; and this period is too short rather than too long.

Tonics should supplement these regiminal measures. They may be hæmatic, stomachic, and nervous—either or all. There is a chain of diseased actions, and it may be attacked at any of its links. Iron stands at the head of the list. It is not only an hæmatic tonic, and in proper conditions a promoter of digestion, but decidedly promotes pelvic congestion, and has therefore an emmenagogue action. The forms at command are so numerous as to meet the requirements of any case or to satisfy any fancy. The standard preparations, as a rule, deserve the preference over more modern ones, in which efficacy is often sacrificed to elegance. Among the best are those which contain the remedy in a nascent state, as the compound mixture or the compound pills of iron of the Pharmacopœia. Dialyzed iron, the tincture of the chloride, and the pyrophosphate are reliable, while the addition of manganese, as in the syrup of the iodide of iron and manganese, is believed by some to increase the efficacy. With iron may be combined nux vomica or strychnia and quinia. In large sections of our country malaria is a constantly-acting depressant of vital force, and the latter medicine may be given for a time with a free hand, and may be followed by or combined with arsenic to great advantage.

Constipation is almost universally present in women. It deserves especial consideration in treating all disorders of the sexual organs. When attention to habits and appropriate laxative food, as fruits, oatmeal, Indian meal, cracked wheat, and salads, do not suffice, resort must be had to enemata or drugs. Aloes has always had a reputation of special virtue in amenorrhœa which is doubtless well founded. In pill form it may be combined with any or all the other medicines. Pills of aloin, one-fifth or one-third of a grain, have the advantage of very small bulk.

Before considering more direct measures for establishing menstruation it may be well to recall to mind the two elements of the function— ovulation and the uterine flow. The first, the prime factor, we can not influence by any medicines nor by any mode of treatment except, perhaps, by electricity. Observation of animals shows that mere proximity of the male influences it plainly, but this only indicates a line along which we cannot prescribe. An opinion may, however, be asked in regard to the propriety or advisability of marriage for a woman who has never menstruated. In such case no advice should be given until after a thorough local examination, and its tenor will then be in accord with the condition of the organs. With such atresia or absence of organs as not to permit sexual intercourse marriage should be positively negatived. In such cases as those of partially-developed or absent uterus the facts should be laid before the parties interested and the decision referred to them. In the former class of cases some hopes of improvement may be entertained.

The second factor of menstruation, the flow, we can influence by such measures as cause a more or less intense pelvic congestion. The ovaries sharing in this congestion, it is not impossible that ovulation is in some degree also promoted, but it can be only to a minor degree and when the ovaries are in a favorable condition. The uterus is the principal organ to be affected, and to it the most of these measures are addressed.

Direct treatment for the establishment of menstruation should be first of a character rather to solicit than to force the flow. These measures act best where, the general health having been restored, the flow does not appear, but the premonitory symptoms are present. Rest in bed, warmth to the pelvic region by poultices or other means, and hot drinks, are to be prescribed; among the latter infusions of pennyroyal, some of the mints, tansy, and cotton-root have a high domestic reputation and should be preferred. Hot pediluvia or hot sitz-baths, prolonged to twenty or thirty minutes, may be taken at bedtime. These may be rendered sufficiently stimulating to irritate the skin by the addition of mustard. More active measures are stimulating enemata and vaginal injections—for the former ten grains of aloes in mucilage, and for the latter liquor ammonia in milk, f℥j–Oj, gradually increasing the strength to production of slight leucorrhœa. Both these have the endorsement of high authority.

Such measures should be used or plied more assiduously about the period, when that is known. During the interval a tonic course is almost always required, and a powerful local influence can be exerted by cold sitz-baths of brief duration, say one or two minutes, once daily, followed by vigorous rubbing with a coarse towel or a flesh-brush.

There are a few drugs known as emmenagogues from the reputation they have of promoting the menstrual flow. They all are powerful stimulants or irritants, and as they are also nearly all abortifacients, their reputation is probably well founded. Modern physiology, by exploding the doctrine of peccant humors to be carried off by menstruation, and by establishing the doctrine of ovulation, has greatly diminished their importance, while the varied conditions and causes of amenorrhœa already given show at a glance how restricted is the field for their administration. To give them when the anatomical conditions are unknown is blind work; to force a function relating to reproduction when the general system is struggling for existence is folly; and to goad diseased organs with special stimulants is certain to do injury. Now and then, however, special stimulants of this class and of the class next to be considered are required. There are some cases which fail to respond to the measures already detailed; there are others, generally recognized by writers, when menstruation is absent without any deterioration of health, known as cases of sexual atony or torpor; and others in which the flow fails or disappears earlier than the usual age. In these latter atrophy of the ovaries may be suspected, but cannot be verified during life, and treatment should be faithfully continued so long as there is reasonable probability of success. One case occurred in the experience of the writer in which the menses appeared occasionally during two years, each time apparently brought on by special stimulants, but ceased at thirty-two, the general health remaining excellent.

The principal emmenagogue drugs heretofore relied on, besides iron, are saffron, apiol, rue, and savin. The first, from impurity and costliness, is rarely prescribed, yet Trousseau says it is a fact of public notoriety that women engaged in picking saffron suffer from frequent attacks of uterine hemorrhage. Apiol may be given in capsules in doses of five or six drops twice daily for a week before the expected flow, or fifteen drops may be administered in the course of the few hours immediately preceding. The oils of savin and rue are generally prescribed in doses of ♏ij–v, three times daily. Ergot and iodine figure sometimes as emmenagogues. The efficacy of the former is denied by very high authority. The latter was esteemed very highly by Trousseau. Its influence upon the scrofulous constitution may possibly explain its action in promoting menstruation.

The permanganate of potassium is a recent addition to emmenagogues, and the testimony in its favor is already sufficient to make it probable that it is the most efficient of the list. The indications for its use are want of action or atony of the organs. It should be administered during a few days or a week preceding the time for menstruation, in doses of from two to four grains three times daily; or two grains three times daily may be administered during the whole month. The union of its elements is but feeble, so that in pills as ordinarily made it would be very likely to undergo decomposition, while in solution it is unpleasant. Compressed tablets of the pure drug are now placed at command of the profession, and are an unexceptionable form for administration. The best time for taking the medicine is toward the close of the digestive process, and each dose should be followed by drinking at least a wineglassful of water. Pain in the stomach has been sometimes observed even when every precaution has been taken. The liability of the remedy to decomposition and its irritating powers are objections to it, but the testimony in favor of its power to bring on or promote the menstrual flow is at present very strong.

More decided measures of local stimulation than those already given may be resorted to, and are far more reliable than drugs. They are—tents, cupping the uterus, and electricity. A sea-tangle or tupelo tent may be kept in the uterus over night just previous to the time of the flow. In cases where stimulation rather than dilatation is needed a tent of slippery-elm bark may be used. Thomas recommends a rubber exhauster for cupping the cervix uteri. Simpson fashioned one for acting on the lining membrane of the body. These measures are most likely to be efficacious just before an expected period.

Electricity is the most reliable emmenagogue, and has such an amount of testimony in its favor as not to permit a doubt as to its value. It is the only direct uterine or menstrual stimulant except permanganate of potassium. Statical electricity is now but little used, although Golding-Bird published striking instances of its efficacy in amenorrhœa at an early day in its therapeutic history. Faradization is now most frequently resorted to. One pole is to be applied to the sacrum and the other above the pubes or over either ovary. The internal application of the current is much more powerful as well as less painful. It is administered by applying a cup-shaped electrode to the cervix, or by introducing an insulated sound into the uterus, the other electrode being external as before. The séances should be repeated every second or third day, and should be more frequent just before the periods when their time is known. Beard and Rockwell insist that general electrization should be administered at the same time, and Mann passes the constant current through the organs during the intervals and the faradic at the periods. Simpson originated a galvanic intra-uterine pessary, which Thomas has modified. It is doubtful whether the feeble current generated by these instruments produces any effect, or whether they act simply as mechanical irritants. When they are used, it should be borne in mind that there is eminent and high authority against the use of intra-uterine pessaries of any kind, and that all agree that a patient to whom one is applied should be kept under careful observation.

It must be stated that good results have been obtained with this class of local remedies in cases which would seem extremely unpromising— even in those in which amenorrhœa depends upon partially-developed organs. There is most positive testimony of the highest character as to good effects obtained in increasing development and promoting the flow.

Cases of acute suppression are to be treated by rest in bed, warmth locally by baths and applications, and hot drinks, as already detailed. Steaming the lower part of the body by placing the patient over the vapor arising from aromatic herbs upon which boiling water has been poured is a remedy which dates back to Hippocrates. Early in the case a drink of spirituous liquor, taken hot, is often efficacious. If, however, there is febrile action, diaphoretics should be administered, such as the liquor ammonii acetatis with spirits of nitrous ether, and aconite if required. Dry or wet cupping may be used if there is evidence of intense uterine congestion. Should internal metritis or inflammation of some pelvic organ result from acute suppression, the treatment will be that for the disease thus caused. If efforts to restore the suppressed flow do not prove speedily successful, special measures should be postponed until the next period, the general health meantime receiving due attention. At the return of the next period such of the remedies for amenorrhœa should be administered as may seem best adapted to the case, considered as to cause, condition of the organs, or constitution of the patient.

Vicarious menstruation is so closely allied to amenorrhœa as to demand some consideration here. The term is applied to a sanguineous flow, recurring at regular intervals, from some organ or part of the body other than the uterus. This flow has taken place from almost every organ or part of the body; most frequently, however, it has been from some mucous membrane, a wound, scar, or some part which by structure is favorable to the exit of blood. Amenorrhœa is frequently present, and is sometimes followed by acute suppression. Puech found 11 cases attended by vaginal atresia congenital, and in 42 others the uterus was absent or but partially developed. The treatment does not differ from that of amenorrhœa. While measures are used to restore normal menstruation, active repression of the abnormal flow should not be attempted, unless the organ from which it proceeds is one likely to be injured by its continuance.

Dysmenorrhœa.

Dysmenorrhœa, according to derivation, signifies a monthly flow with labor or difficulty; its modern synonym is painful menstruation.

In but a very small proportion of women is menstruation painless. Not only general and local distress attends it, but more or less pain.

When the suffering reaches such a degree as to demand relief, the case is one of dysmenorrhœa. In such cases the period generally commences with a more pronounced molimen than ordinary; as it progresses pain makes its appearance and gradually increases in severity. Its seat is the pelvic region, the back and loins, and down the thighs. It may be paroxysmal or continuous; in some cases the flow is accompanied by expulsive efforts like those of labor. The pain may last during the whole period, or relax very much, or even cease as soon as the flow is freely established. In degree it may reach any height, often causing the severest agony, taxing the powers of endurance to the utmost, and requiring the most energetic measures for relief.

The organs in proximity to the uterus, partaking as they do of the menstrual congestion, are also markedly affected. There is rectal tenesmus, and on the part of the bladder frequent micturition and dysuria. Remote organs are influenced either directly or by sympathy. The breasts become tumefied and tender. There is flatulence, nausea, or even vomiting. The nervous system, during normal menstruation in a state of erethism, responds readily to the painful impressions, and presents symptoms of the most varied character and degree, amounting even to general convulsions.

Attacks of severe pain recurring at short intervals cannot but exert a powerful deleterious influence upon the general health. Digestion is interfered with, nutrition and sanguification are imperfectly performed, and there is a continuous chain of deranged function. The results to the nervous system, indirect and direct, and sometimes also from the measures of relief resorted to, are most deplorable. From every point of view this class of cases presents the strongest claims for relief.

The discharge in dysmenorrhœa varies very widely in amount and character. It may be so scanty as to border on amenorrhœa or so profuse as to be menorrhagic. It may be more or less fluid than usual. The expulsion of clots is a frequent feature, and the size and shape of these sometimes give indications of value. Like other uterine derangements, dysmenorrhœa is not a disease per se, but a symptom of some pathological condition the exact nature of which is to be ascertained whenever possible. Cases may be classified as follows: I., Obstructive or mechanical; II., congestive; III., neuralgic; IV., membranous. It cannot be too distinctly kept in view that this classification, like many others, cannot be rigidly followed. The dividing-lines are sometimes but faintly drawn by nature; some cases present the features of more than one class; some by natural progress pass from one class into another. Based upon leading clinical features, this classification will assist in the study of the subject, facilitate diagnosis, and aid in directing therapeutic measures.

Two classes given by some authorities are not included in the above classification. They are spasmodic and ovarian dysmenorrhœa. If by the former is implied painful contractions of the uterus during menstruation, the cases fall into the first class given above, the obstructive; and if irregular nervous action is implied, they belong to the third, the neuralgic. The term ovarian has been applied to those cases in which an abnormal condition of the ovaries exists, such as inflammation, enlargement, or dislocation. Such conditions are not easily ascertained during life; if ascertained, the fact throws light on the etiology of the case; but for treatment the case will range itself, according to the clinical features it presents, among those in which the vascular or the neurotic element predominates.

Obstructive or mechanical dysmenorrhœa is that form in which some impediment exists to the free escape of the menstrual discharge. The genital canal presents no exception to the general rule that when an excretory channel is obstructed violent and painful expulsive efforts are excited.

The causes which give rise to the obstruction are various. Among them are the following: fibroid tumors of the uterus distorting, and polypi obstructing, its cavity or neck; stenosis of the cervical canal, either congenital or acquired, the latter often the result of the injudicious use of strong caustics; a long and conical cervix; a contracted os, sometimes so small as to be justly termed the pinhole os; versions and flexions of the uterus.

The seat of obseruction is almost always uterine, but may be in the vagina or at its entrance. There is much difference of opinion as to the relative frequency of occurrence of obstruction at the internal or external orifice of the cervix.

The pain in this form of dysmenorrhœa generally does not precede the flow. In character it is sometimes like colic, but its leading feature is expulsive effort. It occasionally so nearly resembles abortion as to require care to distinguish between them. It is frequently intermittent, presenting intervals of complete relief. In severity it varies widely. In some cases the patient assumes and maintains a certain position which she has learned affords her some relief. This indicates with great probability uterine distortion from fibroid tumor. The writer has met with a marked instance of this kind.

The flow is more irregular in this than in other forms. It is sometimes extruded drop by drop; more often it appears in gushes, the fluid accumulating and distending the uterus until expulsive efforts are excited. Clots are often thrown off under these circumstances in shape and size corresponding to the cavity of the uterus.

Absence of prodromata, presence of the fluid being necessary to excite the pain, the intermittent and especially the expulsive character of the pain, and the kind of clots, indicate the nature of the case. A certain diagnosis, however, rests alone on physical examination. This should be by the touch, bimanual and rectal, and the sound. Sometimes additional aid will be derived from the speculum. By touch the form, size, shape, and direction of the cervix are ascertained, and its relations to the body of the uterus. The sound will give evidence as to the patency and direction of the cervical canal and uterine cavity.

A diagnosis of obstructive dysmenorrhœa should not be rejected because the patient occasionally passes a period without pain. In the male an enlarged prostate may for a long time interfere but little with micturition, and then all at once completely obstruct the flow of urine. A diagnosis cannot be based alone upon the condition of the cervical canal as found during the intermenstrual period. Two elements are to be considered, each of which may, and doubtless often does, play a part: tumefaction from the congestion attendant on the process, and spasm. The latter, caused by reflex action excited by irritation in the body of the uterus, assumes a leading position with those who claim that obstruction is the sole cause of dysmenorrhœa. That it plays an active part in many cases cannot be doubted; that it is a necessary condition of even spasmodic dysmenorrhœa is disproved by the positive statement of Matthews Duncan, that in some cases he could pass a sound freely into the uterus during the paroxysms.

A due estimate of the part which a uterine flexion plays in producing the dysmenorrhœa is important, but very difficult. Theoretically, the narrowing of the canal at the point of flexion should account for the symptoms, but experience does not accord with theory. All cases of flexion are not accompanied by dysmenorrhœa, and when so accompanied removal of the deformity does not always cure. Siredey in 52 observations found only 22 cases of dysmenorrhœa. Emmet's carefully-prepared tables show that in nearly 50 per cent. of anteflexions menstruation is painless. The conditions necessary seem to be extreme flexion, producing an acute angle. In less-pronounced cases it is maintained by many that the flexion is an unimportant factor, and that the dysmenorrhœa depends upon secondary conditions produced by it, as endometritis and congestion. The problem is difficult, and each individual case requires careful study. The facts indicate that there is much in the pathology of this form of disease not yet fully understood.

Congestive dysmenorrhœa depends upon an advance of the menstrual congestion beyond the physiological limits. In these cases the patient generally suffers for a few days before the period from a sense of fulness, weight, and heat in the back and pelvic region. Pain follows, is more or less severe, and varies somewhat in character, although generally dull and heavy. The hypogastric region usually becomes distended, and is sometimes very tender to the touch over the ovaries, "especially on the left side, without any reason for the difference being known." After a longer or shorter duration of these symptoms the flow appears, and this is often, especially if free, followed by an amelioration of the pain. In many cases, however, there is no remission of the suffering upon the discharge occurring. Not infrequently the general circulation is affected, the face is flushed, the skin hot, and there is more or less fever.

The flow may vary widely as to quantity. It is often at first and for a time more profuse than normal. Leucorrhœa frequently precedes and follows it, persisting during the entire interval. During that time also the patient suffers much from backache and bearing down, with difficulty of walking or of remaining long on her feet.

Upon examination the vagina is found hot and tumefied, and increased arterial action is evident to the touch. The uterus is tender, enlarged, and heavier than usual. In cases associated with or dependent upon chronic inflammation or areolar hyperplasia the increase of size of the uterus during menstruation is marked. The sound may be used to determine the amount of enlargement and also the amount of tenderness. In cases dependent on endometritis touching the interior of the organ causes severe pain. Dyspareunia is frequently a symptom in this class of cases.

The conditions upon which congestive dysmenorrhœa depends are various, and may be either general or local or both combined. Plethora is rare in females, and local congestions are much more frequently dependent upon anæmia, the abnormal condition of the blood favoring them directly and also indirectly by its effect on the nervous system. In past times gout and rheumatism were considered to act frequently as the cause of dysmenorrhœa. They have almost disappeared from view since the era of direct examination began. Malaria, however, as a possible cause or a powerful factor should never be overlooked in regions where it prevails. The sexual instinct plays an important rôle; enforced abstinence, especially when suddenly brought about, and excess, being alike effective etiological factors. Young widows and prostitutes are both subject to this form of disease.

The local causes are numerous. Pelvic inflammations, as cellulitis or pelvic peritonitis, give rise to the disease. Affections of the uterus are frequent causes; displacements, as retroversion or prolapsus; and inflammation, either parenchymatous or of the endometrium. Quite a moderate grade of inflammation, as found during the interval, may, under the increased congestion of menstruation, become extreme. Many cases doubtless depend upon an ovarian influence even when no affection of these organs can be made out. Scanzoni hazards the theory that the maturation of Graäfian vesicles lying deeper than usual in the stroma of the ovary is one cause of this form of dysmenorrhœa.

In neuralgic dysmenorrhœa the neurotic element preponderates. The nerves play a part corresponding to that of the vessels in the congestive form. In some cases of this class no organic lesions can be discovered and they are then termed idiopathic.

This form of dysmenorrhœa depends upon either a peculiar condition of the general nervous system or upon hyperæsthesia of the sexual system, or both combined. Either or both may have been inherited or acquired. It is frequent in subjects of the hysterical temperament, and in those presenting that preponderance of the nervous system so often seen as the result of over-refinement, luxury, habits of idleness, and other violations of hygienic law. Those subject to it often suffer from severe headaches, neuralgia, and other nervous affections. It is often caused by anæmia or chlorosis. Sexual influences, psychical or physical, and especially those that excite without satisfying, are sometimes efficient causes. Ovarian influence is often an important factor; some authorities designate all those cases in which no anatomical change can be found, ovarian. The prodromata of this form are very apt to be some of those nervous attacks to which such patients are liable, as headache or neuralgia, and they may be psychical, as aberration of temper, undue irritability, or tendency to melancholy. In character the pain is generally stated to be more acute than in the other forms. It is subject to great and sudden alternations. In acuteness and irregularity it often justifies the term spasmodic. From these characters and from the absence of anatomical change a differential diagnosis may be made. As in this form the most marked nervous symptoms are witnessed, so are also the most pronounced complications on the part of the general nervous system. They are often hysterical in character, but may be of every kind and degree, even to general convulsions, and mental aberration is sometimes a complication or result.

Membranous dysmenorrhœa is characterized by the expulsion at the menstrual periods of organized membrane, either as a whole or in pieces. In the former case it is like a cast of the interior surface of the uterus. The expulsion of this membrane is accompanied by pain, often of the most severe character. The pain presents well-marked features; it is markedly expulsive, identical with that of the obstructive form, closely resembling an abortion, to which the membrane adds an additional element of similarity. This pain and these expulsive efforts may continue twelve, eighteen, or twenty-four hours, and then cease, to be renewed only at the next period.

This form of disease is rare—so rare that observers having a large field of observation may never meet with over half a dozen cases. In regard to many points very diverse views are held, and the limits of a practical work do not permit even a statement of all of them. The nature of the membrane is one of these points too important to pass over. When thrown off entire, its internal surface is smooth and marked by the openings of the utricular glands; its external or uterine face is rough and villous. It presents the exact shape of the interior of the uterus, with openings corresponding to the Fallopian tubes and the os. It is impossible to escape the conviction that this membrane is the lining membrane of the uterus, thrown off as a whole, instead of by gradual melting down of its superficial layers, as in normal menstruation. The microscope sustains this view, and this is the generally received opinion; yet that the membrane is not always such is testified by competent observers from observations with the same instrument. It seems probable that this disputed point will be settled, as have been so many others in medicine, in favor of both parties. Siredey suggests the possibility of different kinds of membrane in these cases, while Barnes boldly states this as a fact.

Various theories have been advanced to account for the formation of the membrane. An abnormal course of conception, a changed ovarian influence, a peculiar endometritis, have been from time to time favorite terms in which to express our ignorance. Only in regard to the first has unanimity been obtained. That the membrane is always a product of conception is not now maintained by any respectable authority. It is a well-established fact of the utmost importance that such membranes may be expelled when there has never been sexual intercourse.

The membrane of dysmenorrhœa is to be distinguished from fibrinous masses, the remains of blood-clots from which the corpuscles have been squeezed; from mucus coagulated into shreds by astringent injections; and from the products of membranous vaginitis. Neither of these will present much difficulty with the aid of the microscope. The case is very different, however, when the membrane is to be distinguished from the decidua of an early pregnancy. From a single specimen or a single attack a diagnosis cannot be made. Thomas gives an instance of disagreement as to the nature of the same membrane by two of the highest microscopical authorities. The recurrence of the attacks at the regular menstrual periods will establish the diagnosis.

The prognosis of dysmenorrhœa varies in the different classes. In the obstructive form it will depend upon the curability of the lesion upon which it depends, and the same may be said of the congestive. The neuralgic cases do not yield readily to treatment, especially when dependent upon a peculiar and perhaps inherited nervous constitution. Caution should be exercised, however, in expressing an unfavorable prognosis. ·

Like all nervous diseases in the female, it is subject to great mutations without apparent adequate cause, and will sometimes suddenly disappear in an inexplicable manner.

The membranous form affords still less promise of cure: the unsatisfactory results of treatment are generally acknowledged.

During an attack of dysmenorrhœa the patient should remain in bed for the benefit of rest and warmth. In those cases where the flow is not too free, and especially when relief follows its appearance, active measures to promote this end may be instituted by hot drinks and hot fomentations. In married patients a hot sitz-bath, during which the vaginal syringe is used to douche the uterus, is an efficient measure. Pain being the prominent symptom, and remedies for its relief being at hand and reliable, the indication is clear and the treatment can be briefly stated. In execution, however, it is not a simple problem : immediate relief is not alone to be considered. If opiates be resorted to for frequently-recurring pain, a habit will soon be formed that is no less a calamity than the disease itself. While, therefore, opium and its preparations are reliable remedies, and in many cases indispensable, they should be administered as seldom and as sparingly as possible, and always with an appreciation of possible injurious consequences. Many cases can be successfully managed with chloral hydrate, or belladonna, or Indian hemp. When opiates are resorted to, they should be combined as much as possible with other medicines by which their effects are modified, and relief afforded with the smallest possible dose. Thus in cases attended with vascular excitement these ends may be attained by the union of opium with tartar emetic or aconite ; when there is marked disturbance of the nervous system, it may be combined with an antispasmodic, as the compound spirit of ether. Administration by the rectum will produce a local as well as a general effect, and injections of starch and laudanum or suppositories of opium and belladonna may be administered. The speediest and most certain relief is afforded by the hypodermic syringe. Resort to it should, however, be rigidly controlled ; it should be used as a miser uses his gold, and it need scarcely be added that only very exceptional, if any, circumstances will ever justify placing the syringe in the hands of friends or attendants, no matter with what restrictions. Unfortunately, this is sometimes done, but very rarely without great injury resulting.

During the intervals general treatment should be instituted according to the indications. All functions at fault are to be regulated. Anæmia is to be corrected, the debilitating effects of malaria counteracted, good digestion promoted, and a weakened nervous system strengthened. These indications are met by tonics in various forms, notably iron and zinc ; by antiperiodics, as quinia and arsenic ; by stomachics ; and by the judicious use of wine. There are other remedies quite as useful as drugs—cold sponging and shower-baths, followed by vigorous rubbing, general electrization, and, when the patient cannot or will not take outdoor exercise, massage. Change of scene and air is sometimes beneficial or even necessary. In many cases of pronounced neuralgic form, or in which the nervous system has been shattered by the severity or long duration of the attacks, there can be but little hope of amelioration without a thorough change of habits and mode of life in every respect.

The local treatment will be according to the conditions present. In the obstructive form, polypi are to be removed if present, and in stenosis the patency of the canal restored. Dilatation may be accomplished by tents. Should these fail, resort may be had to surgical measures, as the frequent passage of bougies gradually increasing in size, forcible dilatation with steel dilators under an anæsthetic, or by incision. Each of these measures has its advocates, and with all cures have been effected. Flexions should be corrected as far as possible by a vaginal pessary. Intra-uterine pessaries more certainly correct the deformity, but great care should be exercised in their use. If inflammation be present, uterine or pelvic, they will not be tolerated or will do positive injury; nor should a patient with any instrument of this kind ever be allowed to pass out of reach of the physician unless she can herself remove it.

The treatment of many cases of congestive dysmenorrhœa is very similar to that of suppressed menstruation from cold—warm drinks, hot foot- and sitz-baths, fomentations, and douches.

Particular attention should be paid to the bowels, not alone to correct constipation, but to give full relief to a clogged portal system by saline purgatives. If there be prolapsus, a pessary should be adapted so as to keep the uterus up in its place; by this means passive congestion is much relieved. Bromide of potassium is a reliable remedy as a corrector of pelvic congestion. In the congestive cases of anæmic subjects iron will act beneficially; in inflammatory congestion it does injury. Dysmenorrhœa dependent upon hyperplasia or endometritis should receive the treatment appropriate to those affections.

In neuralgic dysmenorrhœa the general treatment is far more important than the local. All those hygienic and therapeutic measures already detailed should be faithfully persevered with. For the relief of pain and control of the nervous symptoms enemata of asafœtida are useful. Chloral may also be administered in the same way or by the stomach, with camphor, valerian, and the æthers as required. In this form apiol has been successfully used; the evidence as to its value is clearer than the explanations of its mode of action. It may be given in capsules, each containing five grains, one, two, or three daily.

Some local measures often render good service: among them is the passage of bougies, which sometimes modify the sensitiveness of the cervical canal, as they do that of the male urethra. The galvanic current, both continuous and Faradic, has effected cures, but the cases to which it is best adapted or in which it is most likely to be good cannot be clearly indicated. A galvanic stem-pessary may be used, observing due caution. This instrument has been modified and much improved by Thomas: being made like a string of metallic beads, it is extremely flexible, and many of its former objectionable features are removed.

A successful treatment of membranous dysmenorrhœa has not yet been promulgated. The great difficulty of its cure is admitted by the highest authorities. Some cases associated with stenosis of the cervix have been cured by dilatation—a fact which but strengthens the general principle of correcting all anatomical changes whenever possible. Strong caustics have been applied to the interior of the uterus with a view of exerting an alterative influence upon the seat of the disease. The course seems correct in theory, but in practice it has not proved fruitful of good results, and treatment in the majority of cases is limited to palliation.

In regard to marriage in females afflicted with dysmenorrhœa, it may be stated to be advisable in many cases of the neuralgic form and in anæmic subjects where the flow is so scanty as to border on amenorrhœa. In cases of the congestive form, if dependent on inflammation or on organic lesions, as fibroids, there is very great probability that the symptoms will be aggravated by this radical change of mode of life.

Menorrhagia.

The term menorrhagia signifies excessive menstrual flow. The excess may be by increased rate of discharge during the usual time, by lengthened duration, or by too frequent returns of the periods.

There are wide physiological limits to the amount of discharge and the duration of a menstrual period. While the average time is from three to five days, and the average amount from three to five fluidounces, both these terms may be doubled, or, on the other hand, they may be diminished to a single day and a single ounce, without detriment to the health. Menorrhagia may be said to exist when the flow is in excess as compared with what is usual with the individual, or when the loss is so great as to affect her general health.

The periodical return of the flow is of prime importance in establishing the existence of menorrhagia. Repetition at periods approximating the menstrual is the keynote of diagnosis. By this menorrhagia is distinguished from the hemorrhage of a miscarriage and from metrorrhagia. A profuse flow of blood after an absence of menstruation for one or two months is held by patients, in perfect good faith, to be the effect of taking cold : with almost absolute certainty such a train of events indicates an abortion. Metrorrhagia is uterine hemorrhage occurring independently of the menstrual periods. More surely indicative of organic disease than menorrhagia, it is often most closely allied to it ; many cases which in the early stages present an increased menstrual flow as a symptom are at a more advanced period accompanied by metrorrhagia.

Thus far the diagnosis of menorrhagia is easy. Not so that differential diagnosis upon which alone can therapeutic measures be based.

This derangement depends upon as many and as widely diverse causes as the others. It is often one expression of affections of the general system, is sometimes caused by disease of organs neither pelvic nor generative, is a common symptom of a number of organic diseases of the uterus, or it may be simply functional. The necessity for a thorough physical examination is apparent. By touch, single and bimanual, by the speculum, and by the uterine sound the condition of all the pelvic organs should be investigated. These means failing to reveal the cause of the menorrhagia, the examination should be pushed farther. The cervix should be dilated by tents and the cavity of the uterus explored. Very frequently this measure, and this alone, will reveal the cause of the derangement. Such an examination is often as valuable for its negative as for its positive results. No practitioner fulfils his duty to his patient or is just to himself who treats a menorrhagia for any length of time without making a physical examination. It may seem unnecessary to emphasize so plain a duty, yet consultants very frequently find cases in which palpable causes of the disease exist and where a direct examination has not even been proposed.

The following schedule will indicate the widely diverse conditions which may give rise to menorrhagia, and will serve as a guide to the study of the subject:

CAUSES OF MENORRHAGIA.—

I. Diseases of the General System:
  Plethora;
  Chlorosis and anæmia;
  Debility, as from excessive lactation;
  The exanthemata and typhoid fever;
  Hæmophilia;
  Scorbutic, uræmic, and malarial cachexiæ.

II. Local Affections, not Uterine:
  Cerebral, as psychical influences;
  Cardiac and pulmonary affections, as valvular disease, emphysema, and phthisis;
  Hepatic diseases, as cirrhosis and the changes produced by residence in tropical climates;
  Splenic and renal disease;
  Abdominal tumors and loaded bowels
  Peri-uterine inflammations;
  Ovarian influences.

III. Uterine Causes:
  Subinvolution;
  Areolar hyperplasia;
  Endometritis, with fungous growths;
  Laceration of the cervix, with eversion;
  Ulceration of the cervix;
  Displacement of the uterus;
  Polypi and fibroid tumors;
  Retention of products of conception;
  Malignant disease;
  Congestion.

I. Menorrhagia, the result of the first class of causes, but rarely occupies more than a subordinate position. The acute affections, as the exanthemata, do not afford time for more than a single flow, and this has been well termed uterine epistaxis. The condition of plethora is manifest. The cachexiæ are generally well marked and evident. An exception may be made in this regard as to the effect of prolonged residence in malarious locations. There can be no question that menorrhagia is frequently of malarial origin, and even when the patient does not present a cachectic appearance. The disease may be produced by hepatic and splenic derangement, by deteriorated sanguinification, or by depression of nervous force. Menorrhagia is not infrequently a result of Bright's disease; an examination of the urine would determine this point. That the opposite conditions of plethora and anæmia should both cause menorrhagia is not difficult of explanation; in the one there is excess of blood with increased vascular pressure; in the other, a changed condition of the blood favoring transudation, with loss of tone of the vessels.

II. That menorrhagia, as well as amenorrhœa, may have a purely emotional origin there can be no question, although this cause is not generally recognized. The following case is an illustration : A healthy young married woman, while menstruating, saw a neighbor's son thrown from his horse; his foot became entangled in the stirrup, and he was trampled to death before her eyes. She was immediately taken with flooding, and profuse menstruation occurred for several succeeding periods. Siredey expresses doubts as to cardiac and pulmonary diseases so frequently causing menorrhagia as they are generally believed to do. In a considerable experience during several years, and paying special attention to this point, he found but one case thus caused. The mechanical effect of disease of the abdominal organs in producing passive congestion in distal parts is more direct and the influence in producing menorrhagia more apparent. The same may be said of accumulations in the bowels and the pressure of abdominal tumors. Peri-uterine inflammations rank very high in the list of causes : their presence and results, direct and indirect, as abscesses, displacements of the uterus, etc., should never be overlooked. Ovarian influence is naturally a potent etiological factor ; menorrhagia is a frequent result of sexual excesses, and is often seen in prostitutes and where there is great disparity of age between the husband and wife.

III. Affections of the uterus itself are by far the most frequent cause of menorrhagia. The necessity of investigating accurately the condition of the great central organ of menstruation, and of ascertaining to what particular disease the derangement of the flow is to be attributed, will bear repetition. That an anatomical or pathological diagnosis can always be made is not maintained, but when examination has failed to reveal a basis for such a diagnosis, the practitioner should distrust his position and consider his diagnosis provisional only, awaiting more information from renewed examination or from further progress of the case. The cases are few in which such a diagnosis cannot be made. They are recognized by the term congestion as a cause in the schedule given above. Congestion is of course the prominent factor in many cases of menorrhagia, as in those from polypi and fibroids, those produced by ovarian influences, and others which are evident. But the class here recognized consists of those cases in which no anatomical or other cause can be found, excess of the congestive element of menstruation alone affording a rational explanation. Such cases occur most frequently at the two extremes of life—at puberty and at the menopause. During both these periods menorrhagia often occurs unexpectedly and inexplicably.

The grosser forms of uterine growths, as malignant disease, polypi, and fibroid tumors, are generally discovered without difficulty. The touch reveals them, or the sound or bimanual examination indicates their possible presence, which is confirmed by dilatation of the cervix and exploration of the cavity of the uterus. This class of cases gives rise more frequently to metrorrhagia ; only exceptionally is the hemorrhage confined to the menstrual periods.

A recent delivery in the history of the patient will indicate with some probability one of several conditions which may give rise to menorrhagia. Especially is this the case if the complete generative cycle has been broken in any part of its course. If there has been a miscarriage, there will be great probability of retained portions of the placenta or membrane if from death of the child or other cause nursing has not been performed, the conditions will be favorable for subinvolution of the uterus; if labor has been instrumental or precipitate, laceration of the cervix may be sus- pected. The first two far exceed in frequency the last as causes of menor- rhagia. Laceration of the cervix exists often without producing this functional disturbance, while subinvolution and retention of products of conception are very often active agents.

Displacements of the uterus, either prolapsus or versions and flexions, often have menorrhagia as a symptom.

The chronic inflammatory affections of the uterus are fruitful causes, and menorrhagia is often found associated with, and sometimes dependent on, the condition known as chronic corporeal metritis or areolar hyper- plasia, with consecutive erosions or ulcerations. Inflammation of the lining membrane of the uterus accompanied by granulations or fungous growths is one of the most frequent causes of menorrhagia. Opinions differ as to the part inflammation plays in producing this condition. Its entire absence in some cases is not improbable, the fungosities springing from the seat of the placenta. By Winckel the affection is termed ade- noma diffusum et polyposum corporis uteri; by Olshausen it is called endometritis fungosa. Under various names the condition is well known and recognized as one of the most frequent of all the uterine causes of · menorrhagia; Siredey believes it to be the origin of nearly one-half the cases. Due consideration of this cause is especially important, because especial investigation is required for its detection. The cervix must be dilated and the blunt curette passed over the internal uterine surfaces. This will furnish ocular and tangible evidence by detaching and bringing away some of the fungous growths, and a diagnosis will thus be made impossible in any other way.

In considering the treatment of menorrhagia the management of the patient during the intermenstrual periods must first engage attention. The general health is to be promoted in every possible way and sound hygienic regimen enforced. Two points demand especial attention— the clothing and the bowels. All tight bandages around the abdomen should be loosened, and all skirts and underclothing which hang upon the hips be supported from the shoulders. The beneficial influence of free action of the bowels cannot be overrated. Regular daily move- ment is required in all cases, but much more is often of decided benefit. In menorrhagia of the menopause in patients who have accumulated con- siderable adipose tissue, especially about the abdomen, in those where there is evident hepatic derangement, and in some others free purgation with salines is one of the most efficient measures of treatment.

During the menstrual intervals cachexiæ are to be treated according to their nature. Chlorosis and anæmia will require iron, quinine, nux vom- ica, and other tonics—the malarial cachexia the same, with the addition of arsenic, which often renders especial service under these circumstances. Then, too, the various uterine lesions giving rise to menorrhagia must be corrected. Subinvolution is to be remedied, polypi removed, the evil effect of fibroids combated by hypodermic injections of ergot, displace- ments corrected by suitable pessaries, the tone of the vessels and tissues of the pelvis increased by cold bathing, and all indications fulfilled· according to the nature of the case. For details of treatment the reader is referred to the articles upon the various general, local, and uterine diseases which have been shown to cause menorrhagia.

Especial attention should be given to girls whose menstrual life begins with menorrhagia, lest a vicious habit become fixed. The evils of school-life or those of sedentary indoor occupations should be corrected, and rest in the recumbent position during menstruation enforced. For the menorrhagia of puberty tonics, especially nux vomica and brief applications of cold to the pelvic region, are particularly indicated.

During an attack of menorrhagia the first remedy, and one without which all others are useless, is rest in the recumbent position. If the attack be severe recumbency should be absolute. Food should be light in quality and moderate in amount, while all drinks are to be taken cold, as ice-water, iced lemonade, or water acidulated with sulphuric acid and sweetened to the taste, the beneficial effect of acids in addition to cold being generally recognized. The bed should be hard and the clothing light, and the foot of the bedstead may be raised some inches. Many cases require no more active measures of repression. In subjects about the menopause, in some cases of malignant tumor, and in some others the hemorrhage seems to be a vent, and in moderate degree is rather beneficial. Such cases are to be watched, but need not necessarily be actively treated, certainly not with repressants and astringent applications, until regimen and mild measures have been tested.

In proceeding to medication the state of the general system first demands consideration. If there be increased vascular action and temperature, with evidences of active congestion of the pelvic region, manifested by pain, distension, and tenderness of the hypogastric region, with heat and throbbing of the passages, arterial sedatives and relaxants will be demanded. Aconite or veratrum viride may be given until an effect is produced on the pulse, and they may be combined to advantage with salines, as the liquor ammonii acetatis. It is in these conditions, of rare occurrence, that nauseants, such as ipecacuanha, are of service.

Medicines having a more direct action in checking uterine hemorrhage produce their effect by exciting contraction of the uterine walls and blood-vessels, moderating congestion, and modifying the condition of the nervous system. They are ergot, digitalis, bromide of potassium, quinine, cannabis indica, and cinnamon.

Ergot stands at the head of the list from its well-known effect in causing uterine contraction, and although reliable in proportion to the increased size of the uterus and the distension of its cavity, it is indicated in almost all cases for its hæmostatic action on the capillaries, as well as for its specific action on the uterus. Digitalis slows the action of the heart and excites the contractility of the arterioles, while experience has proved it to be an efficient remedy for menorrhagia. Bromide of potassium moderates vascular and nervous excitement of the pelvic organs, and is especially indicated in cases having an ovarian origin. Several of the French writers give very strong testimony in favor of the efficacy of cinnamon as a remedy, having tested it in a large number of cases without other medicines. It may always be used as an adjuvant.

All these medicines may be combined in various proportions, and they should be given in full doses. Infusion is the best form for the administration of digitalis. Sulphate of quinia in doses of gr. vj–x is often an efficient remedy, and especially in cases where there have been malarial influences. Cannabis indica is stated, by very high authority, to be one of the best remedies, although its mode of action is not clear. Iron should be administered as an hæmostatic tonic, and not merely because there is some uterine disease or derangement.

The action of medicines may be supplemented by local applications. Cloths wrung out of cold water or vinegar and water may be applied to the hypogastric region or to the vulva. A bladder or rubber bag filled with pounded ice may be laid on the abdomen above the pubes, or applied to the lumbar region for its effect upon the spinal cord. One of the most efficient means of applying cold is by an enema of cold water, or, this failing, of ice-water. The rectum and uterus being contiguous, the cold is applied almost directly. Siredey speaks highly of the cold douche to the soles of the feet, the water being projected in jets from a sprinkler. During the application uterine contractions are felt and the flow stops. This is more especially adapted to debilitated and anæmic patients with loss of vascular tone. Patients will often object to the application of cold to check a flow of blood from the uterus, knowing well the bad effects of suppression of menstruation which often results from exposure to this agent. It is believed that evil results never follow the application of cold when the flow is excessive; perhaps because the system and the organs concerned have been relieved.

The application of heat is also an efficient remedy—hot-water bags to the spine on Chapman's plan, or hot vaginal injections may be administered, as recommended by Trousseau and Emmet, the water being at a temperature as high as the patient can bear. To be properly administered the aid of a nurse is required, as the flow should be kept up for some time, at least a gallon of water being used.

There is only apparent contradiction in the use of both cold and heat to check uterine hemorrhage. Various explanations of the action of both have been given, and much argument presented why one should act better than, or be preferred to, the other. The truth is, that both are efficacious, and the value of both is based upon clinical experience.

The flow in menorrhagia is sometimes, if rarely, so excessive as to demand mechanical means of restraint. A well-applied tampon gives absolute control, and should never be omitted when the hemorrhage is severe and the practitioner is not within easy reach of the patient. Plugging the cervix with a sponge tent, supported by a vaginal tampon, is to be preferred as most reliable, and also because upon its removal the uterus can be explored for diagnosis or is prepared for direct applications. Should a vaginal tampon alone be trusted, it must be thoroughly applied to be reliable. This can only be done through a speculum, preferably with Sims's duckbill. Pledgets or discs of cotton, the first provided with strings to facilitate removal, squeezed out of a carbolized saturated solution of alum, should be packed carefully and firmly around and over the cervix, and the vagina filled. A folded napkin to the vulva, supported by the usual T bandage, sustains the whole. Such a tampon may remain, if necessary, thirty-six hours, the catheter being used to relieve the bladder.

Direct applications to the interior of the uterus are sometimes necessary both to check the flow and, in some cases, especially those dependent upon fungous growths of the endometrium, as a means of cure. They may be either fluid by application or injection, or solid. The former may be by swabbing the interior of the uterus by means of an applicator armed with cotton dipped in the liquid, or by injection. The drugs used for application are carbolic acid diluted with glycerin or pure tincture of iodine, or the stronger tincture known as Churchill's, Monsell's solution, or the liquor ferri perchloridi diluted or of full strength. The preparations of iron are objectionable from the hard, gritty, and disagreeable coagula formed, and the tincture of iodine is generally quite as efficient as a hæmostatic and more active as an alterative.

For efficient application the cervix should be dilated if not sufficiently patulous, and a cervical speculum should be used, or the solution will be squeezed out of the cotton before it reaches the seat of the disease. For injection the same articles are used, beginning with weaker solutions and gradually increasing the strength. They should never be resorted to without the utmost caution. The os should be patulous as a sine quâ non, and the injection carefully administered. In case the os is open the instrument may be the common extra long-pipe rubber syringe bent to a suitable curve by heating. This having been charged with a drachm or so of the liquid, the end is served with cotton like an applicator ; over this several clove-hitch turns with a string are taken, so that the cotton may be withdrawn if pulled off in the uterus. The pipe is then carried to the fundus and the piston very slowly depressed. Buttle's syringe is a more elegant and a safer instrument in cases where the os is not thoroughly opened. The terminal pipe of this instrument is very slender and perforated with minute openings, and the piston is forced in by screw-action of the handle, so that the fluid is expelled drop by drop.

Nitrate of silver is sometimes applied in solid form to the interior of the uterus, both as a means of checking excessive hemorrhage and to effect a cure by modifying the condition of the endometrium. It may be done with a probe, the end of which has been coated with the substance, passed in detail over the inner surface of the organ. A piece of the solid caustic is also sometimes carried into the uterus and left there, the application à demeure of the French, some of whom claim that in their hands this measure has never failed to check the hemorrhage.

In those cases where positive evidence has been gained that the disease depends upon fungous growths of the endometrium there is yet another and a more reliable remedy. It is the curette. By this instrument the growths which are the origin of the menorrhagia can be certainly and safely removed, their return prevented by a thorough application of iodine to the surface from which they spring, and a cure often effected when all other means have failed.

Intra-uterine applications, injections, and surgical measures affecting the interior of the uterus have been detailed, as they are advised and used by authorities. It remains to give an opinion as to their merits, and to state the precautions which should be taken when they are resorted to.

First, it must be said that there is a very considerable difference of opinion as to the safety of these measures. While some do not hesitate to apply to the interior of the uterus fuming nitric acid, and introduce pieces of nitrate of silver to dissolve there, others are extremely careful about making any applications to this part, and reject intra-uterine injections altogether. Nor can it be denied that very severe symptoms have frequently, and death sometimes, followed the application of these remedies. In resorting to them, therefore, the practitioner cannot be too minute in observing every precaution, and they should never be resorted to if evidence of peri-uterine inflammation exists. No intra-uterine injection should be given unless the os be patulous, and the fluid should be thrown in with the utmost gentleness. The milder articles should be tried first, and the severer only as the temper of the uterus is tested. Always treat the patient afterward as the subject of an operation, keep her in bed strictly, and combat the first symptoms of trouble with opium.

While the writer would not be just to the reader if he did not state that some very high authorities are strongly opposed to intra-uterine injections and applications, he would not be just to himself did he not state that his own experience has been favorable to them. While he once saw severe and dangerous symptoms follow syringing the cervix with water to cleanse it of mucus, he never in a single instance saw any evil effects from intra-uterine injections properly administered, nor from nitrate of silver à demeure or the application of nitric acid. But while these measures have often ameliorated cases of menorrhagia where the endometrium was affected, they have seldom cured, as compared with the curette. Indeed, the general statement may be made that as of late years the value of the curette has become more and more recognized, resort to severe intra-uterine applications has proportionally diminished. From his experience he is fully prepared to believe with Courty, that "there are cases of uterine hemorrhage which cannot be mastered in any other way," and with Siredey, that "the operation cures in the great majority of cases." It should be noted, in this connection, that some of the warmest advocates of the instrument explain its beneficial effects otherwise than by the removal of fungosities. Thus, Thomas attributes them to "the fracture of tortuous and distended blood-vessels," and Siredey to "the irritation and excitation produced by its introduction and action during reflex contractions."

INFLAMMATION OF THE PELVIC CELLULAR TISSUE AND PELVIC PERITONEUM.

By B. F. BAER, M. D.

THE subject of inflammation of the tissues surrounding the uterus and its appendages would be very much simplified, especially for the general practitioner, by debarring it of all new and superfluous names and sub-divisions, and by treating it on a broad clinical basis. It will be my aim in this paper to keep that idea constantly in view, rather than to follow the history and varying pathological views by which it has been sur-rounded and complicated.

The importance of this disease is probably greater in its influence on the health and future usefulness of the woman than any other ; and its causes and prevention, as well as its early recognition and treatment, should be fully understood by the physicians who are most likely to be first consulted in the matter, those engaged in general practice. I feel safe in making the statement that were this so, many of the chronic cases of almost incurable displacement of the uterus, Fallopian tubes, and ova-ries, resulting from thickened, indurated, and contracted ligaments, with their distressing symptoms, would never reach the gynecologist, because they would not then exist. In many cases the disease would have been prevented ; in others it would have been arrested in its incipiency.

Whether we understand the primary pathological lesion to be inflam-mation of the cellular tissue, the peritoneum, the lymphatics, or the veins, matters very little, practically, if we recognize the immediate location of the process ; for there can be no doubt that the disease, once started, soon involves to a greater or less degree all of the tissues and organs adjacent to it, and the therapeutic requirements will be much the same in either case.

That inflammation of the cellular tissue can exist without also involving the peritoneum in its neighborhood is scarcely to be conceived, and vice versâ ; but the one has always a predominating influence over the other, and differs somewhat in its cause, course, and consequences. When the inflammatory process has its origin in the cellular tissue, it is more likely to run through a regular course and end in abscess than if it had started as a peritonitis, in which case the course of the disease is often more chronic, resulting in the formation of false membranes which bind the uterus and other pelvic organs in permanent displacement. For these reasons, and for the more systematic study of the subject, I think it best to follow the plan of those authors who describe the disease separately under the two general heads, Parametritis and Perimetritis.

Parametritis.[1]

DEFINITION AND SYNONYMS.—By parametritis is understood an inflammation of the cellular or connective tissue near the uterus and beneath the pelvic peritoneum, including principally the locality close to the lateral margin of the uterus between the layers of the broad ligaments, although embracing also all of the various spaces where connective tissue abounds —viz. between the peritoneal folds which form the utero-sacral and utero-vesical ligaments. I think it a better name than pelvic cellulitis or peri-uterine inflammation, because it more correctly expresses the primary location of the disease than any other. The disease has been described under many other appellations, among which have been pelvic abscess and peri-uterine phlegmon.

ETIOLOGY.—Parametritis does not occur before puberty, and rarely before the great predisposing causes, abortion and injury at parturition, have prepared the parts—opened up the channel—for the more ready advance of the inflammatory process. This is easily understood when we remember how compactly bound together are these ligamentous folds, and how small the cellular-tissue spaces are before impregnation when compared with the condition of the parts after the function of gestation has been performed. Even were no accident to occur to interfere with the perfect involution of the parts which enter into the process of the expulsion of the product of conception, the tissues would probably always remain more vulnerable than before the gestation had occurred. But when the retrograde change which is necessary to perfect involution is retarded, a condition of relaxation and looseness of the parts results which increases many fold the liability to the affection. The blood-vessels and lymphatics remain large, and the connective-tissue cells are not only larger in size, but a cell-proliferation is probably induced as a result of the increased amount of blood-supply. Then a certain low condition of the general nutrition, a diathesis or an inflammatory tendency, no doubt act as predisposing causes of this disease. Now, add to the predisposing causes the injury which probably always attends abortion, and that which so often results from parturition proper, and a condition results which I believe to be the cause of parametritis in the majority of the cases.

Abortion the result of accident or design is a most prolific cause of parametritis, because abortion is so often followed by endometritis, which is frequently the starting-point of the former. Abortion results in a wounding of almost the entire surface of the uterine cavity, from which the placenta is torn, and often also in direct injury to the tissues of the neck of the womb. This almost necessarily interferes with involution; and if nothing worse follows immediately, there is left a strong tendency to a low grade of inflammation or hyper-nutrition, which may practically result in the same condition of induration and thickening of ligaments. It is seldom that the subject of an abortion of this character escapes from a certain degree of parametritis. If it does not manifest itself at the time in violent symptoms, the results are found afterward, when the patient is forced to consult her physician for the relief of suffering the consequence of the thickening and induration mentioned above.

[1] Virchow, Duncan.

Parturition without injury or accident is a predisposing cause, as before mentioned, of parametritis, and renders the patient more susceptible to the disease from cold, fatigue, etc., and from septic influences; but when the labor has resulted in injury to the soft parts, as laceration of the cervix, endometritis, injury to the vessels outside of the uterus, in the l road ligaments from pressure, the disease is far more liable to follow.

Parametritis may result from the various operations on the perineum, vagina, and uterus; from the application of medicines to the uterine cavity; and it is even said that the disease has been excited by the introduction of the uterine sound. I cannot believe that the simple introduction of the sound, when properly done, can be the means of so much harm. If harm follows, it must result from carelessness or want of skill. Of course there are contraindications to the use of the sound, and if these are violated evil will often follow. The use of the instrument ought not to be thought of if a suspicion of pregnancy exists, or when there is marked tenderness of the uterus or of the parts around it, or just before, during, or immediately after menstruation, and certainly not when active inflammation is present. Then the awkward manipulation of the sound when the uterus is fixed as a result of a former inflammation is very apt to relight anew the process.

If the same restrictions are applied and care used in the medication of the uterine cavity, the cases in which parametritis will follow as a result will be almost nil. The same will apply to operations. The danger lies in proceeding with the treatment of cases as they present themselves, by a hurried method and without fully investigating the condition of the tissues and organs outside of the uterus itself.

There is probably no place where experience is of more value than in the manipulations and instrumental measures necessary for the diagnosis and treatment of the various diseases of the pelvic organs—where more depends upon the skill and care of the operator. I believe, with Duncan, that pelvic inflammation and abscess are always secondary, and that these tissues are not specially inclined to idiopathic inflammatory action. But, undoubtedly, certain low conditions of the system or certain individual peculiarities furnish such a strong predisposing influence that a mechanical cause otherwise inactive will be sufficient in some of these cases to produce the disease. We probably see this expressed most fully in the low types of puerperal inflammations which develop gradually and without apparent cause, so far as injury at labor is concerned, and which often persistently progress to a fatal termination. It will be said that these are cases of septic origin; and it may be true, but I believe the poison is developed autogenetically.

COMPLICATIONS.—Parametritis is usually associated with perimetritis, and it may be complicated by ovaritis, endometritis, and salpingitis. Uterine displacement also often complicates this disease; and I wish here to emphasize the statement that no attempt should be made at restoring the organ to its normal position until all evidence of active inflammation shall have subsided. I have seen great harm result from such attempt having been made on the supposition that the symptoms were due to the displacement rather than to the parametritis.

ANATOMY, PATHOLOGY, COURSE, AND TERMINATION.—Everywhere in the pelvis, below the peritoneum, connective tissue is found in sufficient abundance to serve the purposes for which it exists—viz. first, as a bond of union between the pelvic viscera and organs, bladder, uterus, rectum, ovaries, and Fallopian tubes; second, to surround, support, and protect the numerous blood-vessels, lymphatics, and nerves from injury during the mechanical disturbances to which the pelvic tissues are subjected in the performance of their various functions.

If it were not for the padding of the pelvic connective tissue, which allows a free range of movement to the pelvic contents, the ordinary sudden jars from walking, coughing, etc. could not be sustained without pain, nor could the functions of the rectum and bladder be fulfilled properly; much less could the functions of coition and gestation be performed. This cellular tissue most abounds where it is most needed—in the locality or spaces where the vessels and nerves are found in greatest number; viz. at the sides of the uterus and upper portion of the vagina, extending outward between the folds of the broad ligaments toward the pelvic wall and the under surface of the Fallopian tubes and ovaries; next, within the folds of the utero-sacral ligaments and the vesico-uterine space beneath the peritoneum. There is little between the peritoneum and posterior vaginal wall, between the bladder and its peritoneal investment, as well as between the rectum and peritoneum; and there is none between the latter membrane and the posterior, superior, and anterior surfaces of the body of the uterus.

This areolar tissue is the seat of the disease under consideration, and from a priori reasoning it would be inferred that the inflammatory process would be found most frequently and in greatest severity in the locality where this tissue and the vessels most abound; and this is true, for parametritis almost always has its starting-point immediately at the sides of the uterus, in the lower inner edge of the broad ligaments.

But there is another reason why the disease so often begins here. It is the point, which, with the cervix, must bear the brunt of the pressure and injury during parturition and abortion, as well as from many of the operations which are performed upon the uterus. That inflammation of these tissues is secondary to injury is proven by the fact that we so often find the results of it, induration and thickening of the broad ligaments, in the cases of laceration of the cervix which come under our care. I have constantly observed that the inflammatory indurations were greatest on the side on which the laceration was most extensive, and that were the laceration unilateral the evidences of inflammatory action would be unilateral also. I have so frequently met with this condition in connection with laceration of the cervix that I have come to regard its entire absence as quite exceptional. I refer now to the deeper lacerations. Of course these inflammatory products are met with when the cervix is entire and apparently healthy, but this does not disprove the statement that they are probably invariably secondary, and very often secondary to injury at labor; for while the cervix may have escaped laceration, the tissues and vessels may have been so contused from pressure and instrumental measures as to result in the disease. But, however originated, the inflammation and infiltration advance in the direction of least resistance—*i. e.* along the course of the connective-tissue spaces between the various ligaments. The product of the inflammation, the pus, would therefore most likely follow these channels in making its exit. If the primary inflammation arise at the base of the broad ligament, it may travel within the folds of the ligament outward to the lateral wall of the pelvis and upward to the iliac fossa.   This is probably the course which is most commonly taken by the process in puerperal parametritis, and to which is due the induration and tumor which so often exist in that region during the course of the disease. Tumor in the iliac fossa, however, is not at all uncommonly met with in the course of a severe parametritis in the non-puerperal state, and it is doubt-less of the same pathological character.   Or the infiltration may propa-gate in the folds or under surfaces of the utero-sacral ligaments, resulting in the formation of a tumor which may eventually surround the rectum. In rare cases, and probably only in the puerperal, the process may develop higher up and more anteriorly, finally taking the direction and following the course of the round ligaments ; but I have never met with an instance of it.   And it would be impossible to tell correctly in a case opening in the groin—without a post-mortem demonstration, the opportunity for which, fortunately, does not often occur—whether the pus had not de-scended subperitoneally along the pelvic brim toward the inguinal region. Of course the inflammation and infiltration may be general, so that the uterus may be surrounded by exudation tumors, but this is the exception. Inferiorly, the parametritic process is limited by the pelvic fascia which covers the levator ani muscle.

Parametritis, as phlegmonous inflammations elsewhere, has three stages : 1st, that of active congestion ; 2d, that of effusion of serum ; 3d, that of suppuration.   But the disease does not reach the third stage in all cases. It may be arrested in the first stage or end by resolution in the second. I believe, however, that resolution in the second stage is the exception and not the rule.   First, because to end in suppuration is the natural course of the disease ; and secondly, because in many of those cases which are carefully observed the ordinary symptoms of the formation of pus, as chill, etc., are usually manifested, and followed by its evacuation. The fact that pus is not discovered should not be accepted as proof that the disease has not advanced to the suppurative stage ; for it may be so small in quantity as to escape observation, or it may be discharged into the bowel so high up as to mix with the fecal matter, so that its character is lost by the time it is expelled from the anus, or the point of exit may be so small as to allow it to escape guttatim, and thus elude detection.

Further, pus is sometimes formed and reabsorbed harmlessly, or it may remain deeply seated in a cavity—usually, under these circumstances, a number of small cavities — where it may undergo decomposition and result in the absorption of septic material and destruction of the patient before it finds exit.   Then, again, it may become encysted and be retained indefinitely, when it is a source of constant and sometimes obscure suffer-ing, as well as an abiding cause of a renewed attack of the disease.

It is probable also that the process is sometimes arrested in the second stage, neither resolution nor suppuration taking place, the serous por-tion of the liquor sanguinis being absorbed, the remainder undergoing a change to plastic lymph, so called, which proceeds to organization, result-ing in persistent induration of the affected parts ; or, instead of being absorbed, the serum may remain encysted within cavities formed for it by the lymph.   This likewise subjects the patient to the constant menace of a renewal of the inflammation.   The late D. Warren Brickell of New

Orleans has called special attention to what he named the serous form of pelvic inflammation, and which he thought had been too much neglected.[1] I have met with at least one well-marked case which supports Brickell's views.

The usual course, however, of an acute parametritis which has advanced to suppuration is evacuation of the pus by the most favorable channel— *i. e.* through the rectum or vagina. If through the latter organ, the point of perforation is either directly posterior to, or a little to the side of, the cervix. But if the inflammation be located in the vesico-uterine space— which is rare, however—the point of rupture may be anterior to the cervix. Less frequently the bladder is perforated and the pus discharged with the urine. More rarely the abscess is discharged through the abdominal wall, groin, or saphenous opening, and still more rarely through the sacro-ischiatic and obturator foramina. It may also find exit through the floor of the pelvis near the anus, and it may rupture into the peritoneal cavity, but the latter termination is fortunately the least common. This is probably due to the fact that the slightest irritation and pressure, under these circumstances especially, result in adhesive inflammation between the peritoneal surface of the abscess and that of the intestine with which it may be in contact, thus favoring rupture into the intestinal tract. Then, rupture into the intestine is conservative and protective, and the other is not, for should the pus be discharged into the peritoneal cavity the patient would most likely perish.

When the abscess opens at its most dependent portion, which is the rule, it is kept thoroughly drained of the pus, and if a single cavity exists it gradually contracts, and under favorable circumstances soon disappears, the trouble ending by absorption of the wall of the abscess. This is the most favorable termination of a parametritis, and belongs only to the acute form.

When the pus has not been evacuated from the bottom of the sac, or when there is more than a single cavity and only one is drained, or where the pus has taken one of the circuitous routes mentioned above, the disease merges into the chronic form, and may then be indefinitely prolonged by the formation and evacuation of abscess after abscess, until the pelvic cellular tissue becomes involved throughout and riddled by fistulous tracts connecting them.

SYMPTOMATOLOGY.—Pain is probably the first symptom to attract the attention of the patient, and if the attack is sudden or acute the pain is usually attended by a chill of more or less severity. The pain may be so sharp and lancinating as to cause the patient to cry out in agony, or it may be of a throbbing, aching character. If the former, it indicates either intense congestion of the vessels and tissues involved, or that the peritoneum is largely implicated, probably both. Where the pain is of this character the attack is usually of shorter duration, since it is soon followed by the second stage, exudation, when the symptom is at once modified, becoming less acute and resembling now the pain attending an attack of less severity. Of course the location of the pain corresponds to the seat of the inflammatory process. If it is in one or the other broad ligament, the pain is greater in the right or left iliac regions, most

[1] "The Treatment of Pelvic Effusions," *Amer. Journ. of the Med. Sciences,* Philada., April, 1877.

frequently in the left.   Pain is often experienced in the hypogastric and
sacral regions in the beginning of, or preceding, an attack of parametritis,
aud it is due to congestion of the endometrium and uterus, from which
the disease is spreading to the looser cellular-tissue spaces in the ligaments.
If, however, sacral pain persists throughout the course of the disease, or
exists in that region chiefly, it indicates that the inflammation has become
general or has invaded the utero-sacral ligaments.   But it would not be
correct to estimate the extent of the disease by the amount of pain
complained of, for that symptom depends so largely upon the temperament of the patient and her station in life that it is not trustworthy.
Some women suffer so much that they become inured to it or acquire the
habit of suffering in silence; others, from temperament, do not actually
experience pain; whilst others, again, from a love of hardihood, do not
complain, although they may be enduring constant and severe pain.   To
one of these classes those cases must belong which are said to pass through
an attack of parametritis without suffering.   That cases do rarely present
themselves, on account of mild but persistent symptoms, which are found
on examination to contain a large pelvic exudation, I can attest; but I
have so constantly found on careful questioning that the usual symptoms
of pelvic inflammation were present at some time during the course of
the existing illness that I cannot agree with the statement made by some
authors that this disease may develop "without causing any particular
disturbance" (Emmet).

As a rule, the bladder and rectum are reflexly affected, the former
sometimes becoming very irritable, so that there often exists a constant
desire to micturate.   Constipation is the rule, though I have known a
severe diarrhœa to accompany the disease, the result, I thought, of reflex
irritation.   The stomach also is often sympathetically affected, nausea,
and sometimes vomiting of an aggravated form, being present.

With a subsidence of the chill the temperature begins to rise, and continues to increase, with evening exacerbations, until it reaches 102° to 103°,
usually its highest point.   It may, however, rise suddenly and reach as
high as 104° or even 105°—rarely above the latter point.   The pulse is
usually full, and beats from 112 to 120 per minute, sometimes oftener.

In severe cases tympanites exists, with great tenderness in the hypogastric region; the thighs are also flexed upon the abdomen to protect
the parts from pressure and to relieve the abdominal muscles from tension.   But when these symptoms are marked it may be confidently concluded that the peritoneum is extensively involved.

Within a few days to a week from the initial symptoms the stage of
effusion is probably completed or well advanced, when the symptoms are
usually ameliorated.   Pain is diminished and the temperature decreased,
and if, happily, resolution begins, the patient may gradually recover during the succeeding two or three weeks.   But, unfortunately, this very
favorable course is not the usual one.   Instead of it, the disease often
advances to the third stage, that of suppuration.   This stage is very
commonly ushered in and manifested by rigors or chill, followed by a
rise in temperature and an increase in the pulse-rate.   There may now be
daily afternoon exacerbations of temperature, followed by sweating, until
the pus is disposed of, usually by evacuation.

PHYSICAL SIGNS.—If an opportunity is afforded for making a vaginal examination during the first stage, it will be found that the local temper-ature is markedly increased, that great tenderness exists, and that the parts involved are rigid from congestion. A little later this rigidity or erection subsides, and a bogginess may be discovered at the point or points where effusion is now taking place. Still later, a rather firm and, it may be, irregular swelling of variable size and location can be detected, usually in one of the broad ligaments, and from the size of a hen's to that of a goose's egg. If the inflammation has existed on both sides of the uterus, the pelvic roof, so called, may be found as hard and firm as a board. If pus has formed, fluctuation may be felt, and later a softening process may be detected, indicating the point where Nature is attempting to rid herself of the product of the inflammation.

The uterus is usually displaced by the exudation to an extent depending upon the size of the swelling, to which it is fixed more or less firmly. If the effusion has taken place in one of the broad ligaments, the organ will be displaced to the opposite side, but if the inflammatory process has extended to the cellular tissue in the posterior region of the cervix and in the utero-sacral ligaments, the organ may be displaced forward as well as laterally. If the cellular space between the bladder and cervix alone be involved in the inflammation, the resulting effusion may displace the uterus backward, but the disease is rarely met with in this location. Retroversion of the uterus frequently complicates parametritis, but in that case the abnormal position is not necessarily due to displacement by the exudation. It may have existed previous to the attack.

It must not be forgotten, however, that the symptoms and physical signs, as described above, apply only to the acute form of the disease, and that they do not exist in the same degree nor in the same regular order when the inflammatory process has been subacute, as it often is, from its commencement. When the disease is subacute from the start, the patient may be enabled to go about, and even to pursue a laborious occupation, but not without suffering. There will always be more or less pain experienced in the affected region, and the temperature and pulse will be slightly increased. In rare cases the manifestations of the disease may be so slight or so little complained of that the physician is surprised to find, on examination, a large exudation in one or both broad ligaments.

DIFFERENTIAL DIAGNOSIS.—It is of the greatest importance that this disease should be recognized early, so that prompt measures may be taken to arrest it if possible, or at least to modify the severity of its course. Fortunately, as a rule, the subjective symptoms of pelvic inflammation are so marked that the attention is at once directed toward seeking for their confirmation by eliciting the physical signs ; and for diagnosis these local manifestations of the inflammatory process are to be relied upon entirely, as the subjective symptoms of inflammation of the other tissues and organs of the pelvis somewhat resemble those of parametritis.

The diseases the local signs of which approach more nearly those of parametritis are—pelvic hæmatocele, fibrous tumor, the early stage of extra-uterine pregnancy, the early stage of parovarian and ovarian cystic degeneration, and perityphlitis.

In pelvic hæmatocele the symptoms occur suddenly, and often with hemorrhage ; there are also constitutional signs of loss of blood, as pallor and coldness of the surface of the body, and if the hemorrhage is great failure of the pulse and syncope. The tumor caused by the escape of blood into the pelvic cavity is generally post-uterine, distending Douglas's cul-de-sac and crowding the uterus forward toward the symphysis pubis, while that formed by parametritis is oftenest located at the side of the uterus. The hæmatocele at first is soft and compressible, becoming hard within a short time—a few days—as a result principally of the surrounding wall of lymph which nature throws out as a protection. The symptoms of parametritis, on the other hand, are more likely to come on gradually, and to present the pulse- and temperature-signs of inflammation, while the resulting swelling or tumor is rigid at first from congestion of the tissues, then hard, becoming soft later as the process advances to suppuration. Mere location of the tumor, however, cannot be depended upon; we must be guided by the history of the case and the special character of the tumor.

Fibroid tumor is not attended with the usual acute symptoms of parametritis, such as pain, increase of temperature, and accelerated pulse; the tumor is hard from the beginning, or at least never soft; it is circumscribed, usually smooth, and not sensitive to the touch. Its attachment to the uterus is also different from that of the tumor caused by parametritis. The former shows a tendency to pedunculation, while the latter has always a broad surface attachment.

The tumor resulting from the arrest and development of a fecundated ovum in the Fallopian tube or ovary resembles very much in its locality, and somewhat in its characteristics, a parametritic tumor; for usually more or less inflammatory exudation is present in connection with extra-uterine pregnancy, giving at times a fixity and hardness to the gestation-sac not unlike that sometimes observed in a tumor parametritic in origin; besides, there may also be constitutional signs of an inflammatory action. But the presence of some of the ordinary signs of pregnancy and a little time will clear up the difficulty; for as the case progresses the tumor will increase in size and change in character, while the mammary and other signs of gestation will develop. In addition, the pain attending tubal pregnancy is never like that of parametritis: it is more persistent, lancinating, and cramp-like in character, and is unattended by rise in temperature. Soon also the placental bruit may be detected, which of course never exists in parametritis.

The early stage of normal pregnancy is said to have been mistaken for this disease. I can hardly conceive how this mistake in diagnosis could be made, although I have met with several cases where the congestion consequent upon fecundation was so violent as to result in actual pelvic inflammatory symptoms with subsequent exudation.

The following case, which I saw with H. A. M. Smith of Gloucester, N. J., markedly illustrates and confirms this opinion: Mrs. B——, æt. 21, had been married five years, but had never conceived. Her catamenia had always been regular in time, but the flow had been slight in quantity. In the latter part of November, 1884, or about three months before I first saw her, she was attacked with severe pain in the pelvis, accompanied by rise in temperature and accelerated pulse. She was compelled to go to bed, where she had remained up to the time of coming under my care. During this time she suffered from great tenderness over the hypogastrium, some tympanites, and considerable nausea and vomiting. She did not menstruate in November—the period was due when she was first attacked with pain—but in December she had severe uterine tenesmus and a profuse metrorrhagia—symptoms of abortion. Pregnancy had not been suspected, however, as she had been so long sterile, and the inflammatory symptoms had been so violent that the signs of gestation had been masked by them. At the time of my first visit (March, 1885), there was great tenderness of the hypogastrium with slight tympanites; nausea and at times vomiting; great nervous prostration; loss of flesh; menses absent since November, except the uterine tenesmus and hemorrhage in December, as above stated; and at each menstrual cycle afterward she had the symptoms of uterine contraction with a profuse leucorrhœal discharge, but no hemorrhage. The mammary glands showed the usual signs of gestation at about the fourth month; the vagina was purplish; the cervix uteri low down on the floor of the pelvis, and the mucous membrane around the os hypertrophied, soft, and abraded. The body of the uterus was anteverted and symmetrically enlarged to about the size of the organ at the third month of gestation. The uterus seemed to be fixed—incarcerated within the pelvic cavity—by an indurated exudation in the lower portion of the right broad ligament. I diagnosticated pregnancy, and accompanying parametritis as a result. The treatment consisted in painting the right side of the fundus of the vagina opposite the base of the broad ligament with iodine; the application of iodized glycerin on pledgets of cotton, together with the use of the hot-water douche; internally, opium enough to relieve pain and an alterative tonic in the form of the four chlorides, the formula for which will be given at another place. She began to improve at once, but as she was still threatened with abortion and the uterus was still incarcerated within the pelvis, ether was administered for the purpose of attempting to release it. With two fingers of the left hand in the vagina and the right hand upon the hypogastrium to exert counter-pressure, gentle manipulation was made with the view of stretching the adhesions. This resulted in a slight elevation of the womb, and from this time pregnancy went on to full term without further trouble.

This case is introduced chiefly to show the possibility of the existence of parametritis with normal gestation. It is true that the inflammation, which developed simultaneously with fecundation, may have had a latent existence before the occurrence of that event, and that the stimulus of pregnancy served simply to bring about an attack of an active character, but nothing in the previous history of the case indicated such a condition.

Perityphlitis may somewhat resemble in its subjective symptoms, as pain and rise of temperature, an attack of parametritis. A careful study of the physical signs, and also of the exact position of the tumor in each case, however, ought to be sufficient to differentiate between the two diseases. The tumor of perityphlitis is always on the right side, and situated high up in the false pelvis; that of parametritis may be on either side—it is oftenest on the left—and is usually located low down in the true pelvis. The latter is easily reached per vaginam, while the former is almost or quite out of reach from this direction.

Parovarian cystic disease in the early stage, before the tumor has developed sufficiently to rise above the pelvic brim, resembles in its location parametritic exudation; but the history of development and the physical characteristics of each are different. There is an absence of hardness and tenderness to the touch in the former, which always exist in the latter. Parovarian tumor develops without the constitutional phenomena of inflammation; parametritis, I believe, never.

It must not be forgotten, however, that either one or more of these various diseases may exist in connection with, and as complications of, parametritis, rendering the diagnosis at times exceedingly difficult, requiring time and patience to clear the way. A case in point may be stated in brief as follows: Mrs. H—— was sent to me some months ago. She complained of great pain in both iliac regions—more in the right—extending into the pelvis and sacrum and down the limbs. There were also menorrhagia, and profuse leucorrhœa during the intermenstrual periods. She dated the trouble from an abortion which had occurred nine years before, and which was followed by symptoms of acute parametritis, from which she never fully recovered. Physical examination showed the uterus to be considerably hypertrophied and fixed, as in a vise, by an indurated mass on either side of it, which seemed to occupy both broad ligaments or to be closely adherent to them. The cervix uteri was also badly lacerated; its mucous membrane presented a surface so hypertrophied, abraded, and jagged that I was at first strongly impressed with the fear that epitheliomatous degeneration had begun to develop. I pursued a plan of treatment designed to reduce the congestion and hypertrophy of the diseased neck, and at the same time to induce an absorption of the plastic and indurated lymph around the uterus, to render the organ mobile, so that an operation might be made safe. I only partially succeeded, for while the uterus became much more mobile, there still remained a swelling or tumor on either side of it. These tumors had ill-defined borders—were not circumscribed, but elongated and rather cylindrical in form, and fixed to the lateral pelvic walls as well as to the uterus, though not very firmly to either. I now suspected disease of the Fallopian tubes, and probably also of the ovaries. The patient entered my private hospital in February, 1885, when I operated upon the cervix, dissecting away a large quantity of tissue for the purpose of making proper adjustment of the labia and to get rid of the cicatricial tissue; it was not epitheliomatous. I had hoped by this operation to not only restore the cervix to health, but at the same time to induce, by a derivative action, a retrograde metamorphosis in the diseased tissues and organs appended to the uterus. I succeeded in the former, and also in modifying all of the symptoms except the pain in the ovarian regions. This seemed to be made worse, or at least to become more prominent, as the other symptoms were improved. The patient was sent to her home, and advised to rest in the recumbent position for at least a part of every day. Later, when she did not improve, a local treatment, consisting of an application of the tincture of iodine to the fundus of the vagina at intervals of a week, with boro-glyceride tampons almost daily, was renewed. At the same time, counter-irritation, applied to the hypogastrium by means of blistering, was faithfully pursued. But nothing proved of more than temporary avail. She began to lose flesh and to fail in strength. The old fulness at the sides of the uterus, instead of diminishing, had increased. She again entered my private hospital. Under the influence of ether I now determined that the Fallopian tubes were distended to the size of a small sausage, that the ovaries were also enlarged, and that the tubes, ovaries, and ligaments were all adherent to one another by plastic lymph. I now advised laparotomy for the removal of the diseased uterine appendages. The patient very readily assented; indeed, she urged the operation.

A week later I made an incision three inches in length through an abdominal wall fully two inches in thickness, and came upon the omentum, which was very fat. This was adherent by its lower border to the pelvic tissues and organs, so that I was compelled to dissect it off on the right side before I could reach the uterus with my fingers. All the parts—Fallopian tubes, ovaries, broad ligaments, uterus, omentum, and intestines—were so adherent and matted together that it was difficult to differentiate between them. The tubes were greatly distended and contained—the right pus, and the left serum. The fimbriated extremities were glued to the lateral pelvic walls. The ovaries were as large as a good-sized hen's egg, and closely adherent to the posterior surface of the broad ligaments. I dissected with my fingers—two being introduced—until the right tube and ovary were released, when they were drawn to the incision, ligated, and removed. The left ovary and tube were released with still greater difficulty, but I finally succeeded in ligating and removing them.

It will be sufficient to say here that the patient recovered without an untoward symptom, and that she has been entirely free from pain—since her recovery—for the first time within the last nine years.

PROGNOSIS.—A very guarded prognosis should always be given as to the course and termination of a case of pelvic inflammation. The disease may run a very acute course, and result in recovery by resolution or suppuration, or it may become chronic and be indefinitely prolonged. An acute parametritis without complications usually runs its course and ends in recovery in from four to six weeks. But the cases which are acute and uncomplicated are vastly in the minority; certainly this is my experience. The course of the disease, as has been stated above, is often chronic, and requires all the patience and fortitude which can be mustered, both by the patient and physician, to bring about a cure. Generally, the prognosis is good where a rational treatment can be pursued. The tendency of the disease is toward recovery, and comparatively few cases die. It is less favorable in cases occurring just after parturition, and which are probably of septic origin. Where the disease is complicated by peritonitis the prognosis, as to life, becomes less favorable.

TREATMENT.—In the acute form, if the patient is seen during the first stage—*i. e.* before exudation has begun—she must immediately be placed in a warm bed. All sources of excitement must be at once removed, the nervous system quieted, and pain relieved by a full dose of morphia administered hypodermatically. I never give less than a quarter of a grain of the sulphate, and seldom more, but I repeat it within an hour if pain is still severe. If reaction from chill has not yet occurred, it should be hastened by the application of dry heat to the lower extremities in the form of vessels filled with hot water, preferably, while moist heat, in the form of a hot flaxseed poultice or some other convenient vehicle, should be applied to the hypogastrium. Great care must be taken that the moisture from the poultice does not escape and wet the clothing of the patient, for that would not only be a source of great discomfort, but it might also be the means of inducing another chill. The heat and moisture are best retained in the poultice by a covering of waxed paper or oiled silk. At the same time, a hot lemonade, to which may be added a teaspoonful of the sweet spirit of nitre, will often be found useful. According to Emmet, hot water per vaginal injection is a sine quâ non in the treatment of this disease. He says: "It is the only means we possess for aborting an attack of cellulitis, which it will do, if thoroughly employed at the beginning."[1] This is strong language, and doubtless the eminent author feels warranted in its use from his experience with the remedy; but I am sure that I have seen reaction brought about and the disease arrested in the first stage by the plan recommended above, and without the use of hot water by injection. There can be no doubt that the first principle to be carried out in the treatment of this disease is rest—absolute and persistent physical and mental rest. This can be obtained by the use of morphia hypodermically or by opium—administered best by the rectum—and probably by nothing else; certainly by nothing else so well. Hot-water injections are objectionable during the first stage of the disease, because of the fuss and movement of the patient necessarily connected with their administration. Further, I think it is impossible to say of any remedy that it aborted an attack of pelvic inflammation, for the disease cannot be said to be unquestionably established until the stage of exudation has been reached. Indeed, intense pelvic congestion may occur, giving rise to symptoms of the first stage of inflammation, and subside spontaneously.

When it is found that the disease cannot be arrested in the congestive stage, or when it has already passed into the stage of effusion before the patient is seen—which is often the case—exudation should be facilitated by the exhibition of the proper remedies. Happily, the principle to be followed in the treatment of this stage of the disease is the same as that of the first stage—viz. rest, relief of pain, and the local application of heat and moisture, with the addition now of counter-irritation. The first and second are to be obtained by the use of opium. The patient must not be allowed to suffer pain, and immunity can only be secured by the free use of the remedy. This drug is of more value in controlling the heart's action and quieting reflex irritability than all the others combined. The patient should be kept under its influence as long as pain lasts. I usually order twelve suppositories, as follows:

R. Ext. opii aq.,   gr. xij ;
    Ol. theobromæ,   q. s. ;
    M. et ft. supposit., No. xij.

Sig. One to be placed in the rectum every two hours if necessary to quiet pain.

But we should not wait for the rather slow action of the opium administered in this way. It is best to begin with the administration of morphia hypodermically, as stated above, repeating it until the desired result is secured. It is then not difficult to keep up its influence by the use of the suppositories. If the suppositories cannot be obtained, the tincture of opium may be administered by injection into the rectum. The opium should not be given by the mouth where it can be avoided, as it is more apt to interfere with the appetite and digestion when thus

[1] *Prin. and Prac. of Gynæcology*, 3d ed., p. 261.

administered. The proper action of the skin and kidneys should be maintained by the administration of the liquor ammoniæ acetatis in dessertspoonful doses. Irritability of the bladder is often a troublesome symptom during the progress of the disease, and is best relieved, in my experience, by the following formula, which combines a diaphoretic and diuretic as well as an antispasmodic:

R. Tr. belladonnæ, f ʒj ;
Sodii bicarbonatis, ʒiij ;
Spts. etheris nitrosi, f ʒj ;
Mist. potass. citratis, q. s. ad f ʒvj.

M.—Sig. Dessertspoonful three or four times a day, or half the quantity oftener. I have also known this combination to relieve the persistent nausea which often accompanies this disease.

As soon as the skin becomes moist the remedy should be given at longer intervals, and if sweating is induced it should be discontinued entirely for the time, as that only serves to weaken the patient.

If the pulse does not beat oftener than 112, and the temperature does not rise above 102°, nothing more in the way of medication will be required. The patient will recover best if not treated too much. On the other hand, should the pulse be strong and rapid and the temperature high, quinine becomes a valuable remedy. It is more efficient when given in large doses at long intervals than when given in small doses at short intervals. If the temperature rises above 102°, it is my rule to administer ten grains and wait six hours, when, if it has not decreased, the quinine is repeated. If, however, the temperature has increased instead of diminishing, twenty grains are given at the second dose, and the effect carefully noted. Should marked cinchonism result, the remedy must be withheld, even though it has had no influence on the temperature. Quinine is said to have the power of so contracting the capillaries as to prevent the migration of the white blood-corpuscles. If this is true, the remedy ought to have great value in modifying or limiting the third or suppurative stage of the disease.

The tincture of aconite-root is also of value in controlling the pulse and lowering the temperature in certain cases. But its use should be limited to those cases of marked sthenic character, for, as a rule, the tendency of the disease is toward depression. It may be given in doses of two to five drops, repeated every two hours until three or four doses are taken, when, sometimes, the pulse will be found to have decreased ten to twenty beats per minute. The remedy should then be withheld until the effect is shown to have passed off by an increase of pulse-rate, when it may be again exhibited; provided always that the heart continues strong and vigorous and that it has shown no sign of weakness. In the latter circumstance the continued use of the medicine would be extremely dangerous. Under any circumstances its use should be limited to the first and early part of the second stage of the disease.

The diet should be carefully attended to, and should be of the most nutritious character, as milk, eggs, beef-essence, etc.

Locally, in addition to the poulticing, but not to the exclusion of it, counter-irritation by means of iodine will be found useful. The whole surface of the hypogastrium should be painted each time the poultice is changed until the skin shows signs of irritation, when it should be discontinued and the poulticing alone kept up. The abdomen must not be exposed longer than is just necessary to remove one and place another poultice, which should be at hand and not in another room. The poultice must never be permitted to become cool on the patient. Turpentine may be used instead of iodine, and if tympanites is a troublesome symptom it will be found valuable. A few drops should be sprinkled over the poultice, or its action may be more quickly obtained by the use of the remedy in the form of the stupe until marked redness of the surface is produced, when the poultice can be resumed. Tympanites is most troublesome when the disease occurs during the puerperal state, and in these cases I regard the turpentine as a most valuable remedy, not only as a counter-irritant, but also when administered internally. It should be given by enema in teaspoonful doses, repeated every six hours until the desired effect is produced. It improves the secretions and allays pain by relieving distension. If the bowels should move as a result of the enemata, it is all the better. If fecal matter occupies the lower bowel, it should be removed under any circumstances.

Blistering, by means of cantharidal collodion or by the pure cantharides spread in the form of a plaster, I regard as the most efficacious counter-irritant; and if the beneficial effects of the remedy could be obtained without the discomforts, and often positive suffering, attending its action, I would probably employ it to the exclusion of all others. But these cannot be obtained. During the acute stage of the disease, when the pulse and temperature are high and the skin hot, the blister should not be used. It is then more likely to produce strangury; if not that, the other sufferings of the patient are at least increased in the pain and burning produced on the surface of the abdomen. This is not compensated for by relief of pelvic pain, for we have relieved this long since by opium. I think blistering should be confined to the chronic stage or form of the disease.

Resolution by reabsorption of the effused product may now terminate the disease; but that is not the rule when the process has once advanced beyond the first or congestive stage. If it is found that suppuration is likely to take place, that the disease is following its natural course, the third stage must be facilitated. The therapeutic plan laid down above will serve to limit the amount of pus-formation and tend to concentrate it to one point for evacuation. The hot fomentations should be continued, as well as the counter-irritation by the iodine. It will probably be observed that the patient has rigors of more or less severity, followed by rise in temperature. These symptoms should be looked upon as an indication of pus-formation. The patient should be examined from time to time by the digital touch per vaginam and by the combined vagino-hypogastric palpation for the purpose of determining the presence of an abscess and its location, so that the proper treatment may be applied and at the proper time.

These examinations must be conducted with the greatest care and gentleness, and the patient protected from undue exposure. When the disease has advanced to the third stage means for the disposition of the pus should be kept constantly in view, and the case treated as one of pelvic abscess.

Treatment of Pelvic Abscess.—Authorities differ widely as to the proper method of disposing of the contents of a pelvic abscess. Some favor a let-alone plan, believing that Nature is competent to relieve herself more effectually and better than art can do; others, equally eminent, believe that the pus should be evacuated when pointing has positively occurred and made the evacuation easy and safe; while others, again, more radical in their views, believe that much can be gained by liberating the pus as soon as it is known to exist, although it may be deepseated and as yet have shown no tendency toward pointing.

The same therapeutic principle should guide us in the management of a pelvic abscess that we would unhesitatingly apply in the treatment of an abscess in any other portion of the body. It is a settled law in surgery that if a pus-cavity is evacuated and not allowed to burrow, much tissue may be saved, the duration of the disease shortened, and the prognosis rendered more favorable. I believe that the pus should be liberated promptly as soon as it is certain that an abscess has been formed and can be reached without danger to important structures—emphatically so when the way is being pointed out. True, Nature is competent in some instances to discharge the accumulation, and usually by the least dangerous channel. But it is also true that in many other cases she is not. Instead of taking the shortest, most direct, and safest course to the surface, the pus frequently takes the most indirect route, riddling and destroying the tissues in its track; or it may rupture into the bladder or peritoneal cavity, in the latter case to be followed by death from peritonitis. Evacuation of the pus by artificial means when the way has been shown, if done carefully by aspiration, is attended with almost no danger. Where, on the other hand, the abscess is deeply seated and there is no tendency toward pointing, the question of evacuation becomes one requiring great deliberation; for the dangers of puncture increase as the thickness of the tissues to be traversed in reaching the abscess is greater. But, even though the pus be deeply located, when a positive diagnosis of its presence can be made I still favor early evacuation. Mere exploratory puncture in the hope of finding pus is a most dangerous practice, and should not be thought of in connection with pelvic abscess. Delay, even at the risk of spontaneous rupture, is the proper course until the diagnosis can be rendered positive; for when the abscess is deep-seated the progress of the disease is often slow. Of course the condition of the patient should always be taken into account in deciding the question whether or not to interfere. If signs of septic absorption appear, or evidences of constitutional failure become prominent in spite of the means used for staying the progress of the disease, prompt measures must be taken to get rid of the product of the inflammation. The strongest argument in favor of early operative evacuation of the abscess is the danger that the disease may become chronic when the pus is not promptly discharged. Many cases have occurred in which abscess after abscess had been formed and discharged, until the patient became a mere wreck of her former self, and finally died from septicæmia or exhaustion. This is the result of non-interference. I am so fully convinced of the value and necessity of operative measures in the treatment of pelvic abscess that the following questions at once present themselves to me when called upon to decide in a case where spontaneous evacuation has not already taken place: 1st. When shall the abscess be opened? 2d. Where shall the opening be made? and 3d How shall the operation be done?

The first of these questions has been answered in a general way by the preceding remarks, and it is only necessary to add here, by way of recapitulation, that the time for opening the abscess will depend upon its location and the condition of the patient. If the pus is near the surface and can be easily and safely reached, whether pointing has occurred or not, it is ripe for evacuation and should be liberated at once, even though the patient be in the best possible condition and show no evidence of deleterious effect from its presence. Nothing whatever can be gained by permitting it to open spontaneously, but much may be lost. If, however, the situation of the abscess be such that it would be necessary to traverse healthy tissues to a considerable extent in order to reach it, and the patient shows no evidence of septic absorption, it would be highly injudicious to attempt to open the abscess: first, because under the circumstances you could not be positively certain that a collection of pus existed; and, secondly, because it is doing no harm. Delay, with careful observation, is now the proper course. Within a few days the apparent abscess tumor may either show decided signs that it is diminishing in size and undergoing resolution, or it may approach the surface, so that evacuation will become safe. On the other hand, should symptoms of blood-poisoning develop and the patient show signs of rapid exhaustion, our attitude must be one of action instead of delay. The pus must then be liberated even at some risk. I still insist, however, that a positive diagnosis must be established, and that the operative measure shall be in no sense exploratory.

2d. Where shall the opening be made? This question is often decided for us by Nature. The puncture, as a rule, should be made where pointing has occurred. If pointing has not occurred, a position from which the abscess can be most easily reached through the vagina or abdominal wall should be selected. The vagina should be given the preference, because the opening would then be at the most dependent portion. The rectum should not be selected as the channel through which to evacuate the pus artificially, although spontaneous discharge into that tube occurs almost as frequently as into the vagina. The patient does not recover as quickly, however, when the abscess opens into the rectum, and more cases of septic poisoning occur from decomposition of the pus as a result of the entrance of air and fecal matter into the abscess-cavity. Further, it may become necessary to keep the opening patulous and to wash out the cavity of the abscess. This could not be done properly if the opening were in the rectum. I believe it to be the best practice to open from the vagina rather than from the rectum, even at greater risk to intervening structures, because it may greatly facilitate the after-management of the case.

If the tumor should be located high up in the iliac fossa or in the hypogastrium, the point of election for opening must be somewhere on the abdominal surface in the region of the abscess.

3d. How shall the operation be done? The opening of a pelvic abscess should never be regarded as a simple operation. As much care and deliberation should be taken in the selection of the proper method of evacuation of the pus, and in the operation itself, as was previously given to the diagnosis of its presence. Always begin with the administration of an anæsthetic. This not only protects the patient from unnecessary mental agitation and physical pain, but it better enables the physician to confirm his previous opinion of the case, as well as to be more deliberate in the election of the point of puncture. With the patient in the dorsal position, if it be determined that the pus is contained in a single cavity, and there be no evidence of its decomposition, shown by the absence of symptoms of systemic poisoning, it should be liberated by aspiration. By this means a smaller puncture will be required and the entrance of atmospheric air prevented. If, happily, the operation has been performed early, before the formation of the so-called pyogenic membrane, or at least before sinuous tracts have resulted from burrowing, the abscess-cavity may then collapse and disappear. But should the patient not improve after the pus has been removed, or should the cavity again fill up, it is probable either that there is another pus-cavity, which had not been reached by the trocar, or that there has been developed on the internal surface of the sac an unhealthy fungous, granular condition. Under these circumstances a free incision should be made into the cavity of the abscess, so that a drainage-tube may be introduced and the cavity washed out by an antiseptic fluid. The opening should then be kept patulous, so that healing can take place from the bottom of the sac. It . may become necessary to introduce a finger and scrape away with the nail the fungosites from the wall of the sac. But great care must be used in this manipulation, as well as in making the incision, for there is danger of wounding large blood-vessels and of rupturing the wall of the sac. If the cavity be now kept pure by daily injections of a 1 : 1000 solution of the bichloride of mercury or of a $2\frac{1}{2}$–5 per cent. solution of carbolic acid, its surface may become healthy, the secretion diminish, and the sac close up.

The best method of washing out the cavity is by the fountain syringe, to which a long double canula can be attached ; or, probably better, the syphon. It would be unsafe to force water into the sac.

It is well for the patient if the situation of the abscess be such as to render its evacuation through the vagina feasible, for then the opening is made at the most dependent portion, and consequently drainage is more easily and thoroughly accomplished ; but, unfortunately, the location of the tumor may be so high up as to compel the removal of the pus through the abdominal wall.

Almost the same rules as to the selection of the method of operating and of the election of the point for puncture or incision will apply here as in the operation through the vagina, provided pointing has taken place. I am less favorable to aspiration, however, when the puncture must be made through the walls of the abdomen—first, because reaccumulation is almost certain to take place ; and, second, because there is danger of leakage of pus into the peritoneal cavity, since it is difficult by this means to thoroughly empty the sac, and impossible to wash it out and keep it drained.

If pointing has occurred, a free incision should be made at once and the cavity thoroughly emptied, and, if necessary, washed out. The opening must not be permitted to close until the cavity has healed from the bottom.

Where pointing has not occurred and the abscess is so deeply seated that it cannot be safely reached from the vagina, and does not distend the abdominal walls, I would urge greater delay, in the hope that it may approach the surface more nearly. If, however, the condition of the patient be such as to demand immediate action, the operation of laparotomy should be selected as the more thorough and less dangerous method of releasing the pus and of after-treating the abscess.

An incision two inches in length should be made through the linea alba, midway between the umbilicus and pubes, and, after all bleeding is stanched, the peritoneal cavity opened. The index finger should then be passed in and the surface of the abscess-wall explored. It will be a fortunate circumstance if the sac be found adherent to the peritoneal surface, where the incision is made, for it can then be opened without entering the peritoneal cavity. To prevent the escape of pus into this cavity the sac should now be evacuated with great care. For this purpose the aspirator is well adapted, but a small trocar, to which a few feet of rubber tubing has been previously attached, through which to conduct the pus into a convenient receptacle, will answer almost as well. The opening in the sac should next be slightly enlarged by an incision (not torn); it should then be included in the sutures, which are now placed to close the abdominal wound. After the sutures have been introduced the pus-cavity should be washed out with the bichloride or carbolic-acid solution, and a glass drainage-tube placed in the lower angle of the incision, when the edges can be brought together and adjusted around it.

The after-treatment required will be the same as if the opening had been made through the vagina.

The sac must be made to close from the bottom. It may become necessary to stimulate the surface by the injection of a weak solution of nitrate of silver, four to eight grains to the ounce of distilled water, or with the tincture of iodine, one part to four of water.

Cases are sometimes met with in which the pus has burrowed and formed sinuous tracts which are difficult to reach and drain. It may then be necessary to make a counter-opening in the vagina after first cutting through the abdominal wall. These are usually old, neglected, chronic cases, in which the abscess has discharged spontaneously into the bowel too high up to be properly emptied, or which have opened into the bladder or somewhere on the abdominal wall, or possibly taken one of the circuitous routes alluded to under the head of Pathology.

No fixed rule can be set down for the management of these grave cases. Each one must be treated on its individual merits. A ripe experience and judgment are necessary here to decide whether it is best to operate or to pursue a course of masterly inactivity, depending upon the use of hygienic and tonic remedies and time to bring about a cure. I have known instances where patients have recovered spontaneously after having been reduced to the lowest extremity. I have also known others who have died soon after submitting to operative interference. Some of the spontaneous recoveries, however, are only apparent, for the old sinuses often reopen and discharge pus as before, or the pus may be discharged at some new and remote point, the patient finally succumbing to the ravages of a disease from which she flattered herself she had escaped.

The most careful attention must be given to the hygienic surroundings of the patient, the diet liberal and of the most nutritious character. The appetite should be sharpened by the administration of the bitter tonics, the best of which is probably the old tincture of bark (Huxham's). Quinine should be given in doses sufficient to control the temperature when necessary, and for its tonic properties. The blood should be improved by the exhibition of iron, arsenic, and the bichloride of mercury in the form of the mixture of the four chlorides, first used, I believe, by Tilt of London. There can be no doubt as to the value of the combination in cases of plastic exudations. The following is the formula which I am in the habit of using:

R. Hydrarg. chloridi corrosivi,   gr. j ;
Liq. arsenici chloridi,   f3j ;
Tr. ferri chloridi,
Acid. muriatici diluti,   āā. f3iv ;
Syr. simplici,   f3ij ;
Aquæ,   q. s. ad f3vi.

M.—Sig. Dessertspoonful, well diluted, after meals.

The dose of the arsenic and bichloride of mercury can be increased, after it is found that the mixture does not disagree with the stomach, to six drops of the former and a sixteenth to a twelfth of a grain of the latter. The effect of the medicine must be carefully watched, however. After the remedy has been taken two weeks it should be discontinued and some other form of tonic substituted for a week or two. The syrup of the iodide of iron, or the iodide of iron in pill form, will serve well as the substitute. If the patient should tire of the above or the remedies should not agree, some other form of tonic must be given. I have found the following an excellent tonic pill:

R. Strychniæ sulphatis, gr. j ;
Acidi arseniosi,   gr. j ;
Quininæ sulphatis,   gr. xlviii ;
Ferri sulphatis,   gr. xlviii ;
Ext. hyoscyami,   gr. xij ;
Ext. gentianæ,   q. s.

M. et ft. pil. No. xlviii.—Sig. One to two pills after each meal.

As soon as practicable the patient should have a change of air and scene.

Perimetritis.

Having treated the subject of inflammation of the pelvic tissues generally, in the acute form, under the head of Parametritis, with sufficient fulness to answer the purposes of the practical physician, whether the disease dominate the connective tissue or the peritoneum covering it, I shall, under the head of Perimetritis, consider the subject in its chronic aspect principally.

DEFINITION AND SYNONYMS.—I have defined parametritis to be an inflammation of the cellular or connective tissue near the uterus and beneath the pelvic peritoneum, including principally the locality close to the lateral margin of the uterus between the layers of the broad ligaments, although embracing also all of the various spaces where connective tissue abounds—viz. between the peritoneal folds which form the utero-sacral and utero-vesical ligaments. I cannot more clearly or more simply define perimetritis than by stating that it means an inflammation of the peritoneum which serves as a covering and boundary-line for the connective-tissue spaces involved in parametritis. As the term parametritis is used to conveniently express the idea of the existence of an inflammation in the connective tissue near the uterus, so the term perimetritis conveniently and tersely expresses the idea that the inflammatory process exists around the uterus in the pelvic peritoneum. In the acute form it is difficult to differentiate between them clinically, nor is it necessary, from a therapeutic standpoint, to do so. The term perimetritis is synonymous with pelvic peritonitis

ETIOLOGY.—All of the causes which have been enumerated as capable of producing parametritis may be included in the etiology of perimetritis. If, however, the great predisposing causes of the former—abortion and injury at parturition—be absent, the woman be non-parous, the inflammation will affect the peritoneum rather than the connective tissue. Parametritis is rare before pregnancy has occurred, except in so far as the connective tissue always becomes more or less involved when the peritoneum covering it is inflamed. Perimetritis, on the other hand, is frequent in the single and sterile woman. But, as a rule, it does not run the same typical acute course. It is usually subacute or chronic from the beginning, and results in the formation of false membranes which bind the pelvic organs to one another.

Perimetritis of the adhesive form may be produced by the pressure and irritation resulting from displacement of the pelvic organs, as retroflexion of the uterus, incarcerated fibroid or ovarian tumor, prolapse of the ovary and Fallopian tube, fecal impaction, and from ill-fitting and improperly-adjusted pessaries. Under these circumstances the disease usually comes on insidiously, with no acute symptoms, and runs a slow course. It may be discovered accidentally when making an examination on account of pelvic pain obscure in character, or when the attention has not been called especially to it by the presence of specific symptoms.

Perimetritis may result from regurgitation of menstrual fluid through a too patulous Fallopian tube. This is most likely to take place when the egress to the flow has been prevented by a flexion of the uterus sharp enough to practically destroy the calibre of the cervical canal, as when the organ has become retroflexed from subinvolution or some other cause of hypertrophy of the body of the organ. It may, however, occur as a result of the intense engorgement which sometimes attends acute suppression of the catamenia. It may occur from disease in the tube itself, as where a collection of pus or serum has been formed and thrown into the peritoneal cavity either from rupture of the tube or discharge through the natural opening at the fimbriated extremity. Or it may result from hemorrhage following the rupture of a Graafian follicle, especially where the disease of the tube has resulted in the destruction of its calibre or the power of the fimbriæ to grasp the ovary so as to convey the discharge safely to the uterine cavity. Hemorrhage from any other source, as from the rupture of a blood-vessel or of an extra-uterine gestation-sac, usually results in the development of perimetritis.

Coitus is capable of causing perimetritis when the act is awkwardly performed, or where there is a disproportion in the relative sizes of the organs involved, or where the physiological mechanism of copulation is destroyed by displacement of the uterus, free mobility being lost as a result.

According to Noeggerrath,[1] a very common cause of perimetritis is what he is pleased to call a latent gonorrhœa in the male. He believes that the disease, once contracted, is probably never entirely eradicated, but that it always exists in a latent form, and that it is capable of producing a specific inflammation of the pelvic peritoneum years after an apparent cure had been effected. It is of course impossible to positively verify this, although he gives some very striking cases in support of his position. That gonorrhœa in the acute form may extend by propagation from a vaginitis through the uterine cavity and Fallopian tubes to the peritoneum, and produce an inflammation of that membrane, is probable. Cases have been met with where a history of specific infection was undoubted, in which an attack of perimetritis followed soon after the initial symptoms and physical signs of gonorrhœa were manifested. But it is quite another thing to believe that the specific poison may remain latent and harmless in the genital system of the male to be transferred years afterward to that of the female.

Tuberculous or carcinomatous disease of the pelvic organs is nearly always complicated by a certain degree of perimetritis.

Perimetritis may result from external injuries, as blows, kicks, and the like; and under the head of traumatic agencies most of the causes which have been enumerated would stand as examples; but under this head I wish also to emphasize the statement that I believe that perimetritis may result from an unwarranted and unnecessary force used on the part of the physician in his efforts to outline and locate the position of the pelvic organs, especially that of the ovaries and tubes. When the latter organs are in their normal position and not enlarged, it is usually impossible to outline them by the bimanual touch, nor is it necessary. When they are diseased the greatest care in manipulation should be used; and it is often best to administer an anæsthetic, so that less force may be necessary to determine their exact condition. The disease may also result from injury inflicted in the medication of the uterine cavity and in the various operations on the uterus. A most prolific cause is induced abortion.

Recurrent perimetritis should be regarded as the result of the persistence of one of the above-mentioned causes. It sometimes recurs with each menstrual period. Such attacks are often associated with dysmenorrhœa of the congestive type.

PATHOLOGY, COURSE, AND TERMINATION.—When the pelvic peritoneum becomes inflamed, and the disease runs through an acute course, the pathology and termination will be much the same as that described under Parametritis, for the connective tissue will then be involved in the process, as well as the peritoneum; not to the same extent, however, as when the disease begins as a cellulitis. The position of the exudation tumor, should one form, will be more directly posterior to the uterus in Douglas's cul-de-sac; it is sometimes larger, and may displace the uterus far forward. This is more especially the case where the disease has advanced to the third stage and resulted in abscess.

In the subacute and chronic forms of the disease the course is usually a slow one. The exudation soon becomes plastic, or is so from the beginning. This leads to the agglutination of the pelvic organs to one another, and finally to the production of organized pseudo-membrane

---

[1] "Latent Gonorrhœa, etc.," *Trans. Amer. Gynæc. Soc.*, vol. i. p. 268.

of more or less strength. If the Fallopian tubes and ovaries are dis-placed, which is frequently the case under these circumstances, they are bound more or less firmly in the abnormal position. The adhesions are sometimes extremely delicate, and embrace the displaced organs as a net. At other times, or later, they may be so large and firm as to be readily felt through the vagina. Again, the false membranes may be broad and ribbon-like, and occupy a position so as to imprison the displaced organs as though elastic bands were stretched from the anterior to the posterior portion of the pelvic brim. When Douglas's cul-de-sac is bridged over and shut off from the abdominal cavity proper, serum or pus, sometimes both, may collect within it and give rise, from its round, fluctuating cha-racter and rather insidious formation, to the supposition that it is an incar-cerated ovarian cyst; especially so since it may progressively increase in size and attain such dimensions as to distend the abdominal walls. This course of the disease is rare, however.

Under favorable circumstances the course and termination of chronic pelvic inflammation would probably be much the same as where the disease is acute—*i. e.* it would run its natural course and end in resolu-tion by absorption of the effused product. But, unfortunately, the symptoms of the disease are not violent enough to compel the patient to go to bed and remain at rest, so as to place the organs in the most favor-able condition for recovery. The affection comes on so insidiously some-times that when the patient is finally compelled to seek relief it may be found that extensive adhesions and considerable displacement, if not serious disease—especially of the ovaries and Fallopian tubes—exists. The inflammatory process is progressive, and will continue to be so until its cause shall be rendered inactive by the continuous and increasing severity of the symptoms, which force the sufferer to give up the struggle to remain on her feet and pursue her usual round of duties.

SYMPTOMS.—If the attack is acute the subjective symptoms of peri-metritis will differ from those described as belonging to parametritis only in the greater violence of their onset and progress. The pain, which is usually preceded by a chill, is likely to be sudden, sharp, and persistent —sometimes agonizing. The pulse, especially during the first stage of the disease, is small, wiry, and quick, ranging from 120 to 140 beats per minute. But its character is likely to change as the affection progresses, and to become full, as when the connective tissue is the seat of the inflam-mation. The temperature also reaches a higher point, rising frequently as high as 104°–105°, sometimes even higher.

When the disease is chronic from its commencement, the pain is more obscure, and cannot so certainly be relied upon as a diagnostic sign. True, a sharp pain existing low down in the pelvis in either iliac region —pain persistent in character and coming on rather suddenly—should always direct attention to the probable existence of an inflammatory con-dition. The pain of chronic pelvic inflammation is not attended with the rise in temperature and acceleration of pulse which have been described as accompanying the acute form of the disease. There is, doubtless, a slight degree of increase in both, but not enough to attract attention as a rule. There may be many reflex symptoms, chief of which are irritability of the bladder and stomach, the latter manifesting itself in nausea and some-times vomiting.

PHYSICAL SIGNS.—Physical examination may reveal no evidence of exudation or of the presence of an inflammatory condition, and may lead the physician to infer that the attacks are not inflammatory in character, but that they are of a neuralgic nature. As a rule, however, examination will show a thickening or an absence of the usual mobility of the surfaces, and deep pressure may elicit considerable tenderness. On the other hand, the physical signs may be marked, and the surfaces may be felt to be quite thickened and very rigid, so that it will be evident that there is exudation on the surface of the peritoneum. Usually, the vaginal examination reveals a fixation and induration posterior to the uterus. If that organ is retroflexed, it is bound firmly in that position. If the uterus is in its normal position, there will not usually be the same amount of fulness posteriorly. If an ovary and Fallopian tube have been displaced, it will probably be fixed in the post-broad-ligament space or in the cul-de-sac of Douglas. The pelvic roof, so called, may be found as hard and tense as a deal board, as was first described by Doherty. The exudation may be so great as to displace the uterus forward or laterally, and to fix it as though it were surrounded by hardened lymph. This is especially felt in the post-uterine space, gluing the uterus, ovaries, tubes, and broad ligaments together. If there is a small ovarian or fibroid tumor, it may be likewise fixed in this posterior position.

A later examination may show a change in this condition. The exudation material may have been reduced by absorption, or there may have been an increase. If the latter, the disease will probably run an acute course and end by resolution or suppuration—more likely the latter—and practically it will then run the course described under the head of Parametritis.

DIAGNOSIS.—The diagnosis of perimetritis is made with comparative ease. The subjective symptoms are sometimes obscure, but the physical signs are perfectly plain. When there is exudation posterior to the uterus, especially if it has bound the organ in a retroverted position or incarcerated a foreign body, it is almost absolutely certain that agglutination is due to peritoneal exudation. This exudation is, as a rule, not so extensive as that which occurs in parametritis, and if a tumor is present —which is uncommon—its location is different. Where a tumor is present as the result of pelvic inflammation, I think that it may be safely ascribed to connective-tissue inflammation rather than to peritoneal. On the other hand, where there is simply agglutination, and where the effusion seems thin and spread out, the organs and ligaments rigid and thickened, instead of a somewhat circumscribed tumor, the disease may be ascribed to perimetritis rather than to parametritis. Where the condition just described is found there can be no doubt as to the existence of perimetritis.

A small ovarian tumor, abscess of the ovary, pyo-salpinx, fibroid tumor, fecal impaction, and hæmatocele might be mistaken for this disease, but these tumors are, as a rule, more or less circumscribed, while the exudation due to perimetritis is not often so. Perimetritis, however, may coexist with any of the conditions just mentioned. These tumors may be bound to adjacent tissues, forming one large mass, as the result of intercurrent attacks of perimetritis. In such cases the peritoneal inflammation would exist as a complication.

PROGNOSIS.—When the inflammation is acute, or where the peritoneum becomes largely involved, the disease may run a very violent and fatal course. Those cases in which pelvic inflammation is of such severity as to cause death are usually of this character. As a rule, however, the prognosis, so far as life is concerned, is favorable.

The prognosis regarding the restoration of the ligaments and the thickened surfaces to their natural condition, and the restoration of the displaced organs which complicate the disease, will depend upon the extent and duration of the affection and upon the treatment. As a rule, the prognosis is good where the patient has sufficient courage and fortitude to submit to a prolonged course of treatment, with the abstemious habits of life which may be necessary.

TREATMENT.—In order to present systematically the therapeutics of perimetritis it should be divided into the acute and chronic forms, and the treatment of the latter form will necessarily include to a certain degree the management of the complications. All that has been said under the head of the treatment of parametritis will apply to the treatment of acute perimetritis. As the symptoms of acute perimetritis are ushered in with greater violence than where the connective tissue is simply involved, so the remedies for the relief of these symptoms must be more vigorously applied. The patient must be placed at absolute rest, and be kept there, for the favorable termination of the disease will be largely dependent on the faithfulness with which this measure is carried out. The pain, which is usually great and acute in character, must be relieved at once by the administration of morphia subcutaneously in full dose, and the remedy is to be repeated until the pain is under control, when the effect of the drug may be maintained by the administration of opium in the form of suppositories containing one grain of the aqueous extract. As in the treatment of parametritis, so here, I insist upon the administration of the drug by the above method, rather than by the mouth, because nausea and interference with the function of digestion are less likely to follow.

In the peritoneal form of pelvic inflammation the pulse is usually more rapid and the temperature higher than where the connective tissue alone is involved. Both of these symptoms may be controlled by the free administration of opium. If this is not successful, a resort to the tincture of aconite in small and repeated doses will be indicated. If necessary, quinia should be administered. This remedy, however, should not be given unless the temperature remains persistently high ; and, as advised under the head of Parametritis, the dose should not be less than ten grains, repeated in from four to six hours if the temperature is not decreased. The action of the tincture of aconite should be carefully watched, and if its administration is not soon followed by a lowering of the pulse-rate, its use should be abandoned.

If the disease is of a marked sthenic character, the local abstraction of blood by the application of leeches to the hypogastrium is often of great benefit, and poulticing should be most faithfully and persistently carried out, together with hot applications to the lower extremities in the form of hot water, as previously directed. I strongly recommend the application of heat to the hypogastrium in preference to cold. If the patient be seen quite early in the first stage of the disease, which is unusual, the application of cold might be more beneficial than heat; but when the process has advanced toward the second stage, that of exudation, the application of heat will facilitate this process, while cold would probably retard it.

By the above plan of treatment—viz. the immediate relief of pain by full and repeated doses of morphia—it is possible to arrest the disease in the first stage, but this is not the rule. It usually advances to the second stage, that of exudation, if it has not already reached this stage before the patient is seen. A vaginal examination may now show the uterus to be fixed, but there may be an entire absence of tumor. Should an exudation tumor exist, it will probably be found posterior to the uterus, crowding that organ forward rather than laterally, as would be the case were the inflammatory process seated in the cellular tissue; or, what is oftener the case, we have mere fixity of the organ, with thickening of the pelvic peritoneum lining Douglas's pouch and the posterior surface of the broad ligaments. Later an exudation tumor will more likely be found. If this is so, it should be inferred that the connective tissue has become largely involved in the process, and it should rather be expected that the disease will pass through the regular course of pelvic inflammation and advance to the third stage, that of suppuration, as though the disease had originally begun as a parametritis. It should then be treated on the general principle laid down for the management of that form of pelvic inflammation. The case should, however, be regarded with greater solicitude as to prognosis where the peritoneum has been largely involved, and the symptoms should be more carefully watched and counteracted by the application of the proper remedies. There is in such cases more danger of the disease spreading and involving the peritoneum generally, and of course becoming an affection of great gravity. When the peritoneum is largely involved, tympanites, as a rule, becomes a troublesome symptom, more especially if the disease has occurred during the puerperal period, and it requires special attention. The remedy which I have learned to rely upon in the treatment of this troublesome complication is turpentine, administered preferably by enema.

Should the disease advance to the suppurative stage, the case then becomes one of pelvic abscess, and should be managed on the principle enunciated for that stage of the disease. (See Treatment of Pelvic Abscess.)

Treatment of Chronic Perimetritis.—When the disease exists in its chronic form, the uterus, ovaries, and Fallopian tubes may be found fixed either in the normal position or in some form of displacement, usually the latter. The peritoneum lining Douglas's pouch, as well as that covering the uterus, broad ligaments, tubes, and ovaries, will be found more or less thickened, or the ovaries and tubes may be prolapsed and retained by false membranes; or the uterus itself may be retroflexed and fixed by adhesion of the peritoneal surfaces lining Douglas's pouch and that covering the uterus; or false membranes may have been formed so as to roof over the pelvis, thereby incarcerating the uterus and its appendages within that cavity. This condition gives rise to pains which are rather diffused throughout the pelvis, at one time affecting the ovarian region in which the disease exists, and at another being experienced low down in the pelvis and radiating along the course of the sacral nerve down the posterior portion of the thigh, always sharp and distressing in charac-

ter. Where the ovary and tube are involved the pain usually radiates
to the groin and anterior portion of the thigh. Examination should
be conducted with great care, because, although the uterus and its appendages seem to be fixed firmly, there are often new adhesions forming or
weak ones existing which may be easily severed ; and this especially
applies to manipulation of the ovary and tube, the adhesions of which
are, as a rule, not so firm as those fixing the uterus.

The management of these cases must of course be different from that
of the acute form of the disease. The patient often suffers from nervous
exhaustion, indigestion, and loss of flesh as a result of the long suffering
which she has endured during the course of the disease. I believe that here
the most efficacious plan of treatment is that which embraces REST as its
guiding principle, for the disease probably had its origin in over-exertion and derangement of the proper relations of the organs one to another,
as in those cases in which it is developed as a result of prolapse or retroflexion of the uterus or the ovaries, or from the presence of a tumor
incarcerated in the pelvis, which displaces and holds in malposition the
above organs. It is unquestionably true that where the patient is
allowed to exercise and follow her usual avocation the attrition of the
inflamed surfaces upon each other will tend to keep up the inflammatory
condition. It is my plan, where I can get the consent of the patient, to
place her at absolute rest, and begin the treatment by paying strict
attention to the evacuation of the bowels, for constipation is one of
the most troublesome accompaniments of perimetritis. It often stands
in a causative relation, and nearly always as a complication of the
disease ; and of course first attention should be paid to the relief of
this condition.

Strict attention should be paid to the diet. The food should be of the
most nutritious character, calculated to improve the digestive organs, and
through them to build up the general system.

The Local Treatment.—The local treatment should embrace those
remedies which are thought to possess the power of producing absorption of plastic material, either by a counter-irritant or stimulating action.
The persistent use of the tincture of iodine, both to the hypogastrium
and to the fundus of the vagina opposite the seat of exudation, is of great
value. Where the iodine is found to be so irritating to the skin as to
make it necessary to discontinue its use, and also for the relief of pain, I
have found the following formula very useful :

$\qquad$ Ŗ. Tincturæ aconiti,
$\qquad\qquad$ Tincturæ opii, *āā*. ʒj ;
$\qquad\qquad$ Tincturæ iodinii,   ʒvj. Misce.

Sig. Poison. To be applied externally as directed.

This may also be applied to the fundus of the vagina instead of the
iodine alone, either by a camel's-hair brush or by the cotton-wrapped
uterine applicator. The vaginal application of iodine should be made
not oftener than once in three days, and sometimes a longer interval is
advisable, especially if the remedy is used in a concentrated form. If it
is found that irritation or ulceration has been produced, its use must be
discontinued for a time, and remedies of a milder form substituted, as,
for instance, the application of iodoform and glycerin (one drachm to the
ounce), or of glycerin alone on the cotton tamponade.

In the intervals between the application of iodine and the other remedies the hot-water douche should be used daily. When the hot water is administered the patient must be in the recumbent position. I am opposed to indiscriminately advising walking patients to use hot water, because, as a rule, it is not given as intended—that is, hot and in large quantity—and the object for which it has been recommended is not attained. The water is either used at too low a temperature or in too small a quantity, or both. When administered by the patient herself she becomes tired of the pumping and of the position which she must assume, and fails to keep it up during the length of time required for the injection of the quantity of water usually advised—that is, a gallon or two—and the constrained squatting position is of itself injurious. I believe that the long-continued use of hot water is followed by relaxation of the pelvic organs, and this would constitute another objection to the indiscriminate recommendation of this measure, for when it is placed in the patient's hands she is apt to continue its use for too long a period. The remedy is no doubt most efficacious in the treatment of these chronic cases of pelvic peritonitis, and great credit is due Emmet for introducing it to the profession. It should, however, be administered in accordance with fixed rules and under certain restrictions, and these I would class as follows: 1, the patient must always be in the recumbent posture; 2, she must not administer the injection herself; 3, the water should be at a certain temperature, which is best determined by the sensations of the patient. It should be used as hot as can be easily borne, and the temperature gradually increased during the administration of the injection, for the patient will be able to bear it at a higher temperature after the current has been flowing a few minutes than when the application is first made. I believe that the douche is better than pumping, as by Davidson's syringe, because the application is more likely to be thorough and the effect to be maintained longer, for even when the injection is given by the physician or nurse the hand is apt to become tired and the application stopped, for a time at least. It is the continuous application of the remedy which is beneficial. In other words, the organs should be kept as it were in a hot bath. For use in my private hospital I have had constructed a tripod five feet high, with a hook in the centre on which a bucket is easily hung. This bucket holds two gallons of water, and near the bottom is placed a stopcock, to which is attached a tube provided with a nozzle and stopcock at its distal end. The patient is placed on a bed-pan, which is modified after that devised by Meriman. The nozzle is then introduced into the vagina, and the stopcock at the bucket turned by the nurse, the water being at a temperature of at least 110°. The patient can then regulate the flow herself. The water is allowed to enter the vagina, dilating it and flowing off slowly, so that the tissues are in a continuous hot bath, which may be kept up as long as desired—from ten minutes to an hour—care being taken to see that the proper temperature of the water is maintained by the addition of a fresh supply from time to time. The important point is not so much the amount of water as its temperature and constant contact. If the vagina could once be filled to distension and the temperature kept up, it would not be necessary to renew the water, but to keep up the temperature a regular flow of hot water must be provided for. The rapidity of the flow may be regulated by the stopcock. The

application of this remedy should be made once or twice a day, depending on its effect upon the patient.

After all tenderness has subsided much may be accomplished by
gentle massage of the pelvic organs. This is best carried out by the
introduction of one or two fingers of the left hand into the vagina, while
the right hand is placed upon the hypogastrium ; then the contracted
ligaments, thickened membranes, and fixed uterus, ovaries, and tubes
should be gently manipulated and moved from side to side or upward
and downward, care being taken that the force used is not sufficient to
lacerate adhesions or even to so stretch them as to cause their irritation.
The proper amount of force is best regulated by the sensation of the
patient, and if pain is produced by the manipulation it should not be
persisted in. This massage may at first be employed at intervals of two
or three days, but later it may for a time be used almost daily, and it
will almost invariably be found that the organs gradually become more
mobile—that the adhesions become attenuated, and in many cases finally
absorbed. On the other hand, adhesions of such size and strength may
exist that many months may be required to produce any marked effect,
and in some cases the adhesions may be of such a character as to be permanently organized and almost incurably fixed.

I have also found the stretching of the fundus of the vagina by firmly
packing it with absorbent cotton, sometimes repeated almost daily or at
intervals of two, three, or four days, of great benefit in stretching the
adhesions and promoting their absorption. Sometimes, where adhesions
are persistent, the use of the rubber colpeurynter distended with hot water
is of value.

Where there is a foreign body, as a tumor, fixed posteriorly to the
uterus, or where the uterus is fixed in a retroflexed position, the patient
may be placed in the knee-chest position, Sims's speculum introduced, and
the vagina packed with cotton while the patient is in that posture ; or,
instead, the vagina may be simply distended with air. The air may be
admitted by the introduction of Campbell's glass tube or by the separation of the walls of the vagina with the fingers, which may be done by
the patient herself. These measures are often of decided benefit.

I wish to repeat what has already been stated, that the treatment
of chronic perimetritis, to be carried out successfully, requires that the
patient should be in bed and placed under such circumstances and surroundings that the physician may be enabled to pursue personally the
plan of treatment. Of course much will be gained if he is aided by a
trained nurse. This in many cases involves the removal of the patient
from the cares of her home.

Advantage may often be derived from the application of small blisters
to the hypogastric and iliac regions, the counter-irritation being kept up
almost continuously for two weeks at a time. The blisters should not be
larger than two inches square, and should be moved from place to place;
for instance, one blister may be placed on the hypogastrium, and before
this has healed a second should be placed one side of it. This should
be kept up for two weeks at a time, or until four or five blisters have
been applied, when, if benefit is to follow, it will be apparent.

When the organs which are agglutinated to one another become more
mobile, and the thickened membranes more flaccid, much benefit some-

times results from the application of a pessary if a displacement of the uterus, ovaries, or tubes exists and persists; but before the use of this instrument is thought of, it must be positively ascertained that no tenderness remains as a result of the inflammatory process; the inflammation must have entirely subsided, the effects alone remaining. It is sometimes advised that an instrument large enough to constantly stretch and over-stretch the false membranes and adhesions is advisable. It has also been recommended to over-stretch these adhesions by manipulation. Of the two, I much prefer the latter method; that is, stretching by manipulation rather than by continuously acting upon them by means of a pessary large enough to stretch the vagina and through it the adhesions. In stretching by manipulation, with the patient under ether, you have your own sense of touch to guide you, and the action of your efforts ceases with the cessation of the manipulation, while that carried out by means of a pessary is continuous and may result in great harm from irritation, if not from ulceration of the vaginal surface from pressure; or it may result in rupture of the adhesions. If a pessary is adjusted, it should be used, not for the purpose of over-stretching adhesions, but simply for its stimulating effect on the pelvic circulation, or as a support to the pelvic circulation rather than as a support to the uterus. A larger instrument should not be used than one which will occupy the vagina without stretching it—simply unfold any doubling up which may have resulted from retroversion or prolapse of the uterus—and its action should be carefully watched. It should be learned, not from the sensation of the patient, but from actual examination, that it is not making undue pressure; this examination should be made daily at first, and afterward at longer intervals. The use of the pessary should be discontinued as soon as possible. This statement should be qualified by saying that the words as soon as possible mean when all symptoms have subsided, and the uterus and other organs are maintaining a normal or nearly normal position, or when the pessary seems to have ceased to be of value. It may then be removed on trial.

There is a method of using the pessary, in which it is advised that the instrument shall be large enough to span the angle of flexion which may exist, for the purpose of making pressure on the fundus of the uterus, which is incarcerated in the cul-de-sac of Douglas by adhesions between its peritoneal surface and that lining the sac. This I believe to be a bad principle, for an instrument long enough to do this must either take its point of support against the pubic arch or from an external attachment—a principle of using the pessary which should be most emphatically condemned.

The above treatment should be carried out with the patient in bed, if possible, during which time general measures for the improvement of the muscular and nervous system should also be employed. The application of electricity to the thickened peritoneum and adhesions is another measure which should not be allowed to pass without comment. Much good may be done by the daily application of faradism, with one electrode in the vagina and the other on the hypogastrium, and continued for from fifteen to thirty minutes. I have thought that in some cases great benefit followed this application. Galvanism is also of service, and by some is thought to be of more value than the faradic current.

The time for getting up should be determined by the results of treatment; usually a period of from four to six weeks is sufficient to determine whether or not the treatment at absolute rest is going to be of benefit. Of course it is not to be understood that cure will follow in severe and long-standing cases within this period, because if this hope is entertained disappointment will follow nearly always. What we hope and expect to attain is rest, both physical and physiological, during which time local treatment can be carried out with greater facility and thoroughness and the general condition improved. As a rule, the ligaments soften, the false membranes become attenuated, and during the time stated the patient is very much benefited, and sometimes cured. She should now begin to sit up and to exercise moderately; the amount of exercise should be regulated by its effect. If pain follows walking or riding, it should not be persisted in until such time as exercise can be taken without the production of these symptoms.

There are no specific remedies for internal administration. The general medication of the patient should consist in the use of such remedies as we have learned to depend upon as capable of building up the blood and nervous system, embracing especially that class of tonics which are said to have the power of inducing such changes in plastic material as favors its absorption. To this class belong the chlorides, as the chloride of arsenic, the chloride of iron, the chloride of ammonium, and the bichloride of mercury. These remedies should be placed at the head of the class. The next are the iodides, as the iodide of iron, the iodide of potassium, and the bromide of potassium. Whether or not these remedies have the powers ascribed to them is questionable, and their administration for this purpose must always be, to a certain extent, empirical. As tonic remedies the administration of iron and the bichloride of mercury is of course always indicated. Cod-liver oil is also a remedy of much value in some cases where it can be digested. The whole plan of treatment should rather be of a local than of a general character, while at the same time very great importance should be given to the building up of the general system, without which nothing can be gained by local treatment. The patient should have a change of scene and air as soon as practicable. A sojourn at the seaside for a time, and then in the mountains, will be of great benefit always.

The fact should always be borne in mind by the physician and impressed upon the patient that a previous attack of perimetritis will serve as a predisposing and abiding cause for a recurrence of the disease, so that all exciting causes may be avoided as far as possible.

PELVIC HÆMATOCELE.

By T. GAILLARD THOMAS, M. D.

HISTORY.—Prior to the present century the pathological condition which we are about to investigate had no place in the category of diseases peculiar to the sexual organs of the female. Very slowly have its pathogenic features, its etiology, and its importance as a not uncommon factor in pelvic disorders, assumed a systematic basis, and even now considerable diversity of opinion exists upon these points. The reasons for this are not far to seek. In the first place, hæmatocele is a symptom of an accident occurring in the pelvis and resulting in hemorrhage; in the second, the source of the flow which creates the hæmatoma or tumor of blood cannot ordinarily be recognized by any diagnostic measures known to science; and in the third, death rarely occurring from the accident and as a direct consequence of it, autopsic evidence is wanting upon which to base accurate and scientific data.

Although these statements are undoubtedly true, it may nevertheless be asserted with confidence that we are to-day no longer in the dark as to the general pathology of this interesting disorder, and that we are in position to map out a plan of treatment which meets the indications which present themselves in an intelligent and reliable manner. There are, however, several sources of hemorrhage which result in pelvic hæmatocele, and it is highly probable that the day will never come when that one which has created the accident can be ascertained with certainty. But while such accuracy of diagnosis would be gratifying to the ambition of the modern diagnostician, neither the prognosis nor treatment of the disorder would be influenced by it.

Long before our day practitioners had recognized by touch the occasional presence of tumors, more or less marked by fluctuation, which occupied the pouch of Douglas, and by their mechanical influence pushed the uterus out of its normal place; but it was not until the early part of our century that it was discovered that these tumors were sometimes, and that not rarely, composed entirely of coagulated blood; and, curious though it may appear, it was not until the year 1850 that pelvic hæmatocele became a well-recognized disorder.

As early as 1737, Ruysch of Amsterdam appears to have come to the verge of discovering it, but it was left for Récamier, to whom gynecology owes so much besides, to make it known when in 1831 he opened a post-uterine tumor, gave vent to a large accumulation of coagulated blood, and described the case in the *Lancette Française* for that year. In 1850 the

subject attracted the attention of Nélaton, became a recognized pathological condition, and has since received a great deal of attention in all the
civilized countries of the world.

DEFINITION AND SYNONYMS.—Pelvic hæmatocele—which has like
wise received the names of retro-uterine hæmatocele and uterine hæmatoma—may be defined as an effusion of blood into the pelvic cavity of
the female, either into or under the peritoneum. Some authors have
limited this definition to blood escaping from utero-ovarian vessels and
to blood enclosed either by anatomical structures or by previously-exist-
ing inflammatory products. I do not adopt these restrictions, because
their assumption appears to me to be unwarranted and the validity of
the reasons given for their adoption more than doubtful. The location
of the blood-mass differs widely in different cases: sometimes, and usually, it is behind the uterus—high up when obliteration of Douglas's
pouch has occurred, low down and near to the perineum where such
obliteration has not occurred; at other times it exists both behind and in
front of the uterus; and at others still, in front of the uterus alone, adhesions preventing its percolation to the posterior parts of the pelvis.

FREQUENCY.—It may be said, in general terms, that this affection is
by no means rare, every one of large experience in gynecology meeting
necessarily with a large number of cases of it. But no reliable statistics
of its frequency have been collected up to the present time. Olshausen
of Halle declares that in 1145 gynecological cases he saw 34 hæmato-
celes; Beigel in 2000 cases found 38; Schroeder, 7 in 1000; and Seiffert
of Prague reports 66 seen in 1272 cases of female pelvic diseases. Barnes
says that in ten years' practice he met with 53 cases, and in twenty years
Tilt has seen but 12.

Without doubt, the validity of the statistics of this disorder is vitiated
by erroneous diagnosis, as is the case with all affections which generally
end in recovery. Here cases of cellulitis, pelvic peritonitis, imprisoned
cysts, etc. offer prolific sources of error, as I can aver from the results of
my own experience.

PATHOLOGY.—It is a fact, thoroughly proved by physiological experiment, that blood injected into serous cavities very soon encysts itself by
the enveloping influence of lymph which is poured over it, forming false
membranes, or, as the French term them, néo-membranes. The clot,
once formed, clings to the serous membrane in contact with it, and soon
becomes roofed over by lymph, which, according to Vulpian, begins to
show traces of organization as early as the end of twenty-four hours.
Should the effused blood be poor in fibrin, the coagulation and encysting
do not occur, a rapid absorption taking the place of these processes.

Pelvic hæmatocele consists, as has been already stated, in the collection
of a mass of blood in the pelvis, either above or below its roof, without
reference to the source of the flow. Such a flow ordinarily occurs from
one of the three following sources: first, rupture of vessels in the pelvis;
second, reflux of blood from the uterus or tubes; third, transudation of
blood in consequence of dyscrasia or pelvic peritonitis.

From this it becomes evident that hæmatocele is not a disease, but a
symptom which marks a number of different pathological conditions of
quite various significance. As, however, we cannot discover the original
accident or pathological condition, we are forced to compromise with

taking its most prominent sign as the exponent of a state which is beyond the powers of diagnosis.

Autopsic evidence has revealed the following as the special and most frequent sources of the hemorrhage:

1st. Rupture of blood-vessels in the pelvis:
Utero-ovarian;
Varicose veins of broad ligaments;
Vessels of extra-uterine ovisac.

2d. Rupture of pelvic viscera:
Ovaries;
Fallopian tubes;
Uterus.

3d. Reflux of blood from the uterus:
Menstrual blood.

4th. Transudation from blood-vessels:
Purpura;
Scorbutus;
Chlorosis;
Hemorrhagic peritonitis.

It is then clear that the mere presence of a large clot of blood in the pelvis, apart from general symptoms, is a matter of very doubtful significance, since on the one hand it may be the result of a mere regurgitation of menstrual blood due to imperviousness of the cervical or tubal canal, or on the other of the rupture of a Fallopian tube which has become the nidus of an extra-uterine fœtus.

Whatever be the source of the blood which escapes, it coagulates, unless very poor in fibrin, either in the most dependent part of the peritoneum or in the pelvic areolar tissue beneath it. Here the watery portions of the mass are gradually absorbed, leaving a hard, small tumor remaining; or, suppurative action being excited, the hard mass is softened down and discharged into the rectum, vagina, bladder, or peritoneum as a grumous material somewhat resembling currant-jelly in appearance.

CAUSES.—These must be divided into predisposing and exciting, for it is rare to meet with the disease in a woman who has previously been in perfect health. The predisposing causes which can be cited with confidence are—the period of ovarian activity (fifteen to forty-five years); disordered blood-state, plethora or anæmia; the menstrual epoch; chronic ovarian or tubal disease; pelvic peritonitis; and the hemorrhagic diathesis. The exciting causes have been found to be sudden checking of the menstrual flow; blows or falls; excessive or intemperate coition; obstruction of cervical canal; obstruction of Fallopian tubes; violent efforts; and ectopic gestation.

VARIETIES.—The two great classes of the affection are the peritoneal and the subperitoneal. In the former the blood collects in the peritoneal cavity and becomes encysted there; in the latter it collects in the cellular tissue beneath the peritoneum, and there forms a solid mass.

Some authors have opposed the consideration of these two varieties under the same head; among them, Aran, Bernutz, and Voisin. But from a clinical standpoint such a consideration appears to me to be valid. Not only have distinct instances of subperitoneal hæmatocele been recorded by such observers as Barnes, Simpson, Olshausen, and Tuckwell, but cases have been met with in which the subperitoneal variety has ruptured the peritoneal roof of the pelvis, and thus broken down the theoretical barrier which pathologists have been inclined to establish between the two varieties.

Of the two varieties, there can be no doubt that the peritoneal is that which presents itself the more frequently. In 41 autopsies Tuckwell found the tumor to be peritoneal in 38.

SYMPTOMS.—As a rule, long before the occurrence of pelvic hemorrhage the patient will have complained of more or less decided symptoms of disease, or at least of disorder, of the genital system. The symptoms which mark blood-dyscrasia or pelvic peritonitis or menstrual irregularity will probably have attracted attention.

When the accident occurs the gravity of the symptoms will depend in great degree upon the character of the lesion which has taken place. Sometimes the blood-accumulation takes place so insidiously that the existence of the tumor created by coagulation takes the practitioner by surprise. At other times what Barnes has called a cataclysm occurs, and in a few hours puts the unfortunate patient beyond the sphere of hope or the resources of art.

In portraying the symptoms of this affection a writer can therefore merely approximate the truth, satisfying himself with the description of a case of ordinary severity, avoiding the description of cases in either extreme, and guarding the reader against supposing that all attacks give the same intensity of symptoms.

Most prominent among the immediate symptoms are—severe and sudden pelvic pain; pallor, faintness, and coldness of the extremities; a sense of exhaustion; nausea and vomiting; metrorrhagia; uterine tenesmus; enlargement of the abdomen; interference with the bladder and rectum; small and rapid pulse; subnormal temperature.

These are the symptoms of invasion, those which may be termed immediate, and which depend upon loss of blood and a sudden traumatic influence exerted upon living tissues. Very soon, generally within forty-eight hours, a reaction occurs which is sometimes slight, and at other times decided. The secondary symptoms are usually the following: tendency to chilliness; constipation; suppression of urine; tympanites; high temperature; rapid pulse; and tenderness over abdomen.

These symptoms are due to a combination of two causes—loss of vital fluid and the invasion of the peritoneum or pelvic areolar tissue by a mass of blood which becomes coagulated and irritant, on the one hand, and inflammatory processes resulting from such invasion on the other. Half of them might be produced by metrorrhagia, and half by sudden and complete retroversion; but a union of the whole will point toward hæmatocele and prompt a physical examination.

PHYSICAL SIGNS.—A tumor will be felt by vaginal touch, usually, though not always, posterior to the uterus and vagina, and partially occluding the latter. This will, if the examination be made very early, be found to be soft and obscurely fluctuating, but it soon becomes a smooth, dense, and solid body. The uterus is very generally found pressed upward and forward, so that the body lies against the abdominal wall and the cervix is on a level with or a little above the symphysis pubis. In some rare cases the blood-tumor is anterior to or obliquely to one side of the uterus, but these are very rare.

Abdominal palpation reveals the presence of a tumor of varying size, and which sometimes extends up to the navel in peritoneal hæmatocele, but in the subperitoneal variety no tumor whatever may be discoverable by these explorations, unless conjoined manipulation be added to it for the sake of deeper and more thorough search.

DIFFERENTIATION.—Hæmatocele may be confounded with pelvic cellulitis or abscess, retroversion, extra-uterine pregnancy, fibroid tumor, and dislocated ovarian cyst.

The tumor of cellulitis develops slowly, with great pain; is hard at first, and then softens; is tender from the first; does not elevate the uterus or press it forward; and is not often accompanied by metrorrhagia.

Retroversion will readily be detected by the uterine sound, conjoined manipulation, and the absence of anæmic symptoms.

The development of extra-uterine pregnancy is slow and gives the signs of gestation.

Fibrous tumors grow slowly, are painless, and move with the uterus, and they are hard, irregular, and do not lift the uterus against the symphysis.

Displaced cysts are painless, non-hemorrhagic, cause no metrorrhagia, and yield fluctuation readily to palpation.

COMPLICATIONS.—The complications to be feared in this disease are septicæmia, suppuration and abscess, and peritonitis.

COURSE, DURATION, AND TERMINATION.—The hemorrhage may be so severe as to destroy life immediately. Five such instances have been recorded by Voisin; I have met with one; and Ollivier d'Angers mentions two in which death occurred in half an hour from a varicose uteroovarian vein. Such a termination is, however, very rare.

As a rule, absorption takes place unaided by art; in some cases suppuration occurs, and the mass is discharged as if it were a large abscess by the vagina, rectum, bladder, or abdominal walls; and at other times septic absorption, accompanied by septic peritonitis, destroys the life of the patient.

PROGNOSIS.—The prognosis will depend in great degree upon the severity of the constitutional symptoms. As a rule, it is decidedly favorable unless the surgical tendencies of the attending practitioner alter its natural inclination. The prognosis of the peritoneal form is graver than that of the subperitoneal, and when the tumor is very large the danger is greater than when it is small. A large tumor argues great loss of vital fluid, which may in itself destroy life, and the necessity for the absorption of a large amount of coagulated material which may poison the blood.

The usual causes of death are loss of blood, shock from sudden invasion of the peritoneum, peritonitis, secondary discharge of the encapsulated mass into the peritoneum, or septicæmia.

TREATMENT.—Should the physician be called in the inception of the attack, the patient should at once be placed in the recumbent posture, all excitement around her be quelled, the head be kept low, warmth be applied to the soles of the feet, and perfect quiet enjoined. An effort should be made to check the flow by applying bladders of ice or cloths wrung out of hot water over the hypogastrium, pain and tendency to shock met by the use of morphia hypodermically, and ammonia and brandy freely administered by the mouth. This is all that promises benefit, and further efforts should be avoided as calculated to do absolute harm.

After reaction has occurred let it be borne in mind that the factors which tend to the production of death are—1st, peritonitis; 2d, septicæmia; 3d, suppuration and discharge through some dangerous outlet; and let all efforts be directed toward the prevention of these events.

All pain should be quieted by opium or one of its salts, hypodermically or by mouth or rectum; the patient should be thoroughly nourished by milk and strong animal broths, given as often as every two hours; febrile action should be controlled by the coil of running ice-water and quinine; and strict quietude observed, all unnecessary examinations being avoided, as belonging to the most pernicious class of perturbing influences.

Should the case progress favorably, no surgical procedure looking toward the artificial evacuation of the accumulated blood either by bistoury or by the aspirator should be thought of, however large the accumulation be; for experience has proved that cases left to nature, as a rule, do better than those interfered with.

On the other hand, the great value of surgical interference in those cases in which suppurative action occurs, or in which septicæmia develops itself either in acute or chronic form, must not for a moment be lost sight of. Should the case not progress toward recovery, should the symptoms of septicæmia develop as a sharp attack or as the insidious hectic fever, the accumulated blood or pus and blood should at once be evacuated, and the nidus from which it is discharged be thoroughly washed out with a $2\frac{1}{2}$ per cent. solution of carbolic acid or a solution of the bichloride of mercury, 1 to 2000 of water. Should the accumulation be attainable, tuto, cito, et jucunde, by the vagina, an exploring-needle should be carried into it, and as soon as the fluid is seen to flow a sharp-pointed bistoury should be slid along this and a free opening be made, all the contents of the sac evacuated, and antiseptic washing be at once practised by means of Davidson's syringe and a glass tube.

Should the accumulation point toward the abdominal walls, the opening may with perfect safety be accomplished there. I have operated thus upon 3 cases, with recovery in all, but the accumulation had at the time of operation assumed the character rather of an abscess than of an hæmatocele. A. Martin of Berlin has operated by abdominal section upon 8 cases, with 6 recoveries and 2 deaths, and Baumgärtner of Baden Baden has done so upon 1 case, with recovery. Zweifel has collected 30 cases operated upon by free vaginal incision, with a result of 3 deaths, giving a mortality of 10 per cent. Mere puncture through the vagina he found followed by a mortality of 15 per cent.

The question of surgical interference in pelvic hæmatocele is still sub judice. In my judgment, the rule of practice may, with the present light which we have to guide us, be safely formulated thus: So long as the symptoms are good and the case progresses toward recovery, avoid surgical interference of all sorts, however great be the sanguineous effusion. So soon as symptoms of decided septicæmia or septic peritonitis develop themselves, evacuate the accumulation by a free opening practised by the safest outlet which presents itself, and use antiseptic washings thoroughly.

FIBROUS TUMORS OF THE UTERUS.

By WILLIAM H. BYFORD, M. D.

RELATIONS AND STRUCTURE.—These tumors grow from the muscular and connective tissues of the uterus, and consequently partake of the character of these tissues. Sometimes the substance of the tumor consists principally of connective, at others of muscular, tissue. The variations in the relative proportion of these two fibrous substances constitute the main differences in the characters and appearauces of the tumors, and lead to the different terms applied to them, as myomata, fibromata, myo-fibromata, etc. The firmer the tumor the more connective tissue it contains. When we inspect, either ante- or post-mortem, a uterus with a fibrous tumor attached or contained within its wall, it will be found to present a much darker hue than natural. Instead of the normal light rose-color, it is generally dark, sometimes almost of a purplish tint. The time of menstruation makes some difference; just before it is darker than soon after the menstrual flow. The color also varies with the character and size of the tumor. In large solid tumors the color is darker than in the large fibro-cystic variety; indeed, in some of the latter the pearly color strongly reminds one of an ovarian cyst. We cannot therefore depend on the color or shape of surface for a diagnosis. Even after the abdominal cavity is opened the contour of the uterus is usually not regular. If we make an incision into the tumor, we find that it is surrounded by a distinct capsule, which limits and defines its boundaries and separates it from the adjacent substance. This envelope is not a cyst or other form of membrane: it is continuous with, and inseparable from, the muscular structure of the uterine walls. It, in fact, is a condensed layer of the fibrous substance of the uterus. In cases of true encysted tumors the cyst-wall is the generating portion of the growth. In fibrous tumors of the uterus the growth produces the capsule by displacing the surrounding substance in every direction, pressing it strongly against the unaffected fibrous tissue and condensing it into the smooth capsule. It is thus engendered in, and enveloped by, the muscular walls of the uterus. These latter of course grow to dimensions sufficient to keep pace with the increasing tumor. The growth may, as a consequence of such a connection, be hulled out or enucleated, and will not be reproduced. Inflammation or other degenerating processes may occasionally cause adhesion of the capsule and tumor, but this is an accident of uncommon occurrence. To understand this mode of encapsulation we must remember that the uterine muscles are irregularly stratified, and that the tumors are developed between the strata as between the leaves of a book, separating them sufficiently to gain lodgment and room.

The appearances of the substance of the tumor are not uniform. In many cases the color of the interior of the tumor is dark gray; in some it is dull red; again, sometimes almost livid. The surface of the tumor after the capsule has been removed is often marked by sulci denoting a division into lobules. In other cases the tumor is smooth and symmetrical in shape, and the fibres distinctly visible to the naked eye. The smooth tumor is apt to be very dense and comparatively difficult to destroy, while the lobulated variety is less dense and sometimes easily broken to pieces. But the difference of density does not correspond altogether with the color or shape of surface.

We seldom find large tumors of uniform structure. In some places they are of solid fibrous structure; in others there are cavities of greater or less size, containing a tenacious red serum. These cavities, which seem to be made by localized disintegration of the fibrous tissue, are sometimes of great size, containing several pounds of serum (Atlee). Much more frequently they are small and hold a small amount of fluid. I have met with several where the substance of the tumor seemed to be made up of alveoli filled with a tenacious fluid the color of milk.

Besides this effect upon the density of the tumor resulting from what might be called its usual course, there are numerous modifications in it and in the other properties of the tumors arising from spontaneous degeneration.

It may be said, I think, that without adventitious or supplementary vascular supply the life of a fibrous tumor is self-limited, and it ceases to grow after it has attained to a certain size, and that then it either remains stationary or undergoes degeneration. As I shall have occasion to say farther on, the original supply of blood-vessels cannot be increased to an indefinite degree, and the tumor that grows indefinitely derives a supplementary supply of blood by contracting adhesions to the viscera or abdominal walls. Such adhesions are common and mischievous.

After a tumor has attained its growth, degeneration into the more elementary forms of tissue sets in, as the cartilaginous degeneration, and there is often a deposition of earthy material found in it which reduces it to a hard, dense, stationary, and indestructible body. In such cases there is almost a complete loss of vitality in the tumor, and it becomes a calcified mass.

We may easily demonstrate that the structure of these tumors is essentially fibrous. By maceration and careful dissection the fibres are traceable to a greater or less degree in all of them, the proportion and characters of which, as before said, differ greatly. In the smooth, symmetrically-developed tumor the fibres are usually long and distinctly traceable, while in the lobulated light-gray tumor the fibres are more rudimentary and not so easily followed up by dissection.

MODE OF DEVELOPMENT.—It has already been stated that the fibrous tumor of the uterus grows in or on its wall and originates in the fibrous structure of the organ. The point of beginning is in one or more fasciculi of the muscular system or the connective tissue of the uterus. If in one fasciculus, the point of origin is very minute, as indeed it is generally at first.

The development consists in an hypertrophy of the bundle of fibres affected and a deposit of material similar in structure to that first involved. Sometimes there are numerous nuclei, and nearly all the fibrous structure of the uterus is involved in fibrous degeneration. In the case where the deposit is defined and occupies a small space, it should be borne in mind that the future tumor, however large it becomes, must occupy the same nidus in which it first originated. The nidus becomes enlarged sufficiently to accommodate the growing tumor.

The nucleus of development is enlarged by the accretion of substance similar, if not identical, in character to its own proper material. The nature of the tumor is determined by this fact, and its fibres are rudimentary in organization, instead of being hypertrophied and highly developed, as those of the uterine wall by which it is surrounded. As the tumor grows the fibrous structure surrounding it is pressed aside in every direction in such a way as to completely embrace the growth and encapsulate it. The tumor does not incorporate the adjacent fibres and grow by inducing degeneration in them, but, as before said, it presses them aside. As it thus moulds and shapes a bed in the solid substance of the interior wall, it impresses upon the embracing muscular fibres an increased vitality, and they grow by hypertrophy of a character similar to that of pregnancy. The fibres become longer, and apparently, if not really, more numerous. This hypertrophy of the uterine fibres surrounding the tumor is equal to the capacity demanded by the increasing size of the growing tumor. In this description of the method of development and the embracing capacity of the hypertrophied fibres surrounding it the reader will trace the formation of the capsule in which the tumor is contained. The inner surface of the capsule is smooth, and there are many feeble fibres of connective tissue seen to connect it with the surface of the tumor. There is no adhesion proper between the surface of the tumor and its capsule.

I must call attention to another point that governs the extent and limits of the growth of the tumor—viz. the number and distribution of its vessels. The vessels entering the tumor represent the minute twigs that supplied the fasciculus in which it originated. They arrive at the point of morbid deposit from the parts constituting the capsule, and there are always several of them. The number of these vessels always remains the same, and their calibre is increased with the hypertrophy of the surrounding tissues. They cannot grow at the demand of the trophic energies of the tumor to an unlimited degree, but their size is limited by the growth of the surrounding parts. As the tumor grows and its capsule expands, the vessels are separated farther from each other, until after a while the area becomes so large that the supply of blood will not admit of further growth and the tumor comes to a standstill. Thus their growth, from the nature of their supply, is limited; hence the usual history of the tumor is one of self-limitation. It is all-important in forming an opinion in reference to the greater or less vitality of the fibrous tumor, therefore, to remember that it is not supplied by one large arterial trunk entering at one place and spreading over its capsule, but that the supply is by a number of small vessels penetrating the tumor at different points; that their number cannot be increased and their growth is limited; that as the tumor grows their capacity to supply it grows gradually less until entirely exhausted: then the growth stops.

There is another and adventitious source of nutritious supply, and I think it is essential to very large growths: at least, so far as I know, it is always present. I mean the adhesion of the uterus or tumor to the wall of the abdomen, the pelvic or abdominal viscera, or, what is more common, the omentum. When adhesions occur from whatever cause, the vessels of the tumor increase in size and supply it with a vast increase in the amount of blood. All the large tumors I have had an opportunity of examining were to a greater or less extent covered by a network of large vessels contained in the omentum. These vessels penetrate the uterus, carrying a deluge of blood into its substance. These large vascular adhesions are a source of embarrassment in operations for their removal. Operators allude to them and give instructions how to overcome the difficulty presented by them. The uterine vessels alone would never be sufficient to supply the forty- or fifty-pound tumors so often mistaken for ovarian tumors.

EFFECTS UPON THE UTERUS.—I have already said that the fibres immediately surrounding the growth undergo a true hypertrophy, acquiring dimension, susceptibility, and capacity similar to the hypertrophy of gestation. All the fibres of the uterus undergo a similar change, only less in degree; the more remote from the tumor, the less marked the hypertrophy. This remark must be modified somewhat by the consideration of the locality of the tumor. A polypoid tumor growing from the fundus causes universal hypertrophy of the uterine fibres. A submucous tumor will usually cause a general hypertrophy of the uterine fibres, but greater on the side of the tumor. A subserous tumor is attended by a slight hypertrophy, and in a centrally-located intramural tumor the hypertrophy would be much like that in the submucous variety, only less in degree. But this augmentation of tissue is not confined to the fibrous structure: it extends to the vascular and nervous apparatus and to the serous and mucous membranes. With this growth of the tissues comes change in the properties and functions of the uterus itself. It is more sensitive, the secretions are increased, and almost parturient contractility is acquired.

But probably as remarkable and uniform a symptom as any arising from the general hypertrophy is hemorrhage. The mucous membrane of the uterus is hypertrophied in all its constituents and proportions. The membrane acquires larger superfices and greater thickness, its glands are enlarged, and its blood-vessels augmented. Its functions, as a consequence of these changes, are exaggerated. The glands secrete greater quantities of mucus, and the vessels when ruptured in the processes of menstruation pour out a superabundance of blood. Indeed, I know of no other way to account for the hemorrhages so generally present in cases of fibrous tumors of the uterus, except upon the ground that the endometrium, a natural hemorrhagic surface, has its properties and functions enhanced by a general hypertrophy.

LOCATION OF THE TUMOR.—For the purpose of considering the relation of these tumors to the different regions of the uterus we may call that part situated above the entrance of the Fallopian tubes the fundal zone, and that above the internal os uteri the corporal zone; all below this the cervical zone. Fibrous tumors may and do originate in all of these zones or regions, but they spring more frequently from the corporal than either of the others, and less frequently from the fundal zone. The part of the corporal zone in which these tumors more frequently grow is the lower or cervical portion. There is another important view of the relation of the tumors to the uterus. The muscular fibres of that organ run in every direction with reference to the latitude and longitude of the uterine circumference—transversely, longitudinally, obliquely, spirally, etc. There is probably not much more definiteness in the layers constituting the walls of the uterus. If they cannot be completely separated into regular strata, there is sufficient distinctness in the layers to justify us in employing the term strata in connection with their arrangement, and this term will enable us to get a more exact understanding of the language used in the description of tumors. Authorities differ as to the exact number of strata to be found in the body of the uterus, but for clinical purposes it is convenient to describe them as follows: By drawing a line through the middle of the uterine wall longitudinally we will indicate a central stratum of fibres. A tumor originating in that line or stratum is what is usually called an intramural tumor. The number of tumors growing in this stratum is not very great as compared with those situated nearer the two surfaces.

FIG. 25.

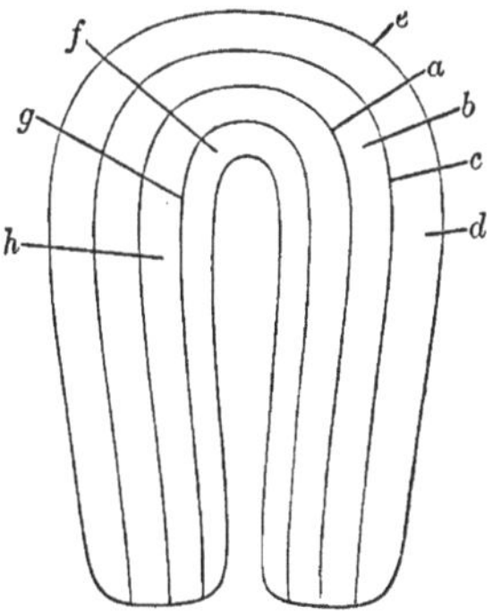

Diagram showing Muscular Strata of Uterus, as divided for clinical purposes.

. If we run one line between the serous and another between the mucous membrane and the central line, as in the diagram, other strata with intervening spaces will be indicated. *a* would represent the centre stratum of the wall; *b*, the space immediately outside of that; *c*, a stratum still farther out; *e*, the subserous; and *d*, a deeper one. When we look at the inner layers of fibres, we find *f* situated immediately beneath the mucous membrane; *g*, farther out; and *h*, next the median line. The nucleus of a tumor may be first manifested in any of the strata or spaces marked by these lines, and its position with reference to the central line will, to a great extent, govern the direction it takes during development. A tumor the nucleus of which is situated in line *a* will, as it develops, press the muscular fibres equally in every direction, and when large, the prominence caused by pressure of the tumor would be equal in the uterine cavity and on the peritoneal surface. In marked contrast to this, when the nucleus is at *f* the growing tumor presses the mucous membrane before it until it becomes pendulous, and then the name of polypus is given to it; or if the origin is at *e*, the serous membrane is pressed before it, and the tumor is called subserous. When the nucleus is at *d*, the tumor elevates the serous membrane and becomes a prominent hemispherical protuberance. It is also called a subserous tumor, although situated some distance from the membrane. When a tumor takes its origin at *g* the mucous membrane is crowded before it, and a marked prominence into the cavity of the uterus is observed. This is the submucous tumor. These illustrations are intended to call the attention of the student to the fact that practically these tumors spring from any one or all the fibrous strata of the uterus instead of only the central, submucous, and subserous layers, and that it is profitable, on account of the difference in their effects upon the shape and functions of the uterus, to study them in this aspect of their growth.

ETIOLOGY.—While we know many of the conditions under which fibrous tumors exist, we have really very little, if any, definite and reliable information as to their causes, either remote or proximate. We know that they occur much more frequently near the time when the uterus begins to undergo senile degeneration, although they do originate in earlier years. They very seldom, if ever, are observed in the fœtus or child, nor is it common for them to commence growing after the menopause. Women belonging to the African race are the most frequent subjects of these tumors.

The married or single status does not seem to have any effect in predisposing to these tumors. We do not know what physiological or pathological states of the uterus or other organs predispose to them. There is probably no tumor in the body strictly analogous in structure, mode of origin, supply, or development to the fibroid tumor of the uterus. There is no other organ in the body that undergoes analogous normal trophic changes. The vast multiplication of tissue that takes place in the uterus during gestation, and the more rapid but equally great changes toward degeneration or atrophy, would naturally suggest pathological possibilities of a peculiar nature. The rhythmical changes of menstruation are like no other functional condition. They too involve the processes of hypertrophy and atrophy. When the menstrual and generative changes are normal every part of the body of the uterus is simultaneously and proportionately hypertrophied and atrophied. Local derangements of these processes of hypertrophy and degeneration must sometimes occur, probably from defective or excessive innervation of loculi in the fibrous structure. Congestion or hyperæmia may thus result, and consequently very great influence be exerted upon the nutrition of the parts concerned after the deposit has begun; its presence increases the hyperæmia and thus perpetuates its growth indefinitely.

CLINICAL HISTORY.—Probably the earliest, most frequent, and constant symptoms connected with fibrous tumors of the uterus are hemorrhage and leucorrhœa. They are both the result of active or arterial hyperæmia, and doubtless come from the endometrium. Polypi, submucous, and intramural tumors are more likely to give rise to these two symptoms. The nearer the mucous membrane, and the greater that membrane is expanded, the greater the amount of hemorrhage and leucorrhœa, and, as a counter-fact, the nearer the serous membrane, the less the amount of these two discharges. While this statement in reference to the effects of the proximity of the tumor to the two membranes is usually true, it is not always so.

Hemorrhage is sometimes not very great, but at others it is appalling, and constitutes an imperative reason for the employment of desperate remedies. The hemorrhage is usually first noticed in connection with the menstrual flow, and it may even be confined to the periods: sometimes it extends over the whole of the interval. The leucorrhœa is generally constant, and sometimes thin and watery, especially after the hemorrhagic paroxysm has subsided, and at others it is constituted mainly of mucus with the débris of the mucous membrane and blood-corpuscles.

Other symptoms are pelvic pressure, vesical and rectal, with tenesmus, distension, and dysmenorrhœa. The pelvic pressure and tenesmus are observed early in the development of the growth, and may be relieved as the tumor becomes large enough to rise out of the pelvic cavity. The abdominal distension of course comes later. Solid tumors do not often attain to such a size as to cause great abdominal distension. The fibro-cystic generally are inconvenient, if not fatal, from this cause.

The above are the more direct and common symptoms. A less frequent yet important effect and symptom is œdema of the lower extremities from pressure upon the venous trunk passing through the pelvis. In rare cases this symptom is aggravated to a degree constituting phlegmasia alba dolens. As the tumor rises and enlarges the pressure may embarrass or interrupt the function of any or all the abdominal viscera.

In many cases none of these symptoms present themselves to an inconvenient degree, and the tumor is discovered by accident. Again, we meet with cases in which the symptoms are formidable for a time, and then entirely subside, leaving the patient free from suffering the balance of her lifetime. While this subsidence may take place at any time during the growth of the tumor, it is very apt to take place at the menopause.

The clinical history of the fibrous tumor may be very much modified by the intervention of various circumstances. As organized bodies they are subject to those affecting the organs of the body. We must regard them as adventitious growths acted upon by organs in a state of disease and reacting in turn upon them. They may become inflamed, undergo suppuration and gangrene, and produce symptomatic fever, hectic fever, prostration, gastric, hepatic, and nervous derangement in a degree sufficient to prove fatal.

When situated near the mucous membrane, nature sometimes turns these organic changes into a means of cure by destroying the portions of the capsule near the uterine cavity and permitting the pus or gangrenous material to escape. They are also subject to pressure from the development of other tumors, and either disappear, become inflamed and adherent, or cause great trouble to adjacent organs. Their clinical history is sometimes modified by complication with pregnancy.

This complication is rare, because the uterus in most cases, on account of the effects produced upon its circulation, nerve-supply, and mucous membrane especially, will not retain the ovum, and conception does not take place. The uterus being more vascular, and subject to congestions that affect the placental attachment injuriously, miscarriages are likely to occur. It is also morbidly sensitive to the pressure of the ovum, while the mucous membrane is rendered incapable of decidual changes. The retentive power of the uterus is further interfered with from the irregularity of its growth: the fibres where the tumor exists, being under a morbid influence, cannot partake of the regular hypertrophy necessary to normal gestation. There is something of uniformity in the circumstances under which the coexistence of pregnancy and fibrous tumor is observed. The nearer the tumor is situated to the mucous membrane, the less likelihood of pregnancy—the more remote, the greater the tolerance of pregnancy. Tumors that occupy the wall of the corporal portion are conducive of sterility. Those in the cervical portion of the corporal and the cervical zone are more likely to be accompanied with pregnancy than those situated in other parts of the organ. While the reader will find these statements borne out by his experience as general facts, he will also discover that pregnancy is occasionally compatible with almost any form, variety, or position of tumor. When this complication occurs, it does not generally influence the process of gestation or the condition of the tumor. The main symptoms depending on it are those caused by pressure. When small this is not very considerable.

Complication with labor generally gives rise to more apprehension than difficulty. Most of the cases of labor terminate spontaneously and happily, and the others are generally within reach of the less destructive modes of delivery. Labor more frequently decidedly affects the growth of the tumor, in the majority of cases causing its disappearance during the process of involution. The cervical polypi affect labor less, and are less affected by labor, than any other variety of the tumor. If small, they are sometimes merely pressed to one side or into the hollow of the sacrum, and the head passes by them; if a polypus is large, the head of the fœtus carries it before it beyond the vulva, where it remains until the child is expelled, when it may recede into the vagina.

DIAGNOSIS.—The history usually includes hypersecretion, hemorrhage, pressure, and enlargement. These, while suggestive, are not conclusive, hence physical examination becomes indispensable to accuracy. The methods of examination vary with the size of the tumor. It is generally near the truth to say that the uterus is enlarged, and may be shown to be so by the introduction of the sound; yet the cavity is not always enlarged, and it is often so tortuous that the ordinary sound may be arrested before reaching the fundus. The sound, therefore, should in such condition be flexible. The fine whalebone or the sound of Jenks will generally pass obstructions caused by tortuosities. The most skilled and dexterous use of the inflexible sound is often delusive. We may generally determine the size by bimanual examination—one finger in the vagina or rectum while the hand is passed down into the pelvis from above. The uterus of normal size cannot be felt with any distinctness from above in this way, while an enlargement of 50 per cent. may be thus determined. The finger below will sometimes recognize the pressure from above when the upper hand will not feel the fundus distinctly. Small tumors of the uterus may be mistaken for many other conditions, and the converse. If one is situated in the posterior wall, it may be mistaken for retroflexion. We may make the distinction by means of the inflexible sound and the finger in the rectum. If the case is one of retroversion, the finger in the rectum will pass behind it and overlap it above. If a retro-uterine tumor is in the cul-de-sac, the finger will not reach above the uterus. If the case is one of retroflexion, a strongly bent sound may be made to enter it, especially if the fundus is slightly raised by the finger in the rectum. If there is a tumor in the posterior wall, the sound with slight flexion will pass above it; which is clearly ascertained by the finger in the rectum. When the sound is introduced in the case of retroflexion, the fundus may be elevated to its proper position by turning the sound upon its axis. In making these examinations with the sound the finger should be made to co-operate with it by being kept in the rectum. A small tumor in the anterior wall may be distinguished from anteflexion by the sound passing upward instead of forward, or into the part lying on the bladder. When a small tumor is intra-uterine, the uterus will occupy its natural position, with the mouth directed slightly backward; and if the polypus is large, the cervix can be moved forward with considerable difficulty. A flexible sound, especially the thin whalebone, may sometimes be made to partially or wholly surround it, and its size or connections be determined. But the diagnosis may be more definitely made out by dilating the cervical cavity and introducing the finger. The difference between a polypus and an intramural submucous tumor may be determined in this way. In the case of a polypus the finger will pass around it, while if the tumor is intramural or submucous the finger will be arrested at the point of attachment. A polypus or intramural submucous tumor presenting at the os externum may sometimes be mistaken for a partial inversion. Such a mistake may be prevented by using the sound. In the case of a tumor the flexible sound will pass to more than the normal depth. In one of inversion the sound will pass very much less or not at all. When a polypus has escaped from the mouth of the uterus and occupies the vagina, the sound will pass beyond it into the enlarged uterus, whereas in complete inversion it cannot be passed into the uterus in any direction. We cannot rely upon consistence or shape as marks of distinction in these two conditions. When the tumor rises above the pelvic brim and is not very large it generally displaces the os from its normal position. If in the front wall, the os will be too far back; if in the posterior, it will be displaced forward. In the former, when a sound is introduced, it will pass backward and upward; in the latter, the sound will pass forward and upward. In both cases the bimanual examination will enable us to determine that the tumor above the pelvis is continuous with or attached to the uterus. With the hands in this position, if we move the uterus the tumor will move with it, and vice versâ. Tumors of this size are usually more or less uneven in their outline, and of greater consistence than the uterus when enlarged from other causes. Tumors of this size may be generally distinguished from the pregnant uterus by the history of pregnancy, by the consistence, and by the size of the cervix. When pregnancy and a tumor are associated, this may be determined by a part of the enlargement being very hard and other parts quite elastic, and by auscultation. I need not caution the reader against the use of the sound where there is any suspicion of pregnancy. When a doubt exists, we should await the progress of the case until pregnancy becomes obvious. We may generally determine whether a tumor is uninuclear by the fact that a single tumor is nearly round, when if there are several points of origin it will be irregular and nodular.

When the tumor is large enough to nearly or quite fill up the abdominal cavity, the flexible sound may be made to pass a great distance into it. It is not often that a solid tumor grows large enough to fill the abdominal cavity. Before it grows to such dimensions it generally undergoes cystic degeneration. When the tumor is solid, generally its very great hardness, and often its irregular shape, will distinguish it from other abdominal tumors. The condition with which I have seen these tumors most frequently confounded is enlargement of the liver or spleen.

In the South and West an enormously enlarged spleen is not infrequently met with. It sometimes spreads over the whole anterior part of the abdomen, completely covering the intestines. Less frequently the liver is found similarly enlarged. In this condition the organ becomes greatly indurated, and sometimes nodular. . The distinguishing features of these enlargements are—first, that the abdomen does not present the prominent rotundity it does when filled by a growth; second, that somewhere in the extent of abdominal surface by careful manipulation the edge may be discovered and the fingers be made to sink beneath and grasp it; third, percussion will elicit general deep resonance, in some parts quite obvious, and in others less so. In the case of tumor none of these signs will be present. Again, the enlarged liver or spleen, while it may reach to the brim of the pelvis, does not reach into that cavity far enough to be recognized by the finger in the vagina, while the tumor does.

Sometimes inflammatory effusions form indurated masses in the abdomen that are mistaken for fibrous tumors. These of course have the history of inflammation, are generally if not always tender, and yield obvious intestinal resonance upon percussion. The large fibro-cystic tumor may be mistaken for pregnancy, ovarian tumor, cystic degeneration of the kidney, and omental tumors. Pregnancy can generally be established by absence of the menses, by the shape, size, consistency, and position of the cervix, together with auscultation. It may be said that in case of fibro-cystic tumor the cervix is greatly displaced in some direction, indurated, and not enlarged. In pregnancy none of these conditions prevail.

The fluctuation of the fibro-cystic tumor is more obscure than that of the ovarian tumor, and, although sometimes noticeable over a large space, it is usually more constricted in extent. There is also usually less regularity in the shape of it. In large ovarian tumors the uterine cervix is not changed in shape and size. The whole organ generally lies beneath the tumor, and the elastic sound will not pass very deeply into the cavity. If the uterus is attached to the anterior part of the tumor, which sometimes happens, the elastic sound will pass into it and the depth will not be very great. The fibro-cystic tumor may be distinguished from the enlarged encysted kidney by the facts that the kidney is traceable to one side more than the other, and it cannot be reached by the finger through the vagina or rectum. Still, if we cannot make the differentiation clear in any other way, we can generally do so by aspiration. In most cases we cannot draw the fluid from the fibro-cystic uterine tumor; in almost all cases the quantity removable in that way is small. When fluid is drawn, it usually coagulates, contains hæmatin, and none of the cells so generally found in ovarian tumors.

The fluid drawn from the kidneys presents epithelial cells, is not coagulable, certainly does not coagulate spontaneously. The abdominal cavity is sometimes more or less filled with peritoneal serum. After this is withdrawn from the peritoneal cavity the uterine attachment of the tumor may be made out by bimanual examination, as above directed, if undertaken immediately after the evacuation.

PROGNOSIS.—Less than twenty years ago the general prognosis to be made upon the discovery of a tumor of the uterus was very grave. The profession knew so little about the clinical history and diagnosis of these tumors that they were invested with many of the bad qualities of other tumors, with which they were so often confounded; and we had so little knowledge of their nature and the measures which would influence their growth that we felt an entire helplessness in the treatment of them. Fortunately, there have been many favorable changes in these respects. We understand their clinical history better, and can make a pretty clear diagnosis. We know that relatively few of them prove fatal even when left wholly to nature. Compared to all other uterine and ovarian growths, they are innocuous. Most of them are self-limited in consequence of the mode of blood-supply. A goodly number not only stop growing, but disappear without the application of any remedial measures. Then, as I shall have occasion to show, they may be often cured by the judicious administration of medicines, and the surgery for their extirpation has become a reliable resort in extreme cases. These considerations render the general prognosis of the true fibrous tumor quite hopeful. The menopause generally starves them out, and thus removes all the bad qualities they may possess.

When they lead to fatal results, they generally do so through three different conditions—viz. hemorrhage, pressure, and complicating inflammations—and probably in the order mentioned. Hemorrhage is by far the most fatal symptom. The kind of fibrous tumor accompanied with severe hemorrhage is usually the submucous variety. The submucous tumor with a broad base is the most mischievous, because it induces great hypertrophy in the vascular system of the mucous membrane especially, and also the vessels of the whole organ. A sessile submucous tumor arising from one nucleus is worse than one in the same situation with several nuclei of origin. The intracorporal polypus or pendulous tumor is almost as bad in this respect as the sessile submucous, especially if it originates at or near the fundus. Fortunately, these forms of the tumor are more amenable to the effects of medicine and more accessible to surgical treatment. The tumors located in the central stratum of fibres are next to these in mischievous qualities. The more remote the tumor is located from the mucous membrane, the less hemorrhage will attend its development.

When the tumor becomes cystic the danger from pressure is very much greater; yet the solid form becomes sometimes so large as to do much mischief from pressure upon the abdominal organs; and any of these, except perhaps the polypoid variety, may be so situated as to cause mischievous if not fatal pressure upon the pelvic organs.

It is rare, however, that the pressure in either of these cavities proves fatal, especially when the case is under intelligent management. The supervention of inflammation in the tumor, even to a moderate degree, is very apt to lead to gangrene and death from peritonitis, shock, or septicæmia. Sometimes subacute inflammation of the peritoneal surface of the tumor gives rise to serous effusion or dropsy in the abdominal cavity that proves fatal; and, as before stated, peritonitis sometimes causes adhesions which result in augmented vascularity and consequent increase of blood-supply. This condition, I believe, often changes a solid to a fibro-cystic growth, a more highly vitalized tumor, and consequently a more mischievous one.

Do these tumors ever become sarcomatous or malignant? I do not believe they have any innate tendency of that kind. Where they are found complicated with malignant growths I believe the malignancy is an independent quality, and is an invasion resulting from some cause extraneous to its organization, and in that respect is analogous to an attack on the cervix or other portions of the uterus.

The prognosis when complicated with pregnancy is of course more grave, but experience has demonstrated the practicability of complete and normal gestation. Conception will not often occur where these growths have attained any great size, but may sometimes. Of the nine cases which I have met and had an opportunity to follow, not one has been attended with abortion or premature labor. In one the pregnancy seems to have been protracted at least four weeks. The fœtus was in a state of decomposition, and had probably been dead four or five weeks before labor began. What is not less remarkable also is that labor did not seem to be seriously affected in but one case, and in that the difficulty was easily overcome by turning.

Until lately there were several supposititious sources of danger at the time of confinement—viz. inefficient uterine contractions, and consequent tedious or impracticable labor, and after expulsion or artificial removal of the fœtus dangerous hemorrhages from the same cause; also, the possibility of the placental connection being made at the site of the tumor, with the imperfect closure of the sinuses that was supposed to follow.

Reports of cases occurring within the last few years, while they have not completely swept away the grounds for such apprehensions, prove that the accidents so greatly feared do not in fact occur. Chadwick reports a case where the placenta was attached to the mucous membrane over the tumor, yet the placenta was spontaneously expelled and there was no considerable hemorrhage. The efficiency of the expulsive efforts were not materially affected in any of the cases I have attended. And this is what we might expect, because conception and gestation would not be perfect where there is not a sufficiency of healthy mucous membrane, upon which a normal decidua could be formed, and of fibrous structure to permit the hypertrophy of gestation.

The apprehension of obstruction from the tumor lying in such a position as to intercept the expulsion of the fœtus is not often realized; for those in the cervix, either pendulous or otherwise, are pressed out of the external parts in advance of the head, while those in the body and fundus are lifted up into the abdominal cavity, where there is plenty of room. It must indeed be rare that the tumor becomes impacted in the pelvis so as to interfere with the passage of the fœtus.

Neither does the puerperal condition seem to be rendered materially more dangerous in consequence of the presence of these tumors.

What effect does pregnancy have upon the growth of these tumors? It might be supposed, from the plentiful supply of blood afforded them by the growth of the vascular system of the uterus, and from the fact of their being situated in and surrounded by tissues in a state of active hypertrophy, that the tumors would grow in a corresponding degree with the uterus itself; but this is not generally, if it is ever, the case. I have not witnessed a decided increase in the size of the tumor in any of my cases. Pregnancy usually produces the opposite effect; and this can be easily understood when we remember that the tumor is subjected to great and uniform pressure, which prevents its own circulation from becoming as great as it otherwise would be; and I think this pressure often inangurates a retromorphosis that results in the final disap,earance of the tumor. Whether degeneration begins during pregnancy or not, the tumor is very apt to disappear after pregnancy and labor. In six of my own cases the tumor disappeared by a slow process of some kind after labor. Speculating as to what might be, another apprehension of danger arises out of the tumultuous excitement and terrible pressure to which it is subjected during the throes of parturition. But this apprehension is rarely if ever realized.

TREATMENT.—The treatment of fibrous tumors of the uterus consists largely of the means calculated to relieve such symptoms as endanger the life of the patient or materially affect her general health. When these are unavailing resort is had to measures calculated to get rid of the tumor. Some remedies necessary to the relief of symptoms act as very powerful curative agents; hence, while it is convenient to speak of the treatment of symptoms under one division of the subject, and the methods employed for radical cure under another, we cannot, in fact, completely separate these two branches.

Hemorrhage is by far the most important of the symptoms connected with these growths, because it is at the same time the most frequent and hazardous. It is also the symptom that leads to most suffering in consequence of depriving important organs of the blood necessary to support them in their functions. Every reasonable means should be made use of, not only to prevent fatal losses, but also to prevent moderate hemorrhage. In the outset, therefore, I would insist upon watching with great vigilance to prevent any unusual loss of blood. It is not advisable to temporize by adopting the milder and less efficient measures as being sufficient, for cases not likely to prove fatal, but we should treat all hemorrhages arising from this cause with promptitude and energy. Fortunately, in many cases we can anticipate the attacks of hemorrhage, because we know when they will occur, and we are generally able to judge of their probable severity. To discharge our duty in this respect effectually, our patient should be properly provided with remedies and fully instructed how to use them. She should be made to understand that unusual hemorrhage at the menstrual period may be checked without endangering her general health. Among the remedies are—dorsal recumbency with the hips elevated, cold to the hypogastric region and cold to the dorsal spine and sacrum, ergot, and some form of tampon. The best fluid extract of ergot in drachm doses, if the stomach will bear it, is probably the most efficacious, but the fresh drug in the form of infusion is also very efficient. Full doses should be given every half hour when there is much loss, until some effect is produced upon the hemorrhage, and then continued every four hours as long as necessary. Compressed sponges saturated with the solution of sulphate of alum make the best tampons for the patient to make use of. These may be made and kept in readiness, so that they can be introduced as soon as they are found necessary. The patient or nurse can make them by taking a fine sponge, large enough to fill the vagina, passing a piece of string through the centre to aid in its removal, and then, after dipping it in the solution, winding it with twine from one end to the other, compressing it into as small a space as possible. The twine should so compress the sponge as to make it assume an elongated form. It should then be laid aside and permitted to dry. Several sponges should be thus prepared. When necessary the twine may be unwound and the sponge introduced. Its size when in the dry condition will allow of an easy passage into the vagina, where the moisture will cause it to expand, and fill up and seal the vagina so as to absolutely check the discharges. If the attending physician is present, he may tampon the vagina with pellets of cotton secured by thread and moistened with a solution of alum. The inconvenience experienced from this plug will be more than counterbalanced by the saving of blood. This form of tampon has the additional advantage of being antiseptic. I have allowed it to remain for three days, and upon removing it satisfied myself that there was no decomposition of the blood or the vaginal secretions. When the tampon is removed it will not be found difficult to wash out all the granular clots caused by its presence. It may be repeated as often as necessary, but usually, if allowed to remain forty-eight hours, the hemorrhage will not return. It may be said that for small losses this is unnecessary, but it is convenient and harmless, and will answer the purpose. In dangerous cases no one will question the propriety of its employment.

Another very important means of arresting hemorrhage which can be used by the physician when necessary is the introduction of a compressed sponge into the cervix uteri. This will temporarily act as a tampon and stimulate the uterine fibres to contraction. The free incision of the cervix, as directed by I. Baker Brown, may be tried between the times of the paroxysms of hemorrhage.

The pressure of the tumor upon the pelvic viscera is another inconvenience which calls for attention. This takes place usually at a time when the tumor has acquired a size sufficient to fill the pelvic cavity. Consequently, the elevation of the tumor above the pelvis is the remedy. This may be done sometimes by placing the patient in the knee-elbow position and pressing the growth upward. The powerful influence of atmospheric pressure called to our aid by the position and opening of the vagina is a very material auxiliary in the process of elevation. If this is not sufficient, we may pass the fingers into the rectum and elevate the tumor. I once succeeded in this operation by using an ivory-headed cane in the rectum when the fingers failed to reach high enough. If we cannot elevate the tumor by any of these means, we may introduce into the vagina or rectum a gum-elastic bag, and by means of a powerful syringe fill it with water to as great distension as the patient will bear, permit it to remain, and thus do the work more gradually.

Dysmenorrhœa is another symptom of fibrous tumors, and sometimes a very distressing one. It depends, no doubt, on the imprisonment of blood in the uterine cavity in consequence of the tortuosity of the canal causing the closure of some part of it. The remedy consists in dilating these narrow places. I know of nothing so well calculated to effect this object as the slippery-elm tent. One or more of these tents, long enough to reach the fundus uteri and of sufficient size, moistened so as to render them very flexible, may be passed up through the tortuous places with great facility. If introduced as soon as the symptom begins to manifest itself, and allowed to remain an hour or two, the relief will be pretty certain. If used once a day for four or five days before the attack, and three or four hours at a time, dysmenorrhœa may be generally avoided.

Curative Treatment.—When we broach the question of the permanent cure of these affections, we find that great difference of opinion exists among the members of the profession as to the value of medicines. One party, perhaps a majority of the profession, believe that no medicine has any direct effect upon them, and these ignore any means of permanent relief but surgical. There is, however, a respectable number of medical men who place great reliance upon the administration of certain medicines, and, if I am not greatly mistaken, recent observation has added greatly to their number. They do not, however, wholly agree as to the therapeutic processes that should be instituted, and consequently do not employ the same kind of medicines. Some gentlemen have more confidence in what I will term the sorbefacient medicines and processes of treatment. They endeavor to institute measures that will cause the absorbents to attack and remove the neoplasm in the same way that tumefactions caused by effusions are removed. This they do by friction, pressure, and the administration of the old-fashioned sorbefacient medicines. The most popular among these are the iodides, chlorides, and bromides of mercury, potassium, sodium, calcium, and ammonium. Reports may be found in books and periodical medical literature of cures by several if not all of these articles and their combinations. The late W. L. Atlee, whose experience was very extensive, had great confidence in the action of hydrochlorate of ammonia. He administered it internally, applied it externally, and used it as vaginal injections. The iodide of potassium has long enjoyed a great reputation in causing the absorption of these and other forms of tumors. There is no professional fairness in assuming that the faith in these remedies derived from the observation of their effects or the promulgation of cures from the use of sorbefacient measures are fallacious. Some of the men arrayed in favor of the opinion that cures may be effected by a patient and long-continued administration of some one of the articles I have mentioned stand high as men of honesty, accuracy of observation, and faithfulness in their records; and therefore I give full confidence to their statements. Yet I must also say that I have not witnessed the good results which I unhesitatingly believe others have seen from the sorbefacient treatment alone.

Others who expect much from medicinal treatment look to that class of medicines which cause contraction of the unstriped muscular fibres as the most promising. With these medicines they expect to diminish the supply of blood to the tumor by causing contraction of the arterioles traversing their substance, and thus disturbing their nutrition to such a degree as to stop their growth, lessen or destroy their vitality, and so render them subject to the influence of the absorbents, whereby they may be removed. Some of the more energetic of these medicines—as ergot and belladonna, for instance—often affect these growths very promptly. Ergot not only lessens the calibre of the small blood-vessels, and thus causes a diminution of their nutrition and disappearance, but it causes strong contractions in the muscular fibres of the uterine walls, which lessen more decidedly their supply of blood. It sometimes squeezes and chafes the tumor until it is disintegrated and rendered a foreign substance.

The capsule finally becomes ruptured, and the tumor is expelled either piecemeal or en masse.

When properly administered, ergot frequently greatly ameliorates some of the troublesome and even dangerous symptoms of fibrous tumors of the uterus—*e. g.* hemorrhage and copious leucorrhœa; it often arrests their growth; in many instances it causes the absorption of the tumor, occasionally without giving the patient any inconvenience: at other times the removal of the tumor by absorption is attended by painful contractions and tenderness of the uterus; by inducing uterine contraction it causes the expulsion of the polypoid variety of the submucous tumor; in the same way it causes the disruption and discharge of the intramural tumor. There are many cases on record to substantiate every one of these propositions.

From what I consider well-authenticated sources, including the cases under my own observation and in the practice of my friends and neighbors, I have collected 136 cases of fibrous tumors treated by ergot. Of these, 25 cases were cured without giving the patients any inconvenience from painful contractions. In 46 cases the tumors were diminished in size and the hemorrhage was cured. In 27 others the hemorrhagic symptom was relieved, while the size of the tumor was not affected. In 8 other instances the tumors were broken to pieces and expelled piecemeal.

For examples of cases in which the first conditions obtained, I would refer to those cured by Hildebrandt; of the other examples, 4 were reported to me by the late J. P. White of Buffalo, N. Y., 1 each by the late Hodder of Canada and Jukes, and 11 that occurred among my immediate acquaintance and in my own practice.

Among those in which the hemorrhage was cured and a diminution of the tumor took place, 11 occurred to Hildebrandt, 2 to Chrobak, 5 to White of Buffalo, and the remainder to gentlemen upon whose veracity I have implicit reliance. The most remarkable case of which I have any knowledge was reported to me by the late G. C. Goodrich of Minneapolis, in which absorption of a large tumor took place under the administration of ergot and belladonna. I subjoin his description: " The treatment was commenced in 1870, and continued two years. The uterus filled the whole space between the ilia, and measured in the transverse diameter twelve inches and in the vertical nineteen inches—extended up under the ensiform cartilage and close up to the margin of the cartilages of the ribs. The treatment was followed by cramps in the uterus, which produced a wild enthusiasm in the mind of the patient and inspired her with strong hopes of recovery. Without consulting me she doubled the dose of medicine, which was administered internally, and as a consequence she was attacked with very strong uterine contractions and symptoms of metritis. This caused me to abandon treatment for about one month, and had it not been for the urgent determination of the patient I would not have resumed it. She insisted that as this was the first medicine which had ever affected the enlarged organ, she believed it would cure her, and promised to obey my directions if I would proceed. She so promptly and rapidly improved that I doubted if it were not a coincidence with, rather than a consequence of, the treatment. Prompted by this doubt, I abandoned the use of the ergot and belladonna and continued alterative treatment. The patient soon assured me that she no longer felt the griping pains caused by the remedy, and that the tumor was softer and larger than when she took the ergot prescription. The ergot and belladonna were again resumed, and in four months she was able to make a trip to Boston alone. While absent she continued to take the medicine. From this time she continued rapidly convalescing, and is now in the enjoyment of fine health." [1]

I subjoin two cases in which the tumors were expelled piecemeal under the administration of ergot, which came under my own observation:

A woman of Sterling, Illinois, called on me December 13, 1875. She was thirty-five years old, married, and had never been pregnant. On the first of the preceding June she noticed a circumscribed hard lump two inches below and to the left of the umbilicus. She was the subject of serious uterine and sympathetic symptoms, for which she had at different times had treatment. She had profuse menorrhagia, leucorrhœa, and great sense of weight in the pelvis. Upon examination I found a hard, round, movable tumor extending up to within two inches of the umbilicus, filling up the whole of the right iliac, the hypogastric, lower half of the umbilical, and more than half of the left iliac regions. The contour of the tumor was somewhat uneven, though not distinctly nodular. The cervix was long, pointed, and thrown backward and to the left. The sound entered the small uterine mouth and passed upward, backward, and to the left five and a half inches. The diagnosis was a fibrous tumor of the right anterior wall of the uterus. I prescribed thirty drops of Squibb's fluid extract of ergot, to be taken three times a day. She went home, but did not commence taking the medicine until the 20th of December. On the 26th of December J. B. Crandall was called to see her, and describes her condition as follows: "The patient was in a state of great nervous prostration and worn out by severe pain and loss of sleep. The pains commenced soon after taking the second dose of ergot, and were excruciatingly severe for about three hours, after which they continued less severely for two days and nights. She had more or less hemorrhage from the uterus after taking the ergot. Her pulse was feeble, 110 to 120 to the minute. The skin was hot and dry, and she complained of great pain and tenderness over the uterus and lower bowels. The feet were drawn up, and the face wore a pinched and peculiar expression." Under these circumstances the doctor administered anodynes, tonics, and nourishment, to the great relief of the patient. On January 11, 1876, the patient began to pass from the vagina small masses of fibrous substance, from the size of a chestnut to that of an English walnut. The substances thus discharged were firm and gray in color, and were exceedingly fetid. This discharge continued up to the 21st of January, when the uterus was very much diminished in size, the tenderness had subsided, and the patient appeared comparatively comfortable. Up to that time she had taken but three doses of ergot—on the 20th of the preceding month—and the doctor ordered it to be resumed again. This time the ergot produced no pain, and after three or four days was discontinued. From the 21st of January there were no more pieces discharged, but up to February 1st a yellowish, thin, offensive fluid passed from the vagina in considerable quan-

[1] The author's address before the American Medical Association at its meeting in 1875.

tities. On the first day of February the ergot was again ordered and continued two weeks, when, as no results ensued, it was finally dropped. Crandall states that on the 14th of February the uterus was reduced to its normal size, and on the 26th the patient was up and about her work, completely cured. He remarked, in this connection, that the first three doses of ergot taken by the patient was the cause of her recovery.[1]

Mrs. L. D. M., aged forty-seven years, had a fibroid tumor in the anterior wall of the uterus, which, with the enlarged uterus, arose to within two inches of the umbilicus. She commenced taking thirty drops of the fluid extract of ergot on the 22d of September, 1876, and was to increase gradually the dose with the object in view of causing the disruption and expulsion of the tumor. The ergot at first produced no perceptible effect until she had taken it ten days, when she began to experience the pain of contraction. The pain became so severe and continuous that it was necessary to omit it for two or three days at a time. The patient was intelligent and understood the object and mode of action of the ergot, and when the pain entirely subsided she courageously resumed it in the smaller doses, and increased again until the pains became intolerable. On the 13th of January, 1877, small pieces of the tumor showed themselves in the vaginal discharges, and by the 26th of the same month the whole of it had been discharged piecemeal. She wrote me on the 30th of January, saying, " I think I wrote one week ago to-day. At that time the tumor was passing. It continued to pass until the 26th, when, I think, the last was expelled. To-day I send you by express a portion of the last that came. I think the whole of it, including the portion I send you, would have weighed one and a half pounds. I do not believe a quart can would hold it if the whole had been preserved. It commenced to come on Saturday, and from Saturday evening to Sunday morning there was a pint or more. After that the stench was so disagreeable that we could not cleanse it; consequently we threw it away. Wednesday and Thursday it seemed to be in one continuous mass. I cannot better describe it than to say that it came like sausage-meat from a stuffer. I would cut off about four inches a day—that is, on Wednesday and Thursday. On Friday morning the last of it came away." During and for some days after the expulsion she suffered slight symptoms of septicæmia, but recovered from them, and in the course of a month afterward she visited me, when I found the uterus measured two inches and a half in depth. She then had some leucorrhœa, but was fast regaining her health. She is now perfectly well, and has passed in safety the menopause.[2]

I have known 9 cases in which the tumors were expelled piecemeal by ergot, with but 1 death. The death occurred in a patient who rode one hundred and fifty miles on a railroad train to see me with pieces of the tumor hanging from the vagina, which she would not allow her physician to remove. When she arrived I passed my fingers up into the contracted capsule and scooped out the remaining portion of the tumor. She was so exhausted, however, by the journey and the sepsis that she died three

---

[1] This case is published in the August (1875) number of the *Chicago Medical Journal and Examiner,* as reported by Crandall.
[2] This case—the abstract of which I have here given—was in the May (1877) number of the *Archives of Clinical Surgery, N. Y.*

days afterward. I cannot help believing that if she had remained at home and submitted to the treatment of her physician, her life need not have been sacrificed.

The influence of ergot over the uterus has been a familiar fact to the profession for a long time. It is not long, however, since we were aware of its effects upon the muscular fibres entering into the formation of other organs. We now know that this medicine acts upon the unstriped muscular fibre wherever found, whether in the viscera or in the vessels of the body.

The fibres of the uterine walls, and the arteries supplying them with blood, both belong to this class; this fact in the formation of the uterus renders it particularly susceptible to the action of ergot. The drug acts upon the uterus[1] in a threefold manner, and causes a diminished flow of blood to the morbid as well as healthy tissues in the uterine structure.

First : the calibre of the arterial tubes is diminished by the contraction of the muscular fibres which enter into their composition. Second : the arterioles are diminished in size by compression from the contraction of the uterine muscular fibres which surround them. Third : these vessels are distorted and drawn in diverse directions by both the contraction and compression, and hence are rendered less fit for sanguineous conduits.

Another consideration of prime importance is that, under the influence of these medicines, the nutrition of fibrous tumors is interfered with, not only from diminution of blood in their tissues, but also from compression of their substance by the proper fibres of the uterus, and are therefore made more susceptible in the process of disintegration and absorption.

The great influence exerted by ergot over the circulation of the uterus is rendered more efficacious in the removal of fibrous tumors of that organ, because of the peculiar organization of the growths. It is now pretty well understood that this neoplasm is not very generously supplied with arterial blood, and that its supply is derived from numerous minute vessels instead of one or two of large calibre. From these circumstances it results that its vitality is very low, its circulation easily disturbed, and consequently its nutrition impaired.

I think we are justified from observation in assuming that the action of ergot may be graded from an almost imperceptible to a very intense degree. Probably the first degree affects the vascular supply ; the second, in addition to this, causes so much contraction as to merely render the fibres tense without causing pain ; and the third prompts the uterine fibres to vigorous and painful contraction.

This inference is plainly deducible, I think, from the several modes by which tumors are made to disappear under its action, as well as from direct observation of the uterine fibres.

I will now venture to call attention especially to the manner of expulsion of the polypoid and submucous intramural varieties. It will be seen that when the uterus contracts all the fibres unite in pressing the polypus through the cervical canal, which is usually already shortened, and rendered dilatable in consequence of its increased vascularity. The cervical canal dilates, and after more or less painful efforts the polypus is expelled entire, covered by the mucous membrane. This membrane is often in a

---

[1] From the author's address before the American Medical Association, 1875.

state of gangrene, but so far as I have observed these cases the tumor is not broken to pieces.

A submucous intramural tumor has a thin layer of fibres separating it from the mucous membrane, and a thick and heavy layer spread over its external hemisphere. A greater part of the muscular wall is therefore applied to the outer side of the tumor. If in this position all the fibres of the uterus vigorously contract, the fibres near the mucous membrane must be overcome by the heavy layer outside. But the opposite wall plays an important part by supporting the weaker layer at the fundus of the tumor, and adding its own force in overcoming the capsule, where it usually gives way. The position of the tumor makes its escape from the concentric action of all the fibres of the uterus impossible, and every one knows that when the resistance is partially overcome the uterus is stimulated to more vigorous action, and the pains will not abate until the mass is expelled. If not too large, it is driven out without undergoing great laceration, but if its size and attachments are such as to make this impracticable, it will be broken into fragments and expelled piecemeal.

In subperitoneal tumors there is, next the uterine cavity, a thick and strong stratum of fibres, while immediately under the peritoneum the layer is very thin and comparatively weak. When the uterus is acting with vigor the former contract forcibly, and the mass becomes pedunculated; but that is all, for the tumor lies outside the field of concentric action and escapes the crushing influence to which the submucous variety is subjected. The amount of force exerted upon it is that exercised by the weaker layer of fibres in a state of conquered antagonism, and the rupture of the capsule is impossible.

In the case of a fibroid tumor situated in the central stratum of fibres the antagonism is equal at all points, and it is evident that there is no tendency to rupture of the capsule, and much less crushing influence exerted upon it than if it were situated slightly nearer the mucous membrane. This variety of the tumor, therefore, yields to ergot only as it may be starved out by diminution of its blood-supply and as the effect of pressure, which we all know are the two conditions most favorable to absorption.

Now I think we have arrived at a point in this investigation where we can draw inferences as to the forms of tumors likely to be effected by ergot in different ways, as well as those that will not be effected by it. We do not expect ergot to cause painful and efficient contractions in the healthy unimpregnated uterus; its fibres are not capable of such contraction, and it is not until the fibres have become greatly developed that they are susceptible to the impressions of ergot. In cases of early abortion its action is very unreliable, but after the fourth month of pregnancy it acts quite efficiently.

In tumors of the uterus the development of the fibrous structure is sometimes so slight that it is incapable of contraction; there may be so many nuclei of degeneration that there are not enough sound fibres left for efficient contraction. Then, where there are many small tumors developed in the uterine walls, the circulation is cut off to such a degree that they degenerate into a cartilaginoid substance, and sometimes they are infiltrated with calcareous material. In none of these cases will ergot cause any appreciable results. When, however, there are but one, two, or three nuclei of morbid growths, as they increase in size the fibres undergo the development necessary to enable them to contract with great efficiency and render them susceptible to the influence of ergot.

Another condition which influences the hypertrophic growth of the fibres is the situation of the tumor. Subperitoneal tumors do not cause as great growth in the fibres of their neighborhood as the intramural or submucous varieties. A single intramural tumor causes great development of the whole uterine tissues, but the development of the wall in which it is situated decidedly predominates. The submucous neoplasm so soon gains the uterine cavity that the development is nearly the same in the whole organ. When, therefore, we administer ergot for the cure of fibrous tumors of the uterus, the beneficial action of the drug will depend upon the degree of development of the fibres of the uterus and the position of the tumor with reference to the serous or mucous surface. The nearer the mucous surface, the better the effects. If the tumor is very near the lining membrane, we may hope for its expulsion en masse or by disintegration.

We can often select the cases in which good results may be expected. There are four conditions which are usually reliable for this purpose: they are—smoothness of contour, hemorrhage, lengthened uterine cavity, and elasticity. A smooth, round tumor denotes, for the most part, uniform textural development, hemorrhage, a certain proximity to the mucous membrane, a lengthened cavity, great increase in the length and strength of the fibres; and elasticity assures us of the fact that cartilaginoid or calcareous degeneration has not begun in the tumor.

An even, nodulated tumor may be composed of many separate solid masses. These displace and prevent the growth of the fibres to such an extent as to render contractions inefficient. When hemorrhage is not present the tumor is probably near the serous surface, and consequently not surrounded by fibres. A short cavity denotes short, undeveloped fibres, while hardness is indicative of unimpressible induration.

Although I have no experience in the use of ergot in such cases, I should expect large fibro-cystic tumors to resist the action of ergot.

From this view of the subject it will be seen that I freely admit that there is a large number of cases in which ergot cannot produce any good results, in consequence of the nature of the cases; but there is another reason of equal moment why ergot may fail to act upon such cases as would seem to be favorable—by the worthlessness of the drug and its preparations. Squibb of New York, a high authority, says in reference to this subject : "The molecular constitution of the active portion of the drug seems, however, in its natural condition to be loose, and, like a slow fermentation, to be undergoing slow molecular changes, so that by age its peculiar activity is slowly diminished until finally lost." And again : "The ergot in the grain, however well kept, is known to become inactive without any known change in appearance, though the sensible properties, such as odor and taste, may and probably do not change. Ergot in powder is known to diminish in activity much more rapidly than when in grain, and probably soon becomes inert. The tincture and wine of ergot are believed to change, though more slowly than the ergot in substance, whilst the extracts and so-called ergotins are all supposed to change more rapidly."

When all these causes of failure are considered, the variety of experience met with in the reports upon its trial in the treatment of these tumors is not surprising. It should not, however, be discouraging, but should prompt us to more care in selecting the cases and securing reliable preparations of ergot. I have implicit faith in the action of ergot when all the conditions I have pointed out are present. I do not believe it to be uncertain in its action.

In addition to the above conditions, I believe perseverance an indispensable condition to success, as it often requires several months to get the best results.

The mode of administration should be governed by the objects to be attained. If we desire to cause the painless absorption of the tumor, the doses ought to be moderate in size and not too frequently administered. Hildebrandt administered by hypodermic injection a preparation containing from fifteen to twenty grains of the crude drug to the dose once daily or once every other day; and once a week will often be sufficient, as proven by cases cited in my address, quoted above. If we desire to have the tumor expelled, we should administer full and increasing doses often repeated, and continued until the object is attained. It will sometimes be necessary to vary the quantity and times of giving it to suit the susceptibility of the patient—less or more according to the amount of pain caused by it.

It is not essential to give it hypodermically, although when it does not produce much inconvenience this is a very efficacious method; it may be given by the mouth, in suppositories, per rectum, etc.

In conclusion, I desire to disclaim any expectation that ergot will supplant other modes of treatment. The expert surgeon will, as he always has done, use his instruments to the neglect of remedies less summary in their effects, and in his hands the maximum of safety will obtain; but there are very few general practitioners who ought or would be willing to undertake enucleation of fibrous tumors of the uterus.

Surgical Treatment.—The surgical processes resorted to for the cure of fibrous tumors of the uterus vary in their nature and gravity with the relations of the growth to the different strata of the uterine fibres. The nearer the mucous membrane, the simpler, safer, and more successful the operation for their removal; the more remote from it, the greater the difficulty and danger. Proximity to the cervix is another element of facility and safety. The removal of the cervical polypus is scarcely ever followed by serious consequences. While a polypus situated at the fundus requires greater complexity in the operation for its removal, and must be regarded as a serious one, the difficulty of removing the submucous tumor more remote from the mucous membrane is increased the higher up in the organ it is situated.

Polypi may be removed by torsion, excision, and écrassement; any one of these operations may be successfully and safely employed. No preparation of the patient is usually necessary for the removal of the cervical polypus, because it is accessible under ordinary circumstances. In very rare instances in the virgin or senile condition the vagina may require dilatation. The polypus attached at the body or fundus is not accessible to any of these operations until the mouth of the uterus is sufficiently dilated to permit the introduction of the instruments in the uterine cavity, or until the tumor is in part or wholly expelled.

It will therefore generally be necessary to completely dilate the cervix with sponge, tupelo, or laminaria tents or the fingers. The fingers, when the object can be accomplished by them, are much the better instruments for dilatation. I have several times accomplished the dilatation of the cervical cavity and removed an intra-uterine polypus in the course of half an hour by the fingers.

I prefer torsion, and believe that when properly performed it is the most simple, expeditious, and safe plan of removing a polypus. The tissues entering into the formation of the neck of a polypus are an extremely thin layer of fibres and mucous membrane. We cannot always be sure of placing the écrasseur or applying the knife or scissors exactly at the point of junction between the substance of the polypus and uterine wall; but, as that is the weakest point, it invariably yields to the force applied in the operation of torsion. The tumor is thus completely removed, and without protracted manipulation. No hemorrhage results, for two reasons: (1) there are no large vessels entering the tumor, and the small ones are torn instead of being cut, as in amputations; (2) septicæmia does not occur, for no portion of the tumor is left to slough. In performing this operation the operator must guide a vulsellum with his fingers high enough on the tumor to enable him to fasten the instrument upon or near the central part of the polypus. In two instances, when the tumor was too large to be firmly held by any forceps at my command, I introduced the hand inside the uterus and detached the tumors by rotating them, afterward making traction with the forceps. I brought them into the vagina and delivered them with the obstetrical forceps. One of these weighed forty-six ounces.

To perform torsion for the removal of a polypus, the surgeon, after fixing the instrument firmly in the desired position, should be careful to twist it enough to be sure of its detachment before commencing traction. Not less than from four to six complete revolutions should be effected. This procedure will prevent the danger of lacerating the tissues of the uterus.

The greatest objection urged against the operation of torsion is the likelihood of lacerating the wall of the uterus at the point of attachment. If we call to mind what was said about the relative thickness of the muscular strata upon each side of the different kinds of fibrous tumors, we will at once perceive the groundlessness of this objection. In the pendulous variety the whole wall of the uterus is outside the point of attachment, and is strong enough to resist the very few fibres that are carried down with it. Indeed, the polypus has almost no substantial attachment except that formed by the investing mucous membrane. If, therefore, the torsion is performed with sufficient thoroughness before traction is begun, laceration of more than the superficial tissues surrounding the neck of the tumor is next to impossible; consequently the operation is perfectly safe.

Hemorrhage is not so likely to occur after torsion as when the tumor is amputated by the knife or scissors, or even by the écrasseur. The danger of hemorrhage, then, is an objection that cannot with any show of reason be urged against torsion. I have never seen hemorrhage succeed torsion. The contractions of the uterus which take place after removing the polypoid growth from the cavity of the uterus in the great majority of cases is as effective in the prevention of hemorrhage as it is when its contents are expelled at the time of labor. I trust that it is not necessary to dilate further upon this part of the subject. However, hemorrhage, although improbable, is yet possible, and we should therefore be prepared for it. After what has been said under palliative treatment about the management of this complication, it will not be necessary to enlarge upon that point. I would therefore refer the reader to the remarks there made.

After an operation of this kind the only treatment necessary is perfect quietude for a few days, cleanliness by injections if needful, and the administration of anodynes to quiet pain. When a tumor has been removed from high up in the uterus, the patient of course should be carefully watched, and if symptoms of inflammation or septicæmia arise they should be treated by suitable remedies.

I will commence what I have to say on extirpation of deeper tumors by assuring the inexperienced that the formidable operations required for their removal are very seldom necessary, and should not be resorted to until all other and less hazardous efforts have been made.

The operation of enucleation is applicable only to cases of sessile submucous tumors, such growths as are nearer the mucous than the serous membrane. If enucleation is practicable in tumors which have their origin in the central stratum of the wall of the uterus, the operation must be regarded as equally hazardous, if not more so, than laparohysterectomy. I am aware that such operations have been recorded, but it is so easy to be at fault with reference to the exact point of origin that I must be permitted to doubt—not the honesty of the operators, but the accuracy of their observations. In many cases of submucous tumors the cervix is dilated so much that immediate dilatation with the fingers or hard-rubber olive-shaped dilators will be practicable. When that is not the case, the cervix must be thoroughly opened by sponge, sea-tangle, or tupelo tents or bilateral incision: the more patent the mouth of the uterus can be made the better. The operation is so serious in its nature that the competent surgeon will study his preparations so carefully as to avail himself of every means that will enable him to perform it in the most expeditious and complete manner. Expedition, rendered possible by thorough preparation, is a most important item; for it must be understood that every superfluous moment spent in enucleation increases the peril of the patient. I would not counsel haste, but the earnest and careful despatch acquired by reflection and experience. When the patency of the mouth of the uterus is secured, the uterus should be drawn to or near the vulva by a strong vulsellum and firmly held by an assistant. The operator may then make an incision with scissors entirely across the most dependent part of the tumor, completely through the capsule. After this is done, another incision is to be made from the centre of this cross-cut upward upon the most prominent part of the tumor, as high as the instrument can be guarded by the fingers. The fingers should then be inserted between the tumor and the capsule, and the latter separated as extensively as possible from the former. In some cases a large part of the tumor may be thus detached from its envelope. When the whole of it cannot be detached by the fingers, Sims's enucleator may be made to finish that task. It can be passed up and around the upper and less accessible portion. The detachment should, when possible, be complete before traction is begun. The traction is affected by a strong vulsellum. By that instrument the tumor, after being firmly seized, can often be rotated upon its longitudinal axis to assure the operator that it is loosened at every point. Simple, firm, but slow traction, aided by pressure of the hand on the upper part, will assist the uterus in expelling the growth. Should the tumor be too large to pass the mouth of the uterus and vagina, it may be divided by well-directed efforts with the scissors or knife and removed in pieces. When the tumor is semi-pedunculated the capsule may be separated by Thomas's serrated spoon in a much more expeditious manner. As the tumor is drawn out of its cavity the uterus usually contracts, and thus prevents the hemorrhage that might otherwise occur. The surgeon, however, must always be prepared with plenty of cotton saturated with the subsulphate of iron with which to plug the uterine cavity. It will very seldom be necessary to use the ironized cotton, and it should not be employed until its necessity is apparent. The after-treatment consists locally in detergent and disinfectant injections, and in such general measures as will aid in reaction where there are symptoms of shock and counteract the tendency to inflammation. For both these purposes a liberal amount of opium will be very useful.

When the symptoms in connection with a tumor situated in or slightly outside the centre of the wall of the uterus are so urgent as to demand surgical interference, the choice of operations lies between laparo-hysterectomy and öophorectomy. In the light of recent observation I have no hesitancy in recommending the former for large tumors and the latter for small ones. As before stated, I regard enucleation in such cases as hardly practicable, and when successful I believe it is attended with as much danger as the entire extirpation of the uterus.

Without entering into details of this operation, I will state that it is so like ovariotomy as to be governed by the same principles and require to a great extent the same methods. The incision should be sufficiently free to permit the removal of uterus and tumor without the necessity of cutting away the tumor in pieces, as thus mutilating it gives rise to great and dangerous hemorrhages and of necessity soils the abdominal cavity. I have always used silk ligatures with which to secure the pedicle. In most instances we will be obliged to ligate the uterus near its junction with the vagina. Extra-peritoneal treatment is probably safer.

Where a small intramural tumor is attended with exhausting hemorrhage, menacing the patient with a probable fatal loss, and other remedies have been found inadequate, öophorectomy may with great propriety be resorted to.

I would refer the reader to the description of this operation as given elsewhere. There is no other surgical operation by which a large fibrocystic tumor can be gotten rid of than laparotomy or laparo-hysterectomy. Recently I have removed a large fibro-cystic tumor that grew from the anterior surface of the fundus and body of that organ without removing the uterus. The tumor was detached by a sort of enucleation, and the detachment left a large bleeding surface. Hemorrhage from that surface was profuse, and seemed to issue from numerous cavernous openings instead of veins and arteries. The hemorrhage was checked by passing silk ligatures one-eighth of an inch beneath the surface from one side to the other of the bleeding surface in several places. When these ligatures were tightened the tissues were so condensed as to entirely control the bleeding.

This was my fourth laparotomy for fibro-cystic tumor of the uterus, and the only one that recovered. In all the other three I ligated the uterus and removed it at the internal os.

Large subserous, fibrous, or fibro-cystic tumors are almost always covered with a network of great vessels, generally furnished by adhesions to the omentum. These vessels should be ligated in bundles by two ligatures around each bundle at least two inches distant from the uterus. If the two ligatures are not thus widely separated from each other, when the division between them is made the collapse and retraction of the vessels will be so great that they will not hold. If in detaching adhesions a bleeding surface is left on the tumor or abdominal wall, the bleeding should be arrested by ligatures applied before the tumor is lifted from its bed. When it is necessary to remove the uterus, a double ligature around its substance should be applied; also, when practicable, before the tumor is lifted out. In this method of securing the vessels we will avoid the terrible hemorrhage that would otherwise follow the removal of the tumor. The pedicle should then be brought out and secured by pins in the wound. The cleansing of the peritoneal cavity and closure of the wound should be done as in ovariotomy. The after-treatment is also the same as in bad cases of ovariotomy.

I have not thus far mentioned the treatment of fibrous tumors by electrolysis; and as the profession has not generally consented to the adoption of this measure as safe and efficacious, I will refer the reader to an account given of that process and its results in my work and other standard works on gynecology.

SARCOMA OF THE UTERUS.

By W. H. BYFORD, M. D.

THIS disease is as much entitled to the clinical definition given to cancer as any of the varieties of that malignant affection. Miller, as quoted by West, says: "Those growths may be termed cancerous which destroy the natural structure of all the tissues; which are constitutional from their very commencement or become so in the natural process of their development; and which, when once they have infected the constitution, if extirpated, invariably return and conduct the person who is affected by them to inevitable destruction." If we substitute the word malignant for cancerous in the above quotation, the definition would include sarcoma as well as carcinoma. It will be found upon comparing sarcoma with fibrous and cancerous tumors that it possesses clinical and histological features common to both. If it is not indeed the result of a transition of fibrous tumors into a malignant form of disease, it is a connecting link between fibromatous and carcinomatous affections, and illustrates in a remarkable manner a relationship of these two forms of growths—viz. the morbid proliferation of the tissue resembling those of the structure in which they originate. Sarcoma has its origin in the fibrous portion of the connective tissue, as do many of the fibrous tumors. It consists of a redundant proliferation of the cells of that tissue, while the fibrous tumor is constituted of a morbid proliferation of the fibrous element of the connective and muscular tissues. Cancer now is admitted to be an excessive production of the cells of the epithelium; this excessive growth of the cells inhabiting these structures, sarcomatous and epithelial, seems to give to them respectively the feature of malignancy. The fibrous tumor is contained in a capsule; both forms of these malignant growths invade the tissues without any such limitation. In this respect the two latter resemble each other and differ from the former. In sarcoma the cells are mingled intimately with the fibres, and are not generally contained in alveoli, or nests, as they are sometimes called. Cancerous cells are always surrounded by alveoli. Sarcoma in many instances resembles very closely the fibrous tumor. In malignancy it is very much like the cancerous tumor.

CLINICAL HISTORY.—The early symptoms of sarcoma are leucorrhœa, hemorrhage, and tumefaction. The discharge from the genital organs resembles that of fibrous tumors. This does not generally possess an offensive odor, but as the disease advances necrosis of the tumor occurs to a greater or less extent, and then the smell of the discharge comes to resemble that of cancer. The necrosis does not take place at the expense of the uterine tissues, but is a process of disintegration going on in the growth. The ulcer resulting does not corrode the uterus, but it eats away the tumor. It in this respect resembles epithelial fungus. The tumor formed by the sarcomatous deposit is sometimes polypoid, and presents the appearance of the fibrous polypus. In other instances it resembles to the touch a submucous fibrous tumor, and again in others it is diffusely disseminated into the whole structure of the uterus. When thus diffused, like cancer it invades the neighboring organs. When the tumor projects from the inner surface of the womb, and has attained a considerable growth, limited necrosis occurs, and sloughs of varying size take place, and offensive sanious discharges occur very similar to the flow observed in cancer.

The general symptoms at first are slight, consisting of obscure pelvic pains and pressure and increased discharge. Gradually septicæmia is developed, and this is the condition in which the patient usually dies.

DIAGNOSIS.—There is nothing in the symptoms by which we can arrive at a correct diagnosis, as in the early periods they resemble those of fibrous tumors so closely as to be undistinguishable from them, and in the latter cancer neither manual nor ocular examination will give us any more definite information. Their qualities in this respect also are in the early stages of development those of fibrous tumors, and in the latter of some forms of cancer. We are therefore reduced to the evidence afforded by microscopical examination.

When the tumor is in such a position and of such a consistence that we can remove a fragment from it, we can study its histology. There are two varieties, as distinguished by the shape and size of the cells. One variety is called the small-celled sarcoma, from the size of the cells; they are round, or nearly so, in shape. The other is called the spindle-celled sarcoma. In some specimens of this variety the cells are much larger than others; and hence there is the large and small spindle-celled sarcoma. The cells are different among the fibres of the tissues affected, and in rare instances some of the cells are contained in imperfectly-formed alveoli, in this respect showing a further analogy to the growth in cancer.

PROGNOSIS.—The malignancy of sarcoma is now universally recognized in the known facts of its persistency in returning when removed, and its simultaneous existence in many organs of the body. This acquired or innate constitutional dissemination is not constant—no more than in cancer, perhaps less so. Hence when the size of the tumor is small and apparently isolated there is some encouragement to attempt a cure.

The comparative prognosis is also probably better than cancer, as it pursues a less rapid course of development, and hence the patient may survive for a longer time.

The local dissemination of the cells cannot always be measured, and that their dissemination into the surrounding tissues may reach much beyond the boundaries of the apparent tumor must be regarded as an important element in considering the subject of prognosis in connection with treatment by ablation or cauterization. The widespread local dissemination of the cells of this growth is doubtless an explanation of the term at first applied to it—viz. recurrent fibroid.

TREATMENT.—It will not be necessary to consume the time of the reader by giving the treatment of sarcoma in detail, as most of it is identical with that of Cancer, and may be found under that head. I will only call attention to the excellent palliative effects of ergot : this drug will often arrest, and generally modify, the hemorrhage so often one of the most annoying symptoms. When the tumor is in a state of progressive necrosis, protrudes like a submucous fibrous tumor, or is pendulous, resembling the fibrous polypus, it may, by inducing contraction of the uterus, be expelled, partially if not completely, and thus for the time being do away with the source of sepsis. I have in several instances been highly gratified with its effects in this way. In one case, when the patient was so overwhelmed with symptoms of septic fever as to cause apprehension of immediate dissolution, the administration of ergot expelled large masses of sloughing tissue, and so cleansed the uterus that the symptoms subsided, the patient rallied, and lived several months in comfort. Not less than four times this process of expulsion was successful in relieving the same patient for long intervals : each time the medicine was administered relief was so marked that both she and her friends anticipated recovery.

CARCINOMA OR CANCER OF THE UTERUS.

By WILLIAM H. BYFORD, M. D.

WHILE it is possible that in very rare instances the scirrhous or colloid form of cancer may attack the uterus, the practitioner will seldom meet with either. I will therefore describe but two varieties—the soft or medullary, and the epithelial. Although there is much difference histologically and microscopically, they are so nearly allied in their clinical history that I feel justified in placing them together. In the clinical description of carcinoma I shall be governed more by what I have seen at the bedside than by the observation of others.

Medullary or Soft Cancer.

I use this term in a comparative sense. By it I mean a tumor caused by a carcinomatous deposit that infiltrates, enlarges, and renders more fragile than natural the parts attacked, which after a greater or less time undergo necrotic ulceration, death, or solution of the morbid growth, giving rise to extensive ulceration. I have never seen this variety convert the uterus into a tumor of encephaloid consistence. The deposit usually begins in the extremity of the cervix and extends up to the body, and without reference to the boundaries of different tissues attacks and involves the fibrous, mucous, and serous tissues, extending to any organ or substance that may be contiguous, thus infiltrating the bladder, rectum, connective tissues in the broad ligaments, and ovaries. The necrotic ulcerations of the part where the disease began, and the extension of the deposit in the more distant parts, progress simultaneously, the one diminishing while the other is increasing the bulk of the parts involved. This kind of progressive local dissemination and necrosis of cancerous matter often results in the more or less complete destruction of the uterus, bladder, and rectum.

Accompanying these morbid processes in the pelvis, cancerous cells migrate to other and distant portions of the body, creating new centres of carcinomatous disease. These multiple centres of disease are probably in all instances caused by the errant products of the pelvic disease. This view of the subject makes the general carcinomatous disease a constitutional infection, the same as the wandering cells of the chancre give rise to constitutional syphilis.

ETIOLOGY.—No one circumstance seems so intimately connected with

274

the origin of cancer of the uterus as age, more than half the cases occurring between the fortieth and fiftieth years, 33 per cent. between the thirtieth and fortieth ; this leaves only 20 per cent. for all other ages. It very seldom attacks the young under twenty-five years or the old over fifty. So far as I have been able to examine statistics, I am not sure that cancer occurs any more frequently among multipara than nullipara. The fact that the number of childbearing women far exceeds those who are not married nor fruitful is likely to mislead us in this respect. Race does not seem to afford even comparative exception. The negro and North American Indians seem to be subjects of cancer as frequently as the European races.

If there is anything in the idea of heredity as a causative influence, it must be rather through physiological similitude of children to parents than the transference of taint from the former to the latter. If cancer is a degeneration of tissues, as the effect of a law that organs in certain individuals undergo dissolution at a particular age, we can understand that the child may inherit such physiological effect from the mother. The cell-formation of the organs of the child will be capable of reaching the same period at which the disease was developed in the mother, when the normal histological changes will be interrupted and dissolution begins. In this view of the subject the child would by virtue of its organization inherit the mode of dying evinced in the mother.

Old writers, assuming that cancer was the result of a peculiar dyscrasia, described the state of general health as a causing condition. It does not seem, however, that the majority of people in whom cancer is developed exhibit any signs of ill-health until the local disease has made sufficient advance to account for their symptoms. Indeed, many present the appearance of a faultless condition of general health until the disease is discovered to have made hopeless progress. The same may be said of the local condition. It so often happens that we are assured by a patient that she had been congratulated by her friends as one especially favored by exemption from female weaknesses. I have yet to witness any evidence that chronic inflammation, congestion, or laceration of the uterus predisposes to malignant disease of any kind.

I do not mean by this to say that patients having chronic uterine ailments may not become the subjects of cancer of the uterus. There is nothing in the gross anatomy or the histological construction of cancer to indicate an analogy to inflammation. The allegation that the long-continued irritation of laceration invites a malignant deposit in the tissues involved is mere assumption, and should rank as an unproved hypothesis.

The location of the primary lesions is usually in the cervix, but occasionally it attacks other parts of the uterus, the body next in frequency to the cervix, and less commonly the fundus.

CLINICAL HISTORY.—The early stage of cancerous development is not marked by obvious symptoms. Judging from my own observation, a bloody discharge more frequently attracts the attention of the patient than any other symptom, and this does not appear until the deposit is somewhat extensive, and it indicates necrosis. The loss of blood is sometimes copious, but generally moderate in quantity. It may be intermittent or continuous. Not infrequently in menstruating women it assumes the form of menorrhagia. The next symptom generally is a discharge of ichor, usually colored, sometimes entirely clear. With the appearance of the serous discharge the cancerous odor becomes apparent and continues. These two exhausting and disgusting symptoms continue alternating with each other with the persistence of fate.

Another symptom of cancer of the uterus is pain. It is not, however, generally an early symptom. Often it is entirely absent until the disease has made great progress. When noticed early, the pain is sharp and lancinating, consisting of recurring twinges rather than of continuous pain. When it does not occur until later in the progress of the case, it is such as arises from the accompanying congestions and inflammations.

GENERAL SYMPTOMS.—No general symptoms are manifest until the disease has made considerable advance, and often not until there begin to be degenerations in the tumor. It would seem, indeed, that the growth of cancer was not a morbifacient process, and that constitutional disturbance results from the septic influence exerted by the necrosis of the tumor.

The absorption and circulation of the products of decomposition at the extremities of the tumor through the nervous centres and secreting organs soon induce nervous ailments and derange the functions of all the important vital organs. A continuance of the derangement thus inaugurated, and kept up, eventuates in fully-developed septic fever, by which the energies of the patient are exhausted. The uniformity with which septicæmia terminates the existence of these unfortunate patients renders the exceptions to the above description very rare indeed While patients think they are being eaten up by cancer of the womb, they are really dying from slow poison caused by absorption of dead tissues.

DIAGNOSIS.—In the great majority of cases the diagnosis of cancer is easily arrived at. For reasons already stated the disease is not suspected until the deposit is extensive and obvious changes in the shape and consistence of the cervix occur. It is enlarged, very hard, and generally irregular in shape. In most instances it is very much enlarged, measuring from one to ten times its natural diameter; the tissues are devoid of elasticity; and nodosities, projections, and sulci deform the cervix in a manner and to a degree that change the shape of the organ as nothing else does. Add to this the stinking sero-sanguinolent discharge, and the diagnosis is complete. By the time these physical changes become diagnostic features of the case the uterus becomes fixed, the immobility being obviously dependent upon the extension of the deposit to the vagina, bladder, and contents of the broad ligament. The invaded tissues become as hard and unimpressible as the uterus. We could hardly mistake cancer in this stage of development for any other disease, and as the general practitioner will seldom see it before the most of these changes have occurred, the diagnosis will generally be easy. When the tissues break down to a considerable extent the ulcers, if they can be so called, are very irregular in shape, greatly excavated, have a hard, rough, granular bottom, and are not tender to the touch. Generally they bleed upon being handled. The hardness, enlargement, irregularity of shape, and fixedness are as conspicuous features during the process of destruction as they are in the stage of deposit.

The demonstrative portion of the diagnosis, however, is derived from the histology of the deposit. "Histological examination of the changed uterine tissues shows, as in every carcinoma, a stroma of small alveoli filled with polymorphous cells, generally arranged without order; sometimes those of the periphery are implanted regularly on the wall of the alveolus. The stroma composed of connective tissues frequently contain also smooth, muscular fibres."[1]

PROGNOSIS.—This form of carcinoma uteri will bear no other than a desperate prognosis. I doubt whether it is ever discovered until the deposit has reached an extent locally that renders complete ablation impracticable. In addition to this consideration the malignant cells are disseminated, if not degenerated, in distant parts.

Nature in an infinitesimal number of cases institutes curative processes. These processes consist of extensive sloughing and a species of atrophy in the morbid growth. The growth ceases to enlarge, becomes smaller, and finally disappears. Very few men are lucky enough to witness the fortunate results of these processes. Art is powerless to cure, but may do much to palliate the suffering connected with the fatal march of carcinoma.

The duration of uterine cancer is greater in the old than in the young. In the former it may last several years; in the latter it often terminates fatally in a few months.

TREATMENT.—Taking the above history of the disease as true, it will not be necessary to say much about curative treatment. If we should find a case of cancer in which the cervix is not enlarged as high up as the junction of the cervix and vagina, I would advise amputation of the cervix and excavation of the uterine tissues as extensively as possible. The amputation and excavation may be performed by means of hooks and scissors, as in epithelioma. Taking the statistics of Freund's operation, as practised and modified by himself and others, as my guide, I am not disposed to sanction or advise the complete extirpation of the uterus for this form of cancer.

The subject of palliative treatment of cancer for the relief of local symptoms, and the amelioration of the general suffering caused by the septic fever, with which the patient usually dies, is more hopeful. The local symptoms requiring palliation are the sometimes disastrous hemorrhages, fetor, acidity of the sanious discharges, and pain.

The tampon made of cotton saturated with the solution of the subsulphate of iron is generally a very effectual means of treating the hemorrhages, while it also temporarily removes the fetor and acridity of the discharges. The tampon saturated with a strong solution of alum is also very effective. Frequent injections and ablutions with a weak solution of carbolic acid or permanganate of potassium will also be very useful in keeping the discharges free from odor. Much comfort may also be derived from small pellets-of absorbent cotton introduced just within the vulva to absorb the discharge. Their frequent removal will of course be necessary, but they will be found to protect the external parts from excoriations that would otherwise occur. Applications of tincture of the chloride of iron or solution of hydrate of chloral carefully made to the raw surface upon the cervix very materially correct the foulness

[1] Cornil and Ranvier, translated by Shakespeare and Simes, p. 696.

of the discharges and lessen the process of necrosis which is continually taking place.

The local and general use of anodynes is about our only means of relieving pain. They may be used locally in suppositories introduced into the rectum or vagina, or hypodermically or by the stomach in such quantities as may be required. Further detail is unnecessary in reference to the use of anodynes, as the quantity, quality, and mode of administering them will depend so much upon the urgency of the pain and the character of accompanying symptoms.

The treatment of the septicæmia is both general and local.

The general treatment consists of such measures as will sustain the vital powers. Tonics of quinine and iron are the remedies that will be of most service, and judiciously used will greatly ameliorate the symptoms of exhaustion. A very important item in the treatment of these prolonged cases of septic fever is a well-selected diet—the more nutritious and easy of digestion the better. It should consist largely of fresh mutton, beef, poultry, game, milk, and butter. The bowels will be generally troublesome in the early part of the time by constipation, and in the later by diarrhœa. For the former a diet containing fruit and coarse flour bread will often enable us to dispense with cathartics, which are generally both exhausting and annoying. For the diarrhœa opiates can be used freely, as also bismuth, pulverized charcoal, etc. etc.

But the most important as well as the most effective measure with which to combat this destructive fever is to keep the raw surface of the tumor as free as possible of necrosed material. This is done most effectively by the sharp curette or Simon's spoon. The whole of the ulcerated surface should be thoroughly scraped off with one of these instruments. The parts completely exposed by Simon's retractors should be scraped energetically until the solid tissue is reached. It should be remembered that the tissues exposed are not sound, but are cancerous deposit. The sacrifice of it, therefore, is not a matter of importance, so that the excavation if not fearlessly should be thoroughly done. An operation of this kind is attended with two dangers. One is the removing so much substance as to open the peritoneal cavity, bladder, or rectum; and the other is hemorrhage. Care will enable us to avoid the former; and, when formidable, the latter may be staunched by the astringent tampon already mentioned.

This operation is only intended as a palliative measure, and it sometimes proves remarkably beneficial. After it the patient will occasionally rally so much and become so comfortable as to indulge in the belief that she is on the road to recovery. The amelioration lasts sometimes months. It will often be profitable to repeat the scraping several times, especially if the case is advancing slowly. It will usually not only make the patient more comfortable, but greatly protract her existence.

Epithelioma of the Uterus.

This malignant disease differs in several respects from the cancer already described. The morbid cell-growth in that form of cancer takes place in the lymph-spaces of the connective tissues of the cervix and uterine body. The lymph-spaces are converted into alveoli or nests in which the cells are developed until they become greatly distended and changed in shape. The lymph-spaces thus occupied freely communicate with each other, and of course with the lymphatic vessels. Hence, the rapid dissemination of the cells locally and the ease with which they find their way to distant parts of the system.

The cells in epithelioma are developed on the free surface of the mucous membrane. From this surface the cells seldom travel to any great distance, and consequently the disease often does not become general. Epithelioma is cancer of the mucous membrane of the uterus, while the other form is interstitial cancer of the uterus. The dense mucous membrane serves as a barrier to the passage of the cells into the surrounding tissues. After the disease has existed for a long time, the surface of the mucous membrane is impaired, and it does not resist the dissemination of the cells. Then the process of cell-dissemination is a result of partial destruction of the membrane. In cancer of the uterus they are disseminated early, and possibly from the beginning, because they are generated within the lymph-spaces, with which the lymphatic vessels are continuous.

Epithelioma of the uterus very rarely assumes the form of an ulcer; generally it is a deposit upon, or growth from, the surface of the mucous membrane. The growth assumes shapes that vary with the different localities. If the extremity or external surface of the cervix is the seat of the disease, it usually projects into the vagina as a fungus which may grow large enough to fill up that cavity. Much more frequently the cervix is enlarged and is covered with a stratum of epithelial deposit very frail in texture that bleeds freely when rudely touched. This fungous growth or deposit does not affect the mobility of the uterus, even when the cervix is considerably enlarged. When the morbid deposit takes place in the cavity of the uterus, it often does not project from the os uteri to any extent, but is confined to the cavity. When the cavity is filled up by an epitheliomatous growth emanating from the entire surface of its lining membrane, we seldom see anything more than an ashy-looking substance filling up the external os uteri. Sometimes the growth covers the whole of the mucous membrane of the body and neck, including the external covering of the latter part.

CLINICAL HISTORY.—The clinical history of epithelioma is essentially the same as that of the other form of cancer, and consequently need not be given in detail. The main symptom is hemorrhage, with an abundant and stinking sanious discharge.

DIAGNOSIS.—In examining with the finger and with both hands it will be found that the uterus is movable and not much, if any, enlarged. If the case is of the ulcerated variety, the finger may not detect the lesion; if, on the contrary, there is a fungus, it will at once detect it. Should the deposit not project from the os externum, the finger may not recognize its presence. Upon exposing the cervix to view in the ulcerative variety an ulcer of a light ash-color will be seen, presenting an irregular outline slightly excavated, and if the probe is applied to it the bottom and sides of the ulcer will be found of the same firmness and consistence as the uterine tissues. It is not indurated. If a fungus exists, it can be seen and examined. When not bleeding it is also ash-colored. The consistency of the projecting mass is sometimes tolerably firm, but more frequently it is quite frail and gives way under moderate pressure. Should the deposit be inside of the uterus, the os will be slightly dilated and filled with a gray substance.

The probe will readily pass through this frail material and enter the uterine cavity. In cases presenting such an appearance the cavity is generally enlarged and filled with this fungous deposit. These facts may be ascertained by the use of the probe while the parts are exposed to view.

The microscope will verify and correct our diagnosis. For microscopic examination some substance from the surface of the ulcer or fungoid projection may be collected and submitted for inspection. The appearances are nests or spaces of greater or less size filled with epithelioid cells.

PROGNOSIS.—Without judicious treatment practised at an early period epithelioma may be said to be invariably fatal. There is, however, much promise of great amelioration in this form of disease with the present improved methods of treatment, and in some cases we may succeed in effecting a permanent cure.

TREATMENT.—The general palliative treatment is the same as that described in the other form of cancer, and need not be repeated. While I have failed to see any other than palliative effects result from amputation of the cervix and excavation of the body of the uterus in the first form of cancer described, I have seen cures of epithelioma effected by thorough extirpation of the diseased mass. One of these cures was in a case where the disease was confined to the posterior lip of the cervix; another, where the deposit apparently occupied the whole surface of the mucous membrane of the body and cavity of the cervix. In other cases I am sure the life of the patient was prolonged and her comfort greatly enhanced. I am persuaded, from a good deal of observation, that the younger the patient the more promising the result of operations. The worst and most rapidly fatal cases of epithelioma I have seen have been in patients beyond the menopause. This is contrary to what I have witnessed in the other form of cancer, as in it the younger the patient the more rapid the progress of the disease and the least beneficial the operations were.

After a trial of the several methods pursued in the removal of epithelioma, and the different instruments used for the purpose, I prefer using the scissors, aided by hooks and vulsellum, to cut away as much of the diseased tissue and the sound structure upon which it is implanted as possible, and then burn the surface with the cautery in some of its forms or the strong caustics. When the disease is confined to the cervix, the whole of the intravaginal portion should be cut away and the excising process carried as high up as possible, carefully avoiding the peritoneal cavity on the one hand and the bladder on the other. With the cervix exposed and fixed by a vulsellum, the sharp-pointed curved scissors may be insinuated beneath the external covering, and the tissues removed by pieces until the operation is completed. When the utmost attainable portion is thus removed, I prefer applying to the whole of the cut surface pellets of absorbent cotton thoroughly moistened with the solution of the pernitrate of mercury (the acid nitrate, as it was formally called), and then filling the upper part of the vagina with dry absorbent cotton, tightly packing it so as to absorb any of the free acid. This last is necessary to defend the sound parts from the superfluous cauterization which would otherwise follow. The dressing may be removed in twenty-four hours, and the whole of the surgical cavity as well as vagina washed out with pure warm water twice a day afterward. If the cavity thus formed does not fill up, and the surface assumes a malignant aspect, it should be scraped out with a view to remove its entire surface and treated again with the acid. This last operation may be repeated again and again. It will sometimes be found that the cavity will grow less after each scraping with the sharp curette, and finally fill up.

If the disease is developed in the cavity of the uterus, Simon's sharp curette should be used to scrape out and destroy the whole mucous membrane. When this is done the cavity should be carefully filled with the cotton pellets saturated with pernitrate of mercury, as recommended for the cervical operation. And this operation should be repeated also with the same thoroughness as at first as soon as evidence of a return is manifested. When the scraping and cauterizing have been beneficial the uterine cavity will become smaller, and when the discharges indicate a reproduction of the morbid deposit the surface to be operated upon will be sensibly diminished, until finally it will be apparently almost closed. I say almost, because one of my patients, while she seems to have been cured, still menstruates.

While I do not pretend that many of these cases can be thus cured, I am sure some of them can be. Hence I do not hesitate to recommend an effort to be made in all cases in which the disease has not spread to the adjoining organs or tissues. When a cure is not thus effected, such great amelioration will so often occur as to make an operation justifiable.

The hemorrhages encountered in these operations are generally unimportant, but occasionally so much blood will be lost as to require hæmostatic measures. The practitioner should therefore be supplied with an astringent tampon and use it if necessary.

If an operation for the complete extirpation of the uterus is ever justifiable for malignant disease, I think it is in this form. The operation which I think the simplest and easiest to accomplish is that performed first in this country, so far as I know, by S. C. Lane of the Medical College of the Pacific, and in Germany by Langenbeck.

DISEASES OF THE OVARIES AND OVIDUCTS.

By WM. GOODELL, M. D.

THE ovaries are two almond-shaped glands attached to either side of the womb by a ligament of contractile tissue called the ovarian ligament, and they are enclosed between the two layers of the peritoneum known as the broad ligament. It has recently been contended that this envelopment in the broad ligament is not a complete one, but that the peritoneum is absent from the posterior surface of the ovary. This has been denied, but even if it be so, the fact does not seem thus far to have any physiological or any pathological bearing.

The ovarian nerves and blood-vessels run between the two layers of the broad ligament, the former coming chiefly from the renal plexuses of the sympathetic, the latter from the spermatic arteries. The ovaries being themselves movable bodies and attached to a movable organ, the exact position of which remains yet a moot question, their own natural situation has not yet been authoritatively determined. His,[1] from an examination of three suicides, holds that the ovary in the adult virgin hangs with its long diameter almost vertical, and with one side against the wall of the pelvis, but below the brim, the free border being behind and the attached end below. Each oviduct is looped over the ovary, rising along the front and falling over behind it. Hence the ovary lies on the fimbriæ which turn back and spread over the summit of the ovary. The ovaries are generally situated on a level with the inlet of the true pelvis, the left one being in front of the rectum, the right one surrounded by a coil of small intestines. When healthy they keep so high up as to be beyond the reach of the examining finger, and consequently they are not impinged upon during coition.

The important and special function of the ovaries—that of secreting and excreting the Graäfian follicles or ovisacs—and their monthly engorgements are the causes of many of the diseases to which they are subject. Hence it is that affections of the ovary, being due most commonly to perverted function, rarely occur before puberty.

Malformations.

Absence of the ovaries is a congenital condition very rarely met with. It is usually associated either with the absence also of the womb or

[1] *British Medical Journal*, Dec. 10, 1881, from *Archiv f. Anat. u. Entwick.*, 1881, Nos. 4 and 5.

with an imperfect development of the other portions of the sexual apparatus. The breasts will be flat, the vagina generally imperforate, the vulva small, the pubic hair absent, and sexual feeling wanting. Menstruation never takes place. Very commonly the growth of the body is arrested, and the stature is dwarfed to that of a child. Occasionally, however, there is an approach to the masculine type in the size, the figure, the voice, and in the growth of hair on the face and on the body.

An arrested development or a rudimentary condition of the ovaries is a more common malformation than the preceding one. The womb is then infantile in size, and the vulva and vagina are small and the pelvis is narrow. Puberty either fails to take place or it is postponed. When menstruation is present it is scant and appears at long intervals. General development is impaired, and the figure and mental characteristics may be those of advanced childhood. Sexual feeling is either wholly absent or very imperfect.

DIAGNOSIS.—Whenever the ovaries are wanting, their absence cannot be positively made out by a digital examination of the parts, for even fully-formed ovaries often elude the finger. The diagnosis depends mainly on the symptoms previously given. If the ovaries are rudimentary, the finger passed high up the rectum while the woman is anæsthetized will sometimes recognize them. But the diagnosis rests usually on some manifestation of puberty, and the greater these manifestations the greater the curability.

TREATMENT.—For the complete absence of the ovaries all treatment is of course useless. Whenever these organs are in a rudimentary condition more can be done for the woman, but success is by no means assured. Every treatment that tones up the body is of service. The rest-cure, with its accessories of massage, general faradization, and over-feeding, promises much. Electricity has done good when one pole is applied directly over an ovary and the other pole placed either on the sacrum or on the cervix uteri. It is still more efficacious when the reophore in the form of a properly insulated sound is passed into the uterine cavity. Should the interrupted current fail to do good, the galvanic current may cautiously be tried.

From the vascular and nervous kinship between the ovaries and the womb all stimulants to the latter tend to invite blood to the former, and from this flux may come growth. It is therefore good practice to irritate the womb by tents, by applications of iodine and of silver to its cavity, and especially by the use of galvanic stems. The marriage relations sometimes quicken dormant ovaries into life, and development, followed by pregnancy, has been the result. But the remedy is a hazardous one, for if the sexual sense be not awakened, as often it will not, the union leads to much unhappiness.

Inflammation of the Ovary; Ovaritis.

Acute inflammation of the ovary rarely exists per se, but it is by no means an infrequent accompaniment of pelvic peritonitis and pelvic cellulitis, the causes of each being the same. It is then so masked by the greater inflammation that its symptoms are lost in the general ones. Following the same course as that of pelvic inflammations, it begins with fibrinous exudation and ends either in resolution or in suppuration, or in chronic hypertrophy.

The TREATMENT of this inflammation is the same as that of pelvic inflammation—viz. rest, poultices, vaginal injections of hot water, and morphia and quinia in large doses. Sometimes the local abstraction of blood will be useful. Should pus form, it must be evacuated by the aspirator, and preferably per vaginam. After such an inflammation, and especially if caused by gonorrhœa, the ovary usually remains permanently injured, its functions being crippled by fibrous bands, adhesions, hardening of its stroma, and thickening of its investing peritoneum. If both ovaries be thus affected, sterility inevitably ensues.

Chronic Ovaritis.

By chronic ovaritis is meant either persistent congestion of the ovaries, or such tissue-changes in the stroma or in the follicles of the ovary, or in both conjointly, as are brought about from a previous attack of acute inflammation or from persistent hyperæmia. In its early stages it appears to be characterized by passive congestion, followed by infiltration of sero-sanguinolent fluid and by increase in bulk. Later on, if the congestion be not dispersed or it passes the health-limit, it becomes formative, or nutritive; the capsule thickens, the follicles enlarge, and a general hypertrophy takes place. According as the brunt of these changes falls on the stroma or on the follicles, the degeneration is termed either interstitial or follicular. When the stroma is chiefly attacked, the ovary becomes hard and rugous; when the follicles are diseased, they increase in size, and one or two of them are usually found to be distended into miniature cysts. There are indeed good reasons for the opinion that an ovarian cyst is a dropsy of many ovisacs, and is caused by ovaritis. The left ovary is the one more commonly affected—a fact accounted for by the pressure of the distended rectum and by the emptying of the left ovarian vein into the renal vein instead of into the vena cava, which is the course of the ovarian vein on the right side. It is a very common form of disease, very rarely coming from an acute attack, but starting subacutely with all the symptoms of chronicity.

CAUSATION.—Whatever induces a lasting congestion of the reproductive apparatus tends to create ovaritis—a torn cervix, a lacerated perineum, an arrest of involution after labor, dysmenorrhœa, and uterine tumors, flexions, and displacements. Barren women are very liable to this disease, and so especially are women who shirk maternity by preventive methods; for in both the menstrual congestions continue without that much-needed break which gestation and lactation bring, and in the latter the sexual congestions arising from incomplete intercourse are not relieved. So repeated erectility from self-abuse, by ending in a passive congestion of the womb and of the ovaries, will tend to produce this lesion. The prevalence of this habit in unmarried women is, I think, very much overrated, and yet I have seen from this cause several cases of ovaritis accompanied with prolapse of the ovaries. In one the ectropion of the cervical mucosa was so marked that it leads me to think that this is the cause of the occasional inversion of the womb in virgins. My notebook shows also cases of ovaritis from such imperfect sexual relations as come from the ill-health or the advanced age of the husband, and not a few from immoderate sexual intercourse. Some of the most common causes of chronic ovaritis are emotional in character, such as long engagements, disappointments in love, single life, the reading of corrupt literature, unhappy marriages, nerve-exhaustion, and hysteria. These causes operate by producing circulatory disturbances which keep up a constant congestion of such exacting organs as the ovaries.

SYMPTOMS.—Pain in one or in both ovarian regions, especially in the left one, is a prominent symptom. It is increased by walking or by standing, and is lessened by the recumbent posture. Starting usually from the ovary, it radiates to the small of the back or down the inner side of the thigh. It often begins from a week to ten days before the monthly period, and goes on increasing until the flow appears, when it commonly abates. Menorrhagia may usher in the disease, and may continue during the remainder of menstrual life, which then is usually prolonged. Ordinarily, however, menstruation becomes scant and irregular, postponing rather than anticipating. Sometimes amenorrhœa takes place. Sterility is usually present, and so almost always is nerve-exhaustion with all its emotional manifestations. Pressure over each ovarian region elicits pain and causes a contraction of the rectus muscle on the affected side. The finger per vaginam or per rectum will often discover behind the cervix uteri or to one side of it the very tender ovary, of the form and size of an almond. Pressure on it gives a sickening pain, very unnerving in its character. Reflex nervous symptoms are very common, especially those of hysteria. In the form of pain they show themselves in backache, spine-ache, nape-ache, and headache; in pain under the left breast, in the scalp on the top of the head, and in the stomach, bowels, womb, and coccyx. Nervous dyspepsia is common, accompanied by costiveness, nausea, vomiting, flatulent distension, and noisy eructation. Wakefulness and bad dreams are not infrequent. Other reflex neuroses may appear, such as paralysis or spasm of the sphincter muscles, the latter producing asthma, dysmenorrhœa, irritable bladder, and painful defecation. Then, again, there may be nervous disturbances, taking the form of low spirits, violent hysterical attacks, epilepsy, hystero-epilepsy, and of positive mental aberration.

PROGNOSIS.—This disease is rarely fatal, but it is always very stubborn, and often incurable. The patient grows anæmic and she tires on the slightest exertion. Very soon nerve-exhaustion with its protean symptoms sets in. She takes to her back and becomes a sofa-ridden invalid. If the patient has contracted the habit of taking stimulants or anodynes, her chances for recovery will be greatly lessened.

TREATMENT.—The pelvic organs should be carefully examined, and any discoverable lesion of the womb and of its annexes be remedied. Pelvic engorgement must be met by keeping the bowels soluble, by scarification of the cervix, by large vaginal injections of water as hot as can be borne, and by vaginal suppositories of belladonna and by rectal ones of iodoform. Tenderness and hardness in either broad ligament is first treated by applications of a strong tincture of iodine both to the roof of the vagina and to the skin overlying the ovarian regions. Flying blisters may also be placed there with benefit. Sexual intercourse should not be indulged in unless the desire for it be strong or there is a possibility of conception, for, by the prolonged rest which it gives to the ovaries, pregnancy usually brings about a cure. The patient should keep on her back during her menstrual period; but, while rest in the recumbent posture should be taken morning and afternoon, she should·be encouraged to move about and exert herself in some light household work, yet not to over-fatigue herself.

As far as medicines are concerned, those should be chosen which lessen the engorgement of the reproductive organs. Thirty grains of potassium bromide and ten drops of tincture of digitalis, given in compound infusion of gentian before each meal, will tend to quench all erectility of these organs. After the patient has been kept for some time on these anaphrodisiacs, alteratives will come into play: very good ones are ammonium chloride and mercuric bichloride, which can be advantageously administered after the following formula:

> ℞. Hydrargyri chloridi corrosivi, gr. j–ij;
> Ammonii chloridi, ʒij–iv;
> Misturæ glycyrrhizæ comp. fʒvj. M.

S. One dessertspoonful in a wine-glassful of water after each meal.

The paregoric in this mixture helps to control the aches; the antimony adds its quota to the needed alterative action; and the licorice disguises the harsh taste of the ammonium chloride.

Another very excellent alterative and nervine is the chloride of gold and of sodium. It is best given in pill and after each meal in doses of from one-eighth to one-quarter of a grain.

As there is in this disease a craving after stimulants and anodynes, which often degenerates into intemperance and into the opium-habit, the physician should be very careful how he prescribes such remedies, reserving their use wholly for emergencies.

In plethoric cases marked with menorrhagia iron is hurtful, but in anæmic cases with scant menstruation it rarely fails to do good, especially when given conjointly with arsenic. An excellent combination is one part of Fowler's solution of arsenic to nine of the syrup of the ferrous iodide. Beginning with ten drops after each meal, the patient increases the dose daily by one drop until thirty drops are reached. She then continues this last dose as long as it does good or it can be borne. In stubborn cases a sea-voyage may prove of lasting benefit.

The best of all treatments, however, and by far the best, is that devised for nerve-exhaustion by S. Weir Mitchell, which goes by the name of the rest-cure. It consists of prolonged rest in bed, seclusion from friends, massage, electricity, muscular movements, and a diet consisting largely of milk. By this treatment the circulation of the blood is made equable and the ovaries and other pelvic organs are thus relieved of their turgescence. I have had wonderful cures from this treatment, and can recommend it with the utmost confidence. Bed-ridden patients have been restored to health and chronic invalids returned to society.

Once in a while, lasting tissue-changes take place in the ovaries which medication cannot reach. The question then comes up, whether the woman shall be doomed to drag out the rest of her menstrual life burdened with distressing ovaralgia, with crippled locomotion, and with pelvic aches and pains and throbs, or whether the source of all these mischiefs, the ovaries themselves, shall be extirpated. This is a very important question, and the removal of these organs should not be decided upon without careful deliberation and without the conviction that the disease is otherwise incurable.

Prolapse of the Ovary.

This displacement of the ovary is almost always one of the lesions of chronic ovaritis, and as such might have been discussed under that genral heading. But as it displays certain symptoms peculiar to itself, and needs a special treatment aside from the general one, it seems to me best to describe it by itself.

At every monthly period the ovaries become turgid with blood, and from their weight sink low down. They can then be often felt, and even outlined, in Douglas's pouch. When this congestive period is over they discharge their over-freight of blood and again float up out of reach. Unfortunately, however, they sometimes keep turgid—blood-logged, so to speak—and consequently become permanently displaced. Accompanying this dislocation there will generally be some uterine lesion which will stand in the relation either of cause or of effect.

Nor could it very well be otherwise, for very close is the vascular and nervous kinship between the two—so close, indeed, that turgidity in the one means erectility in the other. Hence it is not always easy to decide which lesion was primary and which is secondary. When one ovary is displaced, it is usually the left one, because the left ovary, as explained under the heading of Ovaritis, is the one more liable to disease. When both ovaries are displaced, the left one will be the lower and the more easily reached, because the left round ligament is the longer and the left side of Douglas's pouch the deeper.

CAUSATION.—Any condition tending to a lasting congestion of the reproductive apparatus is very likely to lead to a descent of the ovaries. The causes, therefore, are the same as those of chronic ovaritis, to which subject the reader is referred.

SYMPTOMS.—First and foremost is pain in locomotion. Since the ovary now lies between the womb and the sacrum, it is liable at every step to be pinched between them. This pain is referred to the inguinal and sacral regions, and is of a sickening and an unnerving character. It often occurs suddenly, and then runs down the corresponding thigh along the track of the genito-crural nerve. One of my patients would, while walking, be unexpectedly seized with such a pain, which would either momentarily cripple her or else last so long as to compel her to call a carriage. Her left ovary, until cured by treatment, behaved like a loose cartilage in the knee-joint, and slipped down so low as to get pinched.

A second symptom is a throbbing pain while the rectum is loaded, and an agonizing pain during defecation. This arises from the grating of the hardened feces over these tender glands. In one of my cases[1] rectal enemata or the presence of hardened feces kindled up sexual throbs of the

[1] *Lessons in Gynæology,* by W. Goodell, M. D., ed. 1880, p. 332

most painful and exhausting character, which thrilled through the whole body for hours at a time.

A third symptom is painful coition, for the ovaries are now so low down as to be bruised by the male organ. A fourth is gusts of pain radiating from either groin. Lastly, there is usually present a morbid state of the mind, accompanied by low spirits. I have seen suicidal tendencies evoked by dislocation of the ovaries and relieved by their replacement.

DIAGNOSIS.—A digital examination will discover in Douglas's pouch a very tender almond-shaped body on one side of the womb. If both ovaries are dislocated, two such bodies will be found; but the left one, for reasons previously given, will be lower down and more easily defined. Pressure upon one of them produces a sickening pain, like that when the testicle is squeezed. If the pressure be increased, and be so made that one of these bodies slips abruptly away from under the finger, such a thrill of indescribable pain darts through the groin and down the side of the corresponding thigh that the woman screams out and grows pale or becomes nauseated.

A dislocated ovary is sometimes mistaken for a pedunculated fibroid tumor of the womb or for the fundus of a retroflexed womb. But the uterine growth is not sensitive to the touch, and the flexion of the womb can always be told by the sound.

TREATMENT.—Whenever the dislocated ovaries are congested or they display signs of chronic inflammation, the same remedies will of course be useful as those for ovaritis. In addition, pessaries are important adjuvants, and especially in those cases in which the womb has a backward displacement. In the simple, uncomplicated cases of ovarian dislocation, in which the womb is in its proper position, a pessary often does more harm than good. To be of service it must be long enough to obliterate Douglas's pouch, and the pressure on the rectum or on the sacral nerves then becomes unbearable. If, on the other hand, it be too short, the ovary slips down behind it and gets badly pinched. These requirements practically exclude the resort to Hodge's pessary or to any of its modifications, with the exception, perhaps, of Fowler's. In the long run, a thick elastic and soft ring-pessary will do the most good, by offering a broad shelf on which the ovaries will sometimes, but not always, lodge. The air-cushion pessary and Gariel's air-bag will often answer the purpose better than any other, but, being of soft rubber, they soon become fetid and soon collapse.

A very excellent way of keeping up the ovaries is the knee-chest posture devised by H. F. Campbell of Georgia. Two or three times a day, or more frequently if needful, the woman unbuttons her dress, unhooks her corset, and loosens her underclothing. She then kneels on her bed with her body bent forward until her chest is brought down to the surface of the bed, while her head is turned to one side and the lower cheek supported in the palm of the corresponding hand. Her knees should be about ten inches apart and the thighs perpendicular to the bed. The trunk of the woman's body is now supported, like a tripod, by her two knees and the upper portion of her thorax. If she now refrains from straining and breathes naturally, a reversal of gravity will be established. With the fingers of her free hand she next opens the vulva. Air will rush in, distending the vagina, and the contents of the abdomen will at once sink toward the diaphragm. This will, of course, draw the womb and the displaced ovaries out of the pelvic basin. As it is rather awkward for a woman while in this posture to free one hand to reach the vulva, Campbell advises that previously to taking this attitude she should insert into the vagina a small glass tube open at each end and long enough to project externally. This will leave an air-way and dispense with the use of the fingers. After staying in this posture for a few minutes, the woman removes the tube and slowly turns over on her side, where she is to lie as long as she can. Such constant replacements are of great service, for they lessen the throbbing and they give the limp ligaments a chance of shrinking and of keeping the truant ovaries at home.

In this intractable disorder an abdominal brace will sometimes do good. It may not cure, but it often blunts the edge of the aches, and thereby gives much comfort. By pressing the abdominal wall upward and inward the brace forms a shelf on which the viscera rest, and thus it takes off a portion of the load from the womb and from its ovaries. By virtually narrowing the pelvic inlet it lessens the space into which the bowels tend to crowd, and to that extent protects the pelvic organs. By swinging the pelvis backward it makes the axis of the superior strait lie more obliquely to the axis of the trunk, and the sum of the visceral pressure now converges, not in the pelvic basin, but on the portion of the abdominal wall lying between the symphysis pubis and the umbilicus.

There is yet another treatment which, combined with the knee-chest posture, I deem the best of all. It is Mitchell's rest-cure, to which I have before referred. After the patient begins to improve and to fatten, as she usually does under this treatment, she is taught how to replace the ovaries by atmospheric pressure, and the result is that in my experience they finally stay up. The explanation is as follows: By this treatment the circulation of nerve-fluid and of blood is equalized, and the ovaries, relieved of their turgescence, grow lighter. Then the increased deposit of fat in the abdominal walls, in the omental apron, and around the viscera, to say nothing of the needful fat-padding in all the pelvic nooks and crannies, increases the retentive power of the abdomen. Finally, by its gravity the now fat-laden and overhanging wall of the abdomen tends to draw toward itself—that is to say, upward—the movable floor of the pelvis. The behavior is like that of a rubber ball half filled with air, in which bulging at one pole causes a corresponding cupping at the other. This explains the ascent of the womb in women who get fat after the climacteric.

In exceptional cases the hypertrophied glands keep heavy and refuse either to go up or to stay up under any treatment whatever. The only known remedy will then be their extirpation—an operation which will be discussed under its appropriate heading.

Hernia of the Ovary.

This is usually a congenital displacement, and, according to Englisch,[1] is, when double, almost always so. The ovary is then found either in

---

[1] *New Sydenham Soc.'s Biennial Retrospect*, 1871-72, p. 291.

the inguinal canal or outside of this canal in the corresponding labium majus. The oviduct then accompanies it. When the hernia is acquired, the ovary, with or without the oviduct, makes one of the contents of the sac of an inguinal, a crural, a ventral, or an ischiatic hernia. Of these, the inguinal is by far the most common. Thus, out of 67 cases observed in 9 years by Langlou at the Truss Society, all were inguinal with 1 doubtful exception. Of these 67, 42 were congenital, 25 acquired.

The character of the lesion is told by the peculiar tenderness and nausea following pressure, and by the swelling of the tumor just before the menstrual flux. In one case mentioned by Routh[1] pressure on the tumor produced distressing sexual excitement; but this is an unusual symptom, although I have seen it produced by the pressure of hardened feces.[2] It is not always easy to decide whether the displaced glands are ovaries or testicles; and repeated mistakes in regard to sex have thus been made.[3] So difficult, indeed, is it sometimes that the microscope can alone settle the question.

TREATMENT.—In a reducible hernia, taxis and an appropriate truss comprise the treatment. If irreducible, a truss with a concave pad may be used to protect the ovary from injury. If the ovary be fixed by adhesions and it give much discomfort, it should be removed by operation.

Oöphorectomy; Battey's Operation.

There are certain forms of diseases of women peculiar to the menstrual period of life. The attendant lesions are found either in the reproductive organs themselves or outside of them in remote organs, but with such monthly exacerbations as show their participation in the catamenial excitement. They are always very hard to cure, and often prove to be wholly unmanageable until the climacteric has been established.

In this category may be classed fibroid tumors of the womb, chronic pelvic peritonitis and cellulitis, chronic ovaritis and ovaralgia, ovarian insanity, ovarian epilepsy, and, in short, all those phenomena or those lesions which are embraced under the term of pernicious menstruation.

Fibroid tumors of the womb are, fortunately, pretty manageable. Usually, the womb, like a generous host, hospitably entertains them; but once in a while an unwelcome one presents itself which arouses all the resentment of that organ. If, then, it stubbornly resists all treatment, it slowly but surely destroys life by the pain which it evokes and by the loss of blood it gives rise to. In such a case the woman is virtually bed-ridden from her floodings and sufferings, and she looks forward to the climacteric as her only hope. But the change of life is then always postponed for several years beyond the natural term—oftentimes so many years as to be overtaken by the death of the patient.

Then, again, there are those cases in which, despite all treatment, the ovaries remain turgid with blood, acutely neuralgic, and to the last degree sensitive. They become dislocated and lie in Douglas's pouch, or irremediable tissue-changes take place, attended by follicular or by intersti-

---

[1] *Trans. Royal Medical and Chir. Soc., Lancet,* Jan. 28, 1882.
[2] Goodell, *Lessons in Gynæcology,* 2d ed., chap. xxvi. p. 332.
[3] Chambers, *Trans. London Obstet. Soc.,* 1881.

tial degeneration. A woman with such a lesion is usually a helpless invalid, racked with atrocious pains, weakened by exhausting menorrhagia, and wholly unable to fulfil her duties as wife or as mother. Usually she seeks relief in anodynes and becomes a confirmed opium-eater.

There are also many distressing cases of salpingitis or of pelvic peritonitis and pelvic cellulitis which cripple a woman past all hope by monthly exacerbations. Such cases are by no means rare, and the woman, reduced to skin and bone, finally dies, because in spite of all treatment the inflammation is rekindled at every monthly period.

Further, there are cases of epilepsy which seem to come wholly from the sexual organs—cases with an ovarian aura, so to speak. The fits begin at puberty, very generally last through life, and end in impairment of the mind. Often the first convulsion is ushered in by the first menstruation, and ever after it is around ovulation as a storm-centre that future eclamptic attacks revolve. Such an epileptic is the terror of her family and a valueless member of society. Generally she dies insane or with enfeebled mind, and if she marries she is very likely to transmit her infirmities to her children, either in the same form as her own or in kind.

Finally, what insane asylum does not hold incurable women whose mental infirmities seem to depend wholly upon the act of ovulation? Some there are who, indeed, never exhibit symptoms of insanity excepting during the monthly flux.

For these menstrual affections there is a remedy which, while yet in its infancy, promises much—one first proposed and performed by R. Battey of Rome, Georgia. This able surgeon reasoned that, since these disorders are kept up by the monthly afflux of blood to the sexual apparatus, and therefore incurable during menstrual life, the only chance of immediate relief lies in the establishment of an artificial menopause. To bring about this change of life he advocated the extirpation of both the ovaries, and labeled the operation normal ovariotomy. With this name fault has been found, because it does not cover the whole ground, for often the ovaries themselves, together with the oviducts, are found diseased. Now, since it is important to distinguish this operation from that of ovariotomy proper, and since the term spaying, which technically defines the character of the operation, is obnoxious from its association with the lower animals, the terms öophorectomy, or Battey's operation, have been adopted.

In well-selected cases this operation has been followed by wonderful results; but it has been greatly abused. By it I have restored to perfect health cases of otherwise incurable fibroid tumors of the womb, cases of dysmenorrhœa and of menorrhagia, and cases of pernicious menstruation in which the sufferers were reduced to the last degree of emaciation and feebleness. Out of 5 cases of ovarian insanity I have also cured 4; the fifth, while not wholly restored, is yet very much better.

This operation has been performed both by the vaginal and the abdominal section. For some years I was a warm advocate of the vaginal method, but I have wholly given it up, because by this method of operation adherent ovaries cannot be safely dislodged, the ovaries cannot always be reached, the vaginal wound cannot be dressed antiseptically, and because the abdominal mode is more simple and less dangerous. Only when the ovaries are dislocated and low down in Douglas's pouch would I possibly resort to the vaginal incision.

If the abdominal operation be performed, the incision should be made between the navel and the pubes in the median line, and not over each ovary, as advised by some authors. One great caution must, however, be observed, and that is not to wound the intestines. In ovariotomy the cyst is in front of the intestines, and there is very little danger of injuring the latter. But in cases of öophorectomy, no tumor being present, the bowels lie in contact with the wall of the abdomen, and are very likely to be wounded by the knife when the peritoneum is incised. The incision should be long enough to admit two fingers. These, being passed behind the womb, are conducted to the ovary by gliding along the oviduct as a guide. Each ovary, together with its oviduct, is in turn brought up to the opening. It is then seized by a fenestrated polypus-forceps and its stalk transfixed, tied on either side with fine silk, cut off, and dropped back into the abdominal cavity. Should the stalk be so short that ovarian tissue is left behind in the button of the stump, it should be destroyed by Paquelin's cautery, for it is astonishing how small an amount of this tissue will keep up not only menstruation, but even menorrhagia. On the other hand, it will not answer merely to ligate the pedicles without removing the ovaries. This has been tried, and not only did menstruation continue, but in one instance pregnancy took place.[1]

The dressing is precisely the same as in ovariotomy, and, like it, the operation should be performed with every detail of antiseptic surgery.

In the vaginal operation the vagina first should be thoroughly cleansed with a solution of carbolic acid, and the patient placed on her back and not on her side. I am convinced from experience that the usual left-lateral position is a dangerous one, for as soon as the peritoneum is opened the air rushes out and in during every inspiration and expiration —an untoward circumstance which cannot happen in the dorsal position. A duckbill speculum is introduced, and the perineum pulled downward. The cervix uteri is transfixed by a strong thread, by which the womb is drawn downward and forward. The post-cervical mucous membrane is next caught up by a uterine tenaculum and snipped open for about an inch. The index finger of the left hand is then passed in, and each ovary brought down to the incision by the finger-tip hooked into the sling made by the oviduct. The ovary is seized by a fenestrated forceps and brought into the vagina, where its stalk is transfixed by passing a needle armed with a double thread between the ovarian ligament and the oviduct, and each half is securely tied. The ovary and the fimbriated end of the oviduct are then removed, the ligatures cut off at the knot, and the stumps returned into the pelvic cavity. To close the vaginal opening one or two stitches will be needed, and finally the wound is covered with iodoform and the vagina gently packed with pads of carbolated or salicy-lated cotton.

It is a fact worthy of note that during the week following the ablation of the uterine appendages a sanguineous discharge from the womb usually takes place. This is in no wise a menstruation, but a metrostaxis

[1] Murphy, *British Medical Journal,* April 18, 1885, p. 787.

set up by the irritation of the ovarian nerves, caused by the means adopted to secure the pedicles. Candor, however, compels me to say that for some inexplicable reason the removal of the uterine appendages —viz. ovaries and oviducts—does not always bring about the change of life. These cases are exceptional, and they are supposed to be due to either the presence of a third ovary or to some small portion of ovarian stroma left behind.

This operation in no wise unsexes a woman or changes her appearance or character. It simply brings on the change of life with its attendant phenomena. Her instincts and affections remain the same, her sexual organs continue excitable, her breasts do not wither up, and she is no less a mother or a wife.[1]

Extra-Ovarian Cysts.

There is a class of tumors which, while not ovarian, lie so near to the ovary as often to involve it, and usually need precisely the same treatment as cysts of that organ. In their extirpation the ovary is almost always also involved. This close anatomical relationship makes it needful to describe them in conjunction with ovarian tumors. They comprise Cysts of the Parovarium, Cysts of the Oviducts, or Fallopian Dropsy, and Cysts of the Terminal Vesicle of the Oviduct, often called the Hydatid or Vesicle of Morgagni.

Cysts of the Parovarium.

These are formed from the dropsical distension of one of the tubules of the parovarium, or organ of Rosenmüller, which lies between the folds of the broad ligament and between the ovary and the oviduct. Usually, one tubule alone is affected, and the cyst is then unilocular; but exceptional cases have been met with in which several of the tubules have become dilated, and the cyst is then bilocular or even multilocular.[2] These cysts are often called cysts of the broad ligament.

By examining cysts in their early stage Albert Doran has demonstrated that "the vertical tubes of the parovarium are lined with epithelium, sometimes ciliated, but oftener cubical, the original, primitive form of the tubes of the Wolffian body. From these tubes and from the hilum of the ovary, full of Wolffian relics, spring the multilocular papillary cysts which give so much trouble to the operator. At the outer end of the horizontal tube of the parovarium is a cystic dilatation which is lined with a structure resembling endothelium. Apart from the parovarium, between the folds of the broad ligament, minute cysts are frequent. It is from these and from the terminal cyst of the parovarium that the simple unilocular so-called parovarian cyst arises. The terminal cyst of the Fallopian tube never attains a large size, and no true cysts of the broad ligament appear, when young and minute, to arise from that tube."[3]

[1] *Lessons in Gynæcology,* by Wm. Goodell, M. D., chap. xxvi.
[2] "Bursting Cysts of the Abdomen," by Wm. Goodell, *Trans. American Gynæc. Soc.,* 1881, p. 231.
[3] *British Med. Journal,* Oct. 21, 1882, p. 792.

These cysts are more commonly found in young women. From the thinness of their walls and the limpid character of their fluid, they yield very marked waves of fluctuation which are equally distinct at every point. They can usually be distinguished from ovarian cysts either by a lack of that tenseness so characteristic of the latter or by varying conditions of tenseness and flaccidity, as if the fluid were sometimes absorbed more quickly than at other times. They also grow more slowly than the ovarian cyst, and do not exert the same profound constitutional impression. The facies ovariana is absent, and the health of the woman may in no wise be disturbed. They, indeed, in the majority of cases, seem to do no harm, and are merely annoying from their bulk. The fluid they contain is with rare exceptions as limpid and clear as spring-water, but with refractive powers so high as to magnify the fibres of the wooden pail into which it has been drawn off.

Owing to their very thin walls and delicate structure these cysts on very slight provocation are liable to burst. On account of the blandness of the contained fluid this accident is rarely followed by collapse or by peritonitis. The rent heals up and the cyst usually refills; but in a large proportion of cases it does not, and the woman remains permanently healed.[1] Sometimes they are pedunculated, but often they lie between the two folds of the broad ligament, having no proper stalk.

Cysts of the broad ligament must not be confounded with those ovarian cysts which, instead of growing free in the peritoneal cavity, develop between the two layers of the peritoneum—intra-ligamentous ovarian cysts, as Garrigues very aptly calls them in his paper on the "Diagnosis of Ovarian Cysts."[2] In this excellent paper, from which I have gleaned much, he says that sometimes the anatomical relations are so lost that nothing short of a microscopic examination of the outer epithelium can determine the character of the cyst. Thus, "a tumor covered with columnar epithelium is ovarian, and cannot be anything else; while the cyst of the broad ligament, being covered with peritoneum, has flat peritoneal endothelium. In cases of intra-ligamentous development of an ovarian cyst the lower portion is covered by peritoneum, but the upper part has the columnar epithelium characteristic of the ovary." There are, however, certain macroscopic characteristics which will generally tell the nature of the cyst. For instance: usually by a careful examination the corresponding ovary will be found either stretched out and spread out in the wall of the sac, or, what in my experience is more common, elongated and forming a part of the stalk. These cysts are in the vast majority of cases monocysts, while unilocular ovarian cysts are very rarely if ever met with. Their walls are thin, of a conjunctival blue, and fretted with a delicate network of blood-vessels. The oviduct is usually imbedded in the cyst, and by transmitted light its fimbriæ can be traced out in the cyst-walls in long fronds as delicate as those of dried and pressed sea-weed. Then, again, the peritoneal coat is readily stripped off. On the other hand, in an ovarian tumor the oviduct is not ordinarily incorporated in the cyst-wall; in fact, a meso-salpinx usually exists; and, further, the peritoneal coat, being nailed down to the cyst-wall proper by the cicatrices of ovulation, is not capable of being stripped off.

---

[1] "Bursting Cysts of the Abdomen," by Wm. Goodell, *Trans. American Gynæcological Society*, 1881, p. 226. 　　[2] *Am. Journ. of Obstetrics*, April, 1882, p. 394.

TREATMENT.—Since these cysts do not ordinarily affect the general health or grow to a very large size, they should, as a rule, be let alone. Whenever grounds for interference arise the cyst should be aspirated, for sometimes after being wholly emptied it does not refill. Should, however, the fluid return, the cyst must be extirpated in precisely the same way as an ovarian tumor. When it is without a pedicle it will have to be carefully enucleated from between the folds of the broad ligament, which then cover it. If this cannot be done, all of the cyst possible should be removed, the edges stitched to the abdominal wound, and a drainage-tube put in. This is the advice ordinarily given, but I have not yet met with a cyst of this variety which could not be removed. Were such a one to occur in my practice I should be tempted to remove all of the cyst possible, and to close up the adherent portion in the cavity of the abdomen without resorting to a drainage-tube. The fluid secreted by a parovarian cyst is so bland that I believe no mischief would arise. The late Washington L. Atlee was accustomed to make merely a large circular opening in the cyst, without attempting to remove it.

Cysts of the Oviducts, or Fallopian Dropsy.

These tumors may contain either fluid or pus. In the former case the cyst is called hydro-salpinx; in the latter, pyo-salpinx. They are caused by salpingitis, or inflammation of the oviduct, which exists rarely per se, unless of gonorrhœal origin, but is one of the sequels of pelvic peritonitis. The distension of the tube is due to the occlusion of each of its ends. Thus by pelvic inflammation the fimbriæ become glued to the ovary, sealing up the ovarian end, while an endometritis closes the uterine opening. In addition to the dropsy of the tube, I have repeatedly met with small cysts, or bladder-like bodies outside of the tube proper, very analogous to those found on the umbilical cord.

This affection is by no means an uncommon one, every age being liable to it, and it is often the unrecognized cause of ill-health. Since Tait first called the attention of the profession to the frequency of the disease and the means for its cure, many cases have been reported in which obscure pelvic symptoms were cured by the removal of the ovaries and of the oviducts—the uterine appendages, as they are called.

DIAGNOSIS.—This is difficult, because the symptoms are those of pelvic peritonitis or of pelvic cellulitis, the disease of the oviduct being usually associated with that of the broad ligament. In some cases the womb will be found movable, with a sausage-like tumor behind it; the diagnosis is then easy. Usually, the symptoms are negative, and the diagnosis is based upon constant groin-pains and recurring attacks of pelvic inflammation.

TREATMENT.—Like hydrocele of Nuck's canal, hydro-salpinx occasionally heals spontaneously, but more frequently it will need aspiration, together with injections of iodine or of carbolic acid. When pus is present, absorption probably never takes place, and an operation will be needed. If the symptoms are grave enough to warrant an exploratory incision, and dropsy of the tubes be discovered, both the tube and its ovary should be extirpated, for in the great majority of cases the cor-

responding ovary will have undergone follicular or interstitial degeneration. Unless there are very good reasons for adopting a different
course, both ovaries and tubes should be removed, because the sound
ovary, together with its tube, is liable to become diseased. The incision
should always be abdominal, and not larger than to admit two fingers.
The broad ligament is transfixed between the tube and the ovarian ligament by a double ligature and tied on either side. The operation is, in
fact, analogous to that of öophorectomy. When the tubes contain pus,
they are liable to become adherent to the sigmoid flexure, to the rectum,
or to the small intestines, making their removal very difficult—sometimes, indeed, impossible. The separation of such adhesions requires the
greatest care and delicacy.

Cysts of the Terminal Vesicle of the Oviduct.

A little bladder-like body, not larger than a pea, is often found hanging by a thread-like stalk from one of the fimbriæ of the oviduct. It is
a relic of fœtal life, being probably the remains of the Wolffian body,
and sometimes goes by the name of the hydatid or vesicle of Morgagni.
The walls are very thin and covered by peritoneum. What rôle these
vesicles play in the economy is uncertain, but they have been found to
undergo cystic degeneration. They rarely attain to a size larger than that
of an orange, and then either remain stationary or else burst. I have
met with several examples of cysts which, after reaching the above size,
did not grow any larger. I have also met with one case in which, after
attaining the bulk of a small apple, the cyst burst, and immediately
refilled, to burst again and again at intervals of from four to six weeks.[1]
The collapse of the sac was attended each time by colicky pains, but of no
great severity.

Other small cysts I have met with which either burst under the pressure
of the examining finger or were designedly burst by bimanual pressure.
These, I am disposed to think, were cysts of the terminal vesicle of the
oviduct. These cysts are of but little surgical importance, as they rarely
need operative interference. If such should arise, they are to be treated
by aspiration, and if this fails by extirpation.

Solid Tumors of the Round Ligament.

These are occasionally met with, and usually on the right side. They
belong to the connective-tissue group, being either myoma, fibroma, or
sarcoma. They form at any point of the round ligament, and may therefore be either intra-peritoneal, intra-canalicular—that is, in the inguinal
canal—or extra-peritoneal. The symptoms are those arising from pressure, and are not at all diagnostic. The only treatment of these tumors
is removal, but, as their growth is very slow, they are not to be touched
unless the symptoms become exacting.[2]

[1] "Bursting Cysts of the Abdominal Cavity," by Wm. Goodell, *Trans. Amer. Gynæcol.
Soc.*, 1881, p. 228.
[2] *Medical Times and Gazette*, Dec. 1, 1883.

OVARIAN TUMORS.

THE morbid growths of the ovary are conveniently divided into the solid and the cystic.

The solid ones are either benign, under the form of fibroma, or malignant, being then either carcinoma or sarcoma.

Fibroid Tumor of the Ovary.

Fibroid degeneration of the ovary is so rare a form of disease as to be denied by excellent authorities, who contend that all the cases reported under that term were pedunculated uterine fibroids, which had so grown around and so involved the corresponding ovary as to be mistaken for an ovarian fibroid. Yet while such mistakes have undoubtedly been made, there can be no question that ovarian fibroid does occasionally present itself as a rare form of disease.[1] Out of 155 cases of ovariotomy thus far performed by myself, I have met with 4 undoubted cases of ovarian fibroid. The tumors weighed respectively 2, 3, 4, and 15 pounds, and in each, with the exception of the first, abdominal dropsy was the prominent symptom. All but one of these cases promptly recovered.

According to Francis Delafield,[2] "The structure of a fibroid of the ovary resembles that of the ordinary fibroid tumors of the uterus. That is, they are composed of connective tissue and smooth muscular fibre. The tumor, therefore, is a myo-fibroma. There has been some question whether ovarian tumors ever contain smooth muscle, but the best authorities now admit that it does sometimes exist in such tumors."

Occasionally these tumors arise not from a general hypertrophy of the whole ovary, but from a nodule or a tumor growing in and from the stroma of the ovary. Solid ovarian fibroids are of slow growth and rarely attain a large size. When, however, they are of the geode variety, with numerous cystic cavities, they grow rapidly and may reach enormous proportions.

DIAGNOSIS.—The only other abdominal tumor for which it is very likely to be mistaken is a pedunculated fibroid tumor on the peritoneal surface of the womb, and with our present knowledge it seems impossible to tell them apart.

When they float about in ascitic fluid they often give the sign of ballottement in a very perfect manner. From carcinoma of the ovary they can generally be told by their smooth surface.

PROGNOSIS.—Fibroid tumors of the ovary grow so slowly that, like pedunculated fibroid tumors of the womb, they ordinarily do not attain a very bulky size. When the climacteric is reached they tend, like the latter, to stop growing and to undergo a calcareous degeneration. More often, however, they cause by their presence a dropsical effusion of the abdominal cavity, which has to be repeatedly drawn off; and it is for this reason that they usually have to be extirpated. They are removed precisely in the same way as an ovarian cyst, and the prognosis is equally

---

[1] *Brit. Med. Journ.*, March 18, 1882, p. 384.
[2] *Boston Med. and Surg. Journ.*, Nov. 17, 1881, p. 461.

good, but they are liable to have short and broad pedicles which need to be tied very carefully in sections.

Malignant Diseases of the Ovary.

These affections are either primary or secondary. When secondary they follow analogous diseases of the womb or of the pelvic structures. When primary, they appear under different forms, as in other portions of the body, being either encephaloid, scirrhous, melanotic, or papillary. Colloid cancer of the ovary may be practically excluded, because it is of extreme rareness. The term colloid when applied to ovarian cysts refers more to the gluey consistency of the contained fluid than to the question of malignancy. In my experience the most common form is that of papilloma, which, however, like villous growths elsewhere, is not always malignant. I have removed papillary cysts and villous growths of the ovary, yet the subsequent history of the cases proved that the tumors were benign. The only macroscopic distinction between the benign and the malignant form which I have hitherto attempted to make is, that in the malignant form papillary growths will be found in patches upon adjacent structures, or else the womb and the broad ligaments are also involved in one cauliflower-like tumor. But Tait observes that he has had two cases of ovariotomy in which he left large masses of papilloma, fixing the womb, yet in each case these masses wholly disappeared, and the patients are both in perfect health.[1]

There is, however, no question that malignancy lurks in many ovarian cystomata which present to the naked eye an innocent appearance.

The patient recovers promptly from the operation for their removal, but dies a few months later from cancer of the peritoneum or of other organs. Every ovariotomist has met with such examples. In one of my own cases, in which not the slightest sign of malignancy was apparent, the patient wholly recovered from the operation. Shortly after her convalescence an effusion took place in the right pleural cavity. The chest was tapped three times before her death, which was due to cancer of the liver and of the broad ligament at the site of the ablated ovary. In my first case of ovariotomy, one in which the clamp was used, menstruation took place regularly for several months from the cicatrix, which within a year became affected with cancer.

Both ovaries are usually involved in cysto-carcinoma, and this fact should be borne in mind in making a diagnosis. From the marvellous changes often produced progressively in the epithelial linings of ovarian cysts, by which they are transformed into tufts of villous cancer, Tait inclines to the opinion that their growth is associated with a tendency toward malignancy. He believes that tapping hastens on this degeneration, and that after an accidental rupture of such a cyst the peritoneum will be found studded with patches of papillary cancer. Hence he argues that ovarian cysts should never be tapped, and that they should be removed in the earlier stages of their existence, before these malignant transformations have taken place.[2]

DIAGNOSIS.—Since, as has been shown, this cannot always be made

---

[1] *Diseases of the Ovaries,* 4th Am. ed., p. 147.   [2] *Op. cit.,* p. 148.

out, even by the eye, after the removal of the cysts, it follows that in a large proportion of cases the malignant character of the degeneration cannot be recognized.   There are, however, certain symptoms pointing to malignancy which will often throw much light.   These, in the order of their frequency, are—

(*a*) The presence of ascitic fluid or of œdema of the lower extremities when the tumor is too small to produce such pressure symptoms.

(*b*) General cachexia, rapid emaciation, and grave constitutional disturbance out of all proportion to the size of the tumor.

(*c*) The hardness and solidity of the tumor, together with its nodulous and irregular surface.

(*d*) The concurrent development of two ovarian growths.

(*e*) The retraction and burying of the cervix in the vaginal vault.

(*f*) Pain in stabs, starting from the groin and running down the inside of the thigh.   But pain is not a trustworthy symptom, as it is often absent, especially in cysto-carcinoma, and may be caused by benign growths as well.

TREATMENT.—Whenever no doubt exists as to the malignancy of an ovarian growth, an operation looking to its removal should not be urged by the physician.   On the other hand, since a positive diagnosis on this point is rarely attained, and since cancer of the ovary tends for a long time to remain localized, whenever a suspicion of malignancy exists ovariotomy should be performed early, before adhesions have been contracted with neighboring structures.   In such a case I should incline to burn off the pedicle in preference to using the ligature.

In those cases in which, on account of adhesions, no operation is justifiable, palliative treatment can alone be resorted to.   This comprises the removal of the ascitic fluid or the contents of the cyst by the aspirator whenever the pressure becomes uncomfortable.   Symptoms should be treated, and, that of pain being the most urgent, opium will be needed up to the last in increasing doses.

Dermoid Cyst, or Piliferous Cyst of the Ovary.

A dermoid cyst is a congenital tumor having a wall composed of elements like true skin, with its appendages of hairs, sebaceous glands, etc., and contains teeth, hair, bone, cartilage, muscle, and a cheesy material very like vernix caseosa.   These cysts are solitary, two never being found in the same person, and, further, they are always unilocular.   They are either external or internal—that is, they affect either the surface of the body or else the cavities of the body, as "under the tongue, in the pharynx, œsophagus, cranial cavity, peritoneal cavity, lung, ovary, testis, bladder, and kidney."[1]   No tumors are more curious, and none are more puzzling to explain. _ The theories accounting for their origin are very remarkable, and are as follows: Excess of formative nisus.   Parthenogenesis, or virgin birth ; that is to say, imperfect imitation of transmitted fertility—a property peculiar to many insects, by which, without any renewal of fertilization, successive generations of procreating individuals start from a single ovum.   Inclusion of abnormal structures.

[1] Elsner, *Dublin Journal Medical Sciences,* May, 1882, p. 330.

where there is a dipping in of the epiblast to meet the hypoblast during foetal life, and the pinching off of the same. Foetus in foetu—viz. the inclusion of an imperfectly developed ovum within another which matures perfectly. Hypererchesis; which means that "the ovum has in it the origin-buds of certain tissues, which under exceptional hypererchetic action may go on to the rudimental formation of these tissues without a fusion with the male germ."[1] According to Elsner, who has written last on this subject, and to whom I am indebted for much information, "dermoids occur externally and internally in places where the epiblast dips down to meet the hypoblast, and where by processes of grooved involution new bodies are formed, such being, first in order, the testicle and ovary, and that they are therefore all (without exception) embryonal in their first structure."

SYMPTOMS.—These congenital tumors begin early in life, and usually remain dormant until puberty. Then the periodic congestions of menstruation usually stimulate them into growth. Sometimes they need the increased vascularization of pregnancy. They are more liable than ovarian cysts to inflammation and suppuration, but they grow much more slowly, and very rarely reach the large size of the latter. They are also very liable to contract adhesions to every structure they touch, making their extirpation very difficult and sometimes impossible. Often they create pain out of all proportion to their size. Occasionally, they break and empty their contents through fistulous communications with the intestines, bladder, or the abdominal wall. But collapse of the usually thick walls of the cyst does not take place, and a cure results far less frequently than in pelvic abscesses, which empty themselves through analogous channels. The cyst ordinarily does not lessen in size; suppuration goes on with hectic fever and exhaustion, which finally carry off the patient.

DIAGNOSIS.—Quiescent or slow-growing pelvic tumors, semi-solid to the feel, and first discovered at the age of puberty, are usually dermoid cysts. Their small size is also an aid to diagnosis, for they very rarely reach the bulk of the adult head. On several occasions I have found them in Douglas's pouch, fig-shaped and flattened in their antero-posterior diameter. From its attachments to neighboring structures a dermoid cyst is very liable to be mistaken for the cyst of an extra-uterine foetation. But the exclusion of the history of pregnancy and the slow growth of a dermoid cyst, unless suppuration has taken place, ought to distinguish the one from the other.

TREATMENT.—While quiescent the cyst should not be touched, as it is very vulnerable and liable to resent the slightest injury, even from the slender trocar of the aspirator. If suppuration takes place and the tumor points to the surface, it should be treated, like any other abscess, by a free incision, by the evacuation of its contents, by the introduction of a drainage-tube, and by the injection of antiseptic solutions. Small cysts lying in Douglas's pouch can sometimes be cured by aspiration; at least I have twice succeeded in obliterating them in this way. The operation was, however, followed by suppuration of the cyst, the abscess bursting into the vagina. If after an exploratory incision an abdominal cyst turns out to be dermoid, it should be extirpated. But if extensive adhesions

[1] *Diseases of Ovaries*, by L. Tait, 4th ed., p. 177.

preclude such an operation, the cyst should be opened, evacuated, and thoroughly cleansed. The edges of the opening should then be stitched to those of the abdominal wound and a drainage-tube put in. The after-treatment of such a case will be analogous to that of an ovarian cyst under like conditions, to which the reader is referred.

Cystic Tumors of the Ovary.

These represent by far the most frequent variety of ovarian tumors, and as such demand our best attention. They consist, in probably the majority of cases, in a dropsical enlargement of one ovisac or of more— viz. in a follicular dropsy. Indeed, as Cazeaux has aptly said, the ovi-sacs, or Graäfian follicles, are ovarian cysts in miniature. These cysts are divided into three classes, which depend wholly upon the number of ovi-sacs involved. Thus, a single, or barren, cyst, containing merely fluid, is called a monocyst or unilocular cyst. Such a cyst would be due to the dropsical enlargement of but one ovisac. It is extremely rare—so much so that its existence is denied. The probability is that a one-chambered sac does not begin as such, but it becomes so through the breaking of the walls of other contained cysts. A multiple cyst is caused by the simul-taneous growth of two or more ovisacs, one of which usually takes the lead in growth and keeps the others dwarfed. This form of cyst is by far the most common. It grows with great rapidity, and may reach a weight of over one hundred pounds. I have successfully removed one weighing one hundred and twelve pounds. A proliferous cyst is a mother-cyst packed with innumerable child-cysts of varying size. These endog-enous cysts multiply by exogenous and endogenous growth. The pro-liferous cyst rarely attains to the size of the multiple cyst, but surgically it is a solid tumor, because it cannot be emptied by tapping, and therefore often needs a long incision for its removal. It also usually possesses a very thin wall, which is liable to be torn during the needful manipula-tion for its removal. Racemose cysts are occasionally met with. They consist of a number of isolated cysts of varying size attached to one common stalk like a bunch of grapes. I have met with two such exam-ples. Tait thinks that they are "produced by the retention of the ova in the Graäfian follicles, and the distension of their cavities by a contin-uous secretion of the liquor folliculi."

The pedicle or stalk by which an ovarian cyst is attached to the womb consists of the corresponding broad ligament, oviduct, ovarian ligament, and vessels. The pedicle is sometimes long and slender, at other times short and broad. There is one form of ovarian cyst which has no proper pedicle. It grows between the two layers of the broad ligament, and tends to develop downward into Douglas's pouch. It is called the intra-ligamentous cyst, and needs careful and tedious enucleation for its removal. Sometimes, indeed, extirpation is out of the question, and the cyst has to be treated by the drainage-tube, as will hereafter be shown.

The contents of ovarian cysts vary very greatly in color and in consist-ency. In monocysts the fluid is often limpid and colorless. In multiple cysts the contents are usually syrupy, thick, and turbid. Sometimes the color is quite dark, as much so as weak coffee. The surface of the fluid, after standing, will be covered with a pellicle of cholesterin crystals, which sparkle in the sunlight. In proliferous cysts the contents are usually viscid, sometimes as much so as jelly, and to this the term colloid is applied. Foulis, who is an authority on this subject, states that he has "never found that an ovarian fluid, however long kept, ever deposited a precipitate spontaneously. Whereas very frequently in the case of an ascitic fluid such a spontaneous precipitate appeared within a period varying from a few hours to a few days."[1] Again he observes: "After ten years of observation made on fluids withdrawn by the aspirator, I found that ovarian fluids never throw down a precipitate of a fibrinous character. An ovarian fluid was always a pure cellular secretion. An ascitic fluid was always the result of obstruction to the circulation or of inflammatory action in the peritoneum, and ascitic fluids allowed to stand for a short time nearly always showed a precipitate with the character of felted material under the microscope. If they tapped the patient and subjected the fluid to this test, two or three days would suffice to tell in cases in which there was doubt. The deposit in ovarian fluids showed cellular, not fibrinous, elements under the microscope."[2]

Chemically, the contents are mucous and albuminous, the albumen being readily detected by the tests of heat and nitric acid. Microscopically, ovarian fluid is found to contain fat-globules, epithelial, granular, and pus-cells, crystals of cholesterin, blood-corpuscles, and compound granular cells, also called the inflammatory globules of Gluge.

Whether ovarian fluid contains a cell or corpuscle peculiar to itself is yet a moot question. Drysdale contends that it has a characteristic cell. He describes it as "an albuminoid body containing little fatty particles which give it a granular appearance. It resembles in some particulars many other granular cells, but can be distinguished from all other cells found in the abdominal cavity. . . . . The principal test I employ is acetic acid. If the cell is ovarian, the acid changes it but little, perhaps rendering it only a little more transparent. But if it be a white blood-cell, a lymph-corpuscle, or any of those granular cells which resemble them, it will nearly always take on a different appearance, the cells almost vanishing perhaps, and multiple (2–5) nuclei appearing, as in the pus-cell. Then, if the cell be suspected to be fatty, degenerated, or Gluge's cell, ether may be added, by which the fatty materials will be dissolved and disappear. If no fatty degeneration be present, it is sufficient to add acetic acid."[3] Garrigues, on the other hand, contends that the ovarian fluid does not contain a characteristic cell.[4]

If I am not mistaken, the opinion of the best microscopists of Philadelphia is that the Drysdale cell, while not characteristic of ovarian fluids, is not found in any other fluid in such large numbers, and to that extent it is of diagnostic value.

CAUSATION.—In probably the very great majority of cases an ovarian cyst is a dropsy of several ovisacs, but the cause of such growths has never yet been ascertained. In the majority of cases it seems to depend upon some sexual disturbance.

Very recently the relation of the sexual condition to disease has been

[1] *Edinburgh Medical Journal*, July, 1885, p. 76.   [2] *Ibid.*, June, 1885, p. 1131.
[3] *Trans. Amer. Gynæcol. Soc.*, vol. i. p. 195.   [4] *Ibid.*, vol. vi. p. 54.

made the subject of scientific inquiry. From a careful examination of the registrar's tables for France, M. Bertillon shows that marriage, by giving a comparative immunity from diseases of the sexual organs, prolongs life in both sexes. This statement is confirmed by the statistics of ovarian tumor. Of Lee's 136 cases, 88 were married, 37 were unmarried, and 11 were widows. Of Sir Spencer Wells's first 500 cases, 260 were married, 221 were unmarried, and 19 were widows. Out of 155 completed cases of ovariotomy performed by myself, 91 were married, 48 were single, 16 were widows. Of the married, 24 were sterile, 10 had one child, and 26 had but two children, and several confessed to using preventive measures. Out of a total of 791 cases of ovarian tumor, there are, then, 352 without husbands to 439 with husbands. Now, when one considers how small the proportion of single women and of widows is to married women whose husbands are living, the significance of these figures goes to show that childbearing women, and especially the prolific ones, are less liable to cystic degeneration of the ovaries, and that, unless the cycle of reproduction is completed in a woman, she is plainly violating some law of her being.

SYMPTOMS.—There are no symptoms pathognomonic of this affection, for they are mainly those of pressure, and therefore belong in common to all fluid collections in the abdominal cavity. But in proportion as the abdomen swells there is a marked emaciation of the extremities. The limbs waste away, the face becomes pinched, the eyes are hollow and staring, deep wrinkles and furrows appear on the forehead and around the mouth, and the nostrils are wide open. This facial expression is termed the facies ovariana. Sometimes, when both ovaries are simultaneously affected, hair will grow on the chin and on the upper lip.

THE NATURAL HISTORY.—The natural course of an ovarian cyst is to grow rapidly, and in about two years from the time of its discovery to destroy life by exhaustion through the embarrassing pressure which it makes upon the organs of respiration, circulation, and nutrition. Malignant cysts grow more rapidly than the benign, while the latter will, on the other hand, occasionally remain for years in a state of quiescence. I have kept stationary cysts under observation for ten years, and others have been reported which lasted twenty years without change.

As a cyst develops it is very likely to contract adhesions to the organs with which it lies in contact. The most common adhesion is that of the omentum. Next to this is adhesion to the abdominal walls. Then will happen more rarely adhesions to the bowels, womb, bladder, pelvis, liver, and stomach. A loop of intestine will sometimes be found fastened to the front wall of the cyst, but usually the bowels lie packed behind the tumor.

Rupture of the cyst sometimes takes place, either spontaneously, through over-distension, or through violence, as a kick, a rude fall, or from being run over by a carriage. This accident, if the fluid happens to be bland, may be followed by a cure; but more often a violent peritonitis sets in, which carries the patient off in a few hours. From a study of 257 cases, Aronson[1] rates the fatality at 41 per cent.; but without question the very great majority of cases of bursting cysts of the abdomen in which this accident was followed by a cure were cysts of the parovarium, which being

---

[1] *American Journal of Obstetrics*, Nov., 1883, p. 1210.

thin-walled are likely to burst, and which contain a bland, unirritating fluid. Bursting of the sac can be recognized by more or by less collapse and pain, by the disappearance of the cyst, and by the lessened size of the abdomen. If the patient does not at once succumb, excessive diuresis usually occurs.

It happens occasionally that the inner cyst-wall inflames, either spontaneously or in consequence of being tapped or from other injury. Suppuration then takes place, the contained fluid becomes fetid, and offensive gases are generated which give a tympanitic sound on percussion. There will be creeping chills, a red tongue, night-sweats, a frequent pulse, a general rise in the temperature with evening exacerbations: in one word, all the well-known symptoms of blood-poisoning will be present in a greater or less degree. Unless the cyst be at once removed the woman will speedily die.

Ulceration of the cyst, with perforation of its wall, may also occur. The decomposing contents will then be discharged, either into the peritoneal cavity or into any viscus to which the cyst may have contracted adhesions. In this way the purulent contents of an ovarian cyst have been discharged through the bowels, the bladder, the vagina, and even into the womb through the oviducts.

Hemorrhage within the sac is an occasional accident. When it takes place the tumor rapidly enlarges, great abdominal pain is caused by this sudden stretching, the complexion grows pale, the features become pinched; there will be collapse and all the symptoms of internal hemorrhage. If the bleeding does not stop, the patient will die in a few hours. On the other hand, if she survives the immediate danger, she is liable to succumb later to septicæmia, which arises from the decomposition of the now bloody fluid. The immediate removal of the cyst gives the woman, then, her sole chance of life.

Twisting of the pedicle of an ovarian tumor by axial rotation is another serious complication, which leads to its strangulation and gangrene, with consequent fatal peritonitis. The chief factors of this accident are, probably, the filling and emptying of the bladder and rectum, which may rotate an unadherent cyst with a long stalk. The symptoms of axial rotation, as carefully noted by Tait [1] and Aronson, [2] are sudden accession of severe abdominal pain and tenderness, a rapid increase in size, and incessant vomiting, the matter thrown up soon becoming green. The pulse rises, but the temperature is not always affected, and rigors are absent. Such a train of symptoms should lead at once to the abdominal section.

DIAGNOSIS.—The diagnosis of ovarian cysts is often beset with so many difficulties that very humiliating blunders have been made by the best surgeons of the day. Lizars of Edinburgh performed laparotomy on a woman in order to remove a suspected ovarian cyst, and found nothing but fat. Others have done the same thing, and to their dismay have discovered merely an accumulation of wind in the intestines. The great Dieffenbach once opened the belly of a woman for supposed extra-uterine pregnancy, and found neither fat nor wind—not even, indeed, a trace of a tumor. Once an enormously distended bag of waters

[1] *London Obstet. Trans.*, vol. xxii. p. 97.
[2] *American Journal of Obstet.*, Nov., 1883, p. 1211.

broke just as a deservedly eminent British surgeon had rolled up his
sleeves and was about to wheel his patient into an amphitheatre crowded
with spectators to witness an ovariotomy. A surgeon of whom Great
Britain can well be proud once drove his trocar into the shoulder of a
fœtus under the idea that he was tapping one of these cysts. These facts
show the importance of knowing how to make an examination for a suspected ovarian cyst, and how to distinguish such a cyst from other tumors
and other fluid collections in the abdominal cavity.

The usual history of an ovarian cyst is—a tumor first discovered in one
groin, rapidly enlarging, without tenderness or soreness, giving no inconvenience save from its bulk. The general health remains good until the
tumor begins to distend the abdomen; then emaciation takes place, the
strength becomes impaired, and the features begin to assume that pinched
expression described on a preceding page as the facies ovariana. By
inspection and palpation there will be found an elastic but somewhat
irregular tumor, yielding the sense of fluctuation. By percussion a dull
sound will be elicited at every point, except in the flanks, which are more
or less resonant. If the contents of the tumor are colloid or the tumor is
thick-walled or very tense, the sense of fluctuation may be either obscure
or wanting. Sometimes a feeling like that of fluctuation is conveyed by
a fat-laden wall of the abdomen. To muffle this fat-thrill the ulnar edge
of the hand of an assistant is laid along the linea alba while the surgeon
percusses the abdomen. The pressure thus exerted acts precisely like the
damper-wedge of the piano-tuner, which muffles the sound of one string
while its fellow is being tuned. By these means fluctuation can be
detected and the diagnosis of a collection of fluid unhesitatingly made
out.

By the amount of solid and fluid portions of a cyst correct diagnosis
can often be made out, whether it is simple or multiple, compound or
proliferous; but this is a matter of comparatively little practical importance, because when once a growing tumor has been ascertained to be
ovarian, its removal must follow as a matter of course.

There are, however, certain enlargements or tumors of the abdomen
which are very liable to be mistaken for an ovarian cyst, and to these, in
the order of their frequency, we shall call attention.

Ascites.—When the fluid is not encysted, but free, as in ascites, it is at
liberty to go to the most dependent portions of the body. Hence changes
in the posture of the woman will make corresponding changes in the level
of the fluid. These level-changes are made evident by percussion. When
the woman lies on her back the intestines float up to the surface, and the
fluid gravitates to the flanks, making them bulge. In other words, percussion in the dorsal position elicits a clear note in the umbilical region
and a dull note in each flank. In this posture the front surface of the
abdomen is symmetrical and somewhat flattened. But when the woman
sits up the belly becomes convex. Further, ascitic fluid is displaceable
by pressure on the abdomen. But even these signs are not always trustworthy, because the intestines, glued down by adhesions, may not float
up, and there will be dulness over the front of the abdomen, or a distended colon may make each flank resonant. For instance, I have known
a papillary cancer of the omentum attended with dropsy of the abdominal
cavity to give such signs of ovarian cyst as dulness in front and resonance

in the flanks. When the fluid is ascitic the floating or false ribs are not pushed outward. The womb is usually low down and movable; there will also be more or less of bulging in Douglas's pouch.

On the other hand, in an ovarian cyst the womb is usually not very movable, and it is displaced to one side, generally behind the cyst. While the woman lies on her back the front surface of the abdomen is convex and unchanged in form. The floating ribs bulge out, making the chest conical. There will also be dulness in the front wall over the tumor, but usually more or less resonance in the flanks and over the region of the stomach: this clearness on percussion has been aptly termed coronal resonance. These areas of dulness and of resonance remain constant whatever the posture of the woman. Yet in suppurating cysts or after a careless tapping, or in cysts communicating with the intestine, the sac may contain gas, which will give a tympanitic sound over all the elevated portions of the abdominal surface.

It must, however, be borne in mind that ascites may exist concurrently with an ovarian cyst, and especially if the tumor be malignant in character. This can usually be detected by deep palpation, when the cyst will be reached and recognized by the fingers; or by pressing lightly, and then more firmly during percussion, an upper and a lower stratum of fluctuation will be detected.

Pregnancy.—The question of pregnancy is a very serious one, for it is sometimes a most difficult one to decide, especially when dropsy of the amnion (hydramnios) exists. In making a diagnosis nothing must be taken for granted, not even the woman's statement. She may be mistaken, or, indeed, she may be wilfully deceiving in the hope of having a cheap abortion induced by the examination. She may be pregnant and yet menstruate. On the other hand, an ovarian tumor will sometimes arrest menstruation. A healthy, ruddy complexion coexistent with abdominal enlargement should always excite a suspicion of pregnancy. There is sometimes a jaded look in pregnancy—the facies uterina—but never the facies ovariana.

The various signs of pregnancy should be searched for, especially ballottement and the foetal heart-sounds. The cervical region should be most carefully examined per vaginam. A good broad rule to remember is, that when the womb is gravid the cervix is as soft as one's lips; when it is empty the cervix is as hard as the tip of one's nose. In all doubtful cases any operation should be postponed until time has revealed the true condition of things. Of course the introduction of the sound will settle the question of pregnancy, but this procedure is not to be thought of when any doubt exists, and it is therefore useless as a diagnostic agent. An ovarian tumor may coexist with pregnancy, and may have to be tapped or be extirpated before the delivery of the woman. The history of the case, the unusual size of the abdomen, the sulcus between the two tumors, will generally reveal the condition.

Fibroid Tumors of the Womb.—These tumors often reach a very large size, and if of the soft variety give an obscure sense of fluctuation which so closely resembles that of a colloid ovarian cyst or of a tense thick-walled cyst as to make the differential diagnosis very puzzling. The hard myoma gives no sense of fluctuation, but, on the other hand, if pedunculated it can be very readily taken for a solid ovarian tumor. A fibroid tumor of the womb can very generally be told by the history of menorrhagia, by its slow growth, by the uterine souffles and colics, by the effacement of the cervix, and by the tumor being felt to be continuous with the cervix and inseparable from the womb. Then, again, women burdened with a fibroid tumor so far from losing flesh usually become more fat, and their complexion, like that of many pregnant women, is mottled with patches of brown pigment. Further, the uterine cavity is usually much longer than natural, and when the tumor is moved from side to side the motion is communicated to the sound passed within the cavity. But every rule has its exceptions, for when an ovarian cyst has a close attachment to the womb the latter may become elongated and also follow the movements communicated to the tumor.

The positive diagnosis between an ovarian cyst and a fibro-cystic tumor of the womb is impossible, but, fortunately, the latter disease is exceedingly rare. The existence of the latter may be inferred if the woman's face has a jaded appearance and is disfigured by brown patches—the facies uterina—if the growth of the tumor has been very slow, and if the womb is implicated with it. After tapping there will be a partial collapse of the tumor, and the fluid withdrawn is usually bloody and it coagulates on being cooled. After an exploratory incision the tumor presents to the eye a dark-blue and vascular capsule covered with interlacing fibrous bands.

Renal Cysts.—Cysts of the kidney are very commonly mistaken for ovarian cysts. I have made this mistake, and it was not until after breaking up adhesions and emptying the cyst that I discovered the character of the tumor. It was successfully removed. Renal cysts start from below the floating ribs and extend downward and forward, while an ovarian cyst begins from below and grows upward. The former, being generally caused by impaction of a calculus in the ureter, are usually associated with urinary disturbances. They also push the intestines before them, which give a resonant sound on percussion, while the contrary holds good with an ovarian cyst. Since the transverse colon lies between the cyst and the liver, the line of resonance caused by it will show that the cyst is not hepatic. The fluid withdrawn from a renal cyst contains urea and the other constituents of urine, but the urinous odor will be either very faint, or, as in my case, wholly absent. It may as well be stated here that when renal cysts present great difficulties in the way of their removal, they had better be treated by a large drainage-tube.

A floating kidney may be mistaken for a small ovarian tumor. But the latter has a pelvic attachment and can readily be pushed down into the basin, while the former is kept from being pushed very low downward by an upper attachment. Again, the floating kidney usually keeps its peculiar shape, and it is frequently lost by slipping from under the fingers into its natural bed in the flank.

Spina Bifida.—Strange as it may seem, this spinal cyst, when internal on account of a deficiency in the anterior parietes of the lower vertebræ, has been mistaken for an ovarian or a parovarian cyst. I am cognizant of two such errors of diagnosis made by two distinguished gynecologists. In each the sac was emptied by the aspirator, and the patient perished shortly afterward with the same kind of cerebral symptoms which follow the sudden withdrawal of the fluid from the cavity of an external spina bifida.

Phantom Tumors.—In the diagnosis of an ovarian cyst one must be on guard not to mistake for it a phantom tumor. In this imaginary kind of tumor, which hysterical women have the knack of creating, the whole belly will be uniformly distended to the size of the gravid womb at term. This is caused partly by flatus and fat, and partly by the arching forward of the spinal column, with the recti muscles drawn so tense that they cannot be indented. I have frequently had patients with this kind of abdominal enlargement sent to me from a distance, under the impression that it was due to some kind of tumor. But the diagnosis is easily made from the uniform resonance all over the belly; if, moreover, the patient's attention be engaged by conversation, the rigidity of the recti muscles disappears, the abdomen becomes flaccid, and the hand can be made to sink in so as to feel the spine. In very nervous women it may be needful to administer an anæsthetic, when all the tokens of a tumor will promptly disappear.

Obesity.—A large accumulation of fat on the abdominal wall and in the omentum has frequently given rise to the suspicion of the existence of an ovarian cyst. This condition occurs, usually, at the climacteric, and on percussion the vibratile thrill of the fat-laden wall of the abdomen conveys a very misleading impression of fluctuation. Further, to add to the difficulty, if the layer of fat be a very thick one, the abdomen, instead of being resonant on percussion, yields a dull note. But in obesity the fat is not limited to the abdomen, for the breasts, face, and limbs partake of the general enlargement. The abdominal wall hangs in folds when the sitting posture is assumed, and the umbilicus is indented and not protuberant. My own method of making the diagnosis is to grasp the abdominal wall with both hands and ascertain the amount of fat. When this amount is excluded, there will not be found room enough behind it for a tumor of any size, and the enlargement will thus be satisfactorily accounted for.

A dilated stomach, cystic tumors of the omentum, and encysted abscesses of the peritoneal cavity, and, indeed, of the abdominal wall, have been mistaken for ovarian tumors; but these are very exceptional cases. In all doubtful cases an exploratory incision should be resorted to.

SURGICAL TREATMENT OF OVARIAN CYSTS.—In the consideration of this subject it may be divided into the palliative treatment and the radical treatment.

Palliative Treatment.—Tapping either by the trocar or by the aspirator comprises the only palliative treatment of ovarian cysts; yet, as a broad rule with but few exceptions, an ovarian cyst should not be tapped. The objections to this operation are—that, slight as it may seem, it is by no means devoid of danger. Even when the smallest hollow needle of the aspirator has been used inflammation of the cyst may follow, which will compel the immediate resort to ovariotomy and very greatly compromise the success of this radical operation.[1] This has repeatedly happened —once in one of my own cases, in which, however, the removal of the cyst saved my patient's life. Further, the fluid of a polycyst is usually acrid—so much so sometimes as to irritate the hands of the operator— and the escape of a few drops into the cavity of the peritoneum may set

[1] *American Journal of Obstetrics,* Nov., 1883, pp. 1169 and 1189; also *Transactions American Gynæcological Society,* vol. ii., 1877, p. 270.

up a violent and rapidly fatal peritonitis. Then, again, a fatal hemorrhage may take place from some wounded vessel, either in the cyst-wall, or in the adherent omentum, or in the vascular pedicle which may lie spread out in front of the cyst-wall, or, indeed in the abdominal wall itself, for the vessels here are often varicose from impeded circulation. In the fourth place, adhesions are very likely to form after tapping. Fifthly, innumerable child-cysts, which were very small before the tapping, being now relieved from pressure are liable to take on rapid growth and make the tumor more solid; and the more solid the cyst the longer the incision needed for its removal. Sixthly, in polycysts not only are the dangers attending the operation enhanced, but the cyst rapidly refills, and the woman becomes exhausted by the drain on her system. At the very best, 2 per cent. of cases of tapping in polycysts are fatal, even when performed by the most skilled specialists. Seventhly, a cyst once tapped rapidly refills, and soon needs repetitions of the operation. This drain on the system quickly tells upon the woman, and she is sometimes left too weak to have the radical operation performed. The first tapping, indeed, greatly hastens on this crisis, and it should therefore be put off as long as possible. Eighthly, a cyst emptied by tapping tends to rotate on its axis, and torsion of the pedicle may result, ending in gangrene and peritonitis. Ninthly, repeated tappings tend to convert benign papillary growths into malignant. Finally, Lawson Tait[1] draws attention to the fact that "repeated tappings deprive the blood of some element or elements included in the infinite variety of albuminous substances found in ovarian cysts, the deficiency of which predisposes to coagulation of blood." Hence after the removal of the cyst deaths have been "due to the formation of a firm white clot which started from the point of ligature of the pedicle, and slowly traversed the venous system until it reached the heart, death ensuing in from thirty to forty hours after the operation. The symptoms which precede death are swelling of the legs, rapid rise of the pulse, and its disappearance from the extremities some time before death, and breathlessness, ending in suffocation and slight delirium." He has met with several such cases of venous thrombosis starting from the pedicle, and they all occurred in patients who had been previously tapped. There are, however, cases in which tapping cannot be dispensed with; for instance—

1. Many women with ovarian tumors, having heard of cases of abdominal effusion or of cyst in which tapping was followed by a cure, will not submit to the radical operation until repeated tappings have proved to them the futility of the trocar.

2. Cysts of the parovarium and of the broad ligament being often cured by the use of the trocar, it is proper to try the effect of one tapping in slow-growing, unilocular, thinned-walled, and flaccid cysts, which thus exhibit the chief characteristics of these extra-ovarian cysts.

3. When an ovarian cyst develops during the later months of pregnancy, it will often be best to resort to tapping in order to relieve the woman from the pressure of two growing organs and enable her to go to full term. Sometimes labor is made impossible by the presence of a cyst, which will then have to be emptied.

4. In very large tumors which by pressure interfere with the functions of the kidneys, heart, and lungs, thereby causing albuminuria, œdema, or

[1] *Midland Medical Society, Lancet,* Feb. 18, 1882.

dyspnœa, tapping is a useful prelude to ovariotomy. By the relief from pressure afforded to these organs not only will the liability to shock be lessened, but also to hemorrhage, for vessels previously varicose will now contract to their natural calibre.

5. In cases of doubtful diagnosis or in those in which from malignancy, from formidable adhesions, or from other circumstances the radical operation is deemed impracticable, tapping in the first case may clear up the diagnosis, and in the latter ones will prolong the patient's life. But it must always be borne in mind that in a few weeks the fluid will reaccumulate, and the operation will have to be repeated, rapidly exhausting the patient by the drain on her system. It is well, therefore, to put off the first tapping as long as possible.

Tapping may be performed through the abdominal wall, through the vagina, or through the rectum, but, for reasons which will presently be given, the first mode is decidedly the best.

Tapping through the Abdominal Wall.—For this operation either the aspirator may be used or else Wells's trocar with a long rubber tube attachment. Of the two, I much prefer the former. In aspiration, after the bladder has been emptied, the woman lies on her back close to the side of the bedstead with her abdomen exposed. The preferable site of puncture is in the linea alba midway between the navel and the symphysis pubis; that is to say, at a point where the tissues, being tendinous, are most free from blood-vessels, and where the omentum is most out of the way. But if at this point the tumor feels solid, or an underlying knuckle of intestine is discovered by percussion, or the vessels look varicose, any other place in the abdominal wall may be selected where fluctuation is most manifest, provided it lies below the level of the navel. The reason for choosing a low site for the puncture is, that if the hollow needle be plunged in at any point above the navel it will slip out of the cyst as the latter collapses and before it is wholly emptied. The skin is now thoroughly cleansed with soap and water and washed with a 5 per cent. solution of carbolic acid. The painful part of the operation being the penetration of the skin, the selected place for puncture should either be frozen with the ether spray or be benumbed by a lump of ice dipped into some table-salt. After the aspirator-jar has been exhausted of air the hollow needle or canula, armed with its stilette, is lubricated with carbolated oil or vaseline, and rapidly plunged deeply into the cyst. Should the cyst not wholly collapse, the canula has probably become obstructed, and it should be cleared out by one of the blunt stilettes which are made of different sizes to fit the different canulas. Sometimes the flaccid walls of the sac as it becomes empty are sucked up into the end of the canula, and the flow of fluid is suddenly arrested. This accident is recognized by a peculiar valve-like vibration communicated to the instrument, and is overcome by raising up the end of the canula or by directing it to another part of the cyst. Should, on the other hand, other cysts present themselves, they can be emptied without withdrawing the canula by reintroducing the stilette, and by directing its point to each cyst in succession. When the fluid ceases to flow the fore finger and thumb firmly compress the fold of the abdominal wall behind the canula as it is withdrawn, so as to avoid the entrance of air, and the small puncture is covered by a piece of adhesive plaster. A pad of cotton wool is now laid over the scaphoid abdomen and a flannel binder applied. These afford a grateful feeling of support and take away that sense of goneness which is likely to occur. To avoid all risks of inflammation the patient must keep her bed for three or four days and eat sparingly.

When Wells's or any other large trocar is used, the operation should be performed under the spray and with every antiseptic precaution. The skin should be previously incised with a lancet, and, lest air should be sucked up into the sac, the free end of the rubber tubing should touch the bottom of the bucket, so as to be always immersed in the escaping fluid. This rubber tubing acts as a syphon with great suction power, and the cyst is more rapidly emptied by Wells's trocar than by the aspirator. Yet I cannot help believing that the latter by its small size is by far the safer instrument, and I always use it when a simple tapping is aimed at. Should any stubborn bleeding follow the removal of the canula, a hare-lip pin may be passed across the wound deeply enough to get below the wounded vessel, and compression made by a turn or two of silk ligature around the pin. The same means are to be adopted to stop the oozing of fluid which sometimes takes place when a cyst with colloid contents cannot be wholly emptied by the trocar. For it is highly prudent under such circumstances to stop the oozing, as some of the fluid is sure to get into the cavity of the peritoneum, with very generally fatal effects. In such a case the pin ought to include the lips of the wound in the cyst. To avoid as much as possible the escape of irritating ovarian fluid into the cavity of the abdomen, the cyst when tapped should always, if possible, be wholly emptied. This is a rule without an exception. It is therefore very bad practice to remove even with the hypodermic syringe a few drops of the fluid for microscopic examination. Several cases of death from this cause have been reported.[1] I lay stress on this point because in my *Lessons in Gynæcology* I advocate the practice.

Tapping through the Vagina.—This operation is sometimes a very tempting one to perform when one of the cysts of a polycyst is pressing downward behind the bladder and causing dysuria. But it is by no means so safe as the supra-pubic mode of tapping. The reasons for this are—(a) The vessels are larger and lie closer together in the lower wall of the cyst near the stalk; (b) in a polycyst the larger cysts, growing where they have most room, usually develop in the abdominal cavity, while the more solid portion remains below in the pelvic region; (c) other organs, such as the bladder, womb, and rectum, are liable to become dislocated and lie in the track of the trocar; (d) the roof of the vagina responds to every respiratory movement of the diaphragm, and a cyst low down is not, from pelvic adhesions, so likely to collapse when tapped as one higher up: hence the cyst is liable to act as a pair of bellows, sucking in air and forcing it out. This inevitably causes suppurative inflammation with all its attendant evils. For these reasons this mode of tapping is never resorted to, except in cases of pelvic adhesion or in those in which the cyst starts from the lower side of the broad ligament and grows downward. Even then it is done only to relieve the distress caused by the double pressure upon bladder and rectum. In such cases the aspirator should be used, as it lessens all the risks. Should suppurative inflammation set in, the sac must be again emptied, the wound kept open by a

[1] *American Journal of Obstetrics*, April, 1876, p. 146

drainage-tube, and the cavity thoroughly cleansed by daily injections of antiseptic fluids.

Tapping through the rectum has long ago been abandoned by the profession, as it ought to be, except in some very rare cases of atresia vaginæ. It was at one time supposed to possess advantages over the vaginal method, because the subsequent offensive discharges could be retained at will like the other contents of the bowel. But the cavity of the sac always became distended with fecal gas, and fatal septicæmia was pretty sure to set in.

Radical Treatment.—Tapping, followed by the injection of iodine into these cysts, has sometimes been rewarded with a cure, and at one time this mode of treatment had very warm advocates. After the cyst is wholly emptied by aspiration the action of the instrument is reversed, and from two to ten ounces of the officinal tincture of iodine are thrown in. The tincture is used of full strength, because the residual fluid in the cyst will be enough to dilute it. The cyst-wall is next kneaded, and the patient made to turn from side to side and from back to chest, so that the tincture may come in contact with every portion of the secreting surface of the cyst. The fluid is then pumped out, but all cannot be brought away; enough usually remains behind to produce some slight constitutional disturbance. While the canula is being withdrawn, in order to prevent the escape of any of the irritating injection into the abdominal cavity the thumb and fore finger are made to grasp the fold of abdominal wall at the puncture-site and to press it firmly down on to the collapsed cyst-wall. Good and lasting cures have followed such a treatment; but since they can happen only in monocysts, which are almost always parovarian, and not ovarian, it is probable that the mere emptying of the cyst would have done as much. In polycysts such a treatment is not to be thought of, for it would be attended with far more hazard than even the operation of ovariotomy. At the present day injections of iodine are practised only by physicians who do not operate; ovariotomists never resort to them.

Tapping, followed by enlarging the wound in the cyst, stitching its edges to those of the abdominal wound, and permanently keeping it open by tents or by a large drainage-tube, has frequently been attended with success. But since extensive and prolonged suppuration must inevitably ensue, this operation has proved to be a far more dangerous one than that of ovariotomy. It should, therefore, not be resorted to excepting in cases of cysts which are too adherent to be removed. The after-treatment consists in treating the case precisely as if it were an abscess. The cyst is kept empty by draining, and sweet by such deodorizing agents as solutions of iodine, carbolic acid, potassium permanganate, and the liquor sodæ chloratæ. Early this year I had one such case, a patient of C. A. Currie, in which the cyst was wholly adherent to all the pelvic organs and structures, and had besides a communication with the bladder. Not daring, under such circumstances, to remove it, I treated it successfully by incision, drainage, and disinfecting injections; but it was a long time before the drainage-tube could be removed and the woman be released from her bed. Cases, indeed, have occurred in which six months elapsed before the drainage-tube could be taken out and the woman pronounced well.

Another exception in favor of this operation may be made in the case of small cysts growing downward and bulging out the hind wall of the vagina. It may then be advisable to follow Noeggerath's plan. He snips open the vagina transversely behind the cervix to the length of one inch, and makes a corresponding incision in the cyst-wall. The edges of the two incisions are then stitched together and a drainage-tube put in. Thus, the cyst is left with a free and permanent opening into the vagina, through which such antiseptic solutions as have been noted above are thrown up. In time the collapsed cyst-walls adhere to one another and cease to secrete.

Electrolysis has of late also been lauded as a sure and harmless remedy for these cysts. But a careful examination of the subject made by Munde shows that this agent has been greatly overrated as a specific, and that it "can in no wise supplant ovariotomy."[1]

Rupture of ovarian cysts has occasionally taken place, either through over-distension or through such violence as a rude fall or an upset from a carriage. This accident, if the tumor were a monocyst or if the fluid happened to be bland, sometimes ended in a lasting cure. The hint was not thrown away, and several surgeons cut circular openings into the cyst to establish a permanent communication with it and the abdominal cavity. But this practice was soon given up, because it was found that the intrusion of ovarian fluid into the serous cavity usually set up a violent and rapidly fatal peritonitis. For such an accident, when followed by inflammation, there is but one remedy—the immediate removal of the cyst by ovariotomy. Desperate as this remedy seems, it has repeatedly been followed by success. The only cyst in which it might be held warrantable to establish a communication with the abdominal cavity is that of a cyst of the parovarium recurring after repeated tappings, and so bound down by adhesions or so covered by the broad ligament as to be irremovable. The fluid it contains is so limpid and bland as not ordinarily to inflame the peritoneum.

OVARIOTOMY.—The term ovariotomy comes from ὡάριον, ovary, and τομή, an incision. It is a barbarous compound of Latin and Greek, which is forced into meaning the operation for the extirpation of an ovary on account of some disease of its own structures which causes it to increase in bulk. A fibroid or a sarcomatous degeneration of this organ, as has been shown, will sometimes happen, but cystic degeneration is by far the most common form of disease to which the ovary is liable. When both ovaries are enlarged and removed the operation is called double ovariotomy. The terms ovariotomy and öophorectomy (ὡόφορον and ἐκτέμνω, to cut out the ovary) really mean the same thing, the latter word, indeed, being the more appropriate. But by modern usage the former is limited to the operation for the removal of an ovary greatly enlarged by some intrinsic disorder. By öophorectomy is now meant the operation for the removal of both ovaries for the purpose of bringing on the menopause, and thus curing diseases kept up or caused by the functional-existence of those organs, while they themselves may or may not be diseased.

Before the eighteenth century the operation of ovariotomy as a radical cure had been suggested by a number of physicians, but had never been put into practice. Later, John Hunter and John Bell both advocated the operation, but neither ventured to perform it. This honor was

---

[1] *Transactions American Gynæcological Society*, vol. ii. p. 435.

reserved for Ephraim McDowell, a Virginian practising in Kentucky, who had attended Bell's course of lectures delivered in Edinburgh in 1794, and had imbibed the opinions of his teacher. He returned to Kentucky in 1795, and began at once to practise his profession, but it was not until 1809 that he first met with the opportunity for performing ovariotomy. The operation was successful, his patient having lived thirty-two years longer and having died at the end of her seventy-eighth year. Before his own death, which occurred June 25, 1830, in the fifty-ninth year of his age, McDowell had performed 13 ovariotomies, with 8 recoveries.

In spite of McDowell's success, and in spite of a large and growing percentage of recoveries reported by Atlee, Clay, and Spencer Wells, this operation was condemned so violently by the profession that its advocates were fairly ostracised, and fifteen years have hardly elapsed since it has been put upon as firm a basis as any other capital operation in surgery. "In 1843, Dieffenbach, the boldest of all surgeons then living, wrote that ovariotomy was murder, and that every one who performed it should be put into the dock. Now," writes Nussbaum, "we save lives with it by the hundred, and the omission of its performance in a proper case would in these days be looked upon as culpable negligence."[1]

The most common causes of death after ovariotomy are septicæmia or septic peritonitis, traumatic or frank peritonitis, shock, exhaustion, and hemorrhage; and it is against these foes that the operator must from the first aim all his efforts. In no other operation does the issue depend so largely on the experience of the surgeon. Every ovariotomist finds that his success grows with the number of his cases. Of 1000 successive ovariotomies, Wells lost 34 out of the first group of 100 cases, and but 11 out of the last group of 100. Out of his first 50 ovariotomies, Lawson Tait had 19 deaths.[2] The mortality of his last 313 cases was as low as 4.76 per cent.[3] Keith, who began with a mortality of about 20 per cent., lately had a series of 100 cases with 97 recoveries; 70 of these were successive. Schroeder had in the first 100 of his Berlin cases 17 deaths; in the second 100, 18; and in his third 100, 8 deaths.[4] Of my own first cases, I lost about 1 in every 3. Out of my last 22 cases there was but 1 death, and that occurred in a lady operated on at her home, too distant for me to see her again. In July, 1884, Peruzzi collected statistics up to date of Italian ovariotomists. Out of the first series of 100 cases, they lost 61. In the second 100 there were 36 deaths, but in the third series only 26 died.[5]

The statistics of the leading ovariotomists up to January, 1883, are as follows:[6]

	Cases.	Recovered.	Died.	Mortality, per cent.
Clay	93	64	29	31.11
Sir Spencer Wells	1088	847	241	22.15
Keith	381	340	41	10.76
Knowsley Thornton	328	293	35	10.67
Lawson Tait	226	199	27	11.94

[1] *British Medical Journal*, Oct. 26, 1878, p. 617.
[2] *Medical Record*, Jan. 3, 1885, No. 2, and *British Medical Journal*, April 15, 1882, p. 544.
[3] *Medical Record*, Jan. 3, 1885, p 2, and *American Journal of Obstetrics*, July, 1882, p. 547.
[4] *Maryland Medical Journal*, July 1, 1882, p. 110.
[5] *British Medical Journal*, Sept. 16, 1882, p. 528.
[6] *Medical News*, Jan. 27, 1883, p. 117.

The statistics of general hospitals are by no means so good. In the Vienna General Hospital during the year 1881 "ovariotomy was performed 64 times, with 38 complete recoveries, 25 deaths, and 1 woman was discharged with marasmus."[1] Taking the profession at large, out of 5153 cases of ovariotomy collected by Baum, there was a mortality of 29.13 per cent.[2] Out of 2023 cases collected by Younkin, the mortality was 27 per cent.[3] By operative skill, by cleanliness, by wise hygienic measures, and probably by the use of antiseptic precautions, the fatality may be said to have been reduced by skilled specialists to about 10 per cent.; which, considering the size of the wound, the importance of the parts involved, and the delicacy of the exposed structures, is a remarkably low average. The average is indeed ·better than that of amputations. Before 1869, Sir James Y. Simpson stated that the average mortality of amputations of the extremities was 39.1 per cent. In the Glasgow Royal Infirmary the average mortality has been 25.5 per cent.—viz. of thigh cases there were 380 cases, with 113 deaths = 29.7 per cent.; of the leg, 182 cases, with 54 deaths = 29.6 per cent.; of arm cases, 167, with 33 deaths = 19.7 per cent.; of forearm cases, 93, with 12 deaths: mortality = 12.9 per cent.[4]

This brings up the question of simple or of aseptic ovariotomy—a very important question and one not yet fully settled. The objections to Listerism are—that it is very troublesome; that it is liable to poison the patient fatally, as well as to injure the health of the operator; that it is useless, indeed merely a surgical craze; and that it is not the carbolic acid which does good, but the cleanliness enforced by this system. But there is no doubt that since the introduction of antiseptic surgery the mortality has been much lessened in every land. For instance, "in Germany, where the success of ovariotomy has not been so good as in other countries, the mortality by means of the antiseptic treatment has been reduced from 90 to 20 per cent."[5] From an analysis of all the cases of ovariotomies performed by American surgeons, "the percentage of recoveries is overwhelmingly in favor of Listerism."[6] During the year 1881 in the Samaritan Hospital two of the surgeons used the carbolated spray of a strength of 1 in 40, and followed out every detail of antiseptic surgery. They had a mortality of 7 per cent. A third surgeon of that institution, after gradually lessening the strength of the spray until water was alone used, finally gave even it up altogether. He, however, for purposes of cleanliness always covered the instruments in the tray with water. The mortality of his operations showed the high rate of 30 per cent. The house committee, a body of laymen, thereupon "expressed a strong opinion against the performance of ovariotomy for the future without full antiseptic precautions."[7]

On the other hand, Tait of Birmingham and Keith of Edinburgh, with a recent mortality each of only 3 per cent., have abandoned the spray. The latter claims now "to get as good results without it, and better results than any one has yet got with it."[8] My own practice is to adhere

[1] *Medical News*, Dec. 30, 1882, p. 745.   [2] *Agnew's Surgery*, vol. ii. p. 811.
[3] *The New York Medical Record*, Nov. 11, 1882, p. 560.   [4] *Lancet*, Sept., 1882.
[5] *Agnew's Surgery*, vol. ii. p. 800.
[6] H. C. Bigelow *American Journal of Obstetrics*, July, 1882. p. 651.
[7] *British Medical Journal*, May 20, 1882, p. 747.   [8] *Brit. Med. Journ.*, May 27, p. 796.

to the spray and to every detail of antiseptic surgery; and I fully agree with Bigelow that "it would be a grave error to abandon a practice which has achieved brilliant results until something shall be brought forth which shall be as thoroughly protective, and in the use of which there may be no possible dangers. Time alone can demonstrate satisfactorily the relative values of Listerism and of perfect cleanliness without Listerism. The results of a large number of cases in which cleanliness and attention to detail have alone been used are the only criteria upon which we can strike a judicial balance."[1]

Contraindications for Ovariotomy.—An operation should be declined in far-advanced tuberculosis, in cancer of the ovary or of any other part of the body, in grave structural lesions of any of the vital organs, in ascites if caused by disease of the heart, the liver, or the kidney, in gastric ulcer, or in any serious disease of the alimentary canal. Extensive adhesions should not count as a contraindication, nor should age, since young girls and very old women have been successfully operated on. Albuminuria is often due to the pressure of the tumor on the kidneys, and, unless it existed before the appearance of the tumor or is positively known to be caused by Bright's disease, should not preclude the operation. Extreme debility dependent upon the ovarian disease makes the prognosis grave, but it should not prevent a resort to ovariotomy. I have indeed had several recoveries when the patient was so reduced in strength as to make it a very anxious and difficult task to keep her from dying on the table.

Indications for Ovariotomy.—This operation should not, as a rule, be performed when the cyst has first been discovered, but when it has grown so large as to distend the belly, and when the woman has become thin and her health has begun to fail. The reasons for waiting are—that the woman will have lived longer should the operation turn out to be a fatal one; that, the abdominal wall having become thinner both by being overstretched and by the absorption of fat, the incision will be proportionately shorter and shallower; that, the patient being now less full-blooded, both hemorrhage and inflammation will not be so likely to occur; that the bowels are crowded away from the line of incision; and that the pressure and rubbing to which the peritoneum has been for some time subjected will make it less vulnerable, and therefore less likely to take on inflammatory action. When, however, a woman broods over her condition and is anxious to have the tumor removed, the operation should be performed much earlier, especially if the surgeon be experienced.

Again, when an ovarian cyst is complicated with pregnancy it is best to perform the operation in the first half of the period of gestation; for in the last half the broad ligaments receive a large supply of blood, and all the pelvic vessels become varicose. Pregnancy is indeed no bar to the operation, the prognosis being favorable both to the mother and to the child. Schroeder and Olshausen performed 21 ovariotomies in pregnant women, with only 2 deaths.[2]

When septic peritonitis sets in; when the contents of the sac become purulent, as they sometimes do either spontaneously or after an unprotected tapping; when the cyst bursts and serious symptoms arise; when torsion of the pedicle occurs or when a free hemorrhage into the sac takes

---

[1] Am. Journ. of Obstetrics, July, 1882, p. 651.   [2] Brit. Med. Journ., Dec., 1880, p. 1027.

place,—the radical operation should unhesitatingly be performed, and that without any delay.

Preparation of the Patient for the Operation.—The operation having been decided upon, every precaution must be taken to ensure a favorable result. The patient should avoid all exposure to contagious or to zymotic diseases, and she should be put in the very best condition of health possible under the circumstances. If the kidneys be inactive and the urine highly concentrated, depositing mixed urates in abundance, it will be well for the patient to make use of warm baths and to take saline cathartics in quantities sufficient to secure a daily action of the bowels. The alkaline carbonates, largely diluted, will also prove beneficial, and so will also the effervescent citrate of lithia. Sometimes, and especially when anasarca and œdema of the legs occur, it will be advisable to relieve the pressure-congestion of the kidneys by a preliminary tapping. Other organs will also be relieved, and valuable time for the action of medicines is often gained by emptying the cyst. Tonics, iron in the form of Basham's mixture, a generous diet, and fresh air may be needed. A trip to the seashore or to the country will often do much good in preparing a broken-down patient for the operation. If the patient comes from a malarial district, from twenty to thirty grains of quinia should be given during the twenty-four hours for two or three days before the operation, and ten grains a few hours before the time of the operation. If this be not done, a severe explosion of malarial fever after the operation may put the patient's life in jeopardy.

An operation of election should not be undertaken during a monthly period. It should be performed either about ten days before one or about a week after one. The very best time is midway between two fluxes. When, however, through some lesion or some accident, immediate relief is demanded, no regard whatever should be paid to the factor of menstruation. Some surgeons operate, indeed, in any case whether the woman is menstruating or not, and profess to find no difference in the result.[1]

For several days before the operation the bowels should be kept open, and the diet should consist largely of milk, eggs, rice, and of wholesome and easily-digested food. On the day preceding that of the operation the upper portion of the pubic hair should be cut off and the abdomen, if hairy, shaved. In the evening the patient takes a warm soap-bath, and is washed perfectly clean by her nurse, who must be an experienced woman, able to pass the catheter and take the temperature. She then puts on clean clothing and goes to bed, where she stays until the hour fixed upon for the operation. To ensure sleep, I am in the habit of giving at bedtime thirty grains of potassium bromide, combined sometimes with opium. Early next morning a dose of castor oil is administered, and it is much more easily swallowed if disguised in some vehicle and brought to the patient without any previous warning. When oil cannot be taken, I give, at bedtime of the previous evening and in one dose, two compound cathartic and two Lady Webster pills. To avoid ether-vomiting, breakfast should consist merely of one piece of dry toast and a cup of tea, or of a cup of beef-tea or of a goblet of milk, and afterward she must eat nothing more. To calm the nerves another thirty-grain dose of

[1] T. Savage, *Brit. Med. Journ.*, April 14, 1883, p. 712.

potassium bromide may be given, with or without opium as the case may be, and especially if the woman be at all agitated.

A very good time for operating is from noon to two o'clock in the afternoon, for by that time the oil will have acted and the light breakfast will have been digested. Some surgeons operate as early as nine and ten o'clock in the morning, in which case the cathartic will have to be administered in the afternoon of the previous day. At the hour fixed upon for the operation the woman puts on a flannel sacque, warm stockings, and drawers, and her nurse then passes the catheter.

The bedstead on which the woman is to lie after the operation should have a horse-hair mattress, and should be wide enough to permit her attendants to move her on a draw-sheet from one side of it to the other. I formerly placed my patients on narrow single bedsteads, so that they could be reached and be waited upon equally well from either side; but I found that an unchangeable position on the back soon became intolerably irksome. Next, indeed, to the thirst following the operation, my patients complain mostly of the supine posture which they are compelled to assume.

The room in which the operation is to take place ought to be a separate one, so that the lady can be etherized in her sleeping-room, and may not be unnerved by witnessing the needful preparations. Several days beforehand the carpet of the operating-room should be taken up and the curtains taken down. Every useless piece of furniture should be removed, the closets and bureau-drawers emptied, and the whole room thoroughly cleansed and ventilated. Several hours before the time of the operation this room ought to be heated to a temperature of 75°, and the air disinfected and made moist by a solution of carbolic acid kept boiling in a dish on the stove or over an alcohol lamp. Let me here say that, if possible, this operation should not be performed within the walls of a crowded general hospital nor in unhealthy localities, but, as statistics well show, in private houses or, far preferably, in small special hospitals.

Articles Needed for the Operation.—The following articles should be provided by some member of the patient's family. Following the example of the late Washington L. Atlee, I have a printed list of them, which is sent to the family physician some days before the operation:

One yard of rubber plaster; two rolls of raw cotton, made aseptic by being baked in the range-oven just before the operation; two yards and a half of fine white flannel, for two binders; six one-grain rectal suppositories of the watery extract of opium; two pounds of the best ether; two gallons of a 5 per cent. solution of the best carbolic acid, made at least two days beforehand; four ounces of Monsel's solution of iron; twelve ounces of undiluted alcohol for the spray-producer; some old whiskey, with cup, spoon, and sugar; a nail-brush, basin, and soap; a pin-cushion, with large pins; two kitchen tables, or two dressing-tables; one small stand for the spray-producer; one small table for the basins and sponges; one chair without a back for a bucket of hot water; two new tin basins and one tin cup; a new bucket and a jug of hot water; a kettle of boiling water, ready on the range; a small tub and an empty bucket; six bottles filled with hot water and tightly corked; an empty wine-bottle for the aspirator; a rubber ice-cap or two pig's bladders for holding ice; a rubber-cloth one yard and a quarter square, with an oval hole in the centre six inches wide and eight long; one kitchen apron for the operator; one clean blanket for the patient's lower extremities; two large platters or two meat-dishes, to be used as trays for the instruments;[1] clean towels, clean sheets, clean blankets, clean comfortables, and clean pillows.

Instruments.—In simple cases very few instruments are needed; but as one never knows beforehand what complications may be met with, it is best to be always prepared for every emergency. One must therefore have on hand every instrument likely to be wanted in the most formidable operation. The following list comprises all the instruments and other articles that I carry with me in my operating-bag, but it will not suit every surgeon, who will after a few operations choose his own favorite instruments:

One steam spray-producer, which will work two hours; assorted silk ligatures on spools; Lister's antiseptic gauze or salicylated cotton; two dozen straight surgeon's needles; assorted needles with varying curves; two large needles for transfixing pedicles; an aneurismal needle; one needle-holder; one hypodermic syringe; two dozen assorted pressure-forceps; one uterine tenaculum; assorted hair-lip pins and acupressure needles; one grooved director; two scalpels; Baker-Brown's cautery clamp; ten fine surgeon's sponges of different sizes; two long and flat sponges; one wire écraseur; one wire clamp or Koeberle's serre-nœud; Paquelin's cautery or three cautery-irons; one Wells's trocar with rubber tubing; one aspirator; two Nélaton's cyst-forceps; one straight pair of scissors; one pair of scissors curved on the flat; one right-angled pair of scissors; Allis's improved ether-inhaler; one flexible male catheter; three glass drainage-tubes of different sizes and lengths, together with the rubber sheeting and the sponge used with them.

The twenty-four needles should be threaded, two on one thread of fine silk eighteen inches long—viz. No. 1 or 2, of an excellent quality furnished by Messrs. J. H. Gemrig & Son of Philadelphia. To keep these threads from becoming snarled they are rolled up in a strip of muslin gauze, each pair of two needles with their thread being covered up by one fold of the gauze. The two pedicle-needles should also be threaded, but with stouter thread (No. 4), fully two feet long. All these armed needles should be put into a 5 per cent. solution of carbolic acid for several hours before the operation. Assorted needles of varying curves come occasionally into use, and it is always well to have several very fine needles on hand, together with the finest Chinese silk, in order to close a wounded viscus, such as the bladder or the bowels.

As an aid to the memory it is well to have invariably at every operation the same number of sponges and the same number of pressure-forceps, for these are the only articles likely to be left behind and closed up in the abdominal cavity. The cautery-irons should be wedge-shaped; the iron spreader used by apothecaries in making plasters forms an excellent substitute. In my hands the best pressure-forceps is Koeberle's. Its pointed beak catches the tissues far better than that of Wells's forceps, which looks like a crocodile's muzzle. The ordinary hæmostatic bulldog clips, or the serres-fines, must on no account be used, because if

---

[1] These platters are usually too shallow to hold a solution of carbolic acid deep enough to cover the bulkier instruments. It would therefore be well to have a tin tray made especially for the purpose, measuring nineteen inches long, twelve wide, and three deep; or a nest of smaller trays can be carried in the operator's bag.

they should lose their hold and drop into the abdominal cavity they would be too small to be readily discovered, and might indeed be hopelessly lost in the coils of the bowels. Long strings attached to each one would, however, overcome this objection.

The ten sponges must be of the best quality and about the size of one's fist. Two of them should be flat, long, and thin, such as are called by the trade potter's sponges. When first bought, sponges almost always contain sand. To rid them of this they are beaten, then soaked for twenty-four hours in a 3 per cent. solution of muriatic acid, and afterward washed out in clear running water. Sponges should never be put into boiling water, which destroys their elasticity, shrivels them up, and spoils them. After every operation the sponges should be thoroughly cleansed in cold water and immersed for forty-eight hours in a solution of washing soda (sodii carbonas) containing four ounces to the gallon of water. They are then rinsed out in running water, and placed in a 5 per cent. solution of carbolic acid. At the end of a week they are to be taken out and hung up in a bag. Instead of a solution of soda, some prefer an 8-per cent. solution of sulphurous acid, in which the sponges are soaked for from two to four hours. This bleaches the sponges, but does not cleanse them so well as the alkaline solution.

Only three assistants are needed—two are enough if they are experienced—and they and the surgeon should take a soap-bath, and not see on that morning any patient ill from a zymotic or a contagious disease. Their clothes should also be scrupulously clean. To ensure still further protection, each one takes off his coat, waistcoat, and neck-tie if they are of a material which cannot be washed. The nurse must also wear clean clothing which can be washed. A few bystanders may be permitted, but they should wear clean clothing and take off their overcoats. They should also be cautioned not to visit before the operation any case of contagious disease.

Upon arriving at the patient's house the surgeon, together with his assistants and the nurse, proceeds at once to get everything in readiness. The two tables may be arranged in the form of a T, covered with several thicknesses of quilts, and with a pillow on the cross-table. When the tables are thus arranged a third one will be needed for the instruments and the spray-producer. In order to economize room and furniture, I am in the habit of putting one table at right angles to the other—viz. with its short arm to the left instead of to the right, thus: ⌐. The woman lies on the long arm of the ⌐, with her feet directed to the short arm, and on the projecting and free portion of the table forming the short arm are placed the tray of instruments and the spray-producer. As it takes time to get up steam in the necessarily large spray-producer, hot water should be poured into the boiler, and it should be one of the first things attended to. In order not to chill the patient, the spray solution of carbolic acid should also be heated before it is used. The edges of the oval hole in the rubber cloth are next smeared with some adhesive preparation, but a plaster suitable for all seasons of the year is not easy to devise. Keith's formula is the following, but it will not always stick:

℞. Emplastri saponis, ʒiv;
Emplastri resinæ, ʒiij;
Olei olivæ opt., ʒi. M.

After many trials, W. D. Robinson of Philadelphia has succeeded in making for me a very good plaster according to the following formula:

$\mathbb{R}$. Emplastri saponis, 3ij;
Resinæ, 3vi;
Terebinthinæ albæ, 3ij. M.

I must, however, add that I now very rarely use this rubber cloth.

Not all the instruments in one's bag, but only those likely to be needed, are now placed in the tray or in the platters, and covered over with boiling water, to which in a few minutes is added the same quantity of a 5 per cent. solution of carbolic acid. The best plan would perhaps be to pour into the tray a boiling 2.5 per cent. solution of carbolic acid. Into the same tray is also laid the roll of gauze containing the threaded needles. By its side on the table, and within easy reach, is placed a small bottle filled with a 5 per cent. carbolated solution in which are kept two small spools of Nos. 1 and 2 silk. The adhesive or rubber plaster is cut into strips of appropriate length, and the antiseptic dressing put in readiness. The trocar with tubing attached is hung on a nail near by. The sponges are carefully counted and placed in one of two basins arranged side by side on a table to the left of the patient. The other basin is one-third filled with a 5 per cent. solution of carbolic acid, which later on is reduced by the addition of pure hot water to a strength of 2.5 per cent. On a chair is placed a bucket of clean warm water.

Let me here say, once for all, that throughout the operation the assistant who looks after the sponges attends to them in the following way: Every soiled sponge returned to him is first cleaned in the bucket of warm water, next rinsed in the carbolated solution, then squeezed out and placed in the empty basin. This sequence must be rigidly observed, because, if the soiled sponge be plunged first in the carbolated water, the blood and serum which it contains will at once coagulate in its meshes, and become liable to be dislodged in the abdominal cavity as foreign bodies.

Meantime, the woman, in another room, has been inhaling the anæsthetic—the best being, in my opinion, the ether fortior of our leading manufacturing druggists. It should be administered by Allis's inhaler, which largely dilutes it with air. Wells and Thornton employ the bichloride of methylene; Keith uses pure ether; Bantock resorts to chloroform, and Tait to a mixture of two parts of ether and one of chloroform, given by means of Clover's apparatus.[1] When the patient is wholly unconscious her water is drawn off, and she is carried into the operating-room and laid on the table. To this table she is strapped down by a belt over her thighs, and her hands are also secured to the same belt. Her legs are wrapped in warm blankets, and her clothes are drawn up out of the way. Her chest and body are then covered by the rubber sheet, but the edges of its oval opening are made to adhere to the skin from just above the navel to the pubic hair, thus exposing only a limited portion of the abdomen. After this the spray is turned on, and the 5 per cent. solution of carbolic acid in the tray and in the basins is diluted with hot water down to 2.5 per cent. The operator and his assistants now take off their rings and cleanse their hands very carefully with carbolated soap and a nail-brush. They may clean and pare their nails with a penknife

[1] *The Medical Record*, Jan. 3, 1885, p. 2.

before the use of the nail-brush, but not after, because the knife not only does not remove all dirt, but it loosens up that which remains. Arranging themselves in their places, the operator stands to the right of the woman, his chief assistant to her left, the one who gives the ether at her head, while the other, who attends to the sponges, takes his place near the basins at the side of the chief assistant. The nurse holds herself in readiness to hand towels when called for, and especially to see that a third basin always contains warm water, so that at any stage of the operation the surgeon can wash his hands without delay.

When everything is ready the door is locked, and the exposed portion of the abdomen washed with the solution of carbolic acid. An incision about three inches in length is made with a free hand, and not by nicks, in the median line below the navel, where the blood-vessels are few in number. It should end about one inch and a half above the pubes; that is to say, low enough for the pedicle to be easily reached, but high enough to avoid cutting the fold of peritoneum reflected from the bladder to the abdominal wall. The brown line running below the navel is the surface guide, but after cutting through the skin and fat one cannot always hit the linea alba beneath. When the cyst is large the recti muscles have become separated from one another, and there is no difficulty in keeping within the wide tendinous interspace. But when the cyst is small the linea alba is, as its name indicates, a mere line, and the knife will often go astray into the anterior sheath of one of the recti muscles. The red muscular fibres pouting out of the opening will be the danger-signal of one's having got off the track into more vascular regions. To recover it a probe is passed in across the muscle to the right and to the left, and the nearest point of arrest will note the linea alba. The disadvantages arising from the wandering from the linea alba are—that the sheath of the rectus muscle being cut open, or the muscle itself being wounded, there results hemorrhage; that the wound is more jagged, and therefore less easily coaptated; that suppuration in the suture-tracts is more liable to take place; and, finally, that in cases of small cysts with but little abdominal enlargement a spasmodic contraction of the wounded muscle is very likely to embarrass the operator both in removing the cyst and in introducing the sutures.

Again, one cannot on a grooved director cut canonically through the different layers of tissue described with so much precision in the textbooks. On the contrary, all that one needs is to know when the knife is approaching the peritoneum. An excellent landmark is the thin layer of fat overlying the peritoneum. So, after pinching up the abdominal wall to estimate its thickness, the surgeon can boldly cut down through the skin and its underlying fat, but somewhat cautiously through the aponeurotic structures until the second layer of fat is reached. Practically, therefore, he need regard but the following layers: skin with its underlying fat, the intermediate tendinous or muscular structures, the supra-peritoneal fat, and the peritoneum.

Before the abdominal cavity is opened all bleeding is stopped by the use of pressure-forceps, of which one dozen will sometimes dangle from the wound. When the hemorrhage has been wholly stayed, and not until then, the peritoneum is hooked up by a delicate uterine tenaculum and nicked open. On a broad grooved director or on the finger this opening is slit up for a distance of about two inches, either by a right-angled pair of scissors or by a probe-pointed bistoury. A little serum usually escapes and the nacreous wall of the cyst comes into view. This is called an exploratory incision, for by it the diagnosis is confirmed, the presence of adhesions ascertained, and the possibility of completing the operation determined. When it has been decided to go on with the operation, more working room will be needed, and the wound is therefore enlarged by the scissors, the finger being used as a guide to prevent injury to the omentum or to any chance knuckle of bowel that may lie in the way. The size of the incision will depend upon the character of the cyst and on the number of its adhesions. Hence it may range from a length of three inches to the distance from ensiform cartilage to symphysis pubis. An incision contained between the umbilicus and symphysis pubis is technically called a short incision, and one extended above the umbilicus a long incision. Should it be found needful to prolong the wound to a point above the umbilicus, the incision is usually carried to the left of the navel and brought back in a curved line to the linea alba. This is done to avoid the round ligament of the liver and its vessels, which come in there from the right side. Keith, however, cuts directly through the navel; and I find this straight incision to be superior in every respect to the curved one. Other things being equal, the short incision is safer than the long one; but it is a good rule to have an opening large enough for easy manipulation and for the easy withdrawal of the cyst. For instance, a large monocyst without adhesions after being emptied can, like a wet rag, be pulled out, hand over hand, through a very small opening, whereas a much smaller polycyst, which cannot be wholly emptied, and which is more or less adherent, will need a long incision. I once removed an oligo-cyst weighing one hundred and twelve pounds through an incision barely admitting my hand; while I had to open the abdominal cavity from ensiform cartilage to symphysis pubis in order to remove a solid ovarian fibroid tumor weighing but eighteen pounds. Both patients recovered, but the chances were, of course, more against the woman with the long incision. To avoid the escape into the abdominal cavity of any blood from the wound, and to prevent the soiling of the operator's hands, a clean napkin wetted with the carbolated water is doubled over each edge of the incision.

Whenever the cyst-wall in the line of the incision is glued by adhesions to the parietal peritoneum, the latter is liable to be mistaken for the former, and accordingly to be stripped off from the abdominal wall. To avoid this very serious error, either proceed with the cutting until the cyst-wall unmistakably comes into view or is opened, or else extend the incision upward until a point is reached where the cyst is free from adhesions. Adhesions binding the cyst to the abdominal wall are of importance only from the troublesome oozing their rupture often gives rise to. To lessen this risk, they are to be sundered by the finger whenever possible. Should the scissors be used, the adhesion bands must be snipped close to the surface of the cyst, and not to that of the abdominal wall. Thus, a free end is gained, which may, if needful, be subsequently tied or in which the dangling blood-vessels may the more readily constringe. All thick and long bands of adhesion should be tied in two places and be divided between the ligatures. These ligatures should consist either of very fine silk or of gut. For isolated vessels the latter are the better ones, but the silk is more suitable for tying en masse a group of bleeding vessels or for pursing up an oozing surface by an in-and-out stitch. A very important rule, on the observance of which one's success greatly depends, is, never to let a bleeding point or an oozing surface get out of sight. It must either be ligatured at once, or else caught by pressure-forceps and tied later if needful. If the delicate omental apron be found glued to the cyst, it should be carefully detached with as little tearing and splitting as possible, for each shred will bleed, and so will the fork of the split. It should then be turned out of the abdominal cavity on a clean napkin wetted with the carbolated solution. If its bleeding vessels be few, each one may be tied with gut; but if they are many, the torn portion of the omentum should be tied en masse or in sections, and the ligatures cut off close to the knot. All shreds and ragged ends of omentum must be trimmed off, and it is then returned to the peritoneal cavity.

When all the adhesions within reach, and those that do not demand great force, have been severed, it will be time to tap the cyst. This should be done with a large-sized trocar, such as Wells's, which is furnished with spring teeth to prevent it from slipping out of the cyst. Any trocar will do, provided it has a large bore, so that the vent may be free and that none of the acrid fluid can escape along its side into the abdominal cavity. In order to save time, neither Schroeder nor Martin use a trocar. They incise the cyst, and try by pressure and the lateral position to direct the contents externally. Frequently, however, some of the fluid escapes into the abdominal cavity, but they contend that if antiseptic precautions be taken no harm accrues.[1] Although dissenting from this opinion, I must confess to having had the contents of the cyst escape repeatedly into the abdominal cavity without doing any harm whatever. Always tap at the upper angle of the wound, because as the cyst collapses the trocar is drawn downward toward the lower angle. Hence, were the trocar entered low down it could not travel with the collapsing cyst, which would therefore slip off. While the fluid is flowing flat sponges should be packed in between the abdominal wall and the cyst, and the edges of the incision should be pressed firmly against them, so that the peritoneal cavity may not receive a single drop of that which frequently escapes along the side of the trocar. To avoid this accident—which, without being a very serious one, is yet not to be invited—some ovariotomists before tapping turn the woman well over on her belly and over the edge of the table; but this is liable to cause a protrusion of the bowels; which is, in fact, a more dangerous accident than the entrance of some of the fluid into the abdomen. Rosenbach, indeed, reports that during the extraction of biliary calculi through an abdominal incision a cure resulted, although several calculi were lost in the peritoneal cavity.[2] Should the mother-cyst not collapse on account of its containing a few other large cysts, the point of the trocar, without being withdrawn, can be made to enter each one. But if the child-cysts are many and small, the trocar is withdrawn, the opening enlarged, its edge seized by several pressure-forceps, and the hand introduced to break up these cysts.

Before this hand can again be used for separating adhesions it must be

---

[1] *Berlin- klin. Wochenschrift*, 1883, No. 10.
[2] *Medical News*, Feb 3, 1883, p. 130.

carefully cleansed with soap, and dipped into the carbolated solution in the tray of instruments.

The empty cyst is next gently pulled out through the abdominal wound. It is, however, so slippery that this cannot ordinarily be done with the hands alone. A strong forceps with a firm grip is needed, and one of the best is Nélaton's. While the cyst is being withdrawn the bowels are sheltered from the air and the spray by one large flat sponge, and the abdominal cavity must also be packed with smaller ones at every exposed point; and one of them should always be placed between the womb and the bladder.

In the majority of cases there is not much difficulty in freeing the cyst from its ordinary attachments and in reaching its pedicle. But should adhesions bind the cyst to the adjacent viscera, matters will not go on so smoothly. Such adhesions to bladder, liver, bowels, or to other important organs sometimes present difficulties which are insurmountable. The problem here is to sever these bands of adhesion without injuring the viscera to which they are attached. When these adhesions are numerous or very firm, much advantage will be gained by having the assistant put his hand within the cyst and stretch its wall while the operator severs the adhesions over it. By this means the adhesions can be better broken off close to the cyst, which is the all-important course to pursue in visceral attachments. Sometimes it will be needful to peel off the outer and non-secreting layers of the cyst and leave them behind—sometimes to cut off the adherent portion of the cyst and scrape off or strip off the secreting surface. Whenever the stalk of the tumor can be reached before all the adhesions are severed, it will be well to catch it with one or two pressure-forceps, or even to tie it and cut it off between two ligatures, like the umbilical cord. This will prevent bleeding from the torn surfaces of the cyst. When the cyst is closely adherent to the edges of the abdominal incision, either extend the wound upward until a free point is reached, and work downward on the adhesions, or else cut into the cyst, empty it, and seize with strong forceps its inner surface just beyond where the adhesions begin. The sac is then inverted by traction, which will break up its adhesions to the abdominal wall, the last portions to be freed being those attached to the edges of the incision. This prevents the stripping up of the peritoneum. Should the appendix vermiformis be so adherent to the cyst as not to be detached, it must be ligated in two places, between which it is to be cut, in order that its contents may not escape into the abdominal cavity. The fecal plug in each distal end should also be carefully squeezed out. Double ovarian cysts sometimes fuse together, and, rupturing at the point of fusion, form apparently one cyst. Such a cyst will have two pedicles, and will be very puzzling to the inexperienced operator.

When the cyst has been freed from its attachments and turned out of the wound, the very important question comes up of the treatment of the stalk or pedicle. Shall it be secured by a clamp? shall it be burned off by the actual cautery? or shall it be tied, cut off, and dropped back? The first is called the extra-peritoneal method; the others, the intra-peritoneal. For many years the clamp claimed the most advocates, but it has lost ground on account of possessing the following disadvantages: By keeping the wound open it prevents a strictly antiseptic treatment;

the stalk sometimes sloughs below the line of constriction and conveys putrilage into the abdominal cavity; the stalk always becomes united to the abdominal wall, hence when it is short the womb is dislocated or it is too much dragged upon. Then, again, in one-third of the cases the oviduct has a trick of remaining open, and the woman will menstruate indefinitely from the abdominal cicatrix. This is owing to the fact that the clamped portion sloughs off too early for a firm plug of cicatricial tissue to be formed, and the oviduct is therefore liable to stay open. In my first case of ovariotomy this happened, and one year later the cicatrix degenerated into a malignant growth which destroyed the life of my patient. It is, however, probable that in this instance the cystic disease of the ovary was malignant, although the sac did not look so at the time of its removal. Another disadvantage arising from the use of the clamp is the subsequent weakness of the cicatrix at its site, and the liability of ventral hernia to form there. These are the objections to the clamp, and they are so valid that at the present time all distinguished ovariotomists have abandoned its use.

The actual cautery, performed by Paquelin's instrument or by platinum-tipped irons, which do not scale off or discolor the tissues, is theoretically the very best way of dealing with the stalk. No foreign body besides the charred portion of the stalk is left within the abdominal cavity; but, on the other hand, it cannot always be trusted to close the vessels. On this account it is looked upon with disfavor by all ovariotomists with the exception of Keith. His method is as follows: The pedicle is spread out evenly within Baker-Brown's clamp, so as to get equable compression. The cyst is cut off, leaving a stump about an inch in height above the clamp. To protect the parts from heat a folded napkin wetted in the carbolated solution is tucked under the clamp. The stump is next carefully dried, and then burned slowly down to the level of the clamp by wedge-shaped cautery-irons at a brown heat. They give off a whistling sound during the process. The thick end of the stump can be more quickly burned down, but the thin end should be burned very slowly, and the blades of the clamp by prolonged contact with the cautery-iron must also be made hot enough to dry up and shrivel that portion of tissue which they compress. In order not to disturb the stump after it has been cauterized, it is best to clean out the peritoneal cavity first, and to leave this treatment of the pedicle for the last thing. Before removing the clamp, which is to be unscrewed very slowly and carefully, one side of the pedicle is seized by a pressure-forceps, by which it is kept in sight and out of harm's way if the peritoneal cavity needs further cleansing.

The plan of treating the pedicle most in vogue, and the one which I adopt, is that of the ligature—one of fine carbolated silk, the finest compatible with safety. The ends are cut off close to the knot, and the stump is dropped into the peritoneal cavity, where the silk, being animal tissue, will in time become disintegrated and absorbed. Now, when I say silk, I mean silk, and not silver or gut ligature. Silver, being inelastic, cannot bind a shrinking stalk, while the gut is a treacherous ligature, and will sooner or later bring one to grief. It slips in the tying, it is liable to untie, it gives instead of shrinking, and it is too short-lived for the obliteration of large vessels.

The reasonable objection has been urged that since the abdominal cicatrix left by the use of the clamp is liable to reopen every month to give vent to menstrual fluid, the same phenomenon will by this intra-peritoneal method happen within the abdominal cavity and expose the woman to all the risks of a hæmatocele. But fact is here opposed to theory, for it has been found that either the oviduct in the stump atrophies into an impervious cord of fibrous tissue, or that its raw end, by contracting adhesions with the surrounding tissues, becomes hermetically sealed. It might also be supposed that the distal end of the ligatured stalk would slough and expose the woman to septic peritonitis. But such sloughing rarely happens, and for the following reasons : From shrinkage of the stump the constriction is lessened, and the capillary circulation is re-established ; or the peritoneal surfaces on each side of the narrow and deep gutter made by the fine silk will bulge over and touch one another. Adhesion then takes place between the two, and the blood-vessels which shoot over from the proximal or uterine side of the ligatured stump will carry life into the distal end; or lymph exuded by the irritation of the ligature will throw a living bridge across the gutter in the stalk; or, what is the least desirable, the raw end of a long stalk glues itself to any peritoneal surface with which it may come in contact. I say least desirable, because sometimes such an adhesion makes a kink in the bowel, and may so constrict it as to give rise to fatal obstruction. To prevent this accident, Thornton stitches with gut the raw end of the stump to the broad ligament, to which it adheres ; while Bantock catches it up out of harm's way by including it in the lowest abdominal suture, which, being of silkworm gut, can be left in for a long time. If the stump be short, it stands upright, and does not then need this treatment.

If the stalk be a thick one, it is transfixed by a blunt needle threaded with a double ligature, and is tied on either side, each half by itself, and then the whole is further tied by the free ends of one of the ligatures, or the Staffordshire knot, recommended by Tait, may be used. If it be a broad one, it is tied in three or more sections by cobbler's stitches. In thick or in broad stalks it is a good plan to catch the stalk in Dawson's clamp, which compresses it circularly, and to transfix and tie it in the furrow made by the clamp. This lessens the risk of secondary hemorrhage, which is usually caused either by the slipping off of the ligature or by its loosening through tissue-shrinkage. When this clamp is used the pedicle need not be tied until the wound is ready to be closed. The stalk must be cut off at a distance from the ligature of not less than three-fourths of an inch, so as to leave a button of tissue sufficiently large to prevent the loops from slipping off. In short and broad stalks the outer or broad ligament portion, which is thin and membranous and sustains most of the tension strain, is liable to slip out of its ligature and cause a fatal hemorrhage. To avoid this accident the ends of the corresponding ligature may, before being tied, be repassed in opposite directions through the stalk very near its margin to form the cobbler's stitch. Another way is to pass a fine silk thread through the thin portion of the stalk about one-third of an inch from its edge, and tie it. In the notch thus made, and below the knot, is laid and tied the outer ligature.

In anæmic cases Thornton ties the arterial side of the pedicle first, but in young and vigorous women he ties the venous side first, so as to deplete the woman by gorging the tumor with blood. While cutting off the cysts the abdominal cavity must be so protected by sponges that not a drop of blood shall fall into it. A dilated oviduct in the pedicle tends to suppurate; hence in such a case the ligature should be applied as close to the womb as possible, so as to get below the expanded portion. Before the cyst is cut away the pedicle should be seized on one side by a pressure-forceps, and kept more or less in sight until the wound is ready to be closed up. This will also prevent the ligatures from being rubbed off by the sponges while the abdominal cavity is being cleansed.

Sometimes the cyst has no stalk, but lies between two folds of the broad ligament, or else it is bound to the bladder, womb, and the pelvic tissues by intimate adhesions which cannot be safely severed. Formerly, under such circumstances the abdominal wound was hastily closed up and the case abandoned. Now, thanks to Miner of Buffalo, New York, we can fall back on enucleation, and need rarely be foiled.[1] This operation is performed by slitting open the peritoneal capsule of the sac at points close to its attachments, by introducing one finger or more into the opening, and by stripping off this serous and vascular envelope up to where the vessels enter the cyst-wall and become capillary. The artificial stalk thus made is to be treated precisely like a natural one—that is to say, by clamp, ligature, and cautery, or, if it does not bleed, by nothing whatever. This operation I have repeatedly performed, but it is seldom easy, and is always anxious work. Should the cyst be so wholly adherent to the viscera as not to be even enucleated, an incision is made into it. It is then emptied, thoroughly cleansed, and the child-cysts are also crushed by the hand. The edges of the opening thus made in the sac are now included in the stitches of the abdominal wound, but the latter is kept open either by a large cloth tent at the lower angle or by two glass drainage-tubes, one at each angle running down into the sac. Sometimes it may be needful to tie the adherent portion in sections and to cut the free portion away. A drainage-tube must then be inserted at the lower angle of the wound. This expedient has the sanction of Atlee and Olshausen, who have reported successful cases thus treated.[2] My own practice in such cases would be, after breaking up the child-cysts, to gather together the free portion of the cyst and bring it out at the lower angle of the wound. A short nickel-plated steel drainage-tube of large bore is inserted, the sac firmly clamped to it by a small wire écraseur, and the redundant portion cut away. Into this metal tube is passed a glass drainage-tube long enough to touch the lowest portion of the sac.

In such cases, when feasible, I think it would also be well to adopt Freund's plan of tying the pedicle and severing it, in order to lessen the blood-supply to the cyst.[3]

The sac having been removed, the other ovary should be examined, and, if diseased, be tied and cut off. From the sundered bands of adhesion more or less bleeding has been taking place, which must now be attended to. It can usually be stopped by pressure with a sponge or with a finger, or with sponges wrung out of very hot carbolated water. For single vessels torsion will usually succeed, but if it does not, fine

[1] *Transactions International Med. Congress*, 1876, p. 801.
[2] *Monthly Abstract*, July, 1877, p. 334.
[3] *Boston Med. and Surg. Journal*, Aug. 24, 1876, p. 219.

carbolated silk or gut ligatures must be used; and it is wonderful how many can be applied without materially compromising the safety of the woman. I once tied over thirty vessels in a lady sixty-eight years of age, who recovered without any symptoms of peritonitis. The free ends of the ligatures should always be cut off close to the knot. Stubborn oozing surfaces can very generally be stanched by searing them with Paquelin's thermo-cautery, or by passing a needle armed with fine silk under and ligating any vessel that may be detected leading up to the seat of the oozing. In some cases nothing answers so well as the pressure of the finger moistened with alcohol or with a drop or two of the ferric sub-sulphate or of the tincture of iodine. In oozing from inaccessible points in the pelvis a sponge dipped in the undiluted solution of iodine or in Monsel's solution of iron, and afterward well squeezed out, may be pressed firmly down for a few moments into Douglas's pouch. When the oozing comes from a large surface of the abdominal wall, it may finally be arrested by the doubling of the raw surface on itself. The fold thus made is then secured either by a long acupressure needle or by cobbler's stitches passed through from skin to skin. Forty-eight hours after, this needle or these stitches should be removed. For this ingenious device we are indebted to the late Kimball of Lowell, Mass. Should all these measures fail, put in a drainage-tube, close up the abdomen in the manner about to be described, and temporarily lay over the dressings some heavy weights, such as bags of sand or of shot. This plan I have not been obliged to resort to, but it has the sanction of Nussbaum, who uses two large bricks, and it is worthy of being borne in mind.[1] In my hands an elastic flannel binder pinned very tightly over a large roll of cotton wool has made pressure enough to check the hemorrhage.

The toilet of the peritoneum next comes in order. By this is meant the peeling off from the peritoneum of plastic deposits, the removal of the sponges packed into its cavity, and the careful cleansing away of all fluids and of every blood-clot. In the search for all such foreign bodies, or, indeed, for obscure oozing-points, the reflector of the ophthalmoscope or Colin's illuminating lamp will give much aid. Douglas's pouch and the peritoneal fold between the bladder and the womb are favorite localities for the collection of blood or of serum, and should therefore be thoroughly mopped out by small sponges on holders, otherwise peritonitis or septicæmia may result, which are the two great factors of death in unsuccessful cases. When this has been thoroughly done, a clean sponge is placed in Douglas's pouch, another in the sulcus between the bladder and the womb, and a third, a large and broad flat one, is laid over the intestines under the wound to catch the blood that may drop from the needle-tracks. Each needle is passed from within outward a quarter of an inch away from the peritoneal edge of the wound, and is made to emerge at the same distance from its cutaneous edge. If the recti muscles are included in the sutures, there is said to be a liability to the formation of abscesses in the suture-tracks. Hence almost every ovariotomist advises that the peritoneum and skin should be pinched together, and that the needle should be passed through them alone without perforating the muscles. Yet I believe that from a too close observance of this rule come many cases of hernia in the track of the wound, and that were the recti muscles

[1] *British Med Journal*, Oct. 26, 1878, p. 617.

more closely coaptated they would not recede from one another and thus aid in the formation of a rupture.   My own rule is to include these muscles in the suture wherever they are exposed to view.   The sutures should lie about one-third of an inch apart.   The needles should be lance-pointed and held by a needle-holder.   In fat women it is not always easy to get the two surfaces of the wound in exact coaptation; consequently, more or less puckering and eversion of the edges may take place.   To avoid this, it will be well, before passing the needles, to bring the edges of the wound together, and make with a fountain-pen transverse lines at proper intervals across the incision as landmarks for the introduction of the sutures.   These cross-lines are also of advantage whenever the abdominal walls are too tense for accurate coaptation, as after öophorectomy, after the removal of a small abdominal tumor, or after an exploratory incision for a solid tumor which cannot be removed.   In these cases, indeed, it would be well to make the cross-lines the first step of the operation, before even the abdominal incision has been made.

The reasons why the needle is made to enter the peritoneum first are, that the stitches are lodged more evenly on that vulnerable surface, and with less injury to it, such as the stripping of it off from the abdominal wall; and, further, that a stray knuckle of bowel is not so likely to be wounded by the upward as by the downward thrust of the needle.   The object of including the peritoneum in the stitches is to bring in contact two long and narrow ribbon-like surfaces of a membrane, which will quickly unite—so quickly as to forestall any formation of pus in the overlying tissues, and to bar the entrance of this or other septic fluids from the wound in the abdominal wall.   Another advantage is, that this inclusion of the peritoneum by presenting an uninterrupted surface of parietal peritoneum to the visceral peritoneum prevents the adhesion of the omentum and of the intestines to the internal lips of the wound, which otherwise takes place.

When all the sutures have been passed, their ends on one side are loosely twisted together into a single strand, which is securely caught by a pressure-forceps.   The same thing is done with the ends on the other side.   A finger of each hand is now passed down into the centre of the wound, and the middle portion of all the upper sutures and of all the lower ones are separated from one another by being drawn to opposite angles of the wound.   This permits the removal of the sponges, and, if they are stained with blood, the further search for some overlooked bleeding vessel.   To guard against twisting of their convolutions, the bowels, still further disturbed by these final manipulations, are now restored to their natural position, and the omentum, after being again examined for some bleeding vessel, is gently spread out over them.   The forceps and sponges are then counted to see that not one has been left in the abdominal cavity.   The importance of this cannot be too strongly impressed upon the operator, for distinguished ovariotomists have overlooked these articles, and have left them behind in the abdominal cavity—a sponge and a bulldog forceps in one case.[1]   Tait has heard of ten such cases.[2]   It is indeed sometimes no easy task to find a missing sponge when lost in the convo-

[1] Lancet, May 26, 1877, p. 783; British Med. Journ.. Jan. 28, 1882, p. 115; Ibid., Dec. 25, 1880; also, Ovarian and Uterine Tumors, by Spencer Wells, London ed., p. 336.
[2] Diseases of the Ovaries, by Lawson Tait, 4th ed., p. 261.

lutions of the intestines. The sponges therefore should not be much smaller than the fist.

Before closing the wound the operator removes the pressure-forceps and catches in one hand all the ends of the sutures on his side, his assistant does the same thing on the other side, and the edges of the wound are brought together by a firm pressure, which also chases the air out of the abdominal cavity. To stop the bleeding from the needle-tracks as soon as possible, each suture is rapidly tied and by the surgeon's knot. When the whole wound has been closed, and not till then, the ends of all the sutures are gathered together in one hand, and they are cut off about two inches from the knot by one snip of the scissors. This saves precious time, which would be lost were each suture by itself to be cut after being tied. At gaping points of the wound intermediate superficial stitches should be put in. In fat women several such stitches will usually be needed.

Dressing of the Wound.—After the wound has been closed the rubber apron is removed and the abdomen cleansed and dried. The wound may now be dressed according to Lister's plan. This consists, first, of a narrow protective of prepared oiled silk, moistened by a 1 : 40 solution of carbolic acid; next, of one broad layer of antiseptic gauze wetted with the same solution; and over this eight folds more of the dry gauze, having a piece of mackintosh interposed between the seventh and the eighth layer. The lamp is now blown out, and the spray-jet being directed away from the abdomen, the dressing is secured by an elastic flannel binder, the rucking of which can be prevented by tapes pinned to it around each thigh. Most of the leading ovariotomists, however, employ simpler dressings, which have been found equally antiseptic. Wells covers the wound with a dry dressing of thymol cotton, kept in place by long strips of adhesive plaster, going two-thirds of the way around the body. Over all is pinned a flannel binder. The thymol cotton is prepared by steeping absorbent cotton wool in a solution of one part of thymol to one thousand of water, and drying it. Keith dresses the wound with gauze wrung out of a 1 : 8 glycerole of carbolic acid. On this are laid several layers of dry carbolated gauze, next some cotton wool, and over all a flannel binder. Thornton uses Lister's gauze and the mackintosh, but without the protective. This dressing is secured by adhesive straps. On these are laid several folded napkins, and over all a flannel binder is pinned very tightly. Bantock resorts to dry thymol gauze. Tait uses nothing but ordinary absorbent cotton. Salicylated cotton I have found to answer so well that for years I used nothing else. It is made by steeping two parts of absorbent cotton in a solution of one part of salicylic acid to two of commercial ether, and afterward drying the cotton by a low heat. Lately I have been resorting to Keith's dressing, but it probably possesses no greater advantages.

The flannel binder having been pinned on, the night-dress is pulled down and the patient put to bed. The opium suppository containing one grain of the watery extract is slipped into the rectum, the six bottles of hot water are applied to different portions of the body, and she is covered with warm blankets. The tables, tubs, and other articles used in the operation are now removed, the room is darkened, and she is left alone with her nurse, who has positive instructions to admit no one besides the physician.

Drainage.—When blood in small quantities is effused into the peritoneal cavity, coagulation usually takes place, the serum is then absorbed, the clot becomes organized, and no harm results. But when blood in large quantities collects in Douglas's pouch, it may behave as a foreign body and cause mischief. When, also, blood is mixed with serum, coagulation is not so likely to take place ; the blood-corpuscles then are liable to break down, the fluid to become putrid, and septicæmia to set in. For these reasons the removal of these fluids by different modes of drainage has long been put in practice. The best mode is by a glass tube passed down to the bottom of Douglas's pouch through the abdominal wound, and not, as has been recommended, through a special opening made for it in the roof of the vagina. Drainage is at present very rarely resorted to by those operators who use strict antiseptic precautions, for they contend that septic changes in the blood do not then take place. Wells and Thornton have virtually given it up, while Keith, Tait, and Bantock, who have abandoned Listerism, are warm advocates of it. This question is a very important one, because a drainage-tube tends to the formation of a ventral hernia, and, being a foreign body, is in itself hurtful, and therefore should not be resorted to unless it will do more good than harm.

After a careful consideration of the subject I am forced from experience to believe that between the two extremes there lies a golden mean, and that drainage, even when the spray is used, is needed under the following conditions :

(*a*) Whenever a purulent or a colloid cyst has burst, and its contents have escaped into the cavity of the abdomen, either during the operation or some days beforehand.

(*b*) Whenever the contents of the cyst are putrid or purulent, and septic symptoms or those of peritonitis are present.

(*c*) Whenever a large amount of ascitic fluid is found in the abdominal cavity.

(*d*) Whenever four drachms or more of pure blood, or especially of a sero-sanguinolent fluid, can be squeezed out of the sponge in Douglas's pouch when removed just before the closure of the wound.

(*e*) Whenever the operator is in doubt what to do.

Should it be deemed needful for some of the above reasons to make use of drainage, a glass tube, open at both ends and about six inches in length, is passed through the salicylated cotton or other dressing, then between the two lowest stitches, down to the bottom of Douglas's pouch. A wire suture is first introduced between these sutures and left untwisted, its object being to close firmly the opening left by the removal of the tube and to hasten its union. Otherwise, a weak cicatrix results, tending to the subsequent formation of hernia. Keith's drainage-tube of three sizes is the one that I prefer. Its lower end is perforated with holes, and its upper end has a shoulder which keeps it from slipping into the abdominal cavity, and also enables it to hold a piece of thin rubber sheeting about eighteen inches square. In the centre of this a small circular hole is made, which, by stretching, is sprung over the tube. The mouth of the tube is covered by a cup-shaped sponge wrung out of a 5 per cent. solution of carbolic acid, and over this the sheeting is folded four times. The flannel binder may either be pinned over the drainage-tube, or else it may be slit at the site of the tube and passed on each side of it, leaving the sponge and rubber sheeting outside of the dressing. They are then best held in place by a narrow strip of flannel, so as to permit inspection without interfering with the main dressing. Several times a day the sponge is removed, squeezed out, cleansed in a 5 per cent. solution of carbolic acid, and replaced. This in a hospital had better be done under the spray. Bloody serum collecting in this tube is sucked out either by a fine rubber tube attached to a syringe, or else by the long nozzle itself of the ordinary uterine syringe.

To prevent injurious pressure on the rectum, the tube must be lifted up occasionally about half an inch, and allowed to slip back of its own accord. It can be removed whenever the discharge has been reduced to not more than one or two drachms, and this usually happens within the first forty-eight hours. After its removal the opening left in the wound is closed by twisting the free ends of the wire suture placed there for this purpose.

AFTER-TREATMENT.—The subsequent treatment needs the greatest attention. The first care is to establish reaction. This is best done by stimulants, such as brandy and whiskey given in iced soda-water. Enemata of beef-tea and brandy or of milk and brandy will also be of advantage, while artificial heat is kept up. For the vomiting, which comes partly from the anæsthetic and partly from shock, repeated deep inspirations should be tried. They help by getting the blood rid of the anæsthetic as soon as possible. Chloral may also be given, or small lumps of ice may be swallowed. Sips of very hot water, or a tablespoonful every hour of a mixture containing equal parts of lime-water and of cinnamon-water, may also do good. A hypodermic of morphia will often allay vomiting, and I have seen it yield to small doses of atropia, and also to two grains of pure pepsin given every two hours in a tablespoonful of raw-beef juice. Twenty drops of ether given by the mouth will sometimes relieve it, and so also will a few drops of chloroform confined by a watch-glass over the pit of the stomach. In some cases I have tried, with the best results, the following effervescent mixture, recommended by Chèron : [1]

℞. Potassii bicarb. } āā gr. xxxij ;
  Potassii bromidi,
  Aquæ,   f℥ij. M.
℞. Acidi citrici, ʒj ;
  Syrupi,   f℥j ;
  Aquæ,   f℥iv. M.

A dessertspoonful of the former is added to a tablespoonful of the latter, and given every hour. For vomiting, especially of the bilious variety, Lawson Tait recommends Monson's pepsin wine, given every ten minutes in drachm doses with a little ice-water.

Flatus is another annoying symptom, which, however, can very generally be dispelled by turning the patient over on her side and inserting a flexible catheter high up in the rectum. If this fails to relieve it, enemata of turpentine may be tried, or five-drop doses of the tincture of nux vomica may be given every two hours. Should the abdomen become painfully bloated, the binder must be loosened and the adhesive straps

[1] *Archives de Tocologie*, Février, 1883, p. 122.

nicked in several places. The painful tension on the stitches can be relieved by drawing the knees up and supporting them over a pillow doubled on itself. Should the flatus not yield, and symptoms of obstruction set in, the bowels must be opened at all hazards. Castor oil and Epsom salts are good cathartics for this purpose. When vomiting accompanies obstruction, calomel answers best, because it is not so liable to be rejected.

For the first thirty-six to forty-eight hours after the operation nothing whatever should be given to the patient excepting cracked ice, sips of hot tea or of barley-water, and an occasional teaspoonful of old whiskey. After that time tablespoonful doses of milk, of beef-tea, of thin oatmeal gruel, or of barley-water can be given every hour or two. The diet may then be cautiously increased, and especially after wind begins to escape from the rectum, the patient being enjoined not to hold it back from motives of delicacy. If the condition of the patient is such as to demand more nourishment, it had better be taken by the rectum. For a week the urine should be drawn off by the nurse, and the bowels kept quiet by a morning and an evening suppository. No other anodyne need be given unless called for by pain, wakefulness, or restlessness. Should the body-heat indicate a temperature of 101° or over, a bladder filled with broken ice, or, what is far better, a rubber ice-cap, should be kept on the head of the patient as long as it feels comfortable and does not chill her. If the temperature does not fall, and peritonitis or other septic symptoms set in, ice should also be applied to the pit of the stomach. Quinia and morphia must then be given in very large doses, preferably by the rectum, together with ten drops of the tincture of digitalis every hour until the pulse-rate is lessened and the temperature falls.

When a full week has elapsed the bowels should be opened ; and, as this is a matter of importance, and is occasionally attended with symptoms of obstruction and with a good deal of constitutional disturbance, a few words will not come amiss. If the hardened feces can be softened down and dislodged by enemata, this is perhaps the best plan, clysters of ox-gall and water or of glycerin and water being the most efficient. But in my experience enemata have so often failed that I rarely resort to them in the first instance. If the woman's stomach is not irritable, I prefer to give her an ounce of castor oil. This is disguised in the compound syrup of sarsaparilla or in some other suitable vehicle, as warm milk, and is brought to her without any previous warning early on the morning of the eighth day. Should it be deemed unwise to try the oil, two Lady Webster pills and two compound cathartic pills can be given at bedtime of the seventh day, or a pill containing three grains of the compound extract of colocynth with one grain of the extract of hyoscyamus may be swallowed every four hours. The compound licorice powder of the German Pharmacopœia, to which has been added potassium bitartrate, also answers well, provided the patient's stomach will bear teaspoonful doses every four hours. Should these remedies fail to act, they must be supplemented by enemata.

Fatal obstruction of the bowels from matting or from constricting bands of organized lymph has been frequently reported. Thus far, I have met with one fatal case, which, however, passed out of my hands after the operation. But occasionally I see cases of obstinate constipation which give me great uneasiness and put me to my wits' ends. In one case, after the failure of other remedies the obstruction was overcome by broken doses of calomel combined with sodium bicarbonate, and by the distension of the lower bowel with very large enemata slowly given. Another desperate case yielded to repeated doses of tincture of belladonna. A third case, complicated by obstinate vomiting, was saved by ten grains of calomel given every two hours until the bowels were moved. Seventy grains were thus administered before the desired effect was attained, yet salivation did not occur.

When symptoms of obstruction once present themselves, they are likely to recur. The contents of the bowel should therefore be kept fluid, and for this purpose I know nothing better than the German compound licorice powder, given in teaspoonful doses at bedtime.

Suppression of urine sometimes follows ovariotomy, and in cases of diseased kidney is an alarming complication for this condition. For this symptom digitalis and the acetate of potassium should be given. Thornton treats it by baring the arms and packing them in towels which are kept wet with ice-water.

Tetanus may destroy the life of a patient while convalescing from the operation of ovariotomy. J. M. Bennett reports such a case.[1] The symptoms first showed themselves on the sixteenth day, and the woman died two days later. Chloral in drachm doses, administered by the bowel in the yolk of an egg, is perhaps the only remedy from which any good can be expected.

Occasionally, a few days after the operation, without any septic symptoms whatever or without any marked rise in the temperature, the parotid glands grow tender, swell up, and run through a course precisely like mumps, ending in resolution. This complication has been met with so frequently by myself and others that it cannot be a mere coincidence, but must be due to a reverse sympathy between the ovaries and these glands. It does not appear to increase the risk of the patient, for recovery took place in all the reported cases, of which three occurred in my own practice.[2] Parotid bubo may also take place after ovariotomy, but this sign of blood-poisoning, being a general one, happens as well after other grave surgical operations and during the course of specific fevers. Yet from the sympathetic relation between the parotid glands and the sexual organs it seems to occur more frequently in the septicæmia following ovariotomy.

Acute mania sometimes follows ovariotomy, especially when both ovaries have been removed. The attack is usually temporary, but it sometimes ends in insanity, and even in death, as in one of my own patients. Keith, Thornton, Tait, and other leading ovariotomists report analogous cases.[3]

SURGICAL TREATMENT.—The dressings, being antiseptic, need not, as a rule, be removed until the day following that on which the bowels are moved. Every other stitch may then be removed, and especially all that are loose or are cutting the tissues. The wound is then washed with a 2.5 per cent. solution of carbolic acid, and dressed anew with salicylated

[1] *Lancet*, Dec. 3, 1881.
[2] Wm. Goodell, *Transactions of American Gynæcological Society*, 1885.
[3] *The British Medical Journal*, March 21, 1885, p. 597.

cotton. I usually find the first dressing so sweet that I am able to reapply the unsoiled portion of it for a second dressing. A clean binder is now pinned on and the woman's clothing changed. Three or four days later all the stitches should be removed, the wound secured by narrow adhesive strips, and dressed as before. For fear of a weak cicatrix and the formation of a hernia at the site of the wound, the patient should not get out of bed until fully three weeks have elapsed, and should for as many months wear some kind of close-fitting gored binder or abdominal supporter.

If, before the week is over, the dressings become soiled or give out a bad odor, they should be at once renewed. They should also be removed whenever a high temperature, without being accompanied by tympanites, leads to the suspicion of cutaneous abscesses.

THE ACCIDENTS AND COMPLICATIONS OF OVARIOTOMY.—When by the breaking up of adhesions to it the liver is wounded, the bleeding surface can usually be stanched, as Koeberle has shown, by the ferric subsulphate applied to the raw surface by the finger. If this fails the actual cautery at a dull heat should be used.

If, unfortunately, an adherent portion of the bowel is torn open, the wound should be carefully closed with very fine silk by the continuous suture. The sutured portion is then fastened to the lower angle of the abdominal wound as a safeguard in case of the subsequent formation of stercoral fistula.[1] Should the intestine be injured to any extent, the wound must be closed by two sets of fine silk sutures, the first set uniting the mucous edges of the wound by the continuous suture, the other set uniting one serous coat to the other at a line about one quarter of an inch distant from the wound. An ordinary cambric needle with fine sewing-silk will answer admirably for this purpose. In small wounds one continuous suture, carried through all the coats but the mucous, will suffice. A mere puncture can be closed by hooking it up and surrounding it by a single fine ligature.

Wounds of the bladder have frequently happened, but they are by no means necessarily fatal.[2] These accidents are liable to occur when the bladder, being adherent to the cyst and carried upward by it, lies directly under the line of incision, or the bladder may be torn open while adhesions to it are being severed. The wound should at once be grasped by a pressure-forceps, the bladder emptied by the catheter, and the operation proceeded with. When the operation has been completed the wound in the bladder is attended to, and in one of the following ways : Either the vesical wound is brought up within the lips of the abdominal incision, and is closed by being included in the abdominal stitches, or it is closed by the continuous or Glover's suture, without including the mucous membrane in the stitches. A self-retaining catheter, such as the Skene-Goodman, must then be kept in the bladder for at least a week.

One of the ureters will sometimes be torn across while pelvic adhesions are being broken up. This accident is most likely to happen during the enucleation of a cyst growing downward because enveloped in the folds

---

[1] "Discussion on a Paper by Garrigues," *Am. Gynæcol. Soc. Trans.*, 1881.
[2] Eustache, *Archives de Tocologie*, April and May, 1880, pp. 193, 277 ; *Boston Med. and Surg. Journal*, Feb. 16, 1882, p. 153 ; *British Med. Journ.*, Jan. 28, 1882, p. 115 ; *Am. Journ. Med. Sci.*, Jan., 1883, p. 123.

of the broad ligament. It is almost always fatal, and is usually not discovered during the life of the patient, and, I am disposed to think, not often discovered after her death. Sometimes, however, urine will ooze out of the abdominal wound, and in rare cases the patient has recovered with a urinary fistula. In such a case Simon[1] successfully removed the corresponding kidney; Nussbaum[2] constructed an artificial ureter leading from the fistula to the bladder; and Tauffer[3] inserted the upper end of the divided ureter into the bladder by an artificial opening. It, however, failed to unite, and he later made an artificial ureter.

When an umbilical or a ventral hernia of moderate size is present at the time of the operation, efforts should be made for its radical cure. This is done by cutting out the thinned-out sac by two incisions meeting below and above, and by bringing together the thick edges of the abdominal wall in the final closure of the wound.

In cases of ascites complicating ovariotomy the ascitic fluid should not be wholly removed until the cyst has been cut off and the wound is ready to be closed. By this means any blood oozing from broken adhesions, or any fluid escaping from the cyst into the abdominal cavity, being diluted, is less likely to irritate the peritoneum, the cavity of which can also be more readily cleansed.

When a patient seems in danger of dying on the table from shock or from exhaustion the anæsthetic should be withheld while hypodermic injections of ether and enemata of brandy are given. Warmth should also be applied to the body by bottles of hot water, or, what is better, by rubber bags of the same. Theoretically, atropia administered subcutaneously would be the proper remedy, but I have not yet tested it. In all cases of ovariotomy, especially if prolonged, the woman should not be kept profoundly under the influence of the anæsthetic for any length of time, but should be allowed from time to time to come to at least enough to make her flinch or move about. This caution should especially be observed in very feeble patients and in those with very large cysts.

The Removal of Both Ovaries.

Whenever both ovaries are diseased there can be no question about the extirpation. But when only one has undergone cystic or other degeneration the question of the removal of the sound one may come up. There always is a tendency to the subsequent degeneration of the sound ovary after the diseased one has been removed. More especially is this tendency observed in sterile women and in those with malignant affections of the ovary. Many women, therefore, whose lives should have been imperilled but once, have been compelled to face the dangers of a second operation. In view of these facts, it seems to me wise to remove the sound ovary in all cases of sterility, in every case of malignant degeneration of one ovary, and in all women who have either passed the climacteric or are approaching it, provided its removal is not attended with great additional risk. Double extirpation should also be performed whenever the womb con-

[1] *Annales de Gynécologie,* June, 1877.
[2] *Edinburgh Medical Journal,* July, 1876, p. 1.
[3] *Archives de Tocologie,* Avril, 1880, p. 201.

tains a fibroid tumor or whenever it seems desirable to hasten on the climacteric. In these convictions I am further strengthened by the disappointment often expressed to me by my patients that one ovary had been left behind, and by their great fear afterward lest the remaining organ should also become diseased. On the other hand, in women who are in the prime of their menstrual life the sound ovary should be left untouched, unless there exist grave reasons for its removal.

DISEASES OF THE URINARY ORGANS IN WOMEN.

By ALEXANDER J. C. SKENE, M. D.

ORGANIC DISEASES OF THE BLADDER.

Hyperæmia.

THIS is an acute congestion of the mucous membrane due to a disturbance in the balance of the circulation. It may be common to both bladder and urethra, or limited to either; may terminate within a short period of time (a few hours), or it may go on and end in hemorrhage or inflammation. If the mucous membrane is seen with the endoscope, it appears of a bright-red color; the blood-vessels are distended, more prominent, and apparently more numerous. The arteries are the first to be affected. If the cause is transient, this is all that is seen, the membrane returning to its usual color. When the congestion is of a higher grade, rupture of some of the vessels occurs either on the free surface or beneath the epithelium. The venous side of the circulation now becomes more prominent. In a few cases the above order may be reversed, the veins being the first congested, as in the case of a sudden interference with the portal circulation.

SYMPTOMS.—The attack occurs suddenly. Frequent but painless urination is the most prominent feature. There is a sense of heat and heaviness in the bladder, aggravated by standing. When the urethra is involved the patient complains of scalding during urination. The pulse and temperature are practically normal. The composition of the urine is but little changed; there may be excess of mucus and a few blood-corpuscles.

DIAGNOSIS.—This has to be made by exclusion. It is apt to be confounded with a neurosis of the bladder or a displacement.

ETIOLOGY.—The most frequent cause is exposure to cold, especially during menstruation; over-taxation in walking or using the sewing-machine; excessive venereal indulgence; disorders of the portal circulation; and the use of improper articles of food.

TREATMENT.—Every means should be employed to equalize the circulation. The most important element is rest in the recumbent position. Diaphoretics and warm applications to the feet and epigastrium, and, as a rule, a saline laxative. Where there is frequent urination and vesical tenesmus and pain, Dover's powder and camphor should be given, or a suppository of morphia and belladonna by the vagina.

Hemorrhage.

This is a symptom rather than a disease itself. It is usually due to acute congestion or ulceration occurring in advanced inflammations, new growths, or the lacerations caused by foreign bodies and instruments. Hemorrhoids of the bladder due to obstructed circulation is not infrequently the source of the bleeding. The amount of blood transuded varies very greatly, though it is seldom so great as to prostrate the patient. In all cases when it is considerable it is of great importance to localize the bleeding point. The urethra can be excluded if there is no bleeding between the acts of micturition. The differential diagnosis between hemorrhage from the bladder or kidney is less easy. The old rule, that the blood and urine are more intimately mixed in renal hemorrhage than in cystic, is of little service. Sir Henry Thompson's method of detecting the source of pus in the urine may be employed in cases of hemorrhage. He introduces a soft catheter, and then washes out the bladder gently with warm water; if after a time the water comes out clear, the inference is that the bleeding point is higher up. To make sure, he corks the catheter until a drachm of urine has collected; if this is bloody, the diagnosis of its being extra-cystic is tolerably certain. With the endoscope it is occasionally possible, and always desirable, to locate the bleeding point.

The symptoms in hemorrhage from the bladder, besides the actual appearance of blood in the urine, are much the same as those in hyperæmia. Other symptoms liable to arise are from blood-clots forming and either being passed by the urethra, causing its distension and impeding micturition, or else such clots may be retained and accumulate in the bladder, giving rise to still greater functional disturbance, until they are either broken into small pieces by the surgeon and extracted, or else by the slower agency of decomposition they break down and come away.

TREATMENT.—The first thing is to obtain the advantages, both mechanical and physiological, of the recumbent position. A large number of hæmostatics have been used—tannic and gallic acids, ergot, and aromatic sulphuric acid. These are doubtless of some value, but we prefer giving opium in sufficient doses to allay the desire of too frequent micturition, and at the same time to render the urine more bland by alkaline diluent drinks. When the bleeding points can be discovered with the endoscope, they may be touched with caustic acid, nitrate of silver, or persulphate of iron. But such applications must be made with the greatest care, lest inflammation and ulceration result. Ice in the vagina and at the hypogastrium may be tried when other means fail. When the hemorrhage is hemorrhoidal, due to impeded venous return owing to pressure of the gravid uterus, the treatment will have to be purely palliative in the mean time, as the pathological condition of the veins usually rights itself after delivery. When a large blood-clot forms in the bladder, experience has abundantly shown that it is better not to meddle with it, but to let it break down itself and come away, the patient being kept easy—if necessary by opium and alkaline diluents.

Cystitis.

Inflammation may be limited to the bladder alone, in which case we call it cystitis, or to the urethra alone, when it is termed urethritis. But, practically, the pathological processes and the causes of cystitis and urethritis are so closely allied that it will be convenient in our limited space to consider them together. Like inflammation of other mucous membranes, various forms or degrees of cystitis and urethritis are described : these classifications are useful clinically, but .it should not be forgotten that the pathological conditions presented are only different stages of the same process. Inflammations of the bladder are divided according to the cause of the disease and the character of structural lesions into—the acute, including the catarrhal and the suppurative; and the chronic, including the ulcerative, interstitial (and peri-cystitis); and the specific, embracing the gangrenous, croupous or diphtheritic, and gonorrhœal, in which the inflammation is the result of a special poison.

ETIOLOGY.—The causes of cystitis may be classed under four heads : (1) Direct injuries, such as blows in the vesical region, falls, fracture of the pelvic bones, violent copulation, sudden uterine displacements causing pressure, foreign bodies, rough catheterization, over-distension from retention of urine, and, above all, contusions and injuries during labor. (2) Abnormal urine, from improper food or malnutrition and certain irritating drugs (cantharides) and irritating deposits of urine salts. (3) Certain constitutional diseases (eruptive fevers, gout, ague). (4) Inflammation of adjacent organs, hyperæmia due to cold.

PATHOLOGY.—The acute forms always begin with hyperæmia, then follow swelling, perverted or hyper-secretion, then exfoliation of epithelium, giving rise to a roughened and denuded state of the mucous membrane, particularly on the top of the rugæ, the products of inflammation accumulating within the sulci, and finally the formation of pus. A description of these, the ordinary phenomena of inflammation of mucous membranes, it is quite unnecessary to give here, but there are one or two modifying conditions in cystitis that are of great importance and need consideration. The first of these is the effect which the function of the bladder as a reservoir of urine has on the inflammation. Normal urine is irritating to an inflamed mucous membrane, and in cystitis it soon undergoes decomposition, becomes alkaline, and hence more irritating. The main agent in producing this decomposition is mucus, which is secreted abnormally both in quantity and quality. It acts injuriously in two ways, its fixed alkali tending to neutralize the acid of the urine, which in the early stages of cystitis is often hyper-acid, and in promoting the decomposition of the urea and thereby liberating the volatile carbonate of ammonia. As the urine becomes more alkaline the precipitation of the phosphates of lime and magnesia occurs, and the formation of the triple or ammonio-magnesian phosphate.

The irritant effect of these salts, really deposits of foreign bodies, on the inflamed mucous membrane completes the vicious circle, the effect now aiding the original cause.

Another most important point in the pathology of cystitis is the effect of over-distension of the bladder. This is itself sometimes the primary cause of the trouble, as in certain neuroses, but more frequently it is the effect of certain injuries during delivery. The mechanism of its production is not very clearly made out. It usually follows long, tedious deliveries, during which either the child's head or sometimes the forceps crushes the urethra against the unyielding pubic bones, giving rise to an acute urethritis, with swelling of the membrane and blocking up of the canal, causing retention. The primary injury is not done, as a rule, to the bladder in these cases, for if it were we should find the vesical neck the seat of sloughing of the mucous membrane; but, as a fact, this is the part (owing to its more loose connections with the underlying connective tissue) that most frequently escapes. This danger of over-distension is so clearly recognized that the catheter is nearly always used both before and after delivery if there should be retention. But a condition more apt to mislead both the doctor and the nurse is the urine dribbling away either constantly or intermittently. This is too often ascribed to an irritable bladder causing frequent micturition, when it is a sign of over-distension, the dribbling always occurring as soon as the mechanical pressure of the urine is sufficient to overcome the resistance of the swollen parts.

We have already referred to this condition of over-distension as a cause of inflammation; it will suffice to say that it may, if unrelieved, produce a partial or even total slough of the mucous membrane of the bladder; but, fortunately, this is rare.

Thus far we have spoken of the common forms of acute and subacute cystitis; it only remains to say a word with regard to its rarer manifestations. The inflammation may extend to the submucous coats, becoming interstitial cystitis. Again, this may limit itself here, or it may extend still deeper to the serous coat, in which case it is known as peri- or epicystitis. Peri-cystitis is almost always a secondary disease, arising sometimes from deep ulcerations of the inner coats of the bladder, such as occur in chronic cystitis. More frequently it is but a part of a pelvic peritonitis which originated outside of the bladder itself. The final result of peri-cystitis is to form adhesions between the bladder and the neighboring organs, and thereby prevent distension of the bladder.

A very rare form of gangrenous inflammation has been described, but it is more than doubtful if this ever occurs in women except as the result of mechanical violence or pressure, already described. The specific lesion of croupous or diphtheritic inflammation has occasionally been diagnosticated, either from shreds of false membrane passed by the urethra or by means of the endoscope. Gonorrhœal inflammation of the bladder has been less carefully observed in women than in men. Still, it is known that this specific inflammation extends to the bladder in some cases, but it does not differ essentially in its pathology, history, or treatment from that arising from other causes; hence it is unnecessary to dwell upon it here.

The pathology of chronic cystitis is characterized by ulceration and sloughing of the tissues involved. They do not differ materially from the same processes elsewhere, except that the salts of the urine are apt to be deposited upon the shreds of dead tissue the products of destructive inflammation. The hard masses thus formed are passed with great pain. They block up the urethra, and are only expelled by extra strong efforts which cause intense suffering.

Lastly, the ulceration may extend through the bladder into the peritoneal cavity and give rise to septic peritonitis and death, or the perforation may take place into the cellular tissue of the roof of the pelvis, and cause a fatal cellulitis.

SYMPTOMS.—The various forms of cystitis being but different stages and degrees of the same disease, their symptoms may be discussed all together. For convenience we shall consider them under three heads: (1) Referable to the organs themselves; (2) Symptoms referable to the neighboring organs; (3) General symptoms.

(1) In all forms of cystitis there is more or less derangement of function, as shown by pain, tenesmus, and frequent micturition. In the mildest form of the trouble there is a frequent desire to pass water, which often comes with unusual force. Micturition is followed by a desire to strain, as if the organ was not fully emptied. This sensation may pass off in a few moments, and not arise again till the next micturition, but in the severer cases it may last continuously. When urethritis is also present there is the additional and characteristic symptom of painful scalding as the urine passes over the inflamed track.

In urethritis alone there is often a desire to urinate frequently, but if the desire is resisted it passes off, and the patient can retain the urine for a long time. This symptom should not be mistaken for the tenesmus of cystitis. In the more advanced stages of the disease, especially as ulcerative changes occur, the tenesmus becomes more violent. The pains also are more diffused, often shooting to the umbilical region. There is often a dull, aching pain in the perineum, and in nearly all cases there is continuous backache, or, more correctly, sacral pain.

The composition of the urine is of great importance. The specific gravity in cystitis does not present any constant change, except that in the chronic forms it is often a little below the normal. The reaction in acute cystitis, at first at least, is usually acid, whereas in the chronic forms it is almost invariably alkaline. The color at first is not particularly altered; later, unless discolored by blood, it is a pale, dirty yellow. The odor is normal in the acute type, unless where retention has been followed by decomposition, but in the chronic form it is not only ammoniacal, but has a characteristic fleshy or organic smell. The sediment in the acute varieties is mainly light and yellowish, composed of mucus, with some pus generally; in addition there may be blood, epithelium, and the amorphous and triple phosphates. In the chronic forms the sediment is usually heavier and of a darker brownish color. Flakes of pus, shreds of tissue, blood, and epithelium in all stages of growth are more or less present, and in the intensely alkaline conditions of the urine the pus and mucus form a jelly-like, ropy, opaque mass.

Albumen will be found if there is pus in the urine without there being any kidney disease. As the result of a careful analysis of a number of cases of chronic cystitis, the amount of albumen varied from one-sixteenth to one-fifth of the volume of urine. Microscopically, in addition to the pus, mucus, organic shreds, phosphatic and other crystals already spoken of, the most interesting appearances are the various kinds of epithelium. In the advanced stages of chronic cystitis epithelial elements of any kind are very rarely found. It is only in the earlier stages that normal and transitional forms of vesical epithelium are present, and again they reap-

pear on the subsidence of the inflammation. This fact is of great importance, because the transitional forms of bladder-epithelium are often indistinguishable from the permanent forms of the urinary tract higher up.
It is thus often impossible to make a differential diagnosis between pyelitis and cystitis from this symptom alone. When renal disease is superadded to cystitis, the characteristic casts will be found and albumen will
likely be increased in amount.

(2) The symptoms accompanying cystitis in women referable to the
neighboring organs are of some importance, but they very often arise
from some coexisting disease of other pelvic organs. It is therefore
needless to give a list of all the pelvic pains coincident with cystitis
which have been enumerated in the literature of this subject.

(3) The general symptoms are of two classes, toxic and nervous. While
all agree that there is no doubt of direct blood-poisoning in cystitis, there
has been a great deal of difference of opinion as to how this is effected.
I think that there are various agencies at work in this. First, there may
be organic renal disease or sympathetic renal hyperæmia leading to imperfect elimination. In cystitis caused by over-distension from long retention
the kidneys simultaneously take on acute inflammation, which usually
passes off when the bladder is emptied, but it may continue and give rise
to all the constitutional symptoms of renal disease. Again, in chronic
cystitis the thickening of the bladder-walls obstructs the ureters, so that
the urine is dammed back upon the kidneys. This arrests their function,
and in time leads to organic disease with all the consequent derangements
of the nutritive and nervous systems. Secondly, absorption of the products
of decomposed urine, or of pus and other septic materials the result of
decomposing shreds of tissue, may take place.

Anæmia is another of the blood-changes which occur in chronic
cystitis. In its origin and continuance it probably is much like anæmia
due to long-continued inflammation elsewhere. The only peculiar symptom in this connection is the appearance of urohæmatin in the urine.

With this slow deterioration and poisoning of the blood various symptoms are developed. There is an effort made to eliminate urea by the
mucous membrane of the alimentary canal. This is manifested by attacks
of vomiting or diarrhœa. But when it does not come to these explosions,
there is apt to be lack of appetite, especially at the morning meal, or there
are perverted taste and constipation, interrupted by occasional attacks of
diarrhœa. The skin in the chronic cases is at times sallow and clammy,
and at times there is a distinct urinous odor about the body. Various
more or less marked nervous symptoms are apt to be present. One set
is characterized by the sluggishness of the patients, an inclination to sleep,
despondent spirits, and occasionally dizziness and fainting. There can be
little doubt that these and allied symptoms are referable to cerebral
anæmia, for they are much aggravated by bromide of potassium, whilst
digitalis and out-door life improves them. A second set of nervous
symptoms are fairly attributable to blood-poisoning of one kind or
another, and in the most severe cases are often promptly relieved by
diarrhœa. Finally, a number of the irregular, wandering neuralgic pains
and the headache are due to the general depression produced by bladder-
pain and loss of sleep.

DIAGNOSIS.—Cystitis is easily made out, except in certain mild cases.

Similar symptoms, especially frequent urination, occur in prolapsus uteri, often in anteversion and in cases of pelvic adhesions and pregnancy and abdominal tumors, and lastly in certain neuroses. In most of these the recumbent position lessens the desire for frequent urination much more than when cystitis is present. Again, in the neurosis the attacks are irregular. Tenesmus is usually only present in cystitis, and lastly the examination of the urine and exploration of the parts should settle the question. We have spoken above of the method of differential diagnosis of blood coming from the bladder or the kidneys: the same method applies to localizing the source of pus. Urethritis with fissure at the neck of the bladder simulates cystitis in clinical history, and in the fact that pus in small quantity is found in the urine. To differentiate, the urine examined should be taken directly from the bladder with the catheter, when it will be found free from the products of inflammation. In addition to this, in some cases it will be necessary to make use of the endoscope, by which a good view can be obtained of the whole urethra and a portion of the mucous membrane of the bladder sufficient for diagnostic purposes.

TREATMENT.—The female bladder is so accessible, owing to the shortness of the urethra, that it is peculiarly amenable to local treatment. This is by no means, however, all that is required, for in all forms of cystitis, irrespective of the cause, the urine plays a very important part in keeping up the irritation. There are, therefore, always three indications to be met: (1) Removal of the cause; (2) constitutional treatment (diminishing the irritating character of the urine); (3) the cure of the local lesion.

(1) In many cases, of course, the cause is transient. The injury is done, and the inflammation resulting runs its course, longer or shorter according to the modifying influence of treatment. In a smaller number of cases, again, the cause is not removable, as in certain constitutional diseases or permanent pelvic adhesions, tumors, and the like. In such cases of course the treatment is but palliative, and, while relieving the immediate symptoms, aids the organs till a certain amount of toleration of the abnormal conditions is established. But in a large class of cases the cause, though more or less persistent, is removable. This includes the numerous cases of uterine displacement. Lastly, there is a certain number of uncomplicated cases which tend to recovery without treatment.

(2) The constitutional treatment should be first directed to reducing the amount of work the bladder has to do. For this purpose the bowels should be kept rather freely open, saline laxatives being the most valuable for this purpose. The skin too should be kept healthy and active. Next, the character of the urine should be as bland as possible. Food and drugs which are known to cause or keep up cystitis should be carefully avoided. Milk diet has proved successful in the hands of George Johnson. In all cases the diet should be carefully attended to, and should consist largely of fluid foods—milk, yolk of eggs, soups, etc. Lean meat in small amounts and easily-digested solids are allowable. Articles such as asparagus, alcohol, beer, and wine generally are to be avoided. Fruits, such as lemons and oranges, are usually grateful and at least harmless. The alkaline diluents, such as citrate of potassium or the alkaline mineral waters (Vichy), answer an admirable purpose. An infusion of buchu is an excellent agent, and may be combined with nearly

all other drugs employed in treating cystitis. Where pain is an urgent symptom in acute cases, it should be relieved by hot applications and by anodynes. Dover's powder is an excellent form in which to give opium. To relieve tenesmus vaginal suppositories of morphia, with or without belladonna, may be given. But in certain cases twenty-grain doses of potassium bromide every four hours relieve pain where opium fails. Benzoic acid or benzoate of ammonium in ten-grain doses in infusion of buchu, three times a day, is a most valuable remedy. The usual remedies, such as balsam of Peru or copaiba, oil of turpentine, etc., which are given in gonorrhœal inflammation, are very useful in the chronic catarrhal forms of cystitis. To prevent or lessen the decomposition of the urine a vast number of remedies have been employed, all of the astringents and most of the antiseptics, but as a rule these remedies are much better administered locally than constitutionally. In various acute and transitory cases the constitutional remedies above described will be all that is necessary, but in the greater number local treatment is absolutely required.

(3) In local treatment the first point is not to do harm to the parts by the use of instruments. Dirty catheters and rough catheterization so often cause cystitis that it is easy to see that the same causes often perpetuate the mischief. Great care, then, should be used in selecting instruments for injecting. The ordinary metallic catheter with one or two large openings is much more liable to wound the sensitive mucous membrane than one with a number of small holes made either of hard or soft rubber. It should have a stopcock or something similar at the outer end, the better to regulate both the injections and the escape of the solution injected. In ordinary injections only about an ounce at a time should be in the bladder ; this can be repeated four or five times, and the injection should be as slow as possible. To meet these indications I use a double perforated catheter made as follows : A small tube runs from one of the bifurcations to the extreme point. This is the supply-tube, and the catheter acts as the exhaust. The central tube can be removed for the purpose of cleaning the instrument. A piece of rubber tubing attaches the supply-tube to a fountain syringe, and this completes the whole apparatus. The calibre of the supply-tube being small and that of the exhaust large, a great quantity of fluid can pass through the bladder without distending it. The fingers can pinch the rubber tube and act as a stopcock to regulate the entrance and escape of the fluid used.

An injection of borax and water is often highly beneficial, and is alone sufficient in many cases. It should be frequently employed. It should always precede any topical application or medicated injection. Lukewarm water alone is employed, but the addition of a little salt ($\mathfrak{z}$j to Oj) or chlorate of potassium renders it more bland. Very often hot water is a most useful application. Of the medicated injections a vast number might be described, but they are referable to two classes, anodyne and astringent. The painful nature of cystitis suggests the use of opium preparations and chloral hydrate for injections, and they do give some relief. They should be well diluted to prevent their causing irritation.

Of the astringents, acetate of lead, sulphate of zinc, tannic acid, nitrate of silver are the most valuable. Many others—perchloride of iron, chlorate of potassium, hydrastis canadensis, salicylic acid and its preparations, carbolic acid, etc.—have been commended. In all cases the strength of the injection should be short of causing the patient much pain. It is always best to begin with a mild solution and gradually feel the way up to stronger ones. Of all the astringents, I prefer nitrate of silver, which I use in strengths varying from one grain to twenty to the fluidounce. The general rule to be observed, if a strong solution is used, is to employ only a few drops; if a large injection is made, the solution should be weak.

Various antiseptics—iodoform, salicylate of sodium, etc.—have been used to prevent the decomposition which so complicates obstinate cystitis; but, as a rule, I think frequent washings out and astringent applications act much better. One of the most distressing obstacles encountered in making any such injections is where there is a tender or inflamed urethra. It is well then to carry the catheter only up to the sphincter of the bladder (as advised by Braxton Hicks), overcoming its resistance by the pressure of the injection. As a rule, the urethritis will not long survive the cystitis, but in some cases it exists as an independent affection; it is then usually gonorrhœal, and should be treated as in the male. But when not, the same principles apply as in the local treatment of the bladder. Great care is needed, as the female urethra will only hold ten or fifteen drops at a time, and if a large injection is used it is almost sure to enter the bladder. To meet this difficulty I devised a reflux catheter for douching the urethra. It is grooved on the outside, and at the point there is an opening in each groove which lets a jet of the fluid used flow outward, bringing the injection in contact with all parts of the urethra.

In cases of ulceration, such as occur in bad cases of cystitis, applications should be made, if possible, to the part affected only. This can be accomplished by means of the endoscope when the ulceration is seated where it can be reached. Having located the point exactly by means of the endoscope, the inner or glass tube is withdrawn, and the application made directly to the required spot through the rubber tube. A glass pipette properly curved or any ordinary insufflator will answer perfectly, and when a solid is used a delicate long curved forceps will answer.

In chronic cases of cystitis in which all the above methods of treatment fail, it becomes necessary to give the parts complete rest by securing continuous drainage of the urine and products of inflammation. There are two ways of doing this—the one, to use a self-retaining catheter which may keep the bladder empty : this method answers very well when the inflammation is confined to the upper portions of the bladder, but when the neck of the bladder is involved the presence of the catheter gives rise to pain and irritation and cannot be tolerated. The other plan is to establish an artificial vesico-vaginal fistula, and keep it open for some months, until the bladder-walls have become normal again. This secures efficient rest to the inflamed parts ; complete drainage is established, the patient wearing a cup, as she would a pessary, to catch the urine. If the inflammation is limited to the upper portion of the bladder, the drainage by the fistulous opening is all that is required ; but if the neck of the organ is involved, frequent and continued medication will be required. This can be done by injecting through the urethra and letting the fluid escape through the opening in the bladder. This is not the place to discuss the steps of the operation or the indications when and how to close the artificial fistula. For these the reader is referred to works on this department of surgery.

Suffice it to say, in conclusion, that this by no means easy operation should be only undertaken as a last resort, but that if properly done in well-selected cases it will cure where all other known methods of treatment have failed even to relieve.

Hypertrophy of the Bladder.

This lesion may be partial or total, involving any or all three coats of the viscus. But the term usually refers more particularly to increase of the muscular walls. As a rule, the hypertrophic changes are not confined to one portion of the viscus, all being more or less affected. The affection is much less frequent in the female than the male.

ETIOLOGY.—There are two varieties of this affection—one, concentric hypertrophy, in which the bladder is contracted as well as having its walls thickened; the other eccentric, in which there is dilatation. Its principal causes are—obstruction to the outflow of urine from stricture of the urethra, tumors, or foreign bodies; cystocele, preventing complete evacuation; cystitis, causing too frequent or too forcible contraction; and irritable bladder in certain of the neuroses. Accompanying such dilatation diverticulæ are sometimes formed, though rarely in the female.

SYMPTOMS.—There is sometimes present vesical spasm, some pain, and forcible ejection of urine. A certain amount of cystitis is almost always present, aggravating the original disorder. In the eccentric form there are sometimes superadded symptoms of over-distension.

DIAGNOSIS.—This is readily made by measuring the thickness of the bladder-wall between the finger in the vagina and the sound in the bladder. The capacity of the bladder is easily noted by measuring the urine passed at each micturition or by injecting a bland solution of salt and lukewarm water.

TREATMENT.—The treatment should be directed to the removal of the cause. When this is not possible, palliatives may be sought for in the use of the catheter, at regular intervals, to prevent over-distension. Cold baths, astringent injections, and electricity are often of use. By these means the evil results of the disease may be overcome, but the hypertrophy is usually permanent.

Atrophy.

Atrophy of the bladder is a rare disease in early life. In women, in addition to the ordinary decay of age, there is a special predisposition to degenerative changes in the pelvic viscera, the bladder-walls included, after the menopause. Extreme distension of the bladder is usually the exciting cause, giving rise to temporary or even permanent paralysis, and eventually causing either inflammation or atrophy and fatty legencration. Interrupted nutrition, due to impaired circulation, is the immediate cause, but such altered nutrition may be purely nervous and due to atrophy of certain ganglion-cells in the spinal cord.

SYMPTOMS AND DIAGNOSIS.—Patients complain of difficulty in emptying their bladders, the urine coming away in interrupted jets. They are

apt to be irregular in their times of urinating, and are liable in consequence at times to have retention and over-distension.   Pain and sometimes a slight cystitis are present.   Finally, they completely lose the power
of urinating and a catheter has to be used.   The diagnosis is to be made
as in hypertrophy, by a finger in the vagina and a sound in the bladder.

TREATMENT.—Regular catheterization, strychnia in full doses, electricity, and tonics, combined with washing out the viscus.   Where the
atrophy is due to nerve-degeneration these measures are purely palliative, in other cases they are of more avail.

FUNCTIONAL DISEASES OF THE BLADDER.

UNDER the name of functional diseases of the bladder are included a
large number of varied affections of which the pathology is as yet very
obscure.   Where there are marked symptoms of vesical disorder, while
no organic lesions are found in the tissues of the bladder, the affections
must be classed under the name of functional derangements.   As our
knowledge increases the number of these is constantly diminished, and a
still further and more rapid diminution will occur as the physiology and
pathology of the nervous system innervating this viscus become better
known.   These diseases are much more common in children and women
than in men—in children, because the controlling power of habit is only
in process of formation ; and in women, mainly because of the more complex organization of the genito-urinary organs, which are the more easily
exhausted and deranged, especially by the functions of maternity.   True,
neuralgia of the bladder has been described under a variety of names,
irritable bladder, cysto-spasm, etc., but it is rather a rare affection.   The
most prominent symptom is the painful micturition, and attendant on this
a desire to pass water too frequently.

There is no particular change in the character of the urine, and no
appreciable visible alteration in the appearance of the parts, though they
are more sensitive than normal to the touch.   This condition is best met
by warm fomentations locally and sedatives either locally or generally,
while nutrition is improved by appropriate tonics, nervines, and by the
use of the galvanic current.

A much more common class of affections of the bladder accompany
hysteria, sometimes grouped under the name of hysterical bladder.   A
great number of pathological conditions are grouped under this vague
term, but they are held together by all having, as a more or less prominent symptom, varying degrees of incoördination.   The disturbing effect
of strong sudden emotion, as fear, upon the bladder is familiar to all, and
in various organic diseases of the spinal cord and brain, such as myelitis
and locomotor ataxia, a disturbance in the functional action of the bladder
is among the first symptoms.   It then becomes a matter of great difficulty,
and yet of great importance, to make a differential diagnosis.

In hysteria the urine usually diminishes in specific gravity ; it is apt
to be increased in quantity, and, though clear in appearance, is irritating

to the mucous membrane. In such cases frequent urination, sometimes almost continuous, sets in ; but it is an important point that during sleep the patient retains her urine the normal time. In others we get, on the contrary, retention, and this may be due to various causes. In some it is doubtless involuntary, as they say they cannot urinate, but in others it is assuredly will not. Many of these latter derive a morbid pleasure from catheterization. These are the patients who are given to the introduction of hair-pins, slate pencils, etc. etc. into the urethra.

Some authors claim that in the intense sexual excitement of hysteria the chronic erection of the clitoris makes pressure on the urethra, and so prevents the escape of urine, but this seems somewhat apocryphal.

Another class of cases resembling the hysterical in the frequency of urination are those addicted to masturbation ; these are, fortunately, not very common.

In all of these cases the frequency and irregularity of urination is a much more prominent symptom than the pain. This latter is usually a slight scalding from the urine passing over the chafed and irritable urethra, especially at the meatus. (These symptoms sometimes occur in the miasmatic affections.) A number of neuroses of the bladder are reflex and dependent on peripheral irritation elsewhere. A typical example of this class of affections is what has been described under the title of ovarian irritation. In this condition there is very much heightened reflex irritability accompanying the increased tenderness and vascular engorgement of the affected ovary. It is difficult to explain the bladder symptoms which sometimes accompany the recurring crises of this disease, except as due to a nervous excitation spreading from the ovarian centres in the spinal cord to the adjacent bladder centres.

The diagnosis of this group of affections must be made by exclusion. We have some of the same symptoms—increased frequency of micturition, pain during and after the evacuation, tenesmus and shooting pains in the pelvis—as in organic disease. The most important guide is a careful examination of the urine, which shows the absence of abnormal constituents, thereby excluding organic disease. This diagnosis will be much strengthened by a digital examination, by the vagina, of the neck of the bladder, and the passage of a urethral sound, neither causing pain, as they would do in cystitis.

The PROGNOSIS is usually good, but it depends upon the length of time the affection has lasted.

The TREATMENT is mainly tonic and nutritive. The diet should be nutritious and simple, and the bowels regulated by mild purgatives. Constitutionally, small doses of strychnine are most valuable in improving the nerve tone; so also is the constant electric current is of service. Locally, sedative suppositories in the vagina or enemata are advantageous, conium combined with belladonna or hyoscyamus seeming to act best. The liberal use of the bromides gives good results in some hysterical cases.

Paralysis of the Bladder.

This is the most grave of the functional affections, and, like paralysis elsewhere, it may be either peripheral or central. When the latter, as in certain injuries of the brain or in certain well-marked lesions of the spinal cord, it hardly calls for more than mention here. Often, however, the cause is not recognizable in any organic lesion either of the bladder-walls or the central nervous system, and is to be sought for in more temporary and transient influences; thus as a result of over-distension most frequently, of impaired or lost nerve-conduction in fevers involving serious derangements of nutrition, all of which may be described as functional or temporary paralysis.

The invasion is usually gradual, except in apoplexy or traumatism. The patients, who are usually advanced in years, first observe that the urine is expelled from the bladder with less force than usual; the stream is smaller and comes slower, and straining takes place, the aid of the abdominal muscles being invoked. After a while the stream intermits, and finally partial or complete retention occurs. Then, if this condition continues, the sphincteric resistance gives way and constant dribbling occurs. In rare instances dilatation of the bladder-walls takes place, and finally cystitis. Dilatation of the ureters and hydro-nephrosis are not uncommon under these conditions.

Where the condition of retention obtains the DIAGNOSIS ought never to be difficult; the introduction of a catheter will conclusively settle it.

The PROGNOSIS in uncomplicated paralysis is usually good. When accompanying fevers, dysentery, peritonitis, etc. it usually disappears with the original disease. When due to centric lesions the outlook is about hopeless.

In all cases the bladder should be emptied at stated intervals. If the patient cannot do this herself, the surgeon should resort to the systematic use of the clean soft Jacques catheter. A most important point, too often overlooked, is the method of emptying an over-distended bladder. It is not safe to empty the bladder at once: the patient ought to be tapped at intervals, an abdominal binder being gradually tightened meanwhile. The too sudden removal of pressure from the vesicle walls which have been rendered anæmic allows of intense congestion, and in a condition of paralysis is the sure prelude to cystitis. The diet in these cases should be generous and stimulants are not contraindicated.

I cannot agree with those authors who recommend washing out the bladder with medicated solutions and forcibly distending the urethra, nor with those who use tincture of cantharides as a vesical excitant. Both plans are apt to produce cystitis. A far more rational though somewhat impracticable treatment is the use of electricity as recommended by Winckel—one pole (thoroughly insulated up to the point) in the bladder, the other on the symphysis or loins. The sitting should last about five minutes. But by far the most valuable therapeutic agent is strychnia, which should be exhibited in full doses, many of the reported failures with this drug being due to too small doses. In urinating the upright position is generally preferable to lying down, as the pressure of the abdominal organs to some extent compensates for the lack of tonicity in the bladder-walls.

Lastly, in these hopeless cases of complete paralysis an artificial vesico-vaginal fistula and the adaptation of an apparatus to catch the urine may be of service.

Functional disorders of the bladder are frequently met with, due to abnormal constituents in the urine. As was mentioned above, these may be so grave or their irritant action continued so long as to give rise to cystitis. In the slighter forms, due to transient cause, the local trouble will speedily right itself, but in other cases, such as those dependent on functional derangements of other organs, as dyspepsia, the irritation is apt to return at varying intervals. In almost all these cases the immediate mechanism of the trouble is the presence of some urinary deposits. To this may be added the constitutional impairment, as in oxaluria, when the minute octahedral crystals are probably not more to blame for the local difficulty than the impairment of the nervous tone. Similarly, the poison of malaria and of certain of the exanthemata, and of many diseases marked by faults of assimilation and elimination, causes functional disturbance.

The prime indication in treating these cases is to render the urine more bland by dilution. For this purpose water, aided by the salts of potash and the alkaline mineral waters, is the best. This should always be given on an empty stomach, and the addition of infusion of buchu is excellent. In the condition known as oxaluria the alkaline salts are not called for, but instead thereof acids. Nitro-muriatic diluted and tincture nucis vomicæ tend to correct the faults of nutrition, and they should be largely diluted to relieve the local condition.

The last class of functional diseases are caused by lesions of position either of the bladder or of some of the neighboring organs. Here, again, we have conditions which if sufficiently prolonged may lead to organic vesical changes or may simply be temporary or intermittent. By far the greater number of these are dependent on malpositions of the uterus, which either drags or presses on the bladder. Either of these classes may be complicated with adhesions arising from a former cellulitis or pelvic peritonitis, the adhesions resulting therefrom maintaining a fixation of the pelvic organs which impairs the functions of the bladder.

Other causes of displacements are uterine and ovarian tumors, pelvic deformities, and fecal impactions of the rectum. Of the various displacements of the bladder it is needless to speak in much detail. The most important is the downward one. Various degrees of this are found up to complete cystocele, most commonly associated with prolapsus uteri. The bladder naturally sags inferiorly as age advances, and by far the most potent agent in causing this to become pathological is repeated pregnancy and injuries during labor.

It is a well-known fact that the first stage of vesicle prolapsus is apt to be marked by as great discomfort as the third, for after a while the organ seems to become accustomed to its altered relations. The treatment of this condition is difficult. The bladder should be replaced and kept there. As this usually necessitates the reposition and maintenance of the displaced uterus, it is extremely difficult, and in case of existing adhesions it is impossible. A great variety of mechanical means have been tried to furnish an artificial support to keep the parts in position. If the bladder alone is prolapsed, the pessary used for anteversion of the uterus will sometimes answer. The instruments devised by Thomas, Grailly Hewett, and myself are most commonly used.

Acute Urethritis; Inflammation of the Urethra.

This affection may be simple or gonorrhœal, and it is often difficult to tell the one from the other. There is a difference in history when we can get correct testimony from the patient. Simple urethritis usually comes on gradually, and is often preceded by symptoms of uterine or vesical disease, while gonorrhœa comes on rather abruptly, and is preceded or attended by acute vaginitis and vulvitis. The chief symptom is painful urination. Sharp scalding is produced by the urine passing over the tender surface. There is often a frequent desire to urinate, but not so urgent as in cystitis. In some cases the urine is retained for a long time, evidently from a dread of the pain caused in passing it. In quite a number of cases I have noticed hemorrhage, the source of blood being evidenced from the fact that it was not intimately mixed with the urine, and after micturition it oozed from the meatus urinarius.

An examination of the parts will show signs of inflammation about the meatus, with or without the same condition of the vulva. Occasionally there is a discharge seen coming from the urethra, but if the parts have been recently bathed this may not be apparent. Introducing the finger into the vagina and pressing upon the urethra from above downward will cause a discharge, unless the patient has passed water immediately before. The appearance of the discharge corresponds to that of gonorrhœa in its various stages.

Cystitis, which is liable to be confounded with urethritis, may be excluded by using the catheter, and, after letting urine flow for a time, collecting the remainder for examination. The mucous membrane, as seen through the endoscope, is of a deep red, with pus or mucus lodged in its folds. The instrument cannot be used in all cases, owing to the acute tenderness of the parts. Bleeding is very likely to occur in the examination, simply from the contact of the endoscope.

The TREATMENT of acute urethritis, whether specific or not, may be conducted on the same principles as that of gonorrhœa in the male, using the same constitutional remedies, local baths, etc. This will suffice in most cases of acute disease, but when it assumes the subacute form from the beginning, then the use of injections becomes necessary. I have seen much benefit derived from douching the urethra with water as hot as the patient could bear it. For this purpose I use a catheter made like the fluted roller of a crimping-machine. The catheter conveys the water to the rounded point of the instrument. Behind the point of the catheter, where the grooves terminate, there is a perforation in each groove through which the water returns. By this arrangement the water, as it flows back through the grooves, is brought in contact with every portion of the mucous membrane. The instrument is passed up to the neck of the bladder, and a fountain syringe attached to it, and the water as it flows away is caught in a cup.

The injection of solutions of nitrate of silver and sulphate of zinc will often prove useful. It must be borne in mind that the female urethra will not hold more than ten or fifteen drops, and if more is used it will enter the bladder, even where very slight force is employed while injecting. I use a large syringe, placing the nozzle over (not in) the meatus, and inject slowly and without force a small quantity. When the case is of long standing, and the neck of the bladder appears to be involved also, I use a weak injection of one or two grains of nitrate of silver to the fluidounce, and inject it through the urethra with force enough to enter the bladder, and let it remain there, to be passed off when the patient urinates. In old cases which began by a severe acute attack, and where the walls of the urethra are very much thickened and the canal contracted, dilatation with bougies does much good. While the bougie is passed once or twice a week, I apply to the vaginal portion of the urethra oleate of mercury or the unguentum hydrargyri. This will often suffice to stop the gleety discharge, as well as remove the thickening of the urethral walls.

Inflammation of the Urethral Glands.

These glands rarely, if ever, take on inflammation primarily, but vulvitis and vaginitis, especially if gonorrhœal, often extend into them. When they do become inflamed, the disease usually remains without any tendency to subside. More than that, when a gonorrhœa affects these glands the inflammation will remain there after all traces of the disease have left the vagina, vulva, and urethra, and in time the discharge from these glands will light up the original vaginitis and vulvitis again. The symptoms of this inflammation are not diagnostic. The physical signs are the swelling and redness around the mouths of ducts which are located just within the labiæ of the meatus urinarius. This give a general redness to the meatus. By pressure made upon the urethra from above downward a purulent discharge from the ducts will be produced and can be seen escaping. The only effective treatment is to lay open the glands their whole length. They run upward in the posterior wall of the urethra, so that by passing a fine probe-pointed scissors they can be laid open on the vaginal surface. Care should be taken to prevent the incision from reuniting, and if the inflammation does not promptly subside applications should be made, as in the ordinary treatment of inflammation.

Another very troublesome affection of the urethra which usually results from urethritis is granular erosion, as it is called. The mucous membrane is covered with young, imperfectly-developed epithelium ; the papillæ are hypertrophied and extremely sensitive. This gives rise to the most excruciating pain during micturition, and generally keeps up a distressing tenesmus. This disease is rarely seen except among old people. The diagnosis is made from the history and appearance of the urethra. The treatment is cauterization of the whole surface. The milder washes and injections do not accomplish much. Pure carbolic acid may be tried first, brushing it over the surface and repeating it in eight or ten days. This is the least painful application, and generally answers very well. When it fails a solution of nitrate of silver (one drachm to the fluidounce) should be used. In obstinate cases it is desirable, before using strong caustics, to dilate the urethra, and then touch it with a 50 per cent. solution of carbolic acid.

Circumscribed and Subacute Urethritis.

Among the inflammatory affections of the female urethra there are mild forms which fall short of well-marked urethritis. Indeed, some of these attacks amount to little more than congestion or slight catarrh. In others circumscribed patches of the urethra become inflamed, the rest of the canal remaining normal.

The cause of this affection is generally some inflammation of other pelvic organs, such as cellulitis. In one case it occurred in a saleswoman who had been upon her feet many days from early morning until late at night. I found several small ecchymoses on several parts of the mucous membrane with zones of inflammation around them. The long-continued passive congestion had caused some of the small vessels to rupture, and the small blood-clots started the inflammatory process.

These cases tend to recovery if the patient is placed under favorable conditions. If there is much pain, and if the trouble appears to be tending to become chronic, mild injections may be employed.

Dilatation of the Urethra.

Dilatation of the whole urethra is not so common as dilatation of a portion of it. Even when the whole canal is larger than it should be, it is not, as a rule, uniformly so. In general, the urethral walls and the urethro-vaginal septum are usually enlarged, relaxed, and flabby. After a considerable time they may become indurated by infiltration or hyperplasia of the connective tissue. The mucous membrane is usually soft and loosely adherent to the subjacent tissues. Beneath the membrane there are sometimes masses of enlarged veins which give a dark bluish appearance to the parts. If the meatus be distended like the rest of the urethra, the mucous membrane with the large veins beneath it may protrude and form a tumor or tumors, which have quite the appearance of rectal hemorrhoids. This is especially so when the veins are large and numerous and the mucous membrane thin, so that the color of the veins can be seen through it. On the other hand, if the meatus remains normal in size, nothing will be seen by the examiner until the catheter or sound is passed into the urethra, when the distended or distensible condition of the canal will be detected. The dilatation can be easily detected, even when the meatus is normal in size, by observing that the sound can be moved about in the urethra, conveying the same impression obtained when the sound passes into the bladder. By making a digital examination of the vagina the enlarged urethra can be felt, and it is usually elastic and compressible. Through Sims's speculum the abnormal fulness or bulging of the anterior vaginal wall can be plainly seen and distinguished from displacement of the urethra. The points of difference between dilatation and displacement will be brought out more in detail farther on.

When the dilatation has existed for any length of time, the mucous membrane is usually hyperæmic, and sometimes catarrhal, secreting a muco-purulent material, which may be seen escaping from the meatus or lodged in the folds of the membrane, where it can be seen through the endoscope. When the mucous membrane is prolapsed and forms a tumor outside of the meatus, it soon becomes fissured and ulcerated, and consequently very tender and painful. This condition is produced by the retarded circulation, chafing, and the irritation from exposure to the air and the urine passing over it.

Dilatation of the anterior or lower third is the rarest of all forms of urethral dilatation, and occurs usually as a consequence of some enlargement or swelling of the mucous membrane, neoplasm of the urethra, or mechanical dilatation. The dilatation may or may not include the meatus. In rare cases it does not at first, but in time the enlarged mucous membrane slowly, sometimes rapidly, dilates the orifice. The general appearances of the parts are the same as those of which I have spoken under the head of dilatation of the whole urethra. When the dilatation is due to any new growth in the urethra, the tumor can be seen on inspecting the parts.

I have only seen one case where the lower end of the urethra was dilated without any recognizable cause for it. This was a single lady, thirty-five years of age, a school-teacher. She had displacement of the uterus and catarrh of the cervical canal, for which she consulted me. She had no trouble with her urinary organs. While examining the uterus I noticed that the meatus urinarius was peculiarly formed. In place of the concentric corrugations of the mucous membrane which form the closed meatus, the orifice was funnel-shaped and lay open when the labia minora were separated. About half an inch of the lower end of the urethra admitted a No. 21 (Eng.) sound. The remainder of the urethra was normal, and there were no signs of disease about the mucous membrane of the dilated portion. I could obtain no history which pointed to the origin of the trouble, and it caused no discomfort to the patient.

Dilatation of the posterior or upper third occurs in connection with other pathological conditions, such as prolapsus of the bladder and urethra. On this account we will defer what is to be said on this subject until we come to dislocations of the urethra.

Dilatation of the middle third of the urethra is more common than that of any other portion of the canal. In this form the anterior wall of the urethra maintains its normal position, but the central position, being distended, settles down, so that in time the urethra, in place of being a straight or slightly curved canal, becomes triangular, the upper wall being the base, and the central portion of the wall (that is, midway between the neck of the bladder and the meatus) the apex. A sac or cavity is thus formed in the central portion of the urethra.

In the earlier stages of this affection the urethra in front and behind the pouch is really or apparently contracted; but as the disease progresses the upper part of the canal and the neck of the bladder become dislocated downward, and finally the upper portion of the urethra becomes also dilated to some extent.

There is in this as in the other forms of urethral dilatation frequent urination, usually more marked, but, unlike the others, there is difficulty in passing water. This frequency of urinating, and the straining efforts necessary to do so, affect the bladder, producing irritation, and in time hypertrophy of its walls. Cystitis also follows in the order of morbid developments; but whether that comes from the frequent and difficult uimation, or from extension of the inflammation from the urethra to the bladder, is a question.

ÆTIOLOGY.—The hyperæmia of the urethra which occurs in pregnancy, and which tends to produce over-distension of the veins, favors dilatation of the whole urethra. There is an apparent increase of tissue in the walls of the urethra during utero-gestation, and the dilatability of the canal is often increased also. Now, this condition of the parts disappears during the involution which takes place after delivery; but when from any cause the process of involution is interrupted, the enlarged vessels and relaxed condition of the urethral walls remain and sometimes increase. When to this state of the parts a catarrh of the mucous membrane is added, the enlargement of the membrane by swelling still further increases the calibre of the canal.

The dilatation caused by the passage of calculi may remain permanently, and the same may be said of the use of large sounds. Neoplasms obstructing the meatus or stricture at that point may so obstruct the escape of the urine as to cause dilatation at all points above. This is no doubt one of the most important and frequent causes of dilatation.

I have already stated that dilatation of the lower third of the urethra is rare, and is usually due to inflammation of the mucous membrane at that point or to abnormal growths, the distension remaining after the causes that produced it have been removed. This and mechanical dilatation from any cause cover the etiology of this form of the trouble. Baker-Brown says that the meatus is always dilated when there is stone in the bladder.

Regarding dilatation of the upper third of the urethra, I am inclined to believe that it occurs in consequence of a partial prolapsus of the bladder and the upper end of the urethra. The displacement of these parts implies a relaxation of the tissues, caused originally, it may be, by injuries during confinement, and the prolapsus permits an unusual pressure of the urine upon the upper end of the urethra, and dilatation is the result. On the other hand, the prolapsus and accompanying relaxation of the urethral walls may be sufficient to cause the dilatation. In all the cases that I have critically examined there has been displacement as well as dilatation, and the whole trouble could invariably be traced to child-bearing or anteversion of the uterus.

One cause of dilatation of the middle third of the urethra (urethrocele) has been sufficiently dwelt upon in Bozeman's description of the pathology of that affection—that is, narrowing of the lower end of the urethra. This does not explain the etiology of all cases, however, for I have seen this form of dilatation where there was no stricture or hypertrophy of the lower end of the urethra. In such cases I have traced the cause to childbirth, during which the posterior wall of the urethra had been pushed downward and contused, while the upper remained in its normal position. The relaxation caused by this over-stretching of the urethral wall formed a small pocket in the central portion, which gradually dilated more and more by the pressure of the urine until the urethrocele was fully developed. This explanation of the cause may be rather hypothetical, but, so far as my observations go, it agrees with the facts found in those cases which cannot be accounted for by Bozeman's views on the pathology of this affection.

SYMPTOMATOLOGY.—The symptoms vary according to the extent of the dilatation, the portion of the urethra involved, and the condition of the mucous membrane. When the whole urethra is dilated the only symptom present may be frequent urination. When there is inflammation or prolapsus of the mucous membrane, then pain will be caused by passing water, and the desire to do so will be more urgent and frequent. The patient may also be annoyed by a slight loss of control of the water, under the pressure of lifting heavy weights, coughing, or the like.

Dilatation of the lower third of the urethra does not cause any derangement of function, unless accompanied with inflammation or ulceration; then there will be frequent urination possibly, and painful urination certainly. The symptoms in this form of dilatation are less marked than in the other varieties.

When the trouble is located in the upper third of the urethra, the symptoms are sometimes very distressing. In addition to the frequent —it may be constant—desire to pass water, the patient is tormented with partial incontinence. Coughing, laughing, sneezing, stooping to lift anything, a jar on stepping from the curbstone in crossing the street, causes an escape of urine. This distresses the patient very greatly. From the constant wetting of the external parts they become inflamed, unless very great care is taken to keep them dry and clean. In some of these cases the mortification of mind is sometimes more distressing than the physical suffering.

The symptoms occuring in dilatation of the middle portion of the urethra are the same as those already given, with the addition of a slight mechanical obstruction which causes difficult urination; that is, more voluntary effort is necessary on the part of the patient to empty the bladder. The forcing, straining efforts made by some of these patients while urinating are even greater than the mechanical obstruction appears to account for. This may be due to the accumulation of urine in the urethra, which excites extra reflex action in the bladder and urethra out of proportion to the obstruction. This is the only way that we can account for the difficult urination and muscular hypertrophy found in those cases in which there is no great obstruction from stricture.

The constitutional symptoms arising from these urethral troubles are the same as those produced by urethritis, and are not peculiar to this class of affections. In fact, the symptoms here given may all be produced by other pathological conditions, and consequently cannot alone guide to a correct diagnosis. The true character of the trouble can only be discovered by physical exploration.

DIAGNOSIS.—A digital examination by the vagina will detect the increased space occupied by the urethra. The canal encroaches upon the anterior vaginal wall, and feels like a ridge extending from the meatus to the neck of the bladder. This elevation or thickening of the urethra is elastic and compressible in recent cases; in those of long standing the tissues are firm to the touch, but still the canal is compressible. The extent of the dilatation, if general or located in the lower parts, can be measured by the size of the sound that can be easily passed. If at the middle or upper portions, an ordinary female catheter or sound may be used to explore it. By introducing that instrument and pressing it first against the anterior wall and then upon the posterior, the distance between the two can be approximately made out. While the catheter or sound is in the urethra the finger should be introduced into the vagina to ascertain the thickness of the urethral wall. This will differentiate between dilatation and hypertrophy.

When the meatus is dilated and the mucous membrane and enlarged vessels are prolapsed, care is necessary to distinguish that condition from urethral neoplasm. This can be done by observing that in prolapsus the opening is situated either at the upper side or in the centre of the protruding mass, whereas in abnormal growths of the urethra the meatus surrounds the tumor or its pedicle. More than that, by making pressure the distended vessels can be reduced in size and the prolapsed membrane pushed up into the canal. This cannot usually be accomplished with tumors.

PROGNOSIS.—There is no natural tendency to recovery in these affections. If left alone they generally get worse. Recovery under treatment depends upon the location of the dilatation and the duration of the trouble. The conditions upon which an unfavorable prognosis is to be based are—bladder complications, inflammation or ulceration near the neck of the bladder, great varicosity of the veins, and fatty degeneration of the muscular tissue. In the absence of all these complications a complete recovery may be expected. In all cases great relief can be secured by treatment and the patient guarded from getting worse.

TREATMENT.—In the management of all forms of urethral dilatation attention should be given to any inflammation of the mucous membrane that may exist, employing the usual treatment. When there is a relaxed and prolapsed condition of the mucous membrane, astringents should be used. Tannic acid or alum will answer well. When these fail, the redundant membrane should be retrenched, either by touching it with the thermo-cautery or excising a portion with the scissors. In employing the cautery for this purpose the long pointed tip of the instrument should be used, and, having protected one side of the urethra with the speculum, cauterize a narrow strip of the membrane parallel to the axis of the canal. Two or more of these cauterizations may be made at points equidistant on the circumference of the urethra. By operating in this way pieces of normal membrane are left between the portions cauterized, which prevents stricture from occurring after healing—a misfortune which is sure to follow if the mucous membrane is destroyed by cauterization all around.

In excising the prolapsed portion I prefer to remove one or more V-shaped portions on opposite sides and bring the edges together by sutures. This is preferable to clipping off the whole of the protruding mass, because the cicatrices left are less likely to give after trouble.

When the dilatation is caused by varicose veins it may be well to follow the example of Gustave Simon. He exposed the vessels by cutting through the vaginal wall, ligated the largest, and arrested the hemorrhage from the smaller ones by applying liquor ferri perchloridi. He repeated this operation several times on the same patient, who experienced little or no inconvenience from the proceeding and made a good recovery.

Dilatation of the lower third of the urethra is usually secondary to some other trouble, as I have already stated; and all that is necessary to do for such cases is to remove the cause and treat any inflammation that may exist. The dilatation will then disappear; and if it does not, but little if any trouble will be caused by it.

The treatment of dilatation of the upper third consists simply in supporting the parts. This can be effectually done by using the pessary already recommended for the relief of prolapsus of the bladder. It may be necessary to have the instrument so formed as to bring the pressure where it is required. This is done by placing the pessary in position and observing what change of form, if any, is necessary, and then directing the instrument-maker to make the alteration. If the parts are well supported in this way, recovery will follow unless atrophy of the muscular wall has previously taken place. Even then the patient can be kept comfortable by wearing the pessary. If there is urethritis present, it may be necessary to remove that before using the pessary; otherwise the pressure of the instrument may cause pain and aggravate the inflammation.

In dilatation of the middle third Bozeman has proposed to make an opening into the most dependent part of the urethra through the vaginal wall, and maintaining it until all inflammation has been relieved, and then closing the opening by the usual plastic operation. By this means the urethra is perfectly drained of urine and the products of inflammation which accumulated there before. This, with appropriate cleansing and topical applications, soon restores the mucous membrane to its normal condition, and the removal of the redundant tissue during the operation of closing the opening effectually cures the whole trouble. This treatment is admirably adapted to marked cases of long standing, and should be employed. By using the thermo-cautery to make the opening the operation is easily performed. In recent cases of less magnitude I have obtained satisfactory results by dilating the lower part of the urethra and supporting the dilated portion either with a pessary or a tampon of marine lint. This permits the urethra to keep itself empty, and then, by frequently washing it out and applying such remedies as will cure the urethritis, recovery will sometimes follow.

Dislocations of the Urethra.

This is one of the affections most frequently met with in practice. I have found very few cases recorded in medical literature. This neglect of the subject by authors is perhaps due to the fact that in many cases of displacement of the urethra the bladder is also dislocated, and the whole trouble is described under the head of vesicocele or cystocele. Now, it is true that displacement of the two occurs together, but either may take place alone.

The extent of displacement varies exceedingly, but I shall describe only the partial and the complete. A clear comprehension of these two degrees will cover all intermediate forms. In partial displacement downward the upper two-thirds of the urethra are prolapsed, so that the direction of that portion of the canal is backward, instead of curving upward, as in the normal condition. In complete prolapsus the urethra runs from the meatus (which is in its normal position) backward, and rests upon the perineum, or in extreme cases, accompanied with prolapsus of tne bladder and uterus, its direction is backward and downward, the position of the vesical end of the urethra being below the level of the meatus. In this degree of displacement the urethra and bladder can be seen presenting at the vulva or lying between the labia minora. The urethra is usually shortened considerably when the prolapsus is marked.

ETIOLOGY.—Utero-gestation and delivery are the most important causes of this affection. In the advanced months of pregnancy I have observed that while the bladder rose above the pubes the urethra was pushed slightly downward by the settling of the enlarged uterus into the pelvis. In such cases when labor occurs the head of the child dislocates the urethra still more by pushing it still farther down. This process I have often watched in forceps delivery. When there is a partial prolapsus of the urethra existing before labor, the urethra and anterior vaginal wall are forced down before the advancing head, and that, too, while the attendant is making counter-pressure to prevent it. The displacement produced in this way is often restored during convalescence if proper care be taken to push the parts back into place and the patient is kept at rest until the tissues regain their tonicity. But in many cases the trouble is overlooked, and by permitting the patient to get up and be on her feet while there is still prolapsus it will slowly increase until the dislocation is complete. This will surely be the case if there is any loss of perineum. Indeed, rupture of the perineum is an accident which permits the urethra to descend from its place. The perineum supports the vaginal walls, which in turn support the urethra; and if it be lost, even in part, the vaginal walls become relaxed, or perhaps never regain their tonicity after delivery, and, settling down more and more, carry the urethra with them.

SYMPTOMATOLOGY.—The symptoms arising from displacement of the urethra are much the same as those found in dilatation and other urethral diseases. I need not, therefore, repeat them in detail. Suffice it to say that in dislocation of the upper portion of the canal there is, in addition to frequent urination, a partial loss of control of the bladder. Under the extra pressure of coughing, for example, the urine will escape. This loss of control does not exist, as a rule, in complete displacement. On the contrary, there is usually difficult urination, which requires increased voluntary efforts to empty the bladder. In all degrees of displacement the symptoms are increased in the erect position, and are markedly relieved on the patient's lying down.

DIAGNOSIS.—An examination of the vagina, either by touch or speculum, will reveal the downward projection of part or all of the urethra, which will show that there is either dilatation or prolapsus. The change in the direction of the canal will be shown by passing the sound, and dilatation can be excluded by observing that the urethra grasps the instrument firmly at all points. In dislocation of the upper two-thirds of the urethra the sound passes in the normal direction, but is arrested at a half or three-quarters of an inch from the meatus; but by pushing up the vaginal wall and the urethra the sound will then pass into the bladder. When the prolapsus is complete the instrument passes in easily, but takes a downward and backward direction.

PROGNOSIS.—Uncomplicated displacement of the urethra can be remedied in the great majority of cases. By placing the parts in proper position, and holding them there, the relaxed tissues will usually contract sufficiently to support themselves. Should they fail to do so, the patient can at least be made comfortable by wearing some supporter.

TREATMENT.—When the displacement of the urethra is caused by any other trouble, such as defective perineum or prolapsus uteri, then these things should first be attended to. Should there be urethritis, that also should receive appropriate treatment. But the chief indication is to retain the urethra in place ; and this can be easily accomplished by using the pessary which has been recommended for supporting the prolapsed bladder. Prolapsus of the upper part of the urethra can be relieved in this way quite satisfactorily. When the whole urethra is displaced, this pessary, while it supports the upper part, will still permit the middle portion of the urethra to settle down. This difficulty may be overcome by making the anterior portion of the pessary long enough to engage in the introitus vulvæ, and in that way keep the whole canal where it should be. Should this cause the patient much discomfort, a tampon of marine lint should be used to keep the parts in position until some restoration of the parts is obtained, and then the pessary will complete the treatment.

Prolapsus or Inversion of the Urethral Mucous Membrane.

The prolapse may be limited to one side or extend all around the canal. The size and extent of the protrusion vary considerably. If the meatus is of full size, the prolapsed portion will usually preserve its natural color for a time ; but after a little, from chafing when wet with urine, and especially if not kept clean, it will become red and œdematous. When the meatus is small these changes occur sooner and in a more marked degree, because the prolapsed portion is partially strangulated. The longer the membrane remains exposed the more sensitive it becomes, and the frequency of urination and pain attending it increase. It also becomes very tender and painful to the touch. In marked cases the ordinary movements of the body irritate the parts, and in that way render walking painful.

These are symptoms that closely resemble those of irritable growths at the meatus urinarius, and, so far as history is concerned, it is not easy to make a differential diagnosis. To do this it is necessary to make a local examination. The physical signs and the points in the diagnosis between this affection and other diseases have been given briefly but sufficiently under the head of Dilatations of the Urethra, and need not be repeated here.

The causes of prolapsus of the urethral mucous membrane are numerous, but those that are best known are long-continued congestion of the membrane, urethral and cystic irritation causing frequent urination and vesical tenesmus. Chlorotic and greatly debilitated women are said to be predisposed to it, as also old prostitutes. The few cases that I have seen were in women over fifty years of age, and all of them were weak, nervous patients who had suffered from some organic disease or functional derangement of the urinary organs.

PROGNOSIS.—This disease does not yield promptly to mild treatment, unless it is seen early in its progress; and if it does yield to mild, sooth-ing, and astringent applications, it is liable to return. But in case there is no other disease present that tends to keep it up, it can usually be cured by surgical means.

TREATMENT.—When a case is first seen it is well to remove any inflam-mation or other complicating conditions. The prolapsed membrane should be replaced, and the patient kept quiet in bed to favor the retention of the parts in situ. Astringents, such as tannic acid, alum, or persulphate of iron in a weak solution, should also be used. Should these fail, the prolapsed portion of the membrane should be removed. The methods of doing this (by excision and the thermo-cautery) have already been described.

Stricture of the Urethra.

PATHOLOGY.—Obstruction of the urethra by narrowing of its calibre is a much less common affection in the female than in the male. Still, it occurs sufficiently often to demand attention. There are some facts in the pathology of urethral stricture peculiar to women which we will first notice. Passing over congenital narrowing of the urethra by simply say-ing that such a malformation has been known, we find that stricture is developed in the female, as in the male, by the deposit of inflammatory products beneath the mucous membrane, which by gradual contraction constricts the canal. Ulceration of the membrane in a marked degree produces the same results. The inflammation and ulceration which end in the formation of stricture are usually specific in character, but the same may follow from the too free use of caustics and injuries during childbirth. Stricture may also be produced by bands of scar-tissue formed in the anterior vaginal wall and stretching across the urethra. Contrac-tion of the whole canal occasionally occurs in cases of vesico-vaginal fistula of long standing. There the narrowing is simply the result of disuse. The form of stricture that most frequently comes under observa-tion is a contraction of the meatus urinarius, produced in many cases by the too liberal use of caustics in the treatment of abnormal growths at the lower end of the urethra, or from vulvitis. This form of stricture is the least troublesome and is easily relieved. When due to the results of former urethritis or peri-urethritis, the walls of the urethra are thick-ened and indurated at the point of the stricture, and there is usually sub-acute urethritis, sometimes ulceration. In those cases where the calibre of the canal is diminished by cicatrices of the vaginal walls, and in general contraction of the urethra in vesico-vaginal fistula of long stand-ing, the mucous membrane may be perfectly normal.

SYMPTOMATOLOGY.—Frequent and difficult urination are the chief troubles caused by stricture of the urethra. The stream becomes smaller, and may be twisted or flat, but this is rarely observed. Patients, as a rule, only notice that they require to urinate more frequently, and that they have to make more voluntary efforts to empty the bladder than were necessary before. In almost all cases of stricture the subject has at some previous time suffered an injury at childbirth, urethritis, or some-thing to which the origin of the stricture can be traced. The previous history of cases in which stricture is suspected will aid in settling the diagnosis and etiology.

DIAGNOSIS.—A digital examination by the vagina will reveal thickening and induration if the stricture is due to that cause. Cicatrices of the vaginal wall compressing the urethra can be detected in the same way. The use of the sound will determine the location of the stricture and the extent to which the canal is contracted. When the stricture is at the meatus it can be found with facility; but when it is located higher up the largest sound that can be introduced without force should be passed up to the point of stricture. This will localize it; then by using a sound that will pass through it the extent of the constriction will thus be ascertained.

The affections which are liable to be mistaken for stricture are retention of urine or difficult urination from pressure on the urethra by the displaced gravid uterus, pelvic tumors, and dislocations of the urethra. The former can be excluded by a vaginal examination, and the latter can also be detected by the sound, used as directed while discussing the diagnosis of the dilatations.

PROGNOSIS.—Stricture of the urethra usually yields very promptly to treatment, so that the prognosis is good. The only exceptions are where the stricture has existed in a marked degree long enough to cause dilatation of the ureters and disease of the kidneys. Chronic cystitis or urethritis, occurring as a result of the stricture or coincident with it, may so complicate matters as to make recovery slow or even impossible. In cases where the whole urethra is contracted because of the existence of a vesico-vaginal fistula of long standing, it is extremely difficult to restore the tissues of the urethral walls to their normal state.

TREATMENT.—The treatment of stricture will depend upon its location and cause. If it is situated at the meatus, it can be divided by the urethrotome or forcibly stretched with the dilator. When due to bands of scar-tissue in the vagina, they should be divided at several points and the urethra dilated by repeatedly passing the sound. When it is owing to deposition of the products of inflammation in the submucous tissue, forcible and rapid dilatation, as practised on the male subject, will answer well if the proper cases are selected for this form of treatment. Dilatation should be made carefully, with a view to breaking up the constricting tissue without lacerating the mucous membrane. To do this it is not necessary to dilate the urethra to any great extent. As soon as the stricture has given way dilatation should be suspended.

Incising the stricture from within outward, according to the method commended by surgeons for the cure of stricture in the male, will no doubt answer a good purpose. In fact, I am inclined to believe that this plan of treating this affection is the best, but my own experience with this operation on the female urethra is not sufficient to warrant my speaking positively.

In contraction of the whole urethra arising from disuse in cases of vesico-vaginal fistula gradual dilatation with graduated sounds answers very well. This should be attended to before closing the opening in the bladder. In all cases attention should be given to any inflammation that may accompany the stricture or follow the treatment. It is well also to keep such patients under observation, and pass the sound from time to time to see if there is any tendency of the stricture to return. The brilliant results obtained in the treatment of stricture in the male with electrolysis by Robert Newman should warrant a more extended trial of this method.

Stricture at the Junction of the Urethra and Bladder.

This form or location of stricture is, so far as I know, peculiar to women, and its influence on the function of the bladder has not been clearly pointed out. In fact, no distinction has been made between the pathology or clinical history of stricture at the upper end of the urethra and elsewhere in the canal. At least, I am not aware that writers on this subject have mentioned this form of stricture. My own observations have been limited, but sufficient, I think, to warrant me in saying that stricture does occur at the junction of the bladder and urethra, and that it behaves differently from ordinary stricture at other parts of the canal.

The causes are the same which give rise to stricture elsewhere; hence nothing requires to be said on this point. The point of most importance is the fact that stricture at this part of the urethra will cause difficult urination out of proportion to the extent of the narrowing of the canal. Contraction of the canal in a slight degree will cause great difficulty in urination, and frequently retention. This is contrary to the history of stricture of the urethra at other points. In such cases there is no retention of urine until the stricture closes the canal, or very nearly so; but I have seen retention in cases of stricture at the neck of the bladder while a medium-sized catheter could be passed with ease, thus showing that the narrowing of the canal was not alone the cause of the deranged function. It is possible that the original stricture causes spasmodic contraction, or in some way disturbs the normal action of that portion of the canal which performs the function of a sphincter vesicæ.

The symptoms presented in this form of stricture are difficult urination and in some cases complete retention. I have also noticed, in one case, that there was a frequent desire to urinate, but that was accounted for by a slight catarrh of the bladder. These symptoms are such as occur in other conditions, such as atrophy and paralysis of the bladder, obstruction of the urethra from tumors, calculi, the pressure of the displaced uterus, and prolapsus of the bladder.

In this form of stricture there are thickening and induration of the neck of the bladder, which may be detected by digital examination of the vagina. The sound will also reveal a narrowing of the canal at the vesical neck, but the contraction may not be marked. Our main reliance must be placed upon the exclusion of all other conditions which can produce the same symptoms. Pressure upon the urethra and prolapsus of the bladder can be excluded by an examination of the pelvic organs, and the use of the sound will show anything like complete obstruction of the canal.

Having excluded the possible existence of either of these conditions, the only two affections which are to be confounded with this form of stricture are atrophy and paralysis of the bladder. To distinguish these from the stricture, the catheter should be passed when the bladder is well distended, and the character of the flow of urine watched, when it will be observed that in stricture the urine comes away with the usual force. The bladder contracts normally and with its natural vigor, and sends the urine out in a well-sustained stream through the catheter, if there is only stricture. On the other hand, in paralysis and atrophy the stream is slow and without force—so much so that voluntary effort or the pressure of the hand on the abdomen is sometimes necessary to empty the bladder. This is especially so when the catheter is used while the patient is in the recumbent position. Finally, the diagnosis may be confirmed by testing the dilatability of the urethra. This can be done by passing a dilator along the urethra and gently testing the resistance of the walls of the canal. There is a slight yielding at all points except at the stricture, where a decided resistance is met.

Regarding the management of stricture at the junction of the urethra and bladder, I am obliged to say that my experience has not yet been sufficient to enable me to speak definitely. Rapid and free dilatation is not sufficient to effect a cure; at least it has failed in one case. Division of the stricture by incision suggests itself, but I am confident that that operation would be unsatisfactory, because of the great irritation which always occurs when there is a solution of continuity at this point. My practice, therefore, has been to produce slow and gradual dilatation by the use of graduated sounds, and the application of oleate of mercury or iodine to the anterior vaginal wall at the site of the stricture. More extended observation may develop other and better methods of treatment, but for the present that is all that I have to offer on this subject.

DISEASES OF THE VAGINA AND VULVA.

By EDWARD W. JENKS, M. D., LL.D.

DISEASES OF THE VAGINA.

THE subject will be considered in the following order: Anatomy, Vaginitis, Atresia, Prolapsus Vaginæ, Cicatrices, Double Vagina, Growths, and Vaginismus.

Anatomy.

The vagina is a musculo-membranous canal extending from the neck of the uterus—which it embraces—to the vulva. It is usually attached to the uterine neck at a point midway between the os internum and the os externum. This canal is composed of three layers or coats: the outer one is of fibrous and elastic tissue; the middle, of unstriped muscular fibre and fibre-cell; the inner coat or lining is mucous membrane, composed of connective tissue and elastic fibre and covered with squamous epithelium. The outer and middle coats spread out at the upper portion of the perineum, making the perineal septum, and attach themselves to the ischio-pubic rami. One of the peculiarities of the middle coat is that during utero-gestation it becomes much hypertrophied like the same structure in the uterus, and following labor undergoes a similar process of involution. The inner or lining coat extends to the fourchette.

Savage[1] has described the general form of the vagina as similar to that which would be assumed by a flexible tube if shortened to nearly half its length by a cord passed from end to end through one of its sides. The ridge thus formed is called the anterior column of the vagina, and marks the vesico-vaginal septum; it is about two inches long, while the posterior wall or posterior column is twice that length. The anterior column or cord causes the investing mucous membrane to be puckered and thrown into folds or rugæ which run transversely toward the posterior column. "This mucous membrane is studded with papillæ which are covered with pavement epithelium. The papillæ of the vagina, which were first fully described by Franz Kilian, were regarded by him as having for their function the transmission of sensation. He represents them as being thread-like and filiform."[2]

Anatomists have differed regarding the existence of muciparous glands

---

[1] *Anatomy of the Female Pelvic Organs*, London, 1870.
[2] Thomas on *Diseases of Women* Phila., 1880.

in the folds of the vaginal mucous membrane, some asserting that they are present, and others being equally positive that there are none. Notwithstanding this lack of uniformity, the fact that some have discovered muciparous follicles, while others have failed, enables recent writers to state that there is no doubt of their existence.

The vagina is lined with mucous membrane and covered with pavement epithelium, studded with projecting filiform papillæ. This membrane lies in folds, between which are numerous muciparous follicles.

Vaginitis.

DEFINITION.—Vaginitis is a term used to designate inflammation of the mucous membrane of the vagina.

SYNONYMS.—Colpitis, Elythritis.

VARIETIES.—Three distinct varieties of vaginitis are met with—viz. simple, specific, and granular.

ETIOLOGY.—Predisposing Causes.—Young girls are not unfrequently the subjects of vaginitis in consequence of want of cleanliness, exposure to cold, ascarides migrating from the rectum into the vagina, or the introduction of foreign substances. It also frequently appears in consequence of smallpox, measles, and scarlatina. In adults it may be caused by exposure to cold or wet, more particularly at or near a menstrual period. The insertion of a sponge into the vagina, as is not uncommon for the purpose of topical medication or uterine support, acts as an irritant if allowed to remain a few days, which may cause severe inflammation. Pessaries, irritating vaginal injections, gonorrhœal infection, certain conditions of the urine, as in diabetes, acrid uterine discharges, childbirth—more particularly if there has been retention of putrefying secretions—and chemical agents used in treatment of uterine diseases, are sometimes causes. Uterine discharges which cause vaginitis are not generally irritating until they reach the vulva, where by exposure to the air they become changed, first causing vulvitis, and next inflammation of the vaginal mucous membrane.

Some women have slight attacks of vaginitis after each menstrual period, but they are generally slight and soon subside; others will have attacks after each coition or after great physical exertion, but with such patients the disease is not severe, and usually passes off without any signs remaining. It is quite common among prostitutes, independent of specific causes, in consequence of excessive coition. Chronic vaginitis or vaginal leucorrhœa is not uncommon with newly-married women in consequence of excess or awkwardness in coition.

Granular vaginitis is generally caused by pregnancy, but occasionally it seems to be produced by simple or specific vaginal inflammation. A strumous diathesis or a disordered state of the blood, as in phthisis or other constitutional disorders, are predisposing causes.

Mention has been made by some writers of diphtheritic and senile vaginitis. Diphtheritic inflammation of the vagina is sometimes seen during epidemics of the disease or among puerperal women in crowded lying-in hospitals. Senile vaginitis is occasionally met with in women after the climacteric period. Its cause is wholly in consequence of the physiological retrogressive processes incident to the change of life. The epithelium is shed in patches, and, according to Hildebrandt, the raw surfaces adhere, causing contraction of the vagina.

SYMPTOMATOLOGY, COURSE, DURATION, PATHOLOGY, TERMINATIONS, AND COMPLICATIONS.—The subjective symptoms of the three varieties of vaginitis which have been mentioned are nearly identical, but in their physical signs a marked difference is perceptible. In the outset there is a sense of heat and burning in the vagina, a feeling of pain and weight in the perineum, and a frequent desire to urinate. The passage of urine causes pain and a feeling of scalding in the urethra. It is believed by many authorities that the sense of scalding is more pronounced in the specific variety. Not unfrequently there are backache and pain radiating down the thighs into the hips, along the spine, and into the head. Sometimes, with the other symptoms mentioned, there will be a decided febrile disturbance, chilliness alternating with heat, a rapid pulse, and a foul tongue. With such symptoms the thermometer will show an elevated temperature. Coincident with the beginning of pain and irritation the patient has an itching sensation, which sometimes becomes intolerable, and is generally worse at night when she is warm in bed. Emmet states that some cases are so severe as to require anæsthetics before relief can be obtained. After the lapse of from twenty-four to seventy-two hours these symptoms subside, and there is a profuse purulent discharge, yellowish or greenish in appearance and of an offensive odor. In many cases the discharge is of so acrid a character that it excoriates the vulva and surrounding parts. Walking, or even standing, is often painful, particularly the former, owing to the attrition of the inflamed or excoriated surfaces.

A physical examination causes pain, and if the inflammation has extended to the vulva, urethra, or the vulvo-vaginal glands, it will often produce intense suffering. When the vaginitis is acute, the labia are swollen, the vagina assumes a more or less intense red color in place of the light or pale rose-color of health ; it will also be swollen, and at the beginning seem unnaturally dry, but very soon, although still red, it will be covered with a yellowish or greenish-yellow, muco-purulent discharge of an offensive odor. By careful examination with the speculum the vaginal canal will be seen to have a congested appearance, with abraded points, and sometimes follicular ulceration will be found. Generally, the appearance of thick mucus within the os uteri indicates an extension of the inflammatory process into the cervical canal.

Sometimes in gonorrhœal vaginitis the full force of the disease seems to be chiefly expended in the urethra ; when this is the case, and patients complain of intense scalding in passing urine, a finger pressed against the anterior vaginal wall will usually cause pus to exude from the urethral canal.

The duration of vaginitis depends largely upon the treatment. If appropriate treatment is begun early in the course of the disease, a cure can be effected in two or three weeks. On the other hand, it may continue an indefinite length of time or assume a chronic form, constituting a catarrhal condition of the vaginal mucous membrane, or vaginal leucorrhœa.

Sometimes inflammation of the lining of the vagina, more especially specific vaginitis, extends beyond the cervix into the cavity of the uterus.

along the Fallopian tubes to the ovaries and to the pelvic peritoneum, or it may travel along the mucous membrane until it reaches the lining of the bladder, causing a cystitis, or in a similar manner involve the vulvo-vaginal glands.

It is not unusual after all the signs of a vaginitis have entirely disappeared that the inflammation recurs without any apparent exciting cause, but wholly in consequence of a diseased condition of the mucous lining of the cervix uteri, designated cervical endometritis, chronic inflammation, or uterine catarrh. In consequence of this there is an increased and changed secretion, which acts as an irritant and causes vaginitis. These recurrent attacks of vaginitis can be prevented only by a successful treatment of the cervical disease.

Chronic vaginitis or vaginal catarrh occurs after repeated attacks of the acute form in persons of a strumous diathesis, and from uterine disorders, such as catarrh, displacements, or polypi of the uterus.

Vaginal catarrh from any cause may lead to other difficulties; thus, if it is the primary affection it may lead to catarrh of the uterus and of the Fallopian tubes. Its long continuance with or without the co-existence of uterine disorders may lead to relaxation and subsequent prolapsus of the vaginal walls.

In the beginning of vaginitis, as in inflammations of mucous membranes elsewhere, the vaginal lining becomes first very vascular, presenting a congested and swollen appearance, with a diminution in the quantity of normal secretion; but within a few days portions of the epithelium are cast off, leaving abraded spots which sometimes ulcerate and become covered with exudation. Occasionally complete casts of the epithelial lining of the vagina are desquamated. In lieu of the natural secretions, within thirty-six hours after the inception of the disease the vagina is filled with an acrid, foul-smelling muco- or sero-purulent fluid, having the appearance of unhealthy pus. The discharge consists of serum, numerous epithelium cells, pus-corpuscles, blood-globules, and infusorial animalculæ designated Trichomanas vaginalis, and mucus. When an attack is very severe a true phlegmonous inflammation is often developed in consequence of the submucous cellular tissue first becoming involved.

In specific vaginitis it not infrequently occurs that the disease is confined to the vaginal cul-de-sac—a fact which, according to Guérin,[1] explains how sometimes apparently healthy women communicate gonorrhœa to the male.

In granular vaginitis the mucous membrane extending throughout the entire canal and over the neck of the uterus is covered with numerous minute elevations or granulations of about the size and shape of half a millet-seed. Thomas says: "This variety of the disease appears to bear about the same relation to simple vaginitis that follicular vulvitis does to the purulent form of that affection."[2] The same author mentions having seen a patient with granular vaginitis so striking in its features that the family physician believed it to be malignant disease developing, until convinced to the contrary.

Simple acute vaginitis frequently causes and remains associated with

[1] *Mal. des Organes génitaux*, Paris, 1864.
[2] Thomas on *Diseases of Women*, 5th ed., p. 219.

vulvitis, urethritis, and less frequently endometritis, salpingitis, and pelvic peritonitis. The chronic form is not unfrequently complicated with uterine catarrh. Acute specific vaginitis is often complicated with buboes from inflammation of the femoral and inguinal glands and inflammation and abscess of the vulvo-vaginal glands. This variety more frequently than the others is liable to give rise to violent urethritis, cystitis, salpingitis, ovaritis, and pelvic peritonitis.

DIAGNOSIS.—If one is familiar with the symptoms which have been mentioned, the diagnosis of vaginitis is not a difficult task; but it is sometimes not only difficult, but quite impossible, to determine whether a case is one of simple inflammation or of gonorrhœal contagion.

The symptoms which are most liable to lead one to decide that a case is specific are their severity, the sudden development of virulency, the scalding micturition, urethritis with pus in the urethra, the greenish-yellow discharge of a foul odor, the very irritating quality of this causing gonorrhœal ophthalmia if applied to the conjunctiva or gonorrhœa in the male following coition; the occurrence of buboes, inflammation of the vulvo-vaginal glands, peritonitis, and salpingitis. We meet with cases where it is extremely difficult to decide as to the nature of the disease, and especially when we have every reason for believing that the subject herself is chaste; on the other hand, the mere fact of a woman infecting her husband and causing him to have a urethral discharge is not always sufficient proof of her having gonorrhœa, as it is well established that certain forms of leucorrhœa will produce such a result. It is not necessary for us always to express an opinion of the character of the disease, even when convinced that it is specific, but it is always our duty "to lean to the side of charity when the question is one of chastity."[1]

PROGNOSIS.—If appropriate treatment is instituted, the disease will usually subside in the course of a few weeks, or it will assume a chronic form, lasting indefinitely.

Acute vaginitis causes more pain and actual suffering than the chronic variety, but is less rebellious to means of cure. Simple vaginitis, of itself, cannot be considered a grave disease, but the consequences may prove of a most serious character—viz. extension of the inflammation to the bladder, uterus, Fallopian tubes, ovaries, and peritoneum.

Specific vaginitis is more virulent than the other varieties, and consequently there is more tendency to the extension of inflammation than with them. Sterility is not infrequently a sequel of specific vaginitis in consequence of contiguous parts, more especially the Fallopian tubes, being implicated in the disease. Such patients, even long after the acute symptoms have passed, are unfavorable subjects for surgical operations, even of a trivial character.

TREATMENT.—The treatment of acute vaginitis is the same in the different varieties. From the commencement of the attack until the severest symptoms have subsided patients should rest in a recumbent position, walking and coition being forbidden. If the inflammation is severe, with febrile symptoms and a furred tongue, saline laxatives, cooling drinks, and a non-stimulating diet should be prescribed. If pain exists, anodynes of some kind should be given. The best mode of administering

---

[1] Edis, *Diseases of Women*, Philada., 1882.

anodynes is by means of rectal suppositories. Warm hip-baths every six or eight hours for the first twenty-four hours of the disease ought to be employed, and at the same time quite warm water should be thrown into the vagina with a syringe; this is beneficial in curing the disease and contributing to the patient's comfort.

A much better mode of irrigating the inflamed parts is as follows: The patient is to be placed on her back with her hips slightly elevated over a bed-pan, and then by means of a syringe a stream of warm or hot water should be thrown into the vagina for fifteen to thirty minutes. It has been advised by Emmet that the temperature of the water should be raised rapidly from blood-heat to 110° F., or as hot as the patient can well bear. By elevating the hips venous congestion is considerably lessened through gravitation of the blood, and, the hot water causing contraction of the blood-vessels, the mucous membrane will present a blanched appearance. The vagina becomes distended by the weight of water, and somewhat with air, by reason of position, so that with the hips elevated the injection comes in contact with every portion of the vaginal mucous membrane.

In addition to hot water or after its use, other injections are useful, as a decoction of flaxseed alone, or one of the following remedies, either in the decoction of flaxseed or in water: viz. borax, bicarbonate of sodium, hyposulphite of sodium, chlorate of potassium (3j ad Oj), or permanganate of potassium (gr. viij ad Oj). Hydrate of chloral and fluid extract of eucalyptus, either alone or combined, have proved useful quite a number of times in my own practice.

Mild attacks will usually subside in a few days without further treatment than has already been mentioned; but in severe cases, when the disease has got under full headway before treatment is begun, more heroic measures become necessary, especially in specific or granular vaginitis, where there is itching and a greenish offensive discharge. The vagina should be exposed by means of a speculum, the mucous membrane thoroughly dried by the use of absorbent cotton, and a solution of nitrate of silver (gr. xl ad f3j) be applied to every part of the inflamed vagina. Wherever it is applied the mucous membrane presents a whitened appearance. If the vulva is involved, the same application should be made to it. After the parts thus treated become dry a piece of soft linen or a small roll of absorbent cotton should be thoroughly smeared with vaseline or soaked with carbolized glycerin, and inserted within the vagina. The pain caused by the nitrate of silver is usually better borne than the intense itching which it takes the place of. After the lapse of eighteen to twenty-four hours the linen or cotton can be removed and an injection of carbolic acid 3ss, sulphate of zinc and borax each 3j, in a quart of warm water, is to be used three times a day for two or three days; then a weaker solution of nitrate of silver is applied and the tampon inserted as before. This is to be followed the next day by the carbolized injection, and three days later a weaker solution of nitrate of silver is applied. The alternate use of these remedies is to be continued until the mucous membrane appears pale, and the discharge instead of being a greenish-yellow is white, when it should be discontinued, and borax alone or combined with hyposulphite of sodium is to be used as an injection; and immediately after the injection the tampon is inserted, or instead of the injection tannin dissolved in glycerin is to be painted over the vaginal walls and followed by the tampon.

The cure of vaginitis in many instances is obtained by securing rest to the parts. One of the chief objects of the tampon is to give rest to the inflamed walls by keeping them apart, rather than to make it the medium of a topical application. Some gynecologists instead of using a tampon insert one of Sims's glass vaginal dilators to keep the walls from coming in contact, directing that it shall be worn most of the time and that the patient shall rest in the recumbent posture.

The treatment of chronic vaginitis or vaginal leucorrhœa, when caused by acute vaginitis alone, should be essentially the same as in the latter after the severest symptoms have subsided, as clinically the distinction between acute and chronic vaginitis is one of degree.

Generally, vaginal leucorrhœa is an accompaniment of other affections, notably uterine diseases, and hence a consideration of its treatment and its complications would necessarily include everything pertaining to the therapeutics of leucorrhœa.

Atresia.

DEFINITION.—The term atresia ($\dot{a}$ privative, and $\tau\rho\tilde{\eta}\sigma\iota\varsigma$, perforation) means, in its literal sense, an imperforate condition or an entire absence of an orifice or a canal, but custom has sanctioned a more liberal use of the word; thus, atresia is the term sometimes made use of to designate a partial obliteration of a canal; *e. g.* atresia vaginæ, which means literally an absence or obliteration of the vagina, is also applied to a partial imperforation of the canal; hence atresia of the vagina, like that of any other portion of the generative passages, may be either complete or incomplete.

Atresia of the vulva cannot in a strict sense be considered under the head of vaginal malformations or disease, but it seems quite necessary in writing of occlusion of the vagina not to omit a consideration of similar conditions of the vulva. The writer of this article, therefore, has followed the lead of most medical authors in including vulvar under the head of vaginal atresia.

Atresia Vulvæ.

The labia majora may be adherent, and for a long time no suspicion arise of the condition, as such adhesion does not prevent the exit of menstrual blood; but, on the other hand, it does sometimes interfere with micturition, and then calculi are formed, which require surgical interference for their removal. The adhesion of the labia minora, like the same condition of the greater lips, is usually the result of accident or disease, giving rise to the same difficulties in voiding urine. Unlike adhesion of the labia majora, adhesion of the lesser lips may cause retention and accumulation of the menstrual blood. Atresia of either the greater or lesser lips may be consequent upon smallpox, measles, scarlatina, or any constitutional or local disorder that can cause inflammation of these mucous surfaces. Such occurrences are, without doubt, more common in infancy and childhood. This affection is occasionally found to be congenital, and is due to a simple agglutination of the contiguous mucous surfaces of the labia. The nurse in washing the child sometimes discovers that the vulvar orifice is closed, and it is thus brought to the notice of the physician.

Atresia Hymenalis, or Imperforate Hymen.

Although included under the head of Vulvar Atresia, this will be considered chiefly in connection with atresia of the vagina. This is a congenital condition of more frequent occurrence than the other forms of vulvar atresia.

SYMPTOMS.—If the age of puberty has been attained and the subject has all the symptoms of menstruation excepting the characteristic sanguineous flow, an imperforate condition of the genital canal is suspected. Monthly pain of a bearing-down character in the hypogastric region, and pain in the back and thighs or uterine colic, are among the symptoms. At such times the abdomen may become tender and tympanitic, the pulse more frequent, and slight febrile reaction with nausea and vomiting may occur.

These symptoms closely resemble those of an attack of peritonitis, but usually, after a few days of great distress, they gradually disappear. After a lapse of three or four weeks they again return with increased severity. The girl's general health is impaired, the appetite is poor, there is constant nausea and sometimes vomiting, the bowels are constipated, the eyes lose their brilliancy, the skin presents a dirty appearance and is often covered with an eruption. Headache is almost constant. The abdomen is often very prominent from intestinal tympanitis. Later the lower extremities become œdematous, and there are indications of septicæmia, and great constitutional disturbance. The gradual accumulation of menstrual fluid, first filling and then distending the uterus and vagina, causes a gradual enlargement of the abdomen, often giving rise to a suspicion of pregnancy.

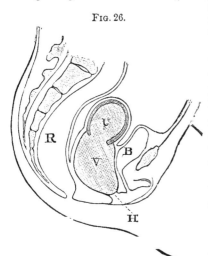

FIG. 26.

Hæmatometra.—Imperforate Hymen, causing distension of uterus and vagina: H, Hymen; V, Vagina; U, Uterus; B, Bladder; R, Rectum.

DIAGNOSIS.—If there is an accumulation of menstrual fluid in consequence of an imperforate hymen, the latter can be observed as an elastic tumor of a red color protruding outwardly between the labia. A rectal examination is necessary in order to complete the diagnosis, as by this means the presence of menstrual fluid is determined, for if it be present in sufficient quantity to distend the hymen a finger in the rectum can detect fluctuation in the vagina.

If there is no escape of the menstrual fluid beyond the vulva on account of an imperforate hymen, the vagina first becomes gradually distended, then the uterus, and finally the Fallopian tubes. As this distension increases, fluid may be forced beyond the fimbriæ of the tubes into the peritoneal cavity, or, instead, one of the tubes may rupture from the pressure within. In other instances the uterus itself ruptures from over-distension and thinning of its walls. Cases are on record where, the accumulation increasing for years, the uterus has become distended to the size attained in the latter months of pregnancy; under such circumstances its walls as well as the walls of the Fallopian tubes become thinned.

PROGNOSIS.—The physician should be careful and guarded in his prognosis. The health may become much impaired, and sometimes this is the case prior to the cause being ascertained. The chief dangers are in connection with the accumulation of menstrual fluid, such as its discharge at the fimbriated extremity of the tubes, or rupture of the tubes or uterus, and consequent escape of the fluid into the peritoneal cavity. There is also great danger in incising the hymen to permit the exit of the fluid, as will be shown under the head of Treatment. Therefore the longer has been the retention, the greater is the liability of rupture and danger in treatment.

TREATMENT.—As this is of necessity surgical, but brief allusion will be made to it. A simple incision of the hymen will permit the escape of the fluid, but the admission of air by this means is liable to cause sudden contraction of the uterus and a reflex escape of the fluid at the fimbriated extremity of the Fallopian tubes, with all the severe consequences of an intra-peritoneal hemorrhage.

The admission of air is liable to cause decomposition of retained fluid, and this in time produces septicæmia. Further, the sudden admission of air where there has been none before is liable to cause inflammation of the lining membrane of the uterus and tubes, resulting in septic peritonitis. To avoid such risks as have been enumerated two plans are recommended by authors—one being a slow draining away of the menstrual fluid and the other its rapid evacuation and washing out of the uterus and vagina. Graily Hewitt makes an opening of a valvular character in the hymen, permitting only a slow escape of the fluid. Others use a small trocar and draw off the fluid slowly, and at different times if there is a large quantity.

The aspirator is to be preferred to the trocar for emptying the vagina, and of late years has been more generally used; either instrument, but especially the former, permits of the discharge of the fluid at different times, and in such quantities as the physician may desire, without the admission of air. The rapid evacuation is best represented by Emmet's mode of procedure. He first cuts the protruding membrane sufficiently to admit the index finger, and tears the tissues enough to allow the fluid to escape rapidly, and then washes out the vagina and uterus with warm water, after which he introduces a glass plug for the purpose of dilatation and to prevent the action of air upon the parts.

Atresia Vaginæ.

Atresia of the vagina may be congenital or accidental, and, like atresia of any other portion of the genital canal, may be partial or complete. In complete congenital atresia of the vagina an examination per rectum with the index finger fails to discover the fluctuation of menstrual fluid, as in atresia from imperforate hymen, but in its place can usually be felt what seems like a hard fibrous cord. If, however, this cannot be discovered, no doubt remains of entire absence of the vagina. Sometimes the cord can be felt a portion of the distance, which indicates that there is a corsponding portion of an undilated vagina.

In case of complete congenital atresia of the vagina an operation should be avoided, unless there is an accumulation of menstrual fluid or a uterus can be distinctly felt by rectal and vesical examination, or the patient is suffering from the absence of menstruation. To these may possibly be added instances, as mentioned by Thomas, where there exists an imperative necessity for sexual intercourse. Where there is no menstrual molimen or distension of the uterus cannot be detected, and there is non-development of the uterus and ovaries, as shown by the condition of the external organs, surgical interference should be indefinitely postponed.

Accidental atresia of the vagina may be produced by causes heretofore mentioned. When the canal, which has previously been pervious, is entirely obliterated from any cause, an operation becomes, as a rule, an imperative necessity by reason of the accumulation of menstrual fluid and consequent distension of the uterus and Fallopian tubes.

In partial or incomplete atresia it frequently happens that a sinuous canal remains which serves as a guide to the surgeon.

The reader is referred to systematic treatises on surgical diseases of women for the details of the various modes of operating for these affections.

Prolapsus Vaginæ.

Displacements of the vagina are usually secondary, either in consequence of relaxation of the walls or of some form of uterine displacement. P olapsus of the vagina is usually associated with prolapsus of the uterus, yet it may exist independently. It may be present for some time without prolapse of the uterus, or exceptionally it may be the exciting cause.

DEFINITION.—When the tonicity of the vaginal walls is from any cause impaired and they protrude downward in the direction of the vulva, the condition is called prolapsus.

SYNONYMS AND CLASSIFICATION.—Owing to the anatomical arrangement, it is impossible, with one exception, for any form of prolapsus of the vagina to occur without the coincident prolapse of some viscera. The single exception is the rare occurrence of prolapsus of the posterior wall without the rectum being similarly displaced. These displacements of the viscera with prolapsus of the vagina are commonly described by medical writers as vaginal herniæ, of which there are three different forms, as follows: cystocele vaginalis, rectocele vaginalis, and enterocele vaginalis or hernia vaginalis posterior.

ETIOLOGY.—The causes of displacements of the vagina and the different varieties of vaginal herniæ can very properly be considered together, as they are identical. Laceration of the perineum, an enfeebled condition of the vaginal structure, and a retarded involution of the vagina and uterus in consequence of pregnancy or childbirth are the most frequent causes. Other occasional causes may be mentioned, as former distension of the vagina from repeated childbirths or by tumors, and senile atrophy. .

PATHOLOGY.—Following childbirth, the vagina, like the uterus, undergoes a process of involution, but if this is retarded from any cause the vagina is rendered more capacious, its tonicity is impaired, and the uterus, being heavy, crowds down upon it and causes it to be displaced. If the vaginal sphincters or the posterior wall are torn or enfeebled or the perineum lacerated, in addition to the presence of a heavy uterus, prolapsus of the vagina, associated with some form of vaginal hernia, is quite sure to follow.

There is a condition which acts as a common cause in producing vaginal and uterine displacements that has failed to receive on the part of medical authors the notice it deserves—namely, a relaxed condition of the vaginal walls and the perineum, in which there may be observed, in many instances, all of the disturbances caused by a laceration, and yet a careful examination fails to reveal where any tearing has taken place. The continuance of this excessive relaxation and atony of the vaginal walls and the perineum for a long time after parturition is, doubtless, due to subinvolution.

SYMPTOMATOLOGY AND COURSE.—The patient will complain of a bearing-down sensation in the vagina, with a sense of fulness and heat in that locality, sometimes extending to the vulva. These symptoms are aggravated by any muscular exertion, particularly by walking. A physical examination will show the presence of an elastic, globular tumor between the labia. In case it protrudes beyond the vulva, it is not unusual to find scattered over its mucous surface excoriated patches of various sizes. Sometimes these become ulcerated. In other instances the tumor has a smooth, shining appearance. Where there is simply prolapsus of the vagina without the coexistence of a hernia, it will, as a rule, be found that it is the posterior wall. If there is a prolapsus of either the anterior or posterior wall with a hernia, there will be additional symptoms to those above mentioned, which will be referred to in connection with cystocele and rectocele.

Cystocele Vaginalis, or Cysto-Vaginal Hernia.

This is sometimes designated as prolapsus of the bladder, and consists of a descent of the bladder and the anterior wall of the vagina, the two being closely adherent to each other. In consequence of such a descent a pouch is formed which becomes filled with urine. The pouch is in the outset quite small, but gradually becomes larger, so that it is not unusual for one to become of sufficient size to protrude beyond the vulva. In consequence of the pouching of the bladder only a portion of the urine is evacuated by the effort of micturition, and, remaining in the bladder, it decomposes, causing cystitis or vesical catarrh.

The SYMPTOMS are a frequent desire to urinate, with tenesmus and scalding; there is also a sense of heat and pain in the bladder. There is usually more or less ropy mucus discharged with the urine. If a uterine sound or catheter is passed into the bladder with its point downward, and can be felt protruding into the pouch, there remains no doubt as to the case being one of cystocele vaginalis.

Rectocele Vaginalis, or Recto-Vaginal Hernia.

This consists in a protrusion inward of the posterior vaginal wall and a pouch of the rectum, which is carried with it. The tendency to rectocele is seen in the natural bulging of the rectum caused by its expansion just above the sphincter ani. This is more readily perceptible in cases where the perineum has been torn. If from perineal laceration or any cause the posterior wall of the vagina fails to give adequate support to the anterior wall of the rectum, the bulging just mentioned increases, forming a pouch which becomes filled with fecal matter. The bowel becomes more distended with feces, which usually accumulate and harden, and, acting as an irritant, produce tenesmus with mucous discharges. The venous circulation being interfered with, hemorrhoids are common, adding to the patient's suffering.

On examination a tumor is found, sometimes as large as a man's fist, which can be felt projecting from the posterior vaginal wall and over the perineum; sometimes it is soft and compressible, while at other times it is quite solid, depending on the absence or presence of hardened feces. To leave no room for doubt in diagnosticating a case of rectocele, the rectum should be explored with the index finger.

Enterocele Vaginalis, or Entero-Vaginal Hernia.

This consists in a portion of small intestine dilating the cul-de-sac so that the peritoneum is carried down with the intestine between the vagina and rectum as far as the perineum, sometimes forming an elastic tumor at the vulva. The chief dangers arising from this form of vaginal hernia are from its being strangulated or lacerated during childbirth.

Enterocele vaginalis is not frequently met with, but it is important for the physician to know that such a condition is possible and difficult to differentiate from some forms of vaginal tumor. A thorough and careful rectal examination is requisite for diagnosis. An enterocele has the peculiar elastic feeling of a tumor distended with air, a tympanitic resonance on percussion, and a peristaltic movement. If there remains any room for doubt, aspiration with the smallest needle will enable the physician to perfect his diagnosis, for if the needle enter the intestine it is not in any sense a dangerous procedure.

TREATMENT.—The treatment of prolapsus and hernia of the vagina is similar to that of prolapsus of the womb.

If a prolapsus of the vagina has existed but a brief period or has come on suddenly, it should be immediately reduced and proper measures taken to prevent its recurrence. To accomplish this the patient should assume the genu-pectoral position, while the physician with well-oiled fingers restores the parts to their normal position. The patient should then lie upon her back with the hips elevated; astringent vaginal injections ought to be used every four or six hours; and quiet secured or discomfort or pain relieved by opiates. Sudden displacements of the vagina not being of frequent occurrence, the physician more frequently meets with cases of long standing which have come on gradually and slowly.

Attention to the general health is an important requisite: with this in view tonics should be prescribed in many cases, the bowels regulated by means of proper diet or if necessary by medicine, and the bladder more frequently evacuated than in health. Astringent injections are fully as useful in cases of long-standing displacements of the vagina as in those of more recent occurrence; among those more generally used are solutions of tannin, sulphate of zinc, or alum (ʒiv ad Oj). Sea-bathing and injections of sea-water into the vagina are beneficial. It is sometimes more convenient to make topical applications with vaginal suppositories containing one of the astringents just mentioned.

Where cystocele exists it is important that the bladder be completely emptied when the patient urinates; to accomplish this she may assume the genu-pectoral position, and at the same time push the tumor up into the vagina. If after this urine remains in the bladder, a catheter should be employed.

If in any form of vaginal displacement the means which have been alluded to fail, then some form of support or some surgical procedure will be necessary. In very fleshy women considerable benefit is sometimes obtained by means of an abdominal band with a perineal pad attached to it. Pessaries, which have been heretofore quite generally depended upon, are now considered as of secondary importance. Sometimes, however, when the hernia is not of great size or when associated with uterine displacement, a pessary proves of service. A Hodge's pessary with a cross-bar, or the one devised by Skene of Brooklyn, will often prove of great benefit in cystocele. For either cystocele or rectocele the most serviceable form of pessary is one like Cutter's or McIntosh's cup pessary, which is retained within the vagina and supported in position by external attachments. To effect a radical cure in either cystocele or rectocele, especially in the latter, some surgical procedure generally becomes requisite.

Of the different operations which have secured the general approval of gynecologists, the most common is perineorraphy: this is the name given to the operation for a torn perineum. Another operation sometimes performed with success is colporrhaphy or elytrorrhaphy, which consists of lessening the calibre of the vagina by removing a portion of the mucous membrane and bringing the edges of the wound together by sutures. This can be performed on either the anterior or posterior wall, depending on which seems to demand it the most; and if the operation on one wall is not likely to be sufficient, it should be made on both. Not unfrequently the most perfect success can be attained by a surgical procedure designated as colpo-perineorrhaphy, which combines the two operations that have been mentioned. Full descriptions of these different operations and the best modes of performing them can be found in all late standard works on surgical gynecology.

Cicatrices.

Cicatrices of the vagina may occur in consequence of lacerations or injuries received in childbirth, surgical operations, wounds from accident, or the use of caustics about the uterus. If any of the causes named excite inflammation, there may be more or less sloughing of the parts, and, as healing must take place by granulation, cicatrices of various dimensions are formed. These cicatrices may be sufficient to cause partial or complete atresia, or they may be merely in the form of projections or bands, dragging the uterus out of its normal position or interfering with its natural mobility, and cause dyspareunia and other discomforts.

Recently, since attention has been directed to the reflex symptoms produced by cicatricial tissue in the neck of the uterus, there has been a growing belief that similar symptoms are often caused by cicatrices in the vagina. Thus it is the opinion of some who have investigated this subject that many cases of remote neuralgia and other nervous disturbances may often be caused in this way.[1]

TREATMENT.—This is of necessity surgical, although some cases can be successfully treated without having recourse to cutting operations, but are treated by pressure. One method is to tampon the vagina with cotton or marine lint previously saturated with carbolized glycerin. The tampon can be left in position four or five days, when the vagina may be washed out and again tamponed. Another method of treating with pressure is by means of a Sims's dilator, either worn continuously or a few hours at a time. Generally a quicker and more effectual mode of treatment is to nick the bands with scissors or a knife in several places sufficiently for the vagina to assume its natural shape, and then insert the dilator. In some instances it is advisable to cut away portions of the adventitious membrane. On account of the tendency to hemorrhage after operations in the vagina the physician should avoid cutting more than is requisite, and must use a finger as a guide in cutting, to inform him when he has cut sufficiently.

If there is considerable hemorrhage it may be necessary to use a styptic, but usually the glass dilator, by putting the walls on the stretch and by pressure, will check the bleeding. It is important that the dilator be worn for several hours each day after the nicking, for fear that there will again be contraction. After each removal of the dilator the vagina should be syringed out with warm carbolized water or a very weak solution of permanganate of potassium (gr. ss ad f℥ij), that no septic matter may be retained and so that healing of the cuts may be more rapid.

Double Vagina.

Among the congenital deformities occasionally met with is a vagina divided by a longitudinal septum, constituting a duplex or double vagina. The septum is not always so situated as to make the passages of equal size, nor does it invariably divide the canal through its entire length. It is stated by most writers on the subject that usually with a double vagina

[1] Vide Skene on "Cicatrices of the Cervix Uteri and Vagina," *Amer. Gynæc. Soc.*, vol. i., 1876.

there will also be a double uterus. The author has met with only two cases of duplex vagina, neither of which was associated with a double uterus. The treatment is of necessity surgical, and consists in dividing the partition with scissors, and inserting a tampon with some styptic or a Sims's dilator for the arrest of the bleeding which invariably occurs from cutting operations in the vagina. If there is persistent hemorrhage, a galvano- or thermo-cautery may be used.

Growths in the Vagina.

New formations of any kind are not of frequent occurrence in this locality. They consist almost exclusively of cystic tumors, fibroid tumors, papillary excrescences or vegetations, sarcomata, epithelioma, and carcinoma.

Cystic Tumors of the Vagina

are sometimes observed, but are by no means common. Their origin and nature has not seemed to be well understood. Hugier and Guérin are of the opinion that they are caused by the mucous follicles being obstructed. In this view they are sustained by Preuschen.[1]

Sinéty remarks that there are two varieties of vaginal cysts—one superficial and the other profound. The superficial are developed in the mucous membrane, are small in size, and contain fluid which is watery or clear and glairy. The profound cysts are developed in the vaginal walls, and are of various dimensions, from the size of a walnut to an orange, and capable of attaining to much greater dimensions than is possible for the superficial variety. Their contents vary greatly; sometimes clear, mucous, and ropy, in other cases they are colored brownish or chocolate.

Cysts of the vagina are not to be confounded with those of the vulva or those which develop in the vulvo-vaginal glands, nor are they as common.

TREATMENT.—Cysts of the vagina can often be cured by laying them freely open with a bistoury and wiping out the cavity with tincture of iodine, carbolic acid, or a solution of nitrate of silver. The tincture of iodine preferred by the author is Churchill's or a saturation tincture, either being much more effective than the simple tincture. Nitric acid and the actual cautery are mentioned by Barnes as having been used for destroying vaginal cysts. Entire removal of these formations can be effected by cutting into or through the mucous membrane and dissecting them out in the same manner as they are removed from other localities.

Fibrous and Sarcomatous Tumors.

Fibrous or fibroid tumors are by no means as common in the vagina as in the uterus. It has been observed that they are frequently but not invariably associated with the latter. They are developed in the mus-

[1] " Die Cysten die Vagina," *Centralblatt für Med.,* 1871, p. 775.

cular or fibrous structure of the vagina in the same manner as similar formations in the muscular tissue of the uterus.

Some authorities assert that they frequently have the point of departure from the uterus, and then descend little by little between the walls of the vagina.

Sarcomatous tumors are developed in the same tissues and similarly to fibrous growths of the vagina. They are, however, of less frequent occurrence. They sometimes appear primarily in the vagina, but more frequently are consecutive to sarcoma of the uterus.

It is a difficult and often impossible task to make out the differential diagnosis of sarcomatous and fibrous growths in the vagina except by means of the microscope. The symptoms of each are similar to those which indicate sarcomatous and fibrous growths of the uterus, it being accompanied by profuse leucorrhœa, more or less sanious, and occasional hemorrhage. If tumors acquire much size, they interfere with the functions of the rectum and bladder, and cause pain and discomfort by their pressure in the pelvis; sexual intercourse is difficult, frequently painful, and followed by a flow of blood.

DIAGNOSIS.—If of a large size, diagnosis is easily made. Uterine tumors and prolapsed uteri have been mistaken for vaginal growths. By using a uterine probe and inserting a finger in the rectum there need be no error in these respects. By careful examination there is little difficulty in diagnosis.

TREATMENT.—This consists of removal by the knife, scissors, écraseur, or galvano- or thermo-cautery. If there are reasons for believing that a tumor is sarcomatous, it is important that every particle be removed. For this purpose scissors or the galvano- or thermo-cautery are preferable to the ordinary écraseur, which by its action crushes and bruises tissues, and is liable to draw into the chain or wire and crush off more than the operator desires. Serious accidents, such as opening into the peritoneal cavity or the bladder, have occurred in this way in the practice of distinguished and experienced surgeons.

Papillary growths and vegetations in the vagina will receive merely a brief allusion, as they are rarely seen even in the practice of gynecologists. They are not commonly limited to the vagina, but are of more frequent occurrence about the vulva and on the cervix uteri. Vegetations of considerable size sometimes develop in consequence of pregnancy or of granular vaginitis. Sometimes papillary growths within the vagina assume a cauliflower shape with well-defined stalks, or about the ostium vaginæ they may take the form of condylomata. These formations may be confounded with epithelioma.

Treatment consists of removal by scissors or with the thermo- or galvano-cautery, and to guard against hemorrhage some styptic and a vaginal tampon will be required.

Cancer of the Vagina.

Carcinoma or epithelioma rarely occurs as a primary affection in the vagina; it is generally secondary, extending from the neck of the uterus. The author has met with only three cases which were primary cancer.

In a recent work Kustner[1] has collected statistics of twenty-two cases of primitive cancer of the vagina. The result of the analysis of these observations is, that nearly always the posterior wall is first affected in primary cancer, while in secondary cancer the anterior wall is the first to be attacked.

The symptoms after the disease is somewhat advanced are similar to uterine cancer—viz. a sanious, watery discharge of an offensive odor or sometimes a veritable hemorrhage. There is no pain peculiar to or pathognomonic of the disease. It is not until infiltration causes pressure on nerves or there is considerable ulceration that pain is experienced; in either of these conditions the sufferings are often excruciating. Occasionally in women of advanced age, in consequence of cancerous infiltration before ulceration has occurred, the vagina is found to be contracted and there is roughness and induration of the walls.

Epithelioma generally occurs in young women. The early symptoms are pain and hemorrhage following coition. A digital examination will show the friable nature of the formation and an indurated base: the examination will cause blood to flow. In the early part of this stage, before there has been much ulceration, the disease is sometimes mistaken for syphilis and the growths for syphilitic condylomata. It is not an uncommon occurrence for the disease to propagate itself by contact, the opposite wall from which it primarily appeared becoming in this way affected. Later, deeper tissues are infiltrated, the bladder or rectum becomes implicated, ulceration occurs, and subsequently perforation. The progress and terminations are similar to uterine cancer.

TREATMENT.—In carcinoma there seems to be no opportunity for anything more than a palliative course of treatment. Medicine or surgery is here of but little avail. If epithelioma be detected sufficiently early, there is some hope of cure, but this lies only in complete removal. For this purpose the knife or scissors or the galvano- or thermo-cautery can be used. When there is much hemorrhage, some styptic, like the perchloride of iron, should be applied, or the cautery or curette may be of service. Unfortunately, the physician is seldom consulted early enough—prior to the cellular tissue being too much infiltrated—for the thorough eradication of the disease.

Death occurs from exhaustion, hemorrhage, septicæmia, uræmia, or from infiltration interfering mechanically with the function of the bladder, kidneys, or intestine.

For the purpose of correcting the offensive odor and lessening pain there seems to be nothing superior to chloral and glycerin ($\mathfrak{z}$j–$\mathfrak{z}$ij ad $\mathfrak{z}$ij) on a tampon of cotton; the fluid extract of eucalyptus combined with the chloral and glycerin ($\mathfrak{z}$ss ad $\mathfrak{z}$ij) has proven an excellent deodorizer in the author's hands.

Vaginismus.

DEFINITION.—This affection, which was first called vaginismus by our distinguished countryman the lamented J. Marion Sims, consists in a hyperæsthesia or peculiar sensibility of the site of the hymen and vaginal

[1] " Ueber den Primären Scheidenkrebs," *Arch. f. Gyn.*, t. ix. p. 279.

outlet, associated with involuntary spasmodic contraction upon irritation of the sphincters of the vagina.

ETIOLOGY.—Predisposing Causes.—This is sometimes an idiopathic affection, but more frequently is symptomatic of some other disorder. When idiopathic, it is due to a diathesis generally termed hysterical, or an excessive nervous irritability affecting the entire system. The symptomatic causes are quite numerous—more frequently some insignificant local disorder than any grave form of disease. The more common causes are irritated or inflamed carunculæ myrtiformes, excoriation, and irritable ulcers and eruptions about the vulva, vaginitis, uterine catarrh, inflammation, growths and fissures of the urethra, disorders of the bladder, fissure of the anus, and inflamed hemorrhoids. Other less frequent causes have been mentioned by writers, as neuromata, an unusually rigid perineum, and a disproportionately large male organ. Neftel of New York asserts that lead-poisoning has been the cause of some cases under his own observation.[1] It is sometimes associated with or apparently caused by congestive dysmenorrhœa and uterine displacements and engorgements.

Emmet's views regarding the etiology and pathology of this affection differ from those of the majority of writers on the subject. He regards it as purely a symptom denoting reflex irritation, and says that with it he has never failed to find some condition, as a displacement, a limited cellulitis, or a fissure in either the rectum or the neck of the bladder, as the exciting cause.[2]

SYMPTOMATOLOGY, COURSE, DURATION, TERMINATION, AND COMPLICATIONS.—The most prominent symptom is excessive pain upon the sexual intercourse; this is often so marked that subsequent attempts, or even a digital examination, will throw the patient into a state of extreme nervous trepidation and apprehension. If attempts at coition are persevered in, the symptoms are further intensified, so that the spasm and violent contraction of the sphincter vaginal muscles induce agonizing pain. Besides having the characteristic pain, patients with this disorder are, as a rule, sterile. If a physical examination be made in a well-marked case of vaginismus, it frequently occurs that the slightest touch on the part of the physician about the site of the hymen will bring on painful contraction of the vagina and sphincters, and cause the patient to spring up and show much nervous disturbance. In the same class of cases it may be brought on by walking. Thomas says that "in some cases a marked tendency to spasm will have been noticed upon sudden changes of position or washing the genital fissure."[3]

Barnes remarks that in some women the irritability of the nervous centres becomes so great, the sensitiveness of the peripheral nerves at the vulva so acute, and reflex action thereby so intensified, that the attempt at intercourse will induce convulsion or be followed by syncope.[4]

One case came under the writer's observation where the sensitiveness was so marked that a slight touch with cotton or a camel's-hair brush would bring on severe painful contraction.

Course and Duration.—This is an affection of indefinite duration;

---

[1] N. Y. Med. Journ., vol. ix. p. 81.
[2] The Principles and Practice of Gynæcology, by Thomas Addis Emmet, M. D., 2d ed., Philada., 1880, p. 607.
[3] Op. cit., p. 206.   [4] Edis, Diseases of Women, p. 533.

unless relieved it may continue through years of discomfort and misery. Cases are reported as lasting twenty-five or thirty years. There is a mild form sometimes occurring among the recently married which will either disappear of itself or yield to simple treatment. More generally, the discomfort and pain continue unless successfully treated, and in well-marked cases attempts at intercourse increase the suffering; there is nervous exhaustion, the health breaks down in consequence and from what has been called "the disappointment of nature under an unfulfilled function."

PATHOLOGY.—In certain morbid conditions the nerves distributed about the outlet of the vagina may possess such a high degree of irritability that a foreign substance coming in contact with them will cause contraction and spasm of the tissue in which they are distributed and connecting muscles.

Sinéty[1] is of the opinion that "in milder forms of the disorder the constrictor vaginal muscles alone may be the seat of the spasm; but more generally all of the muscles forming the floor of the perineum, the constrictors of the vulva and vagina, muscles of the anus and of the urethra, superficial and deep," in truth, "all the muscles of the region," can "simultaneously be the seat of spasm." Emmet[2] considers vaginismus as kindred to neuralgia, for the reason that it more frequently occurs among anæmic and excessively nervous women, and those who have in some manner overtaxed their nervous systems, the locality being determined as it were by accident, and that only in exceptional instances can there be any local exciting cause. Thomas[3] says that it is curious to perceive how, from different standpoints regarding the pathology, "both parties were led to the same surgical resource."

The author's own observation will not permit of his ascribing the majority of cases wholly to morbid constitutional conditions, to the exclusion of local lesions. The reason of his belief is that the greater number of cases he has observed have been treated and cured by surgical measures, having in view the relief of morbid conditions of some pelvic structures.

DIAGNOSIS.—The diagnosis is attended with no difficulty, as there is no other affection presenting similarities.

PROGNOSIS.—Sims remarks that he knows of "no serious trouble that can be so easily, so safely, and so certainly cured." Scanzoni, Tilt, and others, who hold different views as to the pathology and means of cure, express themselves as favorably regarding prognosis. Thomas has never met with a case that he could not relieve or cure. Nearly all gynecologists are of the opinion that a favorable prognosis is warrantable in the majority of cases.

TREATMENT.—In cases where it seems quite difficult to ascertain the etiology and pathology a palliative course may at first be pursued, such as vaginal injections of acetate of lead or borax in warm water ($\mathrecip{z}$j ad Oj), to which may be added carbolic acid or laudanum or the wearing of the vaginal rest or dilator, and total abstinence from any attempts at coition. If the chief cause seems to be in some constitutional trouble, then as complete physiological rest as possible should be enjoined. With

---

[1] *Manuel pratique de Gynécologie*, par L. de Sinéty, Paris, 1879.   [2] *Op. cit.*, p. 607.
[3] *Op. cit.*, p. 205.

this in view, all attempts at sexual intercourse must be discontinued, as it will keep up nervous suffering and local pain and discomfort. The vaginal dilator of Sims secures a rest by keeping the walls apart; it also dilates and benumbs the parts, thus rendering them more tolerant of a foreign body. With every mode of treatment or in cases occurring from any cause the vaginal dilator is required; this is to be worn for two or more hours at intervals of six to twelve hours, according to the degree of tolerance with which it is borne. It should be smeared previous to insertion with some soothing lubricant, as iodide of lead and glycerin (ʒj ad ʒj) or atropia and vaseline (gr. ij ad ʒj) or stramonium ointment. Vaginal suppositories containing morphia, extract of opium, belladonna, hyoscyamus, or stramonium will usually prove of great benefit as local sedatives. In some instances suppositories containing five to ten grains of iodoform may be of service. Copious vaginal injections of warm or hot water alone are beneficial in the majority of cases, as they wash away irritating discharges that aggravate the disease, and by lessening the congestion frequently do away with the necessity of surgical operations.

A careful examination should be made in every case for the purpose of ascertaining whether the vaginismus is not caused or aggravated by fissures, ulcers, or excoriations about the parts; if any are found, they should be properly treated. If any symptoms point toward the rectum or urethra, they should be examined. A patient of the author's suffered from vaginismus during some years, owing wholly to a fissure of the anus, and was cured by an operation for the anal disease alone.

Owing to the pain an ordinary examination produces, it will generally be necessary to etherize the patient before attempting to make a thorough and careful examination.

In anæmic or excessively nervous patients other treatment than local is necessary. Tonics, such as iron, quinia, strychnia, sea-bathing, etc., change of scene, and such kinds of exercise as improve the tone of the nervous organism, should be prescribed. If the trouble is due to some uterine or pelvic disorder, a cure can be effected only by attention to the primary affection.

Some of the modes of treatment that have been mentioned, if persevered in, will succeed in curing many cases without having recourse to any surgical procedure. If, however, a case has not yielded to any of the means heretofore suggested, then some form of surgical operation becomes necessary. The simplest is the one advocated by Scanzoni and Tilt, and consists in a forcible dilatation of the ostium vaginæ with the thumbs, after the manner first practised by Récamier of forcible dilatation of the sphincters in fissure of the anus. Temporary paralysis of the vaginal sphincters is by this means effected, and should be followed by the insertion of a large vaginal dilator, to be worn for several days and held in position by a T-bandage. This sometimes effects a permanent cure, but if a single trial fails to accomplish it, yet the patient is considerably benefited, it ought to be repeated; in the mean time the use of the dilator with one of the ointments previously mentioned should be persevered in.

When the disorder has existed a long time, the muscular power has increased, and the forcible dilatation may require more exercise of strength than can be exerted by the thumbs alone; under such circumstances the writer has been in the habit of using Symes's universal speculum or a tri-bladed rectal speculum, and gradually dilating the vagina to the extent required.

If any of the modes of treatment that have been mentioned fail to effect a cure, or reasons exist for not making use of them, then the radical treatment of Sims or some one of its modifications will be requisite.

A full description of the various surgical procedures and the views of different authorities cannot with appropriateness be presented in this work.

Sims's operation is made as follows : The patient is fully anæsthetized and placed upon her back ; then with curved scissors every vestige of the hymen is removed. It is important that this be most thoroughly done, for it has occurred that by leaving a small portion success has not been complete. As soon as the bleeding has stopped the fourchette is put upon the stretch by inserting the middle and index fingers, and with a scalpel a Y-shaped incision is made through the mucous membrane and part of the muscular fibres on each side of the perpendicular line extending into the perineum. After this a glass vaginal dilator is placed in the vaginal canal and worn two hours each morning and night, or as much of the night as it can be tolerated. This should be continued for about a month. There are several sizes of the dilator, and in selecting one to be worn care should be taken not to use one that is too large. Morphine suppositories per rectum should be used as often as is requisite for the relief of pain. A copious vaginal injection is necessary for the sake of cleanliness after each removal of the dilator.

Sims's dilators are made of glass, the outer end open, the inner closed, and of a conical shape ; on the upper side is a depression to avoid pressure on the urethra.

Fig. 27.

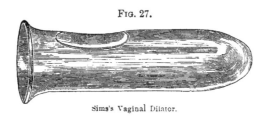

Sims's Vaginal Dilator.

Emmet's operation is a modification of the above, and consists in inserting an index finger in the rectum, and then putting the sphincter on the stretch, when with scissors he divides the fibres encircling the vagina on each side just within the fourchette and about three-fourths of an inch apart. He claims that this method "does not allow a prolapse of the vaginal wall, as when the perineum is lacerated, but does permit of an equal extent of dilatation of the outlet by the glass plug."[1]

The plan of dividing the pudic nerve, as practised by Sir James Y. Simpson, has met with little favor.

The author has been successful in several instances by a less formidable operation than any herein described. His operation has simply consisted of entire removal of every vestige of the hymen or carunculæ myrtiformes with scissors, followed by wearing of the glass plug such length of time

[1] *Op. cit.*, p. 609.

as is requisite.   This procedure is simply the first part of Sims's operation.

Parturition would, as a rule, cure this affection in an effectual manner, but its subjects are generally sterile.   The reason of sterility in vaginismus is often owing to the extreme suffering whenever there is an attempt at coition; this pain prevents its perfect performance, and often all further attempts are abandoned.   When we are convinced that such a condition is the cause of sterility, the patient may be etherized, and while in that condition complete coition may result in fruitfulness and ultimately perfect cure of the vaginismus.

DISEASES OF THE VULVA.

THE subject will be considered in the following order: Anatomy, Vulvitis, Phlegmonous Inflammation of the Labia, Furuncles, Pruritus, Hyperæsthesia of the Vulva, Tumors, Atresia, and Eruptions.

Anatomy.

As regards the anatomy of the generative organs of women in this and the preceding chapter, it has not been deemed necessary by the author to consider the subject in extenso, but to give a brief résumé, as better suited to the needs and wishes of the busy practitioner.

The generative organs of women external to the hymen, in their relative order from before backward, consist of the mons veneris, clitoris, vestibule, meatus urinarius, and orifice of the vagina, and the labia majora and minora on either side.   All these are known under the name of pudendum or vulva.

The mons veneris is a rounded cushion of fatty tissue immediately over the os pubis, and from puberty is covered with hair.

The labia majora are two folds of skin extending longitudinally from the mons veneris to the perineum.   In them are found all the elements of the skin.   The subcutaneous tissue is of loose texture.   A noticeable fact is that here the sebaceous glands are remarkable for their size, some of them being 0.5 millimeters in diameter and opening directly on a free surface.   The labia majora resemble the skin of other portions of the body in that they contain papillæ, nerves, vessels, and Pacinian bodies. Internally they are lined with mucous membrane in which are numerous sebaceous follicles.   A quantity of fat, areolar tissue, and tissue analogous to the dartos of the scrotum, including vessels, nerves, and glands, constitutes the contents of the labia, and gives them a rounded appearance, larger in front and decreasing in size toward the perineum.   The extremities of these folds, joining together, form the anterior and posterior commissures of the vulva.

The labia minora, sometimes called nymphæ, are two membranous folds of erectile tissue within the labia majora, beginning at the anterior commissure and passing down and disappearing midway between the two commissures.   They also contain sebaceous glands.

The clitoris is an erectile organ covered with mucous membrane, and is the analogue of the penis. It arises by two crura, is situated beneath the anterior commissure, and is partially concealed by the labia minora.

The vestibule and the fossa navicularis are triangular spaces on the mucous membrane, the first immediately posterior to the clitoris, the second anterior to the perineum.

The meatus urinarius is the external orifice of the urethra, and is situated in the vestibule about one inch posterior to the clitoris. The mucous membrane is slightly raised above the meatus, giving it prominence, and thus serves as a guide to the introduction of the catheter without exposing the person.

The orifice of the vagina is an elliptical opening just below the meatus urinarius. It is partially covered over in the virgin by a fold of mucous membrane called the hymen.

The vulvo-vaginal glands, or the glands of Bartholin, are two in number, situated anterior to the hymen, each with a single duct opening on the inner side of the nymphæ. They are analogous to the glands of Cowper in the male.

The bulbi vestibuli, on either side of the vestibule, extend downward from the clitoris for about one inch. They consist of a thin layer of fibrous membrane ensheathing a plexus of veins.

Vulvitis.

DEFINITION.—Vulvitis is the term used to designate inflammation of the vulva. It may be purulent, follicular, or occasionally but rarely gangrenous.

ETIOLOGY.—The purulent form may be specific or the result of want of cleanliness, exposure to cold, over-exertion, the strumous diathesis, pruritus, urinary fistula, or cancer. It is also produced by awkward or excessive coitus and masturbation, the irritation of urine, and frequently is caused by pregnancy. Vulvitis is not uncommon with little girls, resulting from some of the innocent causes mentioned, though the symptoms may expose the patient unjustly to the suspicion of having been tampered with.

SYMPTOMATOLOGY, COURSE, AND DURATION.—At first there is heat, dryness, and more or less pain in the affected parts, followed by a profuse flow of yellow pus. There is also tumefaction, hypersensitiveness, and often pruritus. Follicular vulvitis is the term employed to indicate an inflammation of the mucous or sebaceous glands and of the hair-follicles of the vulva. This disease may be the result of any of the causes of purulent vulvitis, as alluded to in the preceding clause. The subjective symptoms are common also to the purulent form. Objectively, the mucous membrane will appear to be very red in spots, resembling in this respect the raised papillæ of the tongue. These spots frequently bleed on slight provocation. The internal surface of the nymphæ and vestibule is the seat of the disease when the mucous glands are involved, but where the sebaceous glands are mainly affected the inflamed papillæ will be found on the surface of the labia and at their juncture anteriorly. In the course of the inflammation a drop of pus will exude from the papules, and they then gradually disappear. Occasionally, collections of exudate from the diseased glands accumulate beneath the labia minora, concealing the diseased surfaces and becoming quickly very offensive. The disorder, though sometimes persistent, is seldom chronic. The acute affection may be the cause of urethritis in the male closely resembling gonorrhœa if coition occurs during its existence, and thus not infrequently giving rise to suspicion of infidelity.

TREATMENT.—In the matter of treatment, touching the inflamed points with carbolic acid or caustic sometimes favorably influences the course of the disease. Cleanliness is the most important item in the treatment of the two forms of the disease, for without it the application of remedies will be of little avail. Strict attention to this, with perfect rest of the parts, will not infrequently be all that is requisite to effect a cure, but in cases that do not yield to this treatment sedative, astringent, or alterative applications are indicated. These should be applied after bathing. In the purulent variety such remedies as the lead-and-opium wash after the following formula will prove serviceable :

$$\text{R}. \quad \begin{array}{ll} \text{Tinct. opii,} & \text{f } \bar{3}\text{j ;} \\ \text{Plumbi acetat.} & \text{3j ;} \\ \text{Aquam ad} & \text{f } \bar{3}\text{viij.} \end{array}$$

Lint may be saturated with this lotion and applied between the labia. If the disease does not yield to the treatment already mentioned in the course of two or three days, a solution of argentic nitrate (gr. x to ʒj) should be brushed upon the parts, and between the intervals of its application bismuth or starch may be kept constantly on the parts. In cases associated with vaginitis a much stronger solution is sometimes required. (Vide chapter on Vaginitis.) The author has used powdered iodoform in some cases with very good results.

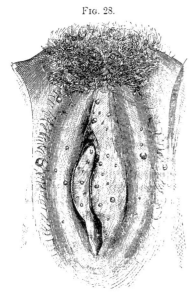

FIG. 28.

Follicular Vulvitis (Hugiuer)

In the follicular variety the disease is more severe and usually of longer duration than the purulent, although the principles of treatment are essentially the same. In this as in the other variety cleanliness is of paramount importance, frequent washing being very essential. To the inflamed follicles such applications as nitrate of silver, persulphate of iron, and carbolic acid are the more frequent remedies used in this disease. After the application of any of these remedies the parts should be rendered dry, and then a piece of soft linen or a roll of absorbent cotton should be smeared with vaseline or soaked with carbolized glycerin and inserted within the vulva in a way to keep the labia apart. Occasionally the practitioner will meet with a chronic form of vulvitis, and the rareness of its occurrence is fortunate, for the reason that it is a very obstinate and intractable variety of the disease. Vulvitis is very frequently associated with vaginitis, owing to the fact that the mucous membrane is continuous in both vulva and vagina. On this account the principle of treatment of inflammation of either locality is essentially the same. To avoid repetition, the reader is therefore referred to the section on Vaginitis for a more detailed description of treatment.

There is a form of this disease described by Vinay[1] as ulcerous or aphthous vulvitis. This is an affection peculiar to childhood, occurring only when the general health is much impaired. It is often a sequel of fevers, and may even become epidemic. It attacks children of any age, but is of more common occurrence in infancy. The disease appears first upon the mucous membrane in the form of small and round patches of a white or grayish-white color, which soon ulcerate, and at a more advanced stage are liable to become gangrenous. This variety of vulvitis has long been known, and is mentioned in the works of Hippocrates. This disease is rarely met with in this country.

Phlegmonous Inflammation of the Labia Majora.

DEFINITION.—The adipose and areolar tissue which compose the greater bulk of the labia majora often become the seat of acute inflammation, in consequence of direct injury, excessive or awkward coition, exposure to cold, from irritating discharges, scratching in pruritus, vulvitis, or that peculiar blood-state which predisposes to the formation of boils or carbuncles.

SYMPTOMATOLOGY AND DIAGNOSIS.—The patient will first complain of heat and pain, increased by standing or walking, and later throbbing and shooting pains in the affected parts. In the outset the part is congested, followed by induration from effusion in the loose tissues, and next suppuration ensues. An examination in the last-named stage will reveal the existence of an abscess in one labium. The diagnosis is by no means difficult, but the physician, however, should bear in mind that this same locality may be the site for pudendal hernia, a dislocated ovary, hæmatocele, or vulvitis.

TREATMENT.—In the outset the inflammation may be caused to disappear by resolution, by means of cold and sedative lotions, such as the lead-and-opium wash, saline laxatives, non-stimulating diet, and perfect rest. In the majority of cases the disease proceeds to suppuration. When it is found that resolution is unattainable, then means should be taken to promote and hasten suppuration. This is best effected by the frequent application of hot poultices. The mistake is often committed of permitting too long intervals to elapse between the application of poultices, and allowing the one applied to become cold before another one takes its place. The patient can be saved many hours of suffering by keeping hot applications constantly on the inflamed labium. As soon as suppuration is detected the abscess should be opened, for two reasons aside from the one of affording relief: First, the tissue resists early natural evacuation; second, owing to the laxity of the tissues, pus will sometimes force itself upward toward and through the abdominal ring.

[1] *Nouveau Dict. de Méd.,* tome xxxiii., 1885.

Furuncles of the Labia.

DEFINITION.—Closely resembling phlegmonous inflammation are the furuncles or boils which are quite common on the labia. They occasion much pain and distress, for the reason that they are very obstinate and apt to recur, one forming as soon as its predecessor has apparently healed. In many instances these boils seem to be consequent upon inflammation of sebaceous glands. They differ in size, some being no larger than a pea, while others are the size of a filbert.

TREATMENT.—This should be constitutional and local. Quinine, arsenic, cod-liver oil, and other remedies of a tonic character should be administered. The bromide of arsenic has been used by the author in a few cases with quite satisfactory results. As soon as one of these furuncles shows that it contains pus, it should be freely opened and a crucial incision made to prevent immediate healing; after which poultices should be applied. These small boils are extremely painful, and are very troublesome, owing, as previously stated, to their liability of recurrence. To prevent their recurrence is one of the reasons why immediate healing of the incisions should be prevented. If contraction of the sacs of the abscesses does not occur, pus will continue to be formed and the tissues in their immediate neighborhood will become indurated. In this way the furuncles may become of a chronic character. To further facilitate healing and aiding their contraction the sacs should have applied to them some stimulating remedy, such as carbolic acid or nitrate of silver. Edis says that painting the surface of the affected labium with tincture of iodine is beneficial in some instances.

One of the most important requisites in treatment is perfect cleanliness.

Pruritus Vulvæ.

DEFINITION.—Pruritus vulvæ, although merely a symptom of disease, characterized by itching of the vulva and contiguous neighborhood at times wellnigh intolerable, has, because of its occasional obscure etiology and severity, always been considered by medical authors as a disease of itself, instead of a symptom of other disorders, in treatises on diseases of women.

ETIOLOGY.—Predisposing and Exciting Causes.—It frequently occurs from external irritation, as animal parasites, or such as may be produced by acrid discharges, particularly in gonorrhœa and uterine cancer, changes in the normal composition of the urine, especially diabetic, and not infrequently during the menstrual flow. Pruritus may occur in connection with inflammation of the uterus and vagina without any irritating discharge; likewise it occurs in diseases of the urethra, bladder, and kidneys. Sometimes masturbation may be the cause as well as the effect of pruritus. Secondarily, there may be an insufferable itching in consequence of the continued titillation or irritation of the parts, although masturbation by no means invariably leads to pruritus. The habitual use of opium or alcoholic drinks often causes intractable forms of this disorder. Edis states "that the custom of immoderate tea-drinking is a by no means infrequent cause of pruritus." But instances of pruritus occur where all of the causes mentioned are lacking, and they are instead purely of a reflex character, such as are met with in women about the time of the change of life and during the latter months of pregnancy, or from the presence of worms in the rectum. If the worms migrate to the vulva, as they sometimes do, the irritation then becomes direct. Interference with the circulation of the vulva by pregnancy and tumors may cause pruritus: unquestionably, certain varieties of the disorder are idiopathic or neurotic.

SYMPTOMATOLOGY AND COURSE.—When the complaint has existed for some time, the itching will be pretty well diffused from the pubis backward, but in more recent cases it may be localized at the perineum, nymphæ, clitoris, or portions of labia. The itching is not always constant, but subject to exacerbations. It is usually much worse when the patient becomes heated from exercise or is warm in bed, thus preventing comfort or sleep, and thereby adding an additional complication to treatment. The sufferer naturally seeks relief by scratching the involved tissues, and for this very transient satisfaction spreads the disease by increasing the irritability of the parts and inducing a condition closely resembling eczema.

TREATMENT.—Inasmuch as the etiology of the complaint is often uncertain, as heretofore stated, it is highly important that the physician should ascertain if possible the cause of the disease, and thereby be better enabled to treat the complaint intelligently. In case the itching can be traced to the animal parasites most common in this region, such remedies as the black or yellow wash, mercurial ointment, or the oleate of mercury will usually prove sufficient; but if it be found that the Acarus scabei is the cause of the itching, the application of the ordinary sulphur ointment will destroy this parasite and the itching will consequently cease. If due to uterine catarrh or any vaginal affection, attention should be directed to the removal of the primary disorder by appropriate means, for it cannot be expected that itching of the vulva can be relieved so long as there is any irritating discharge constantly exciting it. The most important measure of all is perfect cleanliness. This can be secured by sitz-baths, sometimes several being necessary daily. At the same time, the vagina should be syringed with warm water or water with the addition to it of such remedies as are used for the relief of leucorrhœa. The irritated surfaces of the vulva should be prevented from coming in contact by vaseline spread upon absorbent cotton or lint, or by powders, such as bismuth, starch, etc.

In case there is an unmistakable acrid discharge from the uterus causing pruritus, proper topical applications should be made to as much of the endometrium as is diseased; the vagina should be thoroughly douched night and morning, and then there should be placed against or around the neck of the womb one or more tampons of cotton saturated with the boro-glyceride or with glycerin, in which has been dissolved borax or acetate of lead in the proportion of ℥ss of one of these salts to ℥ij of glycerin.

In some instances, where there is a profuse discharge, simply packing the vagina with dry salicylated or borated cotton will suffice. This should never be allowed to remain longer than twelve hours without removal. In those cases where the discharge is less acrid a single tampon saturated with one of the remedies named or glycerin alone, and placed against the cervix daily, will suffice, as it will prevent the discharge from coming in contact with the vulva. In severer forms of this affection a number of tampons saturated in the same manner will be more efficacious, and still permit the patient to move about. When several tampons are used they should be loosely rolled, and each one should have a string attached for convenient removal. In the mean time, topical applications can be made to the vulva, and washing of the parts will not interfere with the tampons. The author has found the following prescription of Thomas very efficacious as a vaginal injection and wash for the vulva:

> ℞. Plumbi acetatis,   ʒij;
> Acidi carbolici,   ϶ij;
> Tr. opii,   fʒj;
> Aquæ,   Oiv. M.

Another prescription which has demonstrated its value is:

> ℞. Bismuthi subnitratis,
> Acaciæ pulv.   āā ʒij. M.

Sig. Add water to the consistency of cream and apply frequently with a brush.

A somewhat similar prescription, to be applied in the same way, is the following:

> ℞. Pulv. acaciæ,   ʒij;
> Bals. Peru,   ʒj;
> Ol. amygdalæ,   ʒiss;
> Aquæ rosæ,   fʒj; M.;

or,

> ℞. Acidi carbolici, ʒij;
> Glycerinæ,   fʒj;
> Aq. rosæ, q. s. fʒviij. M. Ft. lotio.

In all cases of pruritus, except from parasites, much benefit can be derived from washing the parts two or three times daily in a weak solution of bicarbonate of sodium (half a tablespoonful in a quart of water, with a tablespoonful of eau de Cologne).

In pruritus from diabetes some relief may be afforded by the administration of alkaline mineral waters or salicylate of sodium. In pruritus associated with chronic cystitis the last-named remedy is very useful.

In pruritus of a neurotic character a solution of the muriate of cocoaine of the strength of 4 per cent., sprayed upon the parts or applied with a camel's-hair brush, has often in the author's hands afforded relief when every other application has failed.

One of the latest publications relating to the treatment of pruritus vulvæ is a paper by Kustner,[1] agreeing with Schroeder that the results of operative treatment for pruritus vulvæ are encouraging. This author publishes several cases resulting successfully. A synopsis of one will suffice to show his mode of treatment. A patient, unmarried, suffered for a long time from uterine catarrh and pruritus vulvæ: the former was relieved after prolonged treatment, but there still remained two symmetrical spots between the hymen and labia minora which were the seats of most troublesome itching and were exceedingly sensitive to touch. These portions of the mucous membrane were rich in sebaceous glands, and were also studded with small retention-cysts. The author dissected off

[1] *Centralbl. f. Gyn.*, No· 12, 1885.

the two elliptical portions of mucous membrane, each 1 cm. broad and 3 or 4 cm. long, and containing the small retention-cysts, and then united each wound with interrupted sutures. The pruritus entirely disappeared, and did not again return, though some years after the patient again suffered with uterine catarrh. Other cases are related by the same author, notably one case of pruritus where there was a lacerated perineum. The operation for repair of this perineum was performed, with the result of the permanent disappearance of the pruritus. The author does not give any definite rule as to how and in what cases he should have recourse to operative treatment, but, admitting that pruritus may arise from causes heretofore mentioned in this article, he asks whether those cases where secondary pathological changes have occurred in the vulvar mucous membrane cannot be definitely cured by excision of the affected portion. Not enough cases of cure of pruritus by surgical treatment have been reported to fully establish the theory of Küstner, yet it is a matter of sufficient importance to merit our attention and warrant further investigation.

Hyperæsthesia of the Vulva.

DEFINITION.—This is a disorder first described by Thomas under the above caption.[1] It consists of a hypersensitiveness of the nerves supplying some portion of the mucous membrane of the vulva. Sometimes the area of tenderness will be confined to one of the lesser lips or it will be limited to the vestibule, and in other cases a number of parts may be simultaneously affected. "It is a condition of the vulva closely resembling that hyperæsthetic state of the remains of the hymen which constitutes one form of vaginismus," and doubtless is often confounded with the latter.

ETIOLOGY.—It is more common about the time of change of life, and occurs more frequently among women of hysterical diathesis where there exists a morbid mental condition with a tendency to melancholia. In some instances the disease seems to be excited by vulvitis or vascular growths in the urethra.

SYMPTOMATOLOGY.—The slightest friction causes intense pain and nervousness, and even a current of cold air produces very great discomfort. Coition causes such severe pain that for this cause the subject usually consults her physician. As in vaginismus, the mental distress is often of an exaggerated character, in some instances bordering upon monomania.

PATHOLOGY.—In this disorder there are no indications of inflammation except occasional spots of erythematous redness. It is not a neuralgia in a true sense of the term, but an abnormal sensitiveness of diseased nerves supplying the vulva.

DIAGNOSIS.—The affections most liable to be confounded with this are vascular growths (or irritable caruncles) of the urethra and vaginismus, but ocular inspection and digital examination will enable the physician to determine the character of the disease.

TREATMENT.—This is far from satisfactory in many cases. Thomas speaks most discouragingly concerning it, and states that "the treatment of this condition is most unsatisfactory."

[1] *Op. cit.*, p. 145.

The author has at this time a patient with hyperæsthesia of the vulva who has been treated by him for many months, and up to the time of this writing has obtained no relief. Thomas recommends sending the patient "away from home, where, in addition to enjoying changes of air, scene, and surroundings, she would live absque marito."

In this, as in all disorders which depend on or are associated with the hysterical diathesis, galvanism and massage are, as a rule, of decided benefit. In addition, general tonics, such as arsenic, strychnia, quinia, and iron, should be prescribed. If any local affection exist, such as vulvitis or urethral vegetations, it should be cured first. Warm fomentations, the frequent use of warm water, sedative lotions, and ointments consisting of opium or its salts, carbolic acid, chloroform, and iodoform, are useful topical remedies. Much benefit may be derived by the application of a 4 per cent. solution of hydrochlorate of cocaine by means of a spray or soft brush. Strong solutions of alum and tannin have sometimes proved beneficial.

No good results have been derived from the use of the knife or caustics in cases where they have been used.

Tumors of the Vulva.

Under this head will be included any enlargement, neoplasm, or adventitious growth which has the vulva for its site. The most common are the following, which will be considered in the order named: viz. Cysts, Hydrocele, Hernia, Hypertrophy, Elephantiasis, Hæmatoma, Cancer, and Urethral Caruncle. There are other growths of the vulva, such as fibroma, lipoma, sarcoma, lupus, etc., but they are of such rare occurrence that their discussion is necessarily omitted.

Cysts and Inflammation of the Vulvo-Vaginal Glands.

The frequent concomitance of cysts and abscesses in these glands has caused the author to consider them here under the same caption.

The most frequent cysts of the vulva are those springing either from the ducts or glands of Bartholini, or, as more commonly known, the vulvo-vaginal glands, situated near the lower part of the labia. Cysts having their origin in the ducts are single and are invariably of an oval form; such also is the more common shape of those springing from the gland, yet sometimes they are lobulated, of an irregular form, and comprise one or more in number. Inasmuch as this same locality is sometimes the site of hernia, and cysts of the labia often of a similar form, the physician should be positive that the tumor is a cyst before having recourse to any active mode of treatment.

If fluid accumulates in a cyst in such quantity as to cause the subject inconvenience or discomfort, surgical treatment will be required, of which there are three different modes in common use.

The first mode is to remove by scissors a segment of the sac, allowing escape of its contents, after which the cavity is filled with marine lint or carbolized cotton, which is allowed to remain for about forty-eight hours before renewal. By this plan of treatment the sac will usually be obliter-ated. Another method is to freely open the cyst and apply some caustic, preferably the galvano- or thermo-cautery. In the absence of either of the last named nitric acid may be used with good effect. The third and last method has in the author's experience proven the most efficacious, though objection has been made to it on account of its being a more bloody operation—namely, complete extirpation of the gland.

The causes of inflammation of these glands are the same as those that cause vulvitis; in truth, they are often accompanying disorders. The symptoms are pain, heat, itching, and an increased redness, particularly about the opening of the duct. If a finger be pressed over the location of the gland, it will elicit signs of pain.

In the outset of the inflammation it is felt hard and unyielding, but two or three days later a fluctuating tumor may be easily discerned. An abscess of the gland should be easily distinguished and rarely mistaken for a cyst. There are the history and ordinary signs of inflammation to aid in diagnosis. If, on the contrary, there is simply a cyst, it can be rolled about under the finger and no indications of pain pro-duced.

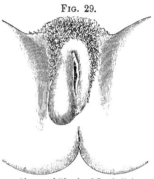

FIG. 29.

Abscess of Glands of Bartholini.

Further, it may exist an indefinite length of time, and unless the gland from some cause become inflamed no great inconvenience is experienced. It is not an infrequent occurrence, from some cause, for inflammation to attack a cyst-wall, in which event the symptoms of inflammation ensue. Where such is the case the treat-ment should be the same as in inflammation of the gland—namely, abso-lute rest and any soothing or anodyne lotions which favor restoration. Should indications of suppuration occur, it should be promoted by the frequent application of hot poultices. If the pain is not severe, the abscess may be left to nature; but if it be severe, then the abscess should be emptied by a free incision at the most prominent point.

Hydrocele, or Cysts of the Canal of Nuck.

DEFINITION.—An accumulation of fluid in the canal of Nuck, consti-tuting a hydrocele or cyst, is of rare occurrence. It is to be found in the upper part of the vulva. Owing to the rarity of this affection the great-est caution should be exercised in its diagnosis. The absence of inflam-matory symptoms, of resonance when percussed, and the ordinary signs of hernia, together with a gradual growth of the tumor without constitu-tional disturbance, would by the exclusive mode of diagnosis leave but little room for doubt as to its character. If, however, the physician still feels uncertain, the means which are used for the cure of this disorder will also aid in diagnosis—namely, aspiration with a fine needle about the size of those used on a hypodermic syringe. Even where hernia exists no harm will be done, for this is not an uncommon practice for the reduc-tion of hernia in this locality.

TREATMENT.—Frequently nothing further is required in the way of treatment than the reduction of the tumor by aspiration. If, however, additional treatment seems to be necessary, it is best to inject tincture of iodine by reversing the action of the syringe. The use of iodine in this manner is for the purpose of obliterating the sac by inducing adhesive inflammation, as is done in the treatment of hydrocele in the male.

Pudendal Hernia.

DEFINITION.—If the process of peritoneum surrounding the round ligaments as they emerge from the inguinal canal to become lost in the dartos-like tissue of the labia is not obliterated at birth, the channel thus formed is known as the canal of Nuck, and furnishes a path for hernia. Besides a loop of intestine or portion of mesentery the ovary or bladder may descend through this canal and constitute an inguinal or labial hernia. The uterus has even been said to have descended by this route. The infrequency of pudendal hernia makes it all the more important to recognize it when it does occur, that serious injury may be avoided when operating on supposed cases of labial abscesses or cysts.

ETIOLOGY.—Pudendal hernia may be produced by blows, falls, coughing, or sneezing, and by violent muscular exertions, as in the male.

SYMPTOMS.—The presence of a part of the intestine can be diagnosticated by the peculiar crackling feeling, the impulse communicated on coughing, and sometimes the disappearance of the tumor on taxis. Occasionally reduction is very difficult, and exceptionally it may become strangulated.

TREATMENT.—The patient being placed on her back with her hips elevated, a gentle taxis will usually suffice to cause reduction. The physician should be positive that the tumor has been returned to the abdomen. After this is accomplished a truss should be adjusted so as to press on the inguinal canal. Usually a perineal band will be necessary to keep the truss sufficiently low to accomplish the purpose for which it was adjusted.

If taxis has proved inefficacious, and strangulation has occurred, a surgical operation will be necessary.

Hypertrophy of the Vulva.

Hypertrophy of the vulva occurs among certain peoples, as the Bushmen and Hottentots, so commonly as to constitute a race-peculiarity, and on account of size and form has been designated as the Hottentot apron. There is also said to be a peculiar deposit of fat in the nates of Hottentot women, but this should not be confounded with the vulvar peculiarity of the same race. Occasionally in our own country hypertrophy of one or more labia will be met with. Sometimes the nymphæ are hypertrophied, so that they hang down much lower than the greater lips; owing to this dependency and their usual pigmentation of a brownish color they bear some resemblance to elephantiasis. In simple hypertrophy the progress is gradual, and there is an entire absence of the inflammatory attacks to which a labium affected with elephantiasis is subject, nor are there any superficial abscesses as in the latter affection. Although there is usually the brown color on the surface in simple hypertrophy, the color is not the same as in elephantiasis. In the latter there is the peculiar pigmentation, also roughness and deep crevices in the skin, so closely resembling in appearance an elephant's skin that there need be no difficulty in the differential diagnosis of simple hypertrophy and elephantiasis of the vulva.

Hypertrophy of the clitoris sometimes occurs as a congenital deformity, and sometimes it is acquired. There has seemed to be quite a general belief that masturbation is one of its most common causes, but there are no substantial grounds for such belief. On the contrary, it has been frequently observed where women were known to have indulged in this habit that no increase in the size of the normal clitoris could be perceived.

TREATMENT.—If a subject of hypertrophy of the vulva suffers any degree of inconvenience therefrom, the affected parts should be removed. A surgical operation for this purpose is an exceedingly simple one and demands no special description.

An operation for the removal of an hypertrophied clitoris is more bloody than one for the removal of the labia; still, with ordinary precautions it need be neither a severe nor dangerous one. Clitoridectomy for the purpose of curing masturbation or various neurotic affections is happily not of as frequent occurrence as formerly. The author is firmly of the opinion that neither in cases of masturbation, epilepsy, nor hysteroepilepsy is the removal of the normal clitoris beneficial or even justifiable.

Elephantiasis of the Vulva.

DEFINITION.—The vulva is sometimes the site of neoplasms known as elephantiasis arabum. The labia may become so hypertrophied that they hang down to the middle of the thighs in the form of tumors; the clitoris and perineum may also be affected. The skin is generally of the peculiar brownish color of an elephant's skin, and hence the name of the disease. The surface of the skin will present many tuberosities due to hypertrophy of the cutaneous papillæ. Superficial abscesses and ulcerations often occur, causing discomfort and pain.

ETIOLOGY.—It is said that elephantiasis of the nymphæ sometimes results from onanism; it is also congenital. Scrofula, malaria, syphilis, and filth are generally considered as among the direct causes of elephantiasis arabum in the countries where it is the most common. Occasionally it is produced by a blow or contusion. Although this disease is not very common in this country, yet a sufficient number of cases have been seen from time to time to call forth a number of articles in the medical periodicals of our country.

PATHOLOGY.—The pathological changes, according to Mayer, consist in a dilatation of the lymphatic spaces and ducts with secondary formation of connective tissue and thickening of the layers of the cutis vera; sometimes the papillæ are specially enlarged, producing swellings which resemble condylomata in form. The labia majora are most frequently affected, next in frequency the clitoris; more rarely are the labia minora hypertrophied. This affection is developed during that period of life when sexual activity is the greatest.

TREATMENT.—The treatment of elephantiasis of the vulva must necessarily be surgical, and therefore will be omitted here, excepting that which is embodied in the following report of cases by the author in the Detroit *Review of Medicine* in December, 1875, and are briefly reproduced here:

Case No. 1.—Fig. 30 shows the condition of Mrs. ——, aged thirty, the

FIG. 30.

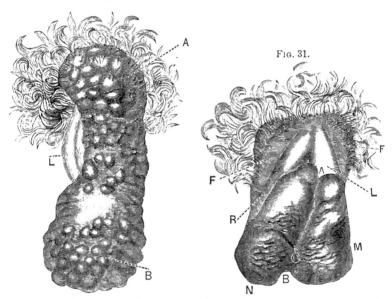

FIG. 31.

FIG. 30.—L, Right labium majus, healthy: A, upper part of pachydermatous tumor, covering a part of the mons veneris; B, lower portion of the tumor, occupying the perineum. This tumor measured from anterior to posterior margins nearly nine inches. In its widest portion it measured three inches.

FIG. 31.—F F, Folds of anterior portion of labia majora, the remaining portion of the great lips being hidden from view; L, anterior part of the left labium minus; R, middle part of the right labium minus; M, enlarged left labium minus: N, enlarged right labium minus. A B, the light line between these letters, is designed to indicate the introitus vaginæ, but the actual opening to the canal had its anterior boundary immediately backward of the nodule seen near the letter B. The urine was voided just above the nodular point, near the letter C. The figure does not well exhibit the elongated clitoris, which was fully an inch and a half long, and could be felt in the mass like a hard cord. The tumor seemed to begin at the clitoris and the anterior portions of the labiæ minora, and as it increased in size the introitus was filled by it anteriorly.

mother of several children and four months advanced in pregnancy at the time she came to my clinic. She walked with difficulty and complained of pain on the left side of the genitalia. She had been troubled with the tumor hereafter described for more than two years, and during her last pregnancy, because of its becoming larger and more painful, it proved a serious impediment to childbirth. For these reasons she wished it removed before being further advanced in pregnancy. The contiguous parts were irritated by fluid discharged from small integumentary abscesses. I removed the tumor by a surgical operation, and the patient made a perfect recovery without any return of the growth. A feature of the case observed during the operation was that an incision made in any portion of the tumor caused a serous discharge to exude, so that at all times it was possible to tell whether I was cutting beyond the diseased tissue or not.

Case No. 2.—Miss ——, æt. twenty-two, a brunette of French parentage, came to the clinic for the purpose of having removed from the vagina a tumor of a year's growth, which she said was still rapidly growing, making it difficult and painful for her to walk or engage in any pursuit. The tumor of which she spoke is the one represented by Fig. 31. The operation for the removal of the tumor simply consisted in excising the entire mass and putting a ligature around the base of the hypertrophied clitoris. Three days after a hard-rubber vaginal dilator was inserted, and ordered to be worn most of the time until the parts were healed.

In the first case here reported there was no evidence of any syphilitic taint, but the woman lived in a markedly malarial district. In the last one there were indications of a syphilitic taint. A microscopic examination of the tumor of each case plainly showed its pachydermatous character. Both women were very dark brunettes, each having a coarse, tawny skin, and neither was over-cleanly in her habits.

An important indication relating to operative treatment in this locality is the use of the galvano- or thermo-cautery, particularly the latter, owing to the great vascularity of the parts and the lack of points upon which to exercise counter-pressure to control hemorrhage.

Hæmatoma.

DEFINITION.—Hæmatoma of the vulva is also designated as thrombus or pudendal hæmatocele. This affection consists of an effusion of blood in subcutaneous or submucous cellular tissue of the vulvo-vaginal region; the effusion occurs usually in one labium or in the cellular tissue surrounding the vaginal walls, and, later becoming coagulated, forms a tumor which may vary in size. The tumors sometimes attain the size of a fœtal head.

ETIOLOGY.—Hæmatoma generally occurs during pregnancy or during labor, usually from some injury, but rarely spontaneously or in the nonpregnant. Muscular effort during childbirth, blows, kicks, falls, the passage of the fœtal head, or anything which can obstruct the return of venous blood or produce rupture of the veins, may be a cause.

SYMPTOMATOLOGY.—The patient will have a feeling of discomfort, later pain of a throbbing character, and often difficult urination on account of the tumor encroaching upon the urethra. If the tumor is very large she will experience some degree of faintness.

DIAGNOSIS.—The sudden appearance of the tumor with the symptoms alluded to usually renders diagnosis an easy task. The affections which may possibly be confounded with this are abscess of the labia, inflammation or cysts of the glands of Bartholini, and pudendal hernia.

TREATMENT.—If the effusion should be small and the symptoms light, but little is demanded except quiet and cooling lotions, like the lead-and-opium wash. If there is effusion in the labia and there are indications of suppuration, it should be treated as phlegmonous inflammation by hot poultices, etc.[1]

[1] Vide Phlegmonous Inflammation of the Labia, p. 391.

It is sometimes necessary during labor, in order to complete it, that a free incision is made in the tumor and the clot turned out with the fingers. This same treatment is often requisite when the tumor is very large and there are good reasons for believing that it will not undergo absorption. It is generally advisable to pursue the same course if a thrombus has existed for some time and there are no signs of absorption or suppuration, by reason of the continued discomfort and pain to which the patient is subject.

After the clot is removed there is often a renewal of the bleeding, in which case the cavity should be plugged with lint or surgical cotton and pressure applied by means of vaginal tampons and external bandages. Sometimes it is requisite to saturate lint or cotton with liquid persulphate of iron, and finally pack the cavity with it in order to check the bleeding. If there is no hemorrhage after the evacuation of one of these tumors, then there is no need of packing or making use of styptics, but it is necessary to prevent phlegmonous inflammation or septicæmia. For this purpose iodoform or carbolic acid should be used and a free outlet provided for the discharge of pus. Washing out the cavity with a weak solution of the permanganate of potassium[1] also serves a good purpose.

Cancer of the Vulva.

Cancer is not a common disease of the vulva, yet as a primary affection it attacks this locality more frequently than the vagina.

Epithelioma is the most common form, and generally appears in the outset near the clitoris or on one labium as a small hard and warty growth, which at first itches and later smarts, but is not painful.

After an indefinite length of time the growth, which has increased somewhat in size, becomes painful, ulcerated, and there is more or less of an offensive ichorous discharge. If the disease pursues its natural course, the ulceration will rapidly extend until neighboring tissue becomes involved; the inguinal glands become affected, and after the characteristic cachexia becomes apparent there is no known remedy or means of treatment that can prevent the progress of the disease to a fatal termination.

If the clitoris becomes affected with this form of malignant disease, it can be detected earlier than epithelioma of any other portion of the organs of generation on account of its more external position, its greater sensitiveness, and the increasing pain which the affection and its enlargement produce.

TREATMENT.—If the disease is detected sufficiently early, an entire removal of all the affected parts, including a wide margin of healthy tissue, will generally effect a cure; but postponement until neighboring parts, more particularly the lymphatic glands, are implicated leaves little or no hope of cure through any mode of treatment. Carcinoma of the vulva is generally an extension of the same disease from the uterus or the inguinal glands, and rarely occurs as a primary affection.

[1] The author usually directs that from 4 to 8 grains of this salt shall be added to each pint of warm water when it is to be used as an injection or wash.

Urethral Caruncle.

This painful affection, commonly included by medical authors as among diseases of the vulva, will be very briefly considered.

DEFINITION.—The most common neoplasm to which the urethra is subject is known as urethral caruncle, vascular tumor, or irritable vascular excrescence of the urethra. These growths consist of all excrescences located at the mouth of the urethra, and sometimes extending within the canal for a short distance. They are of a deep-red color, soft and friable, sometimes regular in shape, but more frequently irregular, and then resemble a small cockscomb. They vary in size from the head of a pin to a raspberry, occasionally attaining that of a walnut.

ETIOLOGY.—No definite cause can be given for the development of urethral caruncle. These growths occur among married and single, old and young.

SYMPTOMS.—The first symptom generally is that the patient experiences a severe smarting pain during or immediately after voiding urine. Pain is also caused by walking, pressure, friction, or even the slightest contact of clothing. Also sleep is frequently disturbed in consequence of slight movements of the body. Coition not only causes a severe pain, but, owing to the friable and vascular character of the growth, it often causes a flow of blood, which leads the subject to believe she has cancer or some other serious disorder. In addition to the foregoing symptoms the patient usually becomes fretful, nervous, hysterical, and melancholy. The severity of one's suffering when thus affected is very much out of proportion to the size of the growths giving rise to it.

Occasionally there will be a feeling of weight and pain in the pelvic region, extending down the thighs. There will also be a muco-purulent discharge from the urethra.

PATHOLOGY.—Urethral caruncles may be briefly defined as consisting of "dilated capillaries in connective tissue, the whole being covered with squamous epithelium."[1]

DIAGNOSIS.—(This has been given in part under head of Symptoms.) If there is protrusion of any portion of the caruncle the diagnosis is easy. Yet a prolapse of the urethral mucous membrane or of the urethra may be mistaken for a vascular tumor, but there will not be the characteristic pain attending either of these conditions that invariably accompanies caruncle of the urethra.

Syphilitic growths are sometimes located here, but they are wart-like and painless, and generally have companions in the same neighborhood.

By placing the patient on her back in the lithotomy position and carefully inspecting the parts a diagnosis is by no means difficult. When the growths are within the meatus slight dilatation may be requisite to see them, for which purpose a pair of ordinary dressing-forceps will usually suffice.

TREATMENT.—Owing to the liability of the recurrence of caruncles their simple removal by a cutting instrument will not, as a rule, suffice. Various modes of treatment have been recommended, but the most efficacious can be very briefly stated as follows: The patient being anæsthetized and placed on her back, the growths are then removed and their bases

[1] Hart and Barbour.

thoroughly cauterized by Paquelin's thermo-cautery at a dull heat; if of a large size it is a better plan to first remove them by scissors and then apply the cautery. If a thermo- or galvanic cautery is not at hand, a knitting-needle heated in the flame of a spirit-lamp will serve a good purpose.

Atresia.

Although the subject is referred to here in its regular order, yet for the greater convenience of the reader vulvar atresia has been included by the author in the preceding section on Diseases of the Vagina (see p. 373).

Eruptions.

The skin and mucous membrane of the vulva may develop eruptions common to such tissues in other parts of the body. Those most often found are eczema, erythema, herpes, and acne. They are not distinguished from eruptions located elsewhere, except it may be their greater obstinacy in responding to treatment.

DISORDERS OF PREGNANCY.

By W. W. JAGGARD, M. D.

"GESTATION," says Mauriceau, "is a disease of nine months' duration." Robert Barnes[1] more truthfully remarks: "Since in pregnancy every organ and the whole organism are specially weighted, undergoing extraordinary developmental and functional activity, so any defect or fault inherited or acquired, however latent, will be liable to be evolved or intensified under the trial. Hence pregnancy is the great test of bodily soundness." The pregnant woman is liable to many disorders which can be distinctly traced to the existence of pregnancy. The study of the natural history of gestation renders it highly probable that these disorders are merely pathological exaggerations of physiological functions. Then, pregnancy confers upon the individual no immunity from the diseases to which the non-pregnant woman is liable. But certain acute and chronic diseases, sustaining the relation of accidental complications, are variously modified in their course and effects by pregnancy, and accordingly are of interest to the general practitioner.

For convenience of discussion the disorders of pregnancy may be classified under two headings: I. The Pathological Exaggerations of Physiological Processes; and II. The Peculiarities of Certain Accidental Acute and Chronic Diseases occurring in the Course of Pregnancy.

I. THE PATHOLOGICAL EXAGGERATIONS OF PHYSIOLOGICAL PROCESSES.

IT is always difficult, frequently impossible, to draw the boundary-line at which normal functional activity becomes pathological. As remarked by Spiegelberg, all the diagnostic penetration of the physician is demanded to recognize this transition. Then, a high exercise of judgment is necessary to determine when to preserve a wise and masterly inactivity, when to adopt measures of active interference.

Alterations in the Constitution of the Blood.

CHLOROSIS AND HYDRÆMIA.

Recent investigations show that qualitative and quantitative changes occur in the constitution of the blood of the normal pregnant woman. The

[1] *Obstetric Medicine and Surgery*, 1884, London, p. 205.

red corpuscles, albumen, and iron diminish, while the white corpuscles, fibrin, and aqueous elements increase. Virchow describes this increase in the number of white corpuscles as a physiological leucocytosis dependent upon the growth of the lymph-vessels and corresponding hypertrophic changes in the pelvic and lumbar lymphatic glands. The total blood-mass is also increased—a change especially notable in the second half of pregnancy. When the number of red blood-corpuscles is abnormally diminished the woman becomes chlorotic. If, in addition, the albumen is abnormally diminished, hydræmia results. Chlorosis and hydræmia can only be regarded as independent affections in the absence of cardiac and renal lesions. They are seldom traceable to pregnancy in the absence of individual predisposition. Effusions into the subcutaneous connective tissue, pleural and peritoneal cavities, are liable to occur. Sudden exudations into the pleural cavity are particularly dangerous, while effusions into the subcutaneous tissue of the abdomen, vulva, and lower extremities are annoying and may interrupt pregnancy.

TREATMENT.—The indications for treatment are obvious. The quality of the blood must be improved, elimination of the aqueous elements attempted, and local disturbances alleviated. Nutritious food, iron in combination with non-irritant diuretics, fulfil the first two indications. Blaud's pill, which Niemeyer and Spiegelberg extol so highly, is an excellent tonic preparation. Basham's iron mixture is admirable in its effects.

PROGRESSIVE PERNICIOUS ANÆMIA.

Gusserow[1] was the first to observe and describe a peculiar form of progressive pernicious anæmia occurring during gestation. The disease is of rare occurrence, and nothing is known as to its etiology. Chlorosis and hydræmia, however, may be mentioned as predisposing causes.

PATHOLOGY.—The alterations in the constitution of the blood are identical with those in anæmia and hydræmia, and produce similar effects. Evidences of fatty degeneration are found in the musculature of the heart, intima of the arteries, and portions of the capillary walls; retinal hemorrhages are constant lesions. The number of white corpuscles is not increased, and signs of leukæmia—splenic tumor, swelling of the lymphatic glands—are wanting. The condition is that of oligæmia or oligocythosis.

The prodromal symptoms occur during the first half of pregnancy, are obscure, and cannot be distinguished from the effects of chlorosis and hydræmia. After the disease has passed through its incipient stages, food, iron, and tonics seem to have no influence upon its course. During the second half of pregnancy abortion or premature labor usually occurs spontaneously. Under these conditons the shock and hemorrhage resulting from parturition are sufficient to cause a lethal issue in many cases.

PROGNOSIS.—Graefe[2] has collected 25 cases of this rare affection: 1 case recovered, 2 cases were discharged improved; the others died before or shortly after labor. The prognosis is obviously grave.

TREATMENT.—As food, iron, and tonics have little or no effect upon the disease after it has passed through its incipient stages, therapeutic resources are limited. The evacuation of the uterine cavity, as shown by

---

[1] *Arch. f Gyn.*, ii. p. 218.   [2] *Diss.*, Halle, 1880.

Graefe's cases, exercises a favorable influence upon the course of the affection. Gusserow advises the artificial interruption of pregnancy when- ever grave symptoms occur, and the weight of professional opinion is very decidedly in favor of such a course. Negative results have attended all efforts at transfusion.

HÆMOPHILIA.

Kehrer[1] has recently called attention to the apparent influence of preg- nancy in the development of the hemorrhagic diathesis. This influence, however, is seldom observed, and then only in cases of distinct, indi- vidual predisposition.

TREATMENT.—The induction of premature labor, or, at times, of abor- tion, is indicated.

PLETHORA.

The experiments and observations of Spiegelberg[2] and Gscheidlen prove the possibility of the occurrence of plethora during gestation. Actual increase of the red corpuscles, albumen, and iron in the blood is observed during the second half of pregnancy, and then only under the most favorable conditions. As described by Spiegelberg, the symptoms are—mammary and cerebral congestions, palpitation, vertigo, constipa- tion, hepatic torpor.

TREATMENT.—Restricted diet, muscular exercise, and an occasional saline purge will relieve the troublesome symptoms. Spiegelberg is con- vinced of the value of bleeding in selected cases.

Circulatory Disturbances.

Among the circulatory disturbances due to pregnancy, mechanical œdema and the varices of the pelvis and lower extremities deserve atten- tion.

De Cristoforis of Milan describes a mechanical inferior venous hyper- æmia, the result of the pressure of the gravid uterus on the iliac veins. The mechanical œdema of the abdominal walls, vulva, and lower extremi- ties, intensified by chlorosis and hydræmia, is usually associated with venous ectasis. The œdema may become so excessive that locomotion is rendered difficult, while the labia are enormously distended and the sub- cutaneous tissue of the abdominal walls becomes pendulous. Toward the end of pregnancy, when the uterus sinks into the pelvic cavity, the œdema and varices frequently abate.

Active measures for the relief of the symptoms produced by œdema are frequently indicated. Threatened gangrene of the skin from hyper- distension may render puncture of the hydropsical regions necessary. It is quite possible to interrupt pregnancy by this little operation, especially if the labia are punctured. ‑ Elevation of the lower extremities, rest in the horizontal position, elastic bandages and stockings, local hot packs, mild diuretics, usually fulfil all indications for treatment.

Varices are observed more frequently among multiparæ, but may occur in primiparæ. They are usually developed during the second half

---

[1] *Arch. f. Gyn.*, x. p. 201. [2] *Lehrbuch d. Geburtshülfe*, Lahr, 1882, p. 58.

of pregnancy. The principal trunk of the saphena is first involved, and subsequently the lateral branches. Congeries of veins are observed on the inner sides of the legs and thighs, especially in the vicinity of the knees. The iliac veins may become dilated, as shown by the condition of the vulvar veins and the occurrence of hemorrhoids. Varices incommode the patient, but seldom cause serious disturbances. Sometimes, however, their tunics are lacerated, and serious even fatal hemorrhage may result. Spiegelberg[1] records four cases of fatal hemorrhage from the rupture of varices in pregnancy. Then there is always the danger of phlebitis and the processes of thrombosis and embolism, even when the loss of blood is insignificant.

TREATMENT.—The regular and gentle evacuation of the bowels will frequently relieve the distressing symptoms due to hemorrhoids. Fordyce Barker points out the fact that aloes is not contraindicated by pregnancy. A pill containing a grain or a grain and a half of powdered aloes, with a quarter of a grain of extract of nux vomica, is a very good remedy. Frequent hot fomentations in conjunction with narcotic ointments will relieve the pain from the congestion of the piles. Attempts at reduction must be instituted with extreme care. It is usually impossible to completely cure the condition during pregnancy, and there is danger of interrupting gestation. Elevation of the lower extremities and equable compression by an elastic bandage or rubber stocking relieve the symptoms caused by varices of the saphena. P. Ruge[2] and A. Martin have seen favorable results from the hypodermatic injection of ergotin.

Disorders of the Alimentary Canal.

THE UNCONTROLLABLE VOMITING OF PREGNANCY.

Nausea, even vomiting, in the morning, before or shortly after meals, during the early months of gestation, is so common and devoid of injurious effect that it is regarded as physiological. Robert Barnes views it as a normal means of discharging superfluous nervous energy. The uncontrollable vomiting of pregnancy, in which the stomach retains absolutely nothing, is a grave disorder. The patient vomits glairy mucus, clear or colored by the bile. Ultimately the vomit is mixed with blood. Violent retching, intense nausea, pyrosis, and hiccough are constant and distressing symptoms. The woman becomes emaciated. The buccal cavity is dry, the tongue red and shining, the teeth and gums covered with sordes, the breath horribly fetid, the skin dry and harsh. Salivation is frequently observed. Constipation and extreme thirst usually coexist. The epigastrium is tender upon pressure. The woman becomes restless and irritable from loss of sleep and painful efforts at vomiting. A fever of typhoid type is developed, with a quick, rapid, thready pulse. The urine is sparingly secreted, concentrated, and contains albumen and tube-casts. Jaundice is frequently noticed. Extreme marasmus supervenes, and the woman succumbs to some intercurrent disease or dies of exhaustion in muttering delirium. Phthisis and diarrhœa are intercurrent affections which may hasten the lethal issue.

[1] *Lehrbuch d. Geburtshülfe*, Lahr. 1882, p. 235.
[2] *Berl. Beitr. z. Geb. u. Gyn.*, Bd. iii. p. 7.

Between the slight nausea upon rising in the morning and the state of extreme marasmus thus briefly sketched every degree of pathological variation may be observed.

It is a remarkable fact that the incessant vomiting, retching, and hiccough seldom interrupt pregnancy until near its end. The muscular effort and loss of blood at this time may precipitate the fatal termination.

Occasionally, spontaneous abortion or premature labor occurs before the patient's condition is desperate. Under these circumstances the severe symptoms may disappear immediately. The same sudden cessation of the vomiting is frequently observed after quickening, rapid excentric hypertrophy of the uterus, and death of the fœtus.

The COURSE of the disorder is chronic. Cases terminate by recovery or death in from two to three months. Alarming symptoms are usually developed from the second to the sixth month—very seldom during the seventh and eighth months.

Fortunately, the uncontrollable vomiting of pregnancy is a rare affection. So few cases are recorded in German medical literature that Hohl[1] has denied the existence of the condition. Carl Braun[2] in a fabulous experience of over one hundred and fifty thousand obstetrical cases has never seen a fatal case.

PATHOLOGY AND ETIOLOGY.—As the essential predisposing cause of this disorder it is necessary to bear in mind the increased functional activity of the nervous system in general, and of the spinal cord in particular, during pregnancy. Increased reflex mobility is apparent in all the so-called sympathetic affections.

Peripheral irritants are not wanting. The growing ovum stretches the uterine fibres, and consequently irritates the uterine nerves. Bretonneau adduces many facts in favor of this theory. Vomiting is severer in first pregnancies, and occurs during the first half of pregnancy. Vomiting is observed in connection with passive distension of the uterus caused by the unusually rapid growth of the ovum, as in hydramnion and multiple pregnancy. Immediate cessation of all symptoms is frequently noted after quickening, rapid excentric hypertrophy of the uterus, death of the fœtus, evacuation of the uterine contents. Henry Bennet directs attention to the importance of congestions, inflammations, and lacerations of the cervix uteri as etiological factors. Graily Hewitt maintains that uterine displacements, with or without incarceration, producing irritation of the uterine nerves, are potent causes. The round gastric ulcer, chronic catarrhal gastritis, are sufficient causes in many cases.

Diseases of the endometrium, decidua, fœtal envelopes, or of the fœtus itself may supply adequate excentric irritants.

Frerichs has pointed out the connection of hyperemesis with the renal insufficiency of Bright's disease. Kiwisch finds a sufficient cause in the relation between the hyperæsthetic gastric nerves and the hydræmic condition of the blood of the pregnant woman. Lebert and Rosenthal are of the opinion that hyperemesis is symptomatic of extreme general inanition of nervous tissue. Numerous other theories more or less ingenious, and adequately explanatory of certain cases, exist in the literature of the subject. Notwithstanding the extent and accuracy of etiological research

---

[1] *Grundriss d. Geburtshülfe*, Kleinwächter, 1881, p. 197.
[2] *Lehrb. d. Gynaekologie*, Wien, 1881, p. 842.

into the uncontrollable vomiting of pregnancy, a large class of cases remains in which no organic change capable of objective demonstration can be found.

DIAGNOSIS.—The diagnosis of the uncontrollable vomiting of pregnancy is not so easy as at first apparent. Guéniot[1] pertinently calls attention to three distinct elements: (1) The diagnosis of pregnancy; (2) the diagnosis of the adjuvant or determining cause of hyperemesis; (3) the differential diagnosis between the uncontrollable vomiting of pregnancy and obstinate vomiting from some other cause entirely independent of the pregnant condition.

Experienced clinicians have committed mistakes, particularly in the third element. Trousseau once made the diagnosis of uncontrollable vomiting of pregnancy in a case in which the autopsy revealed cancer of the stomach. This case was observed by Depaul. Charpentier[2] reports a serious error in diagnosis made by Beau. The case was diagnosticated as hyperemesis of pregnancy. The autopsy showed that the obstinate vomiting was probably due to tuberculous meningitis.

PROGNOSIS.—Severe vomiting in pregnancy is always ground for anxiety, and the prognosis must always be guarded. The majority of cases terminate in recovery without the interruption of pregnancy. Guéniot records 118 cases: of these, 46 died; of the 72 survivals, 42 recovered after the spontaneous or artificial evacuation of the uterine contents. Recovery usually, though not always, rapidly follows the cessation of pregnancy. The prognosis is absolutely unfavorable after the appearance of fever and typhoid symptoms.

TREATMENT.—The treatment of hyperemesis may be effective. Its efficiency, however, depends largely upon the accurate recognition of the adjuvant and determining causes. A rational therapeusis must consist in the elimination of these etiological factors. The treatment naturally resolves itself into (1) hygienic; (2) medical; (3) gynæcological: (4) obstetrical.

Hygienic.—The hygienic treatment is of avail in the minor degrees of the disorder, although not without influence in the more serious cases. Diet is of primary importance. Let the patient breakfast upon a small cup of strong coffee or tea, half a cup of milk and lime-water, a morsel of cracker or toast early in the morning, in bed, and lie quietly for one or two hours following the meal. Small quantities of easily-digestible food at short intervals will be tolerated when the patient has given up all pretence at keeping to regular meals. Liquid foods, as sparkling koumiss, egg-albumen in water, iced milk with lime- or soda-water, commend themselves. Absolute dietetic rules, however, cannot be maintained. The stomach of the pregnant woman is proverbially capricious and fanciful. Charpentier narrates the history of a case suggestive in connection with this subject. The patient, four months advanced in pregnancy, in a critical condition from uncontrollable vomiting, came under the care of Beau in the Hôpital de la Charité. One day she asked for Bordeaux crawfishes. Beau granted her request. On the first day two crawfishes were retained; on the second, six; on the third, crawfishes ad libitum, bouillon, and milk. Within six days

[1] *Thèse Agrégation*, Paris, 1863.
[2] *Traité pratique des Accouchements*, Paris, 1883, t. i. p. 621.

the vomiting disappeared. Cazeaux and Guéniot cite cases in which ham and pâté de foie gras were retained after the rejection of easily-digestible foods. It is necessary to respect these caprices and fancies.

When everything is rejected absolute stomach-rest is indicated. Then nutrient enemata may be tried. Of the great value of rectal alimentation under these conditions there can be no doubt. Henry F. Campbell of Georgia relates the history of a case in which he nourished the patient for fifty-two days by the rectum alone. There is danger, however, of irritating the rectum and causing diarrhœa—a peculiarly unfavorable complication at this time; and this fact must be clearly borne in mind. Of the various nutrient enemata, peptonized milk, cream, defibrinated blood, Leube's beef-and-pancreas mixture, eggs, and beef-tea containing albumens are among the best. From four to six ounces should be exhibited not more frequently than once every six hours.

Inunctions of oil are of undoubted value. Absolute moral and physical rest frequently exercises a favorable influence. Seyfert advised his patients to go home on a visit to their mothers, and return to the conditions to which they were accustomed prior to marriage. Coitus may be a disturbing factor. Rest in the horizontal decubitus exercises as favorable an influence as in sea-sickness.

Medical.—There are few drugs in the Pharmacopœia which have not been vaunted as specifics by some and found utterly worthless by others. This fact indicates, as remarked by Schroeder, that all remedies are unreliable, and that spontaneous cures frequently occur. Various effervescent liquids, as dry champagne, carbonic-acid water containing one drachm of potassium bromide to the siphon, are sometimes grateful. Subnitrate of bismuth and the antacids are of great value in cases of excessive gastric acidity. Oxalate of cerium, a much-vaunted remedy, is of very little value. Small doses of the tincture of nux vomica are useful in cases of gastric catarrh. The various local anæsthetics are of great importance. Small doses of creasote, carbolic acid, tincture of aconite-root, hydrocyanic acid, and the volatile oils have been used with varying degrees of success. Of this class of remedies cocaine hydrochlorate deserves especial attention. On a priori grounds there is much in its favor. Clinical experience with the drug is not such as to warrant very positive deductions. W. Otto[1] has employed cocaine in sea-sickness, especially in pregnant women, with favorable results. Manasseïn[2] reports several cases of hyperemesis of pregnancy cured by its exhibition. The subject is certainly worthy of thorough investigation. G. Gaertner of Vienna states that 0.1 cocainum muriaticum has no toxic effect upon adults. Doses of 0.015–0.02 of the solution (cocain. muriat. sol. Merck, 1.0; aq. destill. 9.0) may be given to an adult three times daily without fear of toxæmia. Goodell recommends drop doses of wine of ipecacuanha and tincture of belladonna, repeated every fifteen minutes.

Of all medical agents, however, opium, the bromides, and chloral are the most reliable. A clyster containing thirty or forty drops of the deodorized tincture, or a half-grain suppository of the aqueous extract of opium, sometimes produces a happy effect. Hypodermatic injections of morphine will frequently allay the distressing symptoms after the failure of other measures. In the German hospitals large doses of the bromides

[1] *Berl. klin. Woch.*, 1885, No. 43.　　　[2] *Ibid.*, 1885, No. 35.

and chloral are exhibited per rectum with gratifying success in many cases.

Flying blisters, the ether spray, and the faradic current applied to the pit of the stomach may give relief in the milder forms of the disorder.

Gynæcological.—Under the gynæcological treatment of hyperemesis quite a number of important operative procedures are included: 1. If bimanual examination reveals a displacement of the uterus capable of producing symptoms, the organ must be replaced if possible, and retained in position by a properly fitting pessary. 2. Henry Bennet suggested the cauterization of the cervix in all cases, basing his therapy upon his peculiar views of the pathology of the condition. Welponer, Sims, and Jones recommend the application of a 10 per cent. solution of argentic nitrate to the vaginal portion of the cervix in all cases, irrespective of the condition of the cervical tissues, when other means have proved useless. Carl Braun[1] bears testimony as to the value of this procedure. 3. As an ultimate resource before artificially interrupting gestation, the plan of dilating the os externum and cervix uteri with the index finger should be tried. Copeman[2] of Norwich, England, desirous of inducing abortion in the case of a patient afflicted with hyperemesis, pushed his finger through the cervical canal to the membranes and attempted to puncture the amnion with a sound. Failing to accomplish his purpose, he went home for assistance, and returned at the expiration of two hours. To his surprise, the uncontrollable vomiting had ceased. Since 1875, when he published the results of this experience, cases have accumulated proving the great value of this method. W. Gill Wylie[3] of New York has devised a steel dilator to substitute the finger. When the os externum is at all patulous, the index finger is the safest and most efficient dilator. The method is a purely empirical one, does not always secure the desired result, and frequently causes abortion or premature labor. Still, as the ultimate gynæcological resort it has important functions.

Obstetrical.—The evacuation of the uterine contents, if effected before the development of the febrile stage, is usually followed by immediate disappearance of all distressing symptoms. In the large majority of cases, however, the same end may be secured by a judicious combination of the hygienic, medical, and gynæcological methods of treatment to which attention has been directed. The weight of professional opinion is decidedly opposed to the procedure. For practical purposes the induction of premature labor may be excluded from consideration. The woman usually recovers or dies before the period of fœtal viability. Carl Braun[4] gives expression to the very general professional conviction upon this subject in the following words: "I myself have never observed a lethal issue in consequence of the uncontrollable vomiting of pregnancy, lay the greatest weight upon the expectant management and more modern medicamentation, and am of the opinion that after a conscientious estimate of all considerations and contraindications, artificial abortion can be omitted, notwithstanding its permissibility from a scientific point of view when extreme danger to maternal life has been determined by several physicians."

[1] *Lehrb. d. g. Gynaekologie*, 1881, p. 841. [2] *Brit. Med. Journal*, 1875, 1879.
[3] *N. Y. Med. Record*, Dec. 6, 1884. [4] *Lehr. d. g. Gynaekologie*, 1881, p. 842.

PTYALISM.

The excessive secretion of saliva is a rare disorder of pregnancy. At all times distressing, it may seriously endanger the patient's life when the quantity of fluid amounts to several quarts per diem. The parotid and submaxillary glands are swollen and tender. The buccal mucous membrane is red and tumid. The absence of fetor serves to distinguish the salivation of pregnancy from the ptyalism of mercurial poisoning. A generous diet and the free exhibition of iron mitigate in some degree the distressing symptoms. Dewees recommends a strictly animal diet. Astringent mouth-washes, small doses of potassium iodide, and subcutaneous injections of atropine over the submaxillary glands are indicated, but seldom influence the condition.

TOOTHACHE.

Toothache in pregnancy may be a purely functional disorder. In the majority of cases, however, actual caries is present. During gestation the secretions of the buccal cavity are sometimes altered, and become sufficiently acid to dissolve the lime salts out of the enamel. Again, when for any reason an insufficient quantity of lime salts is ingested with the food, the foetus is supplied with ossific materials derived in part from the maternal teeth. The condition of pregnancy is not infrequently detected in the dentist's chair from these changes. Popular recognition of these dental changes gave origin to the familiar saw, "For every child a tooth." The indications for treatment are obvious. Quinine and local anæsthetics relieve the symptoms of the functional forms of the disorder. Caries may be prevented, to a certain degree, by extreme attention to the teeth and secretions of the buccal cavity and a free, generous mixed diet. Doubtless, the popular belief, that an absolute fruit diet will limit the deposition of ossific material in the foetal skeleton and render labor easier, is responsible for much of the caries observed in American women. It is needless to say that such a belief is utterly without foundation in fact. When structural changes in the teeth have occurred the decalcified dentine should be excavated, and temporary fillings of oxyphosphates or gutta-percha inserted. This little operation can be performed rapidly, without pain or fatigue, and preserves the contour of the teeth.

CONSTIPATION.

Constipation is a usual, sometimes a troublesome, attendant upon gestation. The etiological factors are mechanical interference of the gravid uterus with intestinal peristalsis, defective innervation of the bowels, and alterations in the intestinal secretions. When the rectum becomes filled with scybalous masses the condition predisposes to abortion or premature labor. Diet is of primary importance in securing regular evacuations of the bowels. Fresh fruits, brown bread, oatmeal porridge are useful to this end. Enemata have obvious advantages over all drugs. In the selection of aperient remedies care must be taken to choose laxatives and avoid drastic cathartics. The compound licorice powder and confection of senna of the U. S. Pharmacopœia, Hunyadi, Friedcrichshalle, and Pullna mineral waters, may be included in the list.

DIARRHŒA.

Diarrhœa is a less frequent but more dangerous disorder during pregnancy than constipation. In the early and latter months of gestation diarrhœa is liable to occur from mechanical compression of the rectum by the gravid uterus. Dysentery, with tormina and tenesmus, is a particularly unfavorable complication. The dangers are apparent. Not only is the blood impoverished, but abortion or premature labor may be induced. Every diarrhœa occurring during pregnancy demands immediate attention. Small doses of argentic nitrate in combination with opium, in pill form, are useful in mild cases of diarrhœa, while the deodorized tincture of opium in starch-water enemata is indicated in dysentery.

Diseases of the Liver.

In normal pregnancy the functions of the liver in the secretion of bile and the excretion of cholesterin are not materially modified. The case is different with the glycogenic function. Blot in 1856 detected the presence of glycogen in the urine of nearly half the pregnant women examined. He concluded that this glycosuria was physiological. Tarnier in 1857 called attention to certain structural changes in the liver occurring during normal gestation. The liver is enlarged in volume, and a peculiar fatty infiltration within the lobule is perceptible. De Sinéty confirmed Tarnier's observations, finding the fatty infiltration within the centre of the lobule, seldom near the periphery. Robert Barnes and Ewart have added corroboratory testimony. Tarnier ascribes the physiological glycosuria announced by Blot to the fatty infiltration observed by himself. Each of these three functions of the liver, the secretion of bile, the excretion of cholesterin, and the glycogenic function, may undergo pathological exaggeration during pregnancy.

ICTERUS.

Icterus is observed with relative infrequency during gestation. Two distinct forms are recognized—simple jaundice, with bright-yellow coloration of conjunctivæ and skin, without fever and cerebral symptoms: and malignant jaundice, with dull-yellow coloration of conjunctivæ and skin, with fever and cerebral symptoms.

Simple Jaundice.—Simple icterus may occur at any time during pregnancy, runs its usual course, and exercises, as a rule, no serious influence upon the maternal health. The effect upon the fœtus is grave. If the icterus is intense and lasts for a considerable period of time, the fœtus dies and gestation is interrupted. All the fœtal tissues are found to be stained with the biliary coloring matters—a condition termed by Lobstein cirrhonosis.

ETIOLOGY.—The causes of simple jaundice in pregnancy are identical with those which produce the condition in the non-gravid state, and are frequently obscure. It is in a high degree probable that pressure from the gravid uterus is without influence, since the symptom may appear at any time during gestation. The pathological condition usually present is catarrh of the mucous membrane of the duct or of the duodenum in the vicinity of the orifice, causing a narrowing of its lumen.

SYMPTOMS.—The conjunctivæ, skin, and urine are colored bright yellow, and there is entire absence of febrile and cerebral symptoms.

The PROGNOSIS and TREATMENT, so far as the mother is concerned, are the same as in the non-pregnant state. In view of the possible causative relation between simple and malignant icterus, and the injurious effect upon the fœtus, medical treatment should be instituted at once. Restricted diet, mercurials or ipecacuanha, followed by saline cathartics, are the more important measures. Artificial abortion or the induction of premature labor has no effect upon the condition. This operative procedure is indicated in the interest of the child, when the icterus is intensive, of long duration, the fœtus living and viable, the frequency of the fœtal heart-beats diminished, and there is reason to fear its death. Carl Braun recognizes very distinctly the force of this indication.

Malignant Icterus.—Malignant icterus, due to the acute yellow atrophy of the liver of the pregnant woman (Rokitansky), is a very rare disease. Carl Braun has observed the condition only once in twenty-eight thousand cases from 1857 to 1863.

ETIOLOGY AND PATHOLOGY.—Very little is known as to the causes of acute yellow atrophy of the liver. Virchow ascribes one case coming under his own observation to compression of the lower half of the liver and gall-bladder by the growing uterus. The rarity of the affection and its occurrence irrespective of the time of pregnancy prove the limited operation of this etiological factor. It is in a high degree probable that the disease may have its starting-point in simple catarrhal icterus.

The liver is ochre-colored, shrunken to one half its volume, and flaccid. On section no signs of lobular structure are visible. Microscopical examination reveals total destruction of the acini and hepatic cells. In the place of the glandular elements, fat-globules, fine granular detritus, crystals of leucin and tyrosin are noted. The spleen is enlarged and the kidneys show acute inflammatory changes. Extensive ecchymoses are observed under the skin, pericardium, and gastric mucous membrane.

SYMPTOMS.—The prodromal symptoms of acute yellow atrophy of the liver are usually overlooked. A trivial jaundice with slight elevation of temperature may precede by several days the development of cerebral symptoms. Difficulty in speech, headache, disorders of the senses followed by delirium, convulsions (cholæmic eclampsia), and coma are the more important symptoms of cerebral origin. The pulse is remarkably frequent and small. The temperature is at first elevated several degrees, but becomes subnormal prior to death. The urine is sparingly secreted, highly colored by the bile-pigments, and contains albumen, tube-casts, leucin, tyrosin, and cholesterin. Urea, uric acid, and the urates are diminished. The combination of symptoms points to the retention within the system of the waste products usually excreted by the liver and kidneys. Ultimately, a condition of complete hepatic and renal insufficiency obtains.

DIAGNOSIS.—The dull yellow color of the skin and conjunctivæ, with fever and cerebral symptoms, is a sign of greatest diagnostic value. Physical exploration reveals tenderness on pressure over the hepatic region, and rapidly diminishing area of hepatic dulness on percussion. Care must be taken to exclude acute phosphorus-poisoning—a toxæmia simulating very closely acute yellow atrophy, and repeatedly confounded with that affection.

PROGNOSIS.—No case of recovery has been recorded up to the present time. The disease pursues a rapidly fatal course, terminating within a few days after the development of the icterus.

TREATMENT.—Therapeutic measures must be addressed to prophylaxis. It is necessary to regard simple icterus as a possible prodrome of the malignant form of the disorder.

DIABETES MELLITUS.

The most superficial discussion of the disorders of pregnancy would not be complete without some mention of diabetes. The existence of physiological glycosuria during pregnancy and lactation has been demonstrated. Bernard has shown that sugar appears in the placenta of calves at an early period, attains its maximum in the third or fourth month, and when the glycogenic function of the fœtal liver is established entirely disappears. The relation between physiological glycosuria and that pathological exaggeration of a normal process, diabetes mellitus, is very obscure. It is, however, a clinical fact that diabetes mellitus occurs more frequently in the pregnant than in the non-gravid woman. Diabetic women are less apt to conceive. When conception does occur, pregnancy is liable to interruption from the death of the fœtus. Under these circumstances glucose is found in the amniotic liquor and fœtal urine. A case related by Bennewitz and cited by Matthews Duncan indicates that diabetes mellitus may be developed during successive pregnancies, and entirely disappear during the intervals. The influence of pregnancy in developing a latent diabetic tendency may be accepted as established. A clinical observation of some importance is that diabetic coma is seldom developed.

PROGNOSIS.—Matthews Duncan[1] has collected the histories of 22 pregnancies in fifteen women varying in age from twenty-one to thirty-eight years: 4 of the 22 pregnancies terminated fatally by collapse, rather than by coma. The majority of the children died during pregnancy after attaining to the age of viability. Two children were feeble at birth, and died a few hours later. One infant was diabetic.

TREATMENT.—The hygienic and medical treatment of diabetes mellitus occurring during pregnancy does not differ from the therapy in the non-gravid state. There is great diversity of opinion upon the subject of the induction of premature labor. On a priori grounds it would seem to be indicated in the interest both of the mother and the child in the graver cases. In the entire absence of authoritative clinical experience, however, the operation must be resorted to with an extreme degree of caution.

Diseases of the Kidneys.

Albumen is found in the urine of from 3 to 5 per cent. of all pregnant women.[2] In parturient women albuminuria is of much more frequent occurrence. Lenbe's researches indicate the existence of physiological

---

[1] *Obstet. Trans.*, vol. xxiv. p. 256.
[2] Schrœder, *Lehrb. d. Geburtshülfe*, Bonn, 1884, p. 373.

albuminuria in the pregnant as in the non-gravid state. It is a matter of great practical difficulty to determine the limits of this normal functional activity. In a large proportion of cases the boundary-line between health and disease is passed. The physiological function undergoes pathological exaggeration, and various forms of nephritis are produced.

ETIOLOGY AND PATHOLOGY.—The types of renal disease to which pregnancy stands in more or less direct causal relation are numerous.

1. Leyden describes a condition, the kidney of pregnancy, which may be regarded as the intermediate stage between health and disease. The amount of albumen is increased; hyaline and granular casts, with renal epithelium, showing fatty changes, appear in the urine. This fatty degeneration of the cells covering the glomeruli and lining the uriniferous tubules is not of an inflammatory nature. Anasarca of the lower extremities is usually present. The condition may last for an indefinite period of time without causing serious symptoms. With the expiration of the term of pregnancy it may disappear, leaving no trace of its former existence. On the other hand, the kidney of pregnancy may be the starting-point of some serious renal lesion.

2. Latent chronic interstitial nephritis, chronic tubal nephritis, and lardaceous degeneration of the kidney are usually influenced unfavorably by pregnancy, and, in turn, may lead to the interruption of that state. Chronic interstitial nephritis and chronic tubal nephritis may have their origin in the kidney of pregnancy. The cirrhotic kidney is distinguished from the other forms by the abundant aqueous urine, containing comparatively little albumen—none at all at times—cardiac hypertrophy, and hard pulse. In the differential diagnosis of chronic tubal nephritis and the kidney of pregnancy chief reliance must be placed upon the history of the case and the course of the affection. Albuminuria is a very inconstant symptom of the lardaceous kidney, especially in the beginning and ultimate stages of the disease.

3. Mixed types of chronic Bright's disease are frequently observed. Thus, the interstitial and tubal forms of the disease may be combined. Lardaceous degeneration may be present with either form, and fatty changes are common in all the types of Bright's disease. Eclampsia is of relatively infrequent occurrence in chronic Bright's disease, although anasarca and its consequences may cause the interruption of pregnancy.

4. Acute Bright's disease is one of the most serious disorders occurring in the course of pregnancy. The urine is diminished in quantity, and contains a large amount of albumen, tube-casts, and red blood-corpuscles. Eclampsia is of frequent occurrence, and usually induces abortion or premature labor.

The causes of renal disease and of its symptom albuminuria are not always evident. In the kidney of pregnancy there is no inflammatory change. The cells covering the glomeruli and the glandular cells lining the uriniferous tubules undergo fatty degeneration, and are cast off as the result of anæmia.

In the acute and chronic forms of renal inflammation there is a variety of probable etiological factors. Mechanical pressure from the gravid uterus may impede the return of venous blood and determine congestion of the kidneys. This explanation is rendered more probable by the fact that albumen usually appears in the urine after the fifth month, when the uterus has attained considerable size. Albuminuria is of comparatively more frequent occurrence in primiparæ with tense abdominal walls. It is frequently observed in cases of large ovarian cysts and uterine fibroids. The increased functional activity of the organs, the elevation of blood-pressure, the alterations in the constitution of the blood, are doubtless potential factors. When any latent tendency to Bright's disease exists, exposure to cold and impeded cutaneous functional activity are more likely to develop the disease in the pregnant than in the non-gravid state. Compression of the ureters is regarded by Halbertsma as a cause of great importance.

SYMPTOMS.—The symptoms of Bright's disease in pregnancy are neither uniform nor constantly present. Anasarca frequently directs attention to the patient's condition long before the appearance of more significant signs. Œdematous swellings of the face, hands, arms, feet, legs, and labia majora are always suspicious, and should lead to an examination of the urine. These œdematous swellings are wandering—appear when the patient is lying down, and disappear when she rises and walks about. Sometimes, toward the end of pregnancy, they become less marked, not infrequently entirely disappearing, while the albuminuria is increasing. The skin covering the œdematous portions of the body is dry, of a chalkish-white appearance, and the surface temperature is depressed.

Anomalous nervous phenomena, such as headache, vertigo, dimness of vision, spots before the eyes, ringing in the ears, sudden deafness, obstinate nausea and vomiting, sleeplessness, neuralgia, are often observed, and should always excite suspicion. These various nervous symptoms may be viewed as produced by the retention within the blood of certain substances normally excreted by the kidneys.

Convulsions, due to renal insufficiency, may occur during pregnancy, but are observed more frequently during parturition and the puerperium.

Attention has already been called to the characters of the urine. It is necessary to remember that in the granular, contracted kidney and lardaceous degeneration albuminuria may escape observation.

Bright's disease strongly predisposes to abortion or premature labor.

PROGNOSIS.—Any organic disease of the kidneys is serious. When the disease is extensive and involves both organs the prognosis is especially unfavorable. Accurate conclusions as to the dangers of Bright's disease during pregnancy are not justified by the present state of our knowledge. It is only possible to say, in a general way, that the prospect of recovery is less favorable than in the non-gravid state. Owing to the strong predisposition to abortion and premature labor, the chances of the fœtus surviving pregnancy are relatively slight. Even if the child is not prematurely expelled from the uterus, it usually succumbs to the influence of the excrementitious products retained within the maternal blood.

TREATMENT.—In view of the serious complications arising in pregnancy from interference with the functions of the kidneys, the absolute necessity of chemical examination of the urine at regular intervals in every case, especially during the latter half of gestation, is apparent. When pathological albuminuria is present, rational therapy will be directed to the removal of the cause. Evacuation of the uterine contents is the only mode of removing the pressure from the gravid uterus, but we have a variety of expedients, hygienic and medical, which must be invoked before resorting to such a radical procedure.

Hygienic.—The diet should be restricted, as far as possible, to milk, and nitrogenous articles of food must be forbidden. The functional activity of the skin can be maintained by frequent baths in lukewarm water, Vapor baths are of still greater value. Hot-water baths are employed on an extensive scale in the obstetrical clinics of the Vienna General Hospital. Carl Braun, Josef Spaeth, and Gustav Braun give testimony to their efficacy. Indeed, in Vienna chief reliance is placed upon the hot-water bath as a prophylactic and remedial agent. Breus[1] has recently described the method usually practised. The patient is placed in a bath-tub filled with water at a temperature slightly above 99° F. The tub is then covered with a heavy blanket, leaving the face free, and the temperature of the water is gradually elevated to 110° or 112° F. She remains in the bath thirty minutes. A towel wrung out of ice-water and placed upon the head relieves any distressing cephalic sensations. While in the bath the patient drinks large quantities of water. Upon emerging from the bath she is covered with a warm sheet and enveloped in an upper and lower layer of thick blankets, so that only the face is exposed. Within a very few minutes free perspiration is observed. The sweating is continued for two or three hours. According to the gravity of the case the hot-water bath may be repeated once daily for an indefinite period. The relief of all threatening symptoms under this simple plan of treatment alone is surprising. Sometimes the hot-water bath acts as an efficient excitant of uterine contractions, and premature labor is induced. A. Sippel[2] calls attention to this fact, and proposes hot-water baths as a harmless method of induction of premature labor. Although such an event is not undesirable, it is unusual, and occurs only when the temperature of the water reaches a great elevation or the baths are frequently repeated, or, finally, when there is a very decided predisposition to the interruption of pregnancy. The lateral or latero-prone posture during sleep serves to relieve in some degree the kidneys of the pressure from the gravid uterus, and should be advised.

Medical.—The exhibition of non-irritating diuretics, such as the acetate and bitartrate of potassium, in large quantities of water, causes an increased secretion of urine and lessens the congestion of the renal vessels. Among the mineral waters Bilin, Giesshübel, Preblau, Selters, and Vichy deserve commendation. Benzoic acid, in conformity with Frerichs' suggestion, is employed in Vienna The tincture of the chloride of iron, alone or in combination with small doses of tincture of digitalis, is an efficient diuretic, and at the same time an excellent tonic.

Cathartics which produce large, watery stools without much irritation supplement the action of diuretics. The compound powder of jalap and the saline purges fulfil this indication. Care must be taken, however, to avoid the drastic effects of too large a dose.

Jaborandi and pilocarpine have been, and are at the present time, extensively used to aid in the elimination by the skin of retained exorementitious matters. The weight of authority is decidedly against the exhibition of this remedy. At best, it is uncertain in its action. It is a cardiac depressant, and frequently stands in a causal relation to pul-

---

[1] *Arch. f. Gynaek.*, vol. xix. p. 219.   [2] *Centralb. f. Gynaek.*, No. 44, 1885, p. 693.

monary œdema. For these reasons the drug has been condemned in unequivocal terms by Carl Braun and Fordyce Barker. The same effect, with less risk, can be produced by the hot-water baths.

Local Treatment.—In the acute forms of Bright's disease various modes of counter-irritation are useful. Wet and dry cups and leeches applied to the loins are indicated. Frerichs recommends pills of the extract of aloes and tannin with the view of restoring the normal tonus to the blood-vessel walls.

By a judicious combination of these varied therapeutic resources, hygienic and medical, threatening symptoms may be averted. Cure of Bright's disease, acute or chronic, is seldom if ever achieved during pregnancy. Not unfrequently, however, notwithstanding all efforts, the amount of albumen steadily increases, hydræmia becomes more pronounced, hydropsies appear with threatening cerebral, cardiac, or pulmonary symptoms. More active treatment is demanded, and the subject of the induction of premature labor must be seriously considered. Without entering into a detailed discussion of the arguments for and against the artificial premature interruption of pregnancy under these conditions, let it suffice to say that clinical experience furnishes overpowering evidence in favor of the operation. The weight of professional opinion is also very decidedly in favor of the artificial induction of premature labor. In the selection of the method for the induction of premature labor it is well to bear in mind the possible excitant effect on uterine contractions of hot-water baths, as pointed out by A. Sippel.[1]

Skin Diseases.

Diseases of the skin occur with comparative frequency during pregnancy. Latent diatheses are roused into activity. The graver forms of skin disease usually disappear during or shortly after the puerperium. These facts point to some causal relation between the diseases and gestation. Under the increased activity of the glandular system the growth of hair may be stimulated, giving origin to a condition termed by dermatologists hirsuties gestationis. Slocum[2] relates the history of a case in which a woman in successive pregnancies grew a full beard. Anomalous deposits of pigment, constituting the condition known as chloasma uterinum, are observed, more especially among pregnant women exposed to sunlight. Chloasma is interesting from a diagnostic point of view, since it is liable to be confounded with pityriasis versicolor, an affection of frequent occurrence during pregnancy. The red nose of acne rosacea may be one of the first signs of pregnancy. General pruritus, a rare affection, belongs to the class of idio-neuroses (Hebra). Spiegelberg relates the history of a case of general pruritus occurring in an old primipara. The affection made its appearance in the second month, and continued without material abatement of symptoms throughout the period of gestation. Pruritus of the vulva is a common disorder of pregnancy. It is usually symptomatic of eczema, some inflammatory condition of the genitalia, or diabetes mellitus. The treatment must be directed to the removal of the cause. Vaginal douches containing vegetable or mineral astringents will

[1] *Centralb. f. Gynaek.*, No. 44, 1885, p. 693.   [2] *New York Medical Record,* 1875

afford relief when the itching is due to acrid vaginal secretions. Dilute solutions of corrosive sublimate in water or alcohol (1 : 100 or 200), followed by compresses saturated with tar-water, are recommended very highly by Spiegelberg.

Pregnancy cannot be regarded as a cause of psoriasis. When that affection exists, however, it is usually aggravated. The elder Hebra[1] in 1872 described a rare form of skin disease occurring in the course of pregnancy which he called herpes impetiginiformis, and of which he encountered five cases. Grouped vesicles upon inflamed bases appear about the genitalia, and subsequently diffuse themselves by successive crops over the body. Great prostration, rigors, and intense fever-accompany the eruption. Four of the five cases terminated fatally. Milton and Duncan Bulkley a few months later described a rare skin affection peculiar to pregnancy which they designated herpes gestationis. Erythema, papules, vesicles, and bullæ are developed. Vesicles predominate, appear on the lower extremities, subsequently spreading over the body. Intense itching and burning attend the vesicles. Urticaria, neuralgia, and other neurotic troubles accompany the affection. The disease appears early in pregnancy, continues until after delivery, and is apt to recur with succeeding pregnancies. The constitutional symptoms are much less severe than in the condition described by Hebra. At the meeting of the American Dermatological Society, 1885, L. A. Duhring[2] called attention to the relation of impetigo herpetiformis, herpes gestationis, pemphigus, and certain other forms of disease to dermatitis herpetiformis. Attention was briefly directed to the identity of the impetigo herpetiformis of Hebra with dermatitis herpetiformis. Herpes gestationis was a misnomer, the affection being found in men as well as in women. The disease was the vesicular variety of dermatitis herpetiformis. The peculiar forms of pemphigus observed during pregnancy, not of syphilitic origin, may be viewed as examples of the same disease. Duhring thinks that "we stand on the threshold of our knowledge of the disease."

Neuroses.

Of all the neuroses occurring in the course of pregnancy, puerperal eclampsia is of chief clinical importance. Puerperal convulsions, however, occur more frequently during labor and the lying-in period than during gestation. For this reason the subject is usually discussed in connection with the pathology of the puerperium. The various psychoses are referred for a similar reason to the same chapter.

TETANUS.

Tetanus, a rare affection, especially in women, is occasionally observed in pregnancy. It occurs with greatest relative frequency in hot climates after abortion and the removal of placental or decidual remains. Sir James Y. Simpson collected 28 cases which sustained some relation to abortion or labor. Mr. Waring[3] has collected 232 cases occurring in a tropical climate.

---

[1] *Wiener Med. Woch.*, No. 48, 1872.
[2] *Journal of Cutaneous, etc. Dis.*, October, 1885, p. 317.   [3] *Indian Annals*, 1855.

The PROGNOSIS is unfavorable. Of Sir James Y. Simpson's 28 cases, only 6 recovered; 2 cases observed by Wiltshire terminated unfavorably.

In the entire absence of knowlege of the pathology of the disease, TREATMENT is empirical. Chloroform, the narcotics, curare, and nitrite of amyl are the remedial agents usually employed.

CHOREA.

Chorea occurs in pregnancy as an accidental complication or as the direct result of that state. It is a rare disorder of pregnancy. Spiegelberg has observed 3 cases; Barnes has collected 56 cases; Fehling[1] brings the number up to 68; altogether, 84 cases are on record.

ETIOLOGY.—The investigations of Robert Barnes show that where chorea arises in pregnancy in the large majority of cases there is a history of chorea in childhood, acquired predisposition prior to pregnancy, or hereditary "nervous diathesis predisposing to chorea." This connection between rheumatism, endocarditis, and chorea is a well-established fact. The precise nature of this relation is unknown. Hughlings Jackson has constructed the theory of "embolism of the small branches of the middle cerebral artery supplying the structures near the corpus striatum." Robert Barnes[2] calls attention to the following facts, which invalidate this ingenious theory: "(1) The frequent recovery of choreic patients; (2) the occasional immediate cessation of choreic fits upon delivery; (3) the progressive character of the disease during pregnancy, convulsions increasing in severity, and the gradual development of mania in some cases; (4) the fact that embolism is rare during pregnancy." In the absence of any definite cause, Spiegelberg refers a large number of these cases to the class of reflex neuroses. All the elements essential to a reflex neurosis are present. We have (1) a predisposition to chorea, inherited or acquired; (2) inanition of the central nervous system incident to the hydræmic state of the blood in pregnancy; (3) various potential peripheral irritants in connection with the sexual organs. Intense emotions, terror and the like, may act as exciting causes.

COURSE AND SYMPTOMS.—Chorea usually makes its appearance in the course of the first half of pregnancy, and continues until the beginning of labor. Sometimes choreic attacks are witnessed during parturition. In only 3 out of the 84 recorded cases the disease continued after the puerperium. Primiparæ are more frequently affected than multiparæ. The disease is liable to recur with succeeding pregnancies, entirely disappearing in the intervals. The choreic movements are the same as in the non-gravid woman affected with the disease. They are usually bilateral. As in chorea in the non-gravid state, transitory albuminuria and glycosuria may be observed. The increase of urates and phosphates in the urine is interpreted as the result of nervous excitement and muscular activity. Pregnancy is interrupted in about one-half the cases. The child may be born alive and affected with the disease.

PROGNOSIS.—Out of the 84 cases, 23 terminated fatally as the result of complications. Mania, loss of memory, grave cerebral and spinal lesions are occasionally traceable to the chorea of pregnancy. The prog-

---

[1] *Lehrb. d. Geburtshülfe*, 1882, p 239.
[2] *Obstetric Medicine and Surgery*, London, 1884, p. 379.

nosis with reference to the child is unfavorable, from the tendency to the premature interruption of pregnancy.

TREATMENT.—The palliative treatment of chorea occurring in pregnancy is unsatisfactory in the extreme. All the specifics of greater or less value in the non-gravid state are frequently without influence during gestation. The diet must be nutritious and easily digestible. Large doses of iron and quinine are indicated. As in other convulsive disorders, during the paroxysms chief reliance is placed upon anæsthetics, subcutaneous injections of morphine, potassium bromide, and chloral. Charcot recommends the exhibition of large doses of bromide of potassium through a considerable period of time. Clifford Albutt extols succus conii. In over one-half the recorded cases the most judicious combinations of hygienic and medical therapeutic resources have proved of no avail. In view of the prognosis, the induction of premature labor is usually indicated, in the interest of both the mother and child, at an early stage of the disease. Sometimes the question of the artificial induction of abortion comes up for consideration. In view of the grave cerebral and spinal lesions which may result from the affection, the mother is justly entitled to the benefit of the doubt. It may not be amiss to add that this indication for the induction of abortion is not generally recognized.

EPILEPSY.

Epilepsy is usually an accidental complication of pregnancy. Spiegelberg[1] is responsible for the observation that in chronic epilepsy pregnancy sometimes modifies the course of the affection in a favorable manner. The seizures occur less frequently and are not so violent in character. Acute epilepsy may be developed as the result of pregnancy when a latent predisposition, inherited or acquired, exists. The epileptogenous zone in acute epilepsy comprehends the distribution of the ischiatic nerve. Acute epilepsy disappears with the cessation of pregnancy, but is apt to recur with succeeding gestations.

The occurrence of acute or chronic epilepsy during pregnancy is of great diagnostic interest from the resemblance of the epileptic seizures to the convulsions produced by renal inadequacy. The urine secreted during or after an epileptic fit is usually free from albumen. In the severest forms of puerperal eclampsia the urine may also be entirely free from albumen and tube-casts. In the ultimate stages of amyloid degeneration[2] and atrophy of the kidney, the most formidable forms of Bright's disease, albumen may not appear in the urine.

The DIAGNOSIS is usually cleared up by the history of the case and the course of the affection.

The PROGNOSIS with reference to mother and child is favorable. Epilepsy rarely leads to the premature interruption of pregnancy.

The TREATMENT is the same as in the non-gravid state.

Disorders of the Special Senses.

Disorders of the special senses usually occur in the course of pregnancy as symptoms of acute or chronic Bright's disease. Amblyopia, amaurosis,

[1] *Lehrb. d. Geburtshülfe*, 1882, p. 241.   [2] Carl Braun, *Lehrb. d. g. Gynaek.*, 1881, p. 827.

ringing in the ears, sudden deafness, loss of taste and smell, may be developed under the influence of renal inadequacy before or after the occurrence of puerperal convulsions. Apart from the disorders of the special senses dependent upon lesions of the kidney, disturbances of vision are of chief clinical interest.

Amblyopia, hemeralopia, and color-blindness are occasionally observed as the result of nutritive disturbances in the retina. Nyctalopia, Spiegelberg says, is not recorded in the literature of the subject.

The PROGNOSIS is favorable as a rule. The disorders of vision usually disappear during the puerperium, and evince no tendency to recurrence.

Generous diet, iron, and a tonic plan of treatment are indicated.

II. THE PECULIARITIES OF CERTAIN ACCIDENTAL ACUTE AND CHRONIC DISEASES OCCURRING IN THE COURSE OF PREGNANCY.

THE older obstetricians believed not only that pregnant women possessed a certain immunity from accidental diseases, but also that the course of such affections was favorably modified by gestation. Modern research has demonstrated the groundless nature of this belief. It is an established fact that pregnancy confers upon the individual no immunity from the disorders to which the non-gravid woman is liable. Moreover, such accessory diseases are usually aggravated by pregnancy, and, in turn, exercise an unfavorable influence upon gestation, frequently leading to its interruption.

Acute Infectious Diseases.

Of all the so-called accessory diseases occurring in the course of pregnancy, the acute infectious diseases are of the gravest clinical significance. These diseases are peculiarly dangerous complications for two reasons:

I. They have a marked tendency to cause the death of the foetus and the interruption of pregnancy, when the loss of blood and the muscular exertion consequent upon the expulsion of the product of conception from the uterine cavity seriously imperil the mother's life.

II. Hemorrhagic endometritis, caused in part by changes in the constitution of the blood, is not an uncommon symptom in the course of acute infectious diseases in the non-gravid state. In pregnancy this symptom is of more constant occurrence, just as it is of graver prognostic moment, both with reference to the mother and to the child.

I. The death of the foetus and the interruption of pregnancy may result from the operation of a variety of etiological factors.

1. The foetus usually dies in consequence of the elevation of maternal temperature. The case is a veritable example of that condition which H. C. Wood of Philadelphia terms heat-stroke. The normal foetal temperature is slightly more elevated than the maternal. The foetus in its membranes, surrounded by maternal tissues, must possess at least the

same temperature as the maternal body. But it has its own heat-producing apparatus in addition. A very slight elevation of the maternal temperature produces a disproportionate rise in the temperature of the fœtal body. Kaminsky[1] has shown that an elevation of maternal temperature to 104° F. imperils fœtal life. Increased frequency of the pulsation of the fœtal heart and abnormally active fœtal movements are followed by diminished cardiac and muscular activity, and the fœtus dies. The autopsy reveals the characteristic lesions of heat-stroke.

2. Runge[2] has demonstrated the occurrence of fœtal death from asphyxia when the maternal blood-pressure is seriously lowered. This lowering of the maternal blood-pressure occurs as the result of diminution in the force and frequency of the heart's action observed in the course of acute infectious diseases or from the sudden loss of blood. Asphyxia may also be caused by structural changes in the epithelium covering the fœtal placenta, due to the state of the maternal blood.

3. The fœtus may perish in consequence of infection with the specific poison of the acute disorder. Death as the result of acute infection has been observed in variola and relapsing fever.

4. Pregnancy may be interrupted, independently of the condition of the fœtus, as the result of the thermic irritation of the uterine muscular fibre by the maternal blood. Spiegelberg on a priori grounds asserted the possibility of this event. Runge[3] has since demonstrated by experimental methods its actual occurrence.

II. Hemorrhagic endometritis in the course of acute infectious diseases complicating pregnancy has been demonstrated by Slavjansky's[4] researches. In cholera this symptom is observed with relative frequency. Following hemorrhage into the decidua, according to the time, extent, and site, pregnancy may be immediately interrupted, or secondarily as the result of the pathological changes in the placenta or membranes induced by the extravasated blood. The hemorrhage may be so severe as to jeopardize the life of the mother.

Of the eruptive fevers, smallpox, scarlet fever, and measles are of especial clinical interest. Smallpox is observed most frequently. The eruptive fevers usually occur early in pregnancy, but the disposition to the severer forms and the mortality, as remarked by Spiegelberg, grow with the duration of gestation.

SMALLPOX.

A mutually unfavorable relation exists between smallpox and pregnancy. A distinct tendency to the hemorrhagic form of the disease is notable. Pregnancy frequently terminates in abortion or premature labor under circumstances which seriously imperil the mother's life from loss of blood. When the disease pursues its course without interrupting pregnancy, the effect upon the fœtus is interesting and instructive. The child may be born alive with characteristic variolous cicatrices or in the eruptive stage. Usually the eruption appears from eight to ten days after birth. Very rarely the child may escape infection altogether. The fœtus may be infected in utero, while the mother

[1] *Moskauer Med. Z.,* 1867, Nos. 13-19.   [2] *Arch f. Gyn.,* Bd. xii. p. 16.
[3] *Volkmann's Sammlung,* No. 174; *Arch. f. Gyn.,* Bd. xii. p. 16.
[4] *Arch. f. Gyn.,* iv. p. 285.

remains apparently unaffected. Fumée of Montpellier narrates the history of a remarkable case of twin pregnancy. Only one of the children showed variolous pustules.

During smallpox epidemics abortions and premature labors, accompanied by abnormally severe hemorrhages, are frequently observed when no exanthem or other sign of the disease is noticeable in the mother. The healthy child of a mother affected with variola in the course of pregnancy is usually insusceptible to vaccinia for a long time after birth.

In the event of a smallpox epidemic the vaccination or revaccination of pregnant women is advisable. The effect of the vaccination of the pregnant woman upon the fœtus is still a subject of controversy. Thorburn in 1870 successfully vaccinated a number of pregnant women, and found no insusceptibility in their children. Behm[1] vaccinated 33 women pregnant in the eighth, ninth, and tenth months. The vaccination was completely successful in 22 cases, partially in 7, and failed in 4. Of the 33 children, 25 were successfully vaccinated. In 8 cases vaccination was not attended with success. Failure was ascribed in 7 cases to bad lymph, leaving only 1 case of presumed protection from intra-uterine vaccination. Bollinger and Burckhardt, supported by the results of Rickett and Roloffs in the inoculation of sheep, maintain that over one-half the infants are protected from vaccinia and smallpox by the vaccination of the mother during pregnancy.

MEASLES.

Rubeola, of infrequent occurrence in the adult generally, is a very rare complication of pregnancy. It is of serious prognostic moment, from the tendency to the hemorrhagic form of the disease, and pneumonia.

SCARLET FEVER.

Scarlatina, like measles, occurs infrequently in the course of pregnancy. Olshausen has collected 7 cases. Pregnancy was interrupted in 4 out of these 7 cases, probably as the result of the elevation of maternal temperature. The renal complications also add an unfavorable element to the prognosis.

TYPHOID FEVER.

Typhoid fever occurs with greatest frequency during the early months of gestation. It is a very rare complication of the puerperium. Pregnancy is usually interrupted. Abortion rather than premature labor is observed. This tendency to the interruption of gestation is more marked than in any of the acute infectious diseases with the possible exception of smallpox. Of 98 cases collected by Kaminsky, interruption of pregnancy occurred in 63; Zülzer reports 14 interruptions of pregnancy in 24 cases; Scanzoni, 6 out of 10 cases. In about 63 per cent. of the cases collected by these observers pregnancy was interrupted. The causes of abortion or premature labor in typhoid fever are found in the elevation of maternal temperature, the hemorrhagic endometritis, and perforation (Kleinwächter). The transmission of the infection from mother to child is a disputed point. The prognosis depends largely upon the stage of the disease in which the interruption of pregnancy occurs. If abortion or

[1] *Centralbl. f. Gynaek.*, 1882.

premature labor occurs early in the course of the disease, before the mother is exhausted, the outlook is naturally more favorable.

RELAPSING FEVER.

Murchison states very positively that pregnancy is invariably interrupted by the occurrence of relapsing fever. Recent investigations, however, indicate that this assertion is entirely too general. Weber[1] has collected 63 cases of pregnancy complicated by this disease. Pregnancy was interrupted in 23 cases, or 36.5 per cent. Hemorrhagic endometritis is of less frequent occurrence than in typhoid fever. In two cases (Wyss-Ebstein and Albrecht) spirilla were found in the fœtal blood, indicating the infection of the child by the mother.

TYPHUS FEVER.

Typhus fever manifests much less tendency to the production of hemorrhagic endometritis than typhoid and relapsing fevers. The interruption of pregnancy is the exception rather than the rule. When abortion or premature labor occurs, it is usually caused by the elevation of the maternal temperature. There is no evidence pointing to the infection of the child with the specific poison of the disease.

MALARIAL FEVER.

The popular belief that pregnant women enjoy a certain[2] immunity from malarial fever seems to have some foundation in fact. This apparent immunity may be due in part to the environment and freedom from exposure to the malarial poison—in part to the condition of pregnancy. In latent, chronic malarial poisoning gestation may be the cause of the explosion or acute exacerbation of the affection. The course and symptoms of malarial fever are materially modified by the coexistence of pregnancy. The attacks lose something of their rhythmical character. Chills are of irregular occurrence, and the fever assumes a remittent or continued type. In the latter months of gestation acute attacks of malarial fever are especially distressing to the patient.

The interruption of pregnancy is not an uncommon event. Göth has recently reported 46 cases, in 19 of which either abortion or premature labor took place. When pregnancy is interrupted hemorrhage is apt to be profuse.

The communication of the disease to the fœtus is a well-authenticated clinical fact. Hubbard reports an interesting case of intra-uterine malarial fever. Autopsies of infants born of mothers affected with acute or chronic malarial poisoning reveal the characteristic lesions of that pathological condition. Malarial paroxysms are usually suspended during labor, but may reappear during the lying-in period. Very rarely the fever assumes a pernicious type, and then may stand in a certain causal relation to the essential anæmia of pregnancy, of which mention has already been made.

In the TREATMENT of malarial poisoning during pregnancy large doses of quinine are indicated. Spiegelberg points out the important fact that, owing to the impairment of the digestive and assimilative functions, only

[1] *Berlin. klin. Woch.*, vii., 1870, p. 22.   [2] Ritter, *Virchow's Archiv*, 1867.

a portion of the quinine is absorbed. There is no ground for fearing any untoward effect from quinine. The researches of Chiara of Milan and numerous other observers prove that even the largest therapeutic doses of quinine are not abortifacient in malarial fever or in health.

CHOLERA.

Pregnant women evince no proclivity to, nor immunity from, cholera. As in variola, the disposition to, and mortality of, the disease grow with the duration of gestation. The prospect of recovery is especially unfavorable during the sixth and seventh months. Pregnancy is usually interrupted when the woman survives the terribly rapid course of the disease. Many women die with the product of conception in the cavity of the uterus. Exceptionally, in the lighter forms of the disease recovery may occur without the interruption of gestation. The causes of premature labor or abortion may be found in the constant hemorrhagic endometritis and the changes in the pressure and constitution of the maternal blood. As the result of the operation of the two latter factors, asphyxia is usually produced. Buhl, Gütterbock, and others are of the opinion that the disease may be communicated by the mother to the fœtus.

Pregnancy undoubtedly exercises an unfavorable influence on the course of the disease, chiefly from the tendency to uterine hemorrhage. Pregnancy is interrupted in over 50 per cent. of the cases. Premature labor is observed more frequently than abortion. The prognosis with reference to the life of the child is absolutely unfavorable.

In very exceptional cases the evacuation of the uterine cavity has seemed to exercise a favorable influence on the course of the disease. Upon this ground the induction of abortion or premature labor has been seriously proposed. The operation, after an extended trial, has fallen into deserved disrepute.

SYPHILIS.

Syphilis is a frequent complication of pregnancy. Sigmund[1] has observed and described the characters of syphilis contracted at the beginning or during the course of gestation. The duration of the stage of incubation is abbreviated. Two weeks is the rule, six weeks the exception. The initial lesions are characterized by an unusual degree of intensity, occasionally involving the vulva, vagina, cervix, nates, and inner surfaces of the thighs. The intensity of the initial lesions is due to the anatomical relations of the genitalia in the pregnant woman and the increased nutritive activity of the parts. The symptoms are marked local reaction, reddening and excoriation of the skin and mucous membrane, swelling, œdema, eczema, follicular abscesses, and necrosis of the connective tissue. Induration is not a characteristic of chancre situated about the genitalia of the pregnant woman. Phagedenic ulceration sometimes attacks the chancre, and then the case may be mistaken for one of phagedenic chancroid. The secondary symptoms are unusually mild. Condylomata appear about the genitalia, and psoriasis is noticeable on the palms of the hands and soles of the feet. Glandular infiltration follows slowly, and alopecia, iritis, laryngitis, and the skin manifestations are observed with comparative infrequency.

[1] *Wien. Med. Presse*, 1873, No. 1, xiv.

Constitutional Syphilis.—The influence of constitutional syphilis upon the fœtus is marked, and always unfavorable. The fœtus may be infected through the medium of the spermatic fluid, the ovum, and by the mother after conception. From an enormous number of carefully-recorded observations it is possible to deduce the following conclusions with reference to the modes of infection and the effect upon the product of conception:

1. When the mother is perfectly healthy, but the father is affected with constitutional syphilis, the fœtus is infected by the diseased spermatozoids. The intensity of the fœtal disease will depend upon the degree of latency and age of the paternal affection. This mode of infection is observed in the severer forms of hereditary syphilis. Usually the mother is not infected. Occasionally the disease is communicated to her by the fœtus in the mode termed by the French syphilographers choc en rétour.

2. When the mother has had constitutional symptoms prior to conception the ovum is infected before its fertilization. The child usually dies in utero, and is expelled in a state of maceration.

3. When the mother is infected during the act of coitus it was formerly believed that the fœtus could only be syphilized during its passage through the parturient canal. Sigmund and Vajda have shown that even under these circumstances the infection may be communicated by the mother to the fœtus in the course of pregnancy. If the father is affected with constitutional syphilis when the mother acquires the initial lesion, the result sketched in the first proposition follows.

4. Infection of the fœtus may occur during its passage through the parturient canal. Weil[1] records a case of this nature.

5. When both parents are affected with constitutional syphilis the disease will be communicated to the fœtus. The intensity of the fœtal syphilis will depend upon the degree of latency and age of the parental affection. When both parents have passed through the tertiary forms an apparently healthy child may be born. Evidences of hereditary syphilis, however, are usually developed before puberty.

According to the intensity of the poison the fœtus dies in utero, causing the interruption of pregnancy; is born alive, with manifestations of hereditary syphilis, seldom acquired; or may give evidence of the inheritance of the disease after a variable interval of from weeks to months.

TREATMENT.—Fortunately, syphilis as a complication of pregnancy is a very tractable affection. The interruption of pregnancy may be prevented and the effect of the syphilitic poison upon the fœtus favorably modified in the large majority of cases by appropriate specific treatment. Mercurial inunctions are preferable to the exhibition of the remedy by the mouth. Iodide of potassium must be used with care, on account of its tendency to provoke uterine contractions.

Attention must be paid to local primary or secondary lesions, since the child may be infected during its passage through the parturient canal.

Cardiac Diseases.

The mutually unfavorable relations between acute and chronic cardiac diseases and pregnancy depend largely upon the seat and character of the affection.

[1] *Deutsch. Zeitsch. f. prakt. Med.*, 1877, No. 42.

ACUTE ENDOCARDITIS,

occurring in the course of gestation, evinces a distinct tendency to the malignant, ulcerative form. This disposition is much more marked during the puerperium. The dangers of the detachment of particles of valvular vegetations, giving origin to the processes of thrombosis and embolism, are obvious.

The PROGNOSIS of acute endocarditis during pregnancy and the puerperium is much more unfavorable than in the non-gravid state.

CHRONIC HEART DISEASES.

The mode in which pregnancy, parturition, and puerperium exert an unfavorable influence on chronic heart diseases is still the subject of controversy. Spiegelberg accounts for the disastrous results attending aortic insufficiency observed in the second half of pregnancy on the ground of the inadequacy of the compensatory hypertrophy of the left ventricle. The intercalation of the placental circulation, the increase of the total blood-mass, the increase in arterial tension, throw an extra amount of work upon the left heart, which it is not able to perform. Irregular heart-action and dyspnœa, sometimes leading to the interruption of pregnancy, are the results.

After labor the placental circulation is eliminated, arterial blood-pressure is lowered, venous blood-pressure is elevated, and the right heart is threatened. In case of mitral insufficiency and dilatation of the left ventricle, without compensatory hypertrophy of the right heart, the effect of· these sudden variations in vascular tension is obviously serious. Dyspnœa, pulmonary catarrh, general œdema, albuminuria, ascites, pleural effusions, occur. Fritsch[1] is of the opinion that these phenomena, sometimes observed in the course of mitral disease after labor, are due to the sinking of intra-abdominal pressure, the accumulation of blood in the great abdominal vessels, and cardiac paralysis from insufficient blood-supply.

During parturition Spiegelberg[2] thinks the chief danger in all forms of valvular defects consists in pulmonary œdema as the result of circulatory disturbances.

Löhlein and Kleinwächter[3] believe that the chief danger of chronic valvular disease occurs during the puerperium, and lies in the tendency to the recurrence of endocarditis.

TREATMENT.—The treatment of acute and chronic heart disease is not materially modified by the coexistence of pregnancy.[4] In threatened asphyxia the induction of premature labor is indicated in the interest of the child. During labor the timely performance of version or application of the forceps lessens the bearing-down efforts, and may prevent alarming complications.

Diseases of the Lungs.

ACUTE LOBAR PNEUMONIA.

This is a rare affection in women at all times, and is a very infrequent complication of pregnancy. Occurring with greatest relative frequency

---

[1] *Arch. f. Gyn.*, viii. p. 373; x. p. 270.   [2] *Lehrbuch* d. *Geburtshülfe*, 1882, p. 248.
[3] *Kleinwächter's Grundriss d. Geburtshülfe*, 1881, p. 190.
[4] Carl Braun, *Lehrb. d. g. Gynaek.*, 1881, p. 708.

in the early months of pregnancy, the unfavorable character of the prognosis grows with the duration of pregnancy. Interruption of pregnancy may occur as the result of a variety of causative agencies. The elevation of maternal temperature, insufficient oxygenation of the maternal blood, placental anæmia from inadequate supply of blood to the left heart, are of chief etiological moment.

The PROGNOSIS with reference to mother and child is always grave.

The TREATMENT is that of pneumonitis in the non-gravid state. Parturition exerts a prejudicial influence by overtaxing the failing heartpower and increasing the hydræmia. The induction of premature labor is therefore strongly contraindicated. In the event of labor every effort must be made by operative procedure to save the mother's strength.

ACUTE PLEURITIS

is nearly as fatal a complication of pregnancy as pneumonitis, and for the same reason. The danger is especially great during labor.

CHRONIC PLEURISY, EMPHYSEMA, AND EMPYEMA

are dangerous complications of pregnancy, limiting respiratory space and producing cardiac complications. The induction of premature labor may be indicated by these conditions in the interest of mother and child.

PULMONARY TUBERCULOSIS.

Pregnancy exerts a prejudicial influence on hereditary or acquired tuberculosis as a rule. Latent tendencies to the disease are developed, and the progress of the existing affection is hastened. These effects upon the course of phthisis, Lusk says, are most frequently observed between the ages of twenty and thirty years, although of not infrequent occurrence between the ages of thirty and forty years. To these general propositions there are occasional rare exceptions. The disease is sometimes—very rarely—observed to make no progress during gestation and the patient may decidedly improve during the lying-in period. The puerperal phases, says Spiegelberg, exercise such varied influences upon the development and course of tuberculosis that it is an imperative necessity to individualize in every case.

When the disease progresses during pregnancy, abortion or premature labor may take place, or the woman may die undelivered. Infants born of tuberculous mothers are usually weak and sickly, and perish during the first months of life.

For these reasons it is an established rule in practice to inform women of the tuberculous diathesis of the dangers entailed by the marital relation. A woman affected with tuberculosis ought never to nurse her own child. As a rule, however, there is seldom any necessity for such a warning, as the function of lactation is rarely established under these conditions.

FUNCTIONAL DISORDERS IN CONNECTION WITH THE MENOPAUSE.

By W. W. JAGGARD, M. D.

DEFINITION AND TERMINOLOGY.—The time of life in a woman when the natural cessation of ovulation and menstruation occurs has received a variety of appellations more or less descriptive of the phenomena which are supposed to precede, attend, and follow that event. Change of life, Turn of life, Critical time, Climacteric, in English ; Das klimacterium, Das aufhören menstrualer Ausscheidung, Das aufhören der Weiblichen Reinigung, in German ; Ménopause, Âge de retour, Âge critique, Temps critique, in French ; Cessatio mensium, Climacterium, in Latin ; Menolipsis, in Greek,—are terms used to mark out a certain period of time commencing with the functional and organic disorders connected with the cessation of ovulation and menstruation in a causal relation, and terminating with the permanent resettlement of health.

DATE OF CESSATION OF MENSTRUATION, AND DURATION OF THE CHANGE OF LIFE.—The function of ovulation, as far as we know, ceases with the discontinuance of menstruation, although immature ova still exist in the ovaries. The date of natural cessation of menstruation and ovulation is variable in different women. It is difficult to determine an average date, because the menopause may be gradually ushered in, and then women are apt to interpret any genital hemorrhage as menstruation. In certain cases the menstrual flow may cease between the ages of thirty and forty years, or even at an earlier period. On the other hand, the function has been noted by competent observers[1] to continue up to and beyond the sixtieth year. According to tradition, Cornelia, the mother of the Gracchi, was confined in her seventieth year. Parvin[2] has recently called attention to another historical instance of alleged late menstruation, recorded in a note to the fifty-sixth chapter of the *Decline and Fall of the Roman Empire*. On the authority of D'Herbelot's great work, *Bibliothèque orientale*, 1777, Gibbon mentions the case of Asima, the mother of Abdallah. When the tidings of the death of her son were borne to Asima her menses reappeared at the age of ninety as the physical effect of her grief. The historian informs us that the flow proved fatal in five days. These anomalous cases of so-called protracted menstruation are frequently examples of pathological hemorrhages dependent upon structural changes, sometimes of a malignant character. Even admitting the

---

[1] Tilt, *The Change of Life*, 4th ed., 1882, p 24.
[2] *The Medical News* 26th Sept., 1885, p. 352.

possibility of the condition of extremely protracted menstruation, such cases, as remarked by Playfair, like examples of unusually precocious menstruation, cannot be regarded as having any bearing on the general rule.

The periodic discharge of blood from the uterus usually ceases between the ages of forty and fifty years. Raciborski[1] concludes, from the observation of a large number of cases, that the average date of cessation is the forty-sixth year. This estimate is confirmed by the observations of Brierre de Boismont, Guy, and Tilt. The average date of cessation in 1082 cases,[2] collected by these three observers, was forty-five years and nine months.

Climate, race, and the various accidental circumstances which exercise such potent influence upon the establishment of the functions of ovulation and menstruation have measurably less effect upon their cessation. Mayer[3] attaches some importance to social condition as determining the date of cessation. From the observation of a large number of cases belonging to the higher classes he determines the average age to be 47.138 years. It is a popular belief that the period of menstrual life is a constant number of years, usually from thirty to thirty-five; that is to say, if a woman commences to menstruate when very young, cessation will occur at an earlier age than in a woman who begins to menstruate in life. Cazeaux, Raciborski, Frank, Dusourd, and Tilt, supported by Guy's[4] analysis of 1500 cases, are of the opinion, on the contrary, that the duration of menstruation is longest in women who have menstruated earliest. In the words of Négrier,[5] "It seems well proved that the ovarian function, creative of germs, is prolonged in life in direct ratio of the volume of the ovaries and of the precocity of ovulation; thus the girl nubile at twelve will continue menstruating until fifty or even fifty-five; whilst the girl who did not menstruate until eighteen or twenty—a fact which reveals feeble development and small energy of the organs— will cease to menstruate at forty, an early age."[6] Cessation occurs later in women who have passed through repeated normal pregnancies than in virgins or sterile females. Cohnstein[7] observed the longest duration of menstruation in women who had menstruated early, married, and borne more than three children, suckled their offspring, and were normally confined for the last time between the ages of thirty-eight and forty-two years. An interesting opinion with reference to the relation between longevity and the date of cessation was expressed by Robert Cowie at the Paris Medical Congress in 1867. According to Cowie, there is a direct and constant relation between longevity and protracted menstruation. A woman who menstruates up to an advanced period of life has more chances of attaining extreme old age than one whose menstrual function has ceased earlier. Cowie derives this opinion from the observation of numerous cases of longevity and coincident protracted menstruation which occurred in the Shetland Islands.

Among the pathological factors which determine the early occurrence

[1] *Traité de la Menstruation*, Paris, 1868.
[2] Tilt, *The Change of Life*, 4th ed., 1882, p. 22.
[3] Schroeder, *Handbuch der Krankheiten der Weiblichen Geschlechtsorgane*, 1881, p. 321.
[4] *Medical Times and Gazette*, 1845.   [5] Barnes, *Diseases of Women*, 1878, p. 194.
[6] T. Gallard, *Pathologie des Ovaires*, Paris, 1885, p. 114.
[7] *Deutsche Klinik*, 1873, No. 5.

of cessation, puerperal atrophy of the uterus, syphilis—especially the graver forms—and chronic alcoholism deserve particular attention (Lancereaux).

The average date of cessation of menstruation may be regarded as the fixed time from which to estimate the duration of the pre-cessation and post-cessation periods of the menopause. The duration of the pre-cessation period—or the dodging-time, as it is popularly termed—is subject to many and extreme variations. Tilt[1] places the limits of normal variation between a few months and six or seven years. The average length of the dodging-time in 275 cases Tilt estimates at two years and three months. The same observer claims to have seen cases of morbid prolongation of the pre-cessation period through ten and even twelve years. Equally variable and indefinite, in point of duration, is the post-cessation period. From the study of his 500 cases, Tilt concludes that cessation of menstruation divides involution into two periods of nearly equal length when no disease of the uterus or adnexa is present. In 383 cases, three or four years after cessation all functional disorders due to the menopause disappeared. But the length of the post-cessation period, as in the case of the dodging-time, is liable to abnormal protraction. Tilt is very positive in the assertion that disturbances directly traceable to the menopause may continue ten or twelve years after cessation of menstruation. The statistical evidence adduced by Tilt in support of his peculiar views as to the possible protraction of the pre-cessation and post-cessation periods (twenty to twenty-four years) may well be questioned. His analysis of cases does not indicate rigid scrutiny. The line between merely coincident phenomena and disorders which are directly traceable to the menopause is nowhere clearly and distinctly drawn. Robert Barnes[1] is of the opinion that the average duration of the change of life, comprehending the pre-cessation and post-cessation periods, is from two to three years—an estimate more in accord with the experience of the majority of clinicians.

THE NATURAL HISTORY OF THE CHANGE OF LIFE.—In order to gain an adequate conception of the dynamic disorders in connection with the menopause, it is necessary to bear clearly and distinctly in mind the alterations in functional activity of a purely physiological character which attend that event. Many of the so-called functional disorders of the change of life are merely physiological processes consequent upon the transition from active ovario-uterine life to sexual decrepitude. There is nothing remarkable in the fact that the cessation of menstruation and ovulation, after functional activity of an average period of time varying from thirty to thirty-five years, is sometimes attended by a series of disturbances of a local and constitutional character. The changes of functional activity under these conditions are in analogy to the course and constitution of nature as observed in connection with dentition, puberty, and other epochs in human life.

The physiology of the menopause is a subject extremely difficult of investigation. The reasons are obvious. Our knowledge of the nature and significance of the function of ovulation and menstruation is very defective. The phenomena in connection with the change of life are numerous and complex. All interpretations of the appearances are peculiarly liable to fallacies and unavoidable sources of error. Correction

1 *The Change of Life*, 4th ed., p. 46 *et seq.*   1 *Diseases of Women*, 1878, p. 287.

and confirmation by anatomical research are usually impossible. Then the number of recorded cases in which the phenomena have been rigidly analyzed is very limited. But, despite the difficult nature of the subject and the poverty of the literature, a solid nucleus of acquired truth exists. Familiarity with these definitely established facts will clear up many obscure points in the pathology of the menopause.

RESPIRATORY CHANGES.—The researches of Andral and Gavarret[1] indicate that the quantity of carbonic acid exhaled by the lungs during the second infancy (eight years to puberty) is increased in man and woman. With the establishment of menstruation the quantity of carbonic acid exhaled by the female becomes constant, and persists in this state throughout her menstrual life. During the pre-cessation period the quantity of carbonic acid exhaled by the lungs is rapidly augmented, attaining its maximum about the time of cessation. During the post-cessation period the quantity gradually diminishes until the resettlement of health is effected. After this period it remains relatively constant. In the male, on the other hand, the quantity of carbonic acid exhaled increases up to the thirtieth year, and then progressively diminishes until the end of life.

During pregnancy the amount of carbonic acid exhaled is approximately the same as at the time of cessation.

Aran[2] recognizes in this augmented excretion of carbonic acid during the change of life a critical or compensating discharge—a waste-gate or outlet, to use the figurative expressions of Tilt and Barnes, for the energy set free in the system by the more or less suddenly suppressed functions of ovulation and menstruation. Gallard,[3] on the other hand, has pointedly called attention to the fact that the menstrual blood carries out of the system a quantity of carbonic acid which during pregnancy and change of life is excreted by the lungs—that, accordingly, the increased exhalation of carbonic acid during the climacterium cannot be regarded in the light of a critical discharge.

ALTERATIONS IN THE FUNCTIONS OF THE SKIN.—It is a matter of common observation that the functions of the skin are profoundly influenced in many cases by the changes consequent upon the menopause. Tilt records 300 cases of more or less profuse perspiration, occurring in 500 women, due in some degree at least to the change of life. This estimate is probably exaggerated. A variety of agents influences the total amount of perspiration, as well as the relation between sensible and insensible perspiration, at all periods of life. The dryness, temperature, and amount of movement of the surrounding atmosphere, nature and quantity of food taken and liquid drank, exercise, mental condition, medicines, poisons, diseases, and the relative activity of the other excreting organs (*e. g.* the kidneys), are factors which deserve due consideration before attributing all increased activity of the sudoriparous glands about the forty-fifth year to the effects of the change of life. In the tables mentioned no distinction is drawn between mere coincidence and causal relation.

---

[1] " Recherches sur la quantité d'Acide carbonique exhalé par les Poumons dans l'Éspèce humaine," *Annales de Chimie et de Physique*, 3e Série, t. viii.

[2] *Leçons cliniques sur les Maladies de l'Utérus et de ses Annexes*, Paris, 1858–60, p. 284.

[3] T. Gallard, *Pathologie des Ovaires*, p. 87, Paris, 1885.

The perspirations due to the change of life may have prodromal signs. These symptoms are—sensations of cold, shivering, chills, sinking or faintness referred to the pit of the stomach. Usually, however, they are not attended by any premonitory phenomena. They are frequently accompanied by dilatations of the skin blood-vessels, corresponding to definite areas of distribution of the vaso-motor nerves, which are popularly known as flushes. When the perspirations following the dilatations of the skin blood-vessels are insensible, women are in the habit of terming the symptoms dry flushes. The number and duration, as well as the time of occurrence, of these sweats and flushes are various in different women. Tilt has observed them to occur as often as five or six times in an hour, and last from two to fifteen minutes. They are usually noticed during the daytime. The regions involved are, in the order of frequency, face, chest, lower portions of the trunk, upper and lower extremities. Very seldom the entire skin surface is affected. In point of intensity the heightened activity of the sudoriparous glands varies from a gentle perspiration to a drenching sweat.

The function of these perspirations and flushes cannot be regarded as definitely settled. The popular opinion is that they constitute an important outlet for the actual energy liberated by the cessation of ovulation and menstruation. Tilt, adopting the popular view, thinks that the relief obtained by increased perspiration is the most important and habitual safety-valve of the system during the change of life. There are certain a priori considerations which render this hypothesis in some degree probable.

The quantity of matter which leaves the human body by the skin, per hour, is considerable. Seguin[1] has estimated it at eleven grains, while the quantity excreted by the lungs is seven grains. It is possible to isolate three factors which directly influence the secretion of sweat : (1) The skin, apart from its glandular apparatus, is a simple animal membrane, and permits a relatively small quantity of water to transude through the portions intervening between the mouths of the glands. As pointed out by Erismann,[2] this function of the skin is a subordinate one. The simple transudation of water is greater through those portions of the skin abundantly supplied with glands than through those in which they are sparsely distributed. (2) Vascular dilatation accompanies, and at least aids, the secreting activity of the cutaneous surface. Bernard's experiments on the division of the cervical sympathetic and clinical observation abundantly demonstrate the operation of this etiological factor. (3) Independently of vascular supply, it is in a high degree probable that there are special nerves directly controlling the activity of the sudoriparous glands. Stimulation of the sciatic nerve causes an increase in perspiration in the toes of the dog, without any concomitant hyperæmia, as shown by the experiments of Kendal and Luchsinger.[3] In a word, the skin is adequate to the regulation of aberrations in nerve-force and blood-supply and to the restoration of equilibrium. If superfluous actual energy is liberated by the cessation of the monthly ovarian stimulus and determination of blood to the uterus, it is not improbable that the perspirations and flushes of the menopause may constitute an efficient means of discharge.

[1] Ann. de Chim., xc. pp. 52, 403.   [2] Zeitschrift f. Biol., xi. p. 1.
[3] Pflüger's Archiv, xiii., 1876, p. 212.

ALTERATIONS IN THE SECRETION BY THE KIDNEYS.—In many cases of the menopause important changes occur in the urine. The secretion becomes turbid and the quantity of sediments is large. These sediments usually consist of the inorganic salts. The phosphates, carbonates, and sulphates are increased, while no change is observed in the quantity of sodium chloride. The quantity of nitrogenous crystalline bodies is apparently not influenced in the great majority of cases. Occasionally the quantity of uric acid is increased,[1] and gives origin to many distressing symptoms. In the absence of accurate data respecting the changes in the constitution of the urine it is useless to speculate about the significance of the occasional increase in the quantity of inorganic salts and uric acid. Doubtless the functional activity of the skin and lungs, diseases of the genito-urinary tract, and diet play an important part in the production of the alterations in the chemical constituents of the excretion. It cannot, however, be denied that the menstrual flow performs some office as an emunctory, and it is not at all improbable that its cessation throws additional work on the kidneys.

ALTERATIONS IN NUTRITION.—Of the various alterations of nutrition consequent upon the change of life, obesity is of greatest clinical interest. It is a matter of common observation that women frequently grow fat coincidently with the cessation of menstruation. Out of 383 cases collected by Tilt, 121 women grew stouter within five years after cessation; 3 women became suddenly fat when the menstrual flow ceased to recur. Barnes, Baillie, Fothergill, and numerous other clinicians abundantly confirm this observation. Adipose tissue is usually deposited in the omentum, abdominal walls, breasts, face, and limbs.

The nature of the relation between the formation of fat and the change of life is obscure. In the attempt to ascribe due influence to the menopause in the production of adipose tissue it must not be forgotten that in males the maximum of weight is attained, according to Quetelet, about the fortieth year. But the accumulation of fat in many of the lower animals after the extirpation of the ovaries, and the frequent occurrence of obesity in women after normal ovariotomy and the Porro-Müller operation of Cæsarean section (Braun, Spaeth), indicate that in some cases, at least, there is a necessary relation between the two phenomena. The generally received view is that the formation of adipose tissue is an outlet for the more or less sudden aberrations in nerve-force and blood-supply following cessation. The weight of probable evidence is very decidedly in favor of this opinion. Physiology teaches that fat fluctuates in bulk more than any other tissue in the body. As remarked by Foster,[2] a large amount of adipose tissue may disappear within a very short space of time, or the quantity in a body may be multiplied many times within an equally short time. Although the direct influence of trophic nerves on metabolic activity has not been demonstrated, there is still evidence of a high order in favor of such a view.

The Mammary Glands.—Apart from the enlargement of the mammary gland from the deposition of adipose tissue, the organ may be the seat of active secretory changes. Tilt observed this phenomenon in 15 out of his 500 cases. The breasts increase in size and become tender. Blue veins are visible through the skin, and changes resembling in kind

---

[1] Barnes, *Diseases of Women*, 1878, p. 285. [2] M. Foster, *Physiology.*

those of pregnancy may be observed about the nipples and areolæ. A milky fluid is sometimes secreted. Semple has described a case in which a monthly discharge of blood continued for five years after cessation. Tilt has published a case in which a painless exudation of red serum, lasting for several days, recurred every three weeks.

In view of the intimate connection between the ovaries and uterus and mammary glands at other periods of life, it is in a high degree probable that many cases of active nutritive disturbances in the mammary glands, occurring about the forty-fifth year, are directly due to cessation. The exact nervous mechanism has not been fully worked out. These nutritive disturbances are probably physiological, and partake of the nature of the so-called critical discharges.

HEMORRHAGES AND MUCOUS AND SEROUS DISCHARGES.—Vicarious hemorrhages are occasionally though rarely observed in connection with the change of life. These more or less regular discharges of blood occur from a great variety of sites. The region is usually so located that the external escape of blood can easily be effected. The more usual forms of vicarious hemorrhage are hæmatemesis, epistaxis, hæmoptysis, and bleeding from hemorrhoids. General hæmatidrosis, bleeding from the nipples, intestinal hemorrhage, bleeding from the alveoli of the teeth, and subcutaneous ecchymoses are more uncommon types. Every case of suspected vicarious hemorrhage deserves most rigid scrutiny. The condition is such a rare one, and so many local causes sufficient to explain the phenomena frequently exist, that a certain amount of scepticism in the concrete case is perfectly justifiable.

The nervous mechanism of these hemorrhages, so far as it has been worked out, may be stated in a very few words. The cessation of menstruation causes an increase in vascular tension, and consequent irritation of the vaso-motor centres. Various local hæmostases result, which cause the symptoms of suffusion of the face, tinnitus, headache, giddiness, etc. In a limited number of cases these local congestions are relieved by the escape of blood. Vicarious hemorrhages seldom lose their physiological character.

Metrorrhagia is a less uncommon event than vicarious hemorrhage during the climacteric. Uterine hemorrhage is regarded as a critical discharge due to the changes brought about by the menopause, when it occurs, in the absence of local disease or constitutional vice, in connection with the perspirations, flushes, obesity, nervous phenomena, and other signs of cessation. In point of time these uterine hemorrhages, or floodings, usually occur after cessation. The causes of the floodings of the menopause are not at all evident. Barnes[1] is of the opinion that they are ultimately referable to imperfect functional activity of the liver and kidneys. Local congestions occur, vascular tension is increased, the heart and blood-vessels are engorged, and a disposition to uterine hemorrhage is created. In many cases flooding seems to exert a salutary influence upon the health of the individual. J. Frank says he has observed cases of critical floodings after cessation in which checking the bleeding caused apoplexy. Tilt[2] confirms this opinion by the citation of two cases. Not infrequently, however, metrorrhagia during the change of life exceeds physiological limits and endangers the life of the individual. In the

[1] *Diseases of Women,* p. 283.   [2] *Change of Life,* p. 197.

large majority of cases flooding after cessation is always a cause for anxiety, and constitutes an urgent indication for a physical examination. By careful indagation it is usually possible to eliminate cases of metrorrhagia due to carcinoma, fibroids, and diseases of the endometrium.

Leucorrhœa.—Closely allied in function to the floodings of the menopause is the profuse flow of mucus, unmixed with pus, from the cervix and vagina. This phenomenon is of frequent occurrence in connection with the other signs of the change of life. In the absence of local disease and constitutional vice it may be regarded as a critical discharge, an effort of nature to relieve pelvic congestion.[1]

Diarrhœa.—The recurrence of a profuse serous diarrhœa at more or less regular intervals during the change of life is common. Gendrin, Brierre de Boismont, and Chambon regard diarrhœa as habitual at this time. It acquires particular prominence as a symptom in the absence of the other critical discharges already mentioned. Indeed, it may constitute the only sign of the menopause apart from cessation of the menstrual flow. Care must be exercised, however, to differentiate in the concrete case between the purely functional serous diarrhœa of the change of life and those forms of the affection which depend upon local or general causes.

The explanation of the serous diarrhœa of the menopause, viewed as a critical discharge, is simple when the intimate connection between the pelvic circulation and that of the mesentery is considered.[2]

FUNCTIONAL DISORDERS IN CONNECTION WITH THE MENOPAUSE.— Vague, indefinite, and speculative as our conception of the physiology of the climacterium is, the deficiency of precise knowledge becomes more apparent when we come to consider the functional disorders of cessation. Many women pass through the change of life without the slightest disturbance of normal functional activity. In such women menstruation has usually been established at an early age and without local or general disorders. Moreover, all traces of disease of the uterus and adnexa are usually absent. Again, it is not an uncommon observation to see hysterical women, afflicted for years with uterine disease, begin to improve in health at an early stage of the pre-cessation period. These facts indicate that the change of life does not necessarily involve morbid phenomena.

In the large majority of cases, however, various functional and organic disorders are observed during this period of life. Under these circumstances it becomes a matter of extreme difficulty to distinguish between accidental complications, dependent up on collateral disease and pathological conditions of the pelvic viscera, and those disorders which stand in some causal nexus with the change of life. The scanty literature of the subject is to a great extent a mass of confused generalizations, in which the distinction between the relation of cause and effect and mere coincidence in point of time is seldom adequately drawn. Tilt's meritorious treatise is not free from this defect. In Table xxi., among the morbid liabilities at the change of life in five hundred women, heart disease, rheumatism, erysipelas, hysteria, epilepsy, cancer of the womb, ovarian tumors, and more than one hundred and fifty other pathological states are mentioned! Any paper on the subject at the present time, to perform a

[1] Emmet, *Gynæcology*, 1884, p. 184.   [2] *Ibid.*

serviceable office, must direct attention to the obscure, confused, inadequate state of knowledge rather than aid in the perpetuation of error by the description of purely hypothetical forms of disease. The comparatively few functional disorders which stand in direct pathological connection with the change of life are, in the large majority of cases, examples of pathological exaggerations of physiological processes. Under these conditions it requires an unusual degree of diagnostic skill and penetration to draw the boundary-line between health and disease. Then in the matter of treatment, as remarked by Spiegelberg, it requires tact to determine how long a purely expectant attitude should be maintained and the time when active interference should be instituted.

The woman passing through the change of life possesses no immunity from accidental diseases. But some of these accidental diseases may be modified in symptoms and course by the changes consequent upon the climacterium.

DISORDERS OF THE ALIMENTARY CANAL.—Salivation.—Ptyalism has been observed by Bouchut and other observers to occur in connection with the other symptoms of the change of life. It is a phenomenon of infrequent occurrence. In the absence of any other adequate explanation it may be regarded as an example of sympathetic irritation strictly analogous to the salivation sometimes observed in pregnancy.

The milder degrees of this affection deserve slight attention. When, however, the flow of saliva is so great as to incommode the individual or seriously endanger her health, active treatment must be instituted. Chalybcate tonics, quinine, hypodermatic injections of atropia over the glands —especially the submaxillary—and iodide of potassium, are among the more reliable remedies. Astringent mouth-washes are grateful and relieve the congestion of the mucous membrane.

Constipation.—The habit of constipation, although not induced, may be aggravated, during the change of life. Interference with the action of the voluntary muscles and intestinal peristalsis by the deposition of adipose tissue in the abdominal walls and omentum, diminution of the intestinal secretions as the result of profuse perspirations and critical discharges, are etiological factors frequently referable to the menopause. Alterations in the innervation of the intestinal walls are probably productive of conditions which tend to constipation. The nature of the changes in the functions of the abdominal sympathetic nervous system during the menopause is a matter of pure speculation. There are many a priori considerations, however, which render probable the view that the constipation in connection with the menopause is, in some degree at least, a visceral neurosis. The prominence of the symptoms, enteralgia and flatulence, lends additional probability to this opinion. The treatment of constipation in connection with the menopause is a subject of the greatest practical importance. Many of the obscure nervous symptoms, distressing perspirations, and critical discharges may be relieved, if not prevented, by attention to the regular daily evacuation of the bowels. The specific hygienic and medical means to be used to secure this end are fully discussed in other portions of this work.

Diarrhœa.—Diarrhœa referable to the menopause and regarded simply as a critical discharge, sometimes, though rarely, passes beyond physiological limits and demands active remedial treatment. This statement holds true especially in cases of chronic diarrhœa aggravated by cessation. It is frequently a matter of extreme difficulty to draw the boundary-line between the physiological process and its pathological exaggeration. Careful attention to the symptoms, however, will usually disclose the fact whether or no the frequent alvine dejections conduce to the patient's well-being. Sometimes the stools are very profuse, and threaten life from the loss of large quantities of serum. Entorrhagia and colic are frequently observed under these circumstances. Rest, restricted diet, opium, the vegetable and mineral astringents, usually suffice to fulfil all the indications.

DISORDERS OF THE LIVER.—Many eminent clinicians unite in the opinion that functional derangements of the liver are peculiarly liable to occur during the change of life. Sir J. Y. Simpson, Robert Barnes, Tilt, Gardanne, Gendrin, Meissner, and Otterburg may be mentioned among the observers who hold that there is some direct relation between certain dynamic disorders of the liver and the menopause. There are also many a priori considerations in favor of this view. Habitual or long-continued constipation—a condition frequently observed in connection with the change of life—interferes materially with the secretion and excretion of bile. Barnes ascribes to the menstrual flow an excretory function. In the absence of this emunctory an increased amount of work is thrown on the liver and other secretory organs. The portal venous system is engorged. Under these circumstances disorders are apt to arise as the result of increased functional activity in an organ which may be undergoing organic change.

Well-pronounced jaundice, however, is of infrequent occurrence during this period in the absence of more potent factors than those just mentioned. It is not more justifiable to speak of the icterus of the menopause than of the icterus of menstruation. Flint[1] has justly said that the occurrence of jaundice at the menstrual periods is too infrequent to suppose that there is any direct pathological connection, as implied in the term icterus menstrualis proposed by Senator.

On the other hand, that condition vaguely described as biliousness, implying the constitutional effects of chronic hepatic hyperæmia, has been noted by many clinical observers. The derangement referred to is aptly described in the words of B. Lane and quoted by Tilt:[2] "Nothing can be more common than to find severe biliary derangement occurring at or about the period of menstrual cessation; and, looking at the great physiological change which then takes place in connection with hepatic development, it is naturally to be expected. A woman will complain of being bilious; there may be a bitter taste in the mouth, a burning in the throat, frontal headache, nausea, and even vomiting, the urine high-colored, the bile abounding in the alvine dejections, and perhaps causing heat and a stinging sensation in the rectum; the tongue furred, a biliary tinge pervading the cutaneous surface." The propriety of ascribing the symptoms so graphically described in these words to excess, deficiency, or vitiation of the biliary secretion, in the entire absence of precise knowledge, may well be questioned. Tilt is of the opinion that the gastro-intestinal disorders produced by functional disturbances of the liver during the menopause are peculiarly obstinate in their resistance to treat-

[1] *Practice of Medicine*, 1881, p. 637.   [2] *The Change of Life*, 4th ed., p. 227, 1882.

ment. Many other clinicians bear testimony to the truth of this statement. This fact increases the importance of the subject of treatment. As this matter is very fully discussed in other parts of this work, it is only necessary to call attention at this time to the importance of directing the therapy to the gastro-intestinal disorders, such as the accompanying subacute gastro-duodenitis and constipation, rather than to the hepatic viscus itself.

Incidentally, it may be remarked that gall-stones are apt to give origin to distressing symptoms during the menopause. The causes in operation are substantially the same as those already mentioned in connection with the functional disorders of the liver.

CLIMACTERIC NEUROSES.—Incidental mention has been made, in the discussion of the physiology of the menopause, of functional changes in the nervous system, as involved in the perspirations, flushes, hemorrhages, and other so-called critical discharges. Knowledge at the present time of the physiological changes undergone by the nervous system during the menopause is limited to these few general statements, all of which are not yet definitely established facts. The field has always been a fascinating one to the medical writer, probably because, in the utter absence of precise information, the widest play is given to the most vivid and fertile imagination. The literature of the subject abounds in vague terms, figurative expressions, and rhetorical forms. Numerous ingenious and interesting speculations may be found in the writings of systematic authors from Gardanne[1] to Barnes and Tilt.

Tilt, following in the wake of the French writers, asserts that the nervous system is in a state of irritability or nervocism. This assertion conveys no information, as irritability may be the expression of weakness as well as of strength. The system is said to be in a condition of nervous plethora. We have seen that the rôle of plethora in recent pathology is insignificant. Cohnheim denies its existence altogether, except as a transitory state. Even admitting the existence of that state, what evidence is there that nerve-force accumulates in the body under the same conditions as the blood?

We have no desire to minify the importance of the physiological and pathological changes in the nervous system connected with the menopause. In comparison with these alterations the other phenomena of the menopause are insignificant. In the absence of precise knowledge, however, it is useless to devote time and attention to empty speculation.

In no part of the subject of climacteric neuroses are notions more obscure or information less precise than in connection with the diseases of the sympathetic or ganglionic nervous system. Under the term gangliapathy Tilt[2] has grouped a number of symptoms frequently observed during the menopause, which have their origin in a condition of " more or less debility associated with paralysis, hyperæsthesia, or dysæsthesia of the central ganglia of the sympathetic system." Gangliapathy includes the functional disorders described by other observers under the terms cardialgia, gastralgia, gastrodynia, and the like.

But it is impossible to view affections of the sympathetic apart from disorders of the general nervous system. It is impossible to distinguish

[1] *Aris aux Femmes entrant dans l'Âge critique,* 1816.
[2] *The Change of Life,* 4th ed., p. 109, 1882.

the conditions described by Tilt as ganglionic shock, paralysis, hyperæs-thesia, and dysæsthesia from abdominal neuralgias and many of the functional and organic diseases of the abdominal viscera. Finally, the connection of these various disorders, entirely irrespective of names, with the change of life has never been demonstrated, nor even rendered in a high degree probable.

Cerebral Hyperæmia.—The older authors dwell with especial emphasis upon hyperæmia of the brain as an important functional disorder in connection with the change of life. The condition is supposed to be apt to occur, in the absence of perspirations, flushes, and the other so-called critical discharges, as the result of plethora. Headache, tinnitus aurium, dizziness, heaviness, drowsiness, suffusion of the face and neck, bounding pulse, are among the symptoms which have been referred to the lighter forms of cerebral hyperæmia. Few systematic writers, however, sustain Dusourd in his assertion that apoplexy and the severer forms of hyperæmia of the brain are frequently caused by the cessation of menstruation.

Under the impression that plethora actually caused cerebral hyperæmia and the symptoms mentioned, and doubtless influenced by the teachings of Broussais (1844), Tissot, Hufeland, and Meissner advocated bleeding in the treatment of climacteric neuroses. Fordyce Barker and Tilt may be mentioned among modern clinicians who retain the old opinion as to the nature and treatment of this condition.

Cohnheim,[1] representing the modern school of pathologists, says "that except as a transitory state polyæmia does not occur under any circumstances." In recent pathology the various appearances of plethora are regarded as caused chiefly by dilatations of the skin blood-vessels, and not by an increase in the total blood-mass. The changes in the character of the pulses are referred to alterations in the vessels or their innervation. Even admitting the existence of the so-called plethora universalis, it does not follow that headache, dizziness, tinnitus aurium, and the like are due to cerebral hyperæmia. Andral has well said that these symptoms might with equal justice be ascribed to qualitative changes in the constitution of the blood.

Whatever view may be accepted as to the pathology of cerebral hyperæmia, and as to the necessary connection with the change of life, two important facts derived from experimental physiology deserve careful consideration before bleeding is performed for the relief of the symptoms mentioned:[2] (1) A high blood-pressure does not imply an augmentation of the total blood-mass. A large quantity of blood may be injected into the vessels without any considerable elevation of pressure. (2) Bleeding does not directly lower blood-pressure unless the quantity of blood removed be dangerously large.

In the lighter cases the so-called derivative treatment fulfils all the indications. Hot, irritating foot-baths, purgatives, saline diuretics, are indicated for the relief of distressing symptoms. Diet, exercise, frequent bathing, and other hygienic resources exercise a most important prophylactic function.

Hysteria.—The occurrence of hysteria during the menopause, as at other periods of life, is a well-established fact. Whether or no there is

[1] Pepper, *System of Medicine,*, Vol. III. p. 886.　　　[2] M. Foster, *Physiology.*

any direct pathological connection of cause and effect between the change of life and the disorder is a question which has been the subject of much controversy, and at the present time is unsettled. Gardanne, Dubois, D'Amiens, Vigaroux, and Beclard think the relation one of coincidence; Charcot, Tilt, F. Hoffman, Pujol, and Meissner are of the opinion that the climacteric may stand in a causal relation. Tilt's tabulated cases bearing upon this subject show nothing more than the coincidence of the two conditions, and contribute nothing to the solution of the problem. There are important considerations which favor the view that while the menopause may influence hysteria favorably or unfavorably, it is only in exceptional cases that the climacteric is the immediate cause of the affection. While hysteria may occur at any time of life, it is most frequently observed between the ages of fifteen and twenty years. It is in a high degree probable that a woman who has arrived at her forty-fifth year without hysterical mansfestations will not be molested during the change of life. It is not an uncommon observation to see hysterical woman rapidly regaining health during the pre-cessation period, and making complete recoveries before the permanent resettlement of health.

Hysteria during the menopause does not differ as to symptoms from the affection at other periods of life. It retains its protean character. Almost all the described forms of nervous disease may be accurately simulated. The severer forms of the disorder are paroxysms characterized by convulsions, coma more or less complete, or delirium. Coma enters to a greater or less degree into the paroxysms characterized by convulsions. Lypothæmia—a term used by the older writers to signify an hysterical semi-unconsciousness with feeble pulse and widely-dilated pupils —is frequently observed. This condition, as well as a state termed pseudo-narcotism by Tilt, may be regarded as a lighter form of coma.

Functional paralyses and pareses of motion or sensation, or both, are occasionally observed. Paraplegia is of relatively frequent occurrence. Not infrequently this condition is of reflex origin, the eccentric irritant residing in the uterus and adnexa or the gastro-intestinal canal. Hemiplegia and general paralysis are observed less frequently.

In the differential diagnosis it is necessary to exclude epilepsy and eclampsia, although it is well to bear in mind the fact that both these conditions may coexist.

The treatment of climacteric hysteria differs in no essential particular from that of the same disorder at other periods of life. The practitioner, however, has the comfortable knowledge that with the resettlement of health all symptoms, in the absence of local disease, will probably disappear.

It may not be amiss, in passing, to notice the value as a palliative measure of that old and well-tried remedy, the hot-water enema containing asafœtida. One to two ounces of the tincture of asafœtida in one quart of hot water, carried well up into the colon, is usually productive of excellent results, moral and physical.

Climacteric Pseudocyesis.—False or spurious pregnancy is a neurosis of not infrequent occurrence at or about cessation. It may justly be regarded as one of the mimetic forms of hysteria. The symptoms which give origin to the illusion may be observed in young, unmarried women or long after the cessation of ovulation and menstruation. In the large proportion of cases, however, the phenomenon is noticed at or about the climacteric. The subjective and objective signs of this curious condition may simulate pregnancy very closely. The breasts are swollen and tender, and a milky fluid may exude from the nipple. Nausea and vomiting in the morning and the various sympathetic disorders of pregnancy may be feigned. The abdomen may become enormously distended from the deposition of adipose tissue in the abdominal walls and omentum and the flatulent distension of the intestines. Fœtal movements are simulated by intestinal peristalsis and irregular contractions of the abdominal muscles. The ensemble of symptoms may be very deceptive, as shown by the famous case of Joanna Southcott. Crichton Browne[1] relates the history of an illustrative case which came under his observation in the West Riding Asylum. A woman long past the menopause claimed to be two months advanced in pregnancy. At the end of seven months she informed her friends that she was about to be confined. Accordingly she went to bed, and the process of simulated parturition lasted four days, terminating with a bloody discharge from the vagina.

The differential diagnosis is easy. The mammary changes, upon close examination, will be found to differ from those of pregnancy. Inspection, palpation, percussion, and auscultation will disclose the fact that the woman is only big with fat and wind, as Barnes puts it. Anæsthesia will facilitate the examination. Bimanual examination usually reveals the characteristic senile changes in the uterus or a pathological enlargement differing essentially from the gravid organ.

The so-called phantom tumors sometimes observed during the menopause are closely analogous to spurious pregnancies.

Epilepsy.—Epilepsy is a relatively uncommon disorder during the menopause. The present state of our knowledge indicates that the climacteric cannot be regarded as a distinct cause of the disease in the absence of previous epileptic seizures or inherited predisposition. Out of 200 cases of epilepsy occurring during the climacteric, observed by Jewell of Chicago, not a single case could be traced by the most rigid analysis to the change of life. Considering the rôle the sympathetic nerve plays in the etiology of epilepsy, it would not seem improbable, on a priori grounds, that the disease should be aggravated at the menopause. Evidence derived from clinical observation, however, is entirely inadequate to settle this question.

Insanity.—Various opinions are held as to the relation between the menopause and insanity. Mania, monomania, dementia, and even idiocy, are among the forms of mental alienation which have been attributed to climacteric influences.

Monomania.—There is much probable evidence in support of the view that the change of life may stand in a direct causal relation to monomania. On the other hand, no proof exists sufficient to establish a necessary pathological connection between cessation and mania, dementia, or idiocy.

Gardanne, Dubois d'Amiens, and Chambon have called attention to the occurrence of melancholia and hypochondriasis at this period. This opinion is confirmed by the results of Battey's operation in the hands of Lawson Tait, Bantock, Thornton, and other operators of large experi-

[1] *British Medical Journal*, 1841.

ence. In many of the cases of artificial induction of the menopause melancholia has been observed as a most distressing sequela. However, in connection with Battey's operation there are numerous and important considerations which must be carefully weighed in order to distinguish between a relation of cause and effect and mere coincidence. The number of women operated upon is now large, and some of the cases of melancholia following ovarian extirpation are probably examples of the return of a disease of earlier life or of the influence of heredity. Then, the fact of disqualification for maternal duties supplies in many cases an adequate psychological cause for more or less complete mental alienation. The important effects of chronic hepatic hyperæmia and the coexisting gastro-intestinal catarrh—conditions so frequently present at cessation—must not be forgotten when disorders of the intellect are referred to the cessation of the ovarian stimulus.

The positive diagnosis of climacteric melancholia and hypochondriasis is always difficult, frequently impossible. After the careful exclusion of all other possible causes, it may be assumed with a certain degree of probability that the intellectual disorder is due to the change of life.

The prognosis of climacteric melancholia and hypochondriasis is not necessarily unfavorable. In a large proportion of cases sanity returns with the re-establishment of health. The treatment, in the absence of a positive diagnosis, must be expectant. Effort must be addressed to the removal of any possible cause. Hygienic measures fulfil all the indications for treatment in the disorder when it is caused by the change of life. Opium and alcohol must be employed with extreme care in view of the great danger of the formation of obstinate habits.

Uncontrollable impulses and perversions of moral instincts are frequently observed during the climacterium, as at other periods of life. There is no reliable statistical evidence sufficient to establish a necessary pathological connection between cessation and uncontrollable peevishness, impulse to deceive, suicidal impulse, nymphomania, dipsomania, kleptomania, and the like. Nor is it possible to assert that these various disorders are of more frequent occurrence during the menopause than at other periods of life.

DISEASES OF THE PARENCHYMA OF THE UTERUS; METRITIS AND ENDOMETRITIS.

By W. W. JAGGARD, A. M., M. D.

Acute Metritis.

THE occurrence of an acute inflammation of the parenchyma of the non-gravid uterus has been denied by many systematic writers. Wenzel[1] says the condition is a figment of the imagination; Duparcque is sceptical; Klob[2] up to 1864 had never seen a case in which a positive diagnosis was possible. Emmet[3] writes in the last edition of his valuable book, "Inflammation of the uterine body never occurs except after parturition."

Comparatively recent investigations, however, have established the fact of occurrence beyond doubt or question. While a relatively uncommon condition, many facts with reference to its causation, pathological anatomy, and clinical course are definitely known.

ETIOLOGY.—Disturbances in connection with menstruation play a rôle of great importance in the production of acute inflammation of the uterine parenchyma. The rapid cooling off of extensive areas of the skin surface, as in wetting the feet in cold water, severe exertion, or the cold-water vaginal douche, may transform the normal menstrual congestion into an acute inflammation. The retention of menstrual blood within the uterine cavity, the result of organic stenoses, flexions, or tumors, occasionally gives origin to acute septic metritis. The inflammatory process frequently extends from the endometrium to the muscular substance. Gonorrhœal endometritis is of chief clinical significance in this connection. Duparcque's observations, confirmed in 1872 by Noeggerath, have recently attracted a great deal of attention. Säuger's statement at Magdeburg, that one-ninth of all gynæcological cases are of gonorrhœal origin, created some surprise at the time. In the light of the recent investigations of Schroeder, Bumm,[4] Lomer,[5] Oppenheimer,[6] and others, it is not considered an exaggeration, although it is still unsettled whether or no the gonococcus of Neisser is the agent of infection.

Under the heading of traumatism a great number and variety of etiological factors are included. Operations on the cervix, curetting the uterine cavity, and other minor gynæcological procedures, in the absence

[1] *Krankheiten des Uterus*, p. 42.
[2] *Pathol. Anatomie der Weibl. Sexualorgane.*
[3] *Gynæcology*, 1884, p. 31.
[4] *Arch. f. Gyn.*, xxiii. 3.
[5] *Deutsch. Med. Wochenschrift*, 22d Oct., 1885.
[6] *Arch. f. Gyn.*, xxv. 1.

of careful antisepsis, may cause traumatic inflammation in the vicinity of the wound, which may involve the entire organ. An ill-fitting pessary, especially the intra-uterine stem, cauterization of the cervix or endometrium with the solid stick of nitrate of silver, intra-uterine injections, the careless passage of the sound, inordinate sexual indulgence,—are all potential causes. Bloeschke[1] relates the history of a case in which a piece of straw penetrated the cervix of a peasant-woman working in the fields. An acute metritis was the result.

Finally, acute inflammations of the muscularis may be lighted up in the vicinity of new growths, as in the case of carcinoma of the cervix or mural fibroids. Such inflammations, however, as remarked by Schroeder, possess only a secondary significance.

PATHOLOGICAL ANATOMY.—The uterus, of a bluish-red color, is enlarged, especially in its upper two-thirds, to the size of a goose's egg, and is thickened in its antero-posterior diameter. Its walls, filled with venous and arterial blood, are soft and succulent from the transudation of serum. The bundles of muscular fibres are swollen, and the inter-muscular tissue is infiltrated with white blood-corpuscles and a few pus-corpuscles. Extravasations of blood, sometimes larger, sometimes smaller, are usually observed in the connective tissue. These changes are most marked in the innermost layers, where there is a greater abundance of connective tissue, and the inflammatory process is propagated toward the periphery. The endometrium, pelvic peritoneum, and connective tissue are usually involved. The tubes and ovaries are less frequently affected except in the case of gonorrhœal infection.

SYMPTOMS.—The attack is usually ushered in by a chill, followed by elevation of bodily temperature—a symptom which is apt to persist throughout the course of the disorder. Pain, referred to the lower portion of the abdomen and sacral region, is constant. The sensation may be dull, gnawing, or boring, like the pains in the first stage of labor or abortion, or sharp and lancinating. Tenderness on pressure, indicating involvment of the perimetrium, is marked. The pain is increased in intensity by standing, walking, coughing, straining at stool, or any act which causes an elevation of intra-abdominal pressure. Distressing symptoms arise in connection with the bladder and rectum. Urination is frequent and painful, while the secretion may contain blood. Griping pains are felt along the colon and rectum; the sensation of fulness or the presence of a foreign body excites a frequent or constant desire to defecate, and the act is accompanied with straining.

When acute metritis is caused by wetting the feet in cold water during the period, the menstrual flow may be suddenly arrested, to return after a variable interval. In very rare cases menstruation is permanently suppressed, and even atrophy of the uterus may result. In other cases profuse menorrhagia may occur. Not infrequently this copious hemorrhage is physiological, relieving as it does the congestion of the organ.

Various sympathetic disturbances, as nausea and even vomiting, are occasionally observed.

Acute metritis is frequently complicated by inflammation of the endometrium, pelvic peritoneum, and connective tissue. Under these circumstances the symptoms peculiar to inflammation of the muscular substance

[1] Säxinger, *Prager Vierteljahrschrift,* 1866, i. p. 130.

are masked. Acute metritis may terminate (1) in resolution, with gradual resorption of the exudation and return of the organ to its normal relations. (2) New connective tissue may be formed, giving origin to induration of tissue and permanent increase in size—the chronic uterine infarct of Kiwisch. The acute inflammation has become chronic. While admitting the possibility of this mode of termination, A. Martin[1] is of the opinion that a causal nexus is only demonstrable in isolated cases. (3) A very rare mode of termination is suppuration and the formation of abscesses in the muscular tissue. In these cases it is necessary, as pointed out by A. Martin,[2] to exclude myomata, which have undergone suppuration in the process of retrograde metamorphosis.

DIAGNOSIS.—The more or less sudden occurrence of a chill, fever, and localized pain and tenderness urgently indicates a careful examination of the pelvic viscera by bimanual palpation. The uterus is exquisitely painful upon the slightest touch, even in the absence of any exudate. The organ is enlarged, especially in its upper two-thirds, and thickened in its antero-posterior diameter. The uterus is softened, resembling in its consistence the organ in the early months of pregnancy. During the stage of active hyperæmia the secretions are diminished in amount ; at a later period profuse leucorrhœa, especially in the absence of menorrhagia, is a prominent symptom. The diagnosis of abscess in the uterine walls is difficult, if not impossible, when the collection of pus is small. The gradual enlargement of the uterus, the presence of fluctuation, the indications of pointing, and the constitutional symptoms are usually sufficient to establish the diagnosis when the pus-cavity has attained a considerable size.

PROGNOSIS.—Under appropriate treatment the prognosis of acute metritis is not unfavorable. It must, however, always be guarded, as it will be governed to a great degree by the causation, clinical course, and complications. Acute metritis from wetting the feet in cold water during the period and the like usually terminates in resolution. It is necessary to bear in mind the fact that in rare cases the function of menstruation may be permanently arrested, and even atrophy of the uterus induced. In acute metritis from traumatism the danger of general sepsis constitutes the unfavorable prognostic element. In gonorrhœal infection the tendency to involvement of the tubes and peritoneum is great; moreover, the condition is apt to recur. In all forms of the disorder the relation to chronic uterine infarct deserves consideration. Finally, death may result from the rupture of an abscess, located in the uterine walls, into the abdominal cavity.[3] Fortunately, these abscesses usually open into the uterine cavity, rectum, or through the abdominal parietes.

TREATMENT.—In general terms, the treatment may be described as vigorously antiphlogistic.

Chrobak[4] has pointed out in a detailed manner the absolute necessity of the most rigid attention to antisepsis in all the minor as well as the major operative procedures in gynæcology. The prophylaxis, a subject

[1] *Pathologie und Therapie der Frauenkrankheiten*, 1885, p. 181. [2] *Ibid.*
[3] Scanzoni, *Krankh. d. Weibl. Sexualorg.*, iv. Aufl. Bd. i., p. 203 ; Lados, *Gaz. médic. de Paris*, 1839, p. 605.
[4] "Untersuchung. der Weibl. Genitalia und Allgem. gyn. Therapie," *Deutsche Chirurgie*, Lief. 54.

of vital importance, is limited, so far as the general practitioner is concerned, to the enforcement of absolute cleanliness in all manipulations of the female genito-urinary tract.

Absolute rest in bed in the dorsal decubitus, with the pelvis elevated or depressed according to the patient's sensations, is a matter of primary importance. Pain demands for its relief the free use of morphine hypodermatically or opium per rectum. Chloral is a valuable adjuvant.

In the absence of menorrhagia free and repeated scarifications of the cervix are indicated to deplete the uterus. Twelve to twenty leeches applied to the abdomen above the symphysis will measurably relieve the congestion of the perimetrium. At a later stage, when the disorder does not occur at a menstrual epoch, mediate cold-water irrigation, by means of Leiter's modification of Petitgard's tubes, over the hypogastric region is an invaluable therapeutic resource. When the affection occurs during the period, hot compresses applied to the abdomen, hot sitz-baths, and even hot-water vaginal injections, are grateful.

The rectum and sigmoid flexure frequently require evacuation. A simple warm- or hot-water enema will usually secure this result. Occasionally a dose of castor oil is indicated, but drastic cathartics are distinctly contraindicated.

When the acute metritis is caused by traumatism, as in the case of operations on the cervix and curetting of the endometrium, the wounded surfaces demand attention. Under these conditions the neck of the uterus and the uterine cavity require careful antiseptic local treatment.

Abscesses in the uterine walls rarely indicate operative interference, except in case of pointing in the direction of the abdominal cavity. When incision is indicated the pus-cavity is usually large and superficial, and its evacuation involves no especial difficulty.

The treatment of the later stages of acute metritis will be considered in connection with the subject of Chronic Metritis.

Chronic Metritis.

SYNONYMS.—Chronic uterine infarct (Kiwisch); Diffuse connective-tissue hyperplasia of the entire uterus (Klob, C. Braun, Wedl); Induration of the uterus (Wenzel); Engorgement (Lisfranc); Hysteritis, Phlegmasie rouge (Duparcque); Congestion ou engorgement hypertrophique métrite (Becquerel); Interstitial metritis (De Sinéty); Congestive hypertrophy (Emmet); Areolar hyperplasia, Diffuse interstitial hypertrophy, Sclerosis uteri (Thomas, Skene); Subinvolution, Irritable uterus (Hodge).

In the absence of exact knowledge with reference to the ultimate pathology of so-called chronic metritis, it is impossible to frame a definition which cannot be justly criticised. Schroeder's definition answers all practical purposes, and probably contains as few objectionable terms as any other in the literature of the subject.

DEFINITION.—Hyperplasia of the connective tissue of the uterus combined with increased sensibility.

ETIOLOGY.—1. Subinvolution of the puerperal uterus is a frequent cause of chronic metritis. But the number of etiological factors which interfere directly and indirectly with the retrograde metamorphosis of the puerperal uterus is immense. Getting up too early from childbed, inability to suckle the child, too early sexual intercourse, retention within the uterine cavity of blood-clots or placental remains, acute inflammations of the uterus during the puerperium, retroversions and flexions of the puerperal uterus, severe exertion and the like,—are some of the more usual causes in this connection. Involution of the puerperal uterus is effected by contractions of the muscular walls, fatty metamorphosis of the uterine substance, and profuse secretion. Disturbance of any one of these processes may defer indefinitely the return of the organ to its normal relations. When pregnancy is prematurely interrupted the operation of each of these factors is materially modified. Uterine contractions are relatively feeble. The stimulus of a nursing child is also lacking. The albuminoids of the muscular protoplasm are not so readily converted into fat capable of easy resorption. A comparatively large quantity of decidua vera—even in the absence of portions of the fœtal envelopes—is retained within the uterine cavity, and the secretory activity of the endometrium is seriously disturbed. Then, women are less careful after miscarriages than labor at term.

Laceration of the cervix uteri—an accident liable to occur in abortion as well as during confinement at term—if at all extensive, usually interferes with the retrograde metamorphosis of the uterus.

2. Continuous or repeated hyperæmia, active or passive, frequently exceeds physiological limits and leads to chronic metritis. Menstrual subinvolution, dysmenorrhœa from organic stenoses, flexions, changes in position with retained menstrual fluid, excessive venery, masturbation, conjugal onanism, chronic endometritis—especially gonorrhœal—inflammations of the pelvic cellular tissue, chronic oöphoritis, new formations as in the case of carcinoma and myoma,—result in the production of active flexion and venous engorgement. The pernicious effects of conjugal onanism in the causation of chronic uterine infarct have been dwelt upon with particular fondness by Wenzel, Scanzoni, Emmet, Goodell, and numerous other ancient and modern gynæcologists of distinction. Van de Warker,[1] on the other hand, is of the decided opinion that the operation of this etiological factor has been exaggerated. His conclusions are based upon an incomplete gynæcological study of the Oneida Community. Onanism was practised on a colossal scale by this strange people for a number of years. Summing up the results of his imperfect investigations, Van de Warker says: "I can discover nothing but negative evidence relating to the effect of male continence upon the health of the community." It is quite possible that too much importance has also been attached to excessive venery. Fritsch[2] does not stand alone when he says, "I have examined puellæ publicæ for years, but have not gained the impression that metritis chronica is of frequent occurrence."

3. Venous stasis from organic hepatic, cardiac, and pulmonary diseases doubtless predisposes to chronic inflammation of the metrium. Consti-

---

[1] Ely Van de Warker, "A Gynecological Study of the Oneida Community," *The American Journal of Obstetrics, etc.*, August, 1884.

[2] Heinrich Fritsch, *Die Lageveränderungen und die Entzündungen der Gebärmutter*, 1885, p. 318.

pation, usually habitual with invalids, and an over-distended bladder, are causes which are more frequently and directly operative in the production of vascular engorgement and displacements of the uterus.

4. Various operative procedures upon the cervix, ill-advised and frequently repeated intra-uterine applications, must be included in the list of causative agencies.

5. Chronic metritis is one mode of termination of acute inflammation of the uterine parenchyma. This method of origin, however, is seldom observed except after repeated attacks of acute inflammation, as in the case of gonorrhœal infection.

The enumeration of possible causes might be indefinitely prolonged. Scanzoni's classical monograph on chronic metritis contains a much larger number. As remarked by Fritsch,[1] "In the elastic bands of his conception of the disease every catarrh, every affection of the uterus, fitted finally snugly into place." The more common efficient causes have been indicated.

PATHOLOGICAL ANATOMY.—Modern pathological doctrines on chronic metritis are largely modifications of the opinions so ably advocated by Scanzoni[2] in 1863. Scanzoni, while fully recognizing the various forms of chronic uterine infarct, simplified the study of the subject by comprehending them all under two stages : I. the stage of infiltration ; II. the stage of induration.

I. In the first stage the uterine tissue is infiltrated with serum, blood, and fibrin (serös-blutige, serös-faserstoffige Infiltration). The organ is in a state of engorgement œdema, the consequence of active and passive hyperæmia. It is enlarged in volume, altered in shape, reddened and more or less sensitive on pressure, soft and doughy to the sense of touch. The uterus may remain in this condition, or, after a longer or shorter interval, pass over into the stage of induration. Long-continued venous hyperæmia leads with comparative infrequency to induration, although intercurrent inflammations, exudations, and new formations of tissue may produce that effect. This stage cannot be invariably viewed as of an inflammatory character. These enlargements of the uterus are frequently examples of the nutritive disturbances commonly observed in other organs in consequence of long-continued venous hyperæmia. The close correspondence of Scanzoni's stage of infiltration with Emmet's congestive hypertrophy is at once apparent.

II. In the stage of induration a luxuriant growth of connective tissue replaces the specific tissue-elements which are destroyed by a chronic inflammatory process. Early in this stage there may be an actual increase in size of the individual muscular elements. Ultimately, the hypertrophy disappears, the soft and succulent connective tissue becomes fibrillated, and the vessels are narrowed, sometimes obliterated, by its contraction. The uterus, though still enlarged and altered in shape, is of a pale color, anæmic, dry, tough, and hard. Ultimately, the uterus is reduced in size by the cicatricial contraction of the firm, fibrillar connective tissue. On section the tissue is white, of cartilaginous consistence, and the knife creaks as it divides the structures. Scanzoni's stage of induration is thus nearly identical with the areolar hyperplasia, diffuse interstitial hypertrophy, sclerosis uteri, of Thomas and Skene.

---

[1] *Op. cit.*, p. 299.   [2] *Die Chronische Metritis*, Wien, 1863.

Klob,[1] a pupil of Rokitansky's, attributes the hyperplasia of connective tissue to nutritive disturbances, considers the terms chronic metritis and chronic infarct anatomically incorrect, and classes the condition among the new formations. Carl Braun[2] and Wedl in 1864 assumed the same position.

Klebs[3] is of the opinion that, although the so-called chronic uterine infarct may be of inflammatory origin, in the majority of cases the clinical and anatomical demonstration is lacking. With Scanzoni and Virchow, he distinguishes two forms of the disease, the one consisting in hyperplasia of the muscular elements, the other in a similar change in the connective tissue.

Birch-Hirschfeld[4] supports the doctrine of Scanzoni, that the stage of induration at least is of an inflammatory nature. The connective tissue is formed out of emigrated white blood-corpuscles. Hypertrophy of the muscular elements is also observed in certain cases.

Fritsch[5] has materially strengthened the position of Scanzoni by his recent anatomical investigations. Mayrhofer[6] subtantially reproduces Scanzoni's doctrines.

Finally, the great majority of modern clinicians have accepted Scanzoni's teachings as originally uttered or as modified in non-essential details. Schroeder,[7] De Sinéty,[8] and A. Martin[9] are notable examples of the truth of this statement.

The hyperplasia of the connective tissue may be diffuse or circumscribed. It may be limited in development to the collum or corpus uteri. The perimetrium is usually thickened, and and other signs of chronic inflammation of that structure are usually present. Chronic endometritis is a constant accompaniment. The pelvic connective tissue is not commonly involved. The plexus pampiniformes and utero-vaginales frequently undergo varicose dilatation.

SYMPTOMS.—The onset of the disease is so insidious and protracted that it is difficult to determine the exact order of occurrence of the symptoms in point of time. Then the complications are so numerous and important that the symptoms of the chronic metritis are frequently masked. A sensation of weight, fulness, or pressure within the pelvis may direct the patient's attention to her condition. This sensation may increase to such a degree that the woman complains of heavy, dull, dragging pains, referred to the centre of the pelvis or the sacral region. Backache is a constant and distressing symptom. Pains radiating up over the abdominal parietes and down the thighs are frequently experienced. Coitus may be productive of acute distress. When the uterus is anteverted, pressing against the bladder, ischuria is the usual result. Constipation, usually present as one of the etiological factors, is aggravated by the retroversion or retroflexion of the top-heavy uterus. Under these cir-

---

[1] Jul. M. Klob, *Pathologische Anatomie d. Weibl. Sexualorgane,* Wien, 1864.
[2] *Lehrbuch d. g. Gynaekologie,* Wien, 1881, p. 351.
[3] *Handbuch der Pathologischen Anatomie,* Berlin, 1873, iv. p. 878.
[4] *Pathologische Anatomie,* p. 1131.   [5] *Op. cit.,* p. 309 *et seq.,* Stuttgart, 1885.
[6] *Entwicklungsfehler und Entzündungen des Uterus.*
[7] Carl Schroeder, *Handbuch der Krankheiten d. Weibl. Geschlechtsorgane,* Leipzig, 1881, p. 91.
[8] L. de Sinéty, *Manuel practique de Gynécologie et des Maladies des Femmes,* Paris, 1879.
[9] *Op. cit.,* Wien, 1885, p. 185.

cumstances one or both ovaries may be drawn down along with the prolapsed, retroverted uterus, and add materially to the woman's discomfort. The act of defecation is painful; the woman avoids the water-closet, days and even weeks elapsing between evacuations.

Disturbances of the menstrual function are constant. All forms of dysmenorrhœa, including dysmenorrhœa membranacea, are liable to occur. Menstruation is usually profuse, giving origin to menorrhagia, which usually results in the production of an alarming degree of anæmia. The periods are irregular in recurrence and duration. The periodic discharge of blood may last from one to three weeks, and then cease, to reappear after a variable interval of from six to eight weeks. In other cases menstruation may last the usual length of time, but recur every two or three weeks. Amenorrhœa may be observed in the stage of induration.

Priestly,[1] Fasbender,[2] Fehling, and numerous other clinicians have called attention to intermenstrual pain (règles surnuméraires) as a tolerably constant symptom of chronic metritis. From fourteen to fifteen days after and before the regular time for menstruation vague intrapelvic pains are complained of, and the woman is of the opinion that the monthly flow of blood is about to begin. The pains, however, are not so severe, and do not last so long, as those of menstruation. Occasionally bloody mucus may escape from the vagina. Fehling ascribes this intermenstrual pain to the swelling of the mucous membrane preparatory to the next monthly discharge of blood. The symptom is not at all pathognomonic, as it occurs in connection with oöphoritis and other pathological conditions.

As the result of the chronic endometritis, which usually follows parenchymatous inflammation, metrorrhagia is frequently observed. Leucorrhœa, more or less profuse, is a constant symptom. Opinions vary extremely as to the systemic reaction following chronic metritis. General failure of nutrition, functional disturbances of the gastro-intestinal canal, hysteria, headache,[3] facial neuralgia (Barnes), coccygodynia, vaginodynia, skin diseases, alopecia (Hebra), and a host of other affections, have been ascribed from time to time to the direct influence of chronic uterine infarct. Doubtless, the condition under discussion plays an important rôle in the production of these and other disorders. But the position is utterly untenable at the present day that chronic parenchymatous inflammation of the uterus is the efficient cause in the absence of all other etiological factors.[4]

Intercostal neuralgia and mastodynia, with swelling of the breasts and darkening of the areolæ, are phenomena of such constant occurrence in connection with chronic uterine infarct that a direct causal nexus is in a high degree probable. The investigations of Krause[5] have established the fact of anastomotic communication between the arteries supplying the mammary gland and those distributed to the uterus. The perforating branches of the internal mammary artery supply in part the mammary gland. The superior epigastric artery, one of the terminal branches of

[1] *Brit. Med. Journ.*, 1872, p. 431.   [2] *Zeitschrift f. Gebürtskulfe und Frauenkrankheiten*, i. 1.
[3] Peaselee, "Uterine Headache," *American Medical Monthly*, 1860.
[4] Fritsch, *op. cit.*, 1885, p. 323.
[5] *Specielle und Makroskopische Anatomie*, Hannover, 1879.

the internal mammary, anastomoses with the inferior epigastric, which arises from the external iliac a few lines above Poupart's ligament. The inferior epigastric sends off a spermatic branch which passes along the round ligament and anastomoses with the ovarian artery derived from the aorta, and the uterine artery derived from the anterior trunk of the internal iliac. The nervous communication is effected through the sympathetic and spinal nerves. There is nothing remarkable, therefore, in the occurrence of intercostal neuralgia, mastodynia, and nutritive disturbances in the mammary gland as the result of chronic parenchymatous inflammation of the uterus. The intercostal neuralgia and mastodynia are examples of reflected neuroses the result of compression of nerve-fibres by the infiltration or of an ascending neuritis (Fritsch).

PHYSICAL SIGNS OF CHRONIC METRITIS.—Bimanual palpation prior to the stage of cicatricial contraction reveals alterations in size, shape, position, consistence, and sensibility of the uterus. Variations in size are extreme. Veit[1] has recorded a case in which the fundus extended two inches above the umbilicus. The uterus is usually thickened, especially in its antero-posterior diameter. As regards position, the organ may be prolapsed, elevated, or remain in situ. The consistence will depend upon the stage of the disease. During the stage of infiltration the organ is soft and imparts a doughy sensation to the examining finger. During an exacerbation of acute inflammation the vagina is hot and dry; the uterus is swollen with blood and very sensitive on pressure. During the intervals between exacerbations no change in sensibility is noticed. The sound demonstrates a varying degree of elongation of the uterine cavity. During the second stage, after cicatricial contraction of the connective-tissue elements, the uterus is relatively small, hard, and insensible.

The cervix is hard or soft according to the time of examination. In virgins or women who have not borne children enlargement is of relatively infrequent occurrence. In multiparæ, especially in cases of bilateral cervical laceration, the increase in volume is great. The mucous membrane of the cervical canal is everted and studded with minute cysts —distended follicles.

The influence of chronic metritis upon conception is not direct. When the endometrium is not seriously involved the condition seems to exercise no untoward influence. However, associated with chronic uterine infarct as complications we have endometritis, salpingitis, oöphoritis, perimetritis, and displacements, pathological states which may obviously cause sterility.

When conception does occur, abortion follows with relative frequency. The reason why is not clear. The chronic endometritis may interfere with the development of the decidua; the parenchyma may not be able to undergo evolution. When pregnancy reaches its normal termination, labor is not materially influenced by the pathological condition of the uterus, but complications are liable to occur during the puerperium. Postpartum hemorrhages which do not readily yield to ergot are observed as the result of the deficiency in muscular elements. The hyperplasia of the connective-tissue elements and destruction of the muscular tissue is a distinct predisposing cause of complete or incomplete uterine inversion. Subin-

[1] *Frauenkrankheiten,* 2 Aufl. p. 367.

volution is increased. Menstruation recurs soon after pregnancy, and the chronic metritis is aggravated.[1]

Occasionally, gestation, parturition, the puerperium, and lactation seem to exercise a favorable influence on the state of the parenchyma. In exceptional cases all traces of the original chronic metritis disappear with the puerperium. The connective-tissue hyperplasia may undergo the same involution to which the hypertrophied muscular tissue is subject. This favorable termination of the disease is seldom observed during the stage of induration.

TERMINATIONS.—I. Chronic metritis may terminate during the stage of infiltration in resolution. This mode of termination is rare. It is observed occasionally as the result of involution in the puerperal uterus. Judicious treatment in favorable cases may reduce the size of the uterus and relieve all distressing symptoms. Recidiva of the disease are liable to occur, however, and all traces of the former condition seldom disappear.

II. Usually, the condition persists, with acute exacerbations, through years, until cessation of menstruation and ovulation occurs. Under the influence of the change of life the symptoms may gradually disappear and the uterus may undergo senile atrophy. In some cases chronic uterine infarct seems to defer the climacteric changes. Finally, the disease may continue after the menopause, usually with abatement in the severity of the symptoms.

III. The morbid condition may terminate in induration. The uterus becomes comparatively small, hard, and insensible. Amenorrhœa may be the result. This process may be viewed as a relative cure, since it is attended, as a rule, with amelioration of all the troublesome symptoms.

DIFFERENTIAL DIAGNOSIS.—It is not always an easy matter to institute a differential diagnosis between chronic metritis and pregnancy and fibroid tumors by bimanual palpation. Alterations in the volume, form, position, consistence, and sensibility of the uterus occur in pregnancy as in chronic metritis. But in pregnancy the uterus, particularly in its vaginal portion, is softer; the organ is not so sensitive; the cyanotic hue of the vaginal mucous membrane is more marked; arterial pulsations in the vagina are more evident; the uterus enlarges more rapidly; finally, there is the history of the case. Pregnancy may occur, however, in a chronically inflamed uterus, and this fact must be borne in mind.

The alterations in the size of the uterus are usually circumscribed in fibroid tumors. One wall is thickened; the other retains its normal relations. In submucous fibroids the cervix is shortened; in chronic metritis it is usually enlarged. In both submucous and interstitial fibroids the cavity of the uterus is encroached upon—a fact to be determined by the use of the sound. The history of the case will throw some light upon the differential diagnosis. Frequently, however, it is impossible to exclude fibroids by any of the means already mentioned. Dilatation of the cervix, and the careful examination of the walls by the finger introduced into the uterine cavity, will clear up the diagnosis in the most obscure case.

PROGNOSIS.—The prognosis with reference to life is favorable. The duration of life however, may be abbreviated in exceptional cases by dis-

[1] A. Martin, *op. cit.*, Wien, 1885, p. 189.

turbances of nutrition, anæmia the result of menorrhagia and metror-rhagia, extension of the inflammation to the peritoneum, and the like—conditions which predispose to some intercurrent affection.

Although the immediate danger of death is minimal, the woman is rendered wretched by the frequent exacerbations of acute inflammation and other symptoms already mentioned. The spontaneous disappearance of the affection with the puerperium or menopause is of such seldom occurrence as to have but slight bearing on the general rule.

Under judicious treatment disappearance of the more distressing symptoms may be confidently expected during the stage of infiltration. The outlook is especially favorable in cases of puerperal subinvolution in the absence of chronic inflammations of the endometrium and parametrium. A perfect restitution of the uterus to its normal condition is so seldom effected by any rational therapy that for practical purposes this desirable result may be excluded from consideration. Recidiva of the disease are liable to occur at any time.

TREATMENT.—Prophylaxis.—Very much can be done to prevent the occurrence of chronic metritis. A careful consideration of the etiology of the disease will at once suggest the principles of prophylactic treatment. The conduct of the second stage of labor, the puerperium, lactation, the hygiene of menstruation, are subjects especially significant in this connection. Antecedent acute metritis and endometritis under a rational therapy usually terminate in resolution, and their pernicious influences as etiological factors may be avoided, or at least modified, in the large majority of cases. The early rectification of uterine flexions and displacement is urgently indicated in view of the probable consequences.

Uncomplicated chronic metritis is such a rare affection that efforts at curative treatment are seldom addressed to the condition of the parenchyma, to the exclusion of the endometrium, perimetrium, and parametrium. Certain special indications, however, exist in the ease of chronic uterine infarct, and the discussion of treatment is limited here to their consideration.

1. Local Treatment.—In view of the pathology of the condition, local treatment, especially in the first stage, is antiphlogistic.

Hot-Water Vaginal Douche.—The irrigation of the vagina with hot water, of different degrees of temperature according to the indications in the concrete case, deservedly occupies the high position in American gynæcological therapeutics which Emmet[1] in particular has assigned it. The smooth muscular fibres of the uterus are excited to contract, and the whole pelvic circulation is directly or indirectly influenced. During the stage of infiltration—Emmet's congestive hypertrophy—hot-water vaginal irrigation is simply an invaluable adjuvant. But to secure the maximum benefit from this remedy it must be rationally employed. With reference to posture, Emmet recommends the dorsal decubitus, with elevation of the hips, or, better, the genu-pectoral position. The temperature of the water should be rapidly elevated from blood-heat to 110° F., or to as high a degree as the patient can tolerate. The quantity of water will vary with the stage of the treatment and the improvement in health of the patient. It is customary to begin the irrigations with one to two

---

[1] *Principles and Practice of Gynæcology,* 3d ed. 1884, pp. 85, 113.

gallons of water, and to increase or decrease the quantity according to circumstances. Two irrigations per diem—one at night before going to bed, one in the morning upon rising—are usually sufficient. Fritsch[1] has tried on an extensive scale the plan of continuous vaginal irrigation with hot water through five and even ten hours, but has obtained better results with the simple periodic vaginal douche as recommended by Emmet.

During the stage of induration, when the muscular elements have been destroyed and replaced by connective tissue, the beneficial effects of the hot-water douche are decidedly less evident. Nor is the plan applicable to all cases during the stage of congestive hypertrophy. General nervous excitement, insomnia, and even positive intrapelvic pain, sometimes, though rarely, may result. The range of therapeutic application of the hot-water vaginal douche is largely empirical.

Local Depletion.—The local bloodletting of from a drachm to one ounce of the fluid, repeated according to the indications every three or four days, ranks next to the hot-water vaginal douche in importance as an antiphlogistic agent. This plan of treatment is of especial value as an adjuvant during the stage of infiltration in cases of menorrhagia, metrorrhagia, exacerbations of acute inflammation, and the like. Local depletion, however, is a double-edged sword. It may cause an increased determination of blood to the uterus and aggravate the pathological condition already existing. This effect is observed when the bloodletting is practised at too short intervals.[2] Thus, frequent scarifications of the cervix constitute a most important therapeutic resource in the treatment of certain forms of atrophy of the uterus.

Local depletion of the cervix is effected by scarification, puncture, leeches, wet and dry cupping. Scarification and puncture have almost entirely superseded the other two methods.

Local depletion has fallen into a state of comparative disuse in America. In the Woman's Hospital of New York[3] it has almost completely passed out of vogue. In Germany, however, it constitutes the basis of all methods of treatment. Schroeder, A. Martin of Berlin, H. Fritsch of Breslau, Carl Braun, Spaeth, and Chrobals of Vienna unite in enthusiastic advocacy of its intelligent employment in suitable cases.

Glycerin Tamponade.—Sims many years ago called attention to the employment of cotton tampons saturated with glycerin in the treatment of chronic metritis and kindred affections. In virtue of its avidity for water the glycerin tampon, when placed in the vagina, provokes a profuse aqueous discharge. The albuminoid constituents of the blood are not affected, while the capillaries are drained of their aqueous elements. Emmet[4] has substituted oakum for absorbent cotton. Oakum, when saturated with glycerin, becomes soft as a sponge, is perfectly antiseptic, and will remain odorless in the vagina a much longer time than cotton. Glycerin dissolves the salts more readily than water. Boric acid (1 : 10), potassium iodide (5 : 100), iodoform, chloral, and a variety of substances may be applied locally by means of this menstruum. Glycerin, employed in conjunction with hot-water vaginal irrigation and scarification, or used

[1] *Op. cit.*, 1885, p. 337.   [2] A. Martin, *op. cit.*, 1885, p. 59.
[3] T. Gaillard Thomas, *Diseases of Women*, 5th ed., 1880, p. 334.
[4] *Gynæcology*, 1884, p. 128.

alone in cases contraindicating these procedures, is an important addition to our therapeutic resources.

Local Alteratives.—Much importance is attached in the United States to the application of various alteratives to the vaginal portion and endometrium in cases of chronic uterine infarct. They may accomplish good results indirectly—for example, by curing the accompanying endometritis —but it is doubtful whether they have any direct effect in hastening the resorption of the infiltration.

The vaginal vault and intravaginal portion of the cervix are usually painted with the compound tincture of iodine; mercury, potassium iodide, iodoform, and other substances are introduced into the vagina by means of vaseline, gelatin, and cacao butter.

Operative Treatment.—1. Repair of Lacerations of the Cervix.—The importance of the repair of lacerations of the cervix for the cure of chronic uterine infarct and allied conditions was recognized by Emmet in 1862. In the autumn of 1862 he devised and performed the operation, which is now known the world over as Emmet's operation. This highly original and valuable surgical procedure has been but little modified in the years which have intervened since its first full description in 1869.

2. Amputation of the Collum Uteri.—Carl Braun[1] and Wedl in 1864 pointed out the fact that amputation of the neck of the chronically inflamed uterus is frequently followed by a more or less complete involution of the whole organ, resembling very closely the reductive metamorphosis of the puerperal uterus. August Martin in recent years has called attention to Braun's observation, and at the Naturforscherversammlung in Cassel described a series of seventy cases in which amputation of the collum uteri had been performed for the relief of chronic metritis. As an ultimate resort in extreme cases, amputation of the neck of the uterus is now a generally well-recognized operative procedure.[2]

3. Castration.—At a comparatively recent date a determined effort has been made to include desperate cases of chronic metritis under the indications for the performance of oöphorectomy. Numerous and distinguished surgeons have taken this advanced position. But at the present time the cases in which the operation has been performed are too few in number and too recent to warrant positive deductions with reference to the effects of the operation.

2. General Treatment.— It is not possible to adequately discuss the subject of the general or constitutional treatment of chronic metritis in the limited space at our command. It is scarcely necessary to add that the subject is of vital importance, and more frequently neglected than the local treatment. The indications for therapeutic aid are usually apparent, and are not always peculiar to the condition. Attention has been directed, in other portions of this work, to the importance of the observation of hygienic laws, in the widest sense of that expression, with respect to diet, rest, clothing, recreation, personal cleanliness, temperance in sexual intercourse, and other bodily habits.

Habitual constipation, involving as it does engorgement of the portal system and pelvic veins, demands especial consideration. In the absence of regular daily alvine dejections the most elaborate plan of local and

[1] *Wiener Med. Jahrbücher*, Wien, 1864.   [2] H. Fritsch, *op. cit.*, 1885, p. 343.

constitutional treatment will fail to effect amelioration of symptoms. Diet, exercise, and the like are not sufficient, as a rule, to correct this most obstinate habit. Among remedial agents, senna, rhubarb, cascara sagrada, and the milder laxatives deserve particular mention. The compound licorice powder and confection of senna of the U. S. Pharmacopœia are comparatively innocent in their effects, even when used through long periods of time. Aloes must be employed with a certain amount of caution. As pointed out by August Martin,[1] when there is a disposition to uterine hemorrhages the drug, in the exercise of its well-known influence on the pelvic circulation, may increase this tendency. Clysters may be employed to advantage in connection with hygienic and medical means.

Ergot, hydrastis canadensis, potassium iodide, ammonium chloride, strychnia, are among the remedial agents which are supposed to have some direct effect upon the condition of the uterine parenchyma. Ergot may be exhibited by the mouth or hypodermatically. Squibb's fluid extract, while an active and tolerably agreeable preparation, is not as effective as the decoction employed on an extensive scale in many of the German hospitals, and the formula of which we append:

R̶. Secalis cornuti recent. pulver., 15.0
Alcohol., 5.0
Acidi sulphurici, 2.0
Aquæ, 500.0
Coque ad 200.0
Ne cola.
Adde Syr. cinnamom., 30.0

Dose: Two to three teaspoonfuls, pro re nata. This unfiltered decoction is extremely distasteful, and its continued use is not without effect upon the gastric mucous membrane. It is, however, physiologically very active. Subcutaneous injections of Squibb's aqueous extract of ergot may be occasionally employed with benefit to keep up the impression of the remedy when exhibition per os is interrupted. Schatz speaks in high terms of the fluid extract of hydrastis canadensis in doses of fifteen to twenty drops two or three times daily.

All European writers ascribe an important influence to the numerous watering-places and baths of the Continent in the treatment of chronic uterine infarct. The rigid observance of hygienic rules, the imbibition of enormous quantities of water more or less impregnated with salines and carbonic acid, the frequent bathings, exercise, and recreation, undoubtedly effect amelioration of symptoms in many desperate cases.

Acute Endometritis.

ETIOLOGY.—An acute inflammation of the mucous membrane of the uterus is a rare affection before puberty. The acute infectious diseases play an important rôle in the production of the condition. The acute exanthems—smallpox, measles, scarlet fever, cholera, typhus, typhoid, and relapsing fever, certain forms of malarial fever—deserve mention in this connection. Probably owing to some change in the constitution

[1] *Op. cit.*, p. 195.

of the blood, these diseases predispose to the hemorrhagic form of acute endometritis. The rapid cooling off of extensive areas of the skin surface during menstruation frequently leads to an acute inflammation of the endometrium, with suppression of the flow as one of the first symptoms. Gonorrhœal infection and sepsis are most important causative factors. Ill-advised therapeutic procedures, as in the case of acute metritis, must be included in the list of causative agencies. Finally, acute endometritis may be caused by various poisons. Among toxic agents which may give origin to the condition under discussion phosphorus is especially noteworthy.[1]

PATHOLOGICAL ANATOMY.—The entire lining membrane of the uterine cavity may be involved in the inflammatory process; usually, the mucosa of the body and fundus is affected, the mucosa of the cervical canal remaining normal. The mucous membrane is of a dark-red color, swollen, softened, and presents a velvety appearance. Its connection with the muscularis is loosened, so that it can frequently be stripped off with the handle of a scalpel. Minute extravasations of blood are visible in the superficial layers and on the surface. The interglandular connective tissue is the seat of the inflammatory process. The glands are involved secondarily. The ciliated epithelium is destroyed and cast off at an early stage. The bloody discharge from the uterine cavity becomes serous, and finally purulent, during the progress of the condition. The cervical secretion becomes thin, turbid, and profuse.

The inflammatory process is seldom limited to the endometrium. It involves, as a rule, the tubal mucous membrane, the uterine parenchyma, and the perimetrium.

DIAGNOSIS.—The symptoms resemble closely in kind, but differ in degree from, the appearances in acute metritis. The uterus is smaller and not so painful on pressure. The endometrium is sensitive to the slightest touch—a fact elicited upon the passage of the sound. The characteristic symptom is the discharge from the uterine cavity of a more or less profuse secretion possessing the character already mentioned. An absolute differential diagnosis is impossible, nor is it necessary, seeing that the treatment of the two conditions is nearly identical.

PROGNOSIS.—Acute endometritis terminates in resolution or chronic inflammation. The latter mode of termination is of more frequent occurrence, particularly in the presence of gonorrhœa, sepsis, and the like as etiological factors. The disease endangers life when the peritoneum is involved by the propagation of the inflammatory process along the tubes or through the uterine parenchyma. Then the acute endometritis may be the starting-point of general septic infection through the media of the veins and lymphatic vessels.

TREATMENT.—Absolute rest in bed, the relief of pain by morphine, the evacuation of the bowels by enemata or mild laxatives, the free imbibition of bland mucilaginous fluids for the vesical tenesmus,—are measures which usually fulfil all indications for treatment. Even in the case of gonorrhœal infections astringent applications to the endometrium are contraindicated. Usually, various complications mark the endometritis, the starting-point of the pathological condition, and these complications demand more active interference.

[1] Hausmann, *Berl. Beitr. z. Geb. u. Gyn.*, Bd. i. S. 265.

Chronic Endometritis.

ETIOLOGY.—Attention has been called to the etiology of chronic metritis in a somewhat detailed manner. The limits of this paper will not admit of adequate mention even of the more common causative factors of chronic endometritis. All the conditions which determine an active fluxion or passive hyperæmia of the uterus may operate as causative factors. Hypersecretion of mucus is frequently observed in chlorotic, scrofulous, and tuberculous females. Syphilis and gonorrhœa are potential causative agents. Climate seems to exercise a more or less direct influence. Thus, we are informed by Schroeder[1] that chronic endometritis is observed with relative frequency in damp, cool regions, such as Holland, Belgium, and certain parts of England. Europeans who reside in hot climates—for example, the Englishwomen living in India—are said to be affected with leucorrhœa to a degree entirely out of proportion to local or constitutional causes.

PATHOLOGICAL ANATOMY.—An analogy of striking character exists between the structural changes in chronic endometritis and chronic metritis. In chronic endometritis, as in chronic metritis, it is possible to clearly distinguish two stages in the inflammatory process. In the first, or stage of infiltration, a more or less acute inflammation is observed, which involves, primarily, the interglandular connective tissue; secondarily, the glands themselves. When the stage of infiltration does not terminate in resolution with the resorption of the exudate, the newly-formed connective-tissue elements contract, and the glands are to a greater or less degree obliterated.

1. Chronic Catarrhal Endometritis.—The endometrium during the first stage is swollen, vascular, soft, and succulent. Small extravasations of blood and pigmentary deposits from ecchymoses are observed in the interacinous connective tissue. The surface of the mucous membrane is smooth or roughened in spots. The orifices of the glands are visible. The mucous membrane of the cervix is infected, its transverse folds distended, the follicles filled with mucus, the canal plugged with tenacious turbid secretion; the vaginal portion is enlarged, spongy, and its mucous membrane exhibits hypertrophic changes in the papillary body. The os externum is frequently patulous. The uterine walls having undergone excentric hypertrophy, the cavity is usually enlarged, and contains a translucent alkaline secretion which resembles mucus.

Microscopical examination of the endometrium reveals a variety of structural changes. A luxuriant development of embryonal connective-tissue elements is observed with relative frequency in the interacinous connective tissue. Olshausen has applied the term chronic hyperplastic endometritis to this condition. The term chronic interstitial endometritis has been more generally accepted. While the newly-formed connective-tissue elements are soft and succulent, hemorrhages are frequent.

Changes in the glandular structures may become more prominent features than alterations in the connective tissue. The laminæ of the glands and the cells of the acini increase in size. The glands branch, frequently resulting in the production of a dendritic network. Schroeder and Carl Ruge have termed this glandular endometritis diffuse adenoma.

---

[1] *Handbuch der Krankheiten der Weiblichen Geschlechtsorgane*, 1881, p. 111.

The thickness of the mucous membrane may increase in spots from three or four millimeters to fourteen or fifteen millimeters, and there is produced a form of chronic endometritis which is known as fungoid or polypoid.

Under the name endometritis villosa Slavianski described in 1874 a condition of the uterine mucous membrane which consists in a papillary growth of the endometrium with myxomatous degeneration of the vessel tunics.

During the stage of induration the ciliated epithelium, destroyed and cast off during the stage of infiltration, is replaced by cells which resemble squamous epithelium. The utricular glands, with dilated cavities, are flattened out, entirely obliterated, or present the appearance of shallow crypts. The secretion is gradually diminished, until finally the endometrium is converted into a layer of connective tissue.

Under the names erosion, ulceration, granulation, and the like a variety of pathological conditions, entirely distinct from, sometimes in connection with, cervical laceration and ectropium, are included. The flattened epithelium covering the vaginal portion may be cast off, and replaced by the dark-red subjacent cylindrical epithelium, giving origin to the condition known as simple erosion. Occasionally, glandular canals, formed out of these cylindrical cells, and penetrating the mucous membrane in every direction, present the appearances of papillary erosion; and the condition has accordingly been termed by Carl Ruge papillary ulcer. Cervical secretions may stagnate in these glandular tubes, retention-cysts appear, and the condition technically termed follicular erosion results. In all forms of cervical erosion or laceration the secretions are increased in amount and altered in physical and chemical characters during the stage of infiltration. In a later stage of the disease the hyperplasia and subsequent contraction of the connective-tissue elements may result in the total obliteration of all traces of glandular structure. There is a certain amount of probable evidence in favor of the view that these changes in the cylindrical cells normally situated beneath the squamous epithelium covering the vaginal portion may terminate in malignant disease. These erosions, in the present state of our knowledge, must be viewed as symptomatic of chronic endocervicitis.

2. Dysmenorrhœa Membranacea.—The exfoliation and casting off of large pieces, or even of the superficial layers, of the entire endometrium during menstruation has been observed from the days of Morgagni up to the present time. Peter Frank pointed out the resemblance between this exfoliation and the membrana caduca. Simpson, recognizing the sieve-like perforations caused by the utricular glands, termed the condition exfoliation of the hypertrophic mucous membrane. Virchow erroneously termed the membrane decidua menstrualis. Olshausen, Wyder, and v. Recklinghausen (1877) have demonstrated the truth of Simpson's view, and have shown that the condition must be regarded as a symptom of a series of endometritic inflammatory processes. In all cases in which a decidual membrane is cast off the diagnosis of abortion must be made, whether the pregnancy be intra-uterine or extra-uterine.

Wyger has reported a case in which syphilis was regarded as an etiological factor. This observation has not been confirmed.

3. Chronic Croupous Inflammation of the Endometrium is sometimes observed in connection with carcinoma of the corpus. It may follow

gangrenous vaginitis in diphtheria and the acute infectious diseases. The interacinous connective tissue is infiltrated with fibrinous materials, and extravasations of blood are everywhere visible. The superficial layers of the mucous membrane become gangrenous, are cast off, and occasionally the entire intra-uterine expanse is converted into a wound surface.

DIAGNOSIS.—The symptoms of chronic endometritis and endocervicitis are usually masked by the appearance of the accompanying chronic metritis. Intrapelvic pains, disturbance of the menstrual function, extramenstrual hemorrhages, the presence of a more or less profuse leucorrhœa, are signs which urgently indicate bimanual palpation.

The catarrhal secretion from the utricular glands may be imprisoned within the uterine cavity by a functional or organic stricture of the internal os, resulting in periodic discharges of a thin, translucent alkaline fluid, readily distinguishable from the thick, tenacious cervical mucus. In certain cases, particularly in old women, the blenorrhœal secretion may be permanently retained within the uterine cavity, constituting the condition hydrometra.

The introduction of a small sharp spoon within the cavity of the uterus will enable the observer to remove sufficient tissue for microscopical examination without entailing the slightest injury on the patient. A positive diagnosis can be made in this way, and a rational therapy instituted.

Digital and specular examinations disclose the condition of the vaginal portion of the cervix. The amount and physical characters of the cervical secretions are items of important diagnostic moment. In suspicious cases of cervical erosion a small bit of tissue may be cut away from the surface and subjected to microscopical examination.

Secondary disturbances in connection with the gastro-intestinal canal and nervous system occur in chronic inflammations of the endometrium, as in the case of chronic uterine infarct.

PROGNOSIS.—Chronic inflammations of the corporeal and cervical mucous membrane seldom threaten life directly. The continuous loss of blood and serum, however, may produce a condition of profound anæmia and render the individual more susceptible to intercurrent disease.

Then the hyperplastic condition of the endometrium is always an occasion for anxiety. The relation between polypoid and fungoid growths of the corporeal mucous membrane, erosions of the vaginal portion of the cervix, and malignant new formations is not settled. The possibility of malignant residua, however, must be admitted.

Sterility, acute and chronic decidual inflammations, adherent placenta, disturbances in the involution of the puerperal uterus, and the like—direct results of chronic endometritic inflammation—are conditions which confer an unfavorable element upon the prognosis.

Finally, while it is possible to effect a material amelioration of all the symptoms by a judicious general and local treatment, a complete restitutio ad integrum is seldom or never achieved. Recidiva are always liable to occur.

TREATMENT.—Prophylaxis.—The remarks made with reference to the prevention of chronic uterine infarct apply with equal force to the prophylaxis of chronic corporeal and cervical endometritis.

Curative.—Of chief importance, in the very large majority of cases, is the subject of general treatment. Many cases of chronic catarrhal endometritis are improved by the regulation of the functions of the gastro-intestinal canal, skin, kidneys, and hæmatopoietic viscera in the absence of all local treatment. This statement holds true with particular force when scrofulosis, tuberculosis, syphilis, and the like are chief etiological factors.

Local Treatment.—The methods of local treatment at the present time are infinitely various. For convenience of description they may be collected under three headings:[1]

I. The washing out of the uterine cavity;
II. The cauterization of the uterine cavity;
III. The curettement of the uterine mucous membrane.

To Schultze, in particular, are we indebted for methods of washing out the cavity of the uterus. The cervical canal is dilated by means of the finger, tents, or metallic instruments, and the mucous membrane lining the cavity of the uterus is cleansed with dilute solutions of carbolic acid, boric acid, bichloride of mercury, and other solvent and antiseptic fluids.

Cauterization is usually effected at the present time by the application of pure tincture of iodine, iodine with glycerin, or carbolic acid, to the endometrium. Bandl's canulæ for the washing out of the uterine cavity with solutions of alum and cupric sulphate are valuable instruments in this connection. The application of the solid stick of nitrate of silver and intra-uterine injections of liquor ferri are gradually passing into disuse.

The curettement of the diseased endometrium has been rapidly gaining ground within recent years, and now constitutes the most reliable method of treatment in obstinate cases in which local interference is indicated at all. Martin, Düvelius, and other clinicians have abundantly established the fact that, after the mechanical removal of the old diseased mucous membrane, a new endometrium of relatively normal functional activity is formed.

The number of operative procedures for the relief of chronic endo-cervicitis is enormous. In the majority of cases occurring among multiparæ it will be found that the condition is aggravated, if not caused, by cervical laceration with ectropium. Under these circumstances, and under the indications and conditions insisted upon by the author of the procedure, Emmet's operation will alleviate, if it does not cure, the pathological state of the mucous membrane.

[1] H. Fritsch, *op. cit.*, 1885, p. 419.

ABORTION.

By GEORGE J. ENGELMANN, M. D.

DEFINITION.—Abortion, the mishap of popular parlance, the fausse couche of the French, is the premature interruption of intra-uterine pregnancy, the expulsion of the non-viable ovum, whether the result of natural causes or criminal interference.

SYNONYMS.—Common as the accident unfortunately is, the nomenclature, both popular and scientific, is somewhat indistinct, the terms abortion and miscarriage being used in a variety of ways, so that the physician is liable to be misunderstood by his professional brethren and in danger of causing serious offence to his patients. A strict definition of the terms is hence of importance, and in order not to add to the confusion we can do no better than adopt the one now adhered to by the authorities of the day. Abortion and miscarriage are strictly synonymous, notwithstanding the popular belief that the term abortion is restricted to the criminal interruption of pregnancy, whilst miscarriage is supposed to designate the accident resulting from natural causes. Again, some make a difference in time between abortion and miscarriage—abortion being the expulsion of the ovum in the first four months of pregnancy; miscarriage, or the partus immaturus, in the next three months, from the fourth to the seventh; and the partus prematurus from the seventh to the ninth month.

CLASSIFICATION.—We might, indeed, in regard to importance, cause, and course of expulsion, designate four different periods of gestation— the first two during the continuance of the chorion frondosum, and the last two during the period of placental development: the first during the first two months of pregnancy, before sufficient adhesions have formed; the second, still during the period of the chorion frondosum, until it begins to disappear, from the second to the fourth month; the third, in the early stages of placental development, before the term of fœtal viability, from the fourth to the seventh month; and the fourth, which is everywhere recognized as the partus prematurus—premature delivery—from the seventh to the ninth month, when the placenta is fully developed with firm adhesions and the child viable.

For practical reasons and simplicity's sake we will distinguish only between abortion and premature labor—miscarriage, abortion, abortus, being the expulsion of a non-viable fœtus, of the ovum before the time of complete placental development, in the first seven months of pregnancy; and premature labor, the interruption of pregnancy in the last two months, from the seventh to the ninth, when the fœtus is viable and formation and attachment of the placenta has been completed. These two classes naturally blend, but are strikingly different in cause, symptoms, and treatment if we consider the type about which they are grouped— abortion proper as most frequent in the third and fourth month, and premature labor in the seventh and eighth. It is abortion or miscarriage of which we shall treat in this article, more especially its characteristic form before the formation of the placenta, whilst we shall touch but lightly upon those forms which approximate premature labor and come within the sphere of the obstetrician; that is, abortion in the sixth or seventh month, when the placenta is more fully developed.

FREQUENCY.—With regard to the frequency with which this accident occurs, we can but form an estimate, as there are but few of the pathological conditions to which the human constitution is subject in regard to which we are more at fault as to statistics: neither the case-book of the physician nor the hospital or post-mortem record permits of more than an indefinite approximation as to the frequency of its occurrence. During the first six or eight weeks of gestation, certainly the first four, the patient herself is often ignorant of her condition, and the ovum passes off amid a more profuse menstruation, with only the symptoms of simple menorrhagia; the same may be true at later periods by reason of coexisting conditions. Some knowingly conceal the fact; many, knowing it, call no assistance; others have midwives, the physician seeing only the more threatening cases; and but few enter the hospital, where our most reliable statistics are gathered.

All points considered, it has been stated that to every 5.5 labors at term we will find 1 case of premature expulsion of the ovum (Busch and Moser). Whitehead asserts that 90 per cent. of married women abort, or that 37 out of 100, somewhat over one-third, of all mothers abort at least once before their thirtieth year. Hegar estimates 1 abortion in the early months to 8 or 10 labors at term, which harmonizes very well with the figures given by Busch and Moser. Multigravidæ abort more often than primigravidæ, although there are certain causes peculiar to primigravidæ which tend to abortion, such as the indiscretions of early married life: uterine disease, perimetritis, and endometritis, on the other hand, are more common in multigravidæ, and, again, the number of multigravidæ is by far greater than that of primigravidæ.

These estimates are all somewhat general, but even if exact statistics could be gathered as to any one locality, they would not hold good in others—true of one region, they would not be so of another. Climate, habits of life, and morals of the community very greatly affect the completion and interruption of pregnancy.

IMPORTANCE.—Frequent as the occurrence of abortion is—common almost as childbirth—its importance is universally underrated. Many of the ills to which women are subject result directly or indirectly from this accident, or, we may justly say, from an undervaluation of its importance. If not criminal or traumatic, it is the result of pathological changes either in the maternal system, in the sexual organs, or in the ovum itself; labor is brought about amid these conditions at a time when neither ovum nor uterus is properly prepared, as in labor at term, and under these conditions, especially in a diseased system or diseased uterus involution will not so readily take place. Morbid conditions of the sexual organs follow, and affect the health of the patient more or less, though death but rarely results, either directly or indirectly. These evils are more commonly the consequence of mismanaged abortion and neglected after-treatment than of the accident itself; hence the result depends rather upon a thorough appreciation of the importance of this condition by both patient and physician, especially the general practitioner, the family physician; if assistance is sought, it is he who is called, and not the specialist—not the gynecologist or the obstetrician. It is the physician conversant with the family secrets whose aid is sought in this matter, which is considered by the mother rather as a delicate and disagreeable than an important affair.

Women should be given to understand more thoroughly the serious results which so often follow neglected abortion or abortions which, for the very reason of their being rapid and favorable in their course, are neglected as to after-treatment. Women must be impressed with the necessity of proper attention during the progress of miscarriage from its very initiation, and the even greater care that is necessary after the ovum is expelled and all is supposed to be over, and involution of the uterus at this period must be guided and guarded as after expulsion at term.

Much suffering would be avoided if women were taught to consider abortion as a disease, a pathological condition, demanding immediate and active attention, and not simply as a disagreeable and disgraceful accident, to be concealed if possible. The patient would then no longer endeavor to worry through without assistance or call in nurse or midwife; and, thoroughly knowing the possible dangers, they would be more cautious, and the frequency of criminal abortions would also decrease : these, above all, cause injury to health, because medical attendance is avoided if at all possible, and care likewise, as the patient is anxious to conceal her indisposition. Then also the practitioner must bear in mind the great importance of this accident, both that he may anticipate and prevent it, and if inaugurated he may guide it to a rapid and successful termination and guard his patient throughout the period of involution. Great temporary pain, and often lifelong suffering, will thus be prevented.

A thorough knowledge of abortion, of its causes, course, and treatment, is equally necessary to the physician, that he may guard his own honor and that of the profession : an abortion, due to uterine disease or malnutrition of the ovum, occurring during some period of medical attendance is often blamed upon the physician by those anxious for offspring, whilst, on the other hand, that large and shrewd class who are seeking to avoid childbirth not infrequently resort to the trick of urging certain methods of treatment during early pregnancy, with the hope that the physician himself may thus induce abortion, or he is called, with all appearance of innocence, by the criminal who has interrupted gestation to complete the abortion once commenced. His own reputation and that of his profession is then at stake : to guard this and to preserve the health of the mother entrusted to his care he must be conversant with the pathological conditions involved and the importance which attaches to them.

Woman requires skilled aid in labor, the physiological termination of pregnancy; more necessary still is this in the premature pathological interruption of this condition, in abortion ! The attendant is often responsible for two lives, as in labor, although under the conditions usually existing medical aid is not summoned until the life of the embryo is already destroyed—a most urgent argument in favor of timely medical advice and of close attention to prevention, a proper management of the pregnant state, and the treatment of threatening abortion, as at this time both lives may still be saved. This accident, so frequent in its occurrence, so disastrous to the health of woman, is important in all its phases, not only in the stage of expulsion and retention, to which attention has been directed on account of the surgical interest, but as well in its incipience, the time of prevention, and its after-treatment; abortion demands, and is worthy of, the most careful study and the best efforts of the physician.

HISTORY.—The history of abortion, it has often been stated, is the history of civilization, but I would rather say that it is the history of races —of their rise and fall. Abortion in consequence of natural causes, as well as criminal, is now, and has at all times been, practised among savage as well as civilized peoples, and develops with the progress of civilization, with the deterioration and fall of races, civilized and savage, as shown by history ancient and modern.

Abortion consequent upon natural causes is by far less frequent among a vigorous and healthy people still struggling for supremacy, full of youth and strength, than among nations who have reached the height of power, who have been enfeebled by indolence and the luxuries of civilization, by vice and fashion. Of criminal abortion this is naturally true to a far greater extent, yet this is common and customary among many primitive, semi-civilized peoples. As nations advance they become debilitated and demoralized amid the brilliancy and luxuriousness of their surroundings, and they rapidly retrograde toward the very worst vices of primitive humanity: they are thus undermined, and succumb to the attacks of their more vigorous neighbors, and magnificent empires are overthrown and extinguished by the youthful vigor of a hardy, simple people. The more civilization progresses, the greater the apparent abhorrence of the crime of abortion, the more numerous the laws enacted to guard against it, the more frequent does the crime become; and, strange though it may seem, it is nowhere punished. Abortionists everywhere are known; in the larger cities of this continent as well as Europe they achieve a widespread fame, are well known, and yet rarely if ever convicted. It is a notorious fact in our community that these worst of criminals almost invariably escape, and even in the states of Germany, where the laws are strict and rigidly enforced, where the crime of abortion is punished by imprisonment of from five to twenty years, that eminent teacher of medical jurisprudence, J. L. Casper, says that " Of all the many accused, never a one was condemned, and in no one case was the crime proven." They are sheltered by the words of the law and the sympathy of the community, which, notwithstanding the abhorrence expressed, still accompanies these criminals, though not to so great an extent as it does those equally forlorn women who are guilty of killing the child when born; for, as Hodge truly says, "There is no class of criminals who meet with so much sympathy as women guilty of fœticide." Greece and Rome when at the height of their power favored by their laws, and almost openly advocated, abortion, whilst among the ancient Germans it was one of the crimes most deeply despised and most severely punished—just as it was condemned by the laws of the Goths. How different is it now among the races sprung from these proud conquerors of Rome, now that they have reached the very acme of their career! The more civilized, the more powerful they become, the more does this crime develop, as in Germany and France, where it is practised upon a most extensive scale, and yet, as we have seen, the criminals escape, notwithstanding the most rigorous laws. Condemned from the bench and the pulpit, the crime still progresses. There is the poor girl who has yielded her honor for the sake of bread for herself or those dependent upon her; there is the lady of fashion, by far more culpable, who cannot give up the time she owes to society to the cares of maternity; or the society belle, who would resort to any and every measure that she may escape maternity for the sake of retaining her beauty and the freshness of her charms, a slender waist and a well-shaped breast; others resort to it that their round of pleasure may not be disturbed. Many an unborn child is executed upon the plea of limited resources, that the family cannot continue to live in their accustomed luxury if an additional member should appear.

Neither the laws of God nor man will affect the hearts of women thus brutalized: it is the physician alone who can interfere; it is to him they come most often; it is he, the trusted family friend, who will do more than judge or priest to change this unfortunate condition of affairs. In crowded countries abortion is looked upon as a necessity of nations, just as it is here considered a necessity in a family too numerous; hence in China, Japan, and Hindostan it is common; in Arabia and in New Caledonia it is produced on account of the scarcity of nourishment and the difficulty of raising children. Among some crude people it is not the wish of the individual, but the law of the land, which determines the course of gestation; so upon the island of Formosa a woman is not allowed to bear a child before her thirty-sixth year, and priestesses fulfil a social law by kicking the belly of the woman who becomes pregnant before the proper age, lest the population grow too large for the resources of the island. So it is among other islanders also—upon the Sandwich Islands, the South Sea Islands, whose population was reduced from two hundred thousand to seven or eight thousand in the course of thirty years. Upon Tahiti and King's Mills Islands it is equally common. Upon the latter a more generous feeling prevails, and the woman is at least allowed to have a family of three, but not beyond that; and upon the Feejee Islands one of every two conceptions is supposed to be destroyed before the period of gestation is completed.[1] So also among the New Zealanders, the Hottentots, and the inhabitants of Madagascar. By the Icelanders this crime is committed as an heirloom left by their Norwegian ancestors.

Not alone upon the islands, but among the inhabitants of states not overcrowded like China and Japan, abortion is legalized; so in Paraguay and La Plata, where it is caused in every family after the birth of two living children. Some of the African negroes produce abortion on account of limitation of resources; among the Buddhists, otherwise so humane in their laws, it is frequent—a wonderful disharmony between

---

[1] Trader. *Criminal Abortion.*

the conduct of individuals and the dictates of their political and religious laws.

Wherever celibacy is demanded crime and abortion result, as among the Buddhists, whose laws condemn large numbers of vigorous subjects to this existence; and in our own civilization we see the same inevitable result in many of the most closely-populated Catholic countries. Thus abortion is frequent among the Anamites and among the Kambysians, who marry late and are frequently obliged to produce abortion before the time of marriage. Among the Brahmans it is a common practice, induced by religious and political arrangements, the direct result of a law which encourages sexual excesses, and frequently of the restrictions placed upon the needs of woman (widows are condemned by law to eternal celibacy); yet this terrible crime is looked upon as most harmless by the people of India, the destruction of a child that has not seen day being, according to their view, less of an evil than the dishonor of a woman. In Turkey it is so common that a certain price is paid for abortion and another for infanticide, and the law is indulgent to the crime, as it can be paid for cheaply. The cost of removing a non-viable fœtus, or even an embryo, is equivalent to a tenth of the price paid for the murder of an infant.

The methods by which expulsion is accomplished are everywhere the same among people civilized and savage, ancient and modern—local and general. Among the local measures external violence is the most simple, as among the Tasmanians, who practise abortion by striking the belly, just as it is done by the priestesses of Formosa; and this is quite common in our day and in our communities. The introduction of instruments and implements into the womb is more intricate, but likewise common; the knitting-needle is a favorite resort in our country, and among primitive peoples a similar practice is resorted to; thus some of the negroes of Africa introduce the sprouting stem of a plant into the uterine cavity. Venesection, the drawing of blood from the vulva, anus, and foot, was often resorted to for the purpose of producing abortion.

Among the more common remedies used in former times are emetics, which are still very often resorted to, cantharides, emmenagogues, sabin, snake-root, and the famous pennyroyal; so also ergot; the compound cathartic pill of the United States Pharmacopœia is a favorite remedy,—all of which maim or kill the patient as often as they produce abortion. In New Caledonia a decoction of red-bud and banana-peel or green fruit is taken boiling: in China aperient medicines are publicly advertised for sale, and aphrodisiacs under the name of remedies to free the stomach and give back virginity. Certain negro tribes bring on abortion by manipulation of the abdomen and the use of purgative substances, such as the bark of the koche and sonnaly, which are also used to facilitate labor. Pen-tsae enumerates a large number of remedies as accelerators of abortion or purgatives according to the dose; many of them have a very doubtful action, however. The natives of India most commonly use the black annin, vulgarly called black anise or fourspice; fifteen grammes is an emmenagogue and larger doses produce abortion. The Arab women seek to produce sterility and escape the annoyance of numerous pregnancies, and imagine that they can arrive at that end by drinking a solution of sal soda, a decoction of peach-leaves, and the sap of the male fig tree.

Among peoples savage and civilized, for good reasons and bad, villains sufficient are found to do the bidding of thoughtless and misguided women; the remedies used, internal and external, local and general, are very often so violent as to be followed by the death of the victim. The plea of limited resources, of the inability of supporting a large family, is one common to people of all races in all stages of civilization: permitted by the unwritten law among some, it is practised with equal frequency by others, though strictly condemned. As we have stated, among many of the American nations it is legalized.

Again, there have been people at all times who have scorned the crime, but this is only among those pure, primitive, and still-developing peoples, as, for instance, the ancient Goths and Germans; and the Noxes of South America, as well as some of the negroes of Africa, even permit the husband without hesitation to kill his wife if she should abort. It is among those of the primitive peoples where the blessing of offspring is held in high esteem that the crime of abortion is most condemned and most rare. With the progress of civilization and religion, of refinement and knowledge, this crime, strange as it may seem, rapidly develops. It is not among the low and ignorant—it is among the educated and refined, among the wealthy—that it is most common; and the plea given in excuse of this crime is one most especially urged by the educated and refined, by the devout Christian, that the embryo is not an animated being, not an individual existence—that it does not attain the dignity of a living being until the time of quickening, until the middle of pregnancy. Religious and scientific reasoning is brought to bear in support of this theory in excuse of the many refined criminals; and it is this very point which the physician must urge: that the ovum, the embryo, from the moment of conception is an animated being, an individual existence with a life of its own. Important as the treatment of abortion, in consequence of natural causes, is, its prevention, and, above all, the prevention of criminal abortion, is still more so; and it is this which lies in the hands of the physician, whose most forcible argument must be in the evident and glaring crime which is committed by the destruction of a living being, as is the embryo from the moment of conception, not to forget the injury resulting to the mother. The former appeals to the moral, the latter to the physical, elements of womanly nature.

Whilst abortion, in consequence of natural causes, is a condition more dangerous than labor at term, the interruption of pregnancy by forcible means—criminal abortion—must necessarily be more grave in its consequences. The interference is often a violent one; the aborting woman is in mental distress, unable to seek the necessary comfort or attention; she is oppressed by the crime in her inner conscience; under unfavorable conditions, physical and mental, for the suffering which is most likely to follow.

With the progress in the practice of medical science the art of the abortionist keeps pace, and in civilized communities of to-day one cause of this growing frequency is in the increased numbers and the increased skill of practitioners ready to pander to all the whims of their degenerated customers; but the greater should be the efforts of honorable physicians to dispel the false illusions by which women seem to justify their doings, and to erase this darkest of all thoughts that lurks amid the noblest sentiments in woman's mind. A strong effort was made not long ago by the American Medical Association to urge the importance of this matter upon the profession, resulting from the earnest efforts of that honored obstetrician Hugh L. Hodge, which culminated in a report of the Committee on Criminal Abortion, read before the American Medical Association in 1871, and a number of papers written upon the subject at that time, prominent among which I would mention those of Van de Warker, Tabor Johnson, and John W. Trader. The wave has swept by: what has been accomplished may be gleaned from the police records of our cities.

PHYSIOLOGY OF EARLY PREGNANCY.—For an understanding of the pathological conditions which determine, precede, and accompany this accident a knowledge of the physiological state is as important as normal anatomy is to the pathologist. But as this subject is treated of in full in other articles, we will confine ourselves to a few of the leading features which are most important for purposes of diagnosis and treatment.

The changes, local and general, resulting from the physiological state of pregnancy are extremely variable, often approximating or simulating pathological conditions, so that we must differentiate and discriminate between such as pertain to the normal condition and such as indicate pathological changes and threatening danger. This is necessary, as prevention is, above all, important, it being often possible thus to save two lives with by far less danger and suffering to the mother than is to be expected from the treatment of abortion once inaugurated after the time of possible prevention has passed. Moreover, a correct post-abortum diagnosis is important for the future welfare of the patient, if not from a medico-legal point of view; and this is equally impossible without a knowledge of the physiological condition. This will enable us to determine whether the ovum expelled is healthy or not—whether the causes are traumatic or criminal, or whether the abortion is due to pathological changes; which, again, must guide us in treatment.

Abortion is the expulsion of an ovum the product of a conception, and can only occur during the period of menstrual life, as conception, the impregnation of the female ovule by the male semen, is the consequence of fruitful intercourse, liable to take place at any time during the period of womanhood, the thirty years of female menstrual life from puberty— the appearance of the catamenia—to the time of their cessation. Its occurrence is followed by intense physiological activity of the maternal organism, lasting throughout gestation to the time of its natural termination with the expulsion of the fully-developed ovum at term at the end of the tenth lunar month. This is made evident by striking changes in the entire system, but especially in the sexual organs, which in the earlier period of pregnancy are entirely progressive, developmental, whilst in the later months, toward term, the character is changed to that of a retrograde metamorphosis, preparatory to the separation and expulsion of the ovum and final restitution of the organs. This hyper-activity inaugurated by impregnation becomes evident by marked changes in the system of the mother, in the sexual organs, and in the ovum itself.

Changes in the Maternal System.—These are most peculiar and varied, differing in repeated pregnancies in the same patient, sometimes entirely absent, at others most distressing, even fatal; sometimes appearing at one period, sometimes at another. Healthy, robust women may suffer throughout the entire period of gestation, whilst those at other times ailing are well only in this condition. The most marked of these symptoms are the hystero-neuroses, disturbances of the entire nervous system, central and peripheral; mental depression, more rarely excitement; gastric disturbances, nausea and vomiting; increased activity, renal and pulmonary, consequent upon changes in the circulation; discoloration of the skin upon the forehead, the linea alba, and areola; œdema and varicosities of the veins upon the lower extremities. All these, and many others still more erratic, may accompany the normal physiological condition.

Changes in the Uterus and Pelvic Viscera.—Whilst the ovum develops in the uterus, this organ, its appendages, and the viscera surrounding it, enclosed together within the pelvic cavity, undergo the most marked changes. The early months of pregnancy are those of greatest physiological activity in the uterine muscle, the period of its hypertrophy. This is inaugurated from the very moment of conception, at first increasing, then gradually lessening, until within the last months, when it becomes passive, the rapidly-growing ovum merely distending the hypertrophied uterus, apparently increasing in size, but merely distended by its contents, as a rubber bag would be. In the earlier months the growth of the uterus is entirely due to muscular development—after the fifth month to distension. The individual muscular cells attain enormous growth, and a large number of pre-existing embryonic cells are developed; so also in the interlacing connective tissue. The blood-vessels as well as the lymphatics increase in size and length; the arteries become tortuous; the capillary circulation is to a great extent supplanted by sinuses.

Weighing in its normal condition, when at rest, little above an ounce, the uterus attains within the first four or five months a weight almost fifteen times greater. Remaining the first four months within the pelvic cavity, the increase in size is not of that diagnostic importance which it attains in the later months, when it is to be felt beneath the abdominal walls, though at the end of this period it is distinctly perceived above the symphysis; about the fifth month, between navel and symphysis; and at the sixth month, at the height of the navel. At the end of the third month the uterus is some 4½ to 5 inches in length, by 4 in breadth and 3 in thickness; at the end of the fourth month, 5½ to 6 inches in length, by 5 in breadth and 4 in thickness; at the end of the fifth month, 6 to 7 inches in length, 5½ in breadth, and 5 in thickness; at the end of the sixth month it is some 8 to 9 inches in length.

The changes which take place in the cervix are a merely passive accompaniment of the uterine hypertrophy, it being enlarged more especially by reason of the succulence of its tissues consequent upon the congestion and activity of the body. It is somewhat enlarged in all its dimensions, thickened, and elongated, soft, velvety to the touch, appearing, however, somewhat shortened by reason of the hypertrophy of the vaginal attachment—a condition that approximates rather that of the vagina and external sexual organs than that of the uterus, softened, succulent, somewhat hypertrophied, congested, of a deeper bluish-red wine color, its cavity occluded by thick tenacious mucus, as the secretions of the mucous membrane of the vagina and external sexual organs are also augmented. In the first and second months the uterus is retroverted. the cervix seems to descend as the enlarged organ, by reason of its weight, settles in the pelvis, the fundus sinking down in the hollow of the sacrum, the cervix consequently pointing more forward; as the organ increases in size and rises above the brim in its endeavor to escape the confining space of the pelvic cavity, the enlarged fundus, meeting with the resistance of the promontory, seeks the point of least resistance, and the uterus begins to . assume that position of anteversion which continues to become more marked as pregnancy progresses: the cervix points backward into the hollow of the sacrum, and rises gradually (as the fundus increases in size and withdraws from the pelvic cavity).

The Uterine Mucosa.—This structure is as interesting as it is important. The wonderful changes which it undergoes go hand in hand with the various changes and stages of female life: it is the nidus for the reception of the impregnated ovum; it serves to shelter and nourish the delicate ovum, and if diseased, affording insufficient nutrition, leads to the death and expulsion of the embryo. Its shreds when expelled are of diagnostic importance, and in early abortions its massive thick tissues, changed by disease, often cause greater trouble than the ovum itself, forming, alone or with the membranes proper of the ovum, what is so commonly but erroneously called the placenta in abortion. The membrane which lines the cavity proper of the uterus, passing at the internal os into the mucous membrane of the cervical canal, is characterized by the absence of even the slightest trace of submucous or areolar tissue—by its peculiar substratum of connective tissue abounding in cells and tubular glands. It is closely and inseparably attached to the muscular coat. In a state of rest it is a little over 0.04 inch in thickness at the fundus,[1] and the anterior and posterior walls diminishing toward the sides, the cervical and tuber ostea. It is traversed by a series of tubular glands, wavy in their upper part, bifurcated toward their base, running more or less parallel to each other. In this membrane, so important for the preservation and development of the ovum, the physiological activity of the system is inaugurated, and seems to centre during the first week of gestation. With the impregnation of the ovule the uterine mucosa, its earliest shelter, begins to hypertrophy: the rapid development which now takes place is owing to the proliferation of the cells of the stroma and the enlargement of the individual cells of all kinds, including those of the glands themselves, as well as the increase of the succulent homogeneous and cellular substance. The glands throughout their greatest extent are enlarged: the increase in thickness is more especially due to the hypertrophy of the superficial layer, the upper half, in which the stroma appears less compact, growing far above the original gland-openings, circumvallating the enlarged ostea, and thus causing those funnel-shaped depressions which give the membrane its sieve-like, cribriform appearance when seen from above. In the third month of pregnancy the mucous membrane attains its greatest thickness, forming a soft succulent lining to the uterine cavity, by its distension closing the various ostea. It is then as much as 0.236 inch in thickness in the anterior and posterior walls, lessening toward the ostea, and begins to present the characteristic layers which become so distinct in the later months—a dense upper and a very loose lower one, comparable to a lax meshwork. Its growth now ceases,

[1] Engelmann *Mucous Membranes of the Uterus.*

and as the uterine cavity increases in size and the ovum in growth, it is distended to cover the rapidly-expanding surface, and becomes thinner and thinner, the upper dense layer remaining as such, whilst the glandular sinuses of the lower layer of the membrane are stretched transversely until they become mere flat meshes like a network stretched along the surface of the womb.

The impregnated ovum, as it rapidly enlarges during the first two or three weeks, becomes imbedded in the thickened succulent decidua: and we may compare this to the sinking of a bullet into soft dough: the soft mass of the dough yields to the weight of the superimposed body, and gradually closes over it, so the tissue of these overlapping folds soon unites, completely surrounding the ovum, the nidus thus formed, in which the ovum settles, being usually in the upper portion of the fundus upon the posterior wall of the right side. We now distinguish in the mucous membrane of the uterus three parts: the decidua vera, the greater part of the membrane lining the cavity of the womb where it is not in contact with the ovum; the decidua serotina, which is that part directly beneath the ovum, between it and the uterine wall, which is in connection with the tufts of the chorion, later in part develops to form the placenta; and the decidua reflexa, that part of the mucosa which overlaps and has overgrown the ovum. This membrane is little known and rarely recognized, though always present. It is of no practical importance; a delicate membrane even at the time when it is the great safeguard of the tender ovum, serving to protect it and hold it within the soft bed formed by the decidua serotina; this function of the reflexa continues until the third month, when the ovum has developed sufficiently to occupy the entire uterine cavity and is everywhere in contact with its walls. The thin tissues of the reflexa become more transparent and delicate as they are distended and compressed between ovum and decidua vera, which now with the muscular wall of the uterus surround the ovum and continue the previous function of the reflexa.

The Development of the Ovum.—Practically, we may distinguish two periods in the development of the ovum: the first, that in which we are here interested, before the development of the placenta, where it is a cyst-like body surrounded by the shaggy chorion, the chorion velosum; and after the development of the placenta, after the fourth or fifth month, when the fœtus is more fully developed and the ovum is covered with the smooth chorion, the chorion levæ.

The period scientifically the first, and the most interesting stage of development, during the first three or four weeks, when segmentation takes place and the form is moulded, we shall in no way consider. The ovum may then be cast off, perhaps at a succeeding monthly period, unbeknown to any one, perhaps not even to the unconscious mother: certainly the services of an accoucheur are not called for. In the third or fourth week it is a delicate cyst-like body of the size of a hazel-nut, some half an inch in diameter, surrounded by its translucent chorion, and is crushed in the passages or disappears amid the clots of blood of an apparently profuse menstrual flow. The following periods of development are, however, of practical importance, as they will serve diagnostic purposes, as well as an understanding of the appearance of the ovum and the symptoms accompanying miscarriage.

The ovum during the first months of pregnancy is an oval cyst-like body surrounded by the chorion, the shaggy tufts of which give it a cha racteristic readily-recognized appearance. Enclosed within is the delicate transparent amnion, and the embryo, attached to the navel-string, floating in the clear liquor. At six weeks the size of the ovum is likened to that of a pigeon's egg; at eight or nine weeks to that of a hen's egg, perhaps 1½ inches in length; at the twelfth week, to that of a goose-egg, some 4 inches in length. In the second month the ovum forms a bulging prominence in the uterine cavity, usually toward the fundus, and reveals all the parts recognized at term with the exception of the placenta and the still distinct umbilical vesicle: its surface is covered by the tufts of the chorion and surrounded by the decidua reflexa. In the third month it is so far developed as to completely occupy the uterine cavity, as yet but slightly adherent, approximated, a part of it agglutinated to the uterine mucosa, to the decidua serotina, the greater mass of the chorion being in no way adherent to the surrounding reflexa. The tufts of the chorion begin to sprout and develop more fully at its point of contact with the uterine wall above the decidua serotina, whilst upon the remaining and greater portion of its surface their growth ceases, and as the membrane distends the delicate filaments gradually disappear. At the end of the third month, in the fourth month, the tufts of the chorion have sufficiently developed in its adherent portion to form the rudimentary placenta, and at the end of the fourth month this is developed still more— has become more dense and large, whilst the remaining portion of the membrane appears smooth and barely shows a few scanty remnants of the once-shaggy tufts.

The growth of the ovum now rapidly outstrips that of the uterine cavity; the membranes are pressed more firmly against its walls, approximated to the decidua vera, but not by any means agglutinated. In the sixth month the placenta has been thoroughly formed—it has become dense and large, the foetal membranes beginning to agglutinate to the uterine wall, and the conditions existing at term are rapidly approached. The embryonic tissues are supplied with the necessary nutriment by endosmosis from the surrounding maternal structures during the first months; the entire surface of the chorion absorbs, whilst this function is delegated to the proliferating villi as they develop and agglutinate with the decidua serotina, foreshadowing the activity of the placenta by which the foetus is nourished to term.

Practically, the most important period in the development of the ovum is the one most dangerous to its existence—in the third and fourth month, that period of intense activity o' chorion and decidua, the time of the formation of the placenta, when hemorrhage is likely to occur from the congestion of the vessels so necessary to the nutrition of the rapidly-growing and delicate tissues. Nutriment is no longer merely absorbed by the succulent embryonic cells of the ovum from the tissue in which they are in contact, but the embryo is forced to seek sustenance through those now fully-developed tufts of the chorion—from the proper site, the decidua serotina and the surrounding vessels—directly from the uterine structures. If hemorrhage interferes or disease prevails, the healthy growth of the ovum is checked, and a morbid development ensues, to result sooner or later in death of the embryo and expulsion.

The embryo in the early months of pregnancy is small as compared to the size of the sac, the membranes, liquor amnii, and navel-string; at the end of the fourth week the embryo measures from $\frac{1}{3}$ to $\frac{1}{4}$ of an inch in length; at the end of the eighth week, from $\frac{3}{4}$ to 1 inch: the arms and legs become visible, the umbilical vesicle, though reduced in size, still exists; the small body with large upper extremity is pendent from the short, thick navel-string. At the end of the twelfth week the embryo measures from 2 to 3 inches in length; fingers and toes can be distinctly seen; mouth and nose are also recognizable. At the end of the sixteenth week, the fourth month, the embryo measures some 4 to 5 inches in length; sex can be distinguished; the head assumes shape, but it is still immense in size, perhaps an inch in length; the features of the face are all formed. At the end of the twentieth week, the fifth month, there is no longer doubt as to sex; the nails, which were previously visible, have become distinct; the soft, woolly lanugo begins to develop; hair may be noticed upon the head; motion, inaugurated weeks before, is felt by the mother. Toward the end of the sixth month, in the twenty-fourth week, the embryo is some 12 inches in length. As has been before stated, with the cessation of the development of individual organs and parts growth in size becomes more rapid. As this was less in the earlier months, it is now very marked. With the seventh month, as the fœtus becomes viable, it is some 12 to 14 inches in length, weighing 2 to 3 pounds; the body is covered with lanugo; the hair on the head becomes quite marked; the papular membrane disappears.

It is well to bear in mind the leading features in the development of the uterus, decidua, and the ovum, and more particularly its membranes, as a guide in the treatment, that we may recognize the parts expelled and know what remains to be removed—as an aid in diagnosis, that we may properly judge the conditions, whether healthy or morbid, and post-abortum, when we may be forced to determine by the corpus delicti, as the all-important evidence in criminal cases, as to the duration of pregnancy and the causes which led to its termination.

ETIOLOGY.—Causes of Abortion.—Interesting as the etiology of disease is to the inquiring mind, to the progressive physician it is of great practical importance as well; and this is eminently true of the causes leading to abortion. More so of (A) spontaneous or accidental abortion, though by no means to be neglected in (B) criminal abortion. Etiology is important in both, as it is a knowledge of cause alone which can lead to prevention, that most valuable of all methods of treatment, and in criminal abortion to detection, thus indirectly to the prevention of recurrence.

A. Accidental or Spontaneous Abortion, or Abortion as the Result of Natural Causes.—The etiology of non-criminal abortion is indispensable to the practitioner, as it is this alone which will enable him to prevent its occurrence and recurrence, thus leading to the preservation of the lives of mother and child, doing away with the danger and suffering of actual treatment, and frequently serving as a guide in the latter. We will meet with some difficulties in our endeavor to analyze these causes, as they are so varied in their nature and differ so greatly in the medium through which they act. There are causes predisposing and exciting, local and general, internal and external, and causes which depend upon father, mother, and ovum. The direct dependence of treatment upon the exciting causes seems to necessitate a simple and practical delineation of the etiology of abortion. A direct reference of the cause to the offending organ is understood most readily, and will point most directly to the necessary measure of relief; hence we will consider such causes as spring from or act through mother and child—more properly, the maternal system and its individual organs on the one hand, and the ovum and its parts upon the other. We cannot, however, pass by these without giving a thought to such causes to which great importance is attached by many, and which it is best to consider separately.

Predisposing Causes.—Almost all abnormal conditions, whether pertaining to the system or external to it, are more or less predisposing causes, whilst direct exciting causes are few; they may or may not be followed by the premature interruption of gestation; they tend to death and expulsion of the ovum, making it likely to occur whenever the exciting cause arises. We may say all those by which the occurrence of abortion is favored are predisposing causes : they are conditions under which we may expect its occurrence; and, knowing them, it is the duty of the physician to guard his patient. The classification is indefinite. Thus Naegele considers as predisposing causes anæmia, congestion local and general of the maternal system, neurotic influences; and as exciting causes—1st, those which tend to sever the amnion from the surrounding uterine structures; 2d, those which cause malnutrition, disease, and death of the embryo or fœtus; 3d, those which directly arouse uterine contraction. Others consider diseases acute and chronic on the part of the mother, local and general, as well as diseases on the part of the father, predisposing causes, whilst traumatism and neurotic influences are considered as exciting causes. All are classifications based upon no strict foundation. I wish, however, to call attention to certain conditions which I look upon as predisposing to abortion : that is, a pregnant woman while under the influence of such condition, such cause, is more liable to abort upon the occurrence of some directly exciting cause. The existence of one or more predisposing causes does not necessitate abortion; pregnancy may continue without interruption if exposed to any of the conditions which we will term as exciting causes.

First. Climate.—We find abortion, both accidental and criminal, prevalent in certain countries and in certain districts, dependent upon climate —in the deltas and valleys subject to malaria, upon barren soil where food is wanting or where the work of woman is particularly laborious.

Secondly. Number and character of the population : this mishap is most common in large cities, where morals are lax, where the ill-fed poor are crowded into tenement-houses and the rich live in the whirl of social dissipation, or in thickly-settled regions where there is an intermingling of sexes, where women are neglected and ill-fed. I may here add an observation which truly shows the difference of locality. Both Playfair and Philippeaux[1] claim that abortion is especially prevalent in the country. This may be true of the rural districts of England, France, and Germany, especially the latter military government, where it is in the country that young, able-bodied women do the hardest and most of the work, as is seen when passing through these regions in harvest-time. In

---

[1] *Annals Gynécologie,* 1881.

America the very opposite is true, as in the country here abortion is most rare.

Third. Certain periods in woman's life eminently predispose to abortion. There are those important epochs in woman's life during which her nervous system undergoes a severe strain wrought by those changes which are all-important to her existence. These are, first, in early married life, when intense hyperæsthesia exists due to changes wrought in the sexual system : the young wife is, moreover, exposed to injurious external influences, certain forms of traumatism; and secondly, toward the approach of the menopause, as the activity of sexual function and the uterine organ diminishes and the nervous system is undergoing those changes with periods of intense neurotic excitement which accompany the menopause. Finally, we may look upon the morbid conditions of the system, all unfavorable changes in the surroundings, as predisposing causes.

Exciting Causes.—We have seen that Naegele considers malnutrition and all causes which lead to separation of the ovum from its surroundings, and even uterine contractions, as exciting causes, whilst Spiegelborg considers hemorrhage so much so that to him the history of hemorrhage during gestation is the history of abortion. As exciting causes I consider uterine contractions and such conditions as directly lead to hemorrhage in the uterine or fœtal membranes; but I cannot class either as exciting causes direct and primarily, both being merely sequents dependent upon some more remote cause. The varied importance of predisposing and exciting causes will be best appreciated if we but recollect the ordeals which a healthy woman may undergo—the direct exciting causes which may act upon her—and yet abortion not occur, provided no predisposing causes exist. Thus we have the well-authenticated statement of a pregnant woman being run over, the wheels of a physician's carriage passing directly over the abdomen, and yet abortion not following. I myself know of the attempts of a husband to produce abortion upon a willing wife by beating the abdomen, finally stamping and sitting down upon it, and yet not succeeding. I have the statement of a reliable physician as to the continuation of intra-uterine application of iodine and astringents to the cavity of a uterus supposed to be diseased, which proved to be pregnant, until the fourth month, and yet abortion not following. We know how women with criminal intent produce local injuries, even such as result in death, whilst the ovum remains undisturbed. These are cases in which no predisposing cause existed. On the other hand, the careless washing of the feet in cold water, a single effort at the wash-tub, a rapid drive, fright, a piece of bad news, coitus, the slightest nervous or physical disturbance, may produce abortion where predisposing cause sufficient does exist. We will here classify the exciting causes of abortion, in reference to the consequent treatment and the possibility of prevention, as maternal and fœtal, dependent upon, acting by means of, the maternal system and organs or those of the ovum. Those dependent upon the mother are amenable to preventive treatment; not so those dependent upon the ovum.

A. Causes of spontaneous or non-criminal abortion :

1. Causes due to pathological changes in the maternal system, general and local. These are by far most important to the practitioner, as they

are amenable to treatment.   His attention should most especially be
directed to—

a. General causes acting through the system.   These are—

(1) Diseases acute and chronic;

(2) Causes acting through the nervous system, neurotic;

(3) Physical or traumatic;

And (4) I shall classify what I might term social causes, such as
result from custom and fashion, which form an important element in
the etiology of abortion, and one more particularly open to and demanding prevention.

b. Local causes on the part of the uterus and its adnexa.

2. Causes on the part of the ovum.

1. Causes Maternal.—These may be general or local.   General causes,
arising either in the maternal system or exterior to it, but acting upon it,
may be either physical or nervous, arising from diseased morbid conditions of the maternal system.

a. General causes acting through or resulting from changes within the
maternal system.

The premature interruption of pregnancy may frequently be traced to
disturbance of the maternal system or external influences which act upon
it, either directly by traumatism or indirectly through the nervous system, and the uterus, hypersensitive in this state of intense physiological
activity, responds.   It is the point of least resistance to which the shock
is conducted : as the electric current invariably passes through the best
conductor in a network of wires to the point of greatest attraction, so
shock follows the course of the uterine nerves, at the time most tense,
and the explosion follows in that organ.

(1) Disease, acute and chronic, on the part of mother and father
interferes with the nutrition and development of the ovum—on the part
of the father, through the semen ; on the part of the mother, by malnutrition of the growing germ.

Acute Diseases.—A vitiated condition of the blood, as well as the
increase of temperature, local and general, which accompanies constitutional disturbance, affects nutrition and development of the ovum.
Zymotic infectious diseases, as well as those accompanied by congestion
of the pelvic viscera, are most liable to affect gestation : the excessively
high temperature of the nutrient fluid and of the surrounding viscera, if
not direct infection of the germ, leads to death of the embryo and consequent abortion in the course of zymotic disease.   The localization of the
morbid affection in the vicinity of the uterus affects the existence of the
embryo by reason of the consequent congestion and irritation, as well as
by depletion of the system, as in dysentery ; direct infection, as in variola
or scarlatina.   This delicate existence is threatened in various ways by
traumatic injury, as may occur in eclampsia.   Fortunately, abortion in
the course of disease is not the rule, but the exception, and usually accompanies morbid conditions of the system only if most intense or if predisposing causes exist ; yet gestation is at all periods endangered by intercurrent disease in the early as well as the later stages.   It is in the later
stages only that the existence of direct infection can be determined, and,
though perhaps not common, well-authenticated cases are recorded : I
have myself delivered a mother, just recovering from a severe case of

variola, of a seventh-month fœtus covered with a typical eruption. That abortion occurs in the course of malarial fever is well known in the valleys and deltas of our great rivers, and it has been most erroneously ascribed by some to the energetic medication which is called for. If the disease attacks pregnant women, its continuance, but not the medication, may lead to abortion : it is not quinine given upon correct indications—it is the existing disease—which causes the accident, and must hence be checked as speedily as possible ; it is the uterus which shelters the developing ovum, congested, hyperæsthetic, which is at the time the centre of physiological activity, and, we may say, the most sensitive portion of the body, most easily affected by an accidentally existing disease, as the non-pregnant woman, one more sensitive or feeble, always suffers most during an accidentally existing disease in that organ which is habitually most sensitive or weak or at the time under an unusual strain; if throat, lungs, or heart is weakened, it is that part which suffers most in the acme of malarial fever ; if a woman is exposed to cold during the menstrual period, the pelvic viscera will respond most readily.

Chronic diseases affect growth and development of the ovum by reason of malnutrition, local and general anæmia. As has before been stated, the impregnation of even a healthy ovule by diseased semen or the semen of a diseased father may result in morbid development, which sooner or later ends in expulsion of the affected ovum. Of the diseases on the part of the father it is more especially—and I may say almost alone—syphilis which exerts a direct influence upon the ovum. Debility of the system is more likely to result in sterility, whilst the ovum, if impregnation takes place by such semen, remains healthy though feeble, and the traces are indelibly marked upon the offspring. The use of liquor, like the morphine habit, may lead to sterility, but not to abortion ; though the offspring of a phthisical father rarely escapes, the disease is inherited, but does not develop during the early stages of gestation, and does not affect the ovum in its growth.

Chronic diseases on the part of the mother would seem as if readily leading to abortion, though the result is comparatively a rare one. The diseased, badly-nourished, often anæmic system offers an unfavorable nidus for the rapidly-developing ovum, which is so much in need of healthy and abundant nutrition ; but as the feeble, sickly mother often has an abundance of healthy milk for the new-born child, a healthy physiological activity seeming to exist in those parts in the time of functional activity, so may the ovum find a sufficiency whilst other parts are affected. The intense activity existing in the uterus attracts an abundance of the circulating fluid ; women low with chronic diseases, phthisis, or cancerous growths, often in the last stages, will bear children, yet they are fortunately not so free to conceive, and if impregnation does occur the healthy growth of the ovum is soon interrupted.

The causes which lead to an enfeebled condition of the system may lead to abortion, whether it be an anæmia, the result of disease or lack of food, of the mode of life, or the locality in which the sufferer lives—of poisonous gases or poisons of other kinds slowly admitted to the system. These poisons, however, whether acute or chronic in the mother, may directly affect the fœtus. Lead and noxious gases, like the infection of variola or smallpox, are examples of the latter ; more rapidly-acting poisons, like strychnia, opium, carbonic oxide gas, and syphilis, of the former.

Death of the fœtus and abortion may result as a consequence of syphilis on the part of either father or mother, or of primary infection during gestation, and are liable to occur at the same period in successive pregnancies; if in the later stages of gestation, the ovum, especially the fœtus, bears its characteristic marks. The effects of treatment and improvement are readily visible: abortion is more and more delayed; if the afflicted parent but slowly improves, abortion will occur at a later period during each subsequent gestation until a fœtus is carried to term, but still-born—the next living, perhaps, for a brief period. If vigorous treatment be applied in the early stages, abortion may cease altogether. The results of disease can be more readily seen in the fœtus than in other parts of the ovum. The gummata of the placenta, the syphilitic indurations, are difficult to distinguish from other conditions, and appear only at later stages. The syphilitic pemphigus, when occurring upon the fœtus, is characteristic, but the mucous membranes are most liable to show its traces. The gummata in the large viscera are frequent, especially in the lungs and liver; but most typical is the osteo-myelitis in the long bones, between epiphysis and diaphysis, a pale-red line in the earlier stages, resulting in a thickening of the parts at later periods.

(2) Causes acting through the Nervous System.—During pregnancy, that stage of intense uterine activity, of gestation and increased growth, we find an increased nervous excitability, motor and vaso-motor, the nerves responding violently to slight causes which would arouse no reaction during the normal condition. There is an increased reflex activity which may lead to a disturbance in the circulation or in the nutrition of the ovum, or to uterine contraction upon some slight excitement. This condition varies exceedingly, the causes which excite these reactions and the extent of the reaction excited differing greatly in degree. Uterine hemorrhage, contractions, and expulsion of the ovum in consequence of neurotic influences are more likely by far to occur during the existence of predisposing causes. Fright, a nervous shock of any kind which in no way affects healthy gestation in a healthy woman, will result in abortion in a person afflicted with uterine disease or in a system otherwise weakened.

The frequent occurrence of abortion in early married life and toward the menopause is mainly referable to nervous influences. Marriage is a period in woman's life comparable to puberty and the menopause—a period of heightened nervous excitability: a change takes place in all the modes of life, and, in addition to the many other causes which at that time unite to interfere with conception, increased nervous excitability is one of the most important, as it is toward the climacterium. We shall consider this period more particularly under the head of Social Causes. As the change of life is approached, the activity of the sexual organs, their nutrition, the blood-supply, and especially the healthy activity of the mucous membrane, are lessened, and hence the growth of the ovum is endangered; but the condition of the nervous system at this period certainly has an equally powerful influence in producing the tendency to abortion. During this hyperæsthesia an existing predisposing cause or some slight additional excitement will arouse the vigorous action of the tensely-strung vaso-motor nerves; coitus even at these periods may be looked upon as dangerous to continued gestation. It is not alone the traumatic influences which must be considered, but the effect upon the nervous system as well, especially the vaso-motor nerves, in the state of intense excitement which accompanies the sexual orgasm. During these periods of increased nervous tension during pregnancy coition is more liable to produce abortion than at other times. It is in the coming together of numerous causes that one more intense than the others, though harmless alone, will be followed by sudden response.

Much has been said as to the injurious effect of coition during pregnancy. Those who look to physical causes as mainly tending to abortion claim the injurious effect to be purely physical, traumatic; whilst others, and I believe more justly, claim that the influence is strictly neurotic. Parvin says that coition is so frequent a cause that he blames upon this half the cases which are termed spontaneous abortions; certainly it has a most unfortunate effect, so that we frequently see the expulsion of a healthy ovum from the second to the fourth month in young women recently married, mainly in the higher walks of life and among delicately organized women, who are more intensely sensitive to the great change which they have undergone. I have repeatedly had occasion to see these unfortunate cases, and almost look for the occurrence of an abortion within the first six or eight months after marriage in the bride of fashionable society. Though the statement of Parvin may seem somewhat forcible, the fact is not to be ignored : the ovum expelled in such an abortion gives evidence of being of healthy growth, so that the cause must not be sought for in malnutrition or local disease. The laws of many peoples are as strict in regard to coition during pregnancy as they are about the care of menstruating women : by some it is forbidden; among the ancient Mexicans it was regulated, it being ordained that sexual intercourse should be exercised to a moderate extent during pregnancy in order that the healthy development might be furthered and strength given to the child. The injurious effect of coition is everywhere acknowledged, and, I can say, not unjustly. Total abstinence was looked upon by the Mexicans and other peoples as likewise harmful.

The changes wrought in the nervous and physical condition of women after marriage and toward the menopause are such that the menstrual periodicity is interfered with, dysmenorrhœa sometimes existing, at times menorrhagia, so that the expulsion of an ovum of from eight to ten weeks is ignored, passing away with the clots of a profuse menstrual flow : it is often not even known to the mother, being considered by herself and family as merely a profuse flow; the accompanying pains are often no greater than those of the dysmenorrhœa common at such times; no precautions are taken, and thus the foundation is often laid for uterine disease.

We know that the emotions—fright, fear, joy—may check the menstrual flow or produce menorrhagia; in the gravid uterus hemorrhage may be caused or contractions aroused, and abortion results. In a misled girl or a young married woman the fear of pregnancy may frequently cause cessation of the menstrual flow : the effect of the mind and nervous system upon these organs is equally evident in the cessation of the menses when pregnancy is longed for, though it does not exist : I have even known of the summoning of midwife and physician by an aged bride with distended abdomen (gastric hystero-neurosis) who longed for pregnancy and thought she felt uterine contraction and the inauguration of labor. As the emotions affect the general health, the ovum may likewise suffer as a part of the maternal system; but when they are sudden, such as by fright or shock, the effect upon the vaso-motor centres by reflex action is so forcible that the uterine vessels are paralyzed, dilated, and hemorrhage follows; or a tetanic contraction of the vessels may result, and then the nutrition of the embryo is checked.

The evil effect of nursing during pregnancy is due in part to the withdrawal of nutrition from the ovum, but in part to the contraction of the uterus and its vessels, which may result as a reflex symptom from the irritation of the nipples, and thus cause abortion. The frequent occurrence of abortion upon ships at sea is due in part to traumatic influence, the vomiting of sea-sickness; in part it is neurotic, due to the changed mode of life, the leaving of a home by the emigrant for foreign lands, just as the menstrual flow is stopped for months and months in the immigrant girl upon her first arrival in a strange country.

(3) Traumatic influences are comparatively rare as a cause of natural spontaneous abortion; and it is true of these as of every other cause that it depends upon existing conditions whether abortion will result or not. The pounding of the belly is an ordinary method of producing abortion among primitive peoples: a fall, a jump from a wagon, may disturb the progress of gestation, while traumatism far more violent may not affect it, as in the case of the woman in the later months of pregnancy over whose abdomen the wheels of a physician's carriage passed without causing any injury whatever.

In the earlier months, while the ovum is still sheltered in the pelvic cavity, injuries are still less liable to cause abortion. I have myself seen a pregnant woman severely bruised about the lower bowels and go to term. I have been told by reliable physicians that local treatment of uterine disease has been continued by reason of the non-cessation of the menses to the third and fourth month, when pregnancy was discovered, and yet abortion did not follow, though I regret to say that quite a number of cases have come to my knowledge where the treatment of supposed uterine disease, especially of uterine tumor—pregnancy in fact—was suddenly terminated by the appearance of the corpus delicti, a four or five months' embryo. The intensity of the resistance is well illustrated in a case which it was my good fortune to see in consultation, where the most brutal local treatment had been resorted to for three or four months and abortion did not occur; the patient had left her persecutor and travelled hundreds of miles to seek treatment. The manipulations had been so violent as to produce metritis and cellulitis, yet the growth of the ovum continued, as demonstrated by the healthy fœtus of five months which was at last expelled. I have but recently examined a lady who has been treated locally for uterine disease, and found her in the beginning of the third month of pregnancy, so far undisturbed.

We may well place the uterine sound and applicator among the traumatic causes. The physician himself, especially the gynecologist, has been sought out by women to aid in relieving them from the product of conception, and it is through sound or applicator that he is expected to accomplish the work. Among the many devices to which women—and, I am sorry to say, those in the most fortunate circumstances, in the best walks of life—resort to attain this end is one which certainly shows knowledge and shrewd calculation, but most villainous intent, which is not unfrequently practised, and against which it is well for the physician to be on his guard. It is that of forcing the attendant to uterine examination and treatment upon the plea of disease, well knowing that the germ must thus be destroyed. The woman calls upon a physician—in preference upon some specialist not attending in her family—upon the plea of uterine suffering, well knowing, either from personal experience or the gossip so common among ladies, some of the more common symptoms of this disease—backache, pains in the side, nervousness, weakness, menstrual suffering. She relates her case; upon questioning states that the period is just passed; and, though the examination may reveal nothing, though no application may be made, she well knows the uterine sound will be used. That is what she desires. If an application of iodine or nitrate of silver follows, all the better. Though for reasons far more important the physician should listen to the history of a patient with distrust, and rely most thoroughly upon his own examination, this course is especially indicated in gynecological cases without distinct sign of disease; and these very cases again point to the importance of a careful bimanual examination, and a resort to all other methods before the sound is used; and that in case of an enlargement of the uterus, discoloration of the cervix and vagina, we should under no circumstances introduce an instrument into the cavity unless it is established with absolute certainty that the congestion and increased size are due to pathological and not physiological causes.

Social Causes.—I wish to call attention more particularly to some of the abuses of modern life which not unfrequently interfere with gestation. These exist among all classes of society, high and low: among the poor they are unfortunately forced; among the wealthy they are the result of devotion to fashion and society. As we have seen that in the Old World abortion is common in the rural districts, it is an evidence of hard labor, especially in the field, at the wash-tub, and labor by which the abdomen is compressed, the abdominal muscles freely exercised. It is not only physical labor, but exposure to cold and wet, cold feet, which are to blame; in those more fortunately situated tight lacing, dancing, and consequent colds have a like injurious influence.

I would again allude to the newly-married, who are so subject to the lighter forms of traumatism, the always greater frequency of coition, the congestion and mechanical insult, the bridal trip being especially injurious. During this period of hyperæsthesia it is too great a strain upon the body as well as upon the nervous system: the young husband, unacquainted with woman's strength and needs, is always liable to judge her powers by his own. Railroad travel, the fatigues of sight-seeing, pleasures, theatre, and the dance, are all borne by the patient bride, anxious to please the groom: upon returning home the cares of the new house, excessive social duties, all combine to undermine the strength of a delicate woman in her first gestation. Enfeebled, often depressed by reason of gestation or nervous changes, excessive pleasures are forced upon her by reason of her condition—i. e, bride—and abortion follows; and, we may say, follows in consequence of traumatism. In other walks of life we find other conditions, still with the same unfortunate developments— excessive labor and pleasure during this period, when rest and care are so necessary. It is in young married women partly the pleasures of society, partly the unaccustomed duties imposed, which lead to injury. Ignorant of their condition, ignorant of the care necessary, even when aware of injury unwilling to acknowledge it, desiring to bear up, to show no weakness, they lay the foundation of much future suffering. The cause of so much uterine and pelvic disease in the unmarried, in the society girl, exists to the same extent in the newly-married, only that the injuries caused are far greater in the first period of married life, as the strain both of body and mind is increased in this most susceptible condition.

Local Causes.—Though the local causes on the part of the mother which lead to abortion, diseases of the uterus, especially of its mucous membrane, are equally frequent and equally amenable to treatment, they are of less practical interest to the general practitioner. Diseases of the uterus itself are not so important etiologically as those of its lining membrane: uterine tumors, unless of enormous size, usually admit of the completion of gestation; flexions and versions rarely interfere with the development of the ovum; a prolapsed uterus may bear the fœtus to term unless the adhesions are unyielding and impregnation is impossible, because the uterus as it develops with the growth of the ovum rises beyond the confines of the pelvic cavity, and the displacement is thus remedied. Anteflexions and anteversions are always rectified; retroversions in rare cases only lead to abortion; adherent retroflexions are most to be dreaded; when the uterine body, bound down to the pelvic floor, expands within the cavity to such a size as to make escape through the brim impossible, abortion must necessarily follow. Deep lacerations of the cervix make conception improbable and interfere with gestation; cervical catarrh in no way affects its progress. Those morbid conditions of the uterine tissues which are unaccompanied by disease of its mucous membrane rarely lead to abortion.

Uterine contractions due to reflex nervous excitability are perhaps the most common of all these causes, yet here the uterus primarily is not at fault. A state of intense excitability is very often due to general causes, to intense febrile action, to congestion or anæmia; high or low temperature, whether due to external or internal causes, and irritation of the surrounding parts,—all of which conditions tend to increased contractility. Such diseases of the uterus as cause induration of the walls may lead to abortion, like the incarceration of the organ in the pelvic cavity, by reason of prevented distension.

Uterine Mucosa, Decidua.—Of far greater consequence than the conditions existing in the muscular tissue of the uterine wall upon the vitality and development of the ovum are those of the uterine mucosa in its state of physiological hypertrophy as the decidua of pregnancy. This soft, succulent tissue, rich in lymphatics and blood-vessels, is the nidus in which the ovum rests, its immediate protecting shelter, and the source from which nutrition is derived; hence morbid changes of this structure react promptly and forcibly upon the ovum — most so in the earliest stages, when it is altogether dependent upon this structure; less so as gestation progresses. As the ovum grows it becomes more resistant, its tissues more dense, and the source of nourishment is gradually changed to the large uterine sinuses at the placental site. Moreover, the decidua after the third and fourth month, when it has served its term, performed its function, gradually diminishes in thickness, until toward•term retrograde metamorphosis is initiated preparatory to the expulsion of this structure, at that time merely forming a line of demarcation in the lax meshwork in its lower layer between the healthy tissue which remains and those structures which are passed off in labor. An inactivity of the mucous membrane, an imperfect development of the deciduous structure due to disease of the mucosa, is a frequent source of abortion. In chronic disease of the uterus or its lining membrane this rapid and healthy development of the decidua after conception is prevented, the delicate membranes of the ovum do not absorb the necessary nutrition, the development of the embryo is checked, morbid conditions of the ovum follow, and abortion results, especially at that time of active development, the period of placental formation. The decidua vera is the least important part of this structure, serving nutritive purposes only in the very first weeks at the site of placental formation, and sheltering the delicate ovum in the nest formed by its soft tissue : it is the decidua serotina, and especially that membrane which holds the ovum in place, the decidua reflexa, which claims attention. But morbid conditions of the vera, the greater part of the mucous membrane, are naturally accompanied by imperfect development of serotina and reflexa, and hence the imperfect imbedding and nutrition of the ovum.

Hypertrophy or excessive morbid development of the decidua may accompany acute infectious diseases, as we find similar conditions in other organs of the body, especially in the larger viscera. These changes, morbid in their character, interfere with development as do the atrophic forms. These hypertrophies may, however, exist independent in their nature, due to local disease of the uterus and its parts, as in chronic endometritis, where in place of the succulent deciduous structure we find an induration and a proliferation of the active tissue usually throughout the entire membrane, rarely localized, of a polypoid form : the chronic catarrhal affections are accompanied by an increase of secretion, morbid in character, which is liable to interfere with the development of the germ. Moreover, hemorrhage more readily occurs under these pathological conditions, usually secondary in character, brought about by minor insults, trivial causes, which would not affect healthy tissues. These hemorrhages, all-important in the early stages, affect development less and less as gestation advances, the importance of the decidua lessening and its functions being superseded. Where a slight extravasation of blood within the deciduous structure may lead to separation and expulsion of the ovum in the first and second months, larger hemorrhages are often without consequence when occurring within the same tissues in the fifth or sixth.

2. The Ovum.—Pathological changes of the ovum itself, of the embryo, of the surrounding membranes are less frequent as primary causes of abortion, and they are of less importance to the practitioner as being in no way amenable to treatment. When they do occur they usually lead to expulsion in the earlier months.

Those conditions liable to lead to abortion are especially diseases of the chorion, placenta, and umbilical cord, rarely of the amnion, the embryo itself, or the amniotic fluid.

Chorion and Placenta.—The chorion being the nutritive organ, supplying the means of communication between mother and child in the earlier stages by the villi over its entire surface, later by the placenta, must necessarily determine the progress or cessation of fœtal development by the conditions existing within its own tissues. One of the most striking and notable changes to which it is subject is the hydatiform degeneration of the villi, leading to a formation of the grape mole or hydatiform mole. This is a cystic degeneration of the terminal sprouts, an hypertrophy of the germinal tissue, the young connective-tissue cells, which usually begins at a very early stage: the vascular development is interfered with, the nutritive material is directed to the morbid activity of the chorion, which in its exuberant growth, usually inaugurated in the first weeks, destroys that of the other structures; the delicate tissues of the embryo are soon absorbed, and even the amniotic sac may disappear, the within-lying cavity, which always remains in every malformation as an unmistakable trace of the ovum—a characteristic which serves at once to mark the product of conception. A mole of this kind usually attains the size of an apple, but may grow to that of a child's head, and the period to which it is carried is much longer than that of the mola carnosa—usually five to seven months, sometimes eight or ten. The appearance is that of a conglomeration of cysts, usually the size of a currant or gooseberry, though they are often from that of a pinhead upward, connected everywhere by thin connective-tissue strands; they consist of a delicate transparent membrane enclosing a pale, colorless fluid: in the earlier stages the amnion with its cavity remains, but with the development of the growth that is destroyed, and the appearance of the hydatiform mole as a product of conception even becomes unrecognizable when no longer surrounded by the decidua; as in cases of excessive development, the morbidly-enlarged villi may even break through the decidua vera in their growth, and we find a dense mass consisting of a conglomerate of small cysts united by connective-tissue shreds enclosed in the cavity of the uterus.

Hemorrhage.—In the third or fourth month, at the time of most active development of the villi at the placental site, primary hemorrhage may occur, due to the active vascular development, and thus lead to abortion, but this is rare; frequent as hemorrhage is, it is almost invariably to be traced to some cause.

The Placenta.—In later stages, when the greater part of the chorion appears as a more firm, non-vascular membrane, that part which in connection with the decidua serotina is developed to the placental formation is the most vulnerable point, as it is the connecting link between the fœtus and the maternal tissues, and the one source of nutrition. Hemorrhage in this structure, whether in its maternal or fœtal portion, if excessive, must lead to a cessation of development, to abortion. Slight hemorrhages, such as must have proved fatal in the earlier stages, no longer interfere with the growth of the ovum, but are absorbed or remain as small hemorrhagic spots, the tufts or cotyledons in which they have occurred appearing as a hard whitish mass of connective tissue. If the hemorrhage is more profuse or widespread, it may lead to abortion directly or to inanition—to death of the fœtus, and secondarily to abortion. Inflammation may occur throughout the entire placental site or localized, as in all other points in the connective tissue of the structure, accompanied by vascular development in the first place, followed by induration and shrinkage; frequently remaining as small irregular or conical indurations between the villi or cotyledons, leading to abortion, either by the tendency to hemorrhage thereby excited or the death of the fœtus if sufficient of the tissue is destroyed to cause inanition.

Fatty degeneration occasionally results in consequence of insufficient nutrition due to hemorrhage, or after death of the fœtus preparatory to premature expulsion—a morbid approximation to the condition upon its maternal surface and in the decidua serotina at term.

Syphilis.—The changes in the chorion and placental tissue accompanying syphilitic disease are rarely the direct cause of abortion or premature expulsion of the ovum ; as a rule, they are mere local manifestations of the morbid condition existing in all the fœtal structures, and frequently in those of the mother. In the early months, during the period of the chorion frondosum, abortion results from insufficiency of the nutriment absorbed by the indurated villi of the chorion, lacking in vascularity and in succulent embryonic tissue; the structures are more dense, the villi hypertrophied, in the more aggravated cases the vessels entirely obliterated, whilst after the formation of the placenta in later months the existence of syphilis is made evident by appearances similar to those which accompany other chronic inflammatory conditions. The appearance presented by a syphilitic placenta is usually that of cellular hypertrophy, the centre in a state of whitish induration or fatty degeneration according to the stage of the disease. But it is hardly possible to diagnose syphilis with certainty from the appearance of the placenta alone, nor is the placenta usually affected to such an extent as to appear as the prime cause of fœtal death. The placenta is usually large as compared to the size of the child, in appearance similar to other inflammatory conditions presented by the placenta, the growth of the fœtus being interfered with, whilst that of the placental structure continues until the retrograde metamorphosis is sufficient to result in expulsion. The placenta in a syphilitic fœtus is larger than ordinary, 1 to 4, whilst usually 1 to 6. Gummata are rare, so also tumors of the placenta. A myxoma developing from the embryonic tissue is occasionally found. If the fœtal portion of the placenta alone is affected, or in the earlier stages the chorion and the decidua healthy, we may with safety infer syphilis on the part of the father alone previous to impregnation.

The Amnion.—The amnion, which serves merely as a container for the preserving fluid, is wanting in vascularity, and consequently but little subject to morbid changes. The only pathological condition which we find in this structure is an inflammatory development, the formation of amniotic bands stretching across this delicate sheath or from some portion of it to the fœtus, crippling or cutting its membranes in such a way as to interfere with gestation. Nor does an abundance or want of amniotic fluid affect the development of the embryo or ovum during the earlier stages. It is no more a cause of abortion than the slight changes occasionally found in the amnion itself.

The Umbilical Cord.—The navel-string, however—the sheath stretching from amnion to fœtus, enclosing the umbilical vessels—is subject to quite a number of changes, frequently the cause of abortion, occasionally mere results of other complications. Excessive or insufficient length of the cord, which may seriously complicate labor at term, in no way affects the development of the ovum; in the third or fourth month the length of the cord is naturally much greater than that of the embryo, and the resulting coils and knots seem in no way to endanger its existence. Knotting of the navel-string may lead to death of the fœtus, but only in the last months, rarely at earlier periods. Stenosis of one or the other of the vessels sometimes occurs, leading to the death of the embryo and consequent abortion: a condition which I have found remarkably frequent is that of torsion of a very long and thin cord in the third and fourth months; but this torsion of the cord seems so frequent in abortion that it must appear as a consequence, movement of the dead fœtus apparently leading to a twisting during inactivity of the tissue. A very striking condition of the cord has frequently attracted my attention—lack of embryonic tissue, the gelatin of Wharton, with excessive torsion; the cord flat, thin, in parts threadlike, and usually very much twisted; the embryo retarded in development as compared to the size of the ovum, no other cause being at the same time discernible, neither disease of the uterus nor affection of the system. The torsion is secondary, often wanting, the cord being very thin and thread-like in places, consisting of the amniotic sheath and the vessels, obliterated entirely or in part. Torsion I believe to be secondary, as I have noticed these excessively twisted cords otherwise healthy in cases of abortion; but this peculiar state, which I cannot term otherwise than atrophy of the cord, appears as a frequent primary cause of abortion in the second to the fourth month; torsion and knots may occur at later periods. Ruge of Berlin,[1] who has investigated this subject, thinks that stenosis of the cord in the vicinity of the umbilical insertion is rarely the primary cause of abortion, though often a secondary, resulting from motion and traction on the inactive, dead vessels; whilst Leopold seems to look upon it as the primary cause.

I have endeavored to call attention to the various conditions which may lead to abortion, but it is almost impossible to place an estimate upon their relative importance. Whilst uterine contractions, hemorrhage, and abortion may result in one case from a slight nervous excitement, a trifling annoyance, the most violent nervous irritation will in no way affect another; whilst a fall, a jump from a buggy, may lead to a mishap in one patient, the crushing of the abdomen beneath its wheels will not affect another; a trifling fever may appear as the cause in one, and again the most severe pneumonia or typhoid condition will not impair development in another; the child may be carried to term by a mother in the last stages of consumption, whilst a very trifling affection may lead to abortion at other times. So it is with remedies taken internally, though as a rule they have but little effect: a violent aperient may cause abortion, and again, as in one instance which I recall, a woman in the fourth month of pregnancy died rapidly of dysentery resulting from the taking of cathartic pills to produce abortion, and the post-mortem revealed a perfectly healthy ovum in a healthy uterus, whilst the dysentery consequent upon the remedy killed the mother. The careful introduction of a sound into the gravid uterus has led to a separation of the ovum, to hemorrhage,

---

[1] *Zeitschrift für Gynäcol. u. Geburtsh.*, vol. i. 1, p. 57.

and to abortion, whilst a knitting-needle has been passed into the uterine cavity and through the womb, causing the death of the criminal mother, without in any way disturbing the ovum. The uterus has been regularly treated for supposed disease for three and five months by internal applications, and gestation has progressed. So it is with all these cases: at one time, especially with pre-existing disposition, a slight interference may result in the cessation of development, and at another the most violent insults in no way disturb gestation.

B. Causes of Criminal Abortion.—The causes proper of criminal abortion are immorality among all classes, high and low—among the wealthy fashion, the pleasures of society, and the desire to limit the number of children—a common cause, strange to say, mostly among those very people who can actually afford the expense. The cause direct, the means by which the crime is accomplished, should be known to the practitioner in order that he may detect the deception which is so frequently practised upon him—that he may prevent it if possible, and at least not, by reason of ignorance, be made particeps criminis.

The means resorted to are either external or internal, traumatic and instrumental, or by medication.

Traumatic.—When produced by the patient herself it is either by violent exercise, running up and down stairs, walking and dancing, occasionally by pressure upon the abdomen or by the use of the knitting-needle, catheter, or similar instrument. The more expert or daring only attempt to enter the uterine cavity, as the organ itself may be pierced; if the catheter is successfully introduced, the attachment of the ovum is severed, and with the knitting-needle the sac is punctured.

These attempts are usually made in the second or third month at the second or third missed period. There is, however, a class of experts among the most elegant who have attained such remarkable dexterity as invariably to introduce the instrument successfully into the uterine cavity; and these are in the habit of regularly practising this dangerous experiment when the first days of the expected period have passed without the coming of the flow.

The abortionist either injects fluid into the uterus or introduces a probe or catheter into the cavity. Customs vary in different countries; so Van de Warker states that in France puncture of the membranes is fashionable, whilst here a syringe or sound is used.

Among the most common—and perhaps most harmless—means is the hot foot- and hip-bath, the "sitz-bath," often with the addition of mustard: this, as well as the steaming of the parts by sitting over a chamber filled with hot chamomile tea, is the first step taken by the nervous wife when the menstrual flow has failed to appear sharp on time and she still lives in hopes that it is but a cold which has interfered with the regularity of its return. Even physicians, respectable men in good practice, who may not venture upon bolder measures and wish to keep their conscience clear, are known to advocate this course, though they well know what such a cold means.

Medication is perhaps more commonly attempted, but less successfully, notwithstanding the injuries caused to the system. To follow Van de Warker's thorough study, the remedies used are mainly of two classes—those which act directly, the emmenagogues, oxytoxics, and reflex abortifacients. Notwithstanding the firm popular belief in their efficiency, they are less harmful to the ovum than to the system of the mother, and, as Van de Warker says, there is more science and skill used than is generally supposed in the various pills and teas, which are less simple, but no less common, than the foot-baths and the gin-bottle. Ergot is almost sure to be called upon to perform its office. Its action is very uncertain, but if persistently used is readily recognized by its effect upon the vascular and nervous system—uterine or ovarian pains and depressed action of the heart where in spontaneous abortion an acceleration is to be expected; the temperature is lowered, and the sphygmograph shows a remarkably flattened apex with an almost senile pulse. Cotton-root is also commonly used, especially in the South, and is marked by its narcotic action.

Among those termed reflex abortifacients, acting more indirectly by their effect upon surrounding organs, we may notice cathartics, principal among them aloes, which, notwithstanding its purgative action, does not appear to deplete the circulation, but, on the contrary, results in pelvic congestion ; but even its excessive use need not in any way affect gestation. I have seen a patient dying amid the resulting dysenteric symptoms, frequent, scanty, and bloody evacuations, accompanied by excessive tenesmus, inflammatory conditions, and abdominal pain, though the uterus did not react and the ovum remained intact. The odor of the drug is imparted, it is said, so intensely to the evacuations that it is unmistakably noticed.

Juniper and black hellebore, the latter especially endangering the life of the patient, are both toxic in their effects. The painful fluid evacuations, accompanied by bearing down, tenderness of the abdomen, pain and sickness at the stomach, dry throat, would characterize the former; the odor the latter, as well as the flushed appearance of the face, with heaviness and pain in the head and frequent micturition. But one of the first and most common remedies to which the desperate woman resorts when she finds a day of the menstrual period passing by without the appearance of the flow is tansy, which seems to act by reason of the uterine congestion which it causes. Though undoubtedly effective at times, it will, like all other drugs thus used, more often cause injury, and even the death of the mother, without disturbing gestation. " Disturbance of the nervous system, profuse salivation, immobility and dilatation of the pupils, and severe strangury," are noted as the symptoms of such poisoning. Hardly less popular is the still more dangerous cantharides.

The female pills and various mixtures more or less openly sold by druggists are, according to the researches of Van de Warker, composed of one or more of the above-mentioned ingredients, and the immense quantities disposed of show how truly abortion is called the crime of the period. Knowledge of the remedies used for these purposes will aid the physician in arriving at a correct diagnosis and enable him to save the child and guard his patient.

PATHOLOGY AND MORBID ANATOMY.—I have endeavored to describe with some accuracy the appearance of the healthy ovum, the sac, and surrounding structures during the various periods of early pregnancy, as it is the comparison with these which will enable the practitioner to distinguish between spontaneous and criminal abortion, enable him to determine the duration of pregnancy, guide him as to the cause, and thus serve to facilitate treatment and perhaps to prevent recurrence. Knowing what has been expelled, whether it is ovum and decidua entire or only in part, the line of action is evident. In all abortions due to an immediate and active exciting cause, whether criminal or resulting from shock or accidental trauma, the ovum is healthy, normal in all its parts, size and development of the embryo corresponding to the period of pregnancy at which the accident occurred; whilst in spontaneous abortions due to accidental causes more or less marked changes exist: the development of the embryo especially is retarded; its life has been destroyed, and growth has ceased, whilst the morbid development of the membranes continues, so that the mass expelled presents more or less of a mole formation—comparatively solid, with thick walls formed by the fœtal membranes infiltrated with blood, the cavity often compressed by the surrounding extravasation, the embryo comparatively small or disintegrated in whole or in part.

The ovum is usually separated in its upper portion by hemorrhage, which comes from that point at which the vessels are most fully developed, the future placental site, though still agglutinated. With the inauguration of uterine contractions separation takes place at its lower pole by dilatation of the os, and retraction of the uterine walls from the ovum proper surrounded by the reflexa; as the abortion progresses, the muscular fibres of the fundus force it down into the dilating cervix through the still partially adherent decidua, and the intact ovum is expelled, the inverted decidua following it as the membranes do the placenta in labor at term. Yet these conditions vary greatly with the existing morbid changes.

In traumatic or criminal abortion the perfectly-formed ovum, the delicate cystic body surrounded by its shaggy chorion, is first expelled, to be followed by the decidua, usually—when in a healthy state—first by its anterior and then by its posterior half; whilst if the abortion has been inaugurated by some slowly-acting cause the decidua is hardened, infiltrated with compressed and clotted blood, the small ovum forming merely a part of the solid mass; and thus a firm oval body, coated with blood upon its rough, irregular exterior, appears.

Up to the third month the ovum is, as a rule, expelled as a whole, often even in the fourth. Later, unless decided pathological changes have taken place, the membranes are mostly ruptured and the embryo separately expelled, as in labor at term. In later months this is always the case, and the progress of abortion is greatly impaired by the adherent tissues: the mass of the ovum, which serves so much to excite uterine contractions and promote expulsion, is destroyed by the collapse of the amniotic sac, and separation and expulsion of the membranes are hindered by reason of the smaller amount of resistance offered. Hemorrhage is most likely to occur in the villi of the chorion, between its tissues and the surrounding decidua; if occurring in the latter structure, it appears thick, hard, infiltrated with blood, and no longer presents that soft, succulent appearance, but is firm and brittle.

The ovum as expelled presents three typical forms: First, as above stated, in accidentally-occurring traumatic or criminal abortion we find a healthy ovum with its shaggy chorion, and the inverted decidua attached or soon following, usually in two sections; most common, however, and almost without exception in spontaneous non-criminal abortion, is the mole formation, rarely the hydatiform mole, which has been described, and results only from the peculiar pathological condition of the chorion. The common form is the flesh mole, the mola carnosa, characteristic in appearance, resembling a polypoid growth, a reddish oval or rather pyriform mass with shreds of tissue (the decidua) adherent to its larger upper extremity, darker clots at the elongated lower pole. Upon section the walls show a brittle reddish structure, that of compressed and inspissated coagula, and in the centre a cavity containing fluid and detritus, if not the embryo, lined with a delicate membrane, amnion or amnion and chorion : the shape of the cavity is rather irregular by reason of the bulging protuberances formed by the contraction of the inspissated mass of blood extravasated between or within the tissues. These moles have very much the appearance of uterine polypi, and are often considered as such by physicians who pride themselves greatly upon curing their patients of tumors and the accompanying hemorrhage by a few doses of ergot. Though the macroscopic resemblance is such as to be quite deceptive, the mole upon section will always reveal a cavity, even if very small, containing fluid ; and this cavity reveals the above-described characteristic slight bulging protuberances lined with a delicate membrane ; whilst the microscopic examination shows the firm walls to consist of nothing but blood-corpuscles : the outer covering, often thoroughly infiltrated with blood, consists of the decidua serotina and reflexa, with more or less of the infiltrated shreds of the vera usually pendent from its upper extremity ; when floated in water and cleansed, the outer or uterine surface of these shreds is ragged, rough, often appearing somewhat like the villi of the chorion, hence looked upon as placenta ; this peculiar appearance is caused by the torn tissue in the line of demarcation in the lower or central meshy layer of the decidua vera, where it is separated from the lowest layer which remains adherent to the uterine wall. The inner surface toward the ovum will show a slightly wavy, cribriform appearance, the openings of the ducts appearing as fine depressions in the surface. (It must be remembered that this smooth inner surface is in the expelled specimen generally the outer one, as the decidua follows the ovum mostly as the membranes do the placenta at term—inverted.) If the disturbance causing the abortion has been of rapid progress, the cavity is large, the embryo approximating in development the period of expulsion ; whilst if the changes have taken place slowly, the walls are thick, the cavity small, and the embryo may appear merely as a small mass pendent from the navel-string, or may have entirely disappeared, and can be traced only by the fine detritus in the amniotic fluid, the cord itself perhaps only in part remaining, and even this may have disappeared. The cavity will always be found toward the pendent pole of the decidua reflexa, as the extravasation takes place mainly in the serotina, giving it the appearance of a thick mass of clotted, compressed blood, and forcing the cavity toward the opposite extremity. These moles are usually more elongated and pyriform, one or two inches in diameter at their upper or larger extremity, three or four inches in length, with a greatly elongated and narrowed lower end, which has been so formed by being first wedged into the slowly-distending cervix.

Such is the appearance in those cases of slow progress in which death of the embryo has probably occurred at an early stage and hemorrhage has been the exciting factor, whether due to disease of the mother or other causes that may have destroyed the vitality of the germ. When resulting from disease of the mucous membrane, especially endometritis or catarrhal affections, it is a more oval tough mass, the main part of which is formed by the thickened and indurated vera; and if this be opened the ovum, in a very early stage of development, will be found within.

The uterus itself presents very much the appearance of the organ after labor; the external os, however, closes more rapidly, less rarely showing the funnel-shaped appearance of the puerperium; the cervix, though somewhat enlarged, is normal in appearance; the cavity is lined by the lower layer of the decidua, soft shreds covered with coagula; but it is lacking in the placental site and the putrid thrombi visible in labor at term.

Involution is slow if we take into consideration the slight distension of the uterus as compared to the process after delivery at term. The organ is in a state of healthy development, not prepared for the following retrograde metamorphosis, unless the expulsion of the ovum has been due to local disease, when some retrograde changes may have been inaugurated; if it results from constitutional causes, the existing depression naturally interferes with restitution. If shreds of tissue, parts of ovum, or decidua remain, absorption or expulsion is retarded. As a morbid or atonic condition so often exists, at least in abortion consequent upon natural causes, subinvolution or inflammatory conditions of the organ itself or the surrounding tissues are hence a frequent sequence.

SYMPTOMATOLOGY.—It will be remembered that abortion is more likely to occur among multigravidæ on account of the greater frequency of disease, especially pelvic affections; that it is most likely to accompany the periodic congestion which recurs at the time of expected menstruation; that it is more frequent in early married life, on account of the greater liability to traumatic injury and the existing nervous disturbance, and toward the menopause in that state of nervous and physical disturbance and lessening uterine activity. The third or fourth month of gestation is the dangerous period, as it is one of change of nutrition for the ovum, of the highest development of the decidua, and intense activity and congestion of the chorion, the rapidly-sprouting vessels finding but little resistance in the embryonic structures of the villi which surround them. Chronic disease of the mother is more likely to interfere with gestation at a later period; and, when knowingly undertaken with criminal intent, the time of choice is either the first month, when the first indications of pregnancy become evident and the menstrual period does not appear at the usual time, or more commonly at the time for reappearance of the third menstrual flow, when the fact of conception has been established to a certainty, and the conscious mother, firm in the belief of the nonviability of the embryo before the fourth month, thinks it harmless to rid herself of the ovum, which she considers a mere growth without life or soul, while she would shrink from destroying what, at a later period, she calls a living being.

SYMPTOMS AND COURSE OF ABORTION.—General Remarks: Preliminary Symptoms.—1. Course of early abortion, first two months.

2. Abortion at the time most common, the third or fourth month: *a*, spontaneous; *b*, criminal and traumatic.

3. Later abortion—in the fifth and sixth months—and hydatiform mole.

The expulsion of the ovum during all periods of pregnancy is characterized by two inevitable symptoms—hemorrhage and pain. It is the time of appearance as well as the relative intensity of these symptoms by which the period of gestation at which the expulsion takes place is at once indicated. In early abortion the hemorrhage is excessive and precedes the pain, the pain being comparatively slight; in labor at term pain is the prominent symptom and precedes the comparatively slight hemorrhage, which does not appear until the pain has almost ceased, and labor is completed after the expulsion of the placenta. Expulsion of the ovum in intervening periods is marked by an approximation of symptoms, though the existing conditions which characterize individual cases greatly modify this typical course.

I have, for the sake of conveniently grouping the symptoms, accepted three periods which serve well to characterize the course which abortion is wont to take in the progressive months of pregnancy. Hemorrhage and pain are the never-failing symptoms—hemorrhage due to the separation of the membranes; pain in the earlier months is due to the dilatation of the rigid, unprepared cervix, which greatly preponderates over the pain which accompanies the expulsion of the comparatively small mass through the once-dilated passage. In the later months, the cervix being gradually prepared, the pain is almost altogether due to the increased effort which is necessary to expel the large mass of the ovum.

1. Early Abortion.—In the first and second months the ovum is small, the vascular development trifling; the decidua preponderates, being greatest in mass and in extent of its vessels; hence this is the most important part. The hemorrhage is considerable, due to the separation of the vascular and hypertrophied mucous membrane, the decidua. The ovum is very small and expelled with comparatively slight pain, the symptoms often resembling those of membranous dysmenorrhœa; no great dilatation of the os is even necessary.

2. In the third and fourth month, the period at which abortion both spontaneous and criminal is most common, the placental formation is inaugurated by the growth of the vascular tufts of the chorion; and it is now that the ovum in toto—or we may perhaps say the membranes, as they are by far the greater part of the ovum—assumes the most important rôle. The abortion is still inaugurated by hemorrhage due to the separation of the vessels, but the pain is greater, as the cervix must dilate more to admit the passage of this larger mass, and an expulsive effort as well is necessary to force the mass out. The greatest amount of pain is caused by the dilatation of the rigid, unyielding cervix, which fortunately remains in this undilatable state until after the period of viability of the fœtus, and serves to a great extent as a check upon its more frequent expulsion.

3. Late Abortions.—Now the ovum and fœtus are of pre-eminent importance; though the parts are still unprepared, hemorrhage continues to be the preliminary symptom, yet pain follows rapidly upon the inaugural flow, because the ovum is now so large that it cannot descend without dilatation: it must have advanced before abortion can progress to any extent, and the expulsive pains assume greater prominence on account of

the increased size of the ovum; the symptoms of labor at term are approximated, and, as the placental formation is developed in the sixth month, pains may at times precede, certainly rapidly follow upon, the preliminary hemorrhage. It is now the placenta which plays the most important part, as in labor at term it is the fœtus which is all-determining, upon which all the efforts of expulsion are centred; the membranes, amnion and chorion, are secondary, and the decidua, which was so important a feature in the first months, has by this time entirely disappeared as a factor in the act. The remaining shreds are partially adherent to the ovum, and in part passed slowly off with the lochial flow. Thus we see how the symptoms, at extreme periods so varying, approximate and interlace, and the various organs gradually yield in importance to newly-developing structures.

In the first period, then, the decidua is all-important, whilst the small and yielding ovum causes but little disturbance, not to mention the embryo. In the second period the membranes of the ovum are more important, and together form what is most erroneously termed the placenta in abortion. Then, as the placenta develops, this with the membranes predominates; finally, in labor at term the decidua, first all-important, has vanished as a factor of consequence, and the embryo, in the first stage a minimum, assumes such dimensions as to concentrate upon itself every effort of the obstetrician.

Pain, especially in the earlier months, is liable to be more excessive in primigravidæ, as the external os is closed, the cervix rigid, the time necessary for the expulsion of the ovum greater. In multigravidæ, with ordinarily more yielding and relaxed cervical tissues, the effort of the uterine muscle is concentrated upon the expulsion of the ovum from the cavity proper; and when it once passes the internal os a path is opened, and little or no force but that of gravity is often necessary to complete expulsion, whilst the cervical canal and external os offer formidable opposition in primigravidæ to the forcing out of the ovum, even though it has passed the os internum. A wide range of varying conditions naturally exists, due to the very different states of the cervical tissues: they may be relaxed in primigravidæ or firm and unyielding in multigravidæ, though the opposite is true in typical cases.

PRELIMINARY SYMPTOMS.—The symptoms which accompany death of the embryo and precede the expulsion of the ovum develop with the growth of the latter and its encroachment upon the cervix; although they vary as strikingly as do the symptoms of pregnancy, yet we may say that the larger the ovum, the greater the fœtal and placental circulation, the more marked must be the effect of their cessation; the larger the uterus and ovum, the more distinct this feeling of fulness, of pelvic dragging, which accompanies the descent of the gravid organ previous to expulsion of the ovum. The larger the ovum, the more distinct the pains which accompany beginning separation, the more the encroachment upon the cervix, the greater the dilatation which gives rise to the earlier symptoms. These symptoms, however, vary so greatly, and are so often altogether wanting, that they are hardly to be considered, especially during the period in which abortions are by far the most common, in the third and fourth month; and as, in all but traumatic and criminal abortions, the disappearance of such symptoms of pregnancy as have existed is indicative of coming abortion, the death of embryo and ovum often precedes expulsion for a considerable period of time, and the symptoms of pregnancy consequently cease. Symptoms of pelvic congestion, bearing-down pains, pressure upon rectum and bladder, are among those frequently preceding abortion. At times we see a rigor, feverishness, rapid pulse, nervous disturbances, lack of appetite, anæmia, fulness of the head, also palpitation, cold extremities, heavy, uneasy feeling at the pubes and coccyx, lumbar pains, and vesical tenesmus—symptoms which are all unusual, with the exception of the latter. The descent of the enlarged and congested uterus in the pelvis, which always precedes the expulsion of any body from its cavity, frequently causes dragging pains in the pelvis, a fulness, heaviness with pressure upon the bladder and rectum, and an uneasiness at the pubes and coccyx or lumbar and vesical tenesmus. Later, the death of the ovum and fœtus will cause more striking symptoms; the cessation of pregnancy will be more marked in mammary changes, but reliable symptoms are rare at all times, and usually wanting in the earlier months.

SYMPTOMS OF ABORTION.—Early abortion is frequently ignored, the symptoms greatly resembling those of profuse and painful menstruation. The course of abortion is inaugurated by hemorrhage, occasionally ceasing: sometimes there is very little pain: again it is quite severe; but the period of expulsion is well characterized; when completed the pain ceases, and with it the hemorrhage. Often the ovum is passed without the knowledge of the mother, even when accompanied by pain, as it is at this time more like that of a dysmenorrhœa.

Abortion in the Third and Fourth Month.—Spontaneous, Non-criminal Abortion.—At this period the ovum usually passes en masse; occasionally, and more often as the fifth month is approached, the membranes are ruptured in the course of its expulsion.

Normal Course.—We have already delineated the normal course of abortion at this period. The death of the embryo has usually preceded, often for weeks, and is characterized by the feeling of pelvic congestion, gastric and vesical irritation, weariness, weakness, and increase of uterine and vaginal secretion; the membranes have developed more or less; expulsion is inaugurated by hemorrhage. If the cause be more violent, the flow of blood is free. Usually there is but a slight oozing, which ceases at times, but gradually increases; the suffering which accompanies uterine contraction is present. Separation of the decidua and dilatation of the cervix are indicated by pain, which is intensified in case of uterine disease, so often present as the cause of abortion: the ovum is expelled as a pyriform mass, its apex imbedded in clotted blood, the inverted decidua adherent to its larger upper pole. If hemorrhage has taken place in the decidua, or the abortion be due to disease of this membrane, it is the most prominent feature and envelops the expelled ovum like a rigid mantle. In traumatic abortion it usually follows; ordinarily the membrane in part or in shreds is expelled with or very soon after the ovum.

Traumatic and Criminal Abortion.—Traumatic, especially criminal, instrumental, abortion varies in its symptoms, so well characterized by Van de Warker, from the spontaneous occurrence. The latter is inaugurated by hemorrhage; constitutional symptoms are wanting, and if they occur usually follow upon injudicious interference. In the former constitutional disturbances are present from the first; so also pains with inflammatory symptoms, mostly in the hypogastric region, abdominal tenderness : the pains of dilatation may even precede hemorrhage, whilst in spontaneous abortion they follow, often after days. The pulse is accelerated from 100 to 120 as a result of the primary insult; tenderness of the sensitive and congested uterus and cervix is rarely wanting; it is, in fact, characterized by Van de Warker as the one almost invariable symptom; vaginal hyperæsthesia, heat, and tenderness of the os are natural results. We have no history of previous accidental or spontaneous abortion: preliminary symptoms are wanting; the occurrence, on the contrary, is inaugurated by violence and shock; constitutional disturbance and hemorrhage follow. The consequences also are liable to be more severe, in accordance with the insults offered.

Recurring Abortion.—Morbid conditions, which interfere with the development of the ovum and lead to abortion, tend greatly to produce similar results if conception again takes place; hence we not infrequently find the repeated occurrence of abortion in a patient once afflicted; and this was formerly looked upon as a habit and known as habitual abortion—a term which must yield to the more correct repeated or recurring abortion, as no such habit exists: it is the continuance of the same cause which brings about a recurrence of the accident in repeated pregnancies. The cause being the same, the results are similar : the abortion will recur at about the same period if conception again take place; if due to a disease of the uterine mucosa, an early interruption is to be expected. The death of the fœtus is usually the indirect cause of the abortion, and always precedes it: in these cases, in most instances, it is due to syphilis; at times to other cachectic conditions of the mother or an affection of the uterus or its mucosa. The development of the ovum continues for some time until abortion takes place, and this occurs, if due to changes in the mucosa or decidua, in the first months; if the result of anæmia or cachectic conditions of the mother, of syphilis, in the sixth or seventh month, or toward term. The death of the embryo is followed by retrograde metamorphosis, thrombosis of placental or uterine vessels, and expulsion from one to three weeks later.[1]

Plethora as well as anæmia may cause this occurrence; thus Campbell relates a case of seventeen successive abortions occurring in an extremely plethoric person, who was finally enabled to bear a child to term by repeated venesections made monthly; and others record cases of a similar nature: lack of nutrition, anæmic conditions, brought about a remarkable increase in the number of abortions during the siege of Paris and in the succeeding year of want. Chronic endometritis with cystic formations has been repeatedly recognized as leading to recurring abortion; so also laceration of the cervix in case conception does take place. The continuation of the same cause should lead to its recognition, as in most cases it is amenable to treatment; syphilis, inflammation of the endometrium, and laceration of the cervix, among the most frequent causes of such repetition, are the very diseases most thoroughly under our control, so that in the present advanced stage of our knowledge we should no longer hear of such a condition as recurring abortion. Ruge of Berlin

[1] Geonbert, *Thèse de Paris,* 1878.

considers syphilis as the cause of death of the fœtus in 83 per cent. of such cases.

VARIATIONS.—A cessation of the symptoms not infrequently occurs: either with or without treatment the oozing may stop; even if hemorrhage and pains have existed all symptoms may cease. Large clots of blood have been expelled, the patient rests quietly in her bed, and gradually becomes easier; contractions and hemorrhage cease altogether, and she recovers, regains her vigor, and begins to move about. At the time of the following menstrual period the same cycle is repeated, and not until then is the ovum expelled. If the membranes are delicate, these may be ruptured by uterine contraction or by artificial or mechanical interference, and with the collapse of the ovum or the expulsion of its greater mass irritation is lessened and the symptoms subside. Exercise or the congestion and irritation consequent upon the return of the menstrual period will again arouse uterine activity, and the remnants are then expelled, a month or two after the inaugural hemorrhage.

These are conditions which are very frequent when the expulsion is left to nature or the aid of the midwife is sought, but they are with equal frequency produced by unskilful interference. The efforts of the physician are not unfrequently directed to a lessening of the hemorrhage, regardless of the existing conditions: applications are made to the abdomen and ergot is given, both methods of treatment which tend to stimulate uterine contraction; the more powerful circular fibres predominate and contract, the os is closed, the symptoms cease, and the conditions above mentioned are produced. Abortion is prevented for the time being, and sooner or later the patient is astonished by a return, which is, however, accompanied by less hemorrhage and more active labor-pains with a more rapid expulsion. If styptic injections are made into the uterine cavity or pieces of the ovum removed with the uterine dressing-forceps, a similar effect is produced, though the result is a more unfavorable one, as parts of the ovum are removed, and the collapsed membranes and shreds which remain are liable to prolong and aggravate the case, as they do not irritate the uterus and stimulate it to healthy action like the intact ovum.

The interval between the period of expulsion and the inaugural hemorrhage is often one of complete rest and health, more usually one of occasional oozing and malaise. As a consequence, we must have putrefaction and sepsis or the development of placental polypi and hemorrhage. Air is often admitted, either during the efforts at removal or later; if the cervix is not fully contracted, the secretions are more copious and liable to putrefy with the retained shreds. The symptoms are, however, unlike those of septic infection after labor at term, on account of the comparatively intact surface, the absence of the large uterine sinuses: they are insidious, not intense and acute—lack of appetite, weakness, slight increase of pulse and temperature—so that assistance may not be sought until increased suffering, putrid discharge, and high fever necessitate interference. This putrefaction is more liable to take place when the greater mass of the ovum has been expelled and parts alone remain, but will also occur when the entire mass is retained. Even without active interference the symptoms may subside as the disintegrating masses pass away as a putrid discharge, intercurrent hemorrhages at times carrying away larger shreds.

The so-called placental polypi result from the retention of parts of the ovum, especially of the placental portion, chorion, or decidua serotina, which, enveloped in fibrinous coagula, are entered by the proliferating vessels of the surrounding tissue. Such growths, sometimes of the size of a hazelnut or walnut, even to that of a small egg, may be unnoticed for months, but sooner or later give rise to oozing and hemorrhage, and in more fortunate cases are finally expelled. The expulsion of these retained membranes is inaugurated by hemorrhage, which may be preceded by more or less oozing: it is rapid in its course, accompanied by that pain which characterizes the last stage of abortion, and terminates with the appearance of the corpus delicti. It is merely the final scene of the abortion, which was but partially completed weeks or months ago, and the task is greatly simplified. Dilatation of the cervix and separation of the tissues were accomplished in the first stages, and during the interval of rest nature has been quietly making the necessary preparations to facilitate and complete the task undertaken, precisely as during the last months of gestation. Consequently, this expulsion is rapidly accomplished: pain and hemorrhage, even if severe for a time, are not of long duration. I have such a mass—which upon section reveals distinctly the villi of the chorion—which was cast off with all the symptoms of abortion four months after the occurrence of the inaugural hemorrhage and partial expulsion. More frequently I have been called to remove these masses, which have given rise to constant oozing and actual hemorrhages, two and three months after the occurrence of abortion, the adhesion to the uterine wall being so firm that the sharp scoop was called for, and sometimes I have been obliged to remove them piecemeal like a small uterine fibroid.

Late Abortion.—All· abortions in the fifth and sixth month approximate in their symptoms those of labor at term; the membranes are ruptured, the ovum is never expelled in toto; the fœtus may either precede the placenta or be expelled with it. It is at this period also that the hydatiform mole usually passes away, though it may be retained for a much longer period of time, even beyond the duration of normal pregnancy, the symptoms resembling those of abortion in the third or fourth month. After complete expulsion of the ovum and membranes more active hemorrhage and pain cease, the uterus contracts, but a slight oozing follows, and this becomes more pale and gradually merges into a serous flow.

DURATION.—The course of abortion varies greatly in its duration, and is usually prolonged, death of the ovum frequently occurring weeks before active symptoms are inaugurated, and even these may be slow in developing: a slight and often interrupted oozing may precede a more profuse flow and the dilatation of the cervix, or, as we have seen, the symptoms may cease for weeks and months even after they have been fully inaugurated; again, the ovum may be expelled in part and the remnants be retained for months—four months being the extent of time in which I have seen such retention terminate in expulsion without interference. By the formation of placental polypi the period may be protracted indefinitely.

The question how long abortion may be delayed, for what length of time the membranes may be retained, is far more important than is generally supposed, both from a social and medico-legal standpoint, and is by no means thoroughly understood. I have recently seen a mole formation, the infiltrated fœtal membranes, and part of the decidua which had been retained nearly four years — three years and nine months.[1] For four consecutive years the foolish woman, who had brought about abortion and expulsion of the embryo, suffered from occasional menorrhagia, and nausea and vomiting like that which had existed in the first months of pregnancy, until the annoyance became unbearable and medical advice was sought. An examination revealed an enlarged anteflexed uterus, from which a peculiar compressed and elongated mole was removed, after which the symptoms ceased. The case is moreover peculiar, as several of the symptoms were those of pregnancy, which do not generally continue after death of the embryo.

For a term of three years a twin embryo has been retained, causing violent epileptiform attacks, always most severe during the menstrual period, which first appeared four weeks after the last labor and continued, to the great detriment of the patient, until the macerated embryo was removed, when recovery took place. This was most probably a twin intramural pregnancy, the twin developing in the tubo-uterine cavity being retained after the expulsion of the one properly located, and then gradually forced into the more commodious uterine cavity.[2] These cases indicate the extent of this still unsettled question.

TERMINATION.—Dangers of Abortion.—Though fatal results are rare and, when occurring, due to sepsis rather than to hemorrhage, much of female suffering is traceable to this accident, the pathological interruption of pregnancy. Uterine and pelvic disease, especially subinvolution and consequent displacement, diseases of the endometrium and cervical tissue, result from abortion; sterility as well—all diseases which leave their traces indelibly marked upon the system of woman. They are not the direct or necessary consequences of abortion, but rather the results of the underrating of this most decidedly pathological occurrence—an underrating which is unfortunately prevalent among the profession and universal among the laity.

The direct consequences of hemorrhage are rarely severe: if harm ensues from loss of blood, it is not from profuse hemorrhage, but from long-continued oozing, generally that which accompanies the oozing following incarceration in the efforts at delivery, by which the system is depleted, and so weakened that years of care may be necessary for perfect restitution: evil results are much more liable to follow upon ill-timed or injudicious interference, the removal of part of the ovum or the checking of hemorrhage, the closing of the os by cold applications or ergot; equally serious consequences arise from sepsis if putrefaction of the parts retained takes place. The indirect results are even more common, and I cannot too often repeat that these, as well as the before-mentioned direct results, are due to a misapprehension of the existing condition— to an underrating of the importance of abortion. It is looked upon by women as no more than a profuse menstruation; some follow their daily vocations, bearing the suffering, or they may remain in bed during

---

[1] Ovum retained nearly four years, E. C. Gehrung, *Weekly Medical Review*, St. Louis, April 25, 1885.
[2] C. K. Patterson, *Weekly Medical Review*. June 13, 1885.

the most profuse flow and the greatest agony, but with the expulsion of
the ovum or after a day's rest they resume their daily toils and pleasures.
Frequently the midwife or nurse is called, and thus after-treatment
neglected; and even the physician too often discharges his patient after
a few days' confinement.

The worst consequences follow upon comparatively rapid and easy
abortions, which are treated lightly, even by the practitioner; and should
he by chance take the proper view of the case, the patient herself is
unwilling to observe the necessary care. If she is prudent, she awaits
the cessation of the discharge; daily work is then resumed by some, the
usual round of pleasures by others. Gradually annoying symptoms appear,
local or general; health fails; backaches, dragging-down pains, appear
after so long a period that so slight a matter as the abortion, which has
occurred months before, is never thought of as the cause of the suffering,
and subinvolution is thus the most common result. As in all but traumatic and criminal abortions pathological conditions precede, especially
of the pelvic viscera, it is often a diseased organ in which the abortion
takes place, and restitution will only be accomplished by time and care,
rest and proper treatment.

Subinvolution, chronic uterine lesion, and sterility are a common result
of the first abortion in young married women, and in most instances it is
the neglect of after-treatment to which these results must be ascribed; it
is the underrating of abortion by the laity, and even by the profession;
and as natural, healthy labor with too rapid getting up is liable to result
in evil consequences slowly developing, so it is true to a far greater extent
of simple abortion. The usual termination is in subinvolution, chronic
cervicitis, and endometritis.

It is the duty of the physician to impress upon his patient the fact that
equal if not greater care is necessary in the management of the pathological condition, of the early termination of pregnancy, than of normal labor
at term, and that abortion is to be compared to a severe labor rather than
to a simple menstruation. Were the physician summoned at once, much
evil would be prevented. But if called at all, it is only when hemorrhage
and pain become alarming; yet I am sorry to say that I have seen those
who have suffered most, ruined in health and sterile, women in the best
walks of life, who have closely followed the advice of able physicians,
who skilfully managed the existing trouble, but undervalued the couse-
quences—not giving the necessary time for involution, comparatively
slow at this period when the system is so unprepared for a process to
which its course is slowly shaped as term approaches.

DIAGNOSIS.—It is of importance to know, when called to a patient,
first whether abortion is threatening or actually inaugurated—that is,
whether the patient is pregnant, and whether the existing symptoms are
those of abortion or of dysmenorrhœa; secondly, whether the abortion
can be prevented, and if not, what treatment is to be pursued; and
thirdly, whether the abortion is completed?

1. Does pregnancy exist and is abortion inaugurated? or are the symptoms those of dysmenorrhœa, metritis, or uterine tumor? The existence of pregnancy is a condition often difficult to discover, especially
in unmarried women intent upon deceit, or in cases where the patient
is herself in ignorance and no cessation of the menstrual flow has oc-

curred. The symptoms of pregnancy must be carefully inquired into, as well as the condition of the patient, local and general, during the previous months and previous pregnancy. Dysmenorrhœa, menorrhagia, and membranaceous dysmenorrhœa may simulate abortion; but the pain in dysmenorrhœa is relieved by the discharge, whilst this is not the case in the pain of abortion: on the contrary, as the flow increases, with the dilatation of the cervix and the separation of the ovum, the pain increases; shreds of membrane accompany the discharge of dysmenorrhœa, whilst in the case of abortion the membranes follow the ovum when pain and discharge have almost ceased. In dysmenorrhœa the pain is ovarian, more violent, and aggravated with the cessation of the discharge, whilst in abortion it is uterine, more particularly referable to the cervix in the period of dilatation and to the fundus in that of expulsion, and lessens or ceases with the cessation of the discharge. The hemorrhage due to fibroids and polypi may greatly resemble that of abortion, especially if mole formations occur, but the pregnant and aborting uterus is greater in size than the congested menstrual organ. In the abortion of a comparatively healthy ovum the uterus approximates in size the period of gestation; the ovum as it descends during the pain becomes more broad, round, and tense, whilst in the case of a growth or clot the part which is forced down during a pain is more pointed at its presenting extremity than in the interval. In most cases of abortion, however, the uterus is rather smaller than it should be at the period of pregnancy at which the interruption occurs, and as the membranes are infiltrated with blood a mole formation is approximated; the ovum is more pyriform, pointed in shape; the apex imbedded in clots of blood, so that it resembles in feel, as it descends during the pain, a clot or polypus. The pregnant uterus, however, is more soft and elastic than the diseased organ.

2. Can abortion be prevented? The presence of an ovum being determined, our attention must next be directed to the possibility of its preservation. The distension of the os, especially the amount of hemorrhage, must guide the practitioner in seeking an answer to this important inquiry, upon which treatment must depend. The amount of hemorrhage is indicative of the separation of the ovum, but a slight flow continued for days is by no means as dangerous to gestation as a profuse instantaneous discharge. The os may be dilated, but if the hemorrhage is slight and the ovum out of reach, the progress of abortion may yet be prevented even after pains have been inaugurated, the first pains being those of dilatation. The appearance of rhythmical pains, indicative of expulsive contractions, leaves little hopes for the practitioner to check the course inaugurated. Even if the ovum can be felt, abortion may still be prevented, but if it protrude through the gaping os, little is to be expected, though even under these circumstances prevention is still said to be possible if the hemorrhage has not been severe. But if the liquor amnii has passed, there is no possibility of saving the ovum at any time, though it is claimed that even this can be done if pain or hemorrhage alone exists and the latter be not too severe. Even if the separation has not progressed so far that abortion is inevitable, the question must arise whether it be judicious to attempt prevention or whether abortion should be furthered. This depends upon the condition of the embryo, whether it is destroyed or not; if no previous abortions have occurred, and no

known cause, especially predisposing or local, exist, if the size of the uterus corresponds to the period of pregnancy, and there are no symptoms of mechanical interference or trauma, an effort should be made to preserve the ovum; but if there be cause sufficient to account for its death, if the uterus be more hard and round, wanting in the elastic oval of normal gestation, if it be smaller than usual at the period of gestation at which the interruption has occurred, death of the embryo and ovum may be supposed, and, notwithstanding the possibility of prevention, abortion should be hastened and completed, the ovum and membranes expelled.

3. Is abortion completed? Difficult as it often is to answer the question whether the ovum has been expelled, it is almost impossible to say whether the abortion has been fully completed, whether the last remnants of tissue have been evacuated. If the physician has been present or the clots have been saved from the time of the inaugural hemorrhage, it may be easy to determine the condition of affairs; but, unfortunately, these are usually thrown away, and the attendant comes at a late period, at one of suffering and exhaustion, when masses of blood, quantities of clots, with whatever of the ovum they may contain, have been removed. If present, he should crumble each clot and float the coagula in water. Fibrin and blood will soon wash away, and the shreds of tissue become separated and remain floating in the fluid.

An examination of all pieces that have passed will readily reveal the existing stage; but ordinarily the physician has no such clue. The hemorrhage has ceased, the uterus is firmly contracted, the os is closed, and the diagnosis is exceedingly difficult, but it must be determined. If left to nature, time will disclose the true condition of affairs: if the ovum has been expelled, the uterus will rapidly diminish in size, the appearance of the discharge will change—it will become more thin and pale; but if the uterus remains firmly contracted, and does not diminish in size, it is probable that the membranes are retained, and the renewal of exertion, of work, or of a succeeding menstrual period—if not the first, the second—will bring about a recurrence of the hemorrhage and the completion of abortion. If the uterus remains large, hard, globular, it is probable that the ovum, or at least the greater part of the membranes, remains in the cavity.

Unless the hemorrhage has ceased and the os be closed for some time previous to the coming of the physician, he will find the uterus low in the pelvis, the os still yielding, except when ergot has been given or ice applied, and by the introduction of the finger into the uterus the condition of the cavity will be determined: this will in all cases be readily accomplished by pressing with one hand firmly upon the fundus and examining with one or two fingers of the other; if not easily done in this way, the entire hand should be introduced into the vagina; the uterine cavity may then be thoroughly swept with the examining finger; but, though this will reveal an enclosed ovum, the membranes can by no means be detected with ease, and will often escape observation; hence the dull curette is in place: it will sever such tissues as may still be adherent. An excellent instrument, especially if the os be small, is the Récamier curette, or the modification which I have devised for the purpose. Should any doubt exist, dilatation should be at once resorted to for curative as well as diagnostic purposes; a rapid dilatation is in place—not instrumental, but by the tupelo or sea-tangle: this affords positive knowledge of the state of the case, and the cavity can then be thoroughly cleansed. Even the sponge tent is harmless if the abortion is completed, as the cervix is still dilatable and yielding, easily expanded. At all events, the diagnosis is unquestioned and the treatment clear. This is by far better than the expectant plan, which is most commonly followed for fear of interference, allowing the patient to continue perhaps for a month or more in ignorance of her condition—allowing her to resume her labors, exposed to sepsis, hemorrhage, and, in the most favorable case, expulsion of the ovum at any time.

If the os is dilated, the finger should be introduced—if necessary the hand—into the vagina, which can easily be done if the fundus be approximated by the other hand; better still, to use the curette, and I would advise the large blade of my instrument; the small one can at all times be passed into the cavity of the uterus during or immediately after abortion, and usually the larger one also. This examination, if with the scoop, consequent upon dilatation, should be followed by an antiseptic injection, but I would unquestionably advocate a correct diagnosis, whatever means may be necessary to obtain it, as appearances are so deceptive. We need but recall those by no means rare cases which to all appearances are those of completed abortion, yet the patient does not perfectly regain health and strength, and if an examination is made the os is found patulous and membranes or parts of the ovum are retained. If examination and dilatation be neglected, a coming menstrual period will discharge the disintegrating mass, or local and constitutional disturbances, even septicæmia, may be looked for.

PROGNOSIS.—As to prognosis, it is the mother whom we must consider, the dangers present and future, the attachment and dimensions of the ovum, and the possibility of continued gestation. The prognosis of traumatic or criminal abortion is worse than that of the spontaneous form, the result of natural causes, because it is inaugurated by shock, by injury, and inflammatory conditions which are aggravated by the congestion and contraction accompanying the expulsion, for which the tissues are entirely unprepared; whilst in natural, spontaneous abortion, usually the result of some morbid condition, some disease of the system, a cachexia, uterine disturbance, or death of the embryo and ovum has preceded, and a retrograde metamorphosis to a certain extent has been inaugurated; some preparation at least has been made for the coming expulsion; hence the separation is more natural, less violent, less liable to be followed by evil results.

The prognosis is invariably favorable if proper medical aid is summoned in the early stages, but actually it varies greatly, as does the course of abortion—whether completed in a reasonable time or of longer duration, more favorable in the former, less propitious in the latter; if hemorrhage has been profuse or comparatively slight, but of long duration, anæmia is liable to result: if expulsion is long protracted, the dangers of subinvolution, metritis, and perimetritis are great: if the expulsive pains cease before the complete expulsion of ovum or membranes, retention, putrefaction, and sepsis may be inaugurated, and subinvolution, endocervicitis, and endometritis will follow.

The embryo is scarce to be considered : it may be saved if the hemorrhage has not been too severe and accompanied by pain, if the ovum does not protrude into the cervix. The inflammation which usually accompanies traumatic or criminal abortion greatly aggravates the prognosis, but, however good it may be in individual cases, the result will depend greatly upon the after-treatment, upon the time allowed for proper involution, and upon the assistance given it. Though the prognosis at the time of abortion may be a most favorable one for the mother, the result is seriously affected by the care taken during the period of involution, the after-treatment, which is by far more important than generally supposed.

TREATMENT.—The successful treatment of abortion requires knowledge, judgment, and resolution on the part of the practitioner, and in importance it is equivalent at least to the management of labor at term. Two lives may even be at stake, though the opportunity of saving the embryo is, as a rule, afforded only during the period of prophylactic and preventive treatment, as vitality is ordinarily destroyed in the embryo when abortion, as the result of natural causes, is once inaugurated : the life of the mother is not in question, as it is in labor at term, but her health is even more endangered. Attention is now forcibly called to the subject by earnest discussions between the adherents of the expectant and those of the progressive method of treatment, but mainly to the treatment of actual abortion; prevention and after-treatment have been neglected. Important as is the method of treatment employed in case of retention of membranes or ovum, the necessity for such interference, especially the frequency of abortion, would be greatly diminished if the family physician were thoroughly imbued with the importance of the subject and could impress the same upon his patients. If the dangers arising from such premature interruption of gestation were appreciated by the laity and medical attention summoned in the early stages, the management of abortion would become more simple and more successful, and the cases of retention which cause such suffering and injury to women would be far less frequent.

Before entering upon the treatment proper it may be well to review briefly the necessary adjuncts, as proper preparation will aid materially the course to be adopted.

Preparations Necessary with Regard to the Patient.—Many of the preparations necessary in the lying-in chamber are desirable in cases of abortion as well. Attention should be paid to the bowels, as a costive condition will interfere to some extent with the manipulations as well as a rapid and favorable course of expulsion and involution ; at best, it is liable to make the patient uncomfortable. The bladder should be evacuated, especially before active measures are resorted to, and the patient should be so clad in night-gown and sacque, with long hose and drawers, that she may be moved and manipulated without exposure.

The bed should be prepared with rubber cloth and quilts, and sufficient quilts, cloths, and towels should be on hand ; a bed-pan is desirable, and also a fountain or bulb syringe ; the bed should be so placed that the physician may be at the right hand of the patient, and convenient to the light when she is placed in Sims's position of the dorsal decubitus for operative interference.

Antisepsis.—Cleanliness and antisepsis should be observed in the management of abortion as strictly as in that of labor or in surgical operations, as sepsis, either in the form of acute infection or an insidious undermining of the constitution, is among the more frequent of the dangerous consequences which follow in the wake of abortion. Circumstances permitting, it is desirable that carbolated vaseline or vaseline with iodoform, carbolated or some similarly prepared soap, be oh hand, and also permanganate of potassium, carbolic or boracic acid, and iodoform. I am in the habit of prescribing carbolic acid for the convenience of use: carbolic acid 2 ounces, alcohol 1 ounce, with 7 of glycerin, which is as concentrated as may be well used (1 to 5, or 20 per cent.), and a proportion readily diluted to $2\frac{1}{2}$ or 5 per cent.

Before and after examinations the hand should be washed in carbolated water or some such disinfectant—permanganate of potassium, corrosive sublimate, or boracic acid—as it appears desirable to use. If carbolic acid is used, the parts should be cleansed with a 2 or 3 per cent. solution. After interference or repeated examinations the vaginal douche should be used, certainly after completion before leaving the patient. If instrumental interference be necessary, and the ovum or membranes forcibly removed, the cavity of the uterus should be washed with hot water, from 115° to 125° F., containing 5 per cent. of carbolic acid, the hot water serving styptic purposes. This may suffice, but it is frequently desirable to mop the cavity with the above-named solution or even the pure liquid after more active interference, especially if some disintegration has taken place and is indicated by odor.

After the use of tampons the vagina should be washed with a 2 or 3 per cent. solution, or 1 : 2000, of corrosive sublimate; and it is even well that the cotton, before being introduced, should be anointed with either carbolized vaseline or carbolized oil (carbolic acid 2 drachms, olive oil 3 ounces). Iodoform serves an excellent purpose for disinfection of tampons, especially such as are packed into or against the cervix, and as an application to the cavity after the removal of the putrid contents following the hot douche. Borated cotton, or even ordinary cotton or prepared tow, should be on hand to use during the after-treatment in place of cloths for the purpose of receiving the discharge: it is warm, soft, forms a good filter, and can be thrown away or burnt when soiled, whilst the cloths ordinarily used, and often very offensive, are kept for the wash.

Medication.—The most important of all the remedies is opium; in preventive treatment it may be called a specific. It is far preferable to the hypodermic injection of morphine, serving to relax and quiet the uterine muscle and to lessen hemorrhage; for the latter purpose it is often combined with acetate of lead—from $\frac{1}{4}$ to 1 grain of opium mixed with $\frac{1}{2}$ to 1 grain of acetate of lead, to be given at a dose and repeated when necessary. Ipecacuanha combined with opium acts well in relaxing the tension.

Viburnum prunifolium has long been used as a uterine sedative in these cases in those States where the plant is endogenous, and its use has been widely disseminated since it has found so able an advocate in Jenks. The preparations are not all equally effective, but in the early stages the fluid extract given in teaspoonful doses, according to the amount of hemorrhage and pain either hourly or every two or three hours, has a most decided effect in allaying threatened abortion, in checking hemorrhage, and in quieting pains. It seems to be a uterine sedative. Several ounces may be taken, and successful cases are reported where the pending expulsion was averted and gestation continued to a successful termination after four ounces had been used. Digitalis combined with acetate of lead also deserves recommendation as an effective remedy in the early stages. Quinine may be given to stimulate the system and further uterine contraction, and is invaluable in an asthenic condition or if disintegrating shreds be present.

Nervines, valerian, asafœtida, valerianate of ammonia, bromide of potassium, are of great service throughout the entire course of abortion, as the patient is usually in a nervous almost febrile state. Alone they may serve to allay the irritating symptoms in the early stages, and answer well in preventing the disagreeable effects of opium. Asafœtida may be given by injection or in pills, from ½ to 2 grains at a dose.

Clysmata tend to irritate, and should not be used as long as we may hope to prevent threatened abortion. Such remedies as are indicated in the treatment of this condition, especially opium and nervines, must nevertheless at times be given by injection, as the stomach may refuse to receive and retain them in the irritated condition which accompanies this state. The clysms should always be warmed, of body temperature: two tablespoonfuls of milk of asafœtida or gum arabic form an excellent vehicle, though water or milk thickened with flour or starch, which is always on hand, will do quite well.

Should it be necessary to move the bowels, castor oil is one of the best remedies, whilst cathartics, especially aloes and similar drugs, must be avoided as long as there is hope of preserving the ovum: they certainly further expulsion. Ergot should not be used until after the uterine cavity is emptied, and is decidedly contraindicated whilst the ovum or any of its parts remain adherent in utero. The dangers arising from the use of ergot in the early stages, whilst the ovum is still intact, are rupture of the membranes and forcible contraction, which always prolongs expulsion of the ovum or its membranes; the circular fibres, which predominate, are stimulated most forcibly to action, more particularly so under the conditions which usually exist in abortion: the muscle of the uterine body is hindered in its contraction by the adhesions of ovum and decidua, especially if these membranes are infiltrated; and, moreover, in cases of abortion the tissues of the womb itself are often more or less diseased; the lower portion of the uterus and cervix alone is free to act, the circular fibres of the internal os contract most readily under the influence of ergot, whilst the activity of the fundus is interfered with; thus closing of the outlet and incarceration of the membranes are liable to result. This popular and dangerous drug must not be given until the tissues are expelled, or, if desirable by reason of excessive hemorrhage, its use may be resorted to under one condition: if the membranes are detached, not only free in the uterine cavity, but entering that of the cervix; they may be found massed together firmly, by compression of the uterine walls, into a conical or pyriform mass; and when this has to a great extent passed the internal os ergot may be given. This drug, so dangerous in obstetric practice, is still used with altogether too much freedom in this country, and it would be far better to do without it than to continue the prevalent abuse. I have insisted that this drug must not be given in labors or abortion until the contents of the uterine cavity have been removed. Although but one of our prominent obstetricians approved of the position I took in 1883, and I was then freely attacked, I now urge the point more earnestly, and the doctrine is more commonly accepted: in Germany such men as Martin, Spiegelberg, and others have succeeded in doing away with this dangerous remedy altogether in the institutions under their care, restricting its use to the non-gravid uterus.

As a styptic, hot water, carbolized, serves the best purpose: in the early stages as vaginal douche, in the later as an intra-uterine injection at 120°, it is an invaluable remedy, preferable to other styptics, as it cleanses and removes the coagula. When the cavity has been emptied, especially after the forcible removal of the membranes, it is well to apply carbolic acid to the surface; and it is better for this purpose than tincture of iodine or perchloride of iron, either of which is only to be used in case that hemorrhage does not yield to the before-mentioned remedies.

Anæsthetics.—Though bromide of potash, morphine, or opium may suffice for the relief of the pain in ordinary cases, the use of an anæsthetic is not only desirable, but necessary, if more active measures are resorted to. For purposes of rapid dilatation and the removal of an adherent ovum or membranes anæsthesia is almost indispensable; without this the suffering of the already nervous, debilitated patient is excessive; the uterine and abdominal muscles are tense, and operations thus greatly impeded. An anæsthetic should be given in a rapid dilatation on account of the pain, as well as the greater facility of operating; and it is most necessary in an attempt at expression, as, if made without an anæsthetic, the abdominal muscles are so tense that the uterus cannot be well manipulated from without. I myself prefer chloroform.

Instruments.—A speculum, a dull curette, a sharp scoop, a vulsellum forceps, and uterine dressing-forceps are essentially necessary. Any speculum may be used. The best is Sims's if the semi-prone position be used, or Simon's in the dorsal decubitus. The Schroeder's or my forceps is necessary to steady and bring down the uterus for the introduction of tent or finger and the use of the scoop or the application of styptics. This is in the main the American bullet-forceps, an instrument far superior to the sharp vulsellum which is so popular. The curette I would most recommend is my own modification of Récamier's instrument of pliable metal, one blade resembling that of Récamier's, but curved somewhat more like the uterine sound—sharp upon one side, dull upon the other—to be used for the purpose of severing the ovum or membranes in the line of their adhesion: this is so narrow that it can be introduced into the os even after contraction if this be not almost tetanic, as after the giving of ergot. The other blade is larger, broad and flat, more spoon-like, to be used in case of moderate dilatation of the os, both, however, being for the purpose of severing the adhesions and leaving the ovum intact. The broad blade serves as a lever to remove the ovum or membranes when detached. But if the membranes be ruptured, it is of service in separating these from the uterine wall, leaving them as complete as possible, which will always facilitate removal or expulsion. The irritation caused by the severing of the adhesions with this instrument frequently suffices to inaugurate uterine contraction; and ovum or membranes, being once liberated, are then compressed by the uterine muscle into one mass, thus affording a resistance which the uterus is enabled to grasp and expel. This method I believe to be far more rational than the removal of the membranes with the sharp instrument: it furthers the process of nature more strictly, separating rather than cutting away the tissues, as does the latter. The sharp scoop is an instrument which is only to be used for firm adhesions in secondary cases, where the progress of abortion has temporarily ceased and the membranes have become more firmly attached, especially where disintegration of such adherent parts has taken place to some extent; it is necessary and cannot be dispensed with where remnants have been retained for months and have become firmly attached, simulating polypoid growths. I object to the use of the sharp scoop in recent cases, because it is preferable to follow the line of demarcation indicated by nature, and separate the membranes or the ovum, if still entire, in this strait; whilst the sharp scoop removes them piecemeal, cutting deep into the mucosa at one place, and possibly leaving pieces of embryonic tissue in another.

Dressing-Forceps.—These are serviceable for the introduction and removal of tampons, the cleansing of the uterine cavity, and the removal of a detached ovum when in the cervical canal or almost extruded; but the very common habit of seizing the ovum with this instrument as soon as the apex appears is a most pernicious one: the membranes are ruptured, the continuity destroyed, the mass collapses, and the resistance offered to the contracting muscle as well as the dilating wedge is thus destroyed, and the course of abortion greatly prolonged. No narrow grasping instruments should ever be used to make forcible traction upon the ovum; the tissues, if healthy, are very often delicate, and if degenerated into mole formations, infiltrated with blood, brittle, breaking beneath the instrument, which is always withdrawn grasping simply what is seized between its blades. I know of none of the many ovum-forceps which I can recommend.

Position of the Patient.—For purposes of instrumental interference the patient may be placed on side or back, in the left-lateral, semi-prone position if Sims's speculum be used; I prefer the dorsal decubitus, using Simon's speculum. The bivalve specula might be used if short, like the operating speculum of Albert Smith, but they are not to be recommended, on account of their small diameter and their usually too great length, by which they push the uterus away. The organ should be approximated as nearly as possible to the vulva and finger by the instrument, and this is best done either by a short, broad Sims's or Simon's speculum. Simon's speculum in the dorsal decubitus has among its other advantages that of greater convenience for the purpose of injections. The patient is transversely brought on the bed, with the hips upon the edge, elevated by a folded blanket or hard cushion; the legs are flexed, the feet placed upon two chairs; an oil cloth directly under the parts is folded into a slop-jar standing underneath, so as to receive all refuse matter, which enables the physician to use the douche freely. Bozeman's catheter, with double current for intra-uterine injection, is a very convenient and valuable instrument, though not an absolutely necessary addition to the armamentarium.

The use of gynecological instruments is even more important in abortion than in labor at term : it is by far more convenient to introduce the tent or dilator, and even to use the scoop through the speculum, than blindly with the aid of the finger, guided only by the hand on the fundus. Knife and scissors, needle and thread, may be of use in difficult cases, or in case of a firmly-contracted os with putrefaction of the membranes, for rapid dilatation. German authorities advocate incision with a knife in preference to rapid dilatation where it must be done quickly for purposes of immediate evacuation ; should this be resorted to, it is very necessary that after abortion is completed the parts should be again carefully united by close sutures—a method which is only to be recommended to the expert in extreme cases. The Récamier or my own curette can be used effectively without dilatation in ordinary cases, even if the os is somewhat contracted ; there is so much relaxation that these instruments can be readily introduced, the os being dilated during the act; and if the sharp instrument be used the particles cut are carried out by the spoon, the douche taking away the remnants. With my own instrument I am in the habit of separating the adhesions and removing the mass more, as with a lever, especially if the ovum be intact. The large blade of the spoon is used to press the ovum down into the hollow of the sacrum, very much as the placenta at term is removed.

PROPHYLAXIS.—In primigravidæ the physician should urge careful attention to all conditions that may further a healthy state. As indicated by the physiology of early pregnancy, this lies mainly in a proper preparation for the changes wrought by the physiological activity of the sexual organs ; free scope must be given for their development, and this guarded against all injuries, nervous and traumatic : the congested developing parts and the sensitive, tensely-strung nervous system must be protected against insult ; a healthy condition of the system must be established, and possibly existing predisposing causes counteracted.

Young married women, above all, are liable to injury from coition, from over-exertion in this period, from amusement or labor, as well as from the demands of fashion. It is the mother, and more often the family physician, who must see that a free and healthy development is permitted : let it be remembered that the close-fitting corset, the heavy dresses suspended from the hips, exertion whether for pleasure or work, frequent intercourse, as well as mental condition, all affect the fate of the ovum. The menstrual congestion, recurring with greater or less periodicity at the usual time of the flow, is a period of especial danger at which still greater care is necessary. As a rule, we can only say that a strict attention to dietetic laws, which should be observed in every gestation, is of the greatest prophylactic importance. In the case of multigravidæ, especially such as have previously aborted, the same rules must be observed, and, in addition, especial attention must be paid to the removal of such causes as may have resulted in previous abortions. The proper prevention, however, lies in treatment of these conditions before the occurrence of conception : as we have seen, these may be either plethora, anæmia, most usually syphilis or uterine disease, and a lacerated cervix, endometritis, pelvic cellulitis, or retroflexion. The treatment of such morbid conditions should be inaugurated as soon after recovery from an abortion as possible, and continued, in case of constitutional disturbance, after conception has again occurred. Though the avoidance of excessive exercise and perfect quiet are desirable, especially during the menstrual congestion and at that period of gestation when abortion has previously occurred, it is ridiculous to confine the patient to bed at this time, without further treatment, with a view of preventing the recurrence of abortion by rest alone. This is a common practice, and can result in good only in isolated cases; it usually annoys and weakens the patient; and it is high time that this antiquated doctrine should be exploded, and that the attending physician take sufficient interest in his patient to urge examination and local treatment by the specialist if he himself cannot detect and relieve the trouble which has caused, and will continue to cause, such serious disturbance. It is a paramount duty of the physician to inquire into the cause of the previous abortion and to prevent recurrence by its removal: if he himself should have attended her, he should examine the ovum most carefully, and later the patient as regards her constitution and the condition of the uterus and pelvic viscera. If the abortion be due to syphilis of mother or father, this must be treated, an existing disease relieved, a retroflexion of the uterus replaced, a lacerated cervix repaired, or the disease of the endometrium overcome; but the confining to bed of the patient during the period of danger, or even during the many months of pregnancy, will aid but little: this is advisable only when the symptoms of threatening abortion again appear. Moderate exercise is conducive to health, and hence to the development of the ovum, and only in rare cases can abortion be prevented by rest alone: confinement to bed may be resorted to as our only means if we are in a state of ignorance, where the original cause has not been detected or treatment is at the time impossible; and this is partially true in pregnancy of a uterus with a lacerated cervix which has not been repaired. An inflamed or irritated cervix is open to treatment, and even a lacerated cervix can be improved during the existence of gestation.

Preventive Treatment.—If symptoms of threatening abortion, or such as resemble them—oozing, hemorrhage, uterine pain—appear in the pregnant woman, however questionable the diagnosis, the treatment must invariably be directed toward the prevention of threatened abortion. If the symptoms are indistinct, the oozing may be merely that of a congested or eroded cervix during the menstrual period or the existing pains —a reflex symptom due to other causes—and should be treated; but then in addition the necessary means must be at once adopted to prevent threatened abortion; and if we are ignorant of the condition of the ovum, whether healthy with a living embryo or pathologically changed, treatment must be directed toward its preservation until absolute knowledge to the contrary is obtained; and this is, above all, necessary in the earlier months, when it is almost impossible to determine as to its condition. Every effort must be made to preserve the ovum as if healthy; and if it be so, success is by far more likely to crown the efforts of the physician, whilst he will strive in vain if it be a healthy effort of the uterus to rid itself of a dead embryo and the diseased membrane surrounding it. Perfect quiet, mental and physical, rest of body and mind, is necessary; the patient is put to bed and kept quiet, excitement and irritation prevented; no coffee, tea, or stimulants should be given, but acids, cool drinks, sour lemonade, aromatic sulphuric acid, opium alone or in combination with other remedies according to the conditions, are in place. If hemorrhage is profuse, we should further vascular contraetion sufficiently to check the flow with chinine, ipecacuanha, or, best, viburnum prunifolium, the fluid extract in teaspoon doses, if very profuse every hour, otherwise every two or three hours; digitalis may be added in case of nervous excitement, which is often intense; so also bromide of potassium, valerian, or asafœtida. Ergot and cold applications to the abdomen must be avoided; the latter are frequently resorted to, as they tend to allay hemorrhage, but at the same time they stimulate uterine contractions too freely. No unnecessary examination must be made, and the patient must be kept in perfect repose until the symptoms have completely disappeared.

TREATMENT OF ABORTION WHICH IS FULLY INAUGURATED AND PROGRESSING.—If all means to overcome the existing conditions and check threatening abortion have failed, if the pains continue, the os dilates, or hemorrhage becomes profuse, the treatment is radically changed. Before this period it was directed to the preservation of the ovum, whilst the object is now to complete delivery. The practitioner must now endeavor to check hemorrhage, allay suffering, and above all empty the uterus at the earliest possible time, and to this latter end all his efforts should be directed. By accomplishing this all other symptoms will be most satisfactorily and perfectly relieved; and though time and patience are remedies which cannot be dispensed with even in this stage, more active interference and local measures are now indicated, which, it will be remembered, were to be avoided if prevention seemed still possible.

The progress of dilatation and separation is often slow, and during this stage one precaution must be observed: whatever measures be adopted, the membranes must be preserved intact. We must avoid all interference with the fœtal sac; after this is ruptured the hemorrhage is liable to become more profuse, as an additional source of bleeding is added by the collapse of the ovum, which causes a diminution of the intra-uterine pressure. The succulent and vascular tissues are no longer compressed between the resistant mass of the ovum and the uterine walls, and ooze freely into the cavity; moreover, the resistance and irritation previously existing, whilst the ovum was unbroken, is removed, and uterine contractions, the expulsive efforts, are diminished or cease entirely.

The prominent indication for interference is given by hemorrhage, and such means must be adopted to check this as will at the same time promote the expulsion of the ovum.

Pain.—Opium must now be most sparingly used. Complete relief of pain is not desirable in this stage; uterine contractions, the dilatation of the cervix, should be furthered; nervous irritation and excessive suffering may be relieved by nervines—valerianate of ammonia, bromide of potash, perhaps a hypodermic injection of morphine; regular pains indicative of uterine contraction must not be interfered with under any circumstances.

Hemorrhage.—The treatment previously inaugurated—rest, quiet, cold iced drinks—may be continued, but in addition more active measures must be employed: our main resort in this stage is in local measures, mainly in the tampon. Ergot must not be given, as it may lead to rupture of the membranes or incarceration of the ovum, or both.

The tampon is all-important in the management of this stage of abortion, as opium is in the first and the curette in that of retention ; according to the method of its use it will serve a variety of purposes, and by skilful manipulation the object desired can be attained with a fair degree of certainty. The cervical tampon is preferable if the os is con- tracted and the cervix not dilating ; pledgets of cotton have been used to plug the cervical canal, but the tent is far preferable ; tupelo or slippery elm should be used. In cases where rapid dilatation as well as relief of hemorrhage is desired the sponge tent may be resorted to, but is, as a rule, to be avoided on account of the dangers of infection and the liabil- ity of adhesion of particles of soft tissues with which it comes in contact within the cavity. The tupelo is preferable to sea-tangle, as it may be had in more serviceable size and shape ; the slippery elm is most excel- lent, is everywhere within reach, especially of the country practitioner, and has no superior : when cut in proper size, the edges slightly smoothed, and placed for a moment in warm water, it is soon covered with mucoid exudation, which makes its introduction extremely easy, and its presence within the uterine cavity decidedly less harmful than any other substance : it will readily find its way between the membranes, and a number of tents can be placed side by side, so that the disadvantages of inferior distension are equalized.

The tent is best introduced through the speculum, the cervix being fixed by a tenaculum, Engelmann or Schroeder forceps, and a tampon of salicylated or carbolized cotton placed in the vagina for the purpose of retention as well as disinfection. Care must always be taken that the tent be of sufficient length and passed well into the uterine cavity, to within a half inch of the fundus, as it will then serve not only to com- press the bleeding vessels and dilate the cervical canal, but to separate the ovum and stimulate uterine contraction. When the tent or cervical tampon is used the vaginal tampon is unnecessary ; each has its proper office to perform.

The Vaginal Tampon.—The vaginal tampon is preferable where the os is patulous and the cervix dilating ; if small, packed merely in the cul- de-sac and directly about the cervix, it irritates but little ; tents should be thus used if it be desirable to check hemorrhage and the possibility of prevention still exists. If larger and the vagina is more thoroughly packed, it is a violent excitor of uterine contractions, and is used in part for this purpose. The rubber bag or colpeurynter, even when filled with hot or cold water, is of little service in checking hemorrhage, though it serves to stimulate uterine contractions ; hence it is of no value in those cases where the vaginal tampon is usually called for. The best method of checking hemorrhage and furthering separation and expulsion of the ovum, when intact, is the thorough packing of the cul-de-sac and larger part of the vagina with balls of cotton ; wads of the size of a walnut should be made, and strong thread or string should be tied to each to facilitate removal : clots should be removed and the vagina cleansed with an antiseptic injection of 2 or 3 per cent. of carbolized water pre- paratory to their introduction. If convenient, salicylated or carbolated cotton should be used ; the ordinary cotton wadding or cotton wool may be taken, but then it is desirable to soak at least the first which are intro- duced in carbolized water, 5 per cent., or carbolized oil, 10 per cent.

Tampons are best placed with the aid of Sims's or Simon's speculum, though the bivalve may also be used. If no instrument is at hand, the vagina may be distended by the fingers, which are so introduced that they separate the parts thoroughly and press down the perineum; the prepared tampons are now seized with the dressing-forceps and securely packed In the cul-de-sac and against the cervix, so that it is firmly surrounded by a compact plug; then the entire vaginal canal is similarly packed to the vulva. Hemorrhage is perfectly checked if the tampon be properly applied; if not, it ceases for a time until the cotton or other material used has been saturated, and then continues as before. If the desired object be attained, the pains will become more severe and rapid and the tampon will be expelled: upon examination the ovum will be found in the vagina or at least within the cervix, and is easily removed. It is stated that the tampon should not be left in place over twenty-four hours: this is certainly the limit, as, saturated with blood and secretions, it is liable to putrefy and thus lead to more unpleasant results. Twelve hours is, as a rule, ample time. If the vagina has been properly packed, hemorrhage is stopped and uterine contractions aroused which should be sufficient to cause dilatation and separation of the ovum. If the desired result be not accomplished at this time, it is best to remove the tampon, and, according to circumstances, introduce another or resort to other measures. After removal of tampons the vagina should always be cleansed by a disinfectant injection. If the os be found closed and uterine contractions have ceased—which is very rarely the case when the vagina has been properly packed—no further measures should be resorted to, as the continuance of gestation may be hoped for.

In case of very profuse hemorrhage the tent or vaginal tampon is necessary, but the hot antiseptic douche is but little inferior as a hæmostatic and excitor of uterine contractions. If carbolic acid is used, 2 or 3 per cent. may be added of corrosive sublimate, 1 : 2000, and the temperature of the water should be at least from 115° to 125° F.—if gauged by the hand, so hot that the fingers can hardly be kept in the water, at least not without moving them about. The external parts, especially the perineum, must be coated with lard, as they are particularly sensitive and liable to be scorched (vaseline washes off too easily). Emetics or purgatives, though still occasionally recommended, must not be given with a view of promoting separation or expulsion of the ovum.

Removal of the Ovum.—The tampon has been expelled by uterine contractions, and the ovum, as before stated, will probably be found within the vagina or separated and easy of removal. Should the tampon, however, have been previously removed by reason of insufficient action, the hot antiseptic douche may be tried and the vagina again packed.

Constitutional symptoms, excessive suffering, nervousness, debility, rise of pulse or temperature, necessitate immediate removal of the ovum. Under ordinary circumstances this is allowable only if the os be patulous, the cervical canal sufficiently dilated, and the ovum detached; and if the above preliminary steps have been taken, this will usually be the case in an abortion during the first three months. If the cervix permits of the introduction of the finger, a satisfactory examination may then be made if the patient be placed in the proper position, with the hips elevated, the limbs flexed, and the uterus approximated to the examining finger by pressure upon the fundus with the other hand. If this be not possible by reason of thick abdominal walls, the fixation of the cervix with Engelmann or Schroeder forceps is called for. Expression is then preferable to extraction. The dressing-forceps, and even the ovum-forceps, are of but little service for this purpose unless the os be dilated and the ovum completely detached, as they are liable to rupture the sac, and thus increase the difficulty of extraction. The broad, blunt blade of my curette, Récamier's instrument, or Munde's, should be passed into the uterine cavity and swept around the entire circumference of the ovum : the uterine sound properly bent may be used for the same purpose, and if liberated it may be removed by using my instrument as a lever, placing it beneath the ovum in case of retroflexion of the uterus, and anteriorly in anteflexion, and pressing it down toward the pelvic outlet. Expression by hand is still recommended, and is very efficient in relaxed or thin abdominal walls, where both hands may be readily used for manipulation. The fingers are pressed against the uterine fundus—anteriorly in case of anterior displacement, posteriorly if the uterus is retroflexed or retroverted—whilst firm counter-pressure is made by the other hand upon the abdominal walls; the ovum being thus, as it were, squeezed out.

In later months greater dilatation is necessary, the importance of preserving the ovum intact is augmented, and the greatest care must be taken that efforts at expression are not made whilst the ovum is still adherent. I have found great difficulty in detaching the membranes, even when the canal is permeable, with the finger, as has been recommended ; and it is for this purpose especially that I have found the large blade of my instrument so valuable. It is readily introduced, pliable, so that it may be bent and properly adapted, and the point of attachment being found it can be passed about the entire ovum in the same plane, loosening without rupturing; and the irritation caused by this manœuvre is often sufficient to stimulate contractions, so that expulsion will follow. In fact, I consider this of less importance than separation, retention being mostly due to adhesions, especially at the point of placental formation. Once separated, it is a foreign body and an irritant, which is readily expelled. Nature thus teaches us the course which we must follow, to complete separation and dilatation before attempting removal.

TREATMENT IN CASES OF RETENTION OF OVUM OR MEMBRANES.— These are by far the more trying conditions, and, unfortunately, the ones to which the physician is most frequently called. Aid is not summoned at an earlier stage on account of that dangerous underrating of abortion or for fear of unnecessary expense, and the position of the practitioner is made a trying one, as he is ignorant of the state of the case. Clots of blood have passed, but as to the precise conditions he is left in doubt; whether the membranes have ruptured, whether the ovum is expelled in whole or in part, he is not told. He may find the os closed ; the size of the uterus reveals but little, as in many cases, at least those of spontaneous abortion, development is retarded ; it is smaller than would be supposed at that period of gestation. It is only in case the uterus corresponds at least approximately in size to the time, or if the os be sufficiently dilated, that he can at once decide positively as to the presence of ovum or membranes.

A closed internal os may usually be looked upon as evidence that the retained masses, whether ovum or membranes, are adherent, though in case of sepsis more or less dilatation exists; yet in the latter case the indications afforded by those symptoms are of little importance, as the constitutional symptoms, with the character and odor of the discharge, clearly indicate the existing conditions, and consequently show the course to be pursued. No question exists as to the necessity of immediate delivery in these cases, but as to the manner of treatment in retention of ovum or membranes not disintegrating there is a wide difference of opinion: able men are still inclined to urge a reliance upon nature, yet it is a dangerous course for the practitioner to pursue: successful as it may prove in many cases, it is certainly fatal in some, and but too often followed by the insidious consequences so frequent in its tracks.

Labor at term may be left far more readily to the powers of nature than abortion: the former is a physiological process, the latter pathological. The expulsion of the ovum at term has been preceded by preparatory changes in maternal and fœtal parts; the separation of the membranes is facilitated by the fatty degeneration of decidua serotina and vera; the hypertrophied uterine muscle is strained to its utmost, its fibres increased and strengthened for the ordeal, but in the early months no such conditions exist. Though expulsion has been anticipated and the preceding hemorrhage frequently serves to separate the structures, and development ceases with the death of the embryo, a retrograde metamorphosis is inaugurated only in certain cases, and then incomplete, and the frequency of intermittent abortion which we find in cases left to nature is evidence of incompetency to fulfil the task attempted: hemorrhage, more or less protracted, and contraction of the uterus cease; the ovum has been partially separated; its growth is checked, and then a retrograde metamorphosis is inaugurated in the tissues which have been in so active a state of development; this continues until a recurring menstrual period or excessive exercise brings about a renewal of the expulsive effort; and if sepsis has not taken place we usually find that the ovum is expelled with rapidity. When the attempt was first made, it proved ineffectual and the effort ceased; the tissues were impaired in their nutrition, underwent a fatty degeneration tending toward disintegration, and the second attempt of nature, with the parts properly prepared, terminates rapidly and effectually. Though the tendency of the profession at large seems toward a more expectant plan, guided by able authorities—such as Parvin, who urges attention to the old-time remedies, rest, time, and laudanum; and Leishman, who advocates this treatment when hemorrhage has stopped and the os is closed, perhaps aiding nature by the use of ergot—I would advise more active interference. It is indeed true that the ovum or some of its parts may remain in utero for months and then be expelled by a healthy effort of nature, without injury to the patient; but this is not the rule. I have seen such cases, but mostly the health of the patient is affected; even if more active symptoms, such as hemorrhage and sepsis, do not appear, subinvolution certainly follows. In cases less severe the patient is nervous, restless, suffers from insomnia, uterine colic, and occasional oozing; perhaps there is an offensive discharge,— all symptoms which are not sufficient to cause great anxiety, but we may with certainty expect them to result in serious inflammations of the uterus and surrounding tissues—metritis, thrombosis, cellulitis, endome-

tritis, peritonitis; hence why should we wait? Why allow these dangerous membranes to remain, as claimed by some, "as long as no injurious
effects appear"? Why wait for these more threatening symptoms when
evil results are almost certain to follow upon the retention of such masses,
even though hemorrhage and sepsis be at the time wanting? I have
removed thoroughly healthy, semi-organized remnants as late as the fifth
month after partial expulsion of the ovum; the patients were suffering
no very serious inconvenience at the time, nor did any grave consequences directly follow; yet it would have been far better for them had
decided steps been taken at the time of the inaugural flow; they were
forced to seek advice in some instances by reason of uterine pains and
oozing, in others by profuse and sudden hemorrhage; and, though decided
injuries were not at the time evident, subinvolution and uterine displacement were certainly threatened.

Various periods are mentioned as preferable for interference. Some say
that there is no need for alarm if the placenta remains in utero for twenty-
four or forty-eight hours, provided the patient be under observation; but
the os is liable to contract, always within a week, sometimes within forty-
eight hours, after preliminary hemorrhage, and it certainly is unreasonable to allow complete contraction of the os and thorough cessation of
the efforts of nature to take place, with the probability of evil results
before us. If the physician is called at a time when the course of abortion seems retrogressive, the os closing, and he is uncertain as to the complete emptying of the uterine cavity, he should satisfy himself of the
existing condition; and there is no reason whatever to the contrary in the
present era of antiseptic gynecology. He should explore the uterine
cavity, determine the state of affairs, and act accordingly. The proper
course is clearly indicated: retained tissues should be removed, though
it is difficult to formulate precisely the conditions by which action should
be guided.

The circumstances permitting of interference and removal are a patulous os, an open cervical canal, and detachment of ovum or membranes:
these existing, removal is easily accomplished, and should be undertaken
even though no threatening symptoms be present. The indications which
at all times determine and obligate immediate removal are—a putrid discharge, hemorrhage and constitutional symptoms, debility, fever or sepsis;
then immediate removal is necessary at all hazards.

Though it does not appear advisable to remove the ovum, as urged by
Fehling, at once, if the tampon fails after ten or twelve hours' trial, the
physician must not wait until threatening local or constitutional symptoms
appear, as various evils develop insidiously long before removal is so loudly
called for. There are no conditions which could, by any possibility, contraindicate immediate interference if the indications above mentioned exist
—not even inflammations, pelvic cellulitis, or fixation of the uterus, as
is claimed by some. The limits of active interference being given by
the above indications, the practitioner must determine by the greatly-
varying symptoms of the individual case, as he does upon the proper time
of applying the forceps in labor at term. If parts of the ovum remain
in utero, they should be removed as irritating and dangerous; and a patulous os must necessarily lead the practitioner to infer the presence of
such a mass; yet this is not a constant symptom: if the os is closed and

the presence of membranes presumptive, he should dilate and satisfy himself as to the true state of affairs, dilatation with antiseptic precautions being entirely harmless. If remnants are found, the first step to their removal has already been accomplished in the diagnostic dilatation. This is best attained with the patient in complete narcosis and in proper position. The dorsal decubitus and Simon's speculum are preferable to the left-lateral semi-prone position, as we are better able to manipulate the uterus both externally and internally, especially to control the fundus. If the os be not too firmly contracted, the finger may be introduced when anæsthesia is established, and sufficient dilatation thus accomplished, or the scoop may be at once used without further preparation. If time is no object, the uterus is best dilated with a tupelo or carbolized sponge tent; where immediate action is indicated, the finger or steel dilator is best. Molesworth's instrument, even if ready for immediate action, is liable to dilate within the cervical and uterine cavity, remaining contracted at the point of greatest importance, the internal os. Incision with the knife, the splitting open of the cervix, is now recommended by German authors.

The tampon can be of service only where a larger mass is retained, not if the membranes alone remain. The use of the tent for the purpose of dilating is of advantage if introduced well into the uterine cavity, stimulating the muscle, so that expulsion frequently follows dilatation; but even then the curette should be used—the dull instrument—for a careful examination of the cavity. I have already stated the conditions indicating a resort to the sharp scoop, the Simon's or Sims's, or the dull curette, such as Munde's or my own. The wire loop of Thomas is too weak, and serves more for the removal of already loose masses than for the separation of the tissues, which I consider by far the most important. Where possible, it is always preferable to use the dull instrument for purposes of separation; and there is no better than Récamier's old instrument, or, in case of a large cavity, the broad blade of my own; both may be used without dilatation if the contraction of the os is not excessive. If firmer masses are found, as is frequently the case when the placental remnants have been retained for several months, Simon's sharp scoop is indicated, and the smaller size can be used without previous dilatation; the speculum is not necessary, but desirable, but for the effective handling of the instrument it is best that the patient be placed in the lithotomy position, upon the edge of the bed, the hips elevated, with a rubber cloth underneath. It is all-important that the movement of the scoop should be thoroughly controlled by the unengaged hand grasping the uterine fundus: this will serve to fix the organ well and prevent its escaping the instrument. Where the fundus is out of reach, as in retro-displacement, the Schroeder forceps, which is always of great service in bringing the uterus within reach, must be used. In case Récamier's or my own instrument is used, it is curved to adapt itself to the cavity, and, with one edge pressing firmly against the uterine wall toward the point of attachment of the membrane, it is carried around the entire space, so as to separate such adhesions as may exist, and the released membranes are then forced or pressed out with the instrument. In case the sharp spoon is used, it must be handled with great care, pressing firmly against, but not too deeply into, the uterine wall, and carried in regular parallel strokes from the fundus toward the internal os. After such manipulation the cavity should be well washed out with hot water containing from 2 to 5 per cent. of carbolic acid, bichloride of mercury, borax, or permanganate of potash, either with the ordinary syringe or Bozeman's catheter; after this the entire inner surface of the uterus is touched with carbolic acid, a little cotton wrapped upon the end of an applicator and saturated with the solution answering the purpose very well.

Hot water and carbolic acid usually suffice to thoroughly contract the organ; should this not be the case, should a flabby, atonic condition exist, it is well to place a tampon of iron cotton in the cavity. The applicator is loosely wrapped with cotton of sufficient thickness to fill the cavity; this is steeped in Monsel's solution or the perchloride of iron, the superabundant fluid expressed, and then introduced. Contraction is sure to follow, and the tampon is left in place for three or four days, when it will either be expelled by the action of the uterus or it will be found, coated with healthy pus, barely held in the grasp of the muscle, and can be removed by the slightest traction: no effort should be made, as it will remain firmly fixed until a healthy granulating surface is established. It may be kept in place by a tampon of cotton carbolated, or, better still, prepared with iodoform, which is always a desirable application after interference. Ergot should then invariably be given, either by hypodermic injection or per os—if the stomach is in good condition, a teaspoonful of the fluid extract every three hours during the first day.

Putrid discharge and septic symptoms unquestionably indicate immediate interference; the method, however, remains the same. In case of beginning putrid discharge without constitutional symptoms, the dull curette is greatly to be preferred to separate the sloughing tissue from the healthy uterine structure without injuring the latter; whilst if the uterine structure itself is affected, it is necessary to resort to the sharp spoon to thoroughly remove all that is diseased.

Constitutional treatment must, of course, follow the local measures above advocated. The danger of the sharp instrument, under these circumstances, is in the possibility of lacerating healthy tissues and opening new ways for infection. It can only be used if all diseased tissue is thoroughly removed and the operation followed by cauterization with pure carbolic acid and intra-uterine injection, that all remaining particles, however small, may be washed away.

An active general treatment must accompany these local measures, but upon this I will not dwell, as it is the same which must be followed in all cases of septic poisoning. Quinine is the main stay, and in addition to the remedies in general use ergot is here indicated to further contraction and expulsion of offensive particles and close the capillary and lymphatic canals to the possibility of infection.

AFTER-TREATMENT.—It cannot be too often repeated that the danger resulting from abortion is not the immediate or primary one, but the secondary, even in case of profuse hemorrhage; it is that of anæmia, of general debility, a slow getting up. After abortion we have conditions analogous to those of the puerperium, the dangers of infection, of septicæmia, the greater liability of the system to surrounding influences, epidemic, infectious, malarial; but even greater than after labor at term is that of incomplete involution with its chain of insidious consequences. In the main, the danger of abortion lies in the lightness of the affection and the indifference to after-treatment. Involution is more questionable than after labor at term, and yet time and opportunity are rarely given nature to accomplish this process of restitution. If the abortion is passed easily, the patient rarely keeps her bed, pays little or no attention to the occurrence, certainly none to her getting up, and subinvolution, by far the most frequent sequence to abortion, follows. Abortion is altogether the most prolific cause of uterine disease, in consequence of the indifference with which it is treated, not only by the patient, but by her physician. With the expulsion of the ovum and the cessation of hemorrhage the case is considered finished; even if a physician is called, proper time is not given for restitution of the parts. Although by far less is to be accomplished by the retrograde metamorphosis than after labor at full term, the parts being not so fully developed, they are not so thoroughly prepared for this restitution: retrograde metamorphosis has not been initiated with the inauguration of the abortion, as it has with the inauguration of labor at term. In the latter fatty degeneration is in progress; the tissues are prepared for the restorative process which is to follow: not so in case of abortion; hence nature must be assisted, must be allowed to perform those functions which are necessary to a healthy restoration of the sexual organs.

In the great mass of cases it is not strictly medical attention which is necessary, medical treatment, but mere ordinary care, precaution, and cleanliness on the part of the patient herself, so as to assist the efforts of nature: a week's rest in bed with healthy nutritious diet should be accorded every woman who has aborted, and this must be followed by at least one more week of quiet and confinement to the room, and not until a month after the accident has occurred should the patient resume her ordinary vocations.

I will not enter into the details of the after-treatment, as it is identical with that after labor at term. No decided treatment is called for unless demanded by symptoms peculiar to individual cases, yet ergot, quinine, and tonics are in place, and the same antiseptic precautions must be observed which are so highly appreciated in the lying-in room.

The patient must be kept in a recumbent position, the room quiet, and visitors excluded; a bed-pan must be used; the food must be easily digestible and nutritious; prepared tow or salicylated or borated cotton should be used in preference to the old-fashioned cloth to receive the discharge, and this must be changed with sufficient frequency: the parts must be washed with a lukewarm antiseptic wash, and vaginal injections of the same given as cleanliness demands, at least once a day; these should be hot ($110°-120°$) to further contraction. Corrosive sublimate 1 : 2000, carbolic acid 2 : 100, or boracic acid or borate of soda, serves a good purpose; intra-uterine injections are called for only in case of putrid or offensive discharge.

After the third or fourth day it is well to add an astringent, such as alum or tannin, to the hot vaginal douche, a teaspoonful to the quart, beginning with less, as some are very sensitive to these remedies, and increasing the strength if desirable.

Iron and chinine are serviceable in aiding the system to regain its tone and in guarding against zymotic and malarial influences, to which it is more subject in this weakened condition. Ergot is here in its proper place : a three-grain pill of the aqueous extract should be given, at least during the first week, three times a day ; I prefer this to the fluid extract in common use, which is nauseating to many. This drug, so much abused during progressing abortion and in labor before the contents of the uterus are expelled, answers an excellent purpose at this stage, and, together with the hot, astringent douche, may be relied upon to prevent subinvolution.

I can but repeat that the after-treatment should be that of the lying-in room after labor at term, modified according to circumstances, but never to be neglected, not even after the most simple cases. We must remember that it is indifference under these circumstances, under-estimation of the accident, which leads to years of suffering, by which subinvolution so insidiously destroys a vigorous constitution.

Rest, peace of mind, and quiet of body should, together with anti-septic precautions and tonic treatment, follow every abortion, intensified according to the severity of the accident. The two most important, and at the same time most neglected, features in the after-treatment of abortion, both of which are called for in even the most ordinary cases, are rest and cleanliness—rest, quiet of body and mind, to afford the proper conditions for the efforts of nature toward restitution and involution ; cleanliness, antisepsis, to prevent external interference with this process and to guard the lacerated cavity of the womb, which offers so ready a receptacle for septic elements, against the dangers which threaten from without and so frequently bring about the rapidly-fatal termination of an apparently simple abortion.

DISEASES OF THE MUSCULAR SYSTEM.

MYALGIA.

PROGRESSIVE MUSCULAR ATROPHY.

PSEUDO-HYPERTROPHIC PARALYSIS.

MYALGIA.

By JAMES C. WILSON, M. D.

DEFINITION.—An affection of the voluntary muscles, of which the chief, and often the only, symptom is pain on movement.

SYNONYMS.—Myalgia as a general term has few synonyms. It is sometimes called myodynia. This affection has no essential relation to rheumatism or the rheumatic diathesis; therefore the common use of the term muscular rheumatism as a synonym for myalgia is an error. This error has occasioned much confusion of thought and mistaken medication, and tends to maintain the obscurity which overhangs the subject of the so-called and often miscalled rheumatic affections in general. That true rheumatic processes may extend from serous or fibrous structures to contiguous muscular masses has, in the absence of demonstration, been assumed by many writers of authority, but that acute or subacute rheumatism, with its recognized characters, ever manifests itself primarily or exclusively as an inflammation of muscle-substance is an assumption wholly without clinical or pathological support.

The term myo-rheumatism is as inapplicable as muscular rheumatism, and lacks the sanction of usage. Myositis is a term used to describe (1) an acute inflammation of muscle, often traumatic, and commonly attended by suppuration, and (2) a chronic indurating inflammatory process, not infrequently due to syphilis. Neither of these conditions resembles the affection under consideration in its clinical aspects, nor is allied to it pathologically.

As manifested in particular muscles or groups of muscles myalgia has been described under the terms cephalodynia, torticollis (myalgia cervicalis), pleurodynia (m. pectoralis seu intercostalis), lumbago (m. lumbalis), dorsodynia, omodynia, scapulodynia (m. dorsalis), etc.

This affection must, in the present state of our knowledge, be classified with the diseases of nutrition in the more narrow sense. It is not a diathetic disease.

HISTORICAL CONSIDERATIONS.—To Inman[1] of Liverpool is due the credit of having first pointed out the frequency of this malady and the ease with which it may be mistaken for other and much more serious diseases—an error in diagnosis which has been followed by serious results, especially in the case of nervous and self-centred females and other hypochondriacal persons. It cannot, however, be denied that this author, carried away by his enthusiasm, exaggerated the importance of this local

---

[1] Thomas Inman, M. D., *Certain Painful Muscular Affections*, 1856; *Spinal Irritation Explained*, 1858; *On Myalgia, its Nature, Causes, and Treatment*, 1860.

affection at the expense of undervaluing the frequency and significance of other painful disorders which have their origin in the nervous system. To Inman we also owe the term myalgia, which has the positive merit of embodying the idea of pain as the chief symptom of the disorder and the muscles as its seat, and the not inferior negative merit of implying no erroneous theory as to its nature and cause.

This affection is described in few even among the recent textbooks; in others it receives merely incidental mention; in the majority of them it is passed over in silence. Yet it is obvious that the descriptions of muscular rheumatism, which are rarely omitted, are based upon and refer to cases of various kinds which for the most part are not rheumatic at all, and very frequently are examples of true myalgia.

ETIOLOGY.—(*A*) Predisposing Influences.—Myalgia is "essentially pain produced in a muscle which is obliged to work when its structure is imperfectly nourished or impaired by disease." Hence all influences which unfavorably affect the nutrition of the muscles, all diseases which directly affect the integrity of their structure, predispose them to this affection. The defect in nutrition may be only relative to the amount of work the muscle is called upon to do, or there may be absolute malnutrition, implicating the whole body. The muscle may be impaired by a local disease which affects it alone, or it may share in morbid processes which also involve other and distant structures.

Sedentary occupations, leading as they do to poor nutrition of the muscular system from want of proper use and exercise; malnutrition from a diet deficient in amount or defective in kind, or in childhood from too rapid growth; the chronic wasting diseases; the state of convalescence from acute maladies; and, finally, degenerative diseases of the muscles themselves,—all favor the development of myalgia. Among the acute diseases which by their derangement of nutritive processes especially render those who have suffered from them liable to this painful affection of the muscles during convalescence, is acute articular rheumatism or rheumatic fever. It is this fact, taken together with the use of a misnomer, that has given rise to the view that the muscles share with the serous and fibrous structures in the lesions of that disease, and that myalgia is rheumatism of the muscles.

There is, however, over and above these defects in nutrition, an especial predisposition or idiosyncrasy, the nature of which is unknown, which renders certain individuals far more liable to suffer myalgic pain than others. This predisposition is encountered in those who have an inherited or acquired gouty habit and in those who are free from gout with perhaps equal frequency. It is not associated with a special liability to true rheumatism.

(*B*) Exciting Causes.—Myalgia is a local affection, and depends for its causation upon a derangement of the balance between the nutrition of the affected muscles and the work they have been called upon to do. Hence the most common exciting cause is (*a*) overwork pure and simple, especially overwork which brings into excessive and prolonged exercise unaccustomed muscles. Next in frequency is (*b*) exposure to cold, and especially to damp cold, when overheated or overfatigued. Finally (*c*), inevitable and incessant contractions, such as are physiological and are performed without consciousness or sensation in a healthy state of the muscles, will, in muscles that are defectively nourished or have undergone fatty, granular, or fibroid degeneration, cause more or less distinct myalgia.

As examples of myalgia due to the first of this group of causes (*a*) I may cite the pain in the adductors of the thighs after a hard ride when out of practice; the epigastric pain in children suffering from measles or other acute affection attended with persistent cough; and the pain of spasm, in particular that which follows tonic spasm, such as occurs from reflex causes in the calves of the legs at night and in bathers. Many of the pains of childhood, which are classed in common parlance together under the name of growing pains, are myalgic in their nature.

Examples of the second form (*b*) may be instanced in the pains of wry neck or lumbago, such as often occur in those who, being very tired, but otherwise healthy, fall asleep in a draught of air, or in those who, coming home at evening in cold weather, find a leaking pipe in the cellar, and stooping over to stop it, or in some other emergency of every-day life, bring into excessive use unaccustomed muscles in an atmosphere that is at once cold and damp.

Examples of the third group (c) are common enough in the flying or fixed muscular pains and soreness that occur in wasting chronic diseases and in the convalescence from acute maladies when prolonged muscular effort is too early undertaken. Certain forms of præcordial pain that occur in degenerative lesions of the muscular substance of the heart are without doubt myalgic in character, and will, when the clinical data of such conditions come to be more fully understood, be recognized as having more or less diagnostic value.

SYMPTOMATOLOGY.—The chief symptom, the one symptom that is common to all the cases, is pain. It is sometimes, especially in acute cases, constant; more frequently it is very slight or wholly absent when the patient is at rest, with the affected muscles in full extension, but it is invariably present or aggravated when the muscles are called into action. It is experienced throughout the muscular mass, but is most intense at or near the point of tendinous insertion. Its character is usually stabbing or stitch-like, but prolonged; sometimes it is acutely dragging or tearing; in others it is like the soreness felt on moving a contused or inflamed part. It is frequently in acute cases, almost always in chronic cases, accompanied by a sensation of stiffness in the affected muscles. The pain is essentially the same in all cases, variations in its character and severity being determined by the opportunities afforded the muscle for physiological rest. It is in accordance with this statement that the most obstinate, and the most severe form of myalgia is that which occurs in the intercostal muscles and their fibrous aponeuroses—pleurodynia. Here the affected muscles are constantly concerned in the movements of respiration, and have no time for physiological rest except in the intervals of those movements. Scarcely less stubborn and severe are the myalgias of the great muscular masses, of which the principal function is to maintain by their nicely-balanced and ever-varying contractions the erect position of the head and trunk. Less painful and of shorter duration are the myalgias of the limbs—less painful because prolonged intervals of absolute rest may be voluntarily secured; of shorter duration, because it is by rest that the balance of the nutrition is most speedily restored.

There is usually some degree of tenderness over the whole extent of the myalgic area, becoming more marked in the regions of tendinous insertion, to which it is, however, in many cases restricted. It is elicited upon moderately firm pressure, and is not associated with cutaneous hyperæsthesia.

Spasm is absent in the acute cases, except when the muscles are brought into use. Its occurrence has much to do with the intensity of the suffering then caused : in chronic cases a condition of tonic spasm or spastic rigidity, with more or less persistent painfulness, comes on, and finally in very chronic cases such tissue-changes take place as result in great impairment or absolute loss of contractile power, with or without atrophy.

Objective signs are absent, except that it is evident that the patient assumes by preference an attitude of repose, and that he keeps the involved structures as much at rest as possible. Pyrexia does not occur ; the appetite and digestion are not impaired ; acid sweats are not present ; the urine shows no constant or characteristic alteration ; there is no tendency to endo- or pericardial inflammation. If constitutional disturbance be present, it is trifling and due to prolonged local suffering and want of sleep. In by far the greater number of instances the patient remains in his usual health except the local malady.

Myalgia may affect the voluntary, and perhaps also the involuntary, muscles of any part of the body. Those most frequently involved are those subjected to continuous and excessive work, and at the same time liable to exposure to cold and damp. Single muscles or groups may be affected. The most common and important varieties are—

(1) Cephalodynia, manifested as a superficial headache, increased by movement of the scalp and attended by tenderness on pressure.

(2) Torticollis ; wry neck, stiff neck—a very common form, involving the muscles of the neck, especially the sterno-cleido-mastoid. The affection is usually limited to one side, toward which the occiput is more or less firmly rotated and flexed. Great pain is experienced in attempting to turn the head in the opposite direction. The position is extremely constrained and awkward ; the head cannot be moved in any direction without moving the whole body, and every effort at motion is accompanied by pain which calls forth involuntary grimaces.

(3) Omodynia, Scapulodynia, Dorsodynia—forms in which the muscles of the shoulders and upper part of the back are affected. They are very common, especially among laboring men.

(4) Pleurodynia, Myalgia of the Chest-walls.—The intercostals, pectorals, and serratus magnus may be involved. The pain is frequently referred to the region of the interdigitations of the serratus magnus with the external oblique. It is very often seated in the infra-axillary region, and is much more common on the left side. It is usually very severe, and is increased by all movements that bring the affected muscles into play. The focus of pain is sometimes a very limited spot, which is exquisitely tender upon pressure. Sometimes the pain alters its position from time to time. It is increased by deep inspiratory efforts and such acts as sneezing and coughing. Extreme flexion of the trunk from side to side also aggravates the pain. Pleurodynia sometimes comes on in consequence of severe and protracted cough, as in patients suffering with phthisis. It is then apt to affect both sides.

This form of myalgia simulates pleurisy, from which it is to be distinguished only by careful physical examination.

(5) Myalgia of the abdominal walls usually affects the recti muscles, and often assumes the guise of an acute, agonizing pain in the epigastric or pubic regions—occasionally so severe as to be mistaken for peritonitis. It is sometimes due to cough, especially in measles, but is more commonly met with in overworked and underfed tailors and cobblers as a result of the excessive action of the recti muscles in maintaining the bent posture assumed by such craftsmen at their toil.

(6) Lumbago, myalgia lumbalis.—The great muscular mass occupying the lumbar region is peculiarly prone to attacks of myalgia. Lumbago is very common in the middle and later periods of life. The attack is usually sudden and severe. Both sides are, as a rule, affected, but not to the same extent. There is constant pain across the loins, dull and aching, rarely absent altogether, always sharply aggravated by such movements as bring the affected muscles into play, and then becoming stabbing in character and almost unbearable in intensity. The spine is held stiffly, and the body is often bent slightly forward. Efforts to stand erect, to rise from the sitting posture, or to recover from the stooping position, such as is assumed in lacing one's shoes and the like, greatly aggravate the pain. In the more severe cases the patient cannot stir in his bed. There is usually tenderness upon pressure, and palpation often discovers a distinct sense of abnormal tension and resistance in the muscles.

(7) The aching, dragging pain in the back of the neck common in poorly-nourished, nervous women and in other cases of neurasthenia, the so-called pain of nervous exhaustion, is myalgia. It is felt chiefly during fatigue, is present in the erect posture, and is almost always relieved when the patient lies down. It is referred sometimes to the base of the skull, sometimes to the whole of the back of the neck, but more commonly to the spinal region just above the level of the upper borders of the scapula, and constitutes a harassing symptom of the cases in which it occurs. In this connection it must be pointed out that many of the pains of that obscure condition to which the term spinal irritation has been vaguely applied are myalgic.

Myalgia manifests itself furthermore in the limbs, in the diaphragm, and occasionally in the muscles of the eyeballs.

The COURSE of the attack is in the simpler forms acute and transient; it frequently, however, becomes chronic, and not uncommonly presents the characters of the chronic form from the beginning. Again, it sometimes attacks in succession several muscles or groups of muscles, and in by far the greater number of individuals it shows a tendency to recur from time to time.

DURATION.—The duration of acute attacks is usually brief, lasting from a few hours to several days; that of the chronic form is indefinite, tending to last years, sometimes, under unfavorable circumstances, a lifetime, with varying periods of exacerbation and remission, which are, after the disease is fully established, much influenced by the phases of the weather.

The TERMINATION of acute myalgia is commonly in full recovery, but the tendency to subsequent attacks is to be borne in mind, and guarded against by the exercise of wholesome precautions in the matter of hygiene. Neglected cases of chronic myalgia not rarely terminate in permanent alterations of the muscular structure, with loss of contractile power and rigidity, with or without atrophy.

COMPLICATIONS.—In the acute forms there are no complications, properly so called. In the more severe cases of the chronic form there is danger of nutritive changes in the tissues entering into the formation of joints, and loss of function from want of use.

SEQUELS.—There are no sequels other than those just pointed out.

PATHOLOGY AND MORBID ANATOMY.—As indicated by the various names by which myalgia has been known, the principal theories advanced to account for the morbid manifestations are three in number: (1) that the malady is a rheumatism of the muscles; (2) a form of neuralgia; (3) an inflammation.

(1) Muscular Rheumatism.—That this affection should be popularly associated with rheumatism is not surprising when the character of the pain is regarded, its aggravation on movement, and the temporary or permanent crippling which it occasions; especially when we call to mind the exceedingly vague and indefinite ideas which prevail in regard to rheumatism. But that it should be looked upon, far and wide, among physicians as a form of rheumatism, and described as such in the systematic works—that it should be regarded as due to the same causes as rheumatism and treated from that point of view—is certainly as remarkable as it is misleading.

Let us look at the facts. Nothing is easier: the two affections are under our daily observation side by side; in this climate and among working people few maladies are more common.

On the one hand we behold a constitutional disease with widespread manifestations—a special joint inflammation, which tends neither to the deposit of urate of soda nor to suppuration; a peculiar acid secretion from the skin; highly acid urine; a notable tendency to inflammatory heart complications; marked pyrexia. We observe also a marked disposition to recurrence and to the hereditary transmission of the diathesis.

The phenomena of rheumatism may be ill defined; that is to say, the attack may be subacute, but the features are the same; or they may linger and assume the chronic form, in which fever is replaced by a peculiar alteration in the fluids of the body, showing itself in a dull anæmic complexion and a greasy skin; but in all cases the seat of the disease-signs is in the joints; it is articular.

On the other hand, myalgia is not a general malady nor the expression of one. It is scarcely a disease at all. It is purely local. A muscle or a group of muscles, overworked, cry out, and this cry is interpreted by the sensation of pain. It is to be borne in mind that the overwork may be absolute, or merely relative to the healthfulness of the muscle at the time. In either case there is a derangement between the balance of work and nutrition in the muscle. The secretions are not altered; there is no sweating; the urine presents no abnormal conditions. Endo- and pericarditis never occur as complications; fever is absent.

The attack is often light, and quickly passes away. If it become chronic, further nutritive changes take place. The muscle becomes rigid, and often atrophies. According to Froriep and Virchow, as quoted by Jaccoud[1] and Niemeyer,[2] the fasciculi are beset here and there with thickened connective tissue. Vogel observed in several chronic cases the neurilemma of the nerves supplying the part to be thickened, hardened, and adherent.

In all cases the affection limits itself to the muscles. The joints remain free. When they undergo changes it is after a long time and as a result of want of use or of reflex disturbances of nutrition through the nervous system. Nothing is known of hereditary predisposition to myalgia. In the manifest tendency to recur in the same individual it and rheumatism are alike. In all essential points their clinical resemblance is of the most superficial kind. It is clear, then, that the processes which give rise to the phenomena of rheumatism do not directly affect the muscular system.

The credit of having first formulated this opinion, previously only vaguely recognized, is due to Roche and Cruveilhier,[3] but Valleix, Garrod, Flint, and other writers, who describe myalgia under the head of muscular rheumatism, coincide in this view. Even the statement that the two diseases are constantly associated is not borne out by the results of extended clinical inquiries. My own observation has not confirmed it. Of 7 cases[4] taken at random to illustrate a point of treatment, 1 had followed an attack of rheumatic fever; 1 occurred in an individual who had many years before suffered from rheumatism; and 5 gave no history whatever of that disease: 1 followed tonsillitis. DaCosta[5] details 2 cases of myalgia—1 in the loins (lumbago), associated with bronchitis or following it, the other occurring during an attack of rheumatic fever and having its seat in the muscles of the neck. In the latter case the constitutional disease yielded to treatment which had no effect upon the local malady. Even were the association much more frequent than it is found to be, the fact would by no means establish a common causation, seeing that myalgia follows other diseases which impair the nutrition of the body. It is worthy of note that the groups of muscles most frequently involved in cases which happen during or after acute diseases are those which must work perforce—those which maintain the equilibrium of the body or carry on respiration, etc. Hence we see wry neck, lumbago, pleurodynia associated with other diseases; affections of the muscles of the extremities after overwork pure and simple.

(2) Neuralgia.—Many observers have regarded myalgia as a neuralgia, having its seat in the muscles. Valleix[6] wrote as follows: " Muscular rheumatism and neuralgia have, in the correspondence of their symptoms, their course, their exacerbations, in the absence of appreciable anatomical lesions, the greatest resemblance to each other. These affections often pass the one into the other. . . . . The pain, which is the capital symptom of neuralgia, expresses itself, according to our observation, in three ways: If it remain concentrated in the nerves, characteristic isolated painful points are found ; here is neuralgia properly so called. If the pain is diffused among the muscles, muscular action is principally painful; we have muscular rheumatism. Finally, if it be spread out upon the skin, an excessive sensibility of the cutaneous surface results, and there exists

---

[1] *Traité de Pathologie interne.* Paris, 1871.
[2] *Lehrbuch der Speciellen Pathologie und Therapie*, Berlin, 1871.
[3] *Dict. de Méd. et de Chir. prat.*, article " Arthrite."
[4] *Philada. Med. Times*, Nov. 7, 1874. [5] *Penna. Hospital Reports*, vol. i
[6] *Loc cit.*

a dermalgia. These three forms of an affection which is the same may all be present at the same time, or two and two—neuralgia and dermalgia, neuralgia and rheumatism, rheumatism and dermalgia." No wonder he found nothing more difficult than to trace with exactitude the picture of this malady.

Flint1 also regards myalgia as closely allied to neuralgia, and states that, " being one of the neuroses, it has no anatomical characters." It is not difficult to trace the results of this teaching in the widespread confusion prevalent in regard to some very common painful affections, as, for example, that painful form of stitch known as pleurodynia, and the still more distressing gastrodynia. Even those observers who refuse to class these affections as rheumatic are too often at a loss as to whether they are neuralgic or purely muscular. Anstie[2] has concisely contrasted the most important characters of neuralgia and myalgia in a way that strongly urges the clinical differences between them, as follows:

NEURALGIA.	MYALGIA.
Follows the distribution of a recognizable nerve or nerves.	Attacks a limited patch or patches that can be identified with the tendon or aponeurosis of a muscle, which, on inquiry, will be found to have been hardly worked.
Goes along with an inherited or acquired nervous temperament, which is obvious.	As often as not occurs in persons with no special neurotic tendency.
Is much less aggravated, usually, by movement than myalgia is.	Is inevitably and very severely aggravated by every movement of the part.
Is at first accompanied by no local tenderness.	Distinguished from the first by localized tenderness on pressure as well as on movement.
Points douloureux, when established at a later stage, correspond to the emergence of nerves.	Tender points correspond to tendinous origins and insertions of muscles.
Pain not materially relieved by any change of posture.	Pain usually completely, and always considerably, relieved by full extension of the painful muscle or muscles.

(3) Inflammation.—That the muscular affection under consideration should have been referred to morbid processes of an inflammatory kind is very natural. The use of the term myositis embodies this view, which is held, among others, by Garrod. This author defines muscular rheumatism as " an affection of the voluntary muscles of an inflammatory nature (?), but unaccompanied with swelling, heat, redness, or febrile disturbance." He assigns the combined influence of cold and damp as a cause, especially when associated with over-use of the muscles.

Though some of the gross characters of inflammation are wanting, and the course of acute cases of myalgia is toward a speedy resolution, there are several features of the affection which strongly suggest its inflammatory origin. At all events, the view that the essential pathological conditions consist in a hyperæmia with slight serous exudation, or a partial paralysis of vaso-motor nerves with escape of serum into the intimate tissues of the muscles, has, from a clinical standpoint, much to support it. In the absence of knowledge derived from the actual investigation of the morbid tissue-changes in all the stages of the affection some

<hr>

[1] *Practice of Medicine.*   [2] *Neuralgia and Diseases that Resemble it*

value is to be accorded to the following facts as confirmatory of this opinion :

It is a local affection ; the onset is usually sudden ; there is often, from the beginning, a slight but obvious fulness of the muscle ; tenderness is present as well as pain ; in chronic cases inflammatory increase of connective tissue occurs, with changes in the nerve-sheaths and fatty degeneration of muscle-substance. Moreover, the permanent contraction (contracture) which sometimes finally sets in is the same as that which follows true inflammation of muscles after injuries (traumatic myositis [1]).

It is uncertain whether the nerves supplying the muscles are thrown into morbid action by changes in the muscular fibres and in their sarcolemma, or by simultaneous changes in their own neurilemma. However it arise, irritation of sensory nerve-twigs is present, giving rise to pain, along with irritation of motor filaments, which occasions spasm.

It is probable that the ultimate cause of the irritation within the muscular mass, whatever it is, is common to all cases, and that when myalgia occurs in a healthy man after extraordinary muscular effort or exposure to cold damp when fatigued, or in a delicate child who has played too long, or in a poorly-fed weaver working long hours over his loom, or in the consumptive whose cough gives him no rest, or in connection with any chronic disease or acute disease, whether tonsillitis or bronchitis or fever or rheumatism, it is the same thing—the expression of muscles or groups of muscles overworked. It is not a disease ; it is not a symptom of disease. It is an accident of many diseases—of any disease that lowers nutrition. And it is not less an accident of health when such muscular effort is demanded as is beyond the capacity of health.

The essential pathology of myalgia is obscure. It is not an inflammation, as that term is generally understood, but there is ground for the opinion that the lesions are of the nature of a subinflammatory process within the muscle. The not uncommon instances in which an injury or contusion—in short, traumatism—has been followed shortly after the recovery by severe myalgia are of further value as illustrating this theory.

The obstacles in the way of precise histological investigation in cases of acute myalgia are so great that it seems probable that further knowledge is to be reached for the most part by way of clinical work.

DIAGNOSIS.—The fundamental question for consideration in this place is whether we are dealing in any given case with local manifestations of a constitutional disease or with purely local phenomena. That the latter is the correct view seems to the writer to admit of no further discussion in this article. This position being assumed, and due regard having already been paid to the differential diagnosis between myalgia and rheumatism, neuralgia and inflammatory myositis, it seems useless to enter upon the consideration of the diagnosis between this and other painful affections to which it bears but slight and superficial resemblances. Spinal irritation, hypochondriasis, locomotor ataxia, alcoholism, syphilis, gout, and lithiasis are on the one hand attended by pains which are clearly not myalgic in character, and on the other hand peculiarly predispose those subject to them to this affection of poorly-nourished and easily-overworked muscles. Each of these diseases, however, presents a complexus of symp-

[1] Erb, *Ziemssen's Cyclopædia*, vol. ix.

toms in which that which is essential and characteristic is readily to be distinguished from that which—as myalgia—is accidental.

A few words concerning the diagnosis of some of the varieties may not be amiss.

In pleurodynia the ordinary physical signs of pleural, pulmonary, and cardiac disease are absent, the painful points characteristic of intercostal neuralgia are not found, and there is little or no constitutional disturbance.

The diagnosis of myalgia lumbalis is, as a rule, unattended by difficulty. The muscular pain in the loins is characteristic. It is greatly increased by efforts to rise or to turn in bed, and is associated with diffused slight tenderness upon pressure, but never with the acute localized soreness of neuralgia or abscess. The practitioner must, however, guard against the danger of mistaking the back pains of more serious affections for lumbago by the careful examination, in all cases, of the back and abdomen, and by the investigation of the condition of the urine. The possibility that pain in this region may be caused by spinal meningitis, lumbar abscess from spinal caries, sciatica, inflammatory affections of the hip-joint, renal calculus, perinephritis, abdominal aneurism, diseases of the pelvic viscera, and the onset of certain of the acute infectious diseases must not be overlooked.

PROGNOSIS.—Under satisfactory conditions as regards hygiene and treatment the prognosis is always favorable. It becomes in chronic cases unfavorable as regards complete recovery when by reason of poverty, unhealthy occupations, unwholesome surroundings, or established wasting diseases the nutrition of the muscles and their physiological rest are permanently interfered with, and the balance between their power and work permanently deranged.

TREATMENT.—The indications are threefold : (a) relief of pain ; (b) physiological rest for the affected muscles ; (c) restoration of the balance between the nutrition of the muscle and the work it has to do.

(a) Relief of pain is often secured by rest in a posture that permits the complete relaxation of the muscles involved. In acute cases due to overwork pure and simple, and where complete rest is attainable, little other treatment is required. In the course of a few hours or days the function of the muscles is fully restored and their contractions are performed without pain. Where, however, complete muscular relaxation is impracticable or fails to afford relief, anodynes are necessary. Morphine hypodermically is very useful, but this altogether independently of any local action. Continuous dry or moist heat by means of flannels, flaxseed poultices, spongio-piline, etc. may be applied. Various anodyne lotions· are useful. Liniments containing aconite, belladonna, chloroform, or chloral also afford relief. The compound belladonna liniment of the British Pharmacopœia is especially to be recommended. So also are plasters of belladonna, conium, and mustard. Galvanism occasionally gives prompt relief. The same statement may be made of the use of static electricity. The pain sometimes disappears under gentle and long-continued massage.

(b) Rest is usually enforced by the intensity of the pain attending movement. In severe cases the bed is a necessity. In affections of the respiratory muscles, as pleurodynia, firm support of the side, by means of overlapping strips of plaster drawn from the spine downward and forward in the direction of the ribs to the median line in front, is sometimes necessary and always comfortable.

(c) The balance of nutrition is restored by rest. Local means to further this end are such as relieve pain—heat, anodyne and stimulating frictions, massage, and galvanism. The parts must be protected from sudden changes in temperature by extra thicknesses of flannel or sheets of wool or cotton batting—if necessary covered with a piece of oiled silk or fine gum-cloth. In old cases prolonged massage with passive movements, shampooing, and the slowly interrupted galvanic current, alternating with rapid faradic currents, are followed by good results.

As a constitutional measure a Dover's powder at night, followed by mild purgation in the morning, is often indicated. Purgation is especially called for in plethoric or gouty persons, in whom also Turkish or vapor baths are of great service, while poorly-nourished, anæmic subjects demand quinine, iron, lime, and cod-liver oil. If the attack linger, full doses of ammonium chloride, and in old eases potassium iodide in moderate doses well diluted and long continued, are advocated; and in stubborn cases Anstie recommends deep acupuncture of the muscle near its tendinous attachment. In cases marked by a tendency to spastic rigidity the repeated hypodermic injection of atropine may often be relied upon as the speediest means of cure.

Where the general nutrition is poor the local trouble is apt to be obstinate, and often yields only to measures that restore the general health.

PROGRESSIVE MUSCULAR ATROPHY.[1]

By JAMES TYSON, A. M., M. D.

SYNONYMS.—Chronic anterior poliomyelitis; Spinal form of progressive muscular atrophy; Adult form of progressive muscular atrophy; Wasting palsy (Roberts); Cruveilhier's atrophy; Amyotrophia spinalis progressiva (Erb).

DEFINITION.—Progressive muscular atrophy is a gradually progressive wasting of a group or groups of voluntary muscles, independent of primary functional inactivity and of local lesion to nerve or muscle.

HISTORY.—We are indebted to William Roberts[2] for the best historical account of this disease up to the date of publication of his monograph. Van Swieten seems to have described the first case, in 1754, but without comment. Cooke in his work *On Palsy,*[3] published 1822, relates a case which had been under the care of Cline—that of an officer, first attacked in 1795. Caleb H. Parry[4] reported another case in 1825, and Sir Charles Bell[5] three cases in 1830. Abercrombie described a marked case in 1828,[6] Dorwall[7] three striking cases in 1831, and Herbert Mayo[8] two evident cases in 1836. In 1849, Duchenne presented to the Institute of France his memoir on *Atrophie musculaire avec Transformation graisseuse.* In the next year Aran published his essay entitled *Recherches sur une Maladie non encore décide du Système musculaire (Atrophie musculaire progressive),*[9] in which he claimed priority in description. He reported in all eleven cases, and regarded it as a primary muscular affection. Aran's researches were very important, and have caused his name to be intimately associated with the disease along with that of Duchenne.

Cruveilhier's studies were commenced as early as 1832, but his results were not published until March, 1853,[10] when he read his memoir before the Academy of Medicine of Paris. He seems to have made the first autopsy, and was much surprised at the absence of any apparent lesion of the

---

[1] From the view taken by the author as to the nature of the disease under consideration, it is evident that its proper position would be under affections of the nervous system. But as this view has not been established to the satisfaction of all who have studied the disease, it seems appropriate to place it in the intermediate position selected for it by the Editor, between muscular and nervous diseases.

[2] *An Essay on Wasting Palsy,* London, 1858.

[3] London, 1822, p 31.

[4] *Collected Works,* London, 1825, p. 523.

[5] *The Nervous System of the Human Body,* London, 1830.

[6] *On the Brain and Spinal Cord,* 1828, p. 419.

[7] *London Medical Gazette,* vol. vii., 1830–31, p. 201.

[8] *Outlines of Human Pathology,* London, 1836.

[9] *Archives générales de Méd.,* t. xxiv., Sept. and Oct., 1850.

[10] *Ibid.,* May, 1853, p. 561.

spinal cord. So enthusiastic and so exhaustive was his study of the disease that his name, too, has become almost inseparably associated with it, and the term Cruveilhier's atrophy is one of those by which it is known. He concluded from his earlier autopsies that the lesions were solely in the muscular system, which is progressively destroyed, while the brain and spinal cord may remain perfectly normal. In a later case (his third), terminating January, 1853, he found atrophy of the anterior roots of the spinal nerves, and then concluded that the disease resided "not in the muscles themselves, but in the anterior roots of the spinal nerves." But after the termination of his fourth case, in which an autopsy was also secured, he placed the primary lesion in the gray matter of the cord, whence he considered the anterior roots take their origin.

Thouvenet,[1] an interne of Cruveilhier's, published in 1851 a thesis based on some cases collected in the Charité, and was the first to claim that the disease resides primarily in the peripheral nerves, and that it must be classed among rheumatic affections.

In December, 1851, E. Meryon[2] read a paper before the Medico-Chirurgical Society of London entitled "Granular and Fatty Degeneration of the Voluntary Muscles." His observations appear to have been made quite independently of any preceding researches. He argues that the primary morbid change is a default of nutrition in the muscular fibres.

Subsequently, cases were published in 1853 by Bouvier, Landry, Burg, and Niepce in France; in 1854 by Chambers in England, Guérin and Robin in France, Cohn, Virchow, and Betz in Germany, and by Schneevogt in Holland; in 1855 laborious essays were published by Oppenheimer, Wachsmuth, and Eisenmann, and cases by Hasse, Valentiner, Virchow, Meyer, and Diemer in Germany, and Gros in France. Duchenne's work on *Local Application of Electricity*, also published in 1855, contains much information on the subject.

Since 1855 the reports of cases and papers on the subject have been so numerous as to make it unprofitable to enumerate them. Among the most notable are those of Eisenmann, published in *Canstatt's Jahresbericht* for 1856; Roberts's classic work on *Wasting Palsy*, in 1858; the papers of Lockhart Clarke in 1866 and 1867,[3] and of Swarzenski in 1867;[4] Kussmaul's clinical lecture[5] and Friedreich's treatise[6] in 1873; and Eulenburg's article on "Progressive Muscular Atrophy" in *Ziemssen's Cyclopædia of Practical Medicine*, published in German in 1875 and in English in 1877. An important case, in consequence of the careful post-mortem study of the nervous tissues, is one recently reported by Wood and Dercam.[7]

ETIOLOGY.—The cause of this affection in a large number of cases is quite unknown. That hereditation plays an important part seems well determined by numerous observations, among which may be mentioned those of Roberts, Friedreich, Hemptenmacher, Trousseau, Meryon,

[1] *Gaz. des Hôp.*, Nos. 143 and 145, 1851.   [2] *Med.-Chir. Trans.*, vol. xxxv. p. 73.
[3] *Med.-Chir. Transactions*, xlix., 1866, p. 171, and l., 1867, p. 489.
[4] *Die Progressive Muskelatrophie*, Berlin.
[5] "Ueber die fortschreidende Bulbärparalyse und ihr Verhältniss zur progressiven Muskelatrophie," *Sammlung klinische Vorträge*, liv.
[6] *Ueber progressive Muskelatrophie, über wahre und falsche Muskelhypertrophie*, Berlin, 1873.
[7] *Therapeutic Gazette*, March 16, 1885.

Eulenburg, Sr. and Jr., Naunyn,[1] Hammond, and Ósler.[2]   In the Farr family, reported by Osler, 13 individuals in two generations have been affected, 6 females and 7 males—a larger proportion of the former than is common in this disease.   Of these 9 had died at date of publication of paper.   With the exception of two, all occurred or proved fatal after the age of forty.   Of the 10 instances in the second generation, 5 are the offspring of males and 5 the offspring of females.   The disease has not yet appeared in the third generation, which promises between forty and fifty individuals, several of whom are over thirty years of age.

The over-use of the muscles involved seems to be a well-determined cause in certain cases of true muscular atrophy.   The following interesting illustrations are given by Eulenburg:[3] Betz observed atrophy of the side three times in the cases of smiths and saddlers, who had to do heavy work with the right hand; Gull, in a tailor after excessive exertion; Hammond reports a case apparently due to excessive use of one thumb and finger in playing faro; Friedreich, one of a dragoon who may have exhausted his left hand in holding the bridle while riding; another in a morocco-leather worker, who used to press hard with his left hand; and a musician who played several hours a day on the bass viol.   Schnee-vogt names two cases of primary atrophy of the shoulder-muscles, especially of the deltoid of the right side—one of a sailor who had to pump for days together on a leaking ship, and the other of the left side in a woman who always carried her child on the left arm while suckling it. Continued threshing and the handling of a musket have both been followed by it in the muscles called into play by these exercises.   Roberts was able to trace the effects of over-muscular exertion in producing the disease in 35 out of 69 cases.   As a determining cause, at least, therefore, we must admit the over-use of muscles.

There is reason to believe, too, that this form of atrophy is one of the consequences of senility—that the tendency to connective-tissue over-growth which characterizes old age operates to produce, in a way to be presently explained, an atrophy of groups of muscles.   In a woman aged seventy, now under my care, the fingers of both hands are clawed—became so inappreciably almost, and the condition is still increasing.

In addition to the above-named causes, long-continued exposure to cold, and especially to the action of very cold water, has been named.   Traumatic influences, such as injuries to nerve and muscle, have been called upon to account for localized and progressive atrophy, but these are excluded by our definition from the category of true progressive muscular atrophy.

Cases have also occurred in the course of convalescence.   Typhoid fever, rheumatism, measles, scarlet fever, cold during salivation, vaccination, childbed, excessive venery, syphilis,—have all been held responsible for a certain number of cases.

AGE AND SEX.—In examining the literature of acute muscular atrophy it is found that cases are reported at all ages.   Thus, Wachsmuth, quoted by Eulenburg, found among 49 cases 13 under the age of fifteen, 8 from fifteen to twenty, 22 from twenty to fifty, and only 6 over fifty years. On the other hand, Roberts—who, following Aran, divides the disease into the general form and partial form—says the latter very rarely falls on indi-

[1] *Berliner med. Wochenschrift*, Nos. 42 and 43, 1873.
[2] *Archives of Medicine*, vol. iv., No. 3, Dec., 1880.   [3] *Op. cit.*

viduals under adult age or over fifty, while the average age of the instances of the partial form studied by him was thirty-two years and four months. In 10 instances of the general form the patients were under twelve, and 2 more are reported as children; 1 was said to be sixty-nine and another fifty-four, the average being twenty-eight years and three months. Of Eulenburg's own cases, 7 acquired the disease before the age of ten, 6 before the twentieth year, 2 before the thirtieth, 8 before the fortieth, 5 before the fiftieth, and none later. The latter observer also finds that whenever the disease is hereditary it occurs earlier, usually before the close of the twentieth year. This was certainly not the case in the Farr family, reported by Osler.

I am inclined to believe, especially in the light of Charcot's[1] and of Erb's[2] recent studies, that the true spinal form of progressive muscular atrophy is a disease of adult life, and that the majority of cases reported as occurring in early life are instances either of what Erb calls the juvenile form of progressive muscular atrophy or of pseudo-hypertrophic paralysis.

As to sex, males predominate. Thus, according to Friedreich's statistics, out of 176 cases but 33 were females, or about 19 per cent. Of Roberts's collection of 99, 84 were males and 15 females. Of 28 cases noted by Eulenburg, 17 were in men and 11 women. This is doubtless owing to the fact that men are subjected to the causes of the disease more than women. For Roberts early noted that women who engage in needle-work, washing, and household service are apparently not less liable than men similarly employed, and he found that of those whose labor did not press excessively on any particular sets of muscles females formed even a majority of cases.

Some singular freaks of selection have presented themselves in the matter of sex, particularly in the cases which have been ascribed to hereditation. Thus it will sometimes attack only the male members of a family. A remarkable instance of this was observed by Meryon, in which four sons were attacked and six daughters remained unaffected; and, again, two boys were attacked and two sisters escaped. This may occur also independent of hereditation. Occasionally the reverse takes place, the sisters only being attacked, while the brothers escape.

PATHOLGICAL ANATOMY AND HISTOLOGY.—Two principal seats of change have been found to exist in connection with progressive muscular atrophy. The first and easiest recognized is, of course, the alteration in muscles; the second, that in the nervous system.

The muscular change is simple, and affords a typical instance of what is known as numerical atrophy. The muscular fasciculi one after another undergo fatty metamorphosis, succeeded by absorption of the resulting fat and substitution of connective tissue. The rate of atrophy varies, but sooner or later the muscle is more or less substituted by fibrous bands and cords, over which may be traced reddish lines which represent muscular tissue in a normal state.

The rationale of these changes has not been always the same. The

---

[1] "Revision nosographique des Atrophies musculaires progressive," *Le Progrès méd.*, No. 10, 1885, i. 314–335.

[2] "Ueber die Juvenile Form der Progressive Muskelatrophie und ihre Beziehungen zur sogenannten Pseudohypertrophie," *Deutsches Archiv für klin. Med.*, xxxiv. 1884, S. 467.

older observers regarded them as the result of a primary fatty metamorphosis of muscular fasciculi, followed by absorption of the resulting fat. Later it was asserted that the atrophy is secondary to a myositis or inflammation of muscle, beginning as a hyperplasia of the interstitial connective tissue in its finest ramifications between the single primitive fibrils. Along with this are seen the results of irritation in the primitive bundles themselves, shown by swelling and multiplication of the muscular corpuscles, proliferation of their nuclei, and sometimes cloudy swelling. Even hypertrophied muscular fasciculi and dichotomous and trichotomous subdivision have been noted by Friedreich.

It sometimes happens that the hyperplastic process in the intermuscular connective tissue is succeeded by a fatty infiltration of the cells of the connective tissue, and there results a lipomatosis which is invariably outside of the muscular fasciculi and between them. This gives rise to an appearance of hypertrophy which is only apparent, for the muscular fasciculi are themselves wasted, and proportionally paralytic. This is seen to occur particularly in the muscles of the calves of the legs, in which is produced an appearance identical with that in the disease known as pseudo-hypertrophic muscular paralysis, with which, indeed, the condition under consideration is considered by some identical. But although we must admit in certain cases a complication of a certain degree of lipomatosis with progressive muscular atrophy, the two diseases are essentially different; and it is quite likely that in some instances pseudo-hypertrophic muscular paralysis has been mistaken for progressive muscular atrophy.

The changes in the nervous system are not nearly so simple. They have been noted in the peripheral nerves, both in their trunks and in their intermuscular branches; in the anterior roots of the spinal nerves; and in different parts of the spinal cord, including the central gray matter, the antero-lateral and posterior columns; also in the sympathetic system. These nerve-changes are not simultaneous, nor have they been discovered in every case. It is a noteworthy fact, however, that as methods of examination have improved and the manipulative skill of observers has increased the number of negative cases has diminished.

First, as to alterations in peripheral nerves in their ultimate distribution: The character of these is of a kind usually described as irritative; that is, there is a hyperplastic process in the connective-tissue sheaths (neurilemmæ) and their internal prolongations, consisting in nuclear proliferation and thickening of the tubular membrane or sheath of Schwann. Varicose distortion of the medullary sheaths and their subsequent disappearance, together with destruction of the axis-cylinders, also occurs.

The changes in the peripheral nerve-trunks, as studied in the median, ulnar, radial, and musculo-spinal, are essentially the same, resulting in thinning of the diameters of the nerves. These changes, however, are by no means constant.

The anterior roots of the spinal nerves exhibit alterations in a large number of instances. Cruveilhier called attention to them in the celebrated case of the rope-dancer Lecomte. At the autopsy, the brain, the cord, and posterior roots were found normal, but the anterior roots, from the point of exit to where they unite with the posterior, were greatly atrophied. In another case the anterior roots were to the posterior in thickness, in the cervical region, in the ratio of 1 : 10, while the normal ratio is 1 : 3;

in the dorsal region as 1 : 5, while the normal is as 1 : 1½ or 2. The posterior roots, brain, and cord were again unchanged. Up to 1876, Eulenburg had collected 26 cases in which this alteration existed, and 19 in which it was absent. In the case of Wood and Dercum, referred to, this atrophy of the anterior nerve-roots existed, making 27 positive cases and 19 negative.

We come, finally, to the spinal cord as the seat of changes, and we are met by Eulenburg's statistics, according to which, up to the date of his article, there were 34 cases of positive disease and 15 negative. To the former we have again to add the case of Wood and Dercum, making 35 against 15. These alterations are by no means constant as to seat and character. Thus, Valentiner, who seems to have been the first after Cruveilhier, in 1853, to record any, found in 1855, in the centre of the cord, in the neighborhood of the three lowest cervical and upper dorsal nerves, that the elements in the region of transition from gray to white substance were obliterated, and the softened place contained numerous compound granule-cells. Schneevogt also found a softening of the cord from the fifth cervical to the second dorsal nerve. Frommann described a red softening from the medulla oblongata downward, involving chiefly the anterior and lateral columns, and especially the commissures and the innermost parts of the anterior columns lying next the commissure.

Luys found the gray matter in the neighborhood of the cervical enlargement full of hyperæmic vessels, which were surrounded with granular masses (compound granule-cells?). The same granular masses, together with numerous corpora amylacea, were scattered throughout the gray substance. The ganglion-cells of the anterior cornua had almost disappeared in the part affected, and appeared to be replaced by the granular masses. Here and there a few ganglion-cells could be recognized in a state of retrograde metamorphosis, pigmented and bereft of their polar prolongations. In this case the degeneration affected principally the left anterior cornu, and it was the left side of the body which was affected by the atrophy. The anterior roots of the spinal nerves on the left side were also atrophied. Lockhart Clarke found essentially the same changes in no less than six cases, and Duménil, Schueppel, Hayem, Charcot (six or seven autopsies), Joffroy, and lately Wood and Dercum,[1] have added others. The last two observers found changes in the lower portion of the cervical enlargement of the cord, and state in the report of their case that "in the anterior cornua of the gray matter there is a marked diminution in the number of nerve-cells. Of the three groups of these cells, the anterior has almost entirely disappeared, the lateral group is represented by but a few individual cells, while the internal group seems to have undergone a less marked change. All of these cells, with the exception of a few in the internal group, appear shrunken, and are evidently much diminished in size. They have lost in great part their polygonal shape, many of them being fusiform, and present but few processes. Only in the internal group are these cells in any way approaching the normal type, and these are few and seen in only a few of the sections. They present the characteristic size and numerous processes of the typical motor-cell, while they disclose a well-defined nucleus and nucleolus. In the atrophied cells the nuclei can only be distinguished with difficulty.

[1] *Loc. cit.*

" The neuroglia of the anterior cornua is increased in amount ; the vessels appear shrunken, with thickened walls and large perivascular lymph-spaces.

" In the lumbar cord the cells in the anterior cornua appear normal: in this respect the lumbar cord is in marked contrast with the cervical."

Another class of cases recorded by Gull,[1] Schueppel and Grimm, Hallopeau and Westphal, consist in dilatation of the central spinal canal with more or less complete destruction of the gray substance, and in Grimm's case hyperplasia of the connective tissue in the white substance along with increase of the axis-cylinders. The nerve-roots were in a state of fatty degeneration, especially the finer fibres of the anterior roots.

Still another set of observations discovers a degenerative atrophy of the white columns only of the cord, sometimes the antero-lateral columns and sometimes the posterior. Virchow, Friedreich, and Swarzenski each found typical gray degeneration of the posterior columns, in one instance recognizable by the naked eye. Atrophy of the antero-lateral columns was noted by Frommann and Baudrimont ; atrophy of the antero-lateral columns, conjoined with inflammatory changes in the gray substance and atrophy of ganglion-cells, by Duménil ; changes in the antero-lateral gray substance and posterior columns by Clarke. Changes have even been found in the posterior cornua and posterior nerve-roots in a few cases, although not confined to them.

Finally, the lesions of this singular disease have been sought also in the sympathetic, and not without some success. Eulenburg's analysis discovered 5 positive observations and 14 negative ones. To the positive must be added the case of Wood and Dercum, who reported a marked increase in the amount of connective tissue and a granular state of the ganglion-cells without diminution in number. Among the changes in the sympathetic were thinning of its trunk and of the two upper ganglia observed by Swarzenski, and advanced fibrous fatty change of the cervical and thoracic portion, with abundant hyperplasia of connective tissue, disappearance of nerve-fibres and regressive metamorphosis of ganglion-cells by Duménil.

PATHOGENY.—We come now to consider the relation of these changes to the muscular atrophy which constitutes the conspicuous symptom of the disease. There are three possible views of the pathology of this affection. According to one, it is a muscular or myopathic disease in the strict sense of the term. Such muscular disease may be primarily inflammatory, a myositis —as Friedreich sought to prove in his great work—followed by fatty metamorphosis of the sarcous substance and subsequent absorption of the fat; or it may be a simple fatty metamorphosis. According to a second view, it is primarily an affection of peripheral nerves or of the anterior roots of the spinal nerves, with secondary muscular atrophy. According to a third, it is a disease of the spinal cord, and more particularly of the anterior cornua of the gray matter—a poliomyelitis anterior.

A careful study of the morbid conditions as described in the various cases reported leads me to adopt the last view. In the first place, the number of instances of positive disease of the spinal cord exceed those of any other seats of alteration, and although the changes do not always involve the anterior cornua, yet it will be noted, from an examination

[1] *Guy's Hospital Reports,* 1862.

of the foregoing paragraphs, that a decided majority involve either the anterior cornua alone or these in connection with the antero-lateral columns, the number of cases of disease of the antero-lateral columns alone or of the posterior columns and posterior nerve-roots being very limited. Again, the number of instances in which lesions of the anterior cornua are found increases as our means of accurate investigation improve.

If we add to these considerations the fact that the symptoms are best explained by such a view, little more seems required to establish it. Recalling the well-known observation of Waller, confirmed by Bernard and others, that after section of the anterior root of a spinal nerve the distal end wastes, while the central end remains intact, because it is still connected with its own trophic centre, we have in this the explanation why atrophy of the anterior roots is also so common a symptom in progressive muscular atrophy. The fibres of the anterior roots arise from the cells of the anterior cornua, and disease of the latter must unfavorably influence the nutrition of the former; hence their atrophy. This atrophy of motor nerve-filaments is continued into the mixed nerves distributed to muscles, but is less easily demonstrable by reason of the gradually diminishing size of the nerve-trunks and by the fact that they are united in the mixed nerve with the sensory fibres from the posterior roots, which do not suffer atrophy. In consequence of the degeneration of these nerves follows degeneration of the muscles to which they are distributed, so that the alterations in the latter are altogether secondary.

From this point of view the disease in question is to be regarded as a chronic form of poliomyelitis anterior, while the essential infantile paralysis of Rilliet and Barthez would correspond to the acute form of the disease.

The association of changes in the anterior roots with others in the spinal cord may be explained either on the ground of extension by continuity to adjacent parts, or on that of coincidence. In illustration of the latter I may refer to a case recently reported from Mendel's clinic[1] in Berlin, in which the symptoms of progressive muscular atrophy were associated with those of tabes dorsalis or progressive locomotor ataxia. Here it is not unlikely that the coincidence is merely accidental; and this was Mendel's opinion in this case. In other instances the involvement of other portions of the spinal cord may be a result of an extension of the disease from its true seat, while many cases described as progressive muscular atrophy are not such at all, but are in part the result of other affections of the spinal cord. It is evident, also, that this order may be reversed, as in a case reported by Eulenburg[2] to the Berlin Medical Society.

SYMPTOMS.—The first distinctive symptom of the disease under consideration is the muscular atrophy or wasting. However general it may subsequently become, it is at first localized. The upper extremity is by far the most frequently involved—7 out of 9 times in Aran's cases. Sandahl out of 62 cases found the right upper extremity attacked 37 times, the left in 14 instances, and both in 11. In Friedreich's statistics it occurred first in the upper 111 times out of 146, while the lower was invaded 27 times,

[1] *Philada. Medical News*, Sept. 12, 1885, p. 188.
[2] *Berliner klin. Wochenschr.*, No. 15, April 13, 1885.

and the lumbar muscles 8. Most frequently it begins in some muscle or group of muscles in the right hand, either the interossei or those of the ball of the thumb. Of the interossei, the external interosseus is usually the first affected. Thence it extends to the other interossei, and soon very striking depressions make their appearance between the metacarpal bones, and the extensor tendons on the dorsum, and the flexors in the palm become as distinct as if dissected out. Succeeding this follows contraction of the flexor tendons until the picture seen in Fig. 32 is produced, in which 1 exhibits the anterior surface of the hand, and 2 the posterior.

FIG. 32.

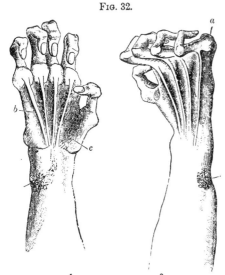

1   2
(1) HAND, PALMAR SURFACE. (2) DORSAL SURFACE (after Duchenne).
a, Ends of the metacarpal bones; b, Tendons of the flexor sublimis; c, Muscles of the ball of the thumb.

Opinion is not unanimous as to whether the atrophy when beginning in the hand involves first the thenar muscles or the interossei. Roberts, Wachsmuth, and Friedreich say that it begins, as a rule, in the thumb; Eulenburg, that it invariably begins in the interossei. From the interossei it may creep up the forearm, and thence to the arm, or it may skip the forearm and pass into the arm, although the triceps extensor muscle is usually spared. It may come to a standstill in either of those places, but may involve the muscle of the shoulder, especially the deltoid. When the latter and the arm are involved, a picture like that of Fig. 33 is produced.

Beginning most frequently in the right, both upper extremities become sooner or later involved.

In other instances in which the upper extremities are previously involved the atrophy begins in the shoulder, in the deltoid—here again the right first. Succeeding the deltoid, the scapular and trapezius muscles may be involved in any order, while a grotesqueness of effect is often produced by reason of certain adjacent muscles retaining their natural size or even being hypertrophied. This is particularly the case with the anterior part of the trapezius, which is almost never involved. With the shoulders first affected, the arm and forearm may retain their usefulness and strength; but the power of lifting the arm from the side, and especially of raising it above the head, is lost. And if the patient wishes to lay hold of anything, he must swing his arm forward with a jerk until it is brought in reach of his fingers, and then it must often be caught up by the pathologically hooked terminations of these.

The muscles of the trunk do, however, become at times involved— the pectorales, the latissimi, serrati, and intercostales, and even the diaphragm and abdominal and lumbar muscles. Life is seriously jeopardized when the intercostals and diaphragm are affected, in consequence of interference with respiration. If the intercostals cease to contract, the upper part of the thorax ceases to move, and if the diaphragm is involved, the epigastric and hypogastric regions are drawn in during inspiration, and talking and singing are interfered with. Even a mild bronchitis is apt to be fatal in consequence of the difficulty in expelling the secretions.

Fig. 33.   Fig. 34.

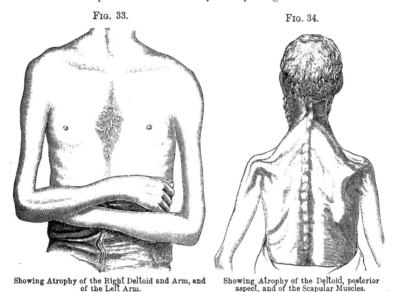

Showing Atrophy of the Right Deltoid and Arm, and of the Left Arm.   Showing Atrophy of the Deltoid, posterior aspect, and of the Scapular Muscles.

The muscular atrophy thus produced is generally accompanied by a corresponding wasting and retraction of the skin, so that this continues applied to the muscles in the usual manner. In some instances, however, this is not the case, and in these a baggy condition of the skin is added, which gives its subject an appearance which has more than once rendered him valuable to the showman as the elastic-skin man, etc. It sometimes happens, on the other hand, that the atrophy is obscured by an accumulation between the muscle and skin of adipose tissue, and an appearance of hypertrophy rather than atrophy may be produced in consequence, analogous to the same state of affairs in pseudo-hypertrophic paralysis, the relations of which disease to progressive muscular atrophy will be considered under the head of Diagnosis.

At almost any stage the disease may come to a standstill, and may continue thus for many years. The time required to attain its various degrees also varies greatly, but the spread is usually slow, requiring, as a rule, years for its completion. A general involvement of the voluntary muscles of the entire body is exceedingly rare.

As stated, the disease may begin in the lower extremity, but much more rarely. It is very seldom that the same order of invasion pursued in the upper extremity is followed in the lower—that is, beginning with the interossei. It may begin in the thigh and involve it alone, or extend to both thighs, or both legs as well. Under these circumstances weakness of the legs is a striking symptom, the patient being unable to stand, often falling down or requiring a cane or crutches to assist him. In illustration of this mode of invasion may be related one of Roberts's cases, that of an adult woman thirty-eight years old, a domestic servant, in whom at thirty-six was perceived a weakness in the right thigh. She first noticed that it grew tired sooner than the left. This gradually increased, until she was compelled to sit much of the day, then to use a stick, and finally crutches. This was accompanied by a gradual wasting of the thigh-muscles. Even in this case the loss of power was greater than would have been expected from the degree of atrophy, the loss of bulk incident to which Roberts believed to have been in part replaced by fat. In other instances, however, the extremest degree of atrophy has been noted where the disease has commenced in the lower extremities.

The deformity produced by the wasting muscle is sometimes further increased—more frequently in the earlier stages—by a painful swelling of the joints, first mentioned by Remak, called by him neuro-paralytic inflammation, and referred to the sympathetic. This may affect the small (phalangeal) as well as the larger joints (shoulder and elbow).

Cases apparently beginning in the face are reported, when the distorted expression resulting is very characteristic.

Aran first, and Roberts afterward, divided cases of the disease into two groups, the partial and general. In the former are included those involving the extremities only; in the latter become involved, sooner or later, the muscles of the trunk, neck, face, mouth, pharynx (muscles of deglutition), thorax (muscles of respiration), and even of the abdomen. Even the tongue is reported as undergoing atrophy.

General wasting palsy, as was early observed by Roberts, is unquestionably a rare disease, and in no case have all the muscles of the body been found implicated in one individual, and a few seem altogether exempted. Such are the muscles of mastication and of the eyeball, including the levator palpebræ.

A second muscular symptom, more or less distinctive, is fibrillar contraction. This consists in a wave-like contraction running along small bundles of muscular fasciculi. The contractions occur spontaneously or are excited by any slight stimulus, as a breath of air or a dash of water, or by tapping the patient, or passing a galvanic current through the parts, and at any stage of the disease, except that they do not occur in muscles wholly destroyed. Sometimes they can be felt by the patient. At other times he is wholly ignorant of them. They are not invariably present, and often they have been observed in muscles atrophied from other causes. They possess, however, a certain amount of diagnostic value, especially when spontaneous.

More rare, and less destructive, are cramps, twitches, and clonic contractions of groups of affected muscles. These, when present, are sometimes exceedingly painful.

Coincident with the wasting of muscles is their loss of function. The power of abducting and adducting the fingers gradually disappears, so also that of flexion and extension, and everywhere the loss of function goes pari passu with the atrophy. As Roberts graphically puts it, "The tailor discovers that he cannot hold his needle; the shoemaker wonders

·he cannot thrust his awl ; the mason finds his hammer, formerly a play-thing in his hand, now too heavy for his utmost strength ; the gentleman feels an awkwardness in handling his pen, in pulling out his pocket hand-kerchief, or in putting on his hat. One man discovered his ailment in thrusting on a horse's collar ; another, a sportsman, in bringing the fowl-ing-piece to his shoulder."

Along with the atrophy of muscle and loss of power comes a gradu-ally diminishing response to electrical stimulus. Direct muscular faradi-zation fails first to excite contraction, and sometimes fails completely even before voluntary mobility is lost. Indirect muscular faradization continues longer to excite contraction, but it also finally fails. Response to the constant current continues still longer, but it also finally fails to elicit con-tractions, stronger and stronger currents being required, until finally all fail. The galvanic excitability of nerve-trunks is maintained for quite a long time, but finally also disappears. Some irregularities present them-selves in this respect.

A singular electrical reaction, first described by Remak, and said by him to be of frequent occurrence in muscular atrophy, was named by him deplegic contraction. He describes it as follows : When the cathode or negative pole is put below the fifth cervical vertebra, contractions can be produced in the atrophied muscles of the arm when the anode or positive pole is placed in an irritable zone, which extends from the first to the fifth cervical vertebra, or, still better, in the carotid fossa or the triangle between the lower jaw and the external ear. The contractions always take place on the side opposite to that at which the anode is placed, while when the electrodes are placed on the median line they occur on both sides, although when the current is very weak they are limited to the muscles most seriously involved. Meyer, Drissen, and Erb confirmed Remak's statement, while Fieber, Benedikt, and Eulenburg failed to do so. Remak interprets these contrae-tions as reflected from the superior cervical ganglion of the sympathetic. He bases this view upon the fact that the patient perceived a sensation behind the ball of the eye when the current was closed. Eulenburg, on the other hand, regards them as genuine reflex contractions, independent of the sympathetic, and caused either by excessive irritability of the central reflex apparatus or by an abnormal excitability of the muscles themselves.

Sensibility is, in many cases, unchanged, the tactile sense being as delicate as ever, and pain, except accompanying the cramps above described, is absent. At times, however, the atrophy is preceded by paroxysms, which may or may not accompany the clonic contractions referred to. It is sometimes in the course of nerve-trunks, but as often diffuse, as though the muscles themselves were its seat. At other times it is variously described as a soreness, an aching, or a rheumatic pain. Accompanying advanced degrees of the atrophy, however, there is very rarely—in 3 out of 105 cases, according to Roberts—a slight diminution of sensibility, especially in the ends of the fingers, while the faradic sen-sibility may be similarly diminished.

Modified sensations, as those of cold, numbness, and formication, may be experienced, and reflex excitability may be increased, while the knee-jerk is said to be absent. Unusual sensitiveness to cold is sometimes noted, and a loss of muscular power under its influence, which is again restored by artificial warmth.

Among more inconstant symptoms, denominated vaso-motor, are, in the early stages, fever and slight elevation in local temperature from 2° to 3° C. Fever is less frequently observed toward the termination of the disease, and at this stage a fall of local temperature, as much as 4° C., has been noted. In the same category of vaso-motor symptoms are classed the skin contractions already referred to, hyperidrosis or excessive sweating, and certain very rare oculo-pupillary symptoms, consisting mainly of contraction of the pupil and slow reaction, but including also, in a case reported by Voisin, flattening of the cornea on both sides and defective sight.

COMPLICATIONS.—Progressive muscular atrophy is not infrequently associated with amyotrophic antero-lateral sclerosis and with labio-glossal or progressive bulbar paralysis. Both affections may result as an extension of the disease from the anterior cornua of gray matter, the former into the antero-lateral columns, the latter into the medulla oblongata, or the affection may be primary in either of these two situations, and extend thence into the anterior cornua of gray matter.

When there is also lateral sclerosis, there is rigidity of the lower limbs in addition to the atrophy of the upper—at first temporary, but afterward permanent. This may extend to the upper also, and the arms become fixed in semipronation and semiflexion.

When there is bulbar paralysis there is difficulty in moving the tongue, in speaking, and in swallowing. The mouth remains open, the lower lip drops, the patient cannot whistle or kiss or blow out a candle; he speaks through his nose. On the other hand, the upper part of the face is natural, the orbicularis palpebrarum muscle and occipito-frontalis acting well. As a consequence, the carrying of the food back into the œsophagus is rendered difficult or impossible; swallowing is imperfectly successful; the food sometimes enters the larynx, and the patient dies of suffocation. The saliva dribbles from the mouth. Later, respiration is embarrassed, and performed principally by the diaphragm; there is difficulty in raising mucus, and if bronchitis supervenes the patient dies of suffocation, because he cannot raise the phlegm. Such was the death of Prosper Lecompte, the historic patient of Cruveilhier.

DIAGNOSIS.—As our knowledge of progressive muscular atrophy increases we realize more and more that there have heretofore been included under this name many cases which must now be relegated to other categories. If we confine the disease, as I think we must, to those cases in which there are degenerative changes in the anterior cornua of the gray matter of the cord, we must endeavor to associate with these lesions a set of symptoms which are sufficiently constant, and exclude all other similar combinations. Such a set of symptoms includes the following: insidious and progressive atrophy of groups of muscles, beginning usually in the hand or shoulder, from which, however, it may extend to others in a diffuse and rarer form of the disease. The atrophy is accompanied by a corresponding loss of power in the affected muscles and partial or complete reaction of degeneration in the same, and by fibrillar twitchings. Along with this, sensibility, the special senses, the reflexes, as a rule, and sphincters always remain normal.

This complex of symptoms is to be distinguished from the so-called juvenile progressive muscular atrophy of Erb, and from pseudo-hypertrophic muscular paralysis. In the first there is also slow, symmetrical, but intermittent and often stationary, wasting and weakness of certain groups of muscles, preferably those encircling the shoulder and upper arm, the pelvis and upper thigh and back—"an atrophy," says Erb, " which is very frequently combined with true or false muscular hypertrophy, with a peculiar toughness of the atrophying muscles, but without fibrillar con- traction or any trace of the reaction of degeneration or other lesion in the body, be it of the nervous system, organs of sense, vegetative organs, or external integuments."[1] The average age in the juvenile form is much less, Erb's cases ranging from seven to forty-six, or an average of twenty- six and a half, while in the spinal form, or true progressive muscular atrophy, although the age is reduced by reason of the admixture of other cases than those of true progressive muscular atrophy, the average age is much greater. Of Roberts's cases, all of which seem true cases, the youngest was twenty, while the age of the remaining four was thirty- nine, forty-seven, sixty-seven, and thirty-eight.

There are certain symptoms in common in progressive muscular atrophy, as heretofore described, and pseudo-hypertrophic paralysis ; and I have already said that Friedreich and others are disposed to consider them one and the same disease ; but such is not the case. First of all, while there is wasting of muscle, although obscured in the lower extrem- ities by the fatty infiltration, and while there is loss of power, there are in pseudo-hypertrophic paralysis absolutely no alterations in the spinal cord. Pseudo-hypertrophic paralysis always begins in the lower extrem- ities, while progressive muscular atrophy begins for the most part in the upper. Pseudo-hypertrophic paralysis is a disease of childhood, and strikingly hereditary ; and while progressive muscular atrophy in its broadest application is also a disease of childhood and hereditary, it is much less so than pseudo-hypertrophic paralysis ; and if, with Erb, we separate the juvenile form from muscular atrophy, progressive muscular atrophy is not a disease of childhood, while heredity is almost entirely removed from it.[2]

[1] "Juvenile Form der Progressive Muskelatrophie," *Deutsches Archiv für klinische Medi- zin*, Bd. xxxiv., 1884, S. 471.
[2] It cannot but help the reader to get a correct notion of this interesting but still some- what imperfectly understood disease to be familiar with Erb's formulated conclusions (*loc. cit.*, p. 510):

"There is a peculiar form of progressive muscular atrophy which is characterized by a definite location, definite course, definite behavior of affected muscles, and definite altera- tion in them, but without alterations in the spinal cord—the condition named by me the juvenile form. It begins in youth or childhood.

"This form agrees in its symptomatology—especially in its localization in the upper half of the body, partly also in the lower—entirely with the so-called pseudo-hypertrophy of muscles, only that in the former a decided lipomatosis leading to an increase in volume is wanting ; on the other hand, true muscular hypertrophy is not infrequent in both forms of the disease.

"If this juvenile form occurs in the earliest childhood, it may in all its details be identical with pseudo-hypertrophy, except that the lipomatosis is wanting.

"The anatomico-histological alterations of the muscles are exactly the same in the juvenile form as in pseudo-hypertrophy.

"The juvenile form not infrequently occurs in entire groups in one family, producing the so-called hereditary—better named family-muscular—atrophy.

"If this juvenile-hereditary form occurs after puberty, it affects most frequently, although not exclusively, the upper half of the body. If it sets in, on the other hand, in

Still another myopathic condition, which in the light of modern knowledge has to be separated from progressive muscular atrophy, is Duchenne's hereditary infantile atrophy. This is characterized by onset at an early age and by its beginning in the facial muscles. Its clinical features are thus described by Charcot[1] and his pupils Marie and Guénon.[2] Although it mostly begins in infancy, it may not come on until adolescence, or even until middle or advanced age; it is often hereditary; the face-muscles are first involved, particularly the orbicularis oris, and there is a peculiar expression of the countenance; whistling is impossible, and the articulation of labials difficult; the eyes cannot be completely closed or the eyebrows raised. Subsequently other muscles become involved, particularly those of the shoulder girdle, except the deltoid, the muscles of the arm, the long supinators of the forearm, and in the lower extremities the muscles of the buttocks, thighs, and of the anterior external aspect of the leg. The muscles of the hands and fingers are spared. Fibrillar tremors are not present, and there is no reaction of degeneration. The distribution of the atrophy is almost identical with that of Erb's form, exceptthat it begins in the face. It is likewise an hereditary or family disease.

PROGNOSIS.—The course of progressive muscular atrophy is never rapid —essentially chronic. Recovery in a well-established case is not to be expected, although it is rare for any one to die of the direct effects of the disease. It is often arrested in its course, and remains at a standstill for years. The wider its distribution and the more numerous the foci of involvement, the more rapid is its course; and when the muscles of deglutition and respiration are involved, and the carrying back of food interfered with, death from asphyxia is liable to be produced by the entrance of food into the larynx or from the accumulation of mucus in what under ordinary circumstances would be a slight catarrh of the respiratory passages.

TREATMENT.—Treatment directed specifically to the cure of the disease is limited. Only where there is reason to believe that syphilis is responsible for it do we find an opportunity to strike at the fons et origo mali by mercurials and iodide of potassium. Yet in Cooke's case, quoted by Roberts,[3] the disease after progressing continuously for five years, during which a variety of modes of treatment was tried, had its further progress stopped by a course of mercury, although no cause of the disease could be assigned.

In the majority of instances treatment must consist merely in efforts to maintain the general health and strength of the patient and to counteract

earliest childhood, it affects preferably the lower extremities and the pelvis. Transitional forms, however, occur also in family groups.

"In the latter form, that occurring in earliest life, we have that which Leyden has proposed to designate as hereditary muscular atrophy.

"Thus, hereditary muscular atrophy is in all essential points identical with pseudohypertrophy, and is distinguished from it only in the slighter degree of lipomatosis of the muscles.

"All of these forms have probably nothing to do with spinal progressive muscular atrophy; they differ from it in localization and course, anatomical changes and clinical phenomena in the muscles, and alterations in the spinal cord."

[1] *Le Progrès médical*, No. 10, 1885.　　　[2] *Revue de Médecine*, October, 1885.
[3] *Op. cit.*, p. 1; also Cooke *On Palsy*, Lond., 1822, p. 31; also quoted by Graves in his *Clinical Lectures*, L. lxxxiii.

the obstinate tendency of the spinal disease to produce wasting of the muscles by depressing their nutrition. The former is accomplished by an abundance of nutritious food, fresh air, and out-door life, by gymnastics, chalybeate and other tonics, including arsenic, strychnine, and quinine. The second is attained by electricity, frictions, and massage. Both forms of electricity are useful, the induced current with rapid interruption with a view to counter-irritate and to stimulate the circulation, or by slow interruptions to stimulate individual muscles to contraction, and thus maintain their nutrition. Duchenne recommended the application of currents of moderate intensity, with not too frequent interruptions, and for a few minutes only at a time, so as not to fatigue the fibres undestroyed. He urged particularly the treatment of important muscles like the diaphragm through the phrenic nerves, of the intercostals, and of the deltoids before they were actually invaded by the disease. He relates the case of a man named Bonnard who had lost many of his trunk-muscles, and who was beginning to suffer with dyspnœa, on whom faradization of the phrenic nerves, repeated three or four times a week, was of great service, enabling him to walk considerable distances and to go up stairs without fatigue. Another patient, whose arms were much wasted, was so far restored that at the end of six months he was again able to support his family.

The direct current—galvanism—is useful in advanced stages of the disease, where even the strongest faradic currents fail to produce response. Even where galvanic currents fail to exert contractions the treatment ought to be persevered in for a long time. It may be necessary to use very strong currents at the outset, which may be gradually weakened as contractility returns.

Remak, who especially advocated the use of the continuous current, advised to place the positive pole in front of one mastoid process and the negative pole on the opposite side of the neck near the spinous processes of the vertebræ, not higher than the fifth cervical, by which he produced the contractions already described as diplegic in the fingers and other paralyzed parts.

Galvanization of the sympathetic has been apparently useful in the hands of some—viz. Roberts, Benedikt, M. Meyer, Guthzeit, Erb, Neseman, and others, while the latter reports a case of complete cure by this treatment. Eulenburg tells us, however, that a relapse is said to have occurred in this case; also that neither he nor Rosenthal have had any results from it.

Massage is equally important, and should be used at the same time with electricity, but at a different time of day. Eulenburg refers to a case which was said to have brought the disease to a standstill. There can be no doubt of the value of the measure as an adjuvant to treatment.

In families in which an hereditary tendency exists prophylactic treatment should be used. It should include hygienic measures of the kind already referred to, and the avoidance of undue fatigue and exposure; and in the selection of an occupation these matters should be kept in view.

On the supposition that the disease is a purely local one, gymnastics, involving the exercise of the groups of muscles prone to attack, would be indicated, but assume less importance from our standpoint that it is a spinal disease. At the same time, the patient should have the benefit of any existing uncertainty in the pathogeny of the affection; and as gymnastics are eminently calculated to improve the general health, and thus indirectly to avert the disease, their use is indicated on these grounds.

PSEUDO-HYPERTROPHIC PARALYSIS.

By MARY PUTNAM JACOBI, M. D.

SYNONYMS.—Hypertrophic paraplegia of infancy (Duchenne); Myosclerosic paralysis (Duchenne); Progressive muscular sclerosis (Jaccoud); Atrophia musculorum lipomatosa (Seidel); Lipomatous myo-atrophy (Gowers); Muscular hypertrophy (Kaulich, Griesinger); Lipomatosis musculorum luxurians progressiva (Heller); Myopachynsis lipomatosa (Uhde); Pseudo-hypertrophic paralysis (Ross); Pseudo-hypertrophy of muscles (Friedreich).

DEFINITION.—Pseudo-hypertrophic paralysis is a rare and predominantly infantile disease, characterized by a considerable increase in the volume of some or all the muscles of the lower extremities, associated with progressive diminution in their functional energy, and accompanied or followed by paresis and atrophy of the muscles of the trunk and upper limbs. Many of the hypertrophied muscles subsequently atrophy; many of the muscles in which atrophy is the most conspicuous lesion pass through a preliminary period of hypertrophy. The proximate cause of these alterations is a profound disturbance in the nutrition of the muscles, attended by great increase of their connective tissue, by wasting of the contractile substance, and by the ultimate replacement of this by fat.

HISTORY.—The honors of the discovery of this remarkable disease may be divided between Duchenne, Meryon, and Griesinger. In 1852[1] the English physician published a series of six cases, four belonging to one family, two to another; but these were described by him under the name of progressive muscular atrophy; and it was left to Duchenne, who in 1861[2] published as a new disease the first case observed by himself, to demonstrate the identity of Meryon's cases with his own.[3] In 1868, Duchenne had collected twelve additional cases, and published an extensive monograph on the subject.[4] But in 1865, Griesinger[5] had excised a portion of muscle from a patient suffering with the disease, and made the first histological examination of its structure. On this account several German writers habitually refer to Griesinger as the earliest authority on the subject. Before Meryon, Partridge in 1847,[6] and Sir Charles Bell in 1830,[7] had described cases of pseudo-hypertrophic paralysis, but without recognizing their separate morbid entity. Bell's case is the following:

[1] Lond. Med. Gaz.
[3] Duchenne at first doubted this identity.
[5] Archiv der Heilkunde.
[7] Nervous System, 2d ed., 1830, p. 163.

[2] De l'Électrisation localisée.
[4] Archives générales, 1868.
[6] Lond. Med. Gaz., 1847.

" A boy at eight years of age began to experience difficulty in rising from a chair. The disease gradually progressed, till at eighteen he had to twist and jerk his body about to get upright. The muscles of the lower extremities, hips, and abdomen were debilitated and wasted. The extensor quadriceps femoris on both sides wasted, but the vasti externi had not suffered as much ; a firm body, remarkably prominent, just above the knee-joint, marked the position of the vastus externus. No defect of sensibility or affection of the sphincters. The upper part of the body, shoulders, and arms were strong." [1]

Autopsies.—The first was made by Meryon : the first which included microscopic examination of the spinal cord was by Cohnheim on a patient of Eulenburg's.[2] Since then autopsies have been made in 12 genuine cases, and in 2 others frequently, though erroneously, ranked with them.[3]

Of cases without autopsies a collection of 80 was made by Friedreich in the monograph on pseudo-hypertrophy which accompanies his longer monograph on progressive muscular atrophy.[4] Mobius has increased this list to 94 ;[5] Gowers describes 24 cases,[6] and refers in an appendix to 20 more—18 observed by Adams, 2 by Clifford Albutt.[7] Hammond in the sixth edition of his treatise on nervous diseases, quotes 17 American cases, of which 6 were observed by himself.[8] Gowers estimated that in 1879 about 220 cases had been reported, divided up among a much smaller number of families.

The material at present on hand is therefore sufficient, if not to solve the problems of the disease, at least to make out a tolerably complete clinical history.

SYMPTOMS.—The early appearance of the morbid symptoms is the first striking peculiarity of the disease. Out of 88 cases whose records I have analyzed, 35 must be considered congenital, since some degree of paresis was observed from the time the child first began to walk ;[9] and the effort

---

[1] *Loc. cit.* This case is quoted in an appendix to Gowers's monograph.

[2] *Vhdlg. der Bul. Med. Ges.*, 1866, Heft 2, p. 191, quoted by Eulenburg in *Ziemssen's Handbuch*, Bd. xii. 2.

[3] Cases of Barth and Müller.   [4] *Ueber Progressiv Muskel Atrophie.*

[5] "Ueber Hereditare Nerven Krankheiten," *Volkmann's Samml.*, 171.

[6] *Clinical Lecture on Pseudo-hypertrophic Paralysis*, Lond., 1879.

[7] Among Mobius's cases is that related by Pick in the *Deutsches Archiv f. klin. Med.*, Bd. vi., and really a case of progressive muscular atrophy in an adult complicated with lipomatosis in the calf-muscles. Of the other cases, 6 are quoted from the Swedish, 6 are hitherto unpublished, and have been collected by the author from several clinics. There remain cases by Davidsohn, *Glasgow Med. Journ.*, 1872 (3 cases) ; Berger, *Schles. Gesellsch.*, 1875 ; Uhde, *Arch. f. klin. Chirurg.*, 1873, Bd. xvi. ; Huber, *Deutsches Arch. für klin. Med.*, 1874 ; Brieger, *ibid*, 1878, Bd. xxii. ; Leyden, *Klinik der Ruckenmark. Krank.*, Bd. ii. S. 529 ; Schlesinger, *Wien. Med. Presse*, 1873.

Many other cases have been published since, but without contributing any special information on the disease. Of importance, however, are — Cornil, accompanied by autopsy, *Bull. Soc. Méd. des Hôp.*, 1880 ; Donkin, followed by recovery, *Brit. Med. Journ.*, 1882, i. ; Albutt, *Med. Times and Gaz.*, 1882 ; Goodridge, *Brain*, 1882 ; Barthélemy, *France méd.*, 1880 ; Suckling, *Med. Times and Gaz*, 1885 ; Dowse and Crocker, *Lancet*, 1881.

[8] These are reported by S. G. Webber, *Boston Medical and Surg. Journ.*, Nov. 17, 1870 ; Wm. Pepper, *Philada. Med. Times*, 1871 ; S. Weir Mitchell, *Photographic Review*, 1871 ; C. H. Drake, *Philada. Med. Times*, 1874 ; C. T. Poore, *New York Med. Journal*, 1875 ; Steele and Kingsley of Missouri (4 cases), *Philada. Med. Times*, Oct., 1875 ; George S. Gerhardt (2 cases), *Alienist and Neurologist*, Jan., 1880.

I have had an opportunity of observing 3 cases of the disease—1 at the Mount Sinai Hospital ; 2, brothers, in a private family.

[9] These cases are the following : Meryon, *Lond. Med. Gaz.*, 1852 (5 cases) ; Partridge,

at walking was unusually late, being deferred till two, three, or even four years of age. In 21 other cases the first symptoms of the disease declared themselves betwen the ages of three and six[1]—at the age of seven 8 other cases began ;[2] between nine and ten, 7 cases ;[3] between ten and six-teen were 8 cases ;[4] finally, in 7 cases, of which 2 are more than doubtful (cases Barth and Müller), the disease seems to have begun in adult life.[5] Thus, 57 cases, or rather more than two-thirds of the whole number, began before the age of six.

The symptoms are of three kinds : 1st, those dependent on alterations in the function of the affected muscles ; 2d, changes in the appearance, consistency, and electrical reaction of these same muscles ; 3d, deformities resulting from their structural alteration.

The first muscles invaded are invariably the gastrocnemii,[6] and there-fore uncertainty of gait is the first symptom observed. The child is usually backward in learning how to walk, even when two, three, or four years intervene between this acquisition and the first decided appear-ance of the disease. In the unquestionably congenital disease the act of walking is always imperfectly performed, and the original imperfection gradually deepens into a noticeable uncertainty of gait, and finally into real paresis. It is noticed that the child falls very frequently—at first only when running, afterward even while standing. He then begins to experience difficulty in going up stairs : pulls himself up by the ban-

ibid., 1847 ; Duchenne, Électris. local., 1861 ; Kaulich, Prager Vierteljahr., 1862, quoted by Friedreich ; Spielmann, Gaz. méd. de Strasbourg, 1862, quoted by Freidreich ; Duchenne fils, Archives gén., 1864 (" De la Paralysie atrophique graisseuse ") ; Griesinger, Archiv der Heilkunde, 1864 ; Sigmund, Deutsches Archiv für klin. Med., Bd. i. Heft 6 ; Wernich, ibid., Bd. ii. Heft 2, 1866 ; Benedikt, Elektrotherapie, Wien, 1868 ; Balthazar Foster, Lancet, 1869 ; Barth, Archiv der Heilkunde, xii. 2, 1871 ; Chrostek, Oesterreich Zeitschrift für prakt. Heilkunde, No. 38, 1871, quoted by Friedreich ; Pekelharing, Arch. Virch., 1882, Bd. lxxxix., quoted by Friedreich ; Knoll, Wien. Medizin Jahrbuch., 1872 ; Friedreich, Pseudo-hypertroph. der Musc., 1878, p. 291 ; Duchenne, Archives gén., 1868 (7 cases) ; Hammond, Treatise Nerv. Dis.; Gowers, loc. cit. (5 cases) ; Ross, Treatise Nerv. Dis., 2, 204.

[1] Cases by Eulenburg, Allgemeine Med. Central Zeitung, Berlin, 1863, quoted by Fried-reich ; Rinecker, Verhand. du Phys. Med. Gesellsch. zu Würzburg, 1860, quoted by Fried-reich ; Heller, Deutsches Archiv. f. klin. Med., Bd. i. H 6 (2 cases) ; Wernich, ibid., Bd. ii., 1866 ; Lutz, ibid., Bd. iii., 1867 ; Benedikt, loc. cit. (5th and 6th cases) ; Russel, Med. Times and Gaz., 1869 (3d case) ; Duchenne, loc. cit. (2d, 3d, 6th, 12th, 13th cases) ; Ham-mond, loc. cit.; Gowers, loc. cit. (6 cases).

[2] Cases by Eulenburg and Cohnheim, Beitr. klin. Woch., 1865 ; Seidel, Atrophia Mus-culorum Lipomatosa, 1867 ; Heller, loc. cit. (2d case) ; Wagner, Berl. klin. Woch., 1866 (8 cases) ; Benedikt, loc. cit. (1st case) ; Duchenne, loc. cit. (9th case) ; Gowers, loc. cit. (7th case).

[3] Seidel, loc. cit. (1st case) ; Coste and Gioja, Schmidt's Jahrb., Bd. xxiv. S. 176 ; Speil-mann, Gaz. méd. de Strasbourg, 1862 ; Boquette, Inaug. Dissert., Berlin, 1868 ; Russel, loc. cit. (2d case) ; Rakowac, Wien. Mediz. Wochen., 1872 ; Brieger, Deutsches Archiv f. klin. Med., Bd. xxii., 1878 ; Pepper, Philada. Med. Times, 1871.

[4] Lutz, loc. cit. (2d case) ; Ross, loc. cit., p. 190 (observed when adult) ; Hoffmann, Inaug. Dissert., Berlin, 1867 ; Russel, loc. cit. (1st case) ; Gowers, loc. cit. (18th and 20th cases).

[5] Benedikt, loc. cit. (2d and 3d cases) ; Dyce Brown, Edin. Med. Journ., 1870 ; Eulen-burg, Archiv Virch., Bd. xlix., 1870 ; Martini, Centralblatt für Med. Wissensch., No. 41, 1871 ; Barth, Archiv der Heilkunde, xii. 2, 1871 ; Müller, Beit. zur. path. Ruckenmarkes, 1871.

[6] Billroth relates an altogether exceptional case of a limited pseudo-hypertrophy with lipomatous degeneration, localized in the hamstring and adductor muscles of one thigh, in a girl seventeen years old. The only generalized lesion was an immense develop-ment of subcutaneous fat (Archiv für klin. Chir., Bd. xiii.).
Dyce Brown (Edin. Med. Journal, 1870) relates a case, also in an adult of twenty-six years, where hypertrophy of the thigh-muscles is said to have preceded by three weeks that of the calves.

nisters, and usually drags one leg completely. After a while it becomes quite impossible for him to go up stairs except on his hands and knees.

These symptoms all point to failure of power in the gastrocnemii muscles, whose function it is to raise the heel from the ground in running, to steady the heel by their tension during the act of standing, and to raise the foot with considerable force during the act of going up stairs. In descending a staircase or any inclined plane great tension is required of these same muscles, and this act should therefore be even more difficult than that of ascension. But it does not seem to have been as carefully studied.

Attention is not often directed to the infirmity at this early stage, especially if the child be very young, since the apparently excellent development of the legs satisfies the parents that nothing serious can be the matter, and the falling is explained by childish awkwardness. Not infrequently, indeed, this is really due to a rachitis which has preceded the degenerative lesion, and at the early stage of the latter a diagnosis from the less severe disease is always required, and is sometimes difficult to make.

The following test may be applied in doubtful cases: The child (if old enough) is requested while standing to rise on the tips of his toes. This act necessitates a powerful effort on the part of the sural muscles, and of this, even at an early stage of degeneration, they are generally incapable.

Functional weakness may precede for several years all visible alteration of the muscles; the child may not learn to walk at all until two or even three years of age; then walks badly until five or six, when, for the first time, the calves begin to enlarge. More often the paresis precedes the hypertrophy by only a few months or weeks, or the symptoms occur simultaneously. A certain amount of hypertrophy will be overlooked; but when the calves enlarge sufficiently to render the child's stockings too tight, attention is forcibly called to the change. The enlargement is more marked at the upper part of the calf, so that the symmetry of the leg is deranged by it. Often, however, the impression of vigor conveyed by the appearance of the child's legs is with difficulty dispelled by the discovery of their functional weakness.

Eulenburg[1] affirms that the consistency of the muscle is soft and doughy, recalling, when grasped in the hand, a lipomatous tumor. This description, however, does not apply to the early stage of the disease; for then the hypertrophied muscles feel extremely hard to the touch; there is even a stony hardness (Duchenne fils); somewhat later, the hypertrophy continuing, these muscles " seem to make hernial protrusions through the skin " (Duchenne). This appearance is most marked when the subcutaneous fat is atrophied; when, as happens especially in the adult cases,[2] the diseased muscles are covered by a thick layer of subcutaneous fat, their protrusion is concealed. A rapid exchange of the hardness characterizing the first stage of the lesions for a lipomatous softening is of bad omen, as indicating a more rapid and irresistible march in the disease (Mobius).

At this early stage the electrical reactions of the enlarging muscles are all intact. Disturbances of sensibility, however, are not uncommon. Especially frequent are pains in the back and loins and stabbing pains in the lower limbs. These pains sometimes follow the track of the

[1] *Ziemssen's Handbuch*, Bd. xii.   [2] See case by Billroth, quoted p. 853, note.

crural or sciatic nerves; at other times they appear in the joints; sometimes are limited to the affected muscles. The pains are diminished by repose and a recumbent position, but are greatly aggravated by movement. Paræsthesias, or a feeling of cold and formication, are also observed—never anæsthesia. Seidel[1] has found the cutaneous sensibility to be intact, as also the sense of space and pressure. The temperature sensibility has not been tested. The temperature of the affected part is, according to Eulenburg, often lowered several degrees. This statement probably refers to the advanced degree of degeneration. At an earlier stage Ord[2] found the temperature of the calves to be increased.

Reflex excitability is maintained, not only in this, but in the second stage of the disease, except in the patellar tendon, where it is abolished after the quadriceps extensor has been invaded. This fact may be of importance in diagnosticating paresis depending on incipient pseudo-hypertrophy from that which would be caused by a mild anterior polio-myelitis.

No symptoms of the third kind (deformity) appear in the first period of the disease. The second is ushered in either by the first perceptible degree of hypertrophy in the calves (Duchenne) or by increase of the hypertrophy, which may have already begun during the first period of paresis, and by extension of this to other muscles.

This extension of the lesion is indicated by further derangement in the functions of station and locomotion. To steady himself the child instinctively widens his base of support by placing the feet far apart, and thus straddles while walking in a manner that is highly characteristic. A second peculiarity is an oscillating movement of the trunk from side to side. The trunk is carried over to the side of the foot planted on the ground, the so-called active limb, and while the passive limb is being swung forward. A third peculiarity of attitude, already exhibited in station, but exaggerated by the act of walking, is lordosis. The lumbar portion of the spine, with the abdomen, is carried forward; the shoulders are carried backward, so that a plumb-line dropped from them falls behind the sacrum. Thus, the walk of the patient becomes highly characteristic —the feet planted so far apart; the lumbar portion of the trunk projecting forward; the body oscillating at each step from side to side.

At this stage the act of rising from a sitting or recumbent position becomes more difficult than walking. If near a support, the child always tries to draw himself up by his arms; if a fixed support be lacking, he first gets on his hands and knees, and then, grasping each thigh alternately with one hand, is enabled to get first one foot and then the other on the floor. He then seizes the thighs by successive grasps, each higher than the other, pressing back the flexed hip- and knee-joint as he does so. By this method of apparently climbing up his own thighs the patient is finally enabled to extend his body and arrive at an upright position.

This attitude of the hands on the knees, and subsequently on the thighs, during the act of rising, is pathognomonic of pseudo-hypertrophy, for it is observed in no other disease.

Corresponding with this increased disturbance in function is the increased visible alteration in the muscles of the lower extremities. The muscles on the anterior part of the legs are not always attacked, but often

[1] *Loc. cit.*, p. 32. [2] *Med.-Chir. Trans.*, 1874, 1877.

become hypertrophied and paretic contemporaneously with the gastroc. nemii. After these, hypertrophy of the glutæi comes next in frequency. The quadriceps extensor of the thighs may become paretic, and even perfectly paralyzed, without showing any sign of enlargement. In many cases, however, hypertrophy proceeds regularly up the limbs, and invades the thighs simultaneously with the buttocks.[1] The exact proportion of cases is difficult to ascertain, because the history is often imperfect, and at the time of observation the quadriceps extensor is frequently atrophied, even when it has been hypertrophied at an earlier date. The thinness of the thighs is then all the more conspicuous from the hypertrophy of the calves below and of the buttocks above. The sacro-lumbales and quadratus lumborum muscles are also frequently enlarged, next in order to the quadriceps extensor femoris, which, as seen, is rather less often hypertrophied than are the gluteal muscles.

The flexor muscles of the leg are much less often affected than these; the adductors and the ileo-psoas rather more frequently. Paresis and moderate hypertrophy of the abdominal muscles, though relatively rare, are observed. Thus, from the foot up to the spinal column the morbid imminence is pronounced on the side of the extensor muscles. The liability to invasion on the part of the flexors is greatest at the foot, where dorsal flexion is early impeded, and diminishes upward toward the abdomen.

Most important for the theory of the disease is the fact that the hypertrophic appearance of the muscles is never accompanied by even a transitory period of increased strength.[2] Some degree of paresis usually precedes the hypertrophy, and becomes intensified when this sets in. The two symptoms, however, are by no means proportioned to one another.

There is another anatomical change in the muscles no less characteristic of the disease than is their hypertrophy, which contributes at least as much to the loss of muscular power. This is atrophy of the muscles, which in the lower extremities is almost invariably secondary to a stage of hypertrophy, but which occasionally in the quadriceps extensor constitutes the primary lesion. On the other hand, the calf-muscles, though occasionally retroceding from a state of exaggerated hypertrophy, never atrophy below the normal dimensions.[3]

It not unfrequently happens that the atrophic and hypertrophic pro-

---

[1] Cases in which the calves and thighs are alone described as hypertrophied: those by Kaulich, Griesinger, Sigmund, Wagner, Wernich (2d), Lutz (1st and 2d), Foster, Stoffella, Eulenburg (2d).

Cases of hypertrophy of calves with atrophy of thighs: those by Eulenburg (1st), Lutz (3d), Adams, Barth (2d), Knoll, Friedreich, Gowers (1st, 4th, 5th, 9th, 10th, 11th, 12th, 14th). In Rakowac's case, as also Barth's, the glutæi were also hypertrophied.

Cases of hypertrophy, calves, thighs, glutæi, and sacro-lumbales muscles: Duchenne (1st, 5th, 6th, 7th, 8th, 12th, the last being the miniature Hercules, in which all the muscles were hypertrophied except the pectorals), Heller (2 cases), Benedikt (1st, 2d, 3d, 4th; in the 5th the sacro-lumbales atrophied), Gowers (13th, 20th), Pekelharing.

Cases with hypertrophy of the calves and glutæi, with atrophy of the thighs: Berend, Duchenne fils (hypert. sacro-lumbales), Duchenne (3d, 4th, 10th).

Cases of atrophy of all but calves: Spielmann, Gowers (7th), Hammond (2 cases).

Cases of hypertrophy of calves and deltoids, atrophy of all other muscles: Ross (2 cases).

[2] In Auerbach's case of true muscular hypertrophy the same paresis was observed.

[3] Hammond relates a remarkable case where the muscles of the calves and thighs, having enlarged progressively during about two years, then began to waste, and continued to do so for three years. Then a second stage of hypertrophy set in, and continued at the time of writing (Treatise on Nervous Diseases, 6th ed., p. 508).

cesses go on simultaneously in the same muscle, and so compensate each other that the muscle varies little or nothing from the normal size. This is especially apt to be the case with the pelvic and lumbo-spinal muscles; and thus functional disturbances will develop for which the mere appearance of the involved muscles seems to furnish no sufficient explanation.

The peculiarities which have been described in station, locomotion, and the act of rising to a vertical position nevertheless all depend on such anatomical lesions of the muscles of the back and lower extremities as render the adequate performance of their functions impossible. Thus, the widening of the base of support by straddling the legs is necessitated by weakness in all the extensor muscles of the limbs—the glutæi, quadriceps, and gastrocnemii—which by their tension should normally provide solid columns for the support of the trunk. The lordosis begins with the first difficulty experienced in steadying the heels, but is increased when the gluteals become incapable of extending the pelvis on the femurs and when the sacro-lumbales are unable to extend the vertebral column on the pelvis. The backward projection of the shoulders, effected by the extensors of the upper portion of the spine, is an instinctive compensation for the lordosis, to prevent the trunk from falling altogether forward in front of the base of support.

The lateral oscillations of the trunk have been variously explained. Duchenne attributed them to weakness of the gluteus medius. This muscle, he asserted, is normally designed to restrain the tendency of the pelvis at each step to incline toward the leg which is off the ground.[1] But, in reality, during the act of walking, the pelvis, and the trunk with it, are inclined toward the leg which is fixed, rotating upon the head of the femur on that side, and being slightly elevated on the opposite side, where the leg is being swung forward. This elevation assists in enabling the swinging leg to clear the ground (Ross, Hueter). The rotation is accomplished by the gluteal abductors on the active or fixed side, the femoral extremity of these muscles being fixed. Weakness of the gluteals must interfere with this rotation, and should therefore diminish lateral oscillation did this depend on the rotary movement.

In a case examined by Ross, in which the lateral oscillation was much marked, contractions of the gluteus medius were distinctly perceptible to the hand placed just above the great trochanter. In another case, where the gluteals were entirely destroyed, the oscillation, on the contrary, was barely perceptible. Ross himself explains the phenomenon more plausibly as a simple exaggeration of what occurs in normal locomotion. In this the centre of gravity is necessarily shifted at each step from the movable to the fixed leg by the inclination of the trunk and shoulders to the side of the latter. When the legs are placed far apart the body must incline farther in order to bring the weight in the same relative position. Moreover, from the weakness of the anterior tibial muscles the dorsal flexion of the foot, which should take place at the moment the leg is lifted off the ground, is impeded or rendered impossible; and the inclination of the pelvis on one side, which necessitates its increased elevation on the other, thus favors the swinging of the leg by leaving more room between the trunk and the ground (Ross).

The curious manner in which pseudo-hypertrophic patients rise from a

[1] *Archives gén.*, 1868, p. 23.

sitting or recumbent position has been carefully studied by Gowers, and minutely analyzed by Ross in an adult case. The act to be accomplished demands a series of extensions of the leg and pelvis on the thigh and of the vertebral column on the pelvis. As the extensor muscles are all paretic, this can only be effected by means of the muscles of the upper extremities and of the weight of the body, which the arms compel to serve as a motor force. Thus, from a recumbent position the patient rolls upon his hands and knees: then, grasping the knee, he lifts the leg upright with the foot planted on the ground. The thighs remain strongly flexed, the trunk bent forward over the thighs. The action of grasping the thighs above the knees, which is so characteristic, serves to extend them by a double mechanism. In the first place, the knee-joints are pressed slowly but directly backward. In the second place, by the intermediary of the arms the weight of the body is transferred from the upper end of the femur, above the power of the quadriceps extensor, to the lower end of the lever, near the fulcrum at the knee. Thus a lever of the third order, with the power between the fulcrum and the weight, is partly transformed into a lever of the second order, with the weight between the fulcrum and the power; and thus the enfeebled quadriceps is able to act to more advantage. Moreover, when the body inclines so far forward that the centre of gravity is carried in front of the knees, it then becomes a force applied to the upper end of the femur capable of extending the knees without any action of the quadriceps.

When extension of the knee-joints is nearly complete, extension of the pelvis on the femurs is effected by grasping the thighs alternately higher and higher. By this manœuvre the femur is pushed back and the trunk is pushed up; and thus is compensated the incapacity of the glutæi to perform their normal action of pulling up the pelvis flexed on the femurs. Enough power remains in these muscles, however, for a long time to complete the extension when, by the pushing movement, this has been nearly effected.

During these actions the patient constantly oscillates the trunk from side to side as he transfers the centre of gravity from one foot to the other. In this, the second stage of the disease, and where the same functional disturbances may arise with very various combinations of hypertrophy and atrophy in the muscles of the lower extremities, a third set of symptoms appears—certain deformities, namely, depending on muscular shrinkage. The earliest, and often the most marked, of these is talipes equinus. The patient becomes unable to plant his heels firmly on the ground, and these are gradually drawn up higher and higher, the patient resting first on the toes, then on the anterior surfaces of the phalanges; ultimately is unable to stand at all, the foot being drawn into a line with the leg, and the astragalus not unfrequently luxated. Some authors explain this deformity by the preponderating action of the gastrocnemius. The paralysis of this muscle, which coincides with its hypertrophy, even when not quite proportioned to it, renders such an explanation highly improbable. The elevation of the heel is due to the gradual shrinkage of the muscular tissue which accompanies the pseudo-hypertrophy; and on this account the talipes is at every stage of its development irreducible.

The other possible deformities in the lower extremities are permanent flexions at the knee- or hip-joints. Both existed in the case recently described by Pekelharing.[1] Before the disease has reached its maximum degree of development in the lower extremities, its progress has usually been marked in another manner—namely, by the invasion of the trunk and arms. In cases 19–22 of Gowers's remarkable series, where four boys out of a family of ten children were affected by the disease, the hypertrophy first involved all the muscles of the lower extremities, and then passed to the trunk and arms.[2]

The description of the disease in the upper half of the body may be distinctly separated from that in the lower half, on account of the remarkable differences observed in the mode of the muscular degeneration. In the lower extremities and pelvis primary pseudo-hypertrophy is the rule; atrophy is almost invariably secondary, and below the hips is rarely excessive.[3] In the upper part of the body primary atrophy is the rule for certain muscles, and succeeds rather early to the pseudo-hypertrophy which affects others. Only a few muscles habitually hypertrophy, and remain enlarged until a somewhat advanced period of the disease. The first in this group is the deltoid, which not unfrequently enlarges simultaneously with the gastrocnemii.[4] In one case the triceps humeri, and after that the biceps, are the next most frequently hypertrophied,[5] in some cases even together with atrophy of the deltoids (2d case Seidel). In exceptional cases all the muscles surrounding the shoulder-joint, especially those covering the scapula, are hypertrophied. Thus in the early case of Coste and Gioga[6] the latissimus dorsi and trapezius were hypertrophied, together with the deltoids, and even the muscles of mastication and the tongue. In this case not only the quadratus lumborum, but also the recti abdominis muscles, were hypertrophied. In Chrostek's case the tongue was hypertrophied, although all the shoulder-muscles, and also the sterno-cleido-mastoids, were atrophied.[7] In Duchenne's third case the temporal and masseter muscles were hypertrophied, while no alteration of size in any direction was observed in the arms or shoulders. In Duchenne's twelfth case all the muscles of the body, including the face, were hypertrophied, with the single exception of the pectorals. In Barth's second case, the left sterno-mastoid, the supra and infra spinali, together with the left deltoid, were hypertrophied.

In the majority of cases, however, at the time the patient came under observation all the muscles above the quadratus lumborum were atrophied, except the deltoids. In the pectoral, which has never been found hypertrophied, the wasting process always sets in the earliest, and advances to the greatest extent. The pectoral muscle is thus the exact antithesis of the gastrocnemius, while the deltoid more nearly resembles

---

[1] *Loc. cit.*   [2] Three other boys in this family, and three girls, remained healthy.

[3] The quadricipites femoris, as already noticed, are not unfrequently wasted.

[4] See cases of Kaulich, hypertrophy of calves, thighs, deltoids; Heller, hypertrophy of all muscles of lower limbs, also of abdomen with deltoids; Benedikt (4th and 6th cases); Friedreich (1st case); Adams; Gowers (4th and 11th); Ross (2 cases); Brieger. In a case by Clarke (*Med.-Chir. Trans.*, vol. lvii.) the deltoids were observed to be large seven years after the beginning of the disease. In a case by Duchenne the enlargement of the deltoids, by great exception, preceded that of the gastrocnemii by several months.

[5] Cases of hypertrophy triceps or biceps: Seidel (2d), Rinecker, Griesinger, Wagner (2d, triceps without deltoid), Knoll, Rakowac, Pekelharing, Spielmann (atrophy deltoid).

[6] *Schmidt's Jahrb.*, Bd. xxiv. S. 196. Other cases are given by Wernich (hypertrophy of rhomboids), Barth, Gowers (11th).   [7] *Oesterreich Zeitschrift f. prakt. Heilk.*, 1871.

the gastrocnemius than any other muscle of the upper extremity. After the pectoral the latissimus dorsi, then the trapezius scapular muscles (including the serratus magnus), those of the arm and fore arm, the muscles of the neck, are found more or less wasted by the time the disease is fully developed. The wasting is sometimes extreme, as in a case described by Gowers, where the patient maintained a permanently crouching attitude, the spinal column being in extreme cyphosis, all its processes projecting, from the extreme emaciation of the trunk.

In Eulenburg's adult case[1] the atrophy began in the hands, and was regarded by him as a combination of true progressive muscular atrophy in the upper, with lipomatosis musculorum luxurians in the lower extremities.[2]

Gowers attaches diagnostic importance to the early signs of atrophy in the latissimus dorsi and great pectoral muscles. The time of their invasion contrasts with that in progressive muscular atrophy, where the process usually begins in the hands and creeps upward to the shoulder-joint.

Neither the atrophic nor the hypertrophic process is necessarily symmetrical on the two sides of the body, but an approximate symmetry is usually observed. The same muscles are usually affected, and in the same way, but not often precisely to the same degree. Fibrillary contractions often occur in the wasting muscles, but not in those which are hypertrophied. The electrical reactions, however, do not differ greatly in the two states. The faradic contractility diminishes in proportion to the diminution in the contractile mass of the muscle, whether this be concealed by the growth of fat and connective tissue or rendered obvious by the general wasting of the whole. But even when contractions can be obtained, these are often abnormally feeble, and by continual diminution in the number of contractile fibres, and increase in the lipomatous masses overlying them, the electrical irritability is ultimately lost. The excitability of the nerves remains intact, and therefore response may be obtained by an indirect excitation after direct excitation of the muscle fails to elicit one.

Eulenburg has occasionally observed one curious phenomenon in the galvanic reaction of nerves. The anode opening contraction grows weaker or even disappears with a progressively stronger current, and then with a still stronger current reappears. This is due to a cross action of the current on the excitability and on the conductibility of the nerve. At a certain moment the increased excitability is compensated by a corresponding increase in the resistance to conduction, and therefore all electrical response ceases. Later, the resistance remaining the same, the excitability is increased and the reaction reappears.

---

[1] Virch. Arch., Bd. xlix., 1870.

[2] Cases of atrophy (often excepting deltoids): 1st case by Seidel, "simultaneous paresis in upper and lower extremities in four years; atrophy of arms and thighs, with hypertrophy of calves and fore arms; in six years, primary atrophy sterno-cleido-mastoids and pectorals; secondary atrophy of deltoids."

Further: case of Kaulich (atrophy of shoulder-muscles, including deltoid, while triceps and biceps hypertrophied); Duchenne fils; Eulenburg and Cohnheim; Heller (2 cases); Wagner (2d case); Wernich (1st case); Lutz (a girl, case much resembling Eulenburg's adult case); Roquette (atrophy of thighs as well); Hoffmann; Russel; Foster (atrophy of muscles of forearm); Chrostek (notwithstanding hypertrophy of tongue); Friedreich (2 cases); Duchenne (2d); Wagner (2d and 3d); Gowers (9 cases) · Ross (2 cases).

The symptoms of the first order (disturbance of muscular function) and of the third (deformity) are for a long time less conspicuous in the upper than in the lower extremities. When the arms begin to be paretic the patient is crippled in the characteristic manœuvres by which, during the earlier period of the disease, he palliates the inefficiency of the lower limbs. When he can no longer push up the trunk by means of his arms, he becomes unable to rise from a sitting position at all. Further progress in the atrophy of the erectores spinæ muscles renders even the act of sitting impossible: the patient can only crouch, and ultimately must remain altogether recumbent. The functions of the hands usually remain unimpaired to the last, so that the unfortunate patient is able to amuse himself with knitting and other light work.

Besides the paralytic cyphosis, scoliosis of a high grade is sometimes, though infrequently, developed. It is due to the lateral oscillations with excessive inclination of the upper portion of the trunk.[1]

It is rare that any researches have been made on the nutritive functions in pseudo-hypertrophic paralysis. Seidel[2] has analyzed the urine in the two cases (brothers) which form the basis of his memoir. He expected to find a marked diminution in the urea, corresponding to the diminution in the mass and in the functional activity of the muscles. This expectation was based on the assumption, at present considered incorrect, that the elimination of urea is modified by muscular contractions. In the cases examined the actual amount of urea was considerable, rising on several occasions to 40, 43, and 69 grammes in twenty-four hours, and offering, in the first boy, a daily average of 41 grammes. But Scherer estimates that the average elimination of urea in children is, per kilogramme, double that in adults; and on the basis of this calculation the amount of urea eliminated by the patient in question should have been 51 grammes. There was therefore a diminution of about one-fifth.

Seidel has also examined the temperature of the diseased muscles during their contraction either under the influence of the will or of the faradic current. The hypertrophied gastrocnemius muscle showed a rise of 1.5° to 2° less than a healthy gastrocnemius similarly excited. The rise of temperature never occurred during the contraction, but during the ten or fifteen minutes which followed it. The duration of this rise of temperature was always longer than in the control experiment performed on a healthy subject. The observation was the same in hypertrophied and in atrophied muscles, and indicated a notable diminution of heat-production in both.[3]

The mental functions are not unfrequently impaired. The defective intelligence exhibited by several of his first patients led Duchenne to attribute a cerebral origin to the disease. The internal hydrocephalus discovered at the autopsy of the case so recently published by Pekelharing suggests that this hypothesis may have been too hastily abandoned, and that it may really prove to be correct for certain cases. In many, however, the intelligence is intact or even precocious, and all suspicion of cerebral lesion must be excluded.

[1] Cases of scoliosis from such cause, where inequality of muscular action cannot be invoked as a cause, help to throw light on the real etiology of the idiopathic deformity so often attributed to irregular muscular action.
[2] *Atrophia Musculorum Lipomatosa*, Jena, 1867   [3] *Loc. cit.*, p. 54.

COURSE OF THE DISEASE.—As already stated, a period of paresis may precede all signs of hypertrophy for several weeks, months, or even years. From the time that the enlargement of the calves has once begun about a year and a half is required before the maximum of hypertrophy is attained. Then the disease usually remains stationary for two or three years before the third period is ushered in by aggravation of paralysis in the lower and by extension of paralysis, together with hypertrophy or atrophy, to the upper limbs.

When, from complete loss of muscular power, the patient has become permanently condemned to a recumbent position, life may nevertheless be prolonged for ten or twelve years, with integrity of all the vegetative functions. Death finally takes place, in all recorded cases, from some acute pulmonary disease, whose effects are intensified by the atrophy of the external respiratory muscles, which often extends even to the intercostals.

The course of the disease, and consequent prognosis, is much modified in the rare cases in which it attacks girls. Two of Duchenne's thirteen cases were girls: in one the disease was spontaneously arrested, in the other apparently cured. Lutz[1] relates the altogether exceptional history of a family in which five female members were affected—two sisters, also one step-sister, daughter of the mother by an earlier marriage, a sister and niece of the mother, of whom a brother also was diseased. The step-sister and niece both died at six years of age, but the aunt lived to be forty-three (the brother to be forty-two), and one of the girls observed by Lutz, who began to suffer at the age of six, was twenty-eight at the time of observation: paresis had only become marked at seventeen, and locomotion impossible at twenty-two. In the other girl the first symptoms appeared at seventeen, and at twenty-two were still moderate and confined to the lower extremities.

In Roquette's female case[2] the disease began at ten; in Hoffman's,[3] at eleven and a half. These cases, with one of Benedikt's, are the only female cases among the 88 I have analyzed.[4] Gowers estimates 30 female cases out of a total of 220, or only 13 per cent. of the whole.

This great preponderance in the male sex is the first of three striking peculiarities which distinguish the clinical history of the disease. The second is its strangely-marked hereditary character. This is not, and indeed hardly could be, shown in a direct line, since the patients are incapable of marriage, or even die before arriving at maturity. But several brothers in a family are usually afflicted. There was, it is true, no trace of heredity in Duchenne's 13 cases, but this author himself recognizes the frequency of hereditary influence in those observed by others. Out of 81 cases analyzed by Friedreich, two or more members of one family were attacked thirty-five times. Thus, the first clinical report, that made by Meryon, described four brothers in one family and two in another. Coste, Griesinger, Wernich, Benedikt, Adams, Russel, Gowers, each relate cases of two members in one family; Heller, Wagner, Billroth,

[1] Deutsches Archiv f. klin Med., Bd. iii., 1867.
[2] Inaug. Dissert., Berlin, 1868, quoted by Friedreich.   [3] Ibid., 1867.
[4] This excludes the adult cases of Eulenburg, where "progressive atrophy of the upper extremities combined with pseudo-hypertrophy of the lower;" the case of Barth, an amyotrophic lateral sclerosis; the case of Müller, a dementia paralytica; and the case of Billroth, where the lesion was localized in the hamstring muscles of one thigh.

Seidel, have seen three : Moore[1] describes three cases out of a family of seven, consisting of five boys and two girls. Two of the cases I myself have seen were brothers. Gowers[2] relates five cases in the families of two sisters who married two brothers. This same writer refers to three other families in which two brothers were affected; to a fourth family described by Clifford Albutt, where two brothers were paralyzed, the third child dying of Hodgkin's disease; finally, to the family of a clergyman, himself living to the age of seventy-four, having always had large calves, and out of whose eight children two boys and one girl were affected.

The families invaded by this singular disease are often remarkably large, and even where several children are affected, many others, even boys, escape. The morbid inheritance is always through the mother, "thus through the ovum—a condition unknown in diseases of the nervous system" (Gowers). This peculiarity belongs to only one other disease, hæmophilia, also almost limited to males. The third fact, which from its all but universality is shown to be of fundamental importance, is that the disease begins during infancy or early childhood. It has been shown that more than two-thirds of all cases began before the age of six. Whether there is ever an intra-uterine origin is still doubtful (Friedreich). This early invasion, often coinciding with the first efforts to walk or to use the muscles which are first attacked, distinctly separates pseudo-hypertrophic paralysis from all diseases which can be traced to definite accidents or to perversion of functions. It implies a profound perversion of nutrition, or rather a misdirection of developmental force.

PATHOLOGICAL ANATOMY.—The anatomical lesions of pseudo-hypertrophic paralysis are to be sought first in the muscles, afterward in the spinal cord, upon which so many peripheric lesions of the nervo-muscular system have recently been shown to depend. The argument from analogy, therefore, has of itself almost sufficed to create a conviction that some disease of the central nervous organs must exist as the real basis of pseudo-muscular hypertrophy.[3] Nevertheless, as will presently be shown, the present evidence in favor of such hypothesis is extremely small.

Muscular Lesions.—In the muscles, however, the anatomical changes are profound and varied. They may be divided into three kinds—those affecting the muscular fibre itself; those touching the connective tissue; and, finally, the fat deposited in this.

The lesions of these different elements are variously combined with each other in different muscles, and also at different stages of the disease. Thus, in the muscles of the trunk and upper extremities affected with primary atrophy the increase of fat is always moderate and quite insufficient to compensate the wasting of the contractile mass, while in the gastrocnemii and gluteal muscles the hypertrophied masses are often found to consist entirely of fat, traversed by bands of connective tissue, and indistinguishable from a lipoma.

The muscles have been examined in two ways—in the course of a general post-mortem examination, and also during life by means of excision or extraction by various instruments. Griesinger in 1864[4] excised a piece

---

[1] *Lancet*, 1880.
[3] This conviction is fully expressed by Hammond, *loc. cit.*
[2] *Loc. cit.*, Appendix.
[4] *Archiv der Heilkunde.*

of the deltoid in a boy of thirteen,[1] and made on it, with Billroth, the first microscopic examination of the diseased muscles. Duchenne, to avoid an operation not devoid of danger for the patient, devised his harpoon, by means of which small fragments of muscles could be torn away. As this instrument is liable to change the relations of the parts separated by tearing, Leech has contrived another, in which the fragment is removed by cutting. By one method or another of harpooning the muscular lesions have been studied during life by Duchenne, Heller, Wernich, Russel, Eulenburg, Martini, Knoll, Rakowac, Friedreich, Ross, Gowers, Auerbach, Hammond, Pepper, in the cases already quoted.

Muscular Fibre.—There are contradictory opinions in regard to the first stage of alteration in the muscular fibres. According to most observers, the fibres are seen to directly atrophy; the transverse striæ become dim and gradually disappear, and the primitive bundles shrink in diameter from loss of some of their fibrillæ (Brieger, Hammond, Pepper). Friedreich[2] adds that the complete collapse of the contractile substance in the primitive bundles often leaves empty or shrunken sarcolemma sheaths, which swell the mass of the connective tissue. Friedreich, however, denies that the striation is modified; and its extreme fineness, commented upon by Duchenne, is considered by Ollivier[3] and Ranvier as devoid of pathological significance.

The real size of the primitive fibres is best estimated by the method of Cohnheim, who isolated the fibres by boiling the muscular fragment from four to six hours in a mixture containing 100 c.c. of 90 per cent. alcohol and $\frac{3}{4}$ c.c. of concentrated muriatic acid. Many were found reduced to one-fifteenth or one-sixteenth their normal size.[4] Between atrophied fibres lay a peculiar striped tissue, probably composed of empty sarcolemma sheaths. Side by side with these atrophied fibres were many normal, and others grossly hypertrophied to two or even three times the normal calibre. These were only found in the hyper-voluminous muscles. Some of these exceeded the largest frog-muscle fibres. They lay in bundles of four to six between the small fibres, and seemed to be about equally distributed through the hypertrophied gastrocnemius and atrophied biceps.[5]

Another alteration observed in the muscular fibres was their dichotomous and even trichotomous division. This same lesion has been seen by Friedreich in progressive muscular atrophy.

The presence of hypertrophied fibres in wasting muscles lends a special significance to the cases of true muscular hypertrophy described by Auerbach[6] and Hitzig.[7] Auerbach's observation related to a soldier aged twenty-one, whose upper arm became rather rapidly hypertrophied and parctio. In a fragment excised from the enlarged biceps the fibres were seen to have a diameter of from 96 to 180 u. (the normal diameter being 33 to 67 u.). The other arm was not enlarged, and yet examination of fibres obtained by means of a similar excision found them also enlarged. Auerbach suggests that this hypertrophy constituted a preliminary stage

---

[1] The wound suppurated for a long time.   [2] Loc. cit., p. 300.
[3] Des Atrophies musculaires, Thèse d'Agrégation.
[4] Berlir. klin. Wochensch., 1865, No. 56.
[5] Hypertrophied fibres have also been seen by Knoll (Medizin Jahrbuch., Wien, 1872), Müller, and Eulenburg.
[6] Virch. Arch., Bd. liii., 1871.   [7] Berlin. klin. Wochen., Dec. 2, 1872.

in the general process of pseudo-hypertrophic paralysis. In it, as when the excessive volume is known to depend upon the presence of non-contractile tissue, the arm, far from increasing in strength, was paretic.[1]

Connective Tissue.—Far more conspicuous than the alterations in the contractile fibre of the muscles are those of its connective tissue. The perimysium internum, between the primitive bundles, proliferates abundantly, and the hyperplasia gradually extends correlatively with the wasting of the muscular fibres, until the hypertrophied mass is mainly composed of connective tissue. Broad bands replace the thin lamellæ normally present between the primitive bundles; the parenchyma of the muscle seems stifled in a sclerosis. It is then that it offers the feeling of stony hardness so often noticed in the clinical history.

Charcot, Knoll, Müller, and Barth describe a rich development of nuclei and of spindle-shaped cells in this new connective tissue, this being especially abundant in the neighborhood of the small vessels and in their adventitia. Eulenburg and Leyden, however, affirm that the connective tissue is unusually poor in nuclei, and thence infer that the hyperplasia is compensatory, and not due to inflammation.

In some cases, as in those of Duchenne examined by Ordonez, the sclerosis and atrophy of contractile tissue constitute the entire lesion of the muscle. Only a few fat-cells are interspersed among the bands of connective tissue or penetrate between the primitive bundles. The fatty infiltration tends constantly to increase, apparently by the same process as governs the growth of normal adipose tissue—namely, the deposit of fat in connective-tissue cells; and ultimately not only muscular fibre, but the hyperplastic connective tissue, is concealed in a yellowish glistening mass indistinguishable from a lipoma.[2]

The growth of fat contributes to the apparent hypertrophy of the diseased muscles, but much less so than does the hyperplasia of connective tissue which invariably precedes it. Great rapidity of fatty infiltration marks a more rapid and irresistible progress in the disease, a lower stage of nutritive degradation. Fat-cells are found penetrating between the primitive bundles of fibres in the atrophied as well as in the hypertrophied muscles; but there the fatty substitution is always much less complete.

In contrast with this fatty infiltration true fatty degeneration of the muscular fibre is as rare in pseudo-hypertrophy as in progressive muscular atrophy. This fact is emphasized by Pepper from observation of the harpooned fragment examined by him,[3] also by Cohnheim.[4] In Meryon's first case,[5] however, the post-mortem examination of the muscular fibres found them "totally degenerated, their substance changed into a mass of granules and oil-globules, while the sarcolemma was destroyed." In Brieger's case[6] the fibres were filled with fat-globules.

The sclerotic process which precedes the stage of fatty infiltration is far from being completed when this latter begins. Both processes, initiated nearly at the same time, continue together, and at the death of the patient may be found existing in about equal proportion, or the one

---

[1] Mobius (*loc. cit.*) declares that neither of these cases bears any relation to pseudo-hypertrophy.

[2] See case of Billroth. [3] *Philada. Med. Times*, 1871. [4] *Loc. cit.*

[5] *Med.-Chir. Trans.*, vol. xv., 1852. [6] *Deutsches Archiv*, Bd. xxii.

markedly predominating over the other. In cases of long duration the hypertrophied muscles, as already stated, are found converted into masses of fat, divided by stripes and bands of connective tissue. With death earlier in the disease the enlargement is found to be due to masses of connective tissue englobing muscular fibres and interspersed with fat-cells.

In the wasted whitish-red muscles the proliferation of connective tissue is sometimes more, sometimes less, marked ; in the pale-yellowish muscles fat accumulates by interstitial deposit, but does not overlay and conceal the remnant of muscular fibre.

Central Nervous Organs.—While the examinations of the diseased muscles have been frequent, post-mortem examinations are still relatively few, although their records are rapidly increasing. The first was made by Meryon[1] on the first of his series of six cases. Charcot has examined a case for Duchenne ; Cohnheim has made a celebrated autopsy for Eulenburg ;[2] Gowers and Clarke have together published a fourth.[3] The cases by Müller and Barth are still habitually—though, as we shall see, erroneously—included among the autopsies of pseudo-hypertrophic paralysis. Ross[4] and Leach have, however, a fifth indubitable case with autopsy ; and more recently Cornil,[5] Brieger,[6] Bay,[7] Schultze,[8] Pekelharing,[9] and possibly Goetz and Drummond,[10] have all described post-mortem examinations. The data for discussion, therefore, are to be derived from 14 cases. Of these, the spinal cord was found perfectly healthy in 7, those related by Meryon, Cohnheim, Charcot, Cornil, Brieger, Bay, Schultze—all most competent observers. The cases by Barth and Müller require some special consideration, for, although rejected as irrelevant by most authors, Hammond still adduces them in proof of the central origin of pseudo-hypertrophic paralysis.

Müller's case[11] is that of a woman thirty-four years of age who at the age of four fell out of bed, and from that time began to walk with difficulty, and ultimately acquired a double talipes equinus. The right leg atrophied, the left remained of tolerable thickness. At the age of thirty-four she was admitted to an insane asylum during the incipient stage of dementia paralytica, and death occurred two years later of pneumonia. The autopsy showed—1st. That the calf-muscles on both sides were converted into masses of fat, streaked with whitish-red remnants of muscular tissue. The short muscles of the feet were atrophied ; all the other muscles of the body normal. 2d. In the brain the blood-vessels showed a thickening of the adventitia by delicate connective-tissue fibrillæ, between whose meshes nucleated cells were strewed. The ependyma of the ventricles was thickened and granular, and their cavity was filled with serous effusion. 3d. In the cord was found diffused degeneration, especially of the lateral columns, consisting in thickening of the interstitial connective tissue, with proliferation of its cells ; atrophy of a part of the primitive nerve-fibres with granular degeneration of the

[1] *Loc. cit.*   [2] *Loc. cit.*
[3] *Med.-Chir. Trans.*, 1874; also monograph by Gowers.   [4] *Loc. cit.*
[5] *Union méd.*, 1880.   [6] *Deutsches Archiv f. klin. Med.*, Bd. xxii. H. 2.
[7] *Virch. Jahresb.*, 1877.   [8] *Virch. Arch.*, 1879, Bd. lxxv.
[9] *Arch. Virch.*, Bd. lxxxix., 11, 2, 1882.
[10] Quoted by Pekelharing—the first from the *Aerztliches Intelligenz Blattmünchen*, 1879; the second from the *Lancet*, 1881, vol. ii, No. 16.
[11] *Beiträge zur pathol. des Ruckenmarkes*, 1871.

medullary sheath, and occasionally atrophy of the axis cylinder. The adventitia of the blood-vessels was thickened, the perivascular spaces dilated. In the central gray substance the ganglion-cells were everywhere intact, but the intercellular substance was thicker, and seemingly composed of a thick net of stout, finely-granular fibres. Traces of an infantile polio-myelitis were found in the lower part of the lumbar enlargement (atrophy of the anterior cornua, especially the right, together with their ganglion-cells).

The final lesion of importance was the obliteration of the central canal, which was moreover surrounded by a dense ring of connective tissue. In this case the suddenness of the original paresis, the atrophy of the right leg, and the lesions of the lumbar cord found at the autopsy prove that the initial disease was an acute anterior polio-myelitis. Upon this a very localized pseudo-hypertrophy seems to have been grafted during childhood, while in adult life a chronic lepto-meningitis and internal hydrocephalus were certainly the cause of the symptoms, and probably of the lesions in the cord.

That such lesions in the cord may be the consequence of chronic hydrocephalus is well argued by Pekelharing in regard to his own recently published case, which in some respects closely resembles that by Müller. The patient was a boy in whom muscular paresis was congenital, and who from birth had exhibited deficient intelligence with an abnormally large head. At the autopsy, made at fourteen, ventricular effusion was found in the brain, and in the cord irregular dilatation of the central canal and great ·dilatation of blood-vessels and accumulation of leucocytes in its immediate neighborhood. Some ganglion-cells in the inner and anterior groups of the anterior cornua were shrunken and deprived of their prolongations. The author suggests that in this case the cerebral hydrocephalus was the primary disease; that the central canal in the spinal cord was dilated by extension of the effusion from the brain; that a partial reabsorption of such effusion had caused hyperæmia ex vacuo in the tissue immediately surrounding the canal; and that the emigration of leucocytes and partial alteration of the ganglion-cells both resulted from this hyperæmia.

In Müller's case the central canal and adjacent tissue were also the part of the cord most diseased; but the canal was obliterated by proliferation of the ependyma, not dilated. In Barth's case also[1] the central canal of the cord was found obliterated. The patient was a man of forty-four, who since the age of forty had suffered from stiffness in the left ankle and difficulty of walking. After a year the stiffness extended to the right ankle; in two years the paresis had mounted to the thighs, and was accompanied by severe pains. Paresis and pain then appeared in the upper extremities, which gradually atrophied. After two years the patient was entirely confined to bed, and two years later was unable even to sit up. Later, the muscles of the neck became hypertrophied. No mention is made of perceptible hypertrophy in other muscles, nor of contractions or tremors other than fibrillary. But at the autopsy was discovered a lateral sclerosis extending the entire length of the cord, associated with partial atrophy of the ganglion-cells in the anterior cornua. In both the gray and white substances the blood-vessels were dilated, and,

[1] *Archiv der Heilkunde,* xii. 2, 1871.

as already stated, the central canal was obliterated. The brain was healthy. The supinators of the upper extremities, the gastrocnemii at the lower, were richly infiltrated with fat streaked with long bands of connective tissue; the remaining muscles were atrophied.

The anatomical lesions in this case are identical with those of the special symptom-complex described by Charcot as amyotrophic lateral sclerosis. Certain symptoms of lateral sclerosis are wanting to complete the clinical history, but at least as many are lacking for a typical history of pseudo-hypertrophic paralysis. Only the muscles of the neck hypertrophied : the gastrocnemii and adductors, primarily atrophied, later regained some of their original size. The fatty infiltration of the calf and muscles was unattended by pseudo-enlargement or by retraction : it resembled a fatty substitution due to nerve-paralysis, rather than the hyperplastic process of pseudo-hypertrophy.

Setting aside the three foregoing cases, three remain which, together with an unimpeachable history of pseudo-hypertrophic paralysis, show positive lesions in the spinal cord. The first and the most famous was made upon a patient of Gowers by Lockhart Clarke.[1] Changes were found scattered through the entire length of the cord. "In the upper cervical region were patches of incipient disintegration in the gray network of the lateral portion of the cord, the lateral white columns being healthy. Here and there in the gray substance of the anterior and posterior cornua the intercellular matrix was wasted and disintegrated, especially in the neighborhood of the blood-vessels and at the bottom of the anterior median fissure. Here were accumulated globules of myeline and other débris of nerve-tissue. The blood-vessels were distended, their perivascular spaces enlarged. Patches of disintegration of nerve-fibres of the lateral and posterior columns were seen in the lower cervical and in the dorsal regions. Globules of myeline and masses of fatty matter were at some points accumulated at the entrance of the posterior nerve-roots, and even, to a much less extent, adjacent to the anterior roots. The most extensive lesion existed in the lowest part of the dorsal region. In the lateral gray substance on each side was an area of softening containing an actual cavity just outside each posterior vesicular column. The latter remained undamaged.

"The anterior cornua throughout the cord were perfectly normal, though the processes of the cells were perhaps less distinct than elsewhere. Further, notwithstanding the spots of disintegration in the lateral columns there was in them no change comparable to that of lateral sclerosis."[2]

The second post-mortem was made by Ross on a patient belonging to Leech : "In the lumbar region of the cord the normal loose and spongy texture of the central column was replaced by a somewhat dense and fibrillated tissue, in which no trace of ganglion-cells could be found. The blood-vessels were enlarged and their walls thickened. In the anterior cornua the ganglion-cells had completely disappeared from the median area, the anterior group, and from the margins of all the other groups. This atrophic process extended into the dorsal and cervical

[1] *Med.-Chir. Trans.*, 1874.
[2] This autopsy was made on a boy of fifteen, in whom the calves began to hypertrophy at three, and reached their maximum size at five.

region, and in the latter the central column was changed in the manner already described."[1]

The third autopsy is recorded by Drummond in the *Lancet* for 1881 (vol. ii.): The subject was a boy of fourteen, who never walked after the age of six. There was found, as the author shows by some good drawings, disintegration in the lateral gray network of fibres halfway between the anterior and posterior horns, extending more or less throughout the cord. In the left lumbar region the tissue had broken down, and a cavity existed filled with serum, which bulged out the wall of the cord, forming an apparent tumor.

Several circumstances are common to all the foregoing five cases. In all, the patients during life had exhibited paresis and atrophy of a large number of muscles (in Barth's case nearly all), with pseudo-hypertrophy of some muscles of the lower extremities. In all, the post-mortem found fatty substitution for muscular fibre in both the atrophied and the hypertrophied muscles. Finally, in all, the lesions found in the cord were principally grouped about the central canal. This was dilated (Pekelharing) or obliterated (Müller, Barth); the hyperæmia was always most intense in its vicinity; and it was in the lateral gray substance adjoining, or in the gray network between it and the lateral white columns, that patches of disintegration were principally noted (Clarke, Ross). Negatively, the absence of any extensive lesion of the anterior cornua is noteworthy in all the cases but one; and here this lesion was evidently secondary to the lateral sclerosis (Barth). On the other hand, the differences between these cases were as numerous as the resemblances. Two resembled each other in the presence of cerebral symptoms and of an internal hydrocephalus to account for them (Pekelharing, Müller); in one alone was there lateral sclerosis (Barth); in one, cavities in the lateral portion of the central gray column (Clarke); in one, traces of an acute polio-myelitis (Müller), Finally, in only three cases (Clarke, Ross, Drummond) was the clinical history perfectly characteristic of the disease.

Comparing these facts with the others, equally significant, where the autopsy in cases of pseudo-muscular hypertrophy has shown the central nervous organs to be perfectly healthy, we should be led to conclude—1st. That if fatty substitution in the muscles is ever to be associated with lesions of the spinal cord, these are to be sought in the central gray substance surrounding the central canal. 2d. That, nevertheless, muscular lesions similar, if not in all respects identical, can develop as the result of an idiopathic process depending on causes at present unknown. 3d. That atrophy of muscular fibre and replacement of it by lipomatous fat are probably determined in several different ways, and must often be regarded as merely secondary processes;[2] but that the muscular lesion characteristic of pseudo-hypertrophy, considered as an idiopathic disease, is the hyperplasia of connective tissue which originates in the perimysium interum of the muscles. This lesion was well marked in the Ross-Leech case, much less distinct in the three we have noted as doubtful (Gowers).

---

[1] *Loc. cit.*, p. 207. Patient was nine years old at time of death; the disease had begun with paresis at two; was well developed at nine.

[2] See Leyden's remarks in his essay "Ueber Polio-myelitis und Neuritis," *Zeitschrift für klin. Med.,* 1880·

PATHOGENY.—These last conclusions, if valid, supersede the necessity for prolonged discussion of the question whether pseudo-hypertrophic paralysis be a peripheral disease or central disease. By the latter term authors almost invariably mean a disease dependent on morbid processes in the spinal cord. Hammond is almost alone in affirming that these exist, and bases his opinion on only three autopsies, of which two are the doubtful cases of Müller and Barth. Mobius,[1] recognizing the frequent absence of spinal lesions, nevertheless claims that the hereditary, frequently congenital, nature of the disease proves that it inheres in the nervous system. Gowers, however, points out that the exclusive inheritance through the mother—that is, from the ovum—is a circumstance unknown in nervous diseases. This mode of inheritance is observed in hæmophilia, which also resembles pseudo-hypertrophy in being almost confined to males.

The pseudo-muscular hypertrophy of children so strikingly resembles in many particulars the progressive muscular atrophy of adults that the theory of their essential identity could not fail to suggest itself. Friedreich unhesitatingly advocates this theory. Many of the facts which support it become for him additional confirmation of the peripheric nature of the adult disease, where, nevertheless, the anterior ganglion-cells of the cord are habitually found atrophied.[2]

Eulenburg thus sums up the relations between progressive muscular atrophy and pseudo-hypertrophic paralysis: In both diseases the fundamental muscular lesion consists in a chronic irritative process, which starts from the interstitial connective tissue, and secondarily affects the muscular fibre. In children, pseudo-hypertrophy of the muscles of the lower extremities is regularly followed by primary atrophy of many of the muscles in the upper half of the body, and secondary atrophy in almost all. In a case of Eulenburg's the two typical diseases seemed to coexist in the same patient, an adult woman. More frequently they coexist in the same family, as in the observation by Russel, where two brothers suffered from progressive atrophy, a third from pseudo-hypertrophic paralysis.

Pick[3] relates a case where a typical atrophy of the upper extremities and of the trunk was accompanied by moderate hypertrophy of the calves, with proliferation in the calf-muscles of the interstitial fat and connective tissue. Charcot admits a special form of atrophia musculorum lipomatosa which complicates progressive muscular atrophy, and is associated, therefore, with atrophy of the anterior ganglion-cells; with which, however, it has no direct connection.

The adult and infantile muscular diseases differ by the remarkable, and sometimes even colossal, apparent development of the calf-muscles through the excessive development in them of fat and connective tissue

[1] *Volkmann's Sammlung,* No. 171.

[2] According to the Friedreich theory, the lesion of the anterior cornua is coincident with or consecutive to degeneration of the other extremity of the nervo-muscular motor apparatus.
Lichtheim, *Arch. f. Psych.,* viii., quoted in *Brain,* 1879, vol. ii., No. 1, quotes a case of progressive muscular atrophy with typical changes in the muscles, but unaccompanied by the slightest change in the nerves or nerve-roots, large ganglion-cells of the anterior cornua, or other part of the spinal cord. The author agrees in regarding the nearly allied pseudo-hypertrophic paralysis as a peripheric affection. See also Hayem.

[3] "Ueber einen Fall von progressive muskel atrophie," *Archiv für Psych.,* Bd. vi., 1876.

—by the fact that the latter disease invariably begins in the lower extremities, and is almost peculiar to childhood, while the progressive atrophy begins in the upper half of the body, and usually the hands, and is as nearly exclusively limited to adult life. For both diseases may be admitted, with Friedreich, "a congenital nutritive and formative weakness of the striated muscle-substance" (Gowers). But, we may add, in progressive atrophy this does not become manifest until the muscles have been for many years subjected to the strain of constant employment: in pseudo-hypertrophy the nutritive failure appears early in the flagging of the developmental forces at the moment that these are strained in muscular growth.

It would perhaps be more correct to ascribe the error of development to a perversion of nutritive forces rather than to their weakness. For there is no arrest in the general development of the limbs, such as occurs after infantile spinal paralysis: the bones grow normally; the initial lesion is hyperplasia of the connective tissue—possibly, also, true hypertrophy of the muscular fibre. The wasting is secondary. Perhaps the terminal nerve-plates, or else the capillary network on the outside of the primitive bundles of muscle-fibre, does not grow in proportion to the increasing mass, and therefore becomes insufficient for its nutrition (Auerbach).

The question arises whether the primitive error of development does not lie in the capillary network. Ranvier has shown that the capillaries of muscles are specially adapted to them, being disposed in quadrangles, at whose corners the vascular canal dilates into little pouches. It is surmised that these pouches serve as reservoirs to hold an extra supply of blood for the moment of contraction.[1] If such specialty of structure be necessary for the proper accomplishment of the muscular contraction, it is evident that any congenital defect in the arrangement of the blood-vessels might disturb in many ways the balance of muscular nutrition. The absence of vascular reservoirs, for instance, would render the supply of blood during the contraction insufficient: the contraction must then be inadequate or exhausting, and the physiological stimulus to the growth of the muscle wanting. On the other hand, the capillaries being, by the hypothesis, adapted to the lower type which nourishes connective tissue, this would become nourished at the expense of the contractile fibre, and the known hyperplasia would result.

That morbid vascularization exists, is shown by the peculiar mottled appearance of the skin, which has often been interpreted as a proof of vaso-motor paralysis (Duchenne). On such an hypothesis, further, the curious and otherwise inexplicable relations between pseudo-hypertrophy and hæmophilia[2] would be explained. The one or the other hereditary disease would be due to imperfection in the blood-vessels—here of structure, there of architecture. This imperfection could be directly traced to the mesoblast in the embryo, in which the vascular tissues exclusively originate. Whether we should admit the bold speculation of His[3] that the tissues of the mesoblast are exclusively derived from the ovum, while

---

[1] *Cours d'Anatomie au Collège de France*, 1880.
[2] Part of which do not exist between pseudo-hypertrophy and progressive atrophy, since the latter disease is not exclusively inherited through the mother.
[3] *Unsere Körper Form.*

the archiblastic tissues—the nervous, muscular, epithelial, and glandular —come from the substance of the spermatozoa fused with it, is beyond the scope of this paper to discuss. But were this speculation well founded, the independent morbid tendencies of the mesoblast would be rendered by so much the more plausible.

The fact that the disease begins in the extensor muscles of the lower extremities is probably to be explained by the rapid development of these muscles during early childhood, and by the functional strain imposed on them during the effort of learning to walk. It is thus really analogous to the début of progressive atrophy in the muscles of the hands of adults —the muscles whose functional activity is the most incessant and the most complex during adult life.

The preponderance of the disease in males remains unexplained, unless it be that the greater extent of muscular development in the male necessitates a greater intensity of developmental force for the muscles, whose deficiency, therefore, would earlier be made manifest.

DIAGNOSIS.—The diagnosis of pseudo-hypertrophic paralysis can never be difficult in typical cases and at an advanced period of the disease. During the early period the diagnosis rests on the gradual diminution of force in the lower extremities, without atrophy or with apparently excellent development of their muscles; the straddling of the legs, lordosis, and lateral oscillation, all at first slight, but constantly becoming more and more emphasized; the peculiar method of rising by placing the hands on the knees and then gradually climbing up the thighs. In the second period the enlargement of the calf or other muscles of the lower limbs, in the third the extension of the paresis to the upper extremities, associated with wasting of the pectorals and usually some of the extensors of the back, confirm beyond question the diagnosis. This may be further established by examination of small fragments of muscular fibre removed by means of the harpoon or trocar, and the repeated examinations, which serve, moreover, to mark the progress of the disease.

Few diseases require to be differentiated. One very rare disease that might be confounded with pseudo-hypertrophy is the infantile form of progressive muscular atrophy. This is distinguished from the ordinary form of atrophy by beginning in the muscles of the face,[1] especially the orbicularis oris, from whose defective contractility the lips become thick and motionless. The morbid process then progresses downward, and is thus in notable contrast with that of pseudo-hypertrophy, which invariably begins in the lower limbs and extends upward, invading the face only by exception.

It is probably after the establishment of talipes equinus and of flexions at the knee- or hip-joint that pseudo-hypertrophy would be most liable to be confounded with infantile atrophic paralysis. In the latter, however, the talipes is much more rarely double, and, if existing, is usually complicated with varus. At an advanced stage of pseudo-hypertrophy the enlargement of the calf is apt to be confined to its upper part, and the retraction of the lower half simulates atrophy, even when this has not really set in. At this stage, moreover, the thighs and gluteal regions are usually atrophied, so that the resemblance to an atrophic paralysis may be considerable. This may be still further increased in those rare

_____
[1] Duchenne has seen seventeen cases of this disease.

cases of extensive polio-myelitis, where paralysis of one or more of the upper extremities coincides with lumbar paraplegia. It is extremely rare, however, that both arms are paralyzed and atrophied,[1] while this is the rule, with approximative symmetry, in pseudo-hypertrophy. In the latter disease, moreover, there are paralysis and atrophy of the muscles of the trunk and abdomen, which is scarcely ever seen, and never to the same extent, in atrophic paralysis. The reflex excitability is lost in the latter disease, as also the faradic; the latter, often intact in pseudo-hypertrophy, rarely is quite abolished. Finally, the history of the case is generally decisive: gradual development in the one, sudden onset, with immediate maximum intensity of paralysis, in the other; primitive wasting of the paralyzed muscles in the spinal paralysis, enlargement preceding the atrophy in the pseudo-hypertrophic paralysis.

Rachitis, with its frequent polysarcia and paretic gait, might sometimes lead to a suspicion of muscular pseudo-hypertrophy, as, conversely, the earlier symptoms of the latter disease may be erroneously referred to rachitis. The error is all the more facile because children afflicted with pseudo-hypertrophy are not unfrequently rachitic, and the symptoms of specific paralysis and muscular sclerosis may easily seem to deepen out of those of muscular inertia and subcutaneous fat which are due to the nutritive diathesis. The consistency of the enlarged limbs is, however, different—soft and flabby in rachitis, hard, even stony, in pseudo-hypertrophy. When in the latter the subcutaneous fat is atrophied instead of increased, the muscles seem to make hernial protrusions through the emaciated skin.

Congenital cerebral disease, due to intra-uterine lesion, causes imperfect walking, and even contraction of the calf-muscles, which may simulate the analogous symptoms of pseudo-hypertrophic paralysis. But the trunk is bent straight forward, and not bent in lordosis; the lower extremities tend to cross in spastic paraplegia; there is no lateral oscillation of the trunk, and the faradic contractility is always preserved. The progress of the diseases suffices to decide all doubts.

TREATMENT.—The excesively bad prognosis of pseudo-hypertrophic paralysis may be inferred from the foregoing description. Duchenne claims to have had two cases brought to him at the early stage of the disease. The first (Obs. 9) was a boy attacked at the age of seven and a half with paresis of the lower extremities. He soon began to walk with a straddling gait, lordosis, and lateral oscillation. Thirty-four months later some enlargement of the calves was noticed, but the disease remained stationary for six months, when the patient was brought to Duchenne. He was treated by hydro-therapeutics, massage, and faradization of the affected muscles. Cure was complete in six months.

The second case (Obs. 13) was a little girl six and a half years old. Paresis of the lower limbs began at the age of four and a half, and rapidly increased. The legs and thighs began to enlarge shortly after the first appearance of the paresis. Treatment began in about a year, and was conducted as in the first case, but in addition cod-liver oil and bitters were administered internally. Cure after a few months' treatment.

Duchenne refers the beneficial effect of the faradic current to a stimu-

---

[1] A patient described by Eulenburg was affected by such general paralysis, but recovered after five months' treatment.

lating action on the vaso-motor nerves and capillary circulation, which he assumes to be paralyzed in this disease. The important point is to exert this stimulus before the hyperplasia of the connective tissue is far advanced.

Benedikt claims to have improved five cases by galvanization of the sympathetic. But the treatment was certainly based on an erroneous theory of the disease, and the alleged results must be received with caution.

Uhde[1] claims to have arrested the progress of the disease in the gastrocnemii muscles by a double tenotomy operation performed for the relief of pes equinus. The patient was a boy of eleven, in whom the disease had begun at the age of five. At the time of observation all the muscles of the legs, as also the glutæi and sacro-lumbales, were hypertrophied. The feet could not be brought to the ground, owing to retraction of the calf-muscles : standing and walking were entirely impossible, and even the power to move the limbs in a recumbent position was very much limited. Faradization during a fortnight produced no effect. Then the tendons were cut, and faradization continued. In a month the patient could execute slight movements in bed ; three weeks later he could walk along the ward ; and four months after the operation he could walk alone and with the soles of the feet flat on the ground. The calves were softer than before, and diminished in circumference. But as the history stops here, it is possible that the two latter changes depended on a substitution of fatty infiltration for sclerosis. By this, moreover, the muscular fibre would be less compressed, and in its temporary liberation would for a while seem to regain part of its force. The last case of alleged recovery that we have seen is by Donkin.[2]

Gowers remarks[3] that treatment must be directed rather against the effects of the morbid process than against the morbid process itself, which, as a primary error of development,[4] must be, to a large extent, beyond our influence. As internal remedies, Gowers recommends arsenic, phosphorus, and cod-liver oil, noting that iron and strychnine seem to have no effect.

Faradization also, which is nearly always used, must have nearly always disappointed expectation, or more cures would be recorded. Systematic muscular exercises are recommended as the appropriate physiological stimulus to muscular growth. But in view of the fact that precisely those muscles are earliest and most profoundly affected which are exposed to the most strenuous influence of this stimulus, it is theoretically doubtful whether this advice be valuable.

[1] *Langenbeck's Archiv für Chir.*, Bd. xvi., 1874.   [2] *Brit. Med. Journ.*, 1882, vol. i.
[3] *Loc. cit.*, p. 52.
[4] Gowers says, "of the muscular tissue," but we have shown reasons why this should rather be sought in the blood-vessels of the part.

DISEASES OF THE SKIN.

DISEASES OF THE SKIN.[1]

By LOUIS A. DUHRING, M. D., AND HENRY W. STELWAGON, M. D.

CLASS I.—DISORDERS OF SECRETION.

Hyperidrosis.

HYPERIDROSIS, or excessive sweating, is a functional disturbance of the sweat-glands characterized by an increased flow of sweat. It may be local or general, slight or excessive. As a local affection, the form which mainly interests the dermatologist, it occurs usually about the hands and feet, especially the palmar and plantar surfaces, and also about the axillæ and genitalia. If the secretion is excessive, maceration of the epidermis results, with tenderness, and even inflammation, of the parts as a consequence: this is not infrequently the result when the feet are involved, a sodden appearance of the parts being not unusual. The affection may be acute or chronic, the latter usually being the case. It is purely a functional disorder, no anatomical changes taking place in the glands or surrounding tissues. There is no change in the nature of the secretion. Debility is usually the fault in general hyperidrosis. The causes of the local varieties are in many cases obscure. Faulty innervation is doubtless frequently an important factor. The nervous system possesses a powerful control over this secretion. The diagnosis presents no difficulties, as there is no other affection with which it could be confounded. Prickly heat and oily seborrhœa are considered to bear some resemblance, but confusion is not likely to occur. Although some cases are readily relieved, the majority prove obstinate. The duration, locality, and extent of the affection, as well as the condition of the general health, are to be considered in pronouncing a prognosis. The disease is liable to relapse.

Concerning treatment, in addition to quinine and the ordinary tonic remedies, belladonna and ergot may be referred to as being useful, particularly the former. Local treatment is always demanded. Dusting-powders are useful, such as starch or lycopodium powder, to which from ten to thirty grains of salicylic acid to the ounce may be added with

---

[1] In the general arrangement and order of diseases the classification adopted by the American Dermatological Association has been followed.

For obvious reasons, personal references are almost entirely omitted in the text, but the authors desire to acknowledge valuable suggestions derived from the writings of J. C. White, R. W. Taylor, L. D Bulkley, J. N. Hyde, W. A. Hardaway, A. R. Robinson. H. G. Piffard, A. Van Harlingen, G. H. Fox, and others.

benefit. They are to be applied freely, so as to absorb the secretions. Astringent lotions are also of value, and constitute the most agreeable method of treatment. One drachm of tannic acid to six ounces of alcohol will be found of service. Solutions of alum and of zinc sulphate may also be employed. Boric acid, either in powder or in the form of a saturated solution, and tincture of belladonna as a lotion, full strength or diluted with alcohol, are both useful. A successful plan of treatment is that by diachylon ointment (unguentum diachyli) as recommended by Hebra. The parts are first cleansed and dried, and then the ointment applied on strips of muslin as a plaster. It is to be renewed twice daily, the parts on each occasion being rubbed dry with lint or a soft towel and lycopodium or starch powder. Water is not to be employed. The treatment must be continued one or two weeks, and then the ointment omitted, and a dusting-powder used night and morning for several weeks. In many cases relief results from one such course; others may require several repetitions. If a good diachylon ointment is not procurable, the same plan may be followed out with an ointment made by melting together equal parts of lead plaster and cosmoline, or with an ointment of tannic acid, a drachm to the ounce.

Anidrosis.

Anidrosis is a functional disorder of the sweat-glands characterized by a diminution or suppression of the secretion. It is the opposite condition of hyperidrosis, and occurs to a slight extent in certain general diseases, and also in some affections of the skin, as ichthyosis. It sometimes occurs as an idiopathic disorder, and may cause much discomfort. Occasionally in nerve-injury localized areas of diminished or suppressed secretion occur. The treatment should be conducted upon general principles, including warm or vapor baths and friction.

Bromidrosis.

Bromidrosis is a functional disorder of the sweat-glands in which the secretion, which may be either normal or excessive in quantity, is of an offensive odor. The quantity is usually excessive, as in hyperidrosis, but occasionally it is normal in amount, while the odor is heavy, strong-smelling, offensive, and disgusting. It may be universal or local in character, more frequently the latter; in either case the odor is rendered more marked by heat and increased perspiration. In smallpox, measles, typhus and relapsing fevers, and in some nervous affections peculiar odors are noticed. Certain drugs, as sulphur, asafœtida, and like substances, taken internally, may be detected in the odor of the sweat. It is as a localized disorder, however, that the affection usually comes under observation, the axillæ, genitalia, and feet being favored localities, the last named being the most common region affected. It occurs about the soles and between the toes, and is generally symmetrical. The sweating, if excessive, causes after a time more or less maceration, and sometimes hyperæmia or inflammation; the skin becomes whitish and sodden, the affected area having a pinkish margin. Both Hebra and Thin consider the socks and soles of the shoes—which become thoroughly permeated by the secretion—and not the feet, the source of the odor. The latter observer states that he has found innumerable bacteria (Bacterium fœtidum) in the fluid in which the sock is soaked. The etiology of the disease is not well understood, but it is without doubt due to some nervous derangement.

The treatment is about the same as that advised for hyperidrosis. In addition, however, to the remedies named for that disorder, there are several other local remedies that have been found useful in this disease, among which may be mentioned a wash of potassium permanganate, two or three grains to the ounce, and chloral, twenty or thirty grains to the ounce of water or dilute alcohol. Thin recommends the use of cork soles, which (and also the socks) are first to be soaked in a boric-acid solution and dried.

Chromidrosis.

Chromidrosis is a functional disorder of the sweat-glands, the secretion being variously colored and generally increased in quantity. The color may be blackish, bluish, reddish, greenish or yellowish, bluish and reddish being the most common. The affection is usually local, occurring in the form of patches, the face, neck, arms, backs of the hands and feet, chest, and abdomen being the favorite localities. The disease is rare. Ferrocyanide of iron, copper, and other substances have been detected in the secretion, to the presence of which doubtless the colors are due. It is generally observed in nervous and excitable persons, chiefly in unmarried women; but it has also been noted in strong men. It tends to recur, and may appear on different parts of the body with each manifestation. The treatment should be directed against the suspected cause, with especial reference to the nervous system.

Uridrosis.

Uridrosis, or urinous sweat, is a functional disorder of the sweat-glands, the secretion containing the elements of the urine, especially urea. This latter is occasionally detected in the sweat of persons apparently in good health. In some cases, however, it exists in such quantity as to be noticeable on the skin, appearing usually on the face and hands as a colorless or whitish saline crystalline deposit or coating. In most of the marked cases reported partial or complete suppression of the renal function has preceded or accompanied the condition.

Phosphoridrosis.

Phosphoridrosis is the rare condition in which sweat is phosphorescent. It is sometimes seen in the later stages of phthisis, also in miliaria, and occasionally in persons who have eaten of putrid fish.

Sudamen.

Sudamen (syn. miliaria crystallina) is a non-inflammatory disorder of the sweat-glands characterized by pinpoint- to pinhead-sized, isolated, superficial, translucent, whitish vesicles. The lesions make their appearance on any portion of the body, but have a predilection for certain regions of the trunk, especially where the epidermis is thin. They show themselves as numerous, closely-crowded, discrete, whitish or pearl-colored minute elevations, in appearance not unlike dew-drops. They form rapidly, remaining discrete, never becoming puriform, and evince no tendency to rupture. They are non-inflammatory, never reddish in color, and are without areolæ. The fluid disappears by absorption and the epidermal covering by subsequent desquamation. The lesions may appear in successive crops or new vesicles may show themselves irregularly from time to time. On the other hand, the first outbreak may disappear rapidly, and no further manifestion show itself. Sudamina occupying the face are usually seen in middle-aged females. The vesicles here are larger, deeper-seated, and more persistent.

Constitutional debility is a predisposing cause of the disease. Diseases accompanied with a high temperature—such, for example, as typhus and typhoid fevers, tuberculosis, and acute articular rheumatism—are frequently responsible for the eruption. The vesicles are produced by the collection of sweat in some part of the sweat-duct or epidermis, usually the latter. As ordinarily seen, the vesicles are situated between the lamellæ of the horny layer, the sweat having made its way from a rupture in an obstructed duct. In those exceptional cases of deep-seated and more persistent sudamina occurring about the face, the vesicles are situated in the corium, and are caused by a dilatation of the duct. The affection is to be distinguished from miliaria by the absence of inflammatory symptoms.

The course and duration of the disease depend upon the cause. In the treatment, removal of the etiological factor is of first importance. For external use some simple dusting-powder, such as equal parts of starch and lycopodium, or frequent bathing of the parts with an evaporating lotion, such as alcohol and water or vinegar and water, may be employed.

Seborrhœa.

Seborrhœa is a disease of the sebaceous glands characterized by an excessive and abnormal secretion of sebaceous matter, appearing on the skin as an oily coating, crusts, or scales. Although most commonly seated on the scalp and face, other parts of the general surface may also be attacked. Upon the trunk the sternal and intrascapular regions are the parts most frequently affected. It may occur at any period of life, although more common in adolescent and early adult age. In newly-born infants it constitutes the vernix caseosa, in which case, however, it is physiological rather than pathological. The course of the disease varies, at times disappearing spontaneously or with simple remedies, and in other cases being rebellious even to judicious treatment. It is in most cases influenced by the tone of the general health. In the majority of instances the disease is non-inflammatory; some cases, on the other hand, show intense hyperæmia and even inflammatory signs, while not infrequently the disease varies from time to time in the activity of the process. Itching and burning in a varying degree are sometimes present; the subjective symptoms are, however, rarely marked. The disease is usually better in warm than in cold weather.

There are two clinical varieties of the disease, depending upon the character of the secretion—seborrhœa oleosa and seborrhœa sicca. Seborrhœa oleosa appears as an oily, greasy coating upon the skin, and is seen most frequently about the nose and forehead. The oiliness may be slight or excessive. Seborrhœa sicca is the more common form of the disease, and is seen usually on the scalp and face, and occasionally on other parts of the body. It consists in the formation of dry sebaceous crusts, usually of a grayish-yellow color, which are slightly adherent. Frequently both varieties are seen together, and present products of a mixed character.

Occurring upon the scalp, constituting seborrhœa capitis, popularly known as dandruff, the disease is commonly of the dry or mixed variety, and usually involves the whole of that region. Sometimes it occurs in disseminate patches. It appears as small, dry, and pulverulent scales, detached and loose, or as thin or thick, greasy, crust-like, adherent masses. In the latter condition the hairs may be matted or pasted to the scalp. The hair sooner or later becomes affected, and in consequence is dry and lustreless, and gradually falls out. The disease, if neglected, finally causes more or less structural change in the follicles, with permanent alopecia as a result. The skin beneath the crusts in chronic cases is often of a dull, grayish or bluish-gray color; sometimes, however, it is hyperæmic. Occurring on other hairy parts, as the bearded region and eyebrows, the same characters are presented, but ordinarily they are less marked. At times a condition is seen on the scalp in which there is a mild degree of inflammation, with the formation of fine, dry epithelial scales, with slight or marked itching and burning.

Seborrhœa when occurring about the nose and face—seborrhœa faciei—is characterized by more or less redness, oiliness, and sometimes with a moderate amount of scaling and crusting. The follicular openings are enlarged and patulous, and are either free or contain sebaceous plugs. On the trunk—seborrhœa corporis—the disease tends to form circular and confluent scaly patches on a pale or hyperæmic base, with the sebaceous covering extending into the follicles in the form of projections. Or the skin may be slightly reddened, the follicles open and enlarged, the scales having been detached by the rubbing of the clothing. Seborrhœa when involving the genital region—seborrhœa genitalium—presents characters somewhat different. The inner surface of the prepuce, the glans penis, and the sulcus in the male, and the labia and clitoris of the female, are the parts commonly affected. A soft, cheesy mass collects about the parts, which, unless frequently removed, rapidly undergoes decomposition. If neglected or if the disease is marked, inflammatory symptoms may arise.

The disease is functional in character, the increased and usually changed oily secretion, with the epithelial scales from the glands and ducts, forming its products. There is no alteration in the gland structure except in long-continued cases, in which there may be slight atrophy. The affection depends usually upon an impairment of the general health. Chlorosis and anæmia are frequently the predisposing causes. Stomachic, intestinal, and uterine derangements are also, not infrequently, factors. Persons of light complexion are more prone to the dry form, while those of a dark complexion usually show the oily variety. It is also to be noted that the affection is not infrequently seen in persons apparently in perfect health, yielding, however, in such cases to simple external treatment.

Seborrhœa occurring on the scalp must be distinguished from eczema and from psoriasis. In eczema the skin is somewhat infiltrated, thickened, and reddened, and rarely involves the whole scalp; there is less scaliness, and at times more or less of the characteristic gummy exudation and marked itching of that disease. Psoriasis occurs usually in well-defined, circumscribed inflammatory patches, and in most cases shows signs of the disease upon other regions. These same points are of value in differentiating when the disease is upon non-hairy parts. From lupus erythematosus, which it may at times, on the face, closely resemble, it is to be distinguished by the absence of infiltration and thickening, of the sharply-defined border and violaceous or reddish color of that disease, as well as by the absence of atrophic scarring. Seborrhœa differs from ringworm, which it occasionally resembles, especially on the trunk, by its history, slow course, and by the greasiness of the scales. In obscure cases the microscope will determine the question.

TREATMENT.—It is a curable disease, but in the majority of cases proves obstinate. The rapidity of the cure depends in a great measure upon the removal of the predisposing causes. In seborrhœa of the scalp, if the process be allowed to continue through a long period, more or less marked permanent alopecia, especially of the vertex, may result. Even in unfavorable cases, however, much may be done toward promoting a regrowth of hair.

Treatment consists in both constitutional and local measures. The former is frequently of importance, with a view of securing, if possible, permanent relief. Iron, quinine, cod-liver oil, and arsenic are useful. In some cases one-tenth to one-quarter grain doses of calx sulphurata, three or four times daily, will prove of benefit. Dyspepsia, if present, is to be relieved. Fresh air and healthful exercise will sometimes aid considerably in effecting a cure.

External treatment is demanded in every case. The crusts and scales are to be removed. If in abundance, oily applications, such as olive or almond oil, are to be made to the parts, and after remaining on for six or twelve hours to be washed off with soap and hot water. In severe cases several repetitions may be found necessary. On the other hand, in mild cases simply washing with castile or ordinary toilet soap and warm water, or with a decoction of soap-bark, will suffice. If scaling and crusting are marked, instead of the plain soap sapo viridis should be used, either alone or in the form of the spiritus saponatus kalinus, consisting of two parts of sapo viridis in one of alcohol, perfumed with an essential oil. A tablespoonful of this poured on the scalp, and then a small quantity of hot water added and the parts rubbed briskly, will produce considerable lather; the scalp is then to be rinsed with warm water, the hair dried, and an oily or fatty substance applied. If after a removal of the crusts the skin is found to be irritated, a bland ointment, such as petroleum ointment, will be the best application. Glycerin and alcohol, one to four, will be of service if the skin is dry and hyperæmic. Subsequently more stimulating applications may be made; in the greater number of cases these are indicated from the start. Chloral, as in the following prescription, may sometimes be used with benefit:

> ℞. Chloralis, ℨij ;
> Glycerinæ, ℳxx ;
> Aquæ rosæ, fℨiv. M.

Gentle friction should be employed in making the application. If the lotion is too drying, more glycerin may be added. An excellent application in many cases is the following :

> ℞. Acidi carbolici, ℳxxx ;
> Olei ricini, fℨij ;
> Alcoholis, fℨj ℨvj. M.

This may be perfumed with a few drops of any essential oil. If greater stimulation is required, then to this last combination one to three drachms each of tincture of cantharides and tincture of capsicum may be added. Liquid applications may be made as follows: An eye-dropper is filled and introduced between the hairs at different points of the scalp, and a few drops pressed out, and subsequently rubbed in by means of a piece of flannel rag; in this manner the application is brought into intimate association with the skin without to any extent soiling the hair.

Ointments are also useful. Sulphur, one or two drachms to the ounce, is one of the best. Ammoniated mercury, twenty to sixty grains to the ounce, red precipitate, five to twenty grains to the ounce, are both valuable. In some cases tannic acid, one or two drachms to the ounce, acts well; also a naphthol ointment twenty or thirty grains to the ounce. Tar is also of decided value, and may be added to any of the above ointments or be prescribed alone in ointment, one or two drachms to the ounce. The tarry oils, as oil of white birch and oil of cade, used pure or in the form of tincture, one or two drachms to the ounce of alcohol, are also valuable. They may also be used with ointments. The treatment of seborrhœa of other parts of the body than the scalp is essentially the same, but the applications should be somewhat weaker. The sulphur preparations are the most useful.

The frequency of applications in seborrhœa will depend upon the activity of the process. Once or twice daily in the beginning may gradually be changed to once every other day, or later even less frequently. The soap-and-water washing is to be regulated in the same manner. It is advisable to intermit external treatment occasionally to see if the disease is entirely removed or merely in abeyance.

Comedo.

Comedo is a disorder of the sebaceous glands, consisting of retention of sebaceous matter, characterized by yellowish or blackish pinpoint- to pinhead-sized elevations corresponding to the orifices of the glands. The affection is seated, for the most part, about the face, neck, and upper part of the trunk ; it may occur, however, wherever there are sebaceous glands. Each lesion is pinpoint to pinhead in size, whitish or yellowish, and usually with a central blackish point.   There is very little elevation unless the amount of retained sebaceous matter is excessive.   They may exist sparsely or in great numbers.   Not infrequently the regions of the forehead, nose, and chin are studded with the lesions, other parts of the face and the shoulders showing them in smaller numbers.   They may be disseminated or grouped.   If they exist in profusion they give the face a soiled, greasy look, as if dirty and unwashed.   Lateral pressure forces out the sebaceous matter in a thread-like form closely resembling a worm, hence the popular terms flesh-worms and grub-worms.   From collection of dust and from other causes the outer ends of the sebaceous plugs become blackened, and this appearance has given rise to the term black-heads.   This coloring may possibly, to some extent at least, as has been suggested, be dependent upon a chemical change caused by the action of the air on the exposed portion of the sebaceous collection.   According to Unna, it is due to pigment matter, either free or contained within epidermal cells.   Krause states that the bluish granules described by Unna are from extraneous sources.   Seborrhœa oleosa is often seen to coexist. At times the retained secretion, either as a result of pressure or in consequence of chemical changes in the mass, excites inflammation, and acne results.   It is not uncommon to find comedones and acne lesions associated together.

The affection is seen most frequently between the ages of fifteen and thirty.   The lesions are sluggish, and are apt to disappear and reappear from time to time, depending upon the activity of the predisposing cause.   As the patient advances in age the affection tends to spontaneous disappearance.   The causes of the disorder are essentially the same as give rise to acne, a disease to which it is, as may be inferred, closely allied.   Thus, disorders of digestion, constipation, chlorosis, scrofulous conditions and menstrual disturbances are often predisposing causes. In addition, the unstriped muscular fibres of the skin lack tone and contract sluggishly.   The infrequent use of soap, especially in those with oily skins (seborrhœa oleosa), favors their formation.   Working in a dirty or dusty atmosphere may cause mechanical obstruction of the ducts, and in consequence the formation of comedones.

Pathologically, the affection has its seat in the sebaceous glands and ducts, consisting essentially of retained secretion and epithelial cells within either the gland or duct or both.   The accumulation gives rise to more or less dilatation, which usually increases the longer the comedo exists.   The mass consists of epidermic cells, sebaceous matter, and sometimes cholesterin crystals, and one or more lanugo hairs.   At times, also, the parasite Demodex folliculorum is found within the mass, but is not responsible in any way for the production of the lesion ; it is also often found in healthy follicles.   The dark points which usually mark the lesions are due to the accumulation of dirt.   The process is an inactive one, occasioning usually no disturbance.   The accumulation may increase until a papule is formed, or, on the other hand, may gradually relieve itself.   The affection is to be distinguished from acne punctata and milium. Acne is a closely-allied disease, but is inflammatory in its nature; comedo is functional in character : the presence or absence of inflammation, therefore, is a decisive differential point between the two diseases. Milium differs from comédo in the facts that it has no open duet, no black point, and the contents cannot be squeezed out.

The result of treatment is usually favorable, several months sufficing for its removal. On the other hand, occasionally cases are met with which prove rebellious. The aim of constitutional treatment should be to remove the predisposing condition. For this purpose cod-liver oil, iron, quinine, arsenic, and various other tonics, and ergot in full doses, are variously prescribed. At times, small doses (about a tenth to a fourth of a grain) of calx sulphurata have a good effect. Saline aperients are often valuable. An aperient tonic pill of iron, aloes, and strychnia is sometimes serviceable. Open-air exercise and other hygienic measures are to be advised.

External treatment is of great importance,—is in fact indispensable. The condition may in many cases be relieved by local applications alone. Removal of the plugs by mechanical means is to be advised. Lateral pressure with the finger-ends, or perpendicular pressure with a watch-key or similar instrument, will be found effectual. Washing the parts with sapo viridis and hot water, with considerable friction and a kneading motion, will aid in dislodging the sebaceous collections. Instead of the sapo viridis its solution in alcohol, two parts of the soap to one of alcohol (spiritus saponatus kalinus), may be employed. Steaming the face or the application of hot water from ten to twenty minutes will aid in softening the secretion, and with friction and kneading will often have a good effect. Friction with sand soap is also valuable. A soap made of equal parts of green soap (sapo viridis) and finely-pulverized marble may also be used. The use of the dermal curette is at times of service, scraping off the tops of the comedones, rendering their expulsion more easy. After the soap-washing and hot-water application ointments or lotions containing sulphur, such as prescribed in acne, may be applied. The following lotion is often valuable :

$$\text{I\!\!R. Sulphuris præcipitati, } \text{ʒij ;}$$
$$\text{Ætheris, } \quad \text{f ʒss ;}$$
$$\text{Alcoholis, } \quad \text{f ʒiijss. M.}$$

S. Shake before using : dab on with a mop for several minutes, allowing it to dry on.

Alkaline lotions containing borax or sodium bicarbonate, ten to twenty grains to the ounce, are often useful. The following paste has been highly spoken of for loosening and dislodging the sebaceous plugs :

$$\text{I\!\!R. Aceti, } \quad \text{ʒij ;}$$
$$\text{Glycerinæ, } \text{ʒiij ;}$$
$$\text{Kaolini, } \quad \text{ʒiv. M.}$$

S. Apply over the surface at night. If applied near the eyes, the lids should be kept closed for a few moments, on account of the pungent fumes of the vinegar. The lotion containing zinc sulphate and potassium sulphide, the formula of which is given in the treatment of acne, is of value. Corrosive-sublimate lotions, one-half to two grains to the ounce, are useful in some cases. In changing from a sulphur to a mercurial application, treatment should be suspended for several days, so that the formation of the black sulphuret of mercury, which may darken the skin and comedo plugs to an annoying degree, may be avoided. If treatment brings about considerable irritation of the parts, a result often desirable, it should be omitted temporarily and soothing applications made.

Milium.

Milium, described also as grutum and strophulus albidus, consists in the formation of small, whitish, roundish, pearly, non-inflammatory elevations situated in the upper part of the corium. The lesions are usually pinhead in size, whitish or yellowish, seemingly more or less translucent, rounded or acuminated, without aperture or duct, and appear for the most part about the face, especially about the eyelids, and occasionally elsewhere. One, several, or great numbers may be present; ordinarily, however, but several are to be seen, usually near the eyes. In our experience the affection is observed most frequently in middle-aged women. The lesions develop slowly, and after a certain size is reached may remain stationary for years. Their presence causes no disturbance, and unless large and numerous the affection is but slightly noticeable. Acne and comedo are often found associated with it. The cutaneous calculi occasionally met with are milia which have undergone calcareous metamorphosis. The etiology of the disease, in a great majority of cases, is not known. In some cases, however, the same causes as are operative in the production of comedo and acne seem to have an influence.

Anatomically, the affection is found to have its seat in the sebaceous glands. The duct from some cause is obliterated and the secretion cannot escape. The retained mass consists of sebaceous matter which tends to become inspissated and calcareous, and, as the lesion is without aperture, it cannot be squeezed out. The epidermis constitutes the external covering. It has also been shown by several authorities that the covering proper is either the gland itself or the wall of the hair-follicle, and that in the larger lesions connective-tissue septa are found. According to the investigations of Robinson, two different conditions have been described as milia—one which evidently has its origin in the sebaceous glands or ducts, and the other in which there is no connection whatever with these structures. The lesions are characteristic and the diagnosis easy. The absence of the duct-opening and black point of comedo serves to distinguish it from that disease. The small lesions of xanthoma—a disease which usually has its seat about the eyelids—may resemble it, but can scarcely be confounded with it, as its nature is entirely different.

As regards treatment, it is usually necessary in all cases to incise the lesions and squeeze out or scrape out their contents; in some, touching the base of the excavation with a minute drop of iodine tincture or nitrate of silver may be required to prevent a reappearance. Electrolysis has also been recommended.

Steatoma.

Steatoma—or, as commonly called, sebaceous cyst, sebaceous tumor, or wen—appears as a variously-sized, elevated, roundish, or semi-globular firm or soft tumor having its seat in the corium or subcutaneous tissue.

One or several may be present. They are cysts of the sebaceous glands, and may exist wherever these structures occur, but are seen most frequently about the scalp, face, back, and scrotum. They develop slowly, are variable as to size, and may exist indefinitely without causing any inconvenience except disfigurement. The overlying skin is either normal in color or whitish from stretching; on the scalp it is usually devoid of hair. Cysts are usually firm, but may be doughy or soft. As a rule, they are freely movable and painless. In some a gland-duct orifice can be seen; in the majority it is absent. Spontaneous suppuration and ulceration may occasionally take place in enormously distended tumors. Anatomically, steatoma is a cyst of the sebaceous gland and duct, produced by retention of secretion. It is in fact an enormously distended duct and gland whose walls have become thickened into a tough sac. The contents vary, in some being hard and friable, in others soft and cheesy or even fluid, with or without a fetid odor, and of a grayish, whitish or yellowish color. The mass consists of fat-drops, epidermic cells, cholesterin, and sometimes hairs. As a rule, the diagnosis is made without difficulty. Gummata, which may have some resemblance, grow more rapidly, are usually painful to the touch, are not freely movable, and tend to break down and ulcerate. Sebaceous cysts can scarcely be mistaken for fatty tumors and osteomata.

In the treatment excision is radical and most satisfactory. A linear incision is made, and the mass and enveloping sac dissected out. A removal of the sac is necessary, or a reproduction usually takes place. As the scalp wound especially should be treated on antiseptic principles, injecting the tumor with a small quantity of tincture of iodine or other irritant has been successfully employed.

CLASS II.—INFLAMMATIONS.

Erythema Simplex.

ERYTHEMA SIMPLEX is a hyperæmic disorder characterized by redness, occurring in the form of variously sized and shaped, diffused or circumscribed, non-elevated patches. The affection is due to various causes, which may be external or internal. Hence it is usual to divide the affection into two classes—idiopathic and symptomatic. Under the head of idiopathic erythema are described the erythemas due to cold, heat, traumatism, poison, etc. Erythema caloricum arises from the action of heat or cold. If the degree of heat or cold is sufficient, a dermatitis, or even gangrene, may result. In a mild degree, however, simple congestion of the skin—erythema—is produced. It is usually bright red in color, later becoming somewhat darker, and at times is followed by slight desquamation. If produced by the action of the sun—erythema solare—the uncovered parts only are affected. Erythema traumaticum is usually seen as a result of the pressure of tightly-fitting clothes, corsets, bandages, etc. It disappears rapidly upon removal of the cause, without scaling. If the cause is long continued, a dermatitis may be produced. Erythema vene-natum is a term applied to the form of hyperæmia resulting from the action of substances poisonous to the skin : such are all irritating chemicals, the ordinary rubefacients, various dyestuffs, acids, alkalies, and the like. The symptomatic erythemas are the more important. The rashes often preceding or accompanying certain of the systemic diseases, such as smallpox, diphtheria, and vaccinia, belong to this class. Disorders of the digestive tract, especially in children, are responsible for many cases. Roseola is a term sometimes applied to the symptomatic rashes. The division-line between simple erythema and dermatitis is often ill-defined.

The indications for treatment in the various erythemata are usually self-evident. A removal of the cause in idiopathic rashes is all that is needed. The same may be stated of the symptomatic erythemata ; but here there is at times difficulty in recognizing the etiological factor. Local treatment is rarely necessary. Dusting-powders, mild lotions, or ointments such as used in acute eczema may be prescribed.

ERYTHEMA INTERTRIGO.—Erythema intertrigo—known popularly as chafing—is a hyperæmic disorder occurring on parts where the natural folds of the skin come in contact, characterized by redness and at times an abraded surface and maceration of the epidermis. The causes are usually local. Thus it appears chiefly about the folds of the neck in fat subjects, the nates, groin, perineum, and axillæ. It is seen usually in hot weather in infants, and others whose skin is tender. The skin becomes red from chafing, and if long continued or untreated the perspiration of the parts causes more or less maceration of the epiderm and a mucoid discharge. If the condition continues, actual inflammation may be developed. The affection may pass away in a few days or last several weeks. There is a feeling of heat and soreness about the affected parts. Occurring between the nates in infants, a favorite locality, from the friction of the parts, and the action of the fæces and urine, it is often persistent. As a rule, it yields readily to treatment. The predisposition to its development, and its continuance are often due in children to derangement of the stomach or intestinal canal.

In the treatment undue moisture and friction of the parts are to be prevented or counteracted. Washing with castile soap and cool water, and cleanliness, should be advised. The folds or parts are to be separated or kept apart with lint, cloth, or absorbent cotton. Dusting-powders are to be used freely, as they constitute the best method of treatment. The following is a good formula :

$$\text{R}. \quad \begin{array}{ll} \text{Pulv. zinci oxidi,} & \text{ʒij ;} \\ \text{Pulv. talci Veneti,} & \text{ʒij ;} \\ \text{Pulv. amyli,} & \text{ʒiv. M.} \end{array}$$

Simple starch and lycopodium powder, alone or together, will both prove efficacious. If the affection prove rebellious to this plan of treatment, astringent and alcoholic lotions may be used. Black wash, diluted, dabbed on the parts several times daily, followed by oxide-of-zinc ointment or a dusting-powder, will be found useful in obstinate cases. A weak solution of corrosive sublimate, a fraction of a grain to the ounce, may also prove valuable in some instances. Lotions of zinc sulphate or of acetate of lead, two or three grains to the ounce, and a weak solution of alum, may also be mentioned. A lotion we have often found of service is the following :

R_f. Pulv. calaminæ,
Pulv. zincl oxidi, *āā.* ʒiss ;
Alcoholis, fʒij ;
Aquæ rosæ, fʒiv. **M.**

Sig. Shake before using. Apply several times daily. The local treatment of rebellious cases is, in fact, that which is found efficacious in acute erythematous eczema.

Erythema Multiforme.

Erythema multiforme is an acute inflammatory disease characterized by reddish, more or less variegated macules, papules, and tubercles, occurring discretely or in patches of various size and shape. Certain regions of the body, such as the backs of the hands and feet and the arms and legs, are the parts mainly invaded. The eruption, as the name signifies, is usually marked by the multiformity of its lesions, although, as a rule, one of the forms is generally predominant. Peculiarities which the lesions assume have given rise to the qualifying terms annulare, iris, and marginatum, etc. Thus, when the erythematous patch is circular, fading in the centre, it is called erythema annulare. At times concentric rings, presenting variegated colors, are formed, giving rise to the term erythema iris. When the eruption consists of sharply-defined marginate patches, it is designated erythema marginatum. Most commonly, the eruption appears in the form of papules and tubercles. Erythema papulosum is the form of the disease usually met with. It consists of discrete or aggregated patches of flat papules, variable as to size and shape. In color they are bright red, violaceous, or purplish, disappearing partly under pressure. They fade rapidly, rarely lasting longer than a few weeks. Erythema tuberculosum is a form of the disease occasionally encountered in which the lesions are larger, but of the same general character as in the papular variety.

Erythema multiforme varies as regards duration, averaging about two weeks. During its course new lesions are apt to develop as the older eruption fades away. As the lesions disappear slight pigmentation and desquamation are noticeable. In addition to the parts already named as commonly invaded, the face is sometimes the seat of the eruption. It may, moreover, attack the mucous membranes. The subjective symptoms are rarely marked : usually-slight burning and itching are complained of. There may be evidences of constitutional disturbance, such as malaise, headache, rheumatic pains, and gastric derangement, especially at the beginning ; as a rule, however, general symptoms are not observed. Relapses, especially from year to year, are not uncommon. The causes of the disease are in most cases obscure. It is most frequent in early adult age. Spring and autumn seem to be predisposing factors, although it is also seen at other periods of the year. Gastric disturbance may give rise to the eruption in some instances. Rheumatism is occasionally associated with it. The affection is more common in the female.

Anatomically, the affection is an exudative disease, resembling urticaria. It is generally regarded as a vaso-motor disturbance. It is closely related to herpes iris and erythema nodosum, and by some these are looked upon as varieties. In regard to the diagnosis, it is to be differentiated from urticaria. In the latter affection itching and burning are prominent and constant symptoms, the lesions are fugacious, and the duration of the disease shorter. It can scarcely be confounded with eczema, in which disease the lesions are smaller and intensely itchy, and the eruption does not assume the different shapes seen in erythema multiforme. Erythema nodosum and herpes iris are also to be differentiated. The prognosis is always favorable, as the affection runs a definite course, usually disappearing at the end of a few weeks. It is rarely influenced by treatment.

Saline laxatives, alkalies, and the bromides may be given and the diet regulated. In the beginning of the attack large doses of quinine may be useful. Locally, applications of alcohol or vinegar and water, or a lotion of carbolic acid, five or ten grains to the ounce of water, will be found of advantage if itching or burning is present. As a rule, active external treatment is not required.

Erythema Nodosum.

Erythema nodosum (syn., dermatitis contusiformis) is an acute inflammatory affection characterized by the formation of variously-sized, roundish or ovalish, more or less elevated erythematous nodes. Febrile disturbance usually ushers in the eruption, often accompanied with gastric derangement, malaise, and rheumatic pains. The efflorescence appears rapidly, having special predilection for the arms and legs, particularly the tibial surfaces. The lesions vary in size, being rarely smaller than a cherry and often as large as an egg, and are ovalish or roundish in shape. They are reddish in color, with a bluish or purplish tinge, which becomes more decided as they grow older. Later, as they are disappearing, yellowish, greenish, and bluish coloration manifests itself, as in the case of a bruise. Not infrequently the lesions are hemorrhagic. When at its height a node has a shining, tense appearance, indicative apparently of beginning suppuration; this latter process, however, does not occur, absorption invariably taking place. Firm and hard at first, as they begin to decline they become softer. They are apt to appear in crops. The lesions are rarely present in large numbers, from five to twenty being the average; occasionally, however, they are much more numerous. The mucous membranes may, as in erythema multiforme, be invaded. They are tender and more or less painful, and are usually accompanied with a sense of burning. Lymphangitis is at times observed. At the end of two or three weeks the affection has usually run its course.

The causes of the disease are not known. It is closely allied to erythema multiforme, and by many observers is regarded as merely a manifestation of that disease. It is generally encountered in the spring and autumn months, and occurs most frequently in children and young persons. It is usually associated with rheumatic pains, and not infrequently with digestive derangement. It is not a common disease. It is regarded by Lewin as an angio-neurosis. According to Hebra, in most cases it is essentially an inflammation of the lymphatics. Bohn regards it as due to embolism of the cutaneous vessels giving rise to inflammatory infarctions. The process is an inflammatory œdema. There is considerable serous transudation, with some blood-corpuscles, and not infrequently with more or less hemorrhage. The lesions usually bear resemblance to bruises, abscesses, and gummata. The rosy hue, the apparently violent character of the process, the number, course, and situation of the lesions, will serve to distinguish it. The prognosis is favorable, as the affection tends to disappear in a few weeks, rarely lasting more than a month.

As spontaneous recovery results, treatment should be conservative. Rest, the more complete the better, sedative applications, as of lead-water and laudanum or of carbolic acid, with the use of saline laxatives and full doses of quinia, are the measures indicated. The diet should be regulated according to the case.

Urticaria.

Urticaria, hives, or nettlerash, is an erythematous affection characterized by the development of wheals of a whitish, pinkish, or reddish color, accompanied by stinging, pricking, and tingling sensations. The advent of the efflorescence is usually sudden ; not infrequently symptoms of gastric derangement precede its appearance. The wheals are of variable size, shape, and color. Ordinarily they are of the size of a coffee-grain or bean, rounded or ovoidal in shape, and whitish, pinkish, or reddish in color. They occur isolated or in the form of patches caused by a coalescence of several lesions, and vary in elevation from half a line to several lines. Instead of the ovoidal or rounded form, the eruption may appear in streaks or irregularly-shaped patches. To the touch the lesions may be soft or firm.

The efflorescence disappears, as a rule, without leaving a trace. Pigment-stains are in some cases left which may be slow to disappear. Burning, tingling, stinging, and itching are prominent subjective symptoms. The individual lesions are fugacious, inclining to disappear at one part and to show themselves at another. They are more apt to appear on parts subjected to pressure by contact of clothes, although no region is exempt. No age is spared, but the disease, especially in its acute form, is more common in the young. Ordinarily, urticaria is an acute disorder, lasting a few hours to several days, in which time frequent exacerbations may take place. On the other hand, it may be chronic in the sense that relapses occur successively, the skin, in fact, rarely being entirely free of the lesions.

At times the wheals are peculiar as to formation or are complicated with another condition, and hence arise the so-called varieties of the disease. The most common of these is urticaria papulosa, which was formerly known as lichen urticatus. The lesions have the form of a papule with most of the characteristics of a wheal. They appear, as a rule, suddenly, and after a few hours or days gradually disappear ; they rarely occur in numbers, and are generally scattered over the trunk and limbs, especially over the latter. They are intensely itchy, and hence their apices are usually excoriated and covered with blood-crusts. The itching usually becomes more marked toward night. This form of the affection is observed particularly in badly-nourished or in ill-cared-for young children. The occurrence of the disease in association with purpura, or as a complication of the latter, has given rise to the names urticaria hæmorrhagica and purpura urticans or urticata. The lesion is of a mixed character—purpurio and urticarial. Sometimes the wheal formation is of such a nature as to give rise to fluid exudation, producing a bulla; hence the name urticaria bullosa. In rare instances large walnut- or even egg-sized nodes or tumors are formed, constituting urticaria tuberosa, or giant urticaria.

The causes of urticaria are numerous. Two that are well known may be classed under the heads of external and internal irritants. Under the former may be mentioned stinging nettle, jelly-fish, caterpillars, fleas, bedbugs, and mosquitoes; among the latter, whatever produces gastric and intestinal derangements. These latter are responsible for most instances of acute urticaria. With some persons indulgence in certain articles of food, as fish, oysters, clams, crabs, lobsters, pork, strawberries, and similar articles, almost invariably calls forth the efflorescence. A number of medicinal substances, such as copaiba, cubebs, turpentine, valerian, chloral, salicylic acid, iodide of potassium, quinine, and others, taken internally, may provoke an attack. Malaria, functional and organic diseases of the uterus, a weak or irritable state of the nervous system, and impaired digestion are common causes of both the acute and chronic forms of the disease. Various nervous, hemorrhagic, and rheumatic diseases are also sometimes associated with urticaria. In fact, an irritation from disease of any internal organ, functional or organic in character, may give rise to the eruption.

Anatomically, a wheal is seen to be a more or less firm elevation, consisting of a circumscribed collection of semi-fluid material exuded into the upper layers of the skin. It has its seat for the most part in the papillary layer. The vaso-motor nervous system is probably the main factor in the production of the wheal. Dilatation following a spasm of the vessels results in effusion; in consequence, the overfilled vessels of the wheal are emptied by the pressure of the exudation, and the central paleness produced, while the pressed-back blood gives rise to the red border.

The features of the disease are so characteristic that there is, as a rule, no difficulty in distinguishing it from other affections. Erythema simplex, erythema multiforme, erythema nodosum, and erysipelas are to be differentiated. Erythema simplex is a simple hyperæmia, while urticaria is a peculiar inflammatory exudation—a point sufficient to distinguish the two. The papular and tubercular forms of erythema multiforme are to be differentiated by their more persistent character, the locality affected, and the absence usually of marked itching and burning. Erythema nodosum may resemble urticaria tuberosa, but the nodes in the former are usually encountered upon the tibial surfaces, are of much longer duration, and are free from itching. It is only when several wheals coalesce, causing swelling and burning, and then only when occurring about the face, that it may be mistaken for erysipelas; but the evanescent character of the eruption in urticaria, its rapid formation, the itching, and the absence of constitutional symptoms usual in erysipelas, are points of difference.

TREATMENT.—Most cases of acute urticaria may be speedily relieved. Relapses may occur, however, upon repeated exposure to the exciting cause. The prognosis of chronic urticaria, on the other hand, is not always so favorable, and will depend in a great measure upon the ability to remove or modify the predisposing condition. The first essential in the management of a case, therefore, is an investigation into its etiological cause.

In the acute disease, where, as in the majority of cases, gastric disturbance is the exciting factor, a purgative — preferably a saline — should be given. In severe cases, if food is still in the stomach, an emetic will be of service, sulphate of zinc, ipecacuanha, and mustard being the best. The diet should be of the simplest kind. Aperients are generally indicated until recovery takes place. In chronic urticaria, where faulty digestion is the exciting cause, remedies appropriate to that condition are to be prescribed. In all cases attention is to be directed to the state of the general health. If there is a suspicion of malaria, quinine and arsenic may be administered. Functional and organic affections should receive proper management, as they may prove to be the active cause of the disorder. If diuretics are called for, acetate of potassium will often best serve the purpose. The alkaline and laxative natural mineral waters are sometimes useful. In obstinate cases, especially in those in which no assignable cause can be detected, pilocarpine, atropia, tincture of belladonna, chloride of ammonium, bromide of potassium, and arsenic may be tried. Change of climate is at times advisable.

On account of the great distress usually attending the affection, local treatment is demanded in almost all cases. Baths and lotions are the most serviceable methods of applying external remedies. Sponging the surface with vinegar or alcohol, pure or diluted, may afford relief. A lotion of carbolic acid, two to four drachms to the pint of water, will frequently give prompt ease. The latter lotion may be improved by the addition of two or three ounces of alcohol and a small quantity (one to two drachms) of glycerin to the pint. A lotion of thymol, one grain to the ounce of alcohol and water, is likewise of value. Benzoic acid and borax, each five to ten grains to the ounce of water; chloral, ten to twenty grains to the ounce; dilute hydrocyanic acid, one to three drachms to the pint; and diluted ammonia-water,—may also be mentioned. Alkaline baths made with carbonate of sodium or potassium, three or six ounces to the bath, are sometimes serviceable. Starch, gelatin, and bran baths may in like manner be used; and acid baths, half an ounce of hydrochloric or nitric acid to the bath, have been recommended. Dusting-powders, especially when applied after baths, will in some cases prove acceptable.

URTICARIA PIGMENTOSA, called also zanthelasmoidea, is an unusual form of the disease, cases of which during the past few years have been reported. It begins usually in infancy, and may continue for a period of months or years. The wheals are intensely itchy, are more or less persistent, and leave yellowish, orange-colored, greenish, or brownish stains. Its nature is obscure: by some observers it is regarded as an urticaria; by others it is claimed that there is a new-growth element in the lesions. Most cases certainly show urticarial lesions and run the course of this affection. It is more than probable that the different cases reported are not examples of one disease. Treatment is, as a rule, unsatisfactory.

Dermatitis.

Dermatitis, although in its general meaning signifying any inflammation of the skin from whatever cause or character, is a term usually applied to those forms which are directly traceable to the action of irritants. Such irritants may act from without, as cold, heat, caustics, etc., or through the medium of the blood, as in the eruptions following the ingestion of certain drugs. The intensity of the inflammation varies from a simple erythematous condition to actual gangrene. Redness, heat, pain, swelling, and at times itching, the common clinical signs of inflammation, are present, but are variable as to degree. The inflammation may be confined to a small area or may be diffused, depending usually upon the cause. The forms of dermatitis are designated according to the causes which produce them.

DERMATITIS TRAUMATICA.—Under this head are included all those inflammations of the skin which are due to traumatism. Contusions and similar injuries, abrasions and inflammation from the pressure of tight-fitting garments, bandages, etc., excoriations, and the like, are common examples of this form. The excoriations from scratching in pediculosis, scabies, pruritus, eczema, and other itchy diseases are to the dermatologist the most frequent examples of traumatic dermatitis. They subside on removal of the cause, leaving often, especially if the scratching has been at all violent and the cause long continued, thickening of the skin and pigmentation, both of which, notably the latter, may be more or less permanent.

DERMATITIS VENENATA.—All inflammatory conditions of the skin due to contact with deleterious substances are classified in this group. Apart from chemical irritants, certain plants, notably those of the rhus family, are capable in some individuals of producing inflammation of the skin. The two well-known plants of this group are the poison ivy or oak and the poison sumach or dogwood. The majority of persons are not affected by these plants, but in many contact, or in some mere proximity to the plant, will be followed by a dermatitis, variable as to degree. The inflammation may simply be of an erythematous character with slight swelling, or, on the other hand, it may be vesicular, pustular, or bullous, with marked hyperæmia, œdema, and swelling. As a rule, the inflammation appears soon after exposure or contact, sometimes within a few hours; not infrequently, however, several days will elapse before the symptoms present themselves. Itching is commonly a prominent symptom, as also heat and burning.

The eruption usually begins as an erythema with heat, swelling, œdema, and itching, remaining for several days, and then subsiding, or, as is frequently the case, vesicles or even blebs are developed, and the affection then is, as a rule, slower in disappearing. Œdema and swelling may be slight, or, as often occurs, so great as to cause marked temporary disfigurement. The face, hands, and genitalia are the parts generally involved, although the disease may extend to other regions, at times involving large areas or even the greater portion of the whole surface. The lesions, either spontaneously or through violence, rupture, and dry to crusts, and subsequently fall off, leaving erythematous spots, which in turn gradually fade. The affection runs an acute course, lasting from one to six weeks. In some cases, especially in those with a tendency to eczema, its duration may be prolonged. The poisonous principle has been found to be toxicodendric acid, and is exceedingly volatile in character.

The eruption is influenced by treatment. Bland astringent lotions or ointments are most serviceable. The fluid extract of grindelia robusta, two to four drachms to the pint of water, dabbed on frequently, or cloths wet with it kept constantly applied, will usually have a remarkably beneficial effect. Black wash, either alone or followed by the oxide-of-zinc ointment, as in acute eczema, and lead-water, are both serviceable. A saturated solution of sodium hyposulphite, a lotion of sodium bicarbonate, one of carbolic acid, one or two drachms to the pint of water, a weak ammonia lotion, and other applications of a similar nature, may also be advised, frequently with good result.

Other substances which at times act on the skin somewhat similarly to the rhus plants are the aniline dyes, mezereon, arnica, and certain other drugs, as savin, croton oil, tartar emetic, mercurials, etc.

DERMATITIS CALORICA.—Both heat and cold are capable of producing serious disturbances of the skin. The condition varies from a simple erythematous inflammation to a state of actual gangrene, depending upon the degree and duration of the cause, and to some extent upon the recuperative power of the exposed parts. Whether due to heat (dermatitis combustionis, combustio, burns) or to cold (dermatitis congelationis, congelatio, frost-bite, chilblain), the clinical symptoms are about the same. Treatment is generally of a soothing character.

In cases of dermatitis due to cold which are seen immediately after exposure, the parts should gradually be brought back to a normal temperature, at first being rubbed with snow or cold water applied. In ordinary chilblains stimulating applications are most serviceable, such as tincture of iodine and frictions with oil of turpentine. Balsam of Peru, camphor, lead plaster, carbolic acid, twenty to sixty grains to the ounce of ointment, camphor, and similar remedies may also be mentioned.

In burns where the inflammation is of a mild degree, sodium bicarbonate, either as a powder or in saturated solution, is effective; while in those of a more severe grade a solution of 2 to 5 per cent. will be of greater advantage. In burns or frost-bites in which the inflammation is vesicular, bullous, pustular, or escharotic the measures advisable in ordinary inflammation are to be employed.

DERMATITIS MEDICAMENTOSA.—Medicinal eruptions are due to the ingestion of certain drugs, some of which produce in a large proportion of individuals, sooner or later, well-defined cutaneous manifestations; on the other hand, many drugs are only exceptionally noted as giving rise to cutaneous disturbance. Of the former, the iodides and the bromides stand conspicuous; while of the latter class, arsenic and quinine may be cited. The glandular structures of the skin are frequently involved, especially in the iodide and bromide eruptions, and apparently the inflammation and resulting pustules are due to the effort at elimination through these structures. In other instances, especially the erythematous and urticarial eruptions, the effects of the drug seem to be due to some action upon the nervous system.

Arsenic.—Exceptionally eruptions are seen to follow the continued administration of arsenic. They are of an erythematous type, resembling the macular syphiloderm and measles; or papular, somewhat similar to the papular manifestation of erythema multiforme. Vesicles, herpetic in character, and pustules have also been observed. An urticarial-like eruption has occasionally been noted. In several instances arsenic has seemed to hold a causative relationship to an attack of herpes zoster. Arsenical dermatitis is most frequently seen about the face, neck, and hands, and lasts usually from a few days to two weeks. Workmen in arsenic-works are occasionally observed to have a pustular, ulcerative, and even gangrenous eruption, due to the local action of the drug.

Atropia or Belladonna.—A scarlatinoid rash is a frequent result of ingestion of belladonna, even a small dose at times sufficing to provoke the eruption. It is seen most frequently in children, face, neck, and chest being usually involved. Dryness of the throat and general malaise may be present. Usually there is no febrile disturbance, and desquamation seldom if ever follows, the rash usually passing away within a few hours or days after the drug has been discontinued.

Bromides.—The eruption from the bromides is usually pustular in type, occasionally furuncular, and at times giving rise to purulent accumulations of a carbuncular character. In some individuals a single dose suffices to call out the eruption; usually, however, it is only after a few weeks' administration that the cutaneous lesions are observed. In rare instances even its prolonged use is unaccompanied by any disturbance of the skin. The face, neck, shoulders, and back are most prone to its effects. The pustules have their seat in and about the sebaceous glands. A small dose of arsenic or bitartrate of potassium with each dose of the bromide will sometimes prevent the eruption caused by the latter.

Cannabis Indica.—An eruption of a vesico-papular type, the lesions pinpoint- to pea-sized, scattered over the entire surface, accompanied with considerable pruritus, has been recorded, following within twelve hours after a full dose of the drug, and disappearing in a few days.

Chloral.—A scarlatinoid or urticarial eruption, dusky-red in color, somewhat itchy, occurring especially about the face, neck, and extremities, occasionally follows the administration of chloral. In some instances, if the drug is long continued, glandular enlargement, vesicles, petechiæ, ulceration, and sloughing, and rarely death with symptoms of purpura hæmorrhagica, result. In a few cases the drug has produced simple purpuric lesions.

Copaiba.—The copaiba eruption is well known. It may follow a single dose, or, as is more often the case, after several days' or a few weeks' use of the drug. It is maculo-papular or papular in type, itchy, and resembles urticaria and erythema multiforme. The extremities are usually invaded, although not infrequently the whole surface is attacked. A scarlatinoid rash has also been observed. The disturbance usually disappears in a few days.

Cubebs.—A diffused erythematous éruption, with milletseed-sized papules, coalescent here and there, occurring over the face and trunk, and to a less extent the extremities, disappearing with furfuraceous desquamation, is occasionally observed.

Digitalis.—A few cases of scarlatinoid and papular eruptions have been recorded as following the administration of digitalis.

Iodides.—Eruptions from the ingestion of the preparations of iodine are not uncommon. They may be erythematous, papular, vesicular, pustular, bullous, or purpuric in character. The erythematous type is not uncommon, appearing in patches chiefly about the forearms, face, and neck. The papular and vesicular forms are rarer, the latter occurring usually about the chest, limbs, scalp, and scrotum. A markedly eczematous eruption, occupying the greater portion of the entire surface, with copious secretion, has been occasionally noted. A pustular eruption, acne-like in character, resembling that seen following the bromides, is the most frequent. It is seen commonly about the face, shoulders, back, and arms. Iodine has been found in the contents of the lesions. A bullous eruption, occurring chiefly about the head and neck, has also been noted. This form is rare. The lesions usually begin as small vesicles or vesico-papules, and develop to blebs, containing a serous, puriform, or sanguinolent fluid. In some cases the eruption does not go beyond the vesicular or vesico-papular formation. Purpura has also, although rarely, been observed, the lesions being small, simple in character, and occurring mainly about the legs ; or exceptionally assuming a grave hemorrhagic type, which may terminate fatally. All of the eruptions of the iodides disappear rapidly after the drug has been discontinued.

Mercury.—An eruption of an erysipelatous character, beginning about the face and extending to other parts, has been occasionally noted to follow this drug. The skin is smooth, shining, red, dry, and itchy.

Opium, Morphia.—An erythematous eruption, scarlatinoid in type, favoring the chest and flexor surfaces of the limbs, with or without itching, is in some individuals caused by even the smallest dose of opium or its alkaloid morphia. It may disappear in a few days or be prolonged and followed by marked desquamation. In some persons one or two doses will give rise to intense itching without any eruption, or if the drug is continued the erythematous condition described is developed. Opium has also rarely caused profuse sweating and sudamina.

Phosphoric Acid.—An instance of a bullous eruption has been recorded as following the administration of this drug.

Quinine.—Quinine rashes are not infrequent, appearing usually first on the face and neck, and then invading other parts. The eruption may be patchy or confluent. The type is generally erythematous. Chill, nausea, and other symptoms of malaise precede its development. There may be œdema and injection of the conjunctivæ, and redness and dryness of the naso-pharyngeal passages. Itching and burning are almost constant symptoms. Desquamation, furfuraceous or lamellar, follows. Eruptions resembling urticaria and erythema multiforme have been observed. A purpuric type has also been noted.

Salicylic Acid.—Dermatitis of an erythematous and urticarial type,

with symptoms of general disturbance, is sometimes seen in patients
taking salicylic acid or its salts.   An efflorescence of vesicles and pustules about the hands and feet, with profuse sweating, has been recorded.
A case in which ecchymotic patches about the back and neighboring
regions appeared from the use of this drug has been reported.

Santonine.—An instance of an urticarial outbreak with œdema of the
eyelids and swelling of the face has been observed following the ingestion
of this drug.

Stramonium.—An erythematous efflorescence has been recorded as following this drug.

Strychnia.—A case is on record in which a rash of a scarlatinoid type
followed a dose of one-twenty-fourth of a grain of strychnia.

Turpentine.—Both erythematous and papular eruptions, usually itchy,
have appeared as the result of large doses of turpentine, occurring principally about the face and upper trunk, the papules being minute in
character.   A vesicular eruption has also been noticed somewhat similar
to vesicular eczema.

DERMATITIS FACTITIA.—Feigned diseases of the skin are not uncommon.   Erythema, vesicles, bullæ, and gangrene have been brought about,
chiefly in hysterical females, to gain sympathy, or, as also in other individuals, for the purpose of deception, by the action of friction, acids, or
strong alkalies.

Dermatitis Gangrænosa.

Dermatitis gangrænosa, or gangrene of the skin, is a rare affection.
It may be idiopathic or symptomatic.   As an idiopathic disease it begins
usually as circular, erythematous, dark-red spots, tending to appear symmetrically, either painful and hyperæsthetic or without sensation. Malaise,
fever, and symptoms of debility usually precede and accompany its development.   The lesions go on to gangrene and sloughing, recovery taking
place or a fatal termination gradually resulting.   There may be several
or as many as thirty or forty patches.   The progress of the disease,
whether terminating fatally or in recovery, is slow, usually of several
months' duration.   Gangrene of the skin as a symptomatic affection is
occasionally seen in grave cerebral and spinal diseases, and also in diabetes.

Furunculus.

Furunculus, or boil, is a deep-seated, inflammatory disease, characterized by one or more variously-sized, circumscribed, rounded, more or
less acuminated, firm, painful formations, usually terminating in central
suppuration.

In the beginning the lesion appears as a reddish spot, small, rounded,
imperfectly defined, inflammatory, and painful to the touch, having its
seat in the corium ; it gradually becomes larger, raised, and with marked
tendency to central suppuration, usually maturing in from one to two
weeks, when it appears as a painful, deep-red, rounded, pointed, inflammatory formation, varying in size from a pea to a walnut, exhibiting
central suppuration, the so-called core.   In some cases there is no tend-

ency to core-formation, such lesions being popularly designated blind boils.

A furuncle is usually painful, of a throbbing nature, which persists until suppuration has taken place and the contents discharged. The intensity of the inflammation gives rise to considerable areolar swelling and hyperæmia. There may be but one lesion present, or, as more frequently happens, several may exist at the same time scattered over different regions. In the latter case, after a partial or complete disappearance of the first crop, a second outbreak frequently occurs, to be followed later by a third, and so on, constituting furunculosis. The lesions are usually isolated. No region of the body is exempt; the face, neck, back, and buttocks are favorite localities. Sympathetic constitutional disturbance, more or less marked in severe cases, is usually present. Boils sometimes occur in association with eczema. In general, they are the result of a depressed state of the system. Friction, a contusion, or similar local irritation is often the exciting cause. They are met with in association with diabetes, pyæmia, uræmia, chlorosis, fevers, and like conditions. Although observed at all periods of life, they are more common during adolescence and in old age. The view has been advanced that a furuncle is due to the presence of a microbe (Torula pyogenica). According to Pasteur, this bacterium is identical with that of abscesses of the soft parts, etc.

The lesion usually has its starting-point in a sebaceous gland in the upper part of the corium, or, deeper, in a sweat-gland or hair-follicle. Beginning in a sweat-gland in the deeper structures it constitutes the so-called connective-tissue furuncle, or hydroadenitis of some authors. The core, or central suppuration, is usually made up of the tissue of the gland in which the boil had its origin, and pus, and when cast off appears as a whitish, tough, pultaceous mass. A more or less permanent cicatrix usually results. There is only one affection with which a furuncle is likely to be confounded—namely, carbuncle. In this latter, however, the lesion is considerably larger, flattened instead of rounded and pointed, the pain of an intense character and in a measure independent of touch or injury. Moreover, a carbuncle has several points of suppuration, the boil having but one, and the former, moreover, is rarely multiple.

When occurring in crops, the affection is often rebellious to treatment. Both constitutional and local measures, especially the former, are demanded. Functional disorders are to be regulated, and any faulty condition of the general health corrected. Tonics, such as quinine, iron, strychnia, mineral acids, and arsenic, are not infrequently of service. The last remedy usually proves of most value in those cases in which the lesions appear in crops. The preparations of sulphur are of positive service in many cases of the disease; hyposulphite of sodium, ten or fifteen grains three or four times daily, is one of the most valuable remedies we possess, and with the same view calx sulphurata, one-tenth to one-half grain five or six times daily, may be prescribed. Alkalies, especially liquor potassæ in ten or fifteen minim doses, are not infrequently beneficial. The compound syrup of the hypophosphites may also be employed with the hope of obtaining relief. In regard to the diet, the most nutritious food, liberally partaken of, is, as a rule, to be advised. At times change of air and scene will act most happily.

Concerning the local treatment, the lesion in the first stage may possibly be aborted, or at least modified in its course, by the application to the forming core of a strong solution or of a crystal of carbolic acid. This procedure is preferable to the actual cautery. If the lesion be farther advanced, a drop of carbolic acid and glycerin, equal parts, will often give instantaneous relief and arrest the progress of the boil. A few drops of a 5 per cent. carbolic-acid solution may also be injected into the apex of the boil with good results. For the same purpose painting the parts with tincture of camphor or tincture of iodine is advised. An ointment of carbolic acid—as, for example, resin cerate an ounce, carbolic acid from fifteen to thirty grains—applied as a plaster will be found useful. The application of poultices affords ease in some cases. As soon as suppuration has been fully established evacuation of the contents will shorten the course of the process. If the boil is open and discharging, boric acid in powder, freely applied, has been recommended.

ALEPPO BOUTON, BOIL, OR EVIL, DELHI BOIL, AND BISKRA BOUTON.—The first of these diseases, the Aleppo bouton, boil, or evil, is observed at Aleppo, Bagdad, and the neighboring regions. Delhi boil is not uncommon in India, and the Biskra bouton is found in Algeria and elsewhere along the African coast. In fact, these diseases are more or less epidemic in these countries. They have been considered as allied to furuncle, but their true nature is somewhat obscure. The three affections are probably examples of the same disease, modified, it may be, by climate, habits, etc. They begin as a papule or tubercle, soon becoming a pustule, and then ulcerate, leaving a cicatrix.

Carbunculus.

Carbunculus (anthrax, carbuncle) is a firm, more or less circumscribed, painful, deep-seated inflammation of the skin and subcutaneous structures, variable as to size, terminating in a slough. General malaise, slight fever, and chilliness precede and usher in the disease. Locally, there appears at first a more or less circumscribed, circular redness, with swelling, tenderness, and pain. Soon a phlegmonous inflammation develops, the surface at times showing vesiculation, the lesion involving an area several inches in diameter and of considerable depth. The progress of the disease is not uniform. At the end of a week or two suppuration is fully established, the first signs of this process appearing about the hair-follicles. The tissues are now soft and boggy ; the skin becomes gangrenous, breaking down at numerous points, disclosing centres of suppuration, giving the lesion a cribriform appearance. Finally, the whole mass sloughs away either as an entirety or in portions, and results in an open, deep ulcer with hard and raised edges, which gradually granulates and heals, leaving a pigmented cicatrix. The area involved varies, and may be extensive, sometimes as much as six or eight inches in diameter. The favorite localities for its development are the nape of the neck, shoulders, back, and buttocks. As a rule, the process ends in three to six weeks. Usually only one lesion exists. When there are several or where they follow each other in succession, the general condition is apt to become markedly depressed, and even a fatal result is not at all uncommon.

The causes which give rise to the affection are similar to those which predispose to furuncle. It is generally observed in those whose health is impaired or broken down. It is more common in men, and is usually encountered in those past middle age. The inflammation starts simultaneously at numerous points, usually from the hair-follicles, sweat and sebaceous glands, extends in all directions, and eventually terminates in gangrene of the whole area. The inflammatory centres break down rapidly, from each of which the collected pus finds its way to the surface, thus producing the cribriform appearance. According to Warren, the pus ascends by way of the columnæ adiposæ to the hair-follicles, and thence to the surface. The process may involve fascia, muscles, and even periosteum and bone. The disease is to be distinguished from furuncle by its greater size, flatness, and the multiple points of suppuration. From erysipelas, to which in the beginning it may have some resemblance, it is to be differentiated by the hardness, painfulness, and circumscribed character of the lesion. It is also to be distinguished from malignant pustule. It is always to be looked upon as a serious affection, especially when occurring in those past the age of fifty or sixty and in those in a debilitated condition. Carbuncle when occurring about the face terminates in a large proportion of the cases fatally.

The treatment is both local and general. The local measures are in the main the same as advised for furuncle. In the early stages the actual cautery may arrest the process. Injections of from eight to twelve drops of a 5 or 10 per cent. solution of carbolic acid will be found valuable, often affording speedy relief. Frequently-repeated paintings with tincture of iodine in the early stage may prove of service. Poultices are of value, and will often diminish the tension and the pain. A dressing of white lead, laid on thick, is highly spoken of by Milton and other English observers. When the purulent collections have broken through the skin the application of a cupping-glass to draw out the pus has been advised. The wound should be dressed with carbolized oil. The use of the moist-sponge dressing, with the view of absorbing the pus, as recommended by McClellan, may be advised. Compression may also be resorted to with good results. The weight of authority is against the practice of incision, although in some cases it is to be recommended, the operation being preceded by hypodermic injections of cocaine. The general treatment should be of a tonic character. Iron—preferably the tincture of the chloride—and quinine in large doses are to be advised. A liberal diet of nourishing food, with a moderate amount of stimulants, is indicated in almost every case.

Herpes Simplex.

Herpes simplex is an acute, non-contagious, inflammatory disease, characterized by the formation of pinhead- to pea-sized vesicles arranged in groups and occurring for the most part about the face and genitalia. Malaise and pyrexia in severe cases may precede the eruption. Usually, however, the efflorescence appears without any systemic disturbance. The lesions are rarely numerous, and appear in the form of one or more clusters. Sense of heat in the part usually signalizes the outbreak. The vesicles show no tendency to rupture. The contents are at first clear, but later become cloudy or puriform, and dry to yellowish or brownish crusts, which subsequently fall off, leaving the skin normal. If broken or rubbed, a superficial excoriation results. The affection is acute, ordinarily running its course, if unirritated, in a week or ten days. It is liable to recur from time to time. Occurring about the face, it is designated herpes facialis. It is usually seen about the lips (herpes labialis), frequently about the alæ of the nose, and occasionally on other regions of the face. The mucous membrane of the mouth may also be invaded. The lesions may remain discrete or may coalesce, forming small blebs.

When the affection shows itself upon the genitalia, it is termed herpes progenitalis; and when on the prepuce, a common site, herpes præputialis. In the female, in whom it occurs here much less frequently, the labia majora and labia minora, as well as the skin about the vulva, are the parts usually invaded. It is seen most commonly in the young and middle-aged. Burning, slight itching, sometimes darting pain, and more or less œdema, may be present. As a rule, the lesions are not numerous, the average number being five or six. They incline to group, and ordinarily but one group is seen. Unless irritated they run the same favorable course as when on other regions. If, however, as often happens, especially when occurring about the inner surface of the prepuce or the glans, or on the inner surface of the labia, the vesicles break down and excoriations resembling ulcers result. The disease is even more prone to recur than when on other parts.

Herpes of the face is often observed in association with lung and febrile diseases. Malaria is sometimes the cause, and digestive and nervous disorders frequently predispose to it. Herpes of the genitalia, it is stated, is seen most frequently in those who have previously had gonorrhœa, chancroid, or chancre, especially the first. It may be that, occurring in such persons, it excites solicitude, and hence medical relief is sought, and the relative frequency of such causes unduly increased. A long prepuce is a predisposing factor.

The characters of the eruption, as it occurs about the face, are so well marked as to preclude an error in diagnosis. About the genitalia, however, the lesions may become abraded or irritated, and may simulate chancroids. The history, course, and character of the two affections should in doubtful cases be carefully considered before expressing a positive opinion.

In herpes facialis, flexible collodion, camphorated cold cream, or the lotion of zinc sulphate and potassium sulphide (see treatment of acne for formula) may be prescribed. In herpes progenitalis cleanliness is of great importance. Liquor gutta-perchæ, a paste composed of equal parts of mucilage of acacia, glycerin, and oxide of zinc, lotions of sulphate of zinc, a few grains to the ounce, and of ammonia-water, may be prescribed. A saturated solution of boric acid and a dressing of borated absorbent cotton are likewise useful, while in some cases dusting the parts with calomel will prove beneficial. Where the affection recurs, if the prepuce is long, circumcision may afford future immunity.

Herpes Iris.

Herpes iris is an acute non-contagious disease, consisting of one or more groups of inflammatory vesicles or blebs, arranged usually in the form of more or less complete concentric rings, the whole efflorescence being somewhat variegated in color.

The eruption most frequently appears on the backs of the hands and feet, especially the former. It begins as a simple papule or vesicle, which soon disappears, a ring of discrete or confluent vesicles now appearing around the periphery. The process may be arrested at this stage, the lesions soon undergoing involution, or still another ring may form. The vesicles may be discrete or confluent, but usually they coalesce, forming small or large blebs. The number of groups or patches in most cases is not large, three or four usually being present at one period; but sometimes as many as a dozen or more exist. The eruption is usually symmetrical. The difference in the age of the several rings that go to form a single patch gives rise to the variegated colors which characterize the disease. In size the vesicles vary from a pinhead to a pea, and the patches from a fraction of an inch to several inches in diameter. They contain a yellowish, clear, or puriform fluid which rapidly dries to crusts. New patches, as a rule, continue to appear in crops for a few weeks, when the process gradually subsides, leaving slight pigmentation, which soon fades away. Variations in the type of the efflorescence are not uncommon. In some instances the lesions barely reach vesiculation, being rather papulo-vesicular, while in others blebs may appear at the beginning in the place of vesicles. The subjective symptoms of itching and burning are either lacking or are not marked. Malaise or slight febrile action may usher in the disease, or, as is usually the case, constitutional disturbance is not observed. The affection is comparatively rare. Recurrences may take place, usually at intervals of a year or more.

It is seen chiefly in spring and autumn, and is met with in both sexes, but is more common in children and young persons. Its nature is obscure. It is probably due to the same causes that are responsible for erythema multiforme, a disease to which it is very closely allied. The process also is intimately identical with that affection, it being, apparently, merely an advanced stage or modification of that disease. It is to be distinguished from ringworm, erythema multiforme, herpes zoster, pemphigus, and dermatitis herpetiformis. In ringworm the process is more superficial, and usually is less inflammatory, the papules or vesico-papules being scarcely distinguishable; in doubtful cases the microscope will decide. Vesiculation will serve to differentiate from erythema multiforme. The absence of neuralgic pain, the distribution, location, and arrangement of the vesicles, are sufficient to exclude herpes zoster. In pemphigus the size, distribution, arrangement, mode of formation, and course of the lesions are different from herpes iris.

The affection tends to spontaneous disappearance in the course of a week or two; nor does treatment seem to influence materially its course. The bowels should be opened with saline laxatives, and other symptoms treated on general principles. Tonics, especially quinine, are in some cases of value. Locally, dusting-powders, such as oxide of zinc, starch, and lycopodium, may be frequently applied. Cooling, antipruritic, or astringent lotions—such, for example, as those used in acute vesicular eczema—will generally prove grateful.

Herpes Zoster.

Herpes zoster, or zoster, popularly known as shingles, is an acute, self-limited, inflammatory disease, characterized by groups of vesicles with inflammatory bases situated along or over a nerve-tract, and accompanied by more or less neuralgic pain.

As a rule, the cutaneous lesions are preceded, usually for several days, by neuralgic or burning pains in the part, and in some cases mild febrile disturbance. An inflamed state of the skin, in the form of one or several patches, is seen, which is soon followed by the formation of vesico-papules, which rapidly become distinct vesicles. They vary in size from a pin-head to a pea, are situated on inflamed bases, and are irregularly grouped. They may occur in small numbers, or, as is usual, be numerous, in which case they are crowded together. In the latter event they may coalesce here and there, forming larger lesions or irregular patches. They continue to appear for five or six days, remain stationary a short time, and then begin to subside. One or more groups may be present; usually a half dozen or more are seen in the one case. The vesicles contain a clear yellowish liquid, which gradually becomes puriform; those that appear last rarely reach full development. They show no tendency to rupture, are distended, subsequently becoming slightly umbilicated, and by the end of two weeks have gradually dried to thin yellowish or brownish crusts, which soon drop off. Except in severe cases, especially the hemorrhagic form, scarring rarely results. A tendency to group is characteristic of the eruption. The disease is acute, and runs its course usually in from ten to twenty days.

In some instances the lesions run an abortive course, barely arriving at the point of vesiculation. On the other hand, small blebs and pustules may be formed. In severe cases the vesicles may become hemorrhagic. The neuralgic pain may accompany the disease, and in severe cases, especially in persons advanced in years, may persist long after the eruption has subsided. In some cases burning is the only subjective symptom complained of. The disease is not confined to any age or sex. It is more common in the winter season. As a rule, it is limited to one side of the body. Moreover, it is rarely seen in the same indvidual twice. The intercostal and lumbar regions show the eruption most frequently. In zoster of the orbital region the eye becomes involved, and the disease may in some instances terminate in loss of sight, and even in destruction of the eyeball. Any nerve-tract or part of the body may be the seat of the eruption, hence the names zoster capitis, facialis, brachialis, pectoralis, etc. The disease is not uncommon.

The eruption is dependent upon an irritable and inflamed state of the ganglia or nerves—a neuritis. Hence any agent that may bring about this condition is capable of producing the eruption. Among such may be included atmospheric changes, sudden checking of the perspiration, compression, nerve-injuries, operations, and similar influences. In some instances the eruption is noted to follow the administration of arsenic.

The primary seat of the affection is usually in the spinal ganglia; they are found softened and altered in structure and the nerves inflamed and thickened. It may, however, have its beginning along the tract of a nerve or in the peripheral branches. In fact, it may be spinal, ganglionic, or peripheral in origin. The vesicles are found to have their seat in the lower strata of the rete. The surrounding corium and papillæ show more or less round-cell infiltration, with dilatation of the papillary blood-vessels. A perineuritis, with cell-infiltration in and about the neurilemma, is also usually observed. The vesicles contain rete-cells, pus-corpuscles, and serum.

The diagnosis is usually unattended with difficulty. The premonitory pain, the appearance of grouped vesicles upon inflammatory bases, with no tendency to rupture, and the limitation of the eruption to one side of the body, are sufficiently characteristic. The vesicles are larger than those of eczema, and lack the well-known tendency of the latter to break and discharge a gummy fluid which rapidly forms to crusts. In erysipelas the line of demarcation, the deep-reddish color, and the constitutional symptoms will serve to differentiate the diseases. It is to be distinguished from simple herpes by its location, number of groups, unilateral distribution, and absence of relapses. The prognosis is favorable, as the eruption usually disappears at the end of two or three weeks; severe cases, however, may last a month or more. When involving the eye, the possibility of its destroying the same, and even of a fatal result, is to be kept in mind. In elderly subjects the neuralgic symptoms are apt to prove persistent.

Treatment is mainly expectant. The disease is self-limited, and hence severe measures are to be avoided. Internal treatment has, so far as experience shows, very little influence upon its course. Phosphide of zinc, in one-third grain doses every three hours, at times seems to have a beneficial effect. Morphia, hypodermically or by the mouth, is required if the neuralgia is severe. The galvanic current, applied once or twice daily, will sometimes quiet the pain and favorably influence the course of the disease. Locally, the parts are to be protected from irritation. For this purpose dusting-powders, to which a small quantity of morphia and camphor may be added, may be employed. The parts should be further protected with a bandage. Oxide-of-zinc ointment, and anodyne ointments containing powdered opium or belladonna, may also be used. Painting the efflorescence with oil of peppermint or with solutions of menthol, thymol, or carbolic acid will be found to relieve the burning and pain; so also, flexible collodion, containing ten grains of morphia to the ounce, will sometimes afford relief. The parts subsequently may be covered with a layer of cotton batting.

Dermatitis Herpetiformis.

This disease is multiform and protean in character, consisting in the formation of herpetic, erythematous, vesicular, pustular, and bullous lesions, occurring separately or in various combinations, accompanied with itching and burning sensations and pursuing usually a chronic course with relapses.

This affection, which until recently has been confounded with other cutaneous diseases, is rare, although as its peculiar features become better known numerous cases will doubtless be reported. It was first described by one of us (Duhring) in a paper read before the American Medical Association in 1884. It is an inflammatory disease of an herpetic character, the various lesions showing more or less tendency to group. In some of its forms it bears likeness to erythema multiforme and herpes iris, while in other cases it is allied to pemphigus. It varies greatly in the degree of development. The causes are varied, though in many cases they are neurotic in their nature; thus, the disease may follow shock to the nervous system. It is also met with accompanying the parturient state. In some cases it is septicæmic in origin. It is also at times due to irregular menstruation. As to sex, while more frequent in women, it is also encountered in men. In severe cases there is more or less constitutional disturbance, consisting of malaise, slight fever, and constipation, accompanying the onset of the disease or its relapses and exacerbations. Increased heat of skin, itching, and burning are also prominent symptoms at such periods.

The disease manifests itself in the erythematous, vesicular, bullous. pustular, and multiform varieties. The erythematous variety is characterized by patches or a diffuse efflorescence of an urticarial or erythema-multiforme-like nature, the similarity to the latter process being sometimes marked. The disease may remain in this form, or, as is usually the case, may pass into other varieties, especially the vesicular. This latter is the usual form of the disease. It is characterized by variously-sized, flat or raised, irregularly-shaped or stellate, glistening vesicles, as a rule without marked areolæ. They are usually firm and distended, are often difficult to detect, and have an herpetic look, being grouped into clusters of two, three, or more. Here and there they are aggregated into patches. When in close proximity they tend to coalesce, forming large irregularly-shaped, oblong, or lobulated vesicles, or even blebs. The eruption is usually profuse. The most striking symptom is the itching, which in most cases is severe or even intense. The vesicles make their appearance, as a rule, slowly, several days or a week being required for their complete development. This variety of dermatitis herpetiformis (formerly described with the name herpes gestationis) is liable to be confounded with vesicular eczema, but the irregularity in the size and shape of the vesicles; their angular or stellate outline, giving them a puckered look; their firm, tense walls, showing no disposition to spontaneous rupture,—will all serve in the diagnosis. In some cases the constitutional disturbance and the magnitude of the eruption, as regards profusion, distribution, and multiformity, will also be apparent.

In the bullous variety the lesions are more or less typical blebs, variable as to size and shape, seated upon a slightly inflamed or non-inflammatory base. They tend to group into small clusters, in which case the skin between them will be red, as occurs in herpes zoster. Together with the blebs, vesicles and small or even minute whitish pustules will usually be found, the combination of these varied lesions being sometimes remarkable. The blebs generally rupture or are broken by injury, and become the seat of yellowish or brownish crusts. This variety of the disease is liable to be confounded with pemphigus, but differs in its marked herpetic and more inflammatory aspect.

The pustular variety is generally less clearly defined than the vesicular, because the lesions are usually intermingled with vesicles, vesico-pustules, and blebs. The pustules are acuminate, rounded, or flat, are variable as to size, and are whitish or yellowish in color. The smallest are generally flat, sometimes being no larger than a pinpoint or pinhead, while those that attain the size of a pea are rounded or acuminate, and are surrounded with a marked red areola. The largest are flat, and incline to spread out and to run together, forming patches which later become covered with greenish crusts. Grouping occurs here as in the other varieties, and is sometimes peculiar in that a central pustule may be surrounded by a variable number of smaller pustules in a circinate form, as in herpes iris. This variety of the disease is the same condition described by Hebra with the title impetigo herpetiformis.

The papular manifestation is an ill-defined form of disease, consisting of small reddish, firm, more or less grouped papules, resembling in general appearance the papular lesions sometimes met with in abortive herpes zoster. They resemble at times also certain phases of relapsing chronic papular eczema. Owing to itching and scratching they are generally excoriated.

Finally, there remains to be described the multiform variety, which consists of several of the foregoing varieties occurring in combination, a phase of the disease which is not infrequent. It comprises erythematous, sometimes slightly raised, urticarial patches of variable size and shape, often marginate or confluent, and of a reddish, yellowish, or variegated color. In addition, there may be present more or less well-defined irregularly-shaped or rounded maculo-papules and flat patches of infiltration, papules, and papulo-vesicles in various stages of evolution. Vesicles, blebs, and pustules may also exist, together with pigmentation. Thus it will be noted there exists a mixture or combination of lesions, calling to mind the peculiarities of eczema, although the process is both more capricious and varied in its behavior.

It must also be stated that the disease may at any period change its type; thus the vesicular variety may exist for weeks or months, to be followed by a crop of blebs or of pustules. The mingling of several varieties at one or another period in the course of the affection is usually a marked feature. It is variable in its course, but is in most cases chronic, and not infrequently is of many years' duration. It inclines to persist and to show itself in distinct crops or attacks at irregular intervals, the patient in the mean time being comparatively free of eruption. Relapses are common. It is in most cases very rebellious to treatment. The prognosis should be guarded. The pustular and bullous varieties are the most grave, and at times may prove fatal, especially in connection with the parturient state.

Concerning the treatment, with the knowledge now at hand but little encouragement can be given. The general state of the patient should receive attention, and the cause inquired into and modified or remedied if possible. The therapeutics must be conducted on general principles. Arsenic and its preparations do not seem to be of value, at least in the cases that have fallen under our observation. Locally, the remedies most useful are those usually employed in chronic eczema and in pemphigus.

Psoriasis.

Psoriasis may be defined as a chronic disease of the skin, characterized by reddish, dry, inflammatory, infiltrated patches, variable as to size, shape, and number, covered usually with abundant whitish, mother-of-pearl-colored, imbricated scales. It varies considerably in the degree of its development, but as a rule the lesions are numerous and their features clearly defined. It is the most uniform in its symptoms of all the diseases of the skin. It is therefore easy to recognize. In the first stage it appears as a small reddish spot, as large as a pinhead or a pea; it grows rapidly or slowly, and from the beginning shows signs of scaling, the scales being whitish, imbricated, and easily detached by scraping. They are reproduced readily, so that the lesion is usually well covered. In their early stages the lesions usually develop rapidly until their determinate size has been attained. The usual course is for the lesion to begin as a pinhead-sized spot, and grow to the size of a small or large coin. Several may appear side by side in close proximity, in which event they tend to coalesce, and to form larger, rounded, ovoidal, or figure-of-eight-shaped patches. Thus in time large surfaces of disease, the size of a hand or larger, may result. In other cases the lesions remain small, but through their great number may involve a considerable portion of the whole integument.

When typically developed, the lesions are of a bright- or dull-red color, and are covered with whitish, grayish, or pale-yellowish scales. The degree of inflammation varies with the case; at times it is slight, causing the lesions to assume merely a pale-pinkish, slightly inflammatory look; at other times it is more active, producing a decidedly inflammatory, strawberry- or raspberry-red hue. The majority of cases show a well-defined dull pinkish-red color of a cold inflammatory hue. The scaling, while usually active and abundant, is likewise variable; where the lesions are numerous and large it is constant, the scales being formed and shed rapidly from day to day; where the process is active, they are large, laminated, of a whitish, silvery, or mother-of-pearl-colored or slightly yellowish hue, varying somewhat with the locality involved. Sometimes they are heaped up. They are, moreover, easily detached, and can be readily picked or scraped off, leaving beneath a dry or very little excoriated, reddish surface. When deeply scratched, minute drops or points of blood, sometimes appear. They never exude serum. The lesions are, as a rule, circumscribed and sharply defined from the surrounding healthy integument, differing in this respect from similar patches of eczema. The skin between the lesions is perfectly healthy. In markedly inflammatory cases they occasionally possess a slightly raised border, and sometimes, especially in certain localities, as the hands, fissures form, as in eczema and syphilis.

The disease pursues an eminently chronic course, often lasting years or even throughout life, disappearing and recurring from time to time. Relapses at intervals of months or years are the rule, sometimes slight, at other times severe. It is a capricious disease. Usually it is better in summer than in winter, and in some cases it makes its appearance only during the latter season. It is generally unaccompanied by marked subjective symptoms, although this depends largely upon the degree of inflammatory action. In most chronic cases the itching and burning are either absent or slight, and when present are generally most annoying during the period that new lesions are appearing or old ones spreading. On the other hand, where the affection is highly inflammatory and running an acute, rapid course, both sensations, especially burning, may exist to an annoying degree. The disease is not contagious.

The eruption takes on different appearances according to the size and outline of the lesions, some of which require mention. They constitute the so-called varieties of the disease, but, strictly speaking, are forms rather than varieties. Thus, when the lesions are pinhead in size the form is termed punctata; when larger, the size of peas, guttata, from their resemblance to a drop of mortar; when still larger, the size of coins, they are designated nummularis, this being the form generally encountered. Sometimes the last-named lesions become more or less clear in the centre, and spread on their circumference after the manner of ringworm of the general surface, the condition being called circinata; at other times, more rarely, they assume a figured or ribbon-like form, causing them to have a serpentine, gyrate, or festooned appearance, termed gyrata. Commonly, however, when they grow to a large size they form, by the coalition of two or more lesions, irregularly-rounded patches, covering, it may be, a considerable area, the condition being called diffusa. The disease shows preference for certain regions, among which may be mentioned the extensor surfaces of the limbs, the elbows and knees, the scalp, and the trunk. The palms and soles and nails may also be invaded alone, or, as is usually the case, in connection with the disease upon other regions. It is usually symmetrical.

The causes of the disease seem to be varied, and are by no means well understood. It is met with, as a rule, in subjects whose general health is of the best, and who have hearty and strong constitutions, with no other ailment than the cutaneous manifestation. But cases are also encountered where the general condition is at fault: sometimes the system is below standard, as during lactation; in other cases the nervous system is depressed, as from some long-continued cause like mental worry. It occurs in both sexes, and usually makes its appearance in early adult life. It is seldom met with before the age of eight, and does not show itself in infants. In some cases it is inherited, but more frequently such is not the case. It occurs in all walks of life, being found among the rich and the poor in about like proportions. Statistics show it to be one of the most common diseases of the skin. It is of more frequent occurrence in some countries than in others. According to White's report of 5000 consecutive cases of skin disease observed in Boston, 152 cases of psoriasis were recorded, while Anderson in Glasgow reports 725 cases among 10,000 cases of skin disease, the difference being more than two to one in favor of Scotland. Diet in the majority of cases possesses but little influence over the disease.

The pathological process is one of the most defined and constant in cutaneous medicine. It is well marked throughout its course, and is subject to little variation. According to the most recent and reliable observations, it is held to be an inflammation induced by a hyperplasia of the rete mucosum. The views put forth by Auspitz and by Tilbury Fox have been substantiated by more recent observers. A. R. Robinson, and later Jamieson and Thin, have investigated the pathological anatomy of the disease with care, and have shown that the disease consists essentially of a hyperplasia of the rete mucosum, the increase taking place in the interpapillary portion of the layer. The growth extends downward, pressing upon the papillæ and corium, and setting up a variable degree of inflammation. In the later stages the superficial blood-vessels become dilated, more or less emigration of corpuscular elements occurring, the connective tissue especially in the neighborhood of the vessels becoming the seat of a round-cell infiltration. Effusion of serum, moreover, takes place, separating the connective-tissue bundles and fibres into an open meshwork. As the disease is vanishing there is a gradual return to the normal state, the hyperplasia, dilatation, and infiltration disappearing without traces. The hair is affected from the beginning in the form of hyperplasia of the external root-sheath, but the sebaceous and sweat glands are not found to be involved.

DIAGNOSIS.—The diagnosis, as a rule, offers no difficulties. The characteristic features are so constant and are usually so well marked that in ordinary cases errors are not likely to occur. When localized, as upon the scalp or upon the hands, it may be, however, readily confounded with other diseases. The general aspect of the eruption, the form of the lesions, the peculiar character of the scaling, the localities invaded, and the course of the process must be kept in view. It may be confounded with squamous eczema, especially where only one or two lesions are present, but the scales are usually more abundant, larger, and whiter than in eczema. The patches of psoriasis, moreover, are circumscribed, often sharply defined, and are always dry. In eczema there is not infrequently a history of moisture; itching is also generally an annoying symptom, much more marked than in psoriasis.

The papulo-squamous syphiloderm at times closely resembles psoriasis, especially as it occurs upon the palms and soles. Symmetry usually exists in psoriasis, but in syphilis it is often lacking, even in connection with disease of the palms and soles. Apart from the question of a history of syphilis, it will be found that psoriasis generally involves more surface, and in a more disseminate form, than the syphilitic eruption; also, that the scales are whiter, larger, and more copious than in syphilis. The color of the lesions in both diseases is similar, but in psoriasis it is pinker or redder, and free from the yellowish, brownish, ham-colored tint that generally characterizes the later syphilitic eruptions. The infiltration and thickening of the skin in a psoriatic patch are less than in syphilis, this observation being a valuable point in the diagnosis. The character of the inflammatory product in the diseases is different, that of psoriasis being simpler and less dense and firm. Finally, the course of psoriasis is peculiar, the lesions always manifesting the same general characters, often disappearing spontaneously and again reappearing.

Seborrhœa, especially of the scalp, sometimes simulates psoriasis, but the patches in the former disease are ill defined, are not so marginate, and are covered with finer, looser, and fatty scales. The lesions of psoriasis are redder and more infiltrated, and will usually be found to exist also in other localities. The disease may also be mistaken for lupus erythematosus in its early stage. The involvement of the sebaceous glands in almost all cases in the latter affection, the character of the scaling, and the fact that the face is the usual locality attacked, will aid in the diagnosis. Ringworm of the general surface may also bear resemblance to psoriasis, especially to the circular form, but the parasitic disease is more superficial and more marginate, is less scaly, and runs a more acute course. In doubtful cases the microscope should always be employed to determine the question.

TREATMENT.—The disease is rebellious to treatment, sometimes even where the lesions are few and small. It must be regarded as one of the most stubborn and persistent of the inflammatory diseases of the skin, for, while many cases yield readily to either internal or external remedies, the majority will often resist the best-directed therapeutics looking toward a permanent cure. It may often be happily dissipated for the time being, but immunity from relapses is a difficult task. To relieve the patient of the lesions, and, secondly, to prevent, if possible, relapses, should be the aim. To accomplish this demands usually both external and internal treatment. Before entering upon therapeutic measures the case should be viewed from a general standpoint. The condition of the general health should be inquired into, and the cause, if possible, determined. The history of the disease in chronic cases should be learned, and, if a relapse, the behavior of the lesions on former occasions. The influence of the several well-known remedies, such as arsenic internally, and tar, chrysarobin, and the mercurials locally, should also be ascertained. Finally, the acuteness or chronicity of the attack, the activity of the process, the amount of disease present, the locality invaded, and the general circumstances of the patient and the time that can be devoted to the treatment, should all receive consideration.

Among internal remedies, arsenic and its preparations occupy the most prominent position. For the majority of cases this remedy will be found valuable, and, if administered when indicated and in suitable doses for sufficient length of time, good results may be expected. It is not indicated in every case, as is shown by the fact that sometimes, instead of relieving, it aggravates the disease. It should be used tentatively at first, with the view of determining its tolerance and effect, not only upon the skin, but on the general system and alimentary canal. It is a powerful remedy, and should always be employed with due caution. At the same time, there need be no hesitation in prescribing it, or even in employing it for a long period, if attention be directed to its effects. Toxic symptoms should never be permitted to occur. In acute stages, whether in first attacks or in relapses, where the process is active, characterized by marked redness, inflammation, and heat, it should be withheld. At these periods it usually aggravates the disease. The more chronic the process, the more useful will the remedy probably prove.

The drug is generally administered in the form of arsenious acid, liquor potassii arsenitis, and liquor sodii arsenitis. A dose of arsenious acid varies from one-fortieth to one-fiftcenth of a grain thrice daily, administered in pill form. The dose of the liquor potassii arsenitis —or Fowler's solution of arsenic, as it is generally termed—varies from one to five minims three times a day, the average dose being two or three minims. It is best to begin with a small dose and gradually to increase the quantity until the maximum dose is ascertained;

after which the regular dose may be instituted. Patients, it will be found, vary as to the amount they can safely and beneficially take: in most cases two or three minims continued for a length of time will prove a full dose, while in others four or five minims will be tolerated. It may be given with water, elixir of calisaya, or wine of iron. The practice of prescribing it pure, directing a certain number of drops to be taken at each dose, is objectionable; it does not ensure an accurate quantity or proper dilution, and, moreover, gives the patient unnecessary trouble. A prescription such as the following possesses practical advantages:

$$\text{R}.\ \text{Liq. potassii arsenitis,} \quad \text{f}\bar{3}\text{iss};$$
$$\text{Elix. calisayæ,} \quad \text{f}\bar{3}\text{iv}.$$

M.—Sig. One teaspoonful with a wineglassful of water thrice daily, after meals. The dose here is three minims; should it prove too strong, a half teaspoonful of the mixture may be ordered. The toxic effects of arsenic should be borne in mind. Some persons are very susceptible to the remedy, half-minim or one-minim doses sometimes causing unpleasant symptoms. The usual ill effects consist of erythema of the fauces, œdema of the eyelids, injection of the conjunctivæ, watering of the eyes, pains in the head, nausea, sharp pains in the bowels, and diarrhœa, coming on within a few days or a fortnight after beginning treatment. As a rule, they pass away in a few days after ceasing the use of the remedy.

The length of time that arsenic should be given will depend upon its effects upon the general system and upon the disease. In most cases improvement is noticeable within a fortnight, though its use from one to three months is generally necessary to bring about complete recovery; and it is best to continue the medicine in small doses for a month or two longer. Arsenic is a nervine tonic. It acts as a stimulant to the skin, exerting a decided impression upon the cells of the rete mucosum; doing this, without doubt, directly through the nerves, which, as is well known, are abundantly supplied to this structure.

Phosphorus has been used by several dermatologists, but with varying results. It is liable to produce gastric disturbance, and is a disagreeable remedy. Tar, in capsule or pill form, will sometimes prove of value where arsenic and other remedies have failed. From one to three capsules, containing from three to five grains each, may be given for a dose. Carbolic acid has also been extolled by some, especially in chronic cases with slight infiltration. Anderson speaks well of it, and gives the following formula for its administration:

$$\text{R}.\ \text{Acidi carbolici,} \quad \text{5iij};$$
$$\text{Glycerinæ,} \quad \text{t}\bar{5}\text{j};$$
$$\text{Aquæ,} \quad \text{f}\bar{3}\text{v}.$$

M.—Sig. One teaspoonful in a large wineglassful of water before meals.

In some cases, more particularly in strong, hearty, plethoric persons, and in those having a rheumatic or gouty habit, the free use of alkalies proves of great value. In these cases arsenic often aggravates rather than improves the condition, whereas the alkali acts most happily. It may be recommended in acute stages of the disease when the lesions are red, heated, and growing. Liquor potassæ, in from ten to twenty drop doses, diluted with a large wineglassful of water, thrice daily, is the form generally prescribed. Improvement is sometimes noted within a few days. Anderson calls attention also to the value of carbonate of ammonium, in from ten to thirty grain doses, in like cases. The acetate of potassium, in thirty-grain doses, may also be referred to as being sometimes useful.

Local treatment may now be considered. This is of great value, and should be instituted in all cases, either alone or in conjunction with internal remedies, according to the case. Sometimes it may be directed alone with good results, more particularly in chronic, sluggish cases where the lesions undergo but little change from time to time and are unaccompanied by subjective symptoms. Before prescribing certain points should be ascertained. The duration of the disease; the extent of the cruption, including the number and size of the lesions, and their acuteness or chronicity; the locality involved; the circumstances and the age of the patient; and the time that can be given to the treatment,—should all be taken into consideration. In this connection it should be remembered that whatever plan of treatment is adopted, the remedies should be applied thoroughly. The disease at best yields stubbornly, and to secure satisfactory results the importance of employing the agents properly should be insisted upon. This requires in most instances considerable time once, and, in some cases, twice a day. The scales are to be removed first. Where they are thick and adherent, inunction with some simple oil, as olive oil, followed by the use of soap and water, may be employed. Ordinarily, soft soap alone, well rubbed into the lesions with a piece of wet flannel and rinsed off with water, will be found sufficient. A 5 or 8 per cent. alcoholic solution of salicylic acid may be employed for the same purpose. The bath, simple or alkaline—the latter containing, for example, borax—is also frequently of service.

In acute, highly inflammatory cases, where the skin is red, hot, scaling profusely, and the lesions spreading from day to day, soothing applications, as of olive oil, will generally prove most valuable. Instances are sometimes encountered where the use of the simple bath, followed by inunctions of olive oil or one of the petroleum ointments, will prove to be the only treatment tolerated. The majority of cases, however, seeking advice show the disease already well developed and in the chronic stage, and here stimulating remedies are demanded.

One of the most valuable and generally useful remedies is tar, employed in the form of ointment or tincture or in combination with other substances, as, for example, the mercurials or sulphur. The tarry products in common use are pix liquida, or common tar, oil of tar, oil of cade, and oleum rusci (oil of white birch). The chief objection to their employment is the penetrating odor, which is almost impossible to banish. The oil of birch is probably the least objectionable in the list. Officinal tar ointment, full strength or weakened, will be found serviceable. It should be applied with a piece of cloth or stiff brush, well rubbed into the skin, and should be used twice daily, the scales having been previously removed by one or another of the methods indicated. Similar ointments, one or two drachms to the ounce, may in like manner be prepared from any of the other preparations of tar, as, for instance, the oil of white birch. Where an ointment is not desired, the oil of tar, oil of cade, or oil of white birch may be employed, the remedy being thoroughly rubbed or worked into the skin. Attention to the mode of application should always be insisted upon.

Other tarry preparations, such as liq. picis alkalinus, liq. carbonis detergens (the formulæ for which have been given in speaking of the treatment of eczema), diluted, may also be prescribed in some cases with benefit. Hebra's modification of Wilkinson's ointment may be referred to as an energetic and useful compound :

> ℞. Sulphuris sublimati,
> Ol. cadini,   āā. ʒiv ;
> Saponis viridis,
> Adipis,   āā. ʒj ;
> Cretæ præparatæ,   ʒijss.
> M. Ft. ugt.

Another method of using tar consists in the so-called tar bath : the patches are deprived of scales by means of soft soap, after which tar ointment or one of the tarry oils is rubbed in, and the patient then placed in a warm bath for several hours. A stimulating tarry mixture, especially useful in circumscribed, infiltrated, obstinate patches, is composed of equal parts of tar, soft soap, and alcohol. Tar should not be applied over extensive surfaces without cautioning the patient that systemic disturbance, produced by absorption, may possibly occur. In ordinary cases, however, such an accident is very rarely noted. Creasote, turpentine, and acetic acid, remedies similar to tar in their action on the skin, may also be mentioned. The first-named may be used in the form of an ointment, from one to four drachms to the ounce. Turpentine may be applied pure or with oil, one to two or three parts. In some cases thymol in the form of an ointment, from five to thirty grains to the ounce, proves of service. The mercurials may also be referred to, but it may be stated that they are not as valuable in this disease as they are in eczema. The most useful is white precipitate in the form of ointment, from forty to eighty grains to the ounce, which is especially valuable in psoriasis of the scalp and of the face. Lotions of corrosive sublimate will also sometimes be found of service.

The treatment of psoriasis by chrysarobin—or chrysophanic acid, as it was originally termed—may now be referred to. It is a very valuable method of treatment. Care should be exercised in the selection of a reliable preparation, there being considerable difference in the strength, and therefore in the results obtained, of the remedy as found in the shops. Its disadvantages must be mentioned: It is liable to irritate and inflame the skin, causing sometimes an acute dermatitis or a follicular or furuncular inflammation and a variegated purplish or mahogany-colored staining of the skin. The hair, nails, and the linen of the patient also become stained. It may be prescribed in the form of an ointment, from ten grains to one drachm to the ounce of lard or petroleum ointment. The most desirable mode of application, that which is least objectionable, is in the form of a pigment, with flexible collodion or liquor guttaperchæ, in the same strength as the ointment mentioned. It should be applied with a brush daily or every other day. The following formula, suggested by G. H. Fox, may be given : Chrysarobin and salicylic acid, each ten parts ; ether, fifteen parts ; collodion, enough to make one hundred parts. Another valuable remedy, having a similar action, to be used in the same manner as chrysarobin, is pyrogallic acid. Like chrysarobin, it stains the skin (a brownish hue), but it possesses the advantage over that substance in not being so irritating. Neither of these remedies, especially the pyrogallic acid, should be applied over extensive surfaces, on account of liability to absorption and systemic poisoning.

Where the patches are not numerous a solution of sulphide of lime may sometimes be used with excellent results, as according to the following formula, known as Vleminckx's solution:

R. Caleis, ʒss ;
Sulphuris sublimati, ʒj ;
Aquæ, fʒx.
Coque ad fʒvj, deinde filtra.

This may be perfumed with oil of anise, five or ten drops to the ounce. It may be applied diluted with two or four parts of water or full strength, and is to be rubbed into the skin with a flannel rag, after which the parts are to be bathed with water and some emollient oil or ointment applied.

Treatment is usually effective in removing the lesions, but, unfortunately, in the majority of cases, relapses sooner or later occur. It may be said relapses are the rule. The prognosis will depend upon the case.

Pityriasis Rosea.

Pityriasis rosea, known also as pityriasis maculata et circinata, is an inflammatory disease, occupying chiefly the trunk, characterized by discrete or confluent pinkish or reddish macular or slightly raised lesions varying in size from a small to a large coin. They are rounded in form, but by coalescence may assume irregular shapes and considerable size, as in the case of psoriasis. They are circumscribed, usually clearly defined, superficially seated, of a bright rosy, pinkish, or reddish hue, which sooner or later fades and is followed by yellowish, salmon-colored, or rusty tints. The surface of the lesions is from the beginning dry, and as the process advances furfuraceous or flaky scaling sets in, similar to that observed in tinea versicolor and in tinea circinata. This feature is more marked about the border, the process inclining to recover in the centre and to spread on the periphery, after the manner of tinea circinata. The skin is only slightly, if at all, thickened. At times there is slight burning or itching, but more frequently subjective symptoms are altogether wanting.

The course of the affection is variable, in many instances lasting from one to several months, while in exceptional cases it is more acute. It tends to spontaneous recovery, and is to be viewed as a mild disease, notwithstanding that the lesions at times, by their redness and size, indicate considerable cutaneous disturbance. It is met with in all ages, in our own experience more frequently in adults than in children, and occurs in both sexes and in those possessing average general health. It is one of the rarer cutaneous diseases, and is not contagious.

It is to be distinguished from ringworm of the body, from tinea versicolor, and from the macular syphiloderm, all three of which diseases it at times closely resembles. It possesses some of the peculiar features which characterize the vegetable parasitic diseases, but in some respects it differs from them in its behavior. The microscope fails to reveal fungus. Concerning treatment there is but little to be said, as the process inclines in most cases to spontaneous disappearance. Mildly stimulating ointments or baths, as in eczema, may be prescribed. When involution sets in recovery usually takes place rapidly.

Pityriasis Rubra.

Pityriasis rubra is an inflammatory disease, usually pursuing a chronic course, characterized by redness and abundant and continuous epidermic exfoliation. It usually develops rapidly, beginning as small, red, scaly patches. It may make its appearance on one or more regions, the spots increasing in size rapidly, and coalescing to form large patches. In a variable time the whole or a large portion of the entire surface is involved, the skin being of a pale or violaceous red color and covered with thin whitish or grayish lamellar scales. These are abundant, and are rapidly formed, cast off and replaced by new, the exfoliation being, as a rule, in the form of flakes. Thickening of the skin seldom occurs. The surface when deprived of the scales is hyperæmic and shining in appearance. The disease usually involves the whole surface. Œdema, especially of the limbs, and stiffness of the joints are sometimes observed. The disease is superficial in character, rarely involving more than the upper cutaneous layers, and is always dry. Fissuring is only exceptionally seen.

As a rule, the subjective symptoms are slight, burning and itching, if present, seldom being violent. Symptoms of constitutional disturbance may or may not be present, but chilliness is often complained of. The disease generally occurs in adults, is acute or chronic, usually the latter, with a tendency to relapses. Being a rare affection, the etiology is obscure. Anatomically, there is found more or less marked cell-infiltration of the cutaneous tissues, especially noticeable in the rete and upper layer of the corium. In severe cases the papillæ are not distinguishable; the same may be said of the sweat and sebaceous glands.

Erythematous and squamous eczema and psoriasis bear resemblance to the disease. Its superficial nature, wide or universal distribution, absence of infiltration, character and rapid formation of the scales, and the slight itching or burning will serve to differentiate it from eczema. In psoriasis the whole surface is rarely if ever involved, while there is more or less thickening of the corium, and the scales are thicker and imbricated. It can scarcely be confounded with lichen ruber or with pemphigus foliaceus.

The disease pursues a variable course. It may last for years, with exacerbations, or outbreaks may occur from time to time. Treatment is, as a rule, unsatisfactory. For external treatment applications of a bland or soothing character afford the most relief. Vaseline, cold cream, and oily substances are generally of most service. Stimulating applications seldom prove useful—in fact, will in most cases give rise to discomfort and positive aggravation. In regard to constitutional remedies general indications are to be followed. There is no drug that seems to exert a specific influence.

Dermatitis Exfoliativa.

This term is employed to designate certain cases in which more or less exfoliation is the prominent characteristic, and which cannot be classified under the head of any of the other diseases in which this symptom is noted. These cases have been variously described under the names of general exfoliative dermatitis, recurring exfoliative dermatitis, desquamative scarlatiniform erythema, recurrent acute eczema, acute general dermatitis, and recurrent exfoliative erythema. The affection is characterized by an erythematous inflammation, rarely vesicular or bullous, acute in type, with desquamation or exfoliation of the epidermis accompanying or following its development. There is also usually more or less marked constitutional disturbance, in some instances of a serious nature, and a tendency to relapse and recurrence. It is possible that in some instances the disease could be properly classified under the head of eczema, psoriasis, pityriasis rubra or pemphigus foliaceus.

Lichen Ruber.

Lichen ruber is an inflammatory disease, characterized by small flat and angular or acuminated, smooth and shining or scaly, discrete or confluent red papules, having a distinctly papular or papulo-squamous course, attended with a variable degree of itching. Two varieties are met with—the plane (lichen ruber planus) and the acuminate (lichen ruber acuminatus), the first of which occurs much the more frequently in this country. The acuminate variety is met with chiefly in Austria, where it was first described by Hebra: it is very rare in the United States, only a few authentic cases being on record. In lichen rüber planus the papules vary in size from a pinhead to a pea, and are peculiar in that they are not rounded, but are quadrangular or polygonal in shape. In their early stage they have a smooth, glazed surface, and are free of scales, but later they become papulo-squamous. They are more or less flattened on their summits, and show slight umbilication with whitish puncta. They are of a dull pinkish, reddish or violaceous color, the hue varying with the individual, age, and locality. As a rule, they are numerous, and occur in variously-sized aggregations, the distribution scarcely amounting to grouping. They tend to coalesce and form patches, which are slightly elevated, flattened, and uneven, the lesions when crowded together having a mosaic pattern. In lichen ruber acuminatus the papules are smaller, pointed, scaly, and disseminated, showing no disposition to group. This variety of the disease spreads rapidly, pursues a chronic course, and is a more serious affection, sometimes terminating fatally.

Lichen ruber planus usually presents itself upon the extremities, especially upon the flexor surfaces, the forearms and wrists and backs of the feet being favorite localities. Not infrequently it appears in the form of short or long narrow bands, following the natural lines of the skin, and sometimes nerve-tracts. The course of the disease is generally slow, extending over months. Occasionally, however, especially where the lesions are acute and very numerous, it is comparatively rapid. New

papules continue to show themselves from to time, the older ones disappearing by absorption, leaving persistent marked reddish or brownish
pigmentation, which is to be regarded as a characteristic symptom.

The etiology of the disease is at times obscure, although, according
to our experience, patients usually show signs of impaired nutrition or
nervous depression, arising from varied causes, as, for example, overwork
or shock.   It occurs at all periods of life, but is usually met with at
middle age, and is more common in women than in men.   Pathologically,
the process is considered an inflammation of a chronic character, accompanied by more or less alterative changes in the structure of the skin,
involving the several layers as well as the follicles.   The lesion is always
of a papular type.   Later investigations (Robinson) into the anatomy of
the lesions of lichen ruber acuminatus and lichen ruber planus are apparently indicative of the distinct nature of the two varieties, the former
being considered a paratypical keratosis, leading to retrograde changes
and atrophy, and the latter an inflammatory process occurring in and
about the papillæ and upper part of the corium.

In the diagnosis of lichen ruber the papular syphiloderm, lichen scrofulosus, psoriasis, and papular eczema are to be excluded.   The irregular
and angular outlines of the lesions of the plane variety, taken with their
flattened, slightly umbilicated, smooth, or scaly summits and the dull-red
or violaceous hue, are sufficiently characteristic.   The evolution of a
patch of psoriasis is entirely different from that of this disease, the former
appearing as small spots and enlarging by peripheral growth, the patches
of the latter resulting from aggregations of lesions.   In papular eczema
the papules are rounded, bright-red in color, intensely itchy, and have a
different history and course.   The prognosis of lichen ruber planus is
generally favorable, although some cases are exceedingly rebellious.
According to Hebra, in the severe forms of lichen ruber acuminatus, if
neglected or improperly treated, a fatal result may ensue.

A general tonic plan of treatment is almost always indicated, such
remedies as iron, quinia, strychnia, and the mineral acids proving of benefit.   Arsenic exercises in many cases a specific influence.   When the
general health is much reduced arsenic fails, as a rule, to benefit until
the patient's condition is brought back to its normal tone.   The remedy
should be given in tolerably large doses, and continued until the lesions
have entirely disappeared.   On account of the itching and discomfort
experienced, external applications are demanded.   The various antipruritic remedies mentioned in the treatment of eczema may be employed.
Alkaline baths are useful.   Unna has reported a few instances of cure
of well-developed cases of the disease by the use of an ointment composed of two ounces of oxide-of-zinc ointment, forty grains of carbolic
acid, and from one to two grains of corrosive sublimate.   Tarry applications, especially in the form of lotions, often prove of service, the liquor
picis alkalinus and the liquor carbonis detergens being the preparations
commonly employed.

Lichen Scrofulosus.

Lichen scrofulosus is a chronic disease characterized by milletseed-sized,
flat, reddish or yellowish, more or less grouped, desquamating papules,

unaccompanied by itching and occurring in those of a scrofulous disposition. The lesions, of a pale red or yellowish color, are usually numerous, are seated about the hair-follicles, and show a decided tendency to group, giving rise to patches of variable size and of a rounded or crescentic shape, which sooner or later become covered with minute scales. They are always small; are seen usually about the abdomen and chest, and exceptionally about the limbs; are chronic in character; and as a rule, are unaccompanied by itching. Pit-like, atrophic depressions may or may not follow the disappearance of the lesions.

The affection is not uncommon in Austria, but in this country it is practically unknown. It was first described by Hebra. It is more common in males, and is seen chiefly in children and young people. Symptoms of a scrofulous habit, such as glandular enlargements, ulcers, bone disease, or lung complaint, are found associated in almost all cases. According to Kaposi, the process is an inflammation and cell-infiltration in and about the hair-follicles, the sebaceous glands, and papillæ around the apertures of the follicles. Each papule, as may be seen on close examination, has its seat about the opening of a follicle, the inflammation beginning around the vessels and at the bases of the follicles and glands, and subsequently the cellular infiltration invading the interior of these structures to such an extent as to give rise to distension and elevation into papules.

It is to be differentiated from papular eczema, lichen ruber, the miliary papular syphiloderm, and keratosis pilaris. According to Hebra, cod-liver oil, employed internally and externally, is the remedy to which the disease readily yields.

Eczema.

SYMPTOMS.—Eczema, known popularly as tetter, is the most important and the commonest of the diseases of the skin. It may be defined as an inflammatory, non-contagious disease of the skin, characterized in the beginning by erythema, papules, vesicles or pustules, or a combination of these lesions, pursuing an acute or chronic course, accompanied by infiltration and itching, terminating either in discharge with the formation of crusts, in absorption, or in desquamation. The disease is multiform in character, and is capable of manifesting itself in a great variety of forms; and for this reason any definition that is attempted must be broad enough to comprise all of its essential features. It may begin as a circumscribed or diffuse small or large erythematous patch, which may remain dry and become scaly, or may pass into a state of moist exudation with crusting. It may also begin with vesicles or pustules, which soon rupture, giving rise to a red, moist, oozing, weeping, excoriated surface pouring forth a scanty or abundant fluid, gummy discharge, which rapidly dries to crusts. Instead of a moist discharging surface the skin may become dry, scaly, thickened, and more or less fissured. In other cases small papules, discrete or confluent, in patches or disseminated, form, constituting papular eczema. Finally, several or all of these lesions may occur together or in the course of the process. Thus, it will be observed, the disease is markedly multiform and protean. Not infrequently it is capricious in its manifestations both as to the nature of the lesions and as to the evolution. Several varieties of the disease may appear simultaneously on one or on different regions.

Infiltration is one of the most marked features, and is present in varying degree. In the discharging varieties the fluid exuded is generally considerable and often excessive, giving rise to abundant crusting. In the papular variety the exudation is plastic in character, causing thickening of the skin, followed by more or less induration. Scaling is also frequently a prominent symptom, giving to the condition known as squamous eczema its peculiar features. Itching, usually marked, is an almost constant symptom, varying in degree. As a rule, it is an annoying feature of the disease, causing the patient to scratch in spite of good resolutions. In some cases, as in the erythematous variety, the sensation is of burning rather than itching, or it may be a combination of the two. Occasionally the locality affected is the seat of pain. The course of the disease is extremely variable. As a rule, it inclines to chronicity. Relapses are common, especially in adults and elderly persons. There are many cases on record, however, where, recovery having taken place, the individual remains free of the disease. The several varieties may now be considered.

Eczema Erythematosum.—This begins as an erythematous spot or macule, or as a patch, variable as to color, size and outline. It is most frequently met with upon the face, occupying a portion or the greater part of this region, usually in the form of several discrete or confluent patches. It generally begins as a coin-sized, ill-defined lesion, rounded or irregular in outline, of a pale-red hue, accompanied by itching and burning. The patch at first may be insignificant, but from time to time it spreads and becomes redder, thicker, and the surface slightly scaly. When fully developed, as is perhaps most frequently encountered upon the forehead, it consists of a more or less broken-up patch of considerably thickened somewhat swollen skin of a mottled or streaked pale-reddish, yellowish-red or violaceous hue. The surface is dry or excoriated and very slightly moist in places, and is covered with a thin film of dried, ragged epidermis or with thin adherent scales. The disease varies from time to time, being paler and less marked one week than another. Scratch-marks and excoriations, punctate or linear, are generally present, indicative of the scratching and rubbing to which the skin has been subjected. As stated, several patches generally exist, the disease tending to symmetry. The forehead, sides of the nose, and cheeks are the localities most frequently invaded, but other regions, as the back of the neck, axillæ, and flexures, are all common seats.

Its course is variable. As a rule, it inclines to assume chronicity, varying in intensity from time to time, or even disappearing and reappearing at irregular intervals. It is exceedingly liable to relapse, perhaps more so than any other variety. Having established itself, it may remain erythematous in character or may pass into other varieties of the disease. Thus, a moist or weeping surface may take the place of the erythema, followed by crusting, giving rise to eczema madidans, or eczema rubrum. Not infrequently the patch becomes markedly scaly, and continues in this form, producing eczema squamosum. When it occurs in regions where two opposing surfaces come in contact, as under the mammæ, between the nates, and about the genitalia, an excoriated moist condition is produced known as eczema intertrigo,. or eczema mucosum.

Eczema Vesiculosum.—This may be regarded as the typical and perfect expression of the disease. It is characterized in the beginning by a diffuse redness with puncta, which rapidly become small pinpoint- to pinhead-sized, more or less perfect vesicles, accompanied with heat and usually intense itching. As a rule, the lesions are small and are discrete or confluent. They soon mature and burst, the fluid oozing forth on and over the surface, forming yellowish honeycomb-like scanty or abundant crusts. The skin of such a patch is generally slightly swollen, and at times considerably infiltrated with serum (eczema œdematosum). The disease may thus develop upon a small surface, or, as is oftener the case, over an extensive area, as, for example, the flexor surface of the forearm. There is no disposition for the lesions to group, but they incline to appear in areas, a large patch being usually composed of several smaller patches. The amount of serous fluid poured forth is often great, large bulky crusts forming which in time completely mask the skin beneath. The exudation may take place rapidly in the course of a few days and cease, or it may continue, oozing slowly from day to day or with intermissions from time to time indefinitely, constituting acute, subacute or chronic vesicular eczema. The amount will, moreover, depend somewhat upon the locality involved and whether the disease be properly treated or irritated.

Vesicular eczema may show itself typically, the whole of the affected skin taking on vesicular formation, or, as frequently happens, it may be associated with other varieties of the disease, more particularly pustules and papules. Abortive vesicles and vesico-pustules and vesico-papules are common, occurring here and there mixed with the vesicles and about the circumference of the patch. The amount of surface invaded varies. The disease often manifests itself in different regions simultaneously, as, for example, upon the neck and flexor surfaces of the forearms or upon the trunk and the thighs. In infants the face is the locality usually attacked, constituting the so-called crusta lactea, or milk-crust, of former writers. While the disease tends to manifest itself upon the thin skin of the flexor surfaces of the extremities and upon the face, such is not always the case, for the hands and fingers are also often invaded.

Eczema Pustulosum.—This variety of the disease (designated by some writers eczema impetiginosum) is closely allied to the preceding variety. The lesions may develop as pustules or may become pustular from pre-existing vesicles ; both lesions are not infrequently found together, although one of the two will usually predominate. In pustular eczema the swelling, heat, and itching are seldom so marked as in the vesicular variety, and the lesions are generally larger and firmer. As in the case of the vesicles, they rupture and dry, forming yellowish or greenish bulky crusts. This variety is most frequently encountered about the face and scalp, and in those—especially young people—who are strumous, ill-nourished, or in a depraved state of health.

Eczema Papulosum.—Eczema papulosum is characterized by small, rounded or acuminated papules about the size of a pinhead. Sometimes they are well defined and circumscribed, but more frequently they possess no sharply-marked outline or form. They are reddish in color, the tint varying with the individual and with other circumstances, and are usually discrete, although not infrequently they are so numerous and so crowded together as to coalesce and form patches or aggregations of disease, which often show considerable infiltration. They begin as papules, and usually preserve this character throughout their course. Vesicles or vesico-papules not infrequently coexist. Sooner or later the lesions disappear, but are usually replaced by others, the process in this manner continuing its course for weeks or months. The itching is in almost all cases severe and persistent, the patient generally scratching himself to the extent of producing excoriations and blood-crusts. Papular eczema shows a preference for certain regions, notably the extremities, especially the flexor surfaces. The face is seldom attacked. It is one of the most obstinate varieties of the disease.

In addition to the principal varieties of eczema, just described, there are other forms of the disease which on account of their peculiar features require mention. Of these eczema rubrum, or eczema madidans, may first be spoken of. It is to be viewed as a secondary condition resulting from one or another of the primary varieties. Thus it usually follows eczema vesiculosum or pustulosum. It is characterized by a reddish, moist or discharging surface, the serum, sometimes bloody, usually exuding freely and forming thick yellowish or brownish crusts, together with more or less thickening of the skin and other secondary changes. In other cases discharge is wanting. The condition varies with the stage of the process and with other circumstances: at one time the red, inflammatory dry or oozing skin is the most striking feature, while in other cases this is completely obscured by large, diffuse masses of crust. It may occur upon any region, but it is most frequently met with on the legs, especially in adults, and more particularly in elderly people. It is usually chronic in its course, and may continue for years, better and worse from time to time, but usually evincing no disposition to spontaneous recovery.

Another clinical form of the disease is known as eczema squamosum, which frequently has been preceded by the erythematous variety, and in many cases is to be viewed as a stage of that variety. It may also follow other varieties. It appears in the form of reddish, dry, more or less infiltrated, scaly patches, the amount of scaling being variable. The scales are usually small or fine, and as a rule are scanty. The condition is generally chronic, and is often met with on the scalp.

Fissures, superficial or deep, are not infrequently met with in eczema, usually in the chronic or recurrent forms of the disease, and may be so pronounced as to give rise to the so-called eczema fissum. This is often seen about the fingers and hands, especially the palms. In localized infiltrated patches of chronic eczema a peculiar warty condition is occasionally met with, which is known as eczema verrucosum; or if simply hard, rather than wart-like, eczema sclerosum.

Eczema is divided into acute and chronic, the several forms of the disease being so different in their clinical pictures as to demand such a division, which relates rather to the pathological changes than to time. Thus the disease may show acute symptoms throughout its course, or, on the other hand, may in the beginning take on a chronic action. As a rule, it tends to chronicity, secondary changes in the skin usually manifesting themselves early in the course of the process.

ETIOLOGY.—Eczema is the commonest of the cutaneous diseases, and seems to be of more frequent occurrence in this country than in Europe. It is met with among all classes of society and at all ages. Individuals with light hair and florid complexions are more often subjects of the disease than those of the opposite temperament. Not infrequently the disease is hereditary, although examples are very common in which no such history obtains. So-called eczematous subjects, in which at longer or shorter intervals throughout life and under variable conditions the disease manifests itself, are of frequent occurrence in practice. The state, though well known clinically, is difficult to define, consisting of a peculiar inherent condition of the system at large and of the skin itself which under favorable circumstances permits the disease to assert itself from time to time. The association in some cases of chronic bronchitis and allied affections of the respiratory tract with eczema, and the clinical observation that as one disease improves the other becomes worse, has led some dermatologists to regard eczema as being catarrhal in its nature.

The constitutional causes which may produce the disease are numerous, and are worthy of careful study as bearing directly upon the treatment. Disorders of the digestive tract, including dyspepsia in its many forms and constipation, are not infrequently found to be the exciting cause of an attack, while faulty excretion through the several emunctories, and the existence of a gouty or rheumatic disposition, may all prove potent factors. Deterioration in the tone of the system, arising from varied causes, with impaired nutrition—as seen, for example, during pregnancy and lactation—is sometimes accompanied with an outbreak of the disease, while nervous exhaustion and other neurotic states, as is now well established, are not infrequently active causes.

In some cases excitants, external or internal—as, for example, cutaneous irritants and intestinal worms—may determine an outbreak. In like manner, dentition and vaccination may call forth the disease. Among the local causes producing the so-called artificial eczemas the preparations of mercury, sulphur, croton oil and tincture of arnica are most notable. Contact with the several varieties of the rhus plant, though usually producing a peculiar dermatitis, may in eczematous subjects provoke a genuine eczema. Heat and cold, especially the rays of the sun, are also factors to be considered, while it is well known that the disease in many instances is influenced by the seasons, being, as a rule, worse in winter than in summer. There are many subjects who suffer only in winter. In sensitive skins water, soap, alkalies and acids, all prove more or less injurious, giving rise to harshness or chapping of the skin, and sometimes to eczema. In the same manner the presence of parasites and the consequent scratching are productive of more or less simple dermatitis, and in eczematous subjects the disease under discussion. Eczema is not contagious, a question which is frequently asked by the patient.

PATHOLOGY.—The changes which occur in the skin in the various eczematous conditions are somewhat different as the process is of short or long duration and mild or intense in character. In all cases hyperæmia and exudation, constant symptoms of all inflammations, are present, varying according to the activity and duration of the process. The rete mucosum is also involved in all cases, being œdematous and infiltrated. In the erythematous form the blood-vessels of the papillary layer are dilated, exudation and congestion as well as increasing activity of the rete taking place. In the papular variety the process is mainly limited, primarily at least, to the follicles. The exudation is confined to small circumscribed areas and gives rise to papular elevations. In the vesicular variety fluid exudation occurs in the upper strata of the corium and in the rete, and the formation of vesicles results. The contents of the vesicles consist of a clear liquid containing a few rete-cells and later some pus-corpuscles. In the pustular form the process is more intense in character, and the cell-emigration and multiplication increased. In the chronic forms of the disease the infiltration involves the deeper parts of the corium and even the subcutaneous tissues, which, in addition to the new connective-tissue formation sometimes taking place, gives rise to considerable thickening. The papillæ are enlarged, and at times are considerably hypertrophied, as exemplified by the so-called verrucous eczema. The exudation and cell-infiltration are especially marked along the blood-vessels. In squamous eczema the blood-vessels of the corium and papillæ are dilated, and these parts infiltrated with round cells and changed connective-tissue corpuscles. Pigmentation may take place in the deeper layers of the rete and in the corium, especially about the vessels. The pathological process in eczema seems to have its starting-point in disturbance of the capillary circulation, the origin and nature of which it is difficult to determine.

DIAGNOSIS.—It must be remembered that the disease is capable of appearing in a multitude of forms, some of which are so dissimilar in their clinical features as sometimes to occasion embarrassment in the diagnosis. No other disease except syphilis manifests itself in such a variety of forms. In all cases where the lesions are varied or where they are ill defined the eruption should be viewed as a whole, when the characters of the process will usually be apparent. Thus a variable amount of infiltration, with swelling or thickening, is almost always present, the skin being more or less red and inflammatory. Moisture or positive discharge, with slight or extensive crusting, is a frequent though by no means a constant symptom, and when present is characteristic. Itching is experienced in almost all cases, and is generally a marked symptom. In some cases heat and burning are complained of.

Cases are occasionally met with in which the eruption bears some resemblance to erysipelas and scarlatina, but the absence of systemic symptoms in eczema would prevent an error in diagnosis. Papular eczema may at times simulate the papular manifestations of urticaria, especially in children, but in ordinary cases there is no likelihood of confounding the diseases. Herpes zoster in its early stage may bear a resemblance to a patch of vesicular or papular eczema, but the grouping of the lesions and the burning or pain in the former disease will generally prove sufficient to distinguish them. Seborrhœa, especially as it occurs upon the scalp, may be mistaken for squamous eczema, but in seborrhœa the scales are greasy, containing more or less sebaceous matter, and the distribution of the disease is usually more uniform than in eczema ; and, finally, in the latter affection the skin is reddish, inflamed, often thickened, and usually itchy.

Psoriasis and squamous eczema frequently simulate each other, and in some instances the resemblance is so close that error in diagnosis may readily occur. Both diseases are common, and are liable to invade all regions. In eczema the patches usually fade away into the healthy skin, whereas in psoriasis their margins are generally sharply defined. In eczema the scales are usually scanty, thin and small; in psoriasis they are abundant, whitish or silvery, large and imbricated. These points, taken in connection with the history of the case, will serve to aid in the diagnosis.

The rare disease pityriasis rubra may be confounded with squamous eczema, but the peculiar abundant, thin, papery scaling of this affection is not met with in eczema. Sometimes papular eczema resembles lichen ruber, but with attention to the characteristics of the lesions in the latter disease the diagnosis in most cases offers no difficulty. The resemblance of tinea circinata to eczema in some cases is to be borne in mind, but in the latter disease there is wanting the tendency to circular and marginate forms so characteristic of the parasitic disease. The microscope should always be employed in doubtful cases. Both tinea sycosis and sycosis may be confounded with eczema of the hairy portion of the face, but the follicular involvement in the former affections is the diagnostic point to be remembered. Scabies in its early stages often looks much like papular, vesicular, or pustular eczema, and care should in all cases be taken to make a correct diagnosis. The history of scabies, the regions involved, the distribution and multiformity of the lesions, and the presence of the parasite, as shown by the extraction of the mite or by the burrow, are all points to be duly inquired into. Eczema seldom simulates syphilis. They are most likely to be confounded one with the other when occurring in chronic forms about the scalp and the hands and feet.

PROGNOSIS.—Under favorable circumstances eczema is always a curable disease. In the prognosis of the affection as regards the probable length of time required to remove it an opinion should be guardedly expressed. It depends upon the extent of the disease, the duration, the attention the patient can give to the treatment, and the ease with which the exciting causes can be removed. Where the disease is the result of nervous prostration, as seen in those who have been mentally overworked from whatever cause, the cure will take place slowly, and many relapses will probably occur before positive recovery sets in.

Where the exciting causes cannot be entirely removed recovery is slow, and a complete or permanent cure is sometimes impossible. Thus in eczema about the hands in those who are obliged to wet or wash the parts frequently, to handle chemicals, dyestuffs, or otherwise expose the parts to the action of deleterious substances, a cure of the affection is exceedingly difficult. The same may be said in regard to eczema of the scrotum and neighboring regions, where the natural heat and moisture are constant and exciting, and to a certain extent irremovable, causes. In eczema of the lower limbs depending upon a condition of varicose veins the disease is obstinate. On the other hand, there are many cases of acute eczema met with which run a rapid course and end favorably. Eczema of the face, lips, and other exposed parts is, for evident reasons, apt to prove rebellious. In each case, then, all these points are to be taken into consideration in rendering an opinion upon the probable duration and termination of the disease.

TREATMENT.—Thete is no other disease of the skin which requires so thorough a knowledge of general medicine for its successful management as does eczema. The exciting cause of the affection is to be ascertained and to be properly treated. It is the specialist who has as the groundwork a comprehensive knowledge of general medicine who is best able to cope successfully with the disease under consideration. In the management of eczema both constitutional and local treatment will be necessary. It is true that some authorities depend upon external applications alone, but, judging from our own experience, a combination of external and internal treatment promises decidedly better results. In those cases in which the exciting cause has disappeared and the eczema persists from habit, as it were, the simplest local treatment may bring about a cure. But these are, unfortunately, exceptional instances. In almost all cases external treatment is indispensable.

Constitutional Treatment.—There are no specific remedies for eczema. Arsenic, it is true, acts in some cases admirably, but these instances are rather exceptional; the proportion of cases in which it may be prescribed with the hope of advantage is not very large. It not infrequently proves positively injurious. It is in the dry, scaly, and papular forms of the disease, and especially those in which the inflammation is of a low grade, that it acts most happily. The drug is to be given in sufficiently large doses to obtain slight evidences of its physiological action; toxic effects are to be avoided. It should never be given in acute cases. In small doses (one or two minims of Fowler's solution) arsenic is frequently of value as a tonic, acting then in the same manner as other tonics. When the physiological effects of the drug are desirable the dose should be gauged accordingly, beginning with two or three minims three times daily, and increasing gradually up to five or six or even more minims; as soon as the action of the drug becomes evident, as shown by a slight conjunctival injection and puffiness about the eyelids, the dose should be diminished and its administration continued for an extended period.

In the management of eczema attention should be given to the subject of diet. The food should be nutritious but plain, avoiding such articles as pork, salted meats, pastry, cabbage, gravies and sauces, pickles, cheese, condiments, beer and wine, etc. In anæmic and debilitated individuals a moderate use of stimulants may prove useful. Fresh air and exercise are often of aid in the treatment. The various remedies to be employed internally will depend upon the cause or causes which have brought about the attack. In robust persons and those of full habit laxatives or purgatives will prove of positive service. A useful formula for such cases, and also for those in whom constipation is present, is the following:

    ℞. Magnesii sulphatis,   ʒiss;
        Potassii bitartratis,   ʒiv;
        Sulphuris præcip.,   ʒij;
        Glyccrinæ,   fʒij;
        Aquæ menthæ pip., q. s. ad fʒiv.

M.—S. A tablespoonful in a tumblerful of water a half hour before breakfast. If this dose of the mixture fails to produce one or two free evacuations daily, then as much as double the quantity may be taken or a dose may be taken morning and evening. In many cases an aperient combined with a tonic is indicated. This is the case in those who are dyspeptic and debilitated, and in whom there is more or less constipation present. The following formula is available for such cases:

℞. Magnesii sulphatis, ℥iss;
Ferri sulphatis, gr. iv;
Acidi sulphurici dilut., f℥ij;
Aquæ menthæ pip., f℥iv.

M.—S. A tablespoonful in a tumblerful of water a half hour before the morning meal. In some cases the acid is contraindicated, and then the mixture may be prescribed without this ingredient. Although this formula is found to agree with most individuals, there are some who are either not able to take it or in whom it is found to aggravate the dyspepsia or to cause more or less gastric disturbance. In these cases the following formula has proved of value:

℞. Ext. cascaræ sagradæ fl., f℥iv;
Acidi muriatici dilut., f℥ij;
Elix. calisayæ, f℥iij ℥ij.

M.—S. A teaspoonful in a large wineglassful of water before or after meals. The laxative effect of the mixture is more marked when it is taken twenty or thirty minutes before meals. In some cases it will be found necessary to increase the proportion of the cascara sagrada, while, on the other hand, not infrequently a less quantity may be sufficiently active. In acute eczema laxatives, especially the salines, are of great service. The various mineral-spring waters may also be mentioned as useful. Of these Friedrichshall, Hunyadi Janos, the Hathorn and Geyser Springs of Saratoga, are the most serviceable. A tonic aperient where there is only slight constipation is the following:

℞. Sodii phosphatis, ℥vj;
Acidi phosphorici dilut., f℥iij;
Syr. zingiberis, f℥j;
Infus. gentianæ comp., f℥iiss.

M.—S. A tablespoonful in a wineglassful of water three times daily.

The following aperient mixtures may be prescribed for children:

℞. Syr. rhei aromat.,
Olei ricini, āā. f℥ij.

M.—S. A teaspoonful two or three times daily, according to the effect.

℞. Ext. cascaræ sagradæ fl., f℥ij;
Syr. aurantii cort., f℥vj.

M.—S. A teaspoonful in water at bed-time.

Occasional laxative doses of calomel are often valuable both in children and adults. Dyspepsia, if present, should receive appropriate treatment. The bitter tonics, mineral acids, alkalies, and the various artificial aids to digestion may be employed as seem indicated. Where malaria is suspected, full doses of quinine and small doses of arsenic should be prescribed. In these cases, as also in those in which there may be anæmia or chlorosis, the preparations of iron may be prescribed. If a gouty diathesis appears to be at the foundation of the attack, purgatives, the alkalies, and colchicum are to be advised. In these cases, if of an acute or subacute type, the following formula is serviceable:

℞. Potassii acetatis, ℥j;
Liquor. potassæ, f℥vj;
Aquæ menthæ pip., f℥iij ℥ij.

M.—S. A teaspoonful in a half gobletful of water an hour before meals.
In cases of a chronic type the following may sometimes prove of benefit:

> ℞. Potassii iodidi, ℨv gr .xx ;
> Liquor. potassii arsenit., f℥iss ;
> Liquor. potassæ, f℥vss ;
> Aquæ, f℥iij.

M.—S. A teaspoonful in a half gobletful of water after meals.

In some gouty and rheumatic cases wine of colchicum may be added to the above two prescriptions with advantage. Where a scrofulous tendency exists cod-liver oil is a valuable remedy ; also in all cases of impaired nutrition, in moderate doses, long continued, it will often prove useful, especially in children.

External Treatment.—The local treatment of eczema is based upon the pathological conditions present. The acute disease requires entirely different management from that employed in chronic cases. The stage of the disease and the amount of skin involved, whether in the form of a circumscribed patch or as a diffuse eruption, are points to be taken into consideration in the selection of a remedy and the mode of its application. The several varieties, the erythematous, papular, vesicular, pustular and squamous, and also the secondary forms rubrum, fissum and verrucosum, all demand applications appropriate to the condition. In acute erythematous or vesicular eczema caution is to be exercised in the selection of remedies. Only the milder applications, as a rule, are tolerated. That which will agree with one may not agree with another. It is advisable to try the remedy upon a small portion of the diseased surface to see if it is acceptable to the skin. In these varieties also soap and water should, as much as possible, be avoided.

For the average case, especially of the vesicular variety, the most successful plan of treatment is with lotio nigra and oxide-of-zinc ointment. The lotion is to be dabbed on by means of a sponge or cloth every three or four hours, ten or fifteen minutes at a time ; as soon as dry a small quantity of oxide-of-zinc ointment is to be gently smeared over. In many instances this method furnishes immediate relief to the itching, and under its use the inflammation is soon relieved. Powdering the surface with dusting-powder will sometimes afford ease, starch or lycopodium powder, either alone or together, equal parts, being useful. Subnitrate of bismuth is also of value, proving a more stimulating powder. In some cases a half drachm of finely-powdered camphor to the ounce may be advantageously added to one or another of the simple powders. Powdered Venetian talc is also sometimes useful alone or in combination with starch, a drachm or two of the former to the ounce of the latter. Dusting-powders should in all cases be used freely and often, their chief object being to afford protection to the inflamed surfaces.

Another lotion frequently employed in acute cases of vesicular eczema with free discharge, especially in cases where there is œdema or where the skin is irritable, is one containing calamine and zinc oxide ; for example,

> ℞. Pulv. zinci oxidi,
> Pulv. calaminæ, āā. ℨiss ;
> Glycerinæ, f℥j ;
> Liq. calcis,
> Aquæ rosæ, āā. f℥iij.

The following may also be mentioned as being useful in similar cases :

℞. Pulv. calaminæ,
Cretæ præparatæ, āā. ʒj ;
Acidi hydrocyanici dilut., fʒss ;
Glycerinæ, fʒij ;
Aquæ,
Liq. calcis, āā. f℥iij.

These lotions, as will be seen, contain more or less insoluble powder, and they are to be applied in the same manner as advised when speaking of the use of black wash.

There are other lotions which are often of service. Carbolic acid, one or two drachms to the pint of water, to which may be added a like quantity of glycerin, is in many cases of value, especially in those in which itching is marked. A saturated solution of boric acid, with or without the addition of glycerin, may also be employed in these cases, especially in erythematous eczema. It is one of the most useful of the milder remedies. In this variety, particularly when confined to the flexures, constituting eczema intertrigo, the following formula containing acetate of lead may be prescribed in some cases with benefit :

℞. Plumbi acetatis, ʒss ;
Acidi acetici dil., fʒij ;
Glycerinæ, fʒiv ;
Aquæ, q. s. ad f℥vi. M.

In those cases where lotions do not seem to act happily a mild ointment of salicylated suet (2 or 3 per cent. strength) will often relieve the condition. The fluid extract of grindelia robusta, one or two drachms to six ounces of water, seems to suit some cases, but it should be applied cautiously, as in some instances it tends to aggravate. Weak alkaline lotions, a drachm of the bicarbonate of sodium or borate of sodium to the pint of water, and a drachm of the solution of subacetate of lead to the pint, may be also mentioned. Tarry lotions of weak strength are sometimes useful. A drachm of the liquor carbonis detergens to two or four ounces of water, or the liquor picis alkalinus, a drachm to the half pint of water, may afford relief. The former tarry preparation is made by mixing together nine ounces of tincture of soap-bark 1 and four ounces of coal-tar, allowing to digest for eight days and filtering. The formula for the liquor picis alkalinus, the other tarry preparation referred to, is as follows :

℞. Potassæ, ʒj ;
Picis liquidæ, ʒij ;
Aquæ, f℥v. M.

A lotion made up of two drachms of zinc oxide, two drachms of glycerin, six drachms of lead-water, and three ounces of infusion of tar is sometimes valuable in the erythematous form.

As a rule, ointments are not so well borne in acute eczema as lotions, but as soon as the more acute symptoms have subsided, and in some instances even during the acute stage, they may be used with benefit. The oxide-of-zinc ointment is well known, and is one of the most soothing ; sometimes it is well to reduce the proportion of zinc oxide.

---

[1] Tincture of soap-bark is made by digesting for eight days one pound of soap-bark in one gallon of alcohol.

Oleate of zinc, in the proportion of one or two drachms to the ounce of vaseline or lard, is somewhat similar to oxide-of-zinc ointment, but is more astringent and stimulating. The oleate of bismuth, pure or with an equal part of vaseline or other fatty base, is also at times of service. The same may be said of the oleate of lead melted with an equal part of lard or vaseline, in this form constituting a soothing and astringent application similar to the well-known diachlyon ointment. The latter ointment, if properly prepared, is in the subacute stage often exceedingly valuable. The same objection to this holds as with the different oleates named— that is, the difficulty of securing properly-made preparations. Many are vaunted as such, but our experience is that good preparations are exceptional, and those furnished, instead of acting as expected, often give rise to irritation or marked aggravation. For the acute and subacute stages of the disease the ordinary cold-cream ointment may be in some cases advantageously prescribed. An ointment of equal parts of diachylon plaster and one of the petroleum ointments, as vaseline, constitutes an elegant preparation, useful when a mild, soothing application is called for.

A paste made up as follows may also be recommended for the subacute condition, and at times suits even during the active inflammatory stage:

> ℞. Pulv. zinci oxidi, ʒss ;
> Mucilag. acaciæ,
> Glycerinæ,   āā. fʒj.

M.—S. Apply with a brush two or three times daily. To this formula, if there is considerable itching present, carbolic acid or salicylic acid in the proportion of 2 per cent. may be added. Glycerite of tannic acid sometimes proves of value, especially in the erythematous varieties of the disease, more particularly when occurring about the face. In like cases glycerite of subacetate of lead may be prescribed. The following is Squire's formula: Acetate of lead, 5 parts ; litharge, 3½ parts ; glycerin, 20 parts, by weight. Mix and expose to a temperature of 350° F., and filter through a hot-water funnel. The fluid resultant contains 129 grains of the subacetate of lead to the ounce, which is to be diluted with from two to six parts of glycerin or with water. This preparation may sometimes be used with benefit in chronic eczema of the legs applied on strips bound on with a bandage. In these cases the following paste, suggested by Unna, proves useful :

> ℞. Kaolini,
> Ol. lini,   āā. ʒvj.
> Zinei oxidi,   ʒss ;
> Liq. plumbi subacetat.,   fʒss.   M.

This is painted on and allowed to dry, and then bandaged for twenty-four hours. In some skins. however, glycerin invariably irritates.

In the papular form the tarry lotions named and carbolic-acid lotion are of most benefit. These cases are from the beginning inclined to take on the chronic type, and the more stimulating applications are well borne. Thymol, one or two grains to the ounce of alcohol and water, is also useful.

In chronic eczema, and, in fact, in all cases of eczema, after the active inflammatory symptoms have more or less subsided—which usually takes place soon after the beginning of the outbreak—stimulating applications are to be resorted to. In fact, the dividing-line between acute and chronic eczema is difficult to define. The products of the disease, be they crusts or scales, must be removed in order that the remedial application may be brought in contact with the diseased surface. Thoroughly saturating the part with oil, and subsequently washing with warm water and soap, will usually suffice to remove the accumulations. On the non-hairy surface a bland oil, lard, or a non-irritating ointment thickly spread on the parts, will soon be followed by softening and removal of the crusts or scales. If these more simple measures are not sufficient, washings with sapo viridis and warm water are to be advised for this purpose, immediately afterward applying a mild unguent. On the scalp, instead of the pure green soap, the spiritus saponatus kalinus is more satisfactory. In patches which are covered with thickened epidermic masses, as in eczema of the palms, strong applications are necessary to remove the accumulations. For this purpose green soap or salicylic acid may be used. Of these, salicylic acid is in most cases to be preferred. It may be applied as an alcoholic solution, 5 or 8 per cent. strength, or in ointment form, fifteen to forty grains to the ounce.

After a removal of the products of the disease the remedies proper are to be applied. The various ointments already named for the treatment of the acute and subacute types may also be employed in the chronic cases. In some instances they may prove sufficient, but in the majority it will be found necessary to have immediate recourse to the stronger ointments and lotions. In small patches washing the parts with green soap and hot water and following with unguentum diachlyi or a similar ointment will be sufficient.

The mercurials are of great value in the treatment of eczema, used either alone or in combination with various other remedies. An ointment of the mild chloride of mercury, twenty to eighty grains to the ounce, is valuable in many cases. Citrine ointment, weakened, and ammoniated mercury, in the same proportion as calomel, are also well-known and very useful preparations, likewise acceptable in many cases. To these ointments tar may often be advantageously added, in the strength of one or two drachms to the ounce. Carbolic acid in ointment, ten to twenty grains to the ounce, may also be mentioned as often proving serviceable. A compound ointment, prized in the Blackfriars Hospital for Skin Diseases, London, is composed of acetate of lead, ten grains; oxide of zinc, twenty grains; calomel, ten grains; citrine ointment, twenty grains; palm oil, half an ounce; benzoated lard, enough to make one ounce. Another mildly stimulating preparation is composed of bisulphide of mercury and red precipitate, each six grains; lard, one ounce.

Tarry preparations constitute the most generally efficacious applications in the treatment of all forms of chronic eczema, where this remedy is at all tolerated by the skin, especially in the squamous variety of the disease. A good formula, and one that is often of service even in the subacute variety, is the following:

    ℞. Picis liquidæ,
      Zinci oxidi, āā. ʒj ;
      Ugt. aquæ rosæ, ʒvj.

M. Ft. ugt.—This is to be gently but thoroughly rubbed into the dis-cased skin. There are three preparations of tar that may be interchange-ably employed : these are the ordinary pix liquida, oleum cadium, and oleum rusci. The oleum rusci is the least unpleasant. They may be employed in the strength of 10 to 50 per cent., either in ointment form or with alcohol. If used upon the scalp, the lotion form, with alcohol, is to be preferred. In the use of a tarry preparation, to be efficient it is to be gently but thoroughly worked into the patches, so that it permeates the skin ; the excess may be wiped off. The liquor picis alkalinus, already mentioned in speaking of the treatment of acute eczema, may be used either in the form of an ointment, in the strength of one or two drachms to the ounce, or in the form of a lotion, in the strength of two to eight drachms to the half pint. This tarry preparation may even be employed in full strength to small and thickened patches, applying care-fully and using no other treatment, or following the application immedi-ately with a simple or tarry ointment. In cases of verrucous eczema or in patches of thickened papular or squamous eczema, used in the manner described, it is often curative. It is a strong remedy, and is to be employed with caution. The liquor carbonis detergens, in the strength of one or two drachms to the ounce of water, is also valuable in these chronic cases. It is a safe plan in the use of these tarry preparations to begin with a mild strength and then increase if advisable. An equally efficacious formula for the thick, leathery patches of chronic eczema is the following :

> ℞. Saponis viridis,
>   Pieis liquidæ,
>   Alcoholis,   āā. ʒiv.

M.—S. Rub in twice daily. There is another mildly alkaline tarry prep-aration, the goudron de Guyot, somewhat similar in composition to the liquor picis alkalinus, which at times seems to suit when the other tarry applications fail to benefit.

In the treatment of eczema rubrum of the legs Hebra was in the habit of employing the following method : A small quantity of the green soap is to be rubbed into the parts with a flannel rag, employing considerable friction, until all the soap has apparently disappeared ; then warm or hot water is to be added and rubbed in in the same manner, an abundant lather being the result. The parts after being rubbed for from five to fifteen minutes, according to the effect, are to be thoroughly rinsed off with simple warm water, and a mild ointment, spread upon cloths, applied. The best ointment for this purpose is the unguentum diachyli, but any mild ointment may be employed. This treatment is to be repeated once or twice daily. In most cases improvement sets in after a few applications. It is an excellent method of treatment, and can be recommended. It requires considerable time and trouble, however, and is therefore not suitable in all cases, for unless the details are properly carried out it may fail.

Salicylic acid is another remedy that is often useful. In thick, leathery patches, an ointment of the strength of thirty to sixty grains to the ounce, applied on cloths or rubbed in, will often produce marked benefit. In the form of a paste it may be used in many cases of subacute and chronic eczema with good effects :

℞. Acidi salicylici, gr. xx ;
Ugt. petrolei, ʒiv ;
Amyli,
Zinci oxidi, āā. ʒij.

M.—S. Apply once or twice daily. If it is used upon the scalp, it should
be used with petroleum ointment or lard, the starch and zinc oxide being
omitted. Boric acid in the form of a saturated solution, as advised in
acute eczema, or in ointment of the strength of a drachm to the ounce,
will prove useful in some instances. Sulphur in the form of ointment
may also be mentioned as being frequently of value in cases of chronic
eczema, especially of the leg. In some cases of subacute and chronic
eczema the lotion containing zinc sulphate and potassium sulphide,
diluted, mentioned in acne, will be found serviceable. In circumscribed
and chronic patches blistering with cantharides is sometimes advisable.
In these cases tincture of iodine is also employed. In thickened patches,
rebellious to the usual remedies, chrysarobin or pyrogallic acid, as used
in psoriasis, may sometimes be applied with benefit.

Mention may here be made of vulcanized india-rubber, used in the
form of bandages, the method proving of most value in eczema of the
lower extremities, especially in those cases which are due to a condition
of varicose veins. It is not suitable in all cases, as in some the disease
is aggravated. Reference may also be made to the use of the so-called
gelatin dressing. The medicinal substance is incorporated with the gelatin basis, which is made by melting together over a water-bath two parts
of water and one of gelatin ; and when the application is made the gelatin
compound is melted over a water-bath and applied while in the fluid
condition ; it rapidly hardens and forms an impermeable coating to the
diseased part. The dressing is liable to crack, to avoid which, in a
measure, a small quantity of glycerin is mixed with the gelatin and water.
Another plan is, after the dressing has dried, to brush over the surface
a few minims of glycerin. It has, however, cleanliness in its favor, and
it is undoubtedly of service in many instances. A good basis formula
for the gelatin dressing consists of eight parts of water, four of gelatin,
and one of glycerin.

Another form of fixed dressing for scaly patches is with collodion.
This may often be made use of when tar is employed, the addition of
one or two drachms of pix liquida or one of the tar oils to enough collodion to make an ounce. Such a preparation may be applied to dry
and scaly patches, and constitutes an excellent method of application ;
but tar so applied is not as efficient as when used in solution or in
ointment. The gutta-percha and muslin plasters[1] constitute excellent
methods of applying remedies ; they are cleanly, easily applied, comfortable to the patient, and efficacious.

Prurigo.

Prurigo is a chronic inflammatory disease, characterized by discrete
pinhead- to small pea-sized, solid, firmly-seated papules, slightly raised,

[1] These plasters were devised by Unna, and are made by Beiersdorf, an apothecary of
Hamburg, Germany. The muslin plasters consist of muslin incorporated with a layer
of stiff ointment; the gutta-percha plasters consist of muslin faced with a thin layer of
india-rubber, the medication being spread upon the rubber coating.

of a pale-red color, accompanied by general thickening of the skin and itching. The disease manifests itself by the development of small firm elevations, which at first are scarcely perceptible; but they may be distinctly felt by passing the hand over the surface. Later, they may be seen as slightly-raised papules, varying in size from a milletseed to a small pea, of the same color as the surrounding skin or of a pinkish hue, and to the touch are found to be well-defined inflammatory deposits. The lesions are discrete, may be present in great numbers and in close proximity, and show no tendency to group, being irregularly distributed. There is rarely distinct scale-formation, but the papules are usually covered with roughened, dry epidermis, and are frequently perforated with hairs.

Itching, usually intense, is a constant symptom, giving rise to scratching, and as a consequence many of the lesions are covered with blood-crusts and the skin is markedly excoriated. In course of time, either as a symptom of the disease or as a result of the scratching and consequent hyperæmia, or more probably resulting from both, the skin becomes thickened and the surface harsh or rough. The extensor surfaces of the legs, especially the tibial regions, and later the forearms and arms, and in marked cases the trunk, are the regions usually invaded. The palms and soles escape, and only in rare cases is the head involved. As a result of strong local remedies or scratching, or of both, a simple dermatitis or an eczema may develop as a complication. In consequence also of the cutaneous irritation the lymphatic glands, especially the inguinal, may become engorged—prurigo buboes (Hebra).

The causes of the disease are obscure. It is common in Austria, and is occasionally met with in France and England, but it is almost unknown in the United States. It is met with, as Hebra states, almost exclusively in poor subjects and those ill nourished in childhood, and so most often in foundlings and beggars' children. The disease is not hereditary. It usually develops, however, in early childhood, and is worse in winter than in summer. Anatomically, the lesions differ but slightly from those of papular eczema. The papillæ and rete show a moderate amount of cell and serous infiltration. Later, as a result of the chronic inflammation, thickening, increased cell-infiltration, atrophied sweat and sebaceous glands, and pigmentation are observed. The process, according to various authorities, begins in the papillary layer.

Prurigo has been, and is still, erroneously confounded with pruritus and pediculosis, diseases which have nothing in common with that affection except the itching and resulting excoriations—symptoms, as is well known, common to many diseases. In pruritus there is no structural change in the skin except that produced by scratching, a point of difference that is diagnostic. The thickening of the skin and the harsh, rough surface encountered in prurigo are absent in pruritus. The latter disease is usually one of middle or old age; prurigo, on the other hand, dates from childhood. In pediculosis the lesions, punctate or papular in form, are consequent upon the wounds of the pediculus, and are most numerous about the trunk, especially the shoulders and hips. Between simple eczema and prurigo the diagnosis is not difficult. It is to be remembered, however, that eczema may exist as a complication, in which case, after its disappearance, the characteristics of prurigo become evident.

Severe cases are said to be incurable, according to Hebra and others, but in the milder forms of the disease a cure may be effected. Good food, hygiene, and tonic remedies, and systematic local treatment similar to that generally employed in chronic eczema, are the measures indicated. Naphthol, in the form of a 5 per cent. ointment for adults and a $\frac{1}{2}$ per cent. ointment for children, has been found by Kaposi to be of value.

Acne.

Acne, or acne vulgaris, is an inflammatory, usually chronic, disease of the sebaceous glands, characterized by papules, tubercles or pustules, or a combination of these lesions, occurring for the most part about the face. There are several so-called varieties of acne, although examples of all these forms may be seen usually in an individual case, and instances in which all the lesions are of the same type or character are practically not encountered. Other disorders of the sebaceous glands, as comedo and seborrhœa, are often seen associated with this affection. In fact, hypersecretion or retention of the sebaceous matter is the exciting cause of the inflammation.

If the retained sebaceous mass causes a moderate degree of hyperæmia or inflammation, a slight elevation with a central whitish or blackish point results, constituting the lesion of acne punctata. If the inflammation is of a higher grade, the elevation is more marked, reddened, and papular, the lesion being known as acne papulosa. If the process is still more active, the central portion of the papule suppurates and acne pustulosa results. The surrounding inflammation of this form is often of a violent type, and the lesion may be situated upon a hard and inflamed base, and then is designated acne indurata. In some cases of acne the disappearing lesions leave more or less atrophy about the gland-ducts in the form of pit-like depressions—acne atrophica. On the other hand, at times there results connective-tissue hypertrophy about the glands—acne hypertrophica. In strumous, cachectic individuals the lesions, which are usually pustular in type, or at times furuncular, almost of the nature of dermic abscesses, may be more general in distribution, and are, moreover, usually of a more sluggish character, constituting the so-called acne cachecticorum. The efflorescence which follows the prolonged ingestion of the iodides and bromides is usually of a more inflammatory type, the glands and follicles being sometimes seriously and irreparably involved. This form of acne, as well as that resulting from the external action of tar, characterized by the formation of all kinds of lesions with a minute central blackish deposit of tar and more or less inflammation of the surrounding skin, constitutes acne artificialis.

The most common form of acne is that in which the pustule predominates. The lesions, in all the varieties, are usually confined to the face, the forehead, cheeks, and chin being favorite localities; not infrequently, however, the eruption also involves the shoulders and upper part of the back. They are irregularly distributed and tend to appear in crops. Sometimes the face and shoulders are spared, and the lesions, being confined to the back, extend as far down as the lumbar region or even to the thighs. In these cases the lesions are usually of a papulo-pustular character and are sluggish in their evolution. As a rule, an acne papule or pustule runs an acute course, disappearing in the course of one or two weeks, and a new lesion appearing at another point to supply its place. The disease is essentially chronic, in the sense that the parts are never or seldom free, new lesions forming and old ones disappearing from time to time, in some cases indefinitely. As a rule, there are no subjective symptoms, but in some markedly inflammatory cases the lesions are painful; in other exceptional instances there is slight itching.

The disease is common about the age of puberty, and occurs in both sexes. Chronic derangement of the digestive apparatus is a frequent factor. Those of a light complexion are more liable to its development, while menstrual difficulties, chlorosis, scrofulosis, and general debility may all predispose to the disease. Medicinal substances, such as the iodides and bromides, and tar externally, are also prone to produce acne-form lesions. The retention of the secretion within the sebaceous gland is the first step in the formation of an acne lesion, and its presence—or it may be its decomposition—gives rise to inflammation, which usually involves the gland-structure and the surrounding tissue. Primarily, it is a folliculitis, the tissue immediately about the follicle subsequently becoming involved, constituting a perifolliculitis. As a result of this latter process, or from inflammation and changes within the gland without much surrounding inflammation, the destruction of the sebaceous follicles may ensue. The hair-follicles at times are also involved in the process. The degree of inflammation determines the character of the lesion; if mild in character, the simple papule or pustule results; if of a severe grade, the lesion of the indurated and hypertrophied forms follows.

Acne resembles at times the papular and pustular syphiloderms. In syphilis the distribution of the eruption, the history of the case, the color, the duration of the individual lesions, the tendency of the papules or pustules to group, and usually the presence of other evidence of the disease, will serve to distinguish it from acne. Tar acne may be recognized by the history, the black points at the follicular openings, and usually evidence of the presence of tar about the patient. Acne resulting from the ingestion of the bromides and iodides is almost always of an acute and markedly inflammatory type, the lesions being scattered over the general surface, and are usually larger and more virulent in character than those of acne vulgaris. From acne rosacea it may be known by the characters referred to in speaking of that disease.

TREATMENT.—Cases of acne vary considerably as to their course and curability. There is in almost every case a natural inclination toward disappearance of the eruption at the age of twenty or thirty. Although the lesions are at any age of the patient generally easily removable by treatment, relapses are the rule; but the older the patient the less probability is there of a recurrence. Even in young subjects, however, the cure may be permanent, depending upon the ability to discover and remove the cause. The disease requires both constitutional and local treatment. For the removal of the existing eruption local applications alone are usually sufficient, but the disposition to the development of new lesions in most cases yields only to appropriate internal treatment.

Each case of acne for its successful management demands careful investigation with a view of discovering the etiological factors. If these can be ascertained and removed, a successful result is assured. As already intimated, disorders of digestion play a most important part in the etiology of this disease, and in a large proportion of cases remedies appropriate to such conditions are required. The diet is to be strictly regulated : all indigestible articles of food, such as pork, salt meats, pastry, cheese, pickles, etc., should be interdicted. If constipation exists, laxatives are to be prescribed. As a rule, salines are more serviceable than vegetable preparations for plethoric individuals, while for others the latter, especially for long-continued administration, are to be preferred. A change from one to the other is often advisable. The dose should be sufficient to produce a free evacuation daily. An excellent tonic aperient mixture is the following :

R̥. Magnesii sulphatis, ℥iss ;
Ferri sulphatis, gr. viij ;
Acidi sulphurici diluti, f℥ij ;
Aquæ menthæ piperitæ, f℥iij ʒvi.

M.—S. A tablespoonful in a tumblerful of water a half hour before breakfast. The tonic effect of such a mixture is best obtained by prescribing one or two teaspoonfuls in a large wineglassful of water before each meal : as a rule, however, when thus given its laxative property is not so well marked. The mint-water may be replaced by a bitter infusion, such as quassia, but the mixture, unpalatable at the best, is not improved by such a substitution. In some cases the acid in the above mixture is contraindicated, and the following, also a valuable formula, may be prescribed :

R̥. Magnesii sulphatis, ℥iss ;
Potassii bitart., ʒiv ;
Sulphuris præcip., ʒij ;
Glycerinæ, f℥ij ;
Aquæ menthæ pip., f℥iv.

M.—S. Tablespoonful in a tumblerful of water a half hour before breakfast. Hunyadi Janos water, in the dose of a large wineglassful thirty or forty minutes before the morning meal, is a useful saline, and is not especially disagreeable. Friedrichshall water is an efficient laxative and cathartic, but has a nauseous taste and odor. The ordinary mixture of rhubarb and soda is of value, not only for its laxative effect, but also for its antacid property where such is indicated. The following formula, containing cascara sagrada, is of service :

R̥. Ext. cascaræ sagradæ fl., f℥iv ;
Acidi muriatici diluti, f℥ij ;
Tincturæ gentianæ comp., f℥iij ʒij.

M.—S. Teaspoonful in a large wineglassful of water before meals. At times this proportion of cascara sagrada is too large, and, on the other hand, in some cases it must be increased. A laxative pill, as the following, containing aloin, belladonna, and strychnia, may be given :

R̥. Aloin, gr. iij ;
Ext. belladonnæ, gr. ij ;
Strychniæ sulphatis, gr. ¼.

M. Ft. pilul. No. xv.—S. one or two at night. If there is torpor of the liver, an occasional dose of blue mass or calomel may be prescribed.

When there is flatulence or other symptoms of fermentative indigestion, a mixture such as the following will be found useful:

R. Sodii hyposulphitis,   ʒijss–ʒj ;
    Ext. nucis vomicæ fl.   fʒij ;
    Aquæ menthæ piperitæ,   fʒiv.

M.—S. Teaspoonful in a large wineglassful of water a half hour before meals. The hyposulphite of sodium contained in the mixture may have a laxative effect in addition to its antifermentative action.

If there is anæmia or chlorosis, a preparation of iron, combined with aloes if there is tendency to constipation, is to be prescribed, the wine of iron being one of the most eligible ferruginous preparations. Ergot in the dose of a half drachm of the fluid extract has been recommended in the acne of females, especially where it seems probable that uterine disturbance is the exciting cause. Possibly its effect is, as has been suggested, due to its action on the unstriped muscular fibres of the skin. After one or two weeks' administration it is apt to cause gastric disturbance and, directly or indirectly, vertiginous symptoms. Calx sulphurata in the dose of one-tenth to one-half grain every three or four hours is of value in some cases, usually proving of most service in the pustular type. In strumous individuals, and in those whose nutrition is below the average, cod-liver oil is a valuable remedy. In like cases glycerin in similar doses may be prescribed, although its action is not so certain.

Arsenic is of decided value in some cases, but proves powerless in others. The sluggish papular forms are often influenced favorably by its continued administration. The alterative effect of mercury is sometimes beneficial, corrosive sublimate in small doses being the most available preparation. Where the inflammation is of a high grade, potassium acetate and other alkalies may be prescribed, as in the following formula:

R. Potassii acetatis,   ʒv gr.xx ;
    Liq. potassæ,   fʒijss ;
    Liq. ammonii acetatis, fʒiij ʒv.

M.—Sig. Teaspoonful in a large wineglassful of water one hour before meals.

Local Treatment.—This is of great importance and is demanded in every case. In acute acne, rarely encountered, mildly astringent applications are to be advised. The disease, as generally met with, however, is of a subacute or chronic character, requiring stimulating measures. External treatment in these cases has for its object the production of hyperæmia and the removal of the superficial layers of the epidermis, thus stimulating the glands and circulation and assisting in the excretion of the sebaceous matter. For this purpose washing the parts energetically with sapo viridis and hot water every night, using a sponge or preferably a piece of flannel, may be advised. After the soap-washing the parts are to be sponged with hot water for several minutes, or the face held over a basin containing steaming hot water. Subsequently, the comedones are to be pressed out by means of pressure with the fingers, or, better, by a watch-key with rounded edges so as not to injure the skin. An application of a simple emollient, such as cold cream or vaseline, may then be made and allowed to remain on over night. This plan of treatment is to be repeated nightly or every other night.

In many simple cases of acne the above method of external treatment, combined with appropriate constitutional medication, will bring about marked improvement and sometimes permanent relief. In the majority of cases, however, a more stimulating plan of treatment is called for. In almost all cases the soap-washing, either with the sapo viridis or a milder soap, and the sponging with hot water, are to precede the nightly remedial applications. Among the external remedies for acne sulphur preparations stand first. Properly managed, they rarely fail to benefit, and often prove curative. Precipitated sulphur is the preparation generally employed, and in many cases the most suitable. It may be prescribed as a powder, in ointment, or in lotion. As a powder it may be applied pure or mixed with starch, and as an ointment the following formula can be recommended :

> ℞. Sulphuris præcipitati,   ʒiss ;
> Adipis benzoati,   ʒiv ;
> Ugt. petrolei,   ʒijss ;
> Olei rosæ,   gtt. iij.

M. Ft. ugt.—Sig. To be rubbed thoroughly into the skin at night. Or, instead of the precipitated sulphur in the above ointment, the sulphur hypochloride may be substituted. As a mild stimulant sulphur soap may often be ordered with advantage in connection with other remedies.

In sluggish, non-inflammatory cases the following may be used :

> ℞. Sulphuris præcipitati,
> Potassii carbonatis,
> Glycerinæ,
> Ugt. petrolei,   āā. ʒij.

M. Ft. ugt.—Sig. Apply at night, rubbing it into the skin. In the above formula the petroleum ointment may be replaced with the same quantity of alcohol. In the form of a lotion precipitated sulphur at times acts more decidedly than as an ointment. There are several useful formulæ which, as a rule, answer equally well, although in some cases differing in their beneficial effects. In the average case the following seems most certain in its results :

> ℞. Sulphuris præcipitati,   ʒij ;
> Pulv. camphoræ,   gr. xx ;
> Pulv. tragacanthæ,   gr. xxx ;
> Aquæ aurantii flor.,
> Liq. calcis,   āā. fʒij.

M.—S. Dab on with a mop or rag ; shake before using.

A similar mixture in the form of a paste may be made with equal parts of mucilage of acacia, glycerin, and sulphur, and is to be applied with a brush, being allowed to remain on the skin over night.

Another sulphur lotion is the following :

> ℞. Sulphuris præcipitati,   ʒij ;
> Glycerinæ,   fʒj ;
> Alcoholis,   fʒj ;
> Liq. calcis,   fʒij ;
> Aquæ aurantii flor.,   fʒj.

M.—Sig. Apply with a sponge or rag, shaking well before using.

The annexed is also a good stimulating lotion :

℞. Sulphuris præcipitati,   ʒij ;
  Ætheris,   f ʒiv ;
  Aquæ cologniensis,   f ʒiv ;
  Alcoholis,   f ʒiij.

M.—Sig. Shake well and dab on with a rag.

Potassium sulphide is a preparation of sulphur which often acts admirably in this disease. It may be employed as an ointment, or, preferably, as a lotion. An excellent formula containing the sulphide, which can be prescribed with advantage in many cases, is the following :

℞. Potassii sulphidi,
  Zinoi sulphatis,   *āā.* ʒj ;
  Aquæ rosæ,   f ʒiv.

M.—S. Apply with a sponge or rag. The resulting lotion from this mixture is a complex one, a double reaction taking place. The salts should be separately dissolved, and then mixed. If properly made, the lotion when shaken is of a milky color and free from odor ; upon standing the particles sink and form a white sediment, the liquid above being clear. If improperly prepared, as is often the case, it is of a yellowish tinge with a decided odor of the potassium sulphide, and has an entirely different effect. Vleminckx's solution,[1] perfumed with an essential oil, is often of service ; it is to be diluted with three to six parts of water and dabbed on every night, the strength gradually increased if necessary.

Another class of external remedies found of service in the treatment of this disease are the mercurials. They are not so valuable as the sulphur preparations. Corrosive sublimate, white precipitate, and calomel are the mercurials commonly used. If sulphur has been previously employed, several days should intervene and the parts be repeatedly cleansed before using a mercurial, otherwise the skin is darkened temporarily by the formation of the black sulphuret of mercury. Corrosive sublimate is prescribed in the form of a lotion, from one-half to two grains to the ounce of alcohol and water, or as in the following formula :

℞. Hydrargyri chloridi corros., gr. ij ;
  Zinci sulphatis,   gr. xv ;
  Alcoholis,   f ʒij ;
  Aquæ rosæ,   f ʒij.

M.—S. Apply with a rag. The zinc sulphate renders the lotion astringent, and is often a valuable addition. Ammoniated mercury, thirty to sixty grains to the ounce of benzoated lard or cold cream, will frequently prove serviceable. If the lesions are numerous and are seated close together, the application is to be made to the entire surface of the part ; on the other hand, if they are sparse, it may be made to the spots only. The same may be said also in regard to the sulphur preparations. A 5 or 10 per cent. ointment of oleate of mercury, rubbed thoroughly into sluggish and indurated lesions, will often shorten their course by promoting suppuration. In many cases puncturing the lesions with a sharp knife or scraping with a curette before applying the hot water will be of assistance in the treatment. In obstinate indurated lesions, in addition to puncturing the lesions, the apices may be treated with carbolic acid. The protiodide of mercury, in the strength of five to fifteen grains to the ounce of ointment, is well spoken of by some authorities ; it is to be used

---

[1] See treatment of Psoriasis for formula.

with care, as it is actively stimulant. In some cases rubbing energetically over the parts a mixture of sapo viridis and sulphur, adding enough hot water to make a lather, and allowing it to remain on over night, will, if repeated nightly until the skin becomes slightly inflamed and then followed subsequently by a mild ointment, produce a decided effect.

Acne Rosacea.

Acne rosacea, or rosacea, is a chronic, hyperæmic or inflammatory disease of the face, invading especially the nose and cheeks, characterized by redness, dilatation and enlargement of the blood-vessels, more or less acne, and hypertrophy. The course of the disease divides itself naturally into three stages. There is at first simply a hyperæmia, due to passive congestion. In young subjects the affection is seen in this stage, and rarely passes beyond it. In other cases, however, sooner or later, dilatation and enlargement of the vessels (telangiectasis) take place, and acne papules and pustules are scattered over the parts, constituting the second stage of the disease. This stage is frequently met with, and illustrates the acne rosacea usually seen. Exceptionally, however, the disease progresses, the vessels increase in calibre, the glands are enlarged, and there is more less hypertrophy of the connective tissue and the third stage is developed. The nose may become much enlarged, even lobulated, and in some portions pendulous (rhinophyma). The nose and its immediate neighborhood are the favorite localities for the development of acne rosacea, but it is not infrequently confined to the cheeks, and sometimes is localized upon the forehead, while all these parts are not infrequently affected simultaneously. As a rule, there are no marked subjective symptoms, although in some instances burning or a sense of fulness is complained of.

It is seen in both sexes, but is more frequent in males; in women it rarely, if ever, reaches the same degree of development as in men. It is most common about middle life. The causes are varied. Chronic stomachic and intestinal derangements, anæmia, and chlorosis are common causes. The habitual use of spirituous liquors is not infrequently a source of the disease. Long-continued exposure to excessive cold or heat is in some cases a causative agent. In women, menstrual and uterine difficulties are often the responsible factors; hence in this sex it is much more common at the climacteric period. When occurring in the young about the period of adolescence, it is frequently associated with seborrhœa, and rarely advances beyond a condition of hyperæmia. Pathologically, in the first stage of the disease there is simply a hyperæmia—a stasis; in the second, hypertrophy and dilatation of the vessels are superadded, together with acne and slight hypertrophy of the sebaceous glands; in the third stage there is, in addition, hypertrophy of the connective tissue of the corium.

Acne rosacea is to be distinguished from the tubercular syphiloderm, lupus vulgaris, and acne vulgaris, to which affections it at times bears resemblance. The tubercular syphiloderm is comparatively more rapid in its course; does not necessarily involve the sebaceous glands; has frequently as a consequence ulceration and crusting; is usually confined to a part of the nose; and is unaccompanied with dilatation and enlargement of the blood-vessels. Its history, the firmer consistence, and the more dusky color of the tubercles, and frequently the presence of other evidences of syphilis, are also points of difference. In lupus vulgaris the characteristic soft, yellowish-red papules, the absence of the hypertrophied blood-vessels, the degeneration, ulceration, and cicatricial-tissue formation, the more or less limited character of the eruption, and the history of the case, will serve to distinguish it. A simple case of acne vulgaris can scarcely be confounded with acne rosacea: in many cases, however, the dividing-line is far from being marked; in fact, the disease under consideration is often acne with hyperæmia and dilated blood-vessels superadded.

TREATMENT.—The affection may in all cases be more or less favorably influenced by treatment. The milder eases, although at times obstinate, are enrable; but when the disease has advanced to marked dilatation and hypertrophy of the blood-vessels and connective tissue, the prognosis is not so favorable. In all stages of the affection, however, as stated, a great deal can be accomplished by appropriate remedies. External and internal treatment are required in the majority of cases. The former usually proves the more valuable.

Concerning internal remedies, there is no drug that exerts a specific influence. The guide to constitutional treatment should be a study of the etiological causes of the disease. Constipation is frequently present, and hence laxatives, especially the salines, are indicated. Chlorosis in the female is often the predisposing cause, and such remedies as iron, quinine, and strychnia will be found useful. Dyspepsia is one of the most frequent causes, and treatment directed toward a removal of that condition will often be of considerable aid in curing the disease. Menstrual irregularities should be inquired into and the appropriate remedies employed.

There are mainly two classes of external remedies which are used in the treatment—namely, the mercurials and the sulphur preparations. The latter are by far the more valuable, precipitated and sublimed sulphur, the hypochloride of sulphur, and the sulphuret of potassium being the most serviceable. They are prescribed either in the form of lotions or ointments. The officinal sulphur ointment, an ointment of the precipitated sulphur and of the hypochloride of sulphur, of the strength of one or two drachms to the ounce, may be referred to as valuable applications. Sulphur may also be used as a dusting-powder or in the form of a paste, as in the following formula:

$$\text{R}. \quad \text{Mucilag. acaciæ,} \quad \text{f}\text{ʒij};$$
$$\text{Glycerinæ,} \quad \text{f}\text{ʒij}:$$
$$\text{Sulphur. præcip.,} \quad \text{ʒiij}.$$

M.—Sig. Use with a brush as a paint.

A lotion containing one to four drachms of precipitated sulphur, twenty or thirty grains of camphor, thirty to sixty grains of tragacanth, in two ounces each of lime-water and orange-flower water, or one of the same quantity of sulphur, two or three drachms of ether, and three and a half ounces of alcohol, will in many cases prove serviceable. A lotion of one or two drachms each of sulphide of potassium and sulphate of zinc, in four ounces of water, is one of great value.

Concerning the mercurials, corrosive sublimate, calomel, and white precipitate are in some cases of service. Corrosive sublimate is prescribed as a lotion of the strength of one-half to four grains to the ounce of water or water and alcohol. Calomel and white precipitate are prescribed in ointment, twenty grains to two drachms of either to the ounce, or they may be used in the form of a powder, full strength or weakened with starch powder, dusted over the surface.

To a great extent, the treatment of acne rosacea is the same as simple acne, and for other formulæ and for the method of applying the various remedies the reader is referred to that disease. When dilated blood-vessels are present, however, other measures, in addition to those advised above, are to be adopted. There are two methods of destroying the blood-vessels. One plan is by the knife, cutting across the vessels at several points or slitting their whole length, permitting them to bleed; subsequently cold water may be applied. The other method is by means of electrolysis, according to the procedure fully described in the treatment of hypertrichosis. If the vessel is long, inserting the needle at several points along its length will be necessary; if short, insertion at one or two points will suffice. While either of these methods will, if properly managed, destroy the vessels, neither will prevent the growth of new vessels. In those cases, however, in which the cause has long ceased to operate destruction of the existing vessels may not be followed by new growth. Excessive connective-tissue hypertrophy may require ablation by the knife.

Sycosis.

Sycosis (syn., sycosis non-parasitica, folliculitis barbæ) is a chronic inflammatory, non-contagious affection, involving the hair-follicles, appearing generally upon the bearded region, and characterized by papules, tubercles and pustules perforated by hairs. The disease is seen, as a rule, only on the bearded part of the face, either about the cheeks, chin, or upper lip, involving a small portion or the whole of these parts. The hairy portion of the neck may also be invaded. The disease may begin by the formation of papules and pustules about the hair-follicles on previously healthy skin, or chronic hyperæmia, or even eczema, may have preceded. The lesions generally occur in numbers, in close proximity, and, together with the accompanying inflammation, make up a patch of disease involving a greater or less area. The pustules are discrete, flat or acuminated, small in size, yellowish in color, perforated by hairs, show no disposition to rupture, and are, as a rule, apt to appear in crops. They dry to thin yellowish-brown crusts. There is more or less swelling and infiltration. Papules and tubercles may usually be seen intermingled with the pustules, or the former may constitute the greater part of the eruption. At first the hairs are firmly seated, but later, when suppuration has involved the follicles, they may be easily extracted. Not infrequently the hair-follicles are completely destroyed, in which case scarring and alopecia result. The process is chronic, it being of a subacute or chronic character, with, usually, acute exacerbations. Burning sensations, and at times pain or itching, accompany the disease.

According to Robinson, the affection is primarily a perifolliculitis, the first changes, which are those usually observed in vascular connective-tissue inflammations, taking place around the follicle. Later, the follicle and its sheath become involved, the pus and transuded serum finding their way into these structures. At times pus does not enter within the follicle, the changes observed therein being due to the transuded serum. The pus reaches the surface by forcing its way through the epidermis close to the hair. The causes of the disease are not understood. It is usually seen in those between the ages of twenty-five and fifty, in all classes of society, and in those in good or bad health. Persons with eczematous skin and those having thick and stiff hair are especially predisposed to the disease. Local irritation may serve as the exciting cause. The affection is not common. It is not contagious.

The disease is to be distinguished from tinea sycosis and eczema. Tinea sycosis usually begins as a circular scaly patch—in fact, as simple ringworm—later invading the hairs and follicles and giving rise to papules and tubercles. These lesions are larger than in simple sycosis, and appear and feel like lumps and nodules. Moreover, the changes in the hairs in the parasitic disease are characteristic: they become opaque, brittle, loose, and can be readily extracted. If necessary, a microscopical examination of the hairs may be resorted to. In eczema there is either an oozing, red, crusted surface, or it is dry and scaly ; the lesions, as a rule, do not remain discrete, are not perforated by hairs, and the eruption is apt to involve other parts of the face. It is scarcely possible to confound the disease with syphilis.

The disease is essentially a chronic one, and under the best management is often rebellious. Relapses are not uncommon. The treatment consists mainly of external measures. Suitable internal remedies are, however, in some cases, as in plethoric or in broken-down subjects, of value. The digestive apparatus is to be looked after. The extremes of heat and cold are to be, as far as possible, avoided. Clipping the hair, or shaving if not too painful, will permit a more thorough application of remedies. If the disease be of an acute type, soothing applications are at first to be advised. If there is crusting, it should be removed by poultices or oily applications. The use of lotio nigra, and subsequently a cloth spread with oxide-of-zinc ointment, as in acute vesicular eczema, may be advised to allay inflammation. Cold cream, vaseline, or applications of lead-water and like remedies, will also be found useful in the acute stage. As a rule, however, astringent and stimulating ointments may be prescribed when the case first comes under observation. As an astringent ointment there is in the average case nothing superior to a good unguentum diachyli. It should be spread thickly on muslin and bound down to the parts, renewing every six or twelve hours. If stimulation is permissible, twenty grains to a drachm of ammoniated mercury or calomel to the ounce of ointment may be prescribed.

If the process be chronic in character, the parts may be washed with sapo viridis and water, and then diachylon ointment applied, repeating the washing every day and the application of the ointment twice or thrice daily. Sulphur, one to three drachms to the ounce of ointment, is a valuable stimulating remedy, and should be applied thoroughly twice daily ; citrine ointment, two or three drachms to the ounce of lard or cold cream, will sometimes have a good effect. Shaving will be found useful in many cases. In some instances epilation proves a valuable adjunct to the treatment. In acute stages the hairs should be extracted from the pustules only—in the chronic stage both from papules and pustules. The operation will be rendered less painful by previously steaming or applying hot water to the parts. After the operation the surface should be dressed with a mild ointment. Epilation at the proper time will often save follicles from irreparable destruction; if for any reason it is not advisable, the pustules should be incised, so that free egress may be given to the pus.

Impetigo.

Impetigo is an acute inflammatory disease, characterized by the formation of one or more pea- or finger-nail-sized, rounded and elevated, usually firm, discrete pustules, seated upon an inflammatory base. The affection is at times preceded by slight malaise. The lesion is pustular from the beginning, and when well advanced may be of the size of a pea or finger-nail, is rounded, or semiglobular, markedly elevated, yellowish or whitish in color, with at first a more or less pronounced areola, which as the lesion matures becomes less and less marked, and finally almost entirely subsides. The pustule is usually distended, shows no disposition to rupture nor to umbilication, and is characterized by but little surrounding infiltration, and even where several exist close together they show no tendency to coalesce. Ten, twenty, or more lesions are usually present, and are most common about the face, hands, feet, and lower extremities. They dry to crusts of a yellowish or brownish color, which are usually thin and drop off, no pigmentation or scar remaining. The process is of brief duration, is benign in character, and is rarely attended with subjective symptoms. It is commonly seen in children under the age of ten.

The disease, apparently, is not related to eczema; occurs, as a rule, in well-nourished subjects, and is not contagious. The lesion is a typical pustule, the process being distinctly circumscribed. The walls are somewhat thick, and are probably made up of both the horny and mucous layers. There is no inflammatory base. Microscopically, the contents are found to be composed of pus-corpuscles, a few red blood-corpuscles, epithelial cells, and cellular débris. The disease is to be distinguished from pustular eczema, impetigo contagiosa, and erythema. The pustules of eczema are numerous, closely crowded together, small in size, tend to coalesce, with a decided disposition to rupture, and are accompanied by itching. The lesions of impetigo contagiosa are vesicular or vesico-pustular, flattened, superficial, thin-walled, often umbilicated; if close together they tend to coalesce, and dry to lamellar crusts of a yellowish color, and the affection is distinctly contagious. The pustules of ecthyma are flat, with an inflammatory base and areola; the crusts are brownish or blackish, and seated upon a deep excoriation; and the affection is, moreover, usually seen in adults and in those whose general health is markedly below the standard.

The affection rarely calls for treatment, as it tends to spontaneous recovery. Incision and evacuation of the matured lesions and a simple protective dressing of a mild ointment, such as oxide-of-zinc ointment, may be advised. If slight stimulation is desirable, ten or twenty grains of ammoniated mercury may be added to the ounce of the ointment.

Impetigo Contagiosa.

Impetigo contagiosa is an acute, inflammatory, contagious disease, characterized by the formation of discrete, superficial, flat, rounded or ovalish vesicles or blebs, which soon become vesico-pustular and pass into crusts. Precursory febrile symptoms, especially in young children, frequently usher in the eruption. The lesions begin as discrete vesicles, small in size, becoming vesico-pustular and increasing by extension peripherally, reaching the size of a pea or developing into blebs as large as a dime or silver quarter dollar. They are flat, slightly or markedly umbilicated, the umbilication being more marked in the older lesions. Several or a few dozen such vesicles or blebs may be present, and if situated close together may coalesce and form patches. There is very little areola, and the covering of the lesion is thin and withered-looking. The superficial character of the process is a striking feature. In a few days the lesions dry to crusts, thin, granular, wafer-like in character, light-yellowish or straw-colored, and but slightly adherent. If the vesicular or bleb wall or the crust is removed, a slightly excoriated surface is disclosed, resembling a superficial burn, secreting a thin fluid. The lesions are seen most commonly about the face and hands, although they frequently occur on other parts. In some cases one or two dozen lesions are scattered over the general surface. In these instances the resemblance of the whole process to an acute contagious systemic disease with cutaneous manifestations is striking. The lesions of the affection as ordinarily encountered appear simultaneously or in crops. As a rule, there is very little itching, and when it exists is usually present only in the beginning of the disease or at night. The affection is contagious and auto-inoculable, and at times apparently epidemic; is seen most frequently in the warm months, and is confined almost exclusively to children. When occurring in adults it is usually of an abortive type. In addition to the cutaneous covering, the mucous membranes of the mouth and conjunctiva are sometimes affected. As a rule, it runs an acute course, lasting ten days or two weeks. In exceptional instances the disease is anomalous, as regards not only its course, but the character and type of the individual lesions.

The causes of the disease are not understood. Some authorities consider it due to the presence of a parasite,—a view in which we are not prepared to coincide. A fungus—in fact, several varieties—may be found in microscopic examinations of the crusts, but the same may be found in crusts of other diseases, and their presence may be considered as accidental. There seem to be two varieties of the disease, in one of which the lesions are for the most part confined to the face and hands, and in the other the lesions are scattered over the general surface. The affection is encountered most frequently among the poor and ill-cared-for. A relationship to vaccination has at times been noted.

In the diagnosis eczema and simple impetigo are to be excluded. The history, course, and characters of the lesions of contagious impetigo are entirely different from those of these two diseases. The size, growth, isolated character, the non-inclination to rupture, and the comparative absence of itching will serve to distinguish it from eczema. The pustule of simple impetigo is prominently raised; that of contagious impetigo is flat and usually umbilicated; the contents of the former are distinctly pustular, and the crusts thicker, smaller, and usually yellowish-brown; of the latter the contents are rarely more than vesico-pustular, the crust thin, light-yellowish or straw-colored, and has the appearance of being stuck on. Those cases which resemble an exanthem may in the early stages be confounded with varicella, but later the lesions are much larger than seen in that disease. In exceptional instances the resemblance to the blebs of pemphigus is more or less pronounced.

As a rule, but little treatment is necessary, as the affection tends to spontaneous disappearance. In some cases, however, in which there is more or less itching, auto-inoculation at the excoriated points takes place, and in this manner the affection may persist. An ointment of ammoniated mercury, ten or fifteen grains to the ounce, rubbed in the lesions, will have a curative effect; likewise an ointment or lotion of carbolic acid, ten grains to the ounce.

Ecthyma.

Ecthyma is characterized by the formation of one or more discrete finger-nail-sized, flat, inflammatory pustules. The pustules are usually few in number, vary in size from that of a pea to a large finger-nail, roundish or ovalish in shape, and are situated on an inflammatory base, with a marked areola of a bright-red color. In the beginning they are yellowish, but later, from an admixture of more or less blood, they become reddish, subsequently drying to brownish but slightly adherent crusts. If the crust is removed, a superficial excoriation, secreting a yellowish fluid, is disclosed. The lesions pursue an acute course, but new pustules are apt to form from time to time. The lower extremities, shoulders and back are favorite localities. The subjective symptoms are usually slight, but burning and pain may be complained of. More or less pigmentation is left to mark the site of the lesions, which sooner or later disappears. The affection is seen in both sexes and at all ages, but is more frequently met with in men.

It is a disease of the poorly-nourished and debilitated; hence it is chiefly seen in the lower walks of life. All causes that tend to reduce the tone of the general health are indirectly responsible for the disease. In such persons external irritants, such as pediculi, bed-bugs, and similar parasites, may provoke the formation of ecthymatous lesions. The affection is not contagious. The process is of a markedly inflammatory type, and tends rapidly to pus-formation. The lesion is a typical pustule, and the excoriation does not extend deeper than the papillary layer. Permanent scarring never results. In the negro, instead of increased pigmentation, loss of pigment results.

The disease is to be distinguished from simple impetigo, contagious impetigo, and the flat pustular syphiloderm. It differs from impetigo in the flat form of the lesion and the character of its crust, and in the more inflammatory nature of the process. The non-contagiousness of the affection, the character and color of the crust, the regions involved, and the course will serve to differentiate it from impetigo contagiosa. In exceptional cases of this latter disease some of the lesions bear considerable resemblance to ecthyma. A striking similarity to the large flat pustule of syphilis is often noticed in ecthyma, and it is here that difficulty in the diagnosis is most likely to be experienced. The local disturbance, such as pain and heat, is generally more marked in ecthyma. The syphiloderm is usually of slower development and runs a more chronic course; moreover, positive ulceration beneath the crusts does not occur in ecthyma. The crusts of syphilis are darker in color, and usually have a greenish hue. Concomitant symptoms of syphilis are almost always present, and are valuable in the diagnosis. Ecthyma can scarcely be confounded with pustular eczema, as the size and discrete character of the pustules and the absence of marked itching are sufficiently distinctive.

Where it is possible for the patient to follow out treatment the result is always favorable. The importance of good food and proper hygiene cannot be overestimated. Tonics may be prescribed as efficient adjuvants. Iron, quinine, nux vomica, and the mineral acids are valuable. As a rule, simple measures are sufficient in the external treatment. If the lesions are numerous and are markedly inflammatory, alkaline baths, six ounces of sodium bicarbonate or of a similar alkaline salt to the bath, will be of service. The crusts are to be removed by poultices or hot-water applications, and the excoriations dressed with an ointment of ten to twenty grains of ammoniated mercury in an ounce of oxide-of-zinc ointment. In some cases a more stimulating ointment is required. Where active stimulation is demanded, touching the parts with nitrate of silver, diluted carbolic acid or a similar agent will prove serviceable.

Miliaria.

Miliaria—popularly known as prickly heat or heat-rash—is an acute inflammatory disorder of the sweat-glands, characterized by pinpoint to milletseed-sized papules or vesicles, attended usually by sensations of pricking, tingling, or burning. In some cases the eruption is almost entirely made up of papular lesions, and constitutes the form of the affection known as miliaria papulosa. In other cases the lesions are vesicular in nature, and miliaria vesiculosa is typified. It is chiefly the papular form to which the name of prickly heat has been applied. This variety begins with the formation of minute elevated, acuminated, bright-red papules, occurring usually in great numbers, more or less crowded together; the individual lesions, however, remain discrete. The affection may be localized, or, as is usually the case, may involve considerable surface. In miliaria vesiculosa the lesions are in the form of vesicles the same in size as the papules, and appear as whitish or yellowish points surrounded with inflammatory areolæ. They are usually crowded so closely together as to give the skin a bright-red look (miliaria rubra). At first the vesicles are transparent and contain a clear fluid, but as they become older they appear opaque and yellowish-white (miliaria alba), and instead of the bright-red appearance the eruption has then a yellowish cast. As in the papular form of the eruption, small areas may be involved or the greater part of the entire surface. The trunk is a favorite locality. The vesicles dry up in a few days, showing no tendency to rupture, and terminate in slight desquamation. In the majority of cases the eruption consists of papular, vesico-papular, and vesicular lesions interspersed. They make their appearance suddenly, usually accompanied with considerable sweat_ ing, and if the cause has ceased to act terminate in the course of a few days. As a rule, the subjective symptoms are mild in character, nothing more than slight tingling, burning, being noted; in others, however, these may be so marked as to give rise to considerable annoyance. Indi_ viduals who are debilitated seem most prone to an outbreak. Hot weather predisposes to it; in fact, excessive heat from whatever cause is apt to provoke an attack. It is especially common in children. The affection as usually met with is essentially an inflammatory disorder of the sweat_ glands, congestion and exudation taking place about the ducts, giving rise to papules or vesicles, according to the intensity of the process.

It is to be distinguished from eczema and sudamen. The papules of eczema are larger, more elevated, firmer, make their appearance more slowly, and are of much longer duration; moreover, the itching of pap_ ular eczema is usually marked. Vesicular eczema differs from miliaria vesiculosa by the larger size of the lesions, their disposition to rupture, their tendency to become confluent, and their greater itchiness, and by the general features of the eruption both as regards its appearance and duration. It is to be noted that miliaria ocurring in children from the conjoint effects of warm weather and superfluous clothing may, if the exciting causes are continued, result in eczema. Sudamen may be differ- entiated by the absence of inflammatory symptoms.

The affection under favorable circumstances runs a rapid course, disap- pearing in a few days or weeks. A removal of the exciting cause will in all cases have a favorable effect. Too active treatment is to be avoided, not only as being useless but prejudicial. Undue perspiration should be guarded against. The patient is for the time to avoid exercise and to be properly clad. Refrigerating diuretics, as citrate or the acetate of potas- sium or simple lemon-juice diluted, may be prescribed. When the erup- tion is kept up or frequently recurs as a result of impaired health, tonics, as quinine, iron, and the mineral acids, will be useful. In the majority of cases local treatment alone is necessary. Dusting-powders and cooling or astringent lotions are of most value. Starch and lycopodium powder, equal quantities or with 20 to 30 per cent. of oxide of zinc added, may be used; the surface is to be kept freely powdered. Astringent lotions may be employed in place of the dusting-powder, or, what is often advisable, may immediately precede the latter, the lotion being first applied, allowed to dry on the surface, and then the powder freely dusted over. A lotion of alcohol and water and sponging with vinegar and water may be pre- scribed.

Pompholyx.

Under this head (and also that of Dysidrosis) a rare disease of the skin has been described, characterized by peculiar vesicles and blebs and an excoriated state of the skin, with subsequent exfoliation of the epidermis. It consists at first of deep-seated vesicular lesions, which resemble small boiled sago-grains implanted in the skin, accompanied by a variable degree of inflammation. As the lesions grow they incline to coalesce, thus forming small or large blebs showing but little if any disposition to rupture. Sooner or later the fluid is reabsorbed or exudes, the epidermis peeling off, usually in large flakes or pieces, sometimes in the form of a cast of the fingers or hand. In most cases burning sensations, tenderness, and soreness are complained of. The disease pursues a variable course. Ordinarily, the process lasts from two to eight weeks. Relapses as well as recurrences of the disease may take place. It attacks by preference the hands, more especially the palms and the sides of the fingers, from which circumstance it was originally designated cheiro-pompholyx; but it may invade the feet and also other regions.

The same disease has been described with the two names given, some observers regarding it as being due to a disordered state of the sweat apparatus, others as being an inflammatory affection. We incline to the latter view, looking upon true dysidrosis as a form of miliaria. The disease under consideration is without question neurotic in origin. It occurs chiefly in those suffering from nervous debility or prostration arising from varied causes. It is due to impaired, faulty innervation. It is most liable to be mistaken for vesicular eczema or pemphigus. The treatment should be general, consisting of such remedies as quinine and arsenic, together with good food and proper hygiene. Local treatment may be prescribed as in the case of eczema, but the result in most cases is not as satisfactory as in that disease.

Pemphigus.

Pemphigus is an acute or chronic bullous disease, characterized by the successive formation of variously sized and shaped blebs. Two varieties are met with—pemphigus vulgaris and pemphigus foliaceus—the symptoms of which differ considerably. Pemphigus vulgaris, the usual form of the disease, appears with or without precursory symptoms. In marked cases headache and fever may precede the cutaneous outbreak. All portions of the body may suffer, but the extremities are more commonly the seat of the eruption. The mucous membrane of the mouth and vagina may also be involved. The lesions, as a rule, are rarely seen in large numbers, a dozen or so usually being present at one time. They vary in size from a pea to a large egg, and are generally rounded or ovalish, fully distended, and according to the size are elevated from a few lines to an inch above the surrounding skin. There is but little inflammation attending their formation. In some cases the blebs arise from erythematous spots or wheals, but generally from apparently normal skin. The fluid is yellowish, later often becoming cloudy or puriform. At times slight hemorrhage occurs, giving the lesions a reddish or purplish color. Spontaneous rupture of the lesions seldom occurs, the contents usually disappearing by absorption. Each bleb runs its course in from two to eight days. Itching and burning are rarely prominent symptoms, in some cases being scarcely noticeable or absent, in others present to a marked degree, constituting pemphigus pruriginosus. In children pemphigus vulgaris is usually attended with systemic disturbance; in adults, as a rule, only in severe cases. The disease may be acute or chronic. Acute pemphigus is rare, and occurs, as a rule, only in children. It usually runs a favorable course, except in ill-nourished children, in whom it may take on a malignant type and have a fatal termination. Chronic pemphigus may be benign or malignant. In the benign form the eruption may persist several months by successive outbreaks, and then disappear, or the blebs may form irregularly and indefinitely. In the former case there may be but the one attack, or, as commonly occurs, relapses may follow after months or years. In the malignant form the disease is more violent, with marked systemic depression and ulcerative action, and may frequently have an unfavorable termination.

Pemphigus foliaceus, the other variety of the disease, is rare. The blebs are loose and flaccid, with milky or puriform contents, rupture, and the oozing liquid dries to crusts, which are cast off, disclosing the reddened corium beneath. The blebs may coalesce and involve considerable surface, and may appear in rapid succession on other regions and on the sites of disappearing or half-ruptured lesions; even the whole surface may become involved, the process continuing for years, undermining the general health and eventually destroying the patient.

Pemphigus is a rare disease, and seems to be of even less frequent occurrence in this country than abroad. It is not contagious, nor is it due to syphilis, the so-called syphilitic pemphigus being a bullous syphiloderm and not a true pemphigus. General debility, overwork, shock, and nervous prostration are influential in producing the disease. Occasionally an hereditary tendency is traceable.

The contents of blebs are at first colorless or yellowish, consisting of serum,—later containing blood-corpuscles, pus, fatty-acid crystals, and epithelial cells, and occasionally uric-acid crystals and free ammonia. The reaction is alkaline, becoming more markedly so as the contents grow older. The lesions are superficially seated, between the horny layer and upper part of the rete and the lengthened cells of the rete and the corium. The papillæ and subcutaneous tissues show round-cell infiltration and dilated blood-vessels.

Herpes iris and the bullous syphiloderm are to be excluded in the diagnosis. In herpes iris the acute course, small lesions, variegated colors, the usually marked areola, the decided tendency to concentric arrangement of the lesions, the seat of the disease,—all tend to distinguish it from pemphigus. The thick, bulky, greenish crusts of the bullous syphilide, with the underlying ulceration, its course, and the presence of concomitant symptoms of that disease, taken with the history of the case, are points of difference. Impetigo contagiosa may at times strikingly resemble pemphigus, but the history of the case, its distribution, the contagious and auto-inoculable properties of the contents of the lesions, and the characteristic crusting of the former disease,—are all available in the differential diagnosis. The blebs of pemphigus are to be distinguished also from the accidental blebs of urticaria and of erythema multiforme. It is to be remembered also that cases sometimes come under observation in which blebs are, for the sake of feigning disease, produced artificially, the subjects being usually hysterical women.

Pemphigus is in most cases a grave disease. The unfavorable symptoms are the presence of numerous bullæ, the rapid and successive development of new lesions, flabby walls, frequent febrile attacks, loss of strength, and marasmus. It is injudicious, even in mild cases, to express an opinion as to the probable duration of the disease. Both constitutional and local treatment, especially the former, are demanded. The general health should receive careful study and faulty conditions corrected. Good food, milk, wine, or ale, eggs and meat are in most cases to be advised. Suitable hygienic regulations should also receive attention. ·Arsenic in appropriate doses, long continued, has in some cases almost a specific action : on the whole, it must be regarded as our most valuable remedy. Quinine in full doses, cod-liver oil, iron, and the mineral acids are also of service. External treatment is of importance, and is in many cases demanded for the comfort of the patient. The blebs are to be opened as soon as developed, and the parts anointed with oxide-of-zinc ointment. Lotio nigra, used as in eczema, will sometimes be found soothing, as also lotions containing liquor carbonis detergens or liquor picis alkalinus. Dusting-powders of zinc oxide with talc and starch are likewise useful. Baths containing bran, starch, or gelatin sometimes afford ease. Corrosive-sublimate baths, one or two drachms to the bath, and alkaline baths in some cases prove of service. After the bath an application of an ointment or mild dusting-powder may be made to advantage. Where baths prove unsuitable or are impracticable, mild ointments may be used, such as diachylon ointment, vaseline, cold cream, or zinc ointment, spread upon cloth and bound down with bandages.

CLASS IV.—HYPERTROPHIES.[1]

Lentigo.

LENTIGO, or freckle, is characterized by irregularly-shaped, rounded or angular, pinhead- or pea-sized, yellowish or brownish spots of pigment deposit, occurring for the most part upon the face and the backs of the hands. They may appear as blemishes scarcely perceptible to the casual observer, or to such an extent and with such intensity of color as to be disfiguring. They may show themselves as discrete or as confluent lesions, and in the latter event the skin presents a spotted, rusty, or dirty appearance. As stated, the face and the backs of the hands are usually attacked, but other regions may also be invaded. They are encountered at all ages, but usually in young persons, especially in those of light complexion, and more particularly in red-haired subjects. They pursue a chronic course, lasting, as a rule, a lifetime, being, however, in most cases much paler in winter than in summer. Sometimes the lesions are blackish rather than brownish, and cases are on record where such were numerous and occupying the general surface. Blackish freckles are also met with in connection with certain rare forms of atrophy of the skin proper complicated with telangiectases, as in the cases reported by Hebra and

[1] Purpura, constituting Class III., appears in Vol. II. p. 186, as a separate article by I. E. Atkinson.

Kaposi, Taylor, and one of us (Duhring), an account of which may be found under atrophy of the skin.

The affection consists of a circumscribed deposit of pigment, which in the majority of cases is due to the influence of the sun's rays, but there are cases in which the lesions cannot be assigned to this cause, as, for example, where they occur upon the trunk or other regions not exposed to light. The treatment will be referred to in connection with chloasma.

Chloasma.

Chloasma may be described as a pigmentary affection, consisting of variously sized and shaped, more or less defined, smooth patches of a yellowish, brownish, or blackish color. The affection is one merely of coloration, the structure of the skin proper being normal. The spots or patches vary much as to size and shape. As a rule, they are irregular in outline, and not infrequently they are angular. They vary in size from a small coin to a hand or larger. At times the affection may develop as a diffuse or even as a universal discoloration. The distribution of the pigment may be uniform, but more frequently it is mottled, giving the skin a thick, muddy, or dirty appearance. Under idiopathic chloasma are included the forms of pigmentation due to various external agencies, as, for example, chemicals, sinapisms, heat, and long-continued scratching. The symptomatic group comprises uterine chloasma and the discolorations occurring in connection with certain general maladies, among which cancer, tuberculosis, Addison's disease, and malaria may be mentioned. Chloasma is also met with as a symptom in certain diseases of the skin proper, as scleroderma, morphœa, leprosy, and syphilis.

Chloasma uterinum, the commonest form, appears in all degrees from a duskiness or swarthiness of the complexion to pronounced patches of mottled yellowish or brownish discoloration, occurring on the face usually of pregnant women. But the same condition is met with also in single women, and at times in men. In women it usually appears as a more or less broken patch invading the forehead, extending from temple to temple, but the nose, cheeks, and chin are likewise very frequently attacked. It is due both to physiological and to pathological changes in the uterus, and also to various disorders of the menstrual function. The nervous system in many cases is without doubt at fault, and to this cause must be assigned those cases occurring in men. It is encountered, as a rule, between the ages of twenty-five and fifty. Its course is variable, depending upon the cause, but, as a rule, it is persistent, and it may continue for a long period. It is liable to be confounded with tinea versicolor, from which, however, it may be readily distinguished by the observation that in the latter disease the surface of the skin is the seat of more or less furfuraceous desquamation, which becomes more evident by scraping. In chloasma the skin is normal in structure. The patches of tinea versicolor are usually more numerous than those of chloasma, and occupy the trunk, a region seldom invaded by the latter affection. The face is the common seat of chloasma, a region practically exempt from tinea versicolor.

The treatment consists in removing the cause where this is possible, or in modifying it by such general remedies as appear indicated. Among the various local remedies corrosive sublimate is one of the most valuable, used in the form of a lotion with water, alcohol, or almond emulsion. Its strength should vary from half a grain to five grains to the ounce, according to the region, size of the spot, sensitiveness of the skin, and the effect produced. Two or three grains to the ounce will generally be found of sufficient strength; and this may be applied, dabbed on lightly for five or ten minutes, twice daily, until irritation or desquamation appears. A lotion recommended by Hardy is the following:

R. Hydrargyri chlor. corros.,   gr. viiss;
Zinci sulphatis,   ʒss;
Plumbi acetatis,   ʒss;
Aquæ,   f ʒiv.   M.

Ammoniated mercury, from forty to eighty grains to the ounce of ointment, may also be referred to as of positive value.

The following formula may also be given:

R. Hydrargyri ammoniati,   ʒj;
Bismuthi magist.,   ʒss;
Ugt. aquæ rosæ,   ʒj.

M.—Sig. Apply at night.

Sulphur ointments, as of precipitated sulphur one or two drachms to the ounce, are also at times useful. The applications may be suspended from time to time should irritation occur. The treatment in some cases is followed by good results, while in others it is unsatisfactory. The discoloration, having been removed, may remain away, or, as often happens, may recur. The treatment recommended for chloasma is that which will be found of most service in lentigo.

There are other discolorations, of a different nature, which may be referred to here, as the staining due to the coloring matter of the bile, and that sometimes following the internal use of nitrate of silver, known as argyria, where the skin assumes a bluish-gray, bronze, or blackish shade. Neumann states that reduced silver is found in all parts of the skin except the lining epithelia of the glands and the cells of the mucous layer of the epidermis. The deposit also occurs in the internal organs.

Keratosis Pilaris.

Keratosis pilaris (also called lichen pilaris and pityriasis pilaris) is an hypertrophy of the epidermis about the apertures of the hair-follicles, forming pinhead-sized, conical epidermic elevations. The lesions are met with usually about the extensor surfaces of the thighs and arms, especially the former, but they may also occur on other parts. They are whitish, grayish, or blackish in color, are rarely larger than a pinhead, each being pierced by a hair, around which are accumulated, in the form of strata, the horny cells of the epidermis. In some lesions the hair is broken off at the apex, appearing as a black central point; in others the hair is not visible, but is found coiled or twisted up within the papules. The skin is dry, harsh, or rough, and together with the papules may feel like a nutmeg-grater. The skin at the base of each papule is of a normal color or slightly reddened. The elevations consist of an accumulation of epidermic cells and sebaceous matter about the orifices of the hair-follicles. The affection in its milder forms is not uncommon, and is encountered usually in cold weather, and especially in those who bathe infrequently. It may occur at any age, but is most common in early adult life. Slight itching is occasionally present. As ordinarily observed, it is a slight disorder, but shows a tendency to persist. It resembles somewhat cutis anserina, the miliary papular syphiloderm in the desquamating stage, and also lichen scrofulosus. In goose-flesh (cutis anserina) the elevations are of a different nature, being due to cold, heat, or nervous excitement. The papules of the syphiloderm tend to group, are firmer, more deeply seated, less scaly, and of a reddish color. In lichen scrofulosus the papules are more solid in character, incline to group, are less scaly, and usually appear about the abdomen.

The disease is readily removable by treatment. Hot baths with the free use of strong soap, as sapo viridis, will usually suffice in ordinary cases; alkaline baths are also serviceable. In rebellious cases oily applications, such as the petroleum preparations, lard, and glycerin, or sulphur ointment, may be used in conjunction with the baths.

Molluscum Epitheliale.

Molluscum epitheliale, also called molluscum contagiosum and molluscum sebaceum, is characterized by rounded, semiglobular, flattened, or verrucous papules or tubercles of a whitish or pinkish color, varying in size from a pinhead to a pea. As generally met with, they are the size and shape of a small split pea; in other cases they are more acuminated or are in the form of a very small pearl button. They have a broad base and are seated close to the general surface. As a rule, they are multiple, three or six or more being present in different stages of evolution. They are unaccompanied by subjective symptons. The skin covering them is stretched, and they have a glistening or waxy look, and at times resemble a drop of wax. In consistence they are usually firm, becoming soft with age. Their summits are sometimes flattened and umbilicated, with a central darkish point representing the mouth of the follicle. Their usual seat is the face, especially the eyelids, cheeks, and chin, but the neck, breast, and genitalia may also be invaded. They grow slowly in most cases, and are unaccompanied by inflammatory symptoms. Later, they become soft and tend to break down, with at times ulceration.

The disease is rare in this country, and is seldom encountered in our experience either in dispensary or in private practice. It occurs chiefly in children, and more especially among the poorer classes. Its cause is obscure. By some authorities it is considered to be contagious, this view being more generally entertained in England (where the disease seems to be more frequently encountered than elsewhere) than in other countries. The evidence for believing it to be contagious, however, does not seem sufficient to warrant such a conclusion. Inoculation has failed to develop the disease. Some observers consider that the process has its origin in the sebaceous glands, while others—ourselves among the number—hold that it is a disease of the rete mucosum. It is to be regarded as a hyperplasia of the rete. If the tumor be cut into, the contents may usually be expressed in the form of a whitish or yellowish rounded mass of a thick or thin cheesy consistence. Under the microscope it is seen to be composed of epithelial cells with nuclei and of peculiar rounded or ovoidal, sharply-defined, fatty-looking bodies—the so-called molluscum bodies, which are to be viewed as a form of epithelial degeneration. The growth probably begins in the hair-follicles, as originally stated by Virchow and more recently confirmed by Thin.

The disease is to be distinguished from molluscum fibrosum, from papillary warts, and from acne. Local treatment, consisting of incision and expression of the contents, with subsequent cauterization with nitrate of silver, is the best procedure. They may also be ligated. As the disease tends to spontaneous cure, the remedies employed should be simple in character.

Callositas.

Callositas (syn., tylosis, tyloma, callus) is characterized by the formation of a hard or horny thickened patch of epidermis, variously sized and shaped, and of a grayish, yellowish, or brownish color. The patches are usually coin-sized, more or less rounded in shape, grayish, yellowish, or brownish in color, somewhat elevated, and of a dense and firm texture. They are most common about the hands and feet, and in a measure are protective to the more sensitive corium beneath. The ordinary surface lines are less distinct than on the surrounding healthy skin, into which the patch gradually merges. The thickening and elevation may be slight or excessive, and are most marked at the centre. The process rarely gives rise to any annoyance or pain, but when excessive the more delicate movements of the parts are restricted. Occasionally, from accidental injury, the underlying corium becomes inflamed, suppurates, and as a result the thickened mass is cast off. When occurring about the joints from motion of the parts, it may, moreover, become fissured and painful. Pressure and friction are the main factors in the production of a callosity—on the hands from the use of tools and implements, and on the feet from ill-fitting shoes. But cases are seen exceptionally in which there has been no apparent external cause; moreover, the same amount of pressure or friction in different individuals may give rise to different degrees of callosity; hence there must in some cases be other causes which at times enter into its production, as, for example, altered nerve-supply. The epidermis is the only part involved; fissuring and suppuration, it is true, involve the deeper structures, but these conditions are accidental and secondary. A section of a callosity shows a thickening of the horny layer, the corium remaining normal.

Unless the callosity is excessive or gives rise to inconvenience, treatment is rarely demanded. When advisable, the parts are to be softened by means of hot-water applications or poultices, solutions of caustic potash, or sapo viridis used as an ointment; after which the callus may be removed by scraping with a dermal curette or shaving with a sharp knife. An excellent method of treatment consists in the continuous application for some days of a plaster of salicylic acid of 10 or 12 per cent. strength, the same to be renewed every few days; at the end of a week or two the parts should be soaked in hot water, and the mass will readily come away. A solution of salicylic acid in collodion of the same strength or stronger, applied frequently for five or six days, will often act in like manner.

Clavus.

Clavus, or corn, is a small, circumscribed hypertrophy of the horny layer of the epidermis, painful upon pressure, situated usually about the feet. As commonly met with, it is about the size of a pea, with a smooth and shining surface, having a hard and horny feel. Corns are seen most frequently upon the outer surface of the little toe, but are often met with also upon the other toes and on the soles of the feet. Occurring between the toes, the moisture and friction of the part have a softening effect, and as a result the corns are soft and spongy, constituting soft corns. One, several, or more may be present. When slightly developed they cause very little disturbance or discomfort, but if large or irritated they may become sensitive and render walking painful. Continued pressure and friction, as from badly-fitting shoes, are the active factors in their production. Anatomically, a corn is a localized epidermal hypertrophy, consisting of a horny mass, cone-shaped, with the base externally and the apex pressing upon the rete and corium; the cone being made up of concentrically-arranged, closely-packed layers of epidermic cells. The corium upon which this cone-shaped mass presses may be atrophied or hypertrophied.

The first essential in the treatment is a removal of the cause. The feet should be properly fitted. The corn is to be softened by means of continuous or repeated soaking in hot water or by poulticing, after which it may be pared down or extracted. Salicylic acid, either in solution or in the form of a plaster, 15 or 20 per cent. strength, applied for several nights, will often give relief. A well-known and efficient formula is the following:

℞. Acidi salicylici, gr. xxx ;
Ext. cannabis Indicæ, gr. x ;
Collodii, f℥ss. M.

Sig. Paint on every night and morning. At the end of several days or a week the part is soaked in warm water and the epidermic mass, or greater portion of it, is readily detached. Nitrate of silver is useful after softening of the growth has been brought about, and is also of advantage n the treatment of soft corns. Caustic potash, thirty to sixty grains to the ounce of water or alcohol, is also of service, but is to be employed cautiously. Considerable relief to the soft formation is obtained by separating the toes with a thin layer of raw cotton. A ring of rubber, wadding or felt should be employed to prevent pressure and friction upon a corn, and, as this removes the exciting cause, permanent relief may follow.

Cornu Cutaneum.

Cornu cutaneum (syn., cornu humanum, horny tumor) is characterized by the development of a true horny formation of variable size and shape, arising from the skin. The growth bears a striking similarity to the horns of the lower animals. It is a solid, dry, harsh, somewhat brittle formation, usually more or less tapering, conical, or rounded, crooked or twisted, with a laminated, irregular, and fissured surface, and of a grayish-yellow or brownish color. Horns vary as to size and form, being a few lines or several inches in length, with a broad base, and tapering toward the end. They may be broad and flat or elongate. They have a flattened or concave base resting directly upon the skin, with the underlying and surrounding tissue normal, slightly elevated, or inflamed and undergoing epithelial degeneration. In some cases the papillæ are much enlarged and extend up into the growth. Ordinarily, there is present but one growth, but in some instances several or a dozen or more have been observed in a single case. The face and scalp are favorite regions, and to a less degree the male genitalia. As a rule, the horns are painless, but if injured more or less pain is usually experienced about the base. They rarely develop before middle age, attain a certain size, and then tend to loosen and fall off, disclosing an ulcerating base, from which a new growth is usually reproduced. Epitheliomatous degeneration is not an uncommon sequela.

Anatomically, the growth has its origin in the deeper layers of the stratum mucosum, either from that lying directly over the papillæ or from that lining the follicles and glands. It is essentially an epidermic hypertrophy, similar or closely related to warty formation. A variable degree of papillary hypertrophy, the papillæ running up into the base of the horn, is invariably present, and precedes, doubtless, the horny outgrowth. The horny cells are massed together to form columns, and in the columns themselves are concentrically arranged. Blood-vessels also appear in the base of the growth. There can be no difficulty in the diagnosis. In regard to prognosis the possibility of degeneration into epithelioma is to be kept in view. If the horn becomes detached or is knocked off, it is almost invariably reproduced. Properly managed, horns are easily removed and permanent freedom assured. The possibility of epitheliomatous degeneration, as well as their unsightliness, demands active treatment. The formation is to be detached and the base thoroughly scraped with the dermal curette, and pyrogallic acid or arsenious acid applied, as in epithelial cancer ; or it may be cauterized with zinc chloride or caustic potash. The galvano-cautery is also efficient, while in some cases excision may prove the best method of treatment. If the base is properly treated, a return of the growth rarely occurs.

Verruca.

Verruca, or wart, is a hard or soft, rounded, flat, or acuminated, circumscribed epidermal and papillary formation. There are several forms of warts. The most common varietiy, verruca vulgaris, is seen mostly upon the hands. It is usually split-pea-sized, elevated, circumscribed, rounded, with a broad base. At first there may be epidermal hypertrophy, but later this in a measure disappears, and the hypertrophic papillæ constitute the growth and are seen as minute elevations. It is firm, hard, or horny, and the color is ordinarily the same as the surrounding skin, but at times it is darker. The papillæ forming a wart are some-times so irregularly developed as to make it appear lobulated, causing a cauliflower-like form. One, several, or great numbers may be present. Another form is verruca plana, or flat wart, differing from the ordinary wart described above in being flat and broad. It is usually the size of a split pea or finger-nail; occurs most frequently upon the back, especially in elderly people; and is usually brownish or blackish in color, constituting verruca senilis and keratosis pigmentosa. Verruca filiformis, a third variety, is a thread-like formation, usually about an eighth of an inch in length, occurring singly or in groups, and generally about the face, eyelids, and neck. Verruca digitata, another form, is mostly observed upon the scalp, and occurs as a slightly elevated formation, varying in size from a pea to a finger-nail, and marked by digitations, especially noticeable about the border.

Verruca acuminata (syn., venereal wart, pointed wart, moist wart, fig wart, pointed condyloma, cauliflower excrescence; verruca elevata) consists of one or more groups of acuminated or irregularly-shaped elevations, usually so closely packed together as to form a more or less solid mass of vegetations. At times they present an appearance of granulation tissue. In color they are usually pinkish or reddish, and are seen mainly about the genitalia, more particularly about the glans penis, on the inner side of the prepuce, and about the labia, and more rarely about the arms, axillæ, umbilicus, and toes. They are dry or moist according to the regions about which they occur and to other circumstances. The secretion from the moist formation is yellowish and of a puriform character, undergoing rapid decomposition and giving rise to a penetrating and often disgusting odor. They are seen both in men and women, especially in young people; develop rapidly, at times attaining the size of a fist; and variously resemble the cauliflower, cock's-comb, fungi, or raspberries.

The etiology of warts is not known. They are common to both sexes, and are much more frequent in the young. The various causes which, in the popular mind, are capable of producing these growths are merely conjectural, and in most instances have no foundation in fact. The acuminated wart is usually caused by irritating secretions. Anatomically, a wart consists of a connective-tissue growth as a basis, with papillary and slight epidermic hypertrophy, the interior of the growth containing vascular loops. In the acuminated or venereal wart there is considerable connective-tissue growth, the papillæ being markedly enlarged, the cells of the mucous layer highly developed, and the vascular supply abundant.

There is rarely any difficulty in the diagnosis, as the formations are well known and their characters pronounced. Prognosis is favorable; as a rule, the growths respond rapidly to treatment; at times, however, they prove obstinate. When they exist in numbers it is best to remove a part only of the whole manifestation at a time. Occasionally removal of several will be followed by spontaneous disappearance of the others. In some cases, indeed, after existing a shorter or longer period, they tend to disappear without treatment.

Excision by means of the curved scissors or a knife in some cases will be found the best method of dealing with them, their bases immediately after the operation being touched with nitrate of silver.

Caustics, such as potassa, chromic acid, nitric acid, and acetic acid, may be employed, but strong remedies should be applied with care. Touching the growths frequently with a 10 to 20 per cent. solution of salicylic acid or a salicylic-acid plaster of the same strength, constantly applied, will be found useful. Multiple flat warts may be treated with a paste of precipitated sulphur and equal parts of acetic acid and glycerin, prepared at the time of using. In obstinate and relapsing cases the internal use of arsenic has been recommended. Stimulating powders and lotions, such as calomel, burnt alum, powdered savine, solution of chlorinated soda, and carbolic acid, may be used in the acuminated variety.

Nævus Pigmentosus.

Nævus pigmentosus, commonly called mole, is a circumscribed pigmentary deposit in the skin. In addition to hypertrophy of pigment there may also be hypertrophy of one or of all of the other cutaneous structures, especially of the hair. When the surface of the nævus is normal and smooth it is termed nævus spilus; if there is a growth of hair upon it, nævus pilosus; if the connective tissue is increased, forming growths of variable dimensions, it is designated nævus lipomatodes; if the surface is rough and warty, nævus verrucosus. Moles may be congenital or acquired, usually the former. As ordinarily met with, they are rounded, of the size of a coffee-grain, the color varying from a light yellowish-brown to a chocolate or black. The trunk, neck, back and face are favorite localities. One or more may be present, usually upon different parts of the body, or in exceptional cases following nerve-tracts. When once formed there is little tendency to change. They occur with equal frequency in both sexes. Anatomically, there is found an increase in the natural coloring-matter of the skin, and in almost all cases variable degrees of connective-tissue hypertrophy. Enlargement of the papillæ gives rise to nævus verrucosus, and an increase in size and numerically of the hair-bulbs constitutes nævus pilosus.

Treatment of a nævus consists in its removal by means of caustics or the knife. The small and flat lesions may be removed with potassa or the ethylate of sodium; a 1 per cent. solution of corrosive sublimate, applied for a few hours by means of compresses, causes blistering and usually the removal of the pigment. Excision or thorough cauterization may be employed for nævus verrucosus and nævus lipomatodes. The galvano-caustic has also been advocated.

Ichthyosis.

Ichthyosis, also called xeroderma and fish-skin disease, is a chronic, hypertrophic disease, usually occupying the whole surface, characterized by dryness or scaliness of the skin, with a variable amount of papillary growth. There are two varieties of the disease,—ichthyosis simplex and ichthyosis hystrix, arbitrary divisions, however, employed to designate the milder and more severe forms respectively.

The milder variety is that which is usually encountered. In this form the disorder may be so trifling in character as to give rise to simple dryness or harshness of the integument,—a condition to which the term xeroderma has been given. In others the process may be more developed, and the scales somewhat thick, having a polygonal or plate-like form. When the latter is the case, the form and size of the plates are usually determined by the natural lines or furrows of the parts. The scaling may be merely thin and bran-like or thick and horny, resembling fish-scales. In the milder forms of this variety the color of the scales may be light and pearly ; when more or less thickly developed, may be dark, even olive-green or blackish. This color cannot be attributed entirely to extraneous matter, pigment-granules having been demonstrated in the scales. The amount of scaling depends somewhat upon the age of the patient, the severity of the disease, and also the frequency of ablutions. If the scales are allowed to accumulate, they may become enormously thickened. The disease is found most developed upon the extensor surfaces of the upper and lower extremities, especially the latter, the flexor surfaces in mild cases being free. The scales are firmly attached, but can usually be removed without injury to the underlying parts.

In the other variety of the disease—ichthyosis hystrix—in addition to excessive formation of scales there is marked papillary hypertrophy, at times the papillary outgrowths reaching several lines, bearing resemblance to the quills of a porcupine. This resemblance has given rise to the qualifying term hystrix. This variety of the disease is not apt to be so generalized as the milder variety. It is not infrequently seen to occur as one or more rounded, irregular or linear patches, solid, corrugated, warty or spinous in character. The patches may exist close together or widely separated or along nerve-tracts, and the other parts of the surface may exhibit the milder variety.

Ichthyosis is usually first noticed in the early months of childhood, from which time it becomes progressively worse until it reaches a certain point, and then usually remains stationary throughout life. It is common to both sexes. The scalp and face usually escape. The condition is affected favorably by warm weather, so much so that the milder forms of the disease disappear entirely during the summer, to reappear as soon as the cold season begins. Even the severer forms of the affection disappear to some extent during the warm months. This change is due to the activity of the glands in the summer, the secretions macerating the epidermis, rendering the removal easy and thus relieving the patient. Unless the affection is well marked subjective symptoms rarely exist, but slight itching is sometimes present. In the well-developed cases, however, the scales may become so thick and the hypertrophy so marked as to interfere with the natural mobility of the parts, or as a result of motion fissures may occur. The general health of patients suffering with ichthyosis is usually noted to be good.

The causes of the disease are not clearly understood. An hereditary tendency is frequently traceable. The affection is to be looked upon more in the light of a deformity than as a disease. Although it does not manifest itself, as a rule, until the end of the first or second year, it is nevertheless to be considered, in most instances at least, as born with the individual. The disease is so slight in the beginning that in view of the repeated ablutions that infants are subjected to it might exist slightly in the first months of life without being noted. Race and climate have been stated as important factors in its production. It will be found, however, that where it exists in any great proportion, as in Paraguay and in the Moluccas, for various reasons intermarrying among the natives is the practice, and it is unquestionably a natural consequence that a distinctly hereditary disease should become frequent under such conditions. In this country the disease in its marked form is comparatively rare.

Anatomically, a constant feature of the disease is epidermic hypertrophy. This may be slight or marked according to the severity of the process. There is usually also considerable hypertrophy of the papillæ. In some cases, in addition to these conditions the rete may found hypertrophied, the blood-vessels dilated, the hair-follicles and the sweat and sebaceous glands more or less involved. The features of the disease—the harsh, dry skin, the hypertrophy of the epidermis and papillæ, the furfuraceous or plate-like scaliness, the greater development of the affection upon the extensor surfaces, and the history—are so characteristic that a diagnosis is a matter of no difficulty. From psoriasis, scaly eczema, and the other inflammatory scaly disorders it may be distinguished by the absence of inflammation.

The prognosis of the affection, as already intimated, is unfavorable as regards its cure. In only a few cases has a cure been noted. Hebra reports two such cases, the disappearance of the affection having followed an attack of one of the exanthematous fevers. Internal treatment is very rarely, if at all, of any benefit. Some good has been stated to follow the administration of linseed oil. In a few cases under observation jaborandi in moderate doses has temporarily influenced the disease favorably, probably by increasing the action of the sweat-glands. Although the prospect of a cure is entirely unfavorable, the affection may be, in almost all cases, kept in abeyance by external measures. Oily applications, soaps, and frequent bathing are the measures to be advised. In mild cases simple baths, frequently repeated, will suffice. In others it may be necessary to make the bath alkaline by the addition of bicarbonate of sodium, three to six ounces to the bath: the patient should soak in the bath for thirty minutes or longer. Where the alkaline baths seem unsuitable or fail to benefit sufficiently, the hot bath and washing with sapo viridis may be employed. The vapor bath is particularly serviceable in these cases. Rubbing in some mild ointment, allowing it to remain a few hours or longer, and then following it with a hot bath and green-soap washing, subsequently rinsing with simple warm or hot water, and then again anointing the surface with the ointment, will be found valuable in the more severe cases. An ointment such as the following may be employed for this purpose:

℞. Adipis benz., ℨj ;
Glycerinæ, ℨj ;
Ugt. petrolei, ℥j.

M. Ft. ugt.—Apply after bathing.
Or, ℞. Potassii iodidi, ℈j ;
Glycerinæ, ℨj ;
Adipis benz.,
Ol. bubuli, āā. ℥ss.

M. Ft. ugt.—Apply once daily.

Or any simple oil or salve may be substituted. In the more severe cases of the hystrix variety, in addition to the measures already described, it may be necessary to employ caustics, or even the knife, for the removal of the horny patches which form. For localized patches a 10 to 20 per cent. salicylic-acid plaster will be found useful. For the general scaliness the same drug in ointment form, 5 to 10 per cent., will prove of benefit.

Onychauxis.

Onychauxis (syn., onychogryphosis, hypertrophy of the nail) is seen as an idiopathic affection and also as a consequence or accompaniment of other diseases. The hypertrophy may consist in excessive length, width, thickness, or all combined. In addition to the increase in size, the nails may be abnormal as regards their shape, being twisted, conical or curved, their surface roughened, uneven or furrowed, and may also be attended with changes in color and consistence. If the hypertrophy increases the width to any marked extent, the parts encroached upon become irritated and inflamed, resulting in paronychia. At times the matrix may be the seat of inflammation, giving rise to structural changes in the nail-substance,—onychia. One, several, or all the nails, both of the fingers and toes, more frequently the latter, may be involved. Hypertrophy of the nail is met with in eczema, psoriasis, ichthyosis, leprosy and syphilis, and also as a result of the invasion of the vegetable parasites of tinea trichophytina and favus. The rare diseases lichen ruber and pityriasis rubra may also involve the nails. In syphilis infiltration of the matrix gives rise to the changes in the nail-substance. The nails in eczema and psoriasis are thickened and brittle, with an uneven surface. In some cases, especially those due to the vegetable parasites (onychomycosis) softening occurs.

Treatment depends upon the cause. Both constitutional and local means are in most cases employed. The nail should be softened and trimmed by means of the scissors or knife. Inflammation of the surrounding tissues is to be combated by the ordinary methods, and all sources of irritation avoided. Ingrowing nails should be cut transversely and not rounded, and the soft parts may be relieved of pressure and irritation by placing a piece of lint or cotton between the nail and skin-fold. In hypertrophy due to syphilis, psoriasis, and like diseases appropriate constitutional treatment is essential. In onychomycosis the parasiticides are to be applied.

Hypertrichosis.

Hypertrichosis (hirsuties), or hypertrophy of the hair, is a term applied to unnatural growth of hair, either as regards region, extent, age, or sex. It may be slight or excessive; thus, it may be universal, as in the so-called hairy people (homines pilosi), or limited, as upon a wart or nævus (nævus pilosus). The hairs themselves may be fine, coarse or of the average thickness. The hair of the scalp, eyebrows, axillæ, pubes, and beard in men may show excessive development either in thickness or length. Increased activity of hair-growth may take place in the fine downy hairs present over the greater portion of the surface. It may occur in the very young —in fact, may be congenital—and the growth may also appear on the face, arms, and other parts of females, resulting, of course, from a hypertrophy of the natural lanugo hairs.

It is difficult to give any definite or satisfactory explanation of the causes which give rise to unnatural growth of the hair. It is seen more frequently in persons of dark complexion, and may be congenital or acquired ; if the latter, the tendency to excessive development manifesting itself, as a rule, toward middle life. It is frequently associated in women with other masculine peculiarities, appearing especially at the climacteric period, and also noted in connection with the diseases of the utèrus and ovaries. It is sometimes seen in sterile women, also on the faces of insane women. Local stimulation or irritation will at times have a curative influence.

For general hirsuties there is no remedy. Hairy nævi, if small, may be treated by excision, or, if large, the hairs may be removed by electrolysis, as described below. The excessive growth seen about the faces of women is an annoying disfigurement, and such patients will submit to almost any treatment with the hope of relief. Extraction of hairs and shaving are frequently employed, but give only temporary relief. The method of removal by electrolysis is the only plan which promises permanent success. A fine needle in a suitable handle is attached to the negative pole of a galvanic battery, introduced into the hair-follicle alongside of the hair to the depth of the papilla, and the circuit made by the patient touching the sponge electrode attached to the positive pole. At the point of insertion the parts become blanched, and frothing appears at the aperture of the follicle, a result of the decomposition of the tissues at the point of the needle. The action should be continued for several seconds or longer, and then the circuit broken by the patient removing the hand from the sponge electrode, after which the needle is to be withdrawn. If the papilla has been destroyed, the hair may be readily extracted by the forceps with very little traction. In most cases, after the needle is withdrawn, or at times even before this, a wheal-like elevation appears at the point of insertion. In some cases the follicles may suppurate. Scarring, which is liable to take place, is to be guarded against. It occurs more markedly in some subjects than in others. Noticeable scarring, however, may generally be prevented if the operator is skilful. The operation is somewhat painful, the amount of pain varying with different persons, in some being slight, while in others it is severe. A current from four to twelve cells of a freshly-charged battery usually suffices.

Removal of hairs by the use of depilatories is considerably practised, but, as they are caustic in their nature, they should be employed with care. If prescribed, one made up of two drachms of barium sulphide and three drachms each of oxide of zinc and starch may be recommended. Enough water is added to the powder to make a paste, which is thinly laid on the parts for ten or fifteen minutes. Heat of skin or a burning sensation soon occurs, upon the advent of which the paste is immediately to be scraped off, the parts thoroughly cleansed, and a mild ointment applied. As with extraction and shaving, this method is only temporary in its effects.

Sclerema Neonatorum.

Sclerema neonatorum, or sclerema of the new-born, is a disease of infancy manifesting itself usually at birth, characterized by a diffuse stiffness, rigidity or hardness of the integument, accompanied by coldness, œdema, discoloration, lividity, and general circulatory disturbance. Frequently it is congenital. It usually begins on the lower extremities, extending upward and invading the trunk, arms, and face. The skin is reddish, purplish or brownish, glossy, and tense or stretched, causing more or less rigidity and stiffness. The surface is usually cold, and upon pressure œdema, together with an infiltrated state of the tissues, is noted. When the disease is general the body bears resemblance to a half-frozen corpse. The child is unable to move, respires feebly, and usually perishes in a few days. The disease is very rare. It is in most cases found associated with pneumonia or with affections of the circulatory apparatus. The causes are obscure. After death the condition of the skin undergoes but little change, the induration remaining; on incision a considerable quantity of serous fluid is poured out, when the tissues become softer and resemble ordinary œdematous tissue. The treatment should consist of warm applications, frictions, and like measures. The prognosis is unfavorable.

Scleroderma.

Scleroderma, known also as sclerema and scleriasis, is an acute or chronic disease, characterized by a diffuse, more or less pigmented, rigid, stiffened or hardened, hide-bound condition of the skin. It was first described by Alibert with the name sclérèmie des adultes, since which time many cases have been recorded. The first symptoms consist of more or less rigidity or induration of the integument, which may increase rapidly, or, as is usually the case, slowly, until the region affected becomes hard and bound down to the tissues beneath. In some cases febrile symptoms, œdema, and pigmentation precede the induration, but usually the process asserts itself insidiously, the first symptom noted by the patient being the sclerosis. In marked cases the skin is rigid, tight, or immovable, and is firm or positively hard to the touch, as though frozen, but without the sensation of cold. In some cases it may seem wooden or as though undergoing petrifaction. It is hide-bound, and cannot be made to glide over the structures beneath, nor can it be taken up between the fingers. The skin, owing to the immobility, becomes set or fixed, the natural lines and wrinkles disappearing, causing persons to look younger. The induration is diffuse, being neither circumscribed nor defined, and generally occupies a considerable area, the face, neck, back, chest, and upper extremities being the regions most frequently involved. It may occupy variously sized and shaped areas, for the most part irregular in outline, or it may appear in the form of narrow or broad bands or elongated patches, which usually become more or less shrunken and sunken atrophic lesions.

The surface of the integument in scleroderma is usually on a level with the neighboring healthy skin, except in the later stages where atrophy has occurred, and is generally smooth and shining. Pigmentation is in

most cases a marked symptom, being yellowish or brownish, in the form
of patches, giving a dirty, chloasmic appearance to the part. Subjective symptoms are usually wanting, although there may be numbness or cramp-like pains, especially when the limbs are the seat of the
disease. The skin in all cases feels contracted, tightly stretched or too
short. The disease may be limited, as is generally the case, or it may
occupy the greater portion, or even the whole, of the body. It is usually
symmetrical. It pursues a variable course, at times acute, but more frequently chronic, extending over a period of years or throughout life.
Sooner or later resolution and recovery set in, or atrophic changes take
place, characterized by a wasting or a condensation of the integument
and of the subjacent tissues, causing contraction and deformity, which are
especially marked when occurring about joints. As a rule, the general
health remains good. The disease in some cases is accompanied by
patches of morphœa, which affection is regarded by some authors as being
merely a circumscribed variety of scleroderma.

The causes are obscure. The disease is rare, and is encountered oftener
in women than in men, and occurs usually in early adult or middle life.
Sudden changes of temperature, exposure to wet or cold, and violent
impressions on the nervous system have been cited as causes. The
anatomy of the disease has been studied by various observers, but with
different results, in the majority of cases slight structural changes only
having been found. Both the true skin and the subcutaneous connective tissue are the seat of the process, showing a marked increase of
the connective tissue, with thickening and condensation of the fibres.
The disease may be viewed as a tropho-neurosis. The diagnosis, as a
rule, presents no difficulty. From morphœa, to which it is closely allied,
it may be distinguished by its tendency to involve large areas, occupying
sometimes the greater portion or the whole of the integument, whereas
morphœa usually appears in smaller lesions. Scleroderma manifests
itself diffusely and without lines of demarcation; morphœa is circumscribed, and in its early stage is surrounded by a pinkish border. Scleroderma is always characterized by stiffness or hardness, whereas morphœa
is usually soft or firm. In scleroderma the skin is merely rigid or hard
in the beginning, whereas in morphœa there is hyperæmia and only slight
induration.

Concerning the treatment of this disease there is but little to be said.
Constitutional remedies, such as arsenic, quinine, and cod-liver oil, together
with the employment of stimulating oily or fatty applications, frictions,
and electricity are indicated, though it is difficult to state their intrinsic
value. The course and termination of the disease varies. In some cases
spontaneous involution sets in sooner or later, while in other instances the
process continues to progress, and lasts throughout life.

Morphœa.

Morphœa, formerly known as keloid of Addison, is characterized by
one or more rounded, ovalish or elongate, coin-sized patches, which, as a
rule, are circumscribed and clearly defined. At first they are hyperæmic
and pinkish, becoming as the process advances pale yellowish or whitish,

with a faint pinkish or lilac border made up of very minute injected capillaries. The patch may be slightly elevated or puffed in the beginning,
but later is on a level with the surrounding skin, or even somewhat
depressed. When typically developed it is either soft or firm to the
touch, or, more rarely, leathery or brawny. The surface is usually smooth,
and may be shining and have an atrophic appearance. Not infrequently
it resembles in color and in look a piece of cut bacon or ivory laid in the
skin. Around the patch there is usually, in addition to the hyperæmic
border, more or less diffuse, mottled yellowish or brownish pigmentation.
The disease exhibits no disposition to symmetry, but not infrequently it
manifests itself over nerve-tracts. The regions commonly invaded are
the face, neck, chest, mammæ, back, abdomen, arms, and thighs. The
lesions pursue a variable though usually chronic course, lasting, as a rule,
years. There is always a marked tendency to varied atrophic changes,
which in most cases appear early, the skin becoming thin, shrivelled, or
parchment-like, later being bound down to the tissues beneath, forming
cicatriform, keloidal lesions, which may cause contraction and deformity,
with, in some cases, wasting and general atrophy, more particularly of
the extremities.

In addition to the usual characteristic circumscribed patches described,
there may exist distinctly atrophic lesions consisting of small pit-like
depressions resembling scars; also, reddish or bluish, tortuous, short or
long, large and minute, dilated, superficial cutaneous blood-vessels and
telangiectases, together with smooth, glazed, whitish, slightly-depressed
spots or grooved streaks—true maculæ et striæ atrophicæ. Accompanying
these various lesions there is usually considerable diffuse or patchy yellowish or brownish pigmentation. The process in some cases is simple
as regards the lesions, but not infrequently it is complex, being characterized, as indicated, by a variety of lesions in different stages of evolution. The course is chronic, extending in the majority of cases over
years. The disease in some cases eventually tends to spontaneous
recovery; and this is all the more remarkable considering that atrophy
has existed. The disease is met with more frequently in females than in
males. Impaired nerve-power is without doubt the important factor in its
production. Concerning the relation of morphœa to scleroderma, it may
be said that these affections are closely allied, and that they may occur
together. The pathological anatomy of the characteristic patches varies
with the stage of the disease. In the early stages there is shrinkage or
atrophy of the papillary layer, with condensation of the connective tissue
of the corium. Crocker further noted marked cell-infiltration around
the sebaceous glands, hair-follicles, and vessels, and in the later stages the
transformation of these cells into fibrillar tissue, its contraction, and the
consequent obliteration of blood-vessels, with atrophy of the sebaceous
and sweat glands.

Morphœa is to be distinguished from scleroderma, from vitiligo, and
from the anæsthetic patches of leprosy. In appearance morphœa and
leprosy possess features in common, and it is probable that they are both
due to the same cause—namely, perverted innervation. As a rule, no
difficulty will arise in the diagnosis, for the reason that in leprosy other
symptoms of that disease will almost invariably be present.

To be viewed as a variety or form of morphœa, we may mention hemiatrophia facialis, or unilateral atrophy of the face, which affection consists of a variable degree of atrophy of the skin and deeper structures, the cutaneous lesions being the same as those in morphœa. The neurotic origin of the disease in this case is plain.

A general tonic treatment, with the long-continued use of such remedies as arsenic, quinine, cod-liver oil, iodide of potassium, and electricity, is called for, most reliance being placed upon arsenic. Good results sometimes follow its administration. The prognosis should always be guarded

Elephantiasis.

Elephantiasis, or elephantiasis arabum (also called pachydermia, Barbadoes leg, elephant leg), is a chronic hypertrophic disease of the skin and subcutaneous tissue, characterized by enlargement and deformity of the part affected, accompanied by lymphangitis, swelling, œdema, thickening, induration, pigmentation, and more or less papillary growth. The legs and genitalia, especially the former, are favorite localities for its development; about the latter, the penis, scrotum, and clitoris are most frequently involved. It begins with an inflammation of the parts, erysipelatous in character, attended with febrile disturbance, swelling, pain, heat, redness, and lymphangitis. The inflammation may have its starting-point in a local lesion, as a wound or scar, or, as is usually the case, manifests itself without any apparent cause. Similar attacks occur more or less frequently, after each of which the part remains increased in size. After a year or longer, during which time repeated attacks may have taken place, considerable increase in size is noted : the part is swollen, œdematous, and hard, and the skin hypertrophied, fissured, pigmented, and the papillæ enlarged and prominent. Later, the hypertrophy becomes still more marked ; the part is often enormously enlarged and swollen, the skin rough, fissured, and warty. In Eastern countries the disease assumes huge proportions. Eczematous inflammation may coexist and complicate the appearance. The fissures may be slight or large and deep, the normal lines and folds of the surface exaggerated, with more or less maceration of the epidermis taking place, especially about the folds. Ulcers sooner or later tend to form, developing usually from varicose veins, while scales and crusts may also be present. Pain varies, being usually marked during the inflammatory attacks.

Elephantiasis is met with in all parts of the world, but much more frequently in tropical climates, especially about the West Coast of Africa, Brazil, the West Indies, and particularly India, and to less extent in Mediterranean regions and Arabia. In our own country, and also in Europe, it is not common. It rarely occurs before puberty. Heredity has no influence, nor is it contagious. It is commonly observed among the poor and neglected.

The immediate cause of the disease is to be found in inflammation and obstruction of the lymphatics. This obstruction is, according to late investigations, probably due to the presence in the lymphatic vessels of the parasite filaria and its ova. The filaria—a microscopic thread-worm —has been found in large numbers adhering to the walls of the lymphatics and blood-vessels, but is discoverable only during certain hours of the day. The parasite has also been found in lymph-scrotum, a disease closely related to, if not identical with, elephantiasis.

The great mass of the growth in the disease is made up of hypertrophic connective tissue and connective-tissue new growth. All parts of the skin and the subcutaneous tissues share in the hypertrophy. Papillary enlarge. ment is usually a marked feature. The lymphatic glands are swollen and enlarged and the lymphatic vessels prominent. There is marked œde. matous infiltration, lymphatic in character. As a result of pressure, the glandular structures of the skin are atrophied or destroyed, the fat atrophied, and the muscles degenerated. The walls of the blood-vessels are thickened.

In well-developed cases of elephantiasis the symptoms are so character. istic that the disease is readily recognized. Recurrent attacks of ery. sipelatous inflammation of the leg or genitalia will point, with prob. ability, to a development of the disease, even before marked hypertrophy or the clinical features are developed. As regards the outcome of the disease, if the case comes under treatment in the early months of its development the process may be checked or held in abeyance; later, after the affection has become well established, but little more than palliation can be effected.

The inflammatory attacks are to be treated with rest in bed, hot or cold applications, lead-water, and similar measures. Quinine and iron internally, especially the former, are of value. Potassium iodide has also been well spoken of. Climatic change, especially in the early stages, may prove of marked advantage. After the acute symptoms of the erysip. elatous attacks have subsided inunctions of iodine or mercurial ointments may be employed to soften the skin and promote absorption. The parts should also be firmly bandaged, either the roller bandage, or, preferably, one of rubber, being used. Instrumental compression and ligation of the main artery of the limb have been employed, at times, with diminution in the size of the part; also excision of a portion of the sciatic nerve was practised in a single case by Morton with reduction in the size of the limb, but these methods of treatment are not to be recommended. Lately, the use of the strong, constant current has been extolled as having a beneficial effect. Elephantiasis involving the genitalia is, if the disease is well advanced, to be treated by the knife, amputation of the parts being practised.

Dermatolysis.

Dermatolysis consists of a more or less circumscribed hypertrophy of the cutaneous and subcutaneous structures, characterized by softness and looseness of the skin and a tendency to hang dependently. It may be slight or extensive, and may be limited to a certain region or show itself simul-taneously in several different parts. The integument is thickened, bulky, superabundant, and to a greater or less extent hangs down in folds. The hypertrophy is general over the area affected; the glandular structures, connective tissue, muscular fibres, pigment, and the subcutaneous areolar tissue share in the process. The surface is usually soft and pliable to the touch, but is uneven, in consequence of the hypertrophy of the follicles and the natural folds and rugæ. As a result of the increase in pigment the skin is more or less brownish in color. The tissues may develop to an enormous size, and the redundant parts may hang down in several folds, overlapping one another and forming a cloak to the parts below.

Dermatolysis may be congenital or may not develop until after puberty. It is a simple hypertrophy involving the integument and all its component parts, especially the subcutaneous connective tissue. The causes which bring about this condition are not known. It appears to be closely allied to molluscum fibrosum, the two diseases sometimes occurring together. It is not malignant, but its presence impedes locomotion and its weight is a discomfort.

The affection is classified under the head of elephantiasis by German writers, but the clinical features and course of the two diseases are entirely different. Elephantiasis telangiectodes is a term that has been given to a form of simple hypertrophy of the skin in which a marked new growth of vascular tissue takes place. In connection with this disease mention may be made of the condition characterizing the so-called rubber or elastic-skin man. In this condition there is no hypertrophy. The mobility and elasticity of the skin are probably due to a peculiar and abnormal looseness of the subcutaneous areolar tissue. It is to be looked upon as a congenital deformity. The treatment of dermatolysis is by excision when this operation is practicable.

CLASS V.—ATROPHIES.

Albinismus.

ALBINISMUS is a term employed to designate that condition in which there is congenital absence of the normal pigment. It may be localized (albinismus partialis) or general (albinismus universalis). Persons in whom it is universal are called albinos. They are characterized by more or less complete absence of pigment in the skin, hair, iris, and choroid. The skin is milky-white, with, usually, a pinkish tint; the hair is white or yellowish, fine, thin, soft, and silky. The eyes are sensitive to light, the pupils appear red and contract and dilate continuously; oscillation of the eyeballs is noted, and also rapid and constant winking. These individuals are usually physically and mentally deficient, with a tendency to pulmonary disease.

Partial albinismus is seen more frequently in the negro. There may be one or more whitish or pinkish-white patches, variable as to size and shape, occurring upon any region. The skin is normal with the exception of loss of pigment. The hairs existing upon the spots are blanched. The eyes show no loss of pigment. The negroes in whom the patches occur are termed pied, or piebald. In exceptional instances a redeposit of pigment has been observed. Albinismus is not confined to any race or climate, and is comparatively rare. Its causes are not known. It is frequently inherited.

Vitiligo.

Vitiligo (known also as acquired leucoderma or leucopathia) is a disease consisting of one or more usually sharply-defined, rounded or irregularly-shaped, variously-sized and distributed, smooth, whitish spots, whose borders usually show an increase in the normal amount of pigmentation. The patches may appear on any region, the backs of the hands and the trunk being favorite localities. The disease begins by the appearance of small pale spots, which gradually increase in size, new patches showing themselves from time to time. They are well defined in outline, the pale milky whiteness of the patches contrasting markedly with the surrounding pigmented skin. The increased pigmentation of the borders is almost an invariable accompaniment of the disease, and may be slight or excessive, gradually becoming less intense as the healthy skin is approached. The patches are smooth, on a level with the surrounding skin, rounded, ovalish, or irregular. They may be small or large, depending upon their age and also upon the rapidity of their growth. If several coalesce, as is frequently the case, large irregular patches are formed. The secretion of the sweat and sebaceous glands and the sensibility of the skin are not disturbed. With the exception of the loss of color the skin is normal. Hairs included in the patches may or may not be whitened. There are no subjective symptoms.

As a rule, the progress of the disease is slow, years frequently elapsing before the patches attain a large area. In some instances, after reaching a certain size, they remain stationary, either for a time or permanently. In most cases, however, the disease is progressive. In rare instances the skin has been known to become normal again. The sole annoyance the disease occasions is the disfigurement, and this is often striking. The spots are but little, if at all, affected by the sun, except that they are rendered more conspicuous by the bronzing of the normal skin which its rays cause. As a rule, the affection first shows itself in early adult life, although it may appear earlier or later. Both sexes, whether of a light or dark complexion, are attacked. The general health is usually good. It is attributed to a disturbance of innervation. Alopecia areata and morphœa have been seen in association with it.

Anatomically, it consists of both an atrophy and a hypertrophy of the normal pigment of the skin, the pale patch resulting from the former, and the pigmented border from the latter. There is no textural change in the skin. It may be mistaken for chloasma, tinea versicolor, and morphœa. In the former diseases, when several patches are close together, the normal skin between appears, in comparison, pale, and if cursorily examined might be mistaken for the pale patches of vitiligo, while the surrounding yellowish patches of tinea versicolor or chloasma may appear as the pigmented borders. - In tinea versicolor the patches are slightly scaly. In morphœa there is always structural change.

Treatment in most cases is unsatisfactory. The functions and the state of the general health must receive attention. In some cases arsenic long continued proves of benefit. It is the only known remedy of any value. The disfigurement produced by the patches can in a measure be removed. For this purpose the darkened border should receive appropriate applications, such as are used in the removal of patches of chloasma. The white spots sometimes may be made darker by the application of cantharides, promoting capillary congestion.

Canities.

Canities is a term applied to grayness or blanching of the hair. Loss of pigment in the hair may be partial or general. It may occur early in life or, as is commonly the case, as the result of old age. The change in color may take place throughout the entire hair or in parts. The color varies from slight blanching to white. It is usually grayish. In rare instances the color is to a moderate degree regained in summer. Grayness of the hair in the young—canities præmatura—is exceptional; in the old —canities senilis—it is constant, individuals differing considerably, however, as to the time of life at which the change begins. After the hair has become gray it rarely recovers its coloring matter, although occasionally in the young, after the lapse of years, the hair may again become dark. In those of a dark complexion the loss of pigment occurs, as a rule, much earlier than in those whose hair is of the lighter shades. Usually considerable time is required in the complete change to gray or white, but authentic cases are on record in which the change has taken place in the course of a night or within a few days. The pathology is obscure.

Canities, as may be readily inferred, depends upon a deficient production of pigment. The causes which gives rise to this deficiency are not understood. Hereditary influence is often noticeable. Conditions which impair the general nutrition, such as chlorosis, anæmia, fevers, etc., and those that hinder the local nutrition, as seborrhœa and inflammatory diseases of the parts, may possibly have some influence. In sudden blanching of the hair fright, intense anxiety, and the like are the usual causes. Treatment, whether internal or external, has no effect in preventing the loss of pigment or in restoring it. Dyeing, however, may be practised, and the condition masked; but it is not to be recommended, as the skin of the scalp becomes discolored and the nutrition of the hair interfered with.

Alopecia.

Alopecia consists of partial or complete deficiency of hair, irrespective of cause. There are several varieties, named according to the causes which have produced the affection. Thus, congenital alopecia consists of a partial or complete absence of hair, either over the entire surface or confined to a portion. In some instances there is scantinesss or irregular development. In rare cases there is complete absence of the hair, microscopical examination failing to show the existence of hair-bulbs. In cases of congenital deficiency there usually exists an hereditary predisposition.

Senile alopecia and senile calvities are terms applied to the baldness of advanced years. With the loss of hair there is usually atrophy of the other cutaneous structures. In these cases the hairs, as a rule, first turn gray, become dry and thin, and fall out, with no tendency to a new growth. The condition is seen upon the scalp, beginning usually at the crown; in occasional instances other parts of the body may also sooner or later show more or less atrophy of the hairy appendage. Upon the scalp, the skin, which is more or less free of the hair, becomes atrophied, smooth and glossy. The alterations in the cutaneous structures in senile baldness consist of marked atrophy of the sebaceous glands, of the hair-follicles and of the skin itself. The affection is common in men, but is compara-tively infrequent in women. No satisfactory reason can be assigned for this. Idiopathic premature alopecia is the term applied to the baldness which begins to manifest itself about the age of twenty-five or thirty. The hairs may fall out rapidly or the loss may take place slowly. In these cases the normal hairs are usually replaced with finer, thinner, and shorter hairs, but finally even these eventually cease to be reproduced, and more or less alopecia results. There is no sebor-rhœa, and the skin shows no other atrophic change. As a rule, sev-eral years elapse before the condition becomes marked. The location affected is the same as in senile alopecia, and the same statement may be made as to its frequency in the two sexes. According to microscopical examination, there is an increase in the connective tissue, compressing the blood-vessels, and thus interfering with the blood-supply of the parts.

Symptomatic premature alopecia includes all those forms of alopecia which are the result of disease, either local or general. Falling of the hair is frequent after fevers and other systemic diseases. Mental anxiety, ner-vous exhaustion, and depraved conditions of the general health may also cause varying degrees of alopecia. In these cases the shedding of the hair usually takes place rapidly, constituting defluvium capillorum. With a disappearance of the exciting cause there is usually a regrowth, but this is not always the case, as not infrequently the baldness is permanent. Among local diseases which give rise to baldness, chronic seborrhœa is the most important. As a result of the seborrhœa, atrophy of the glands occurs, and alopecia sooner or later sets in. Many other local affections, as lupus erythematosus, erysipelas, variola, tinea tonsurans, and tinea favosa, are at times attended with loss of hair. Syphilitic alopecia may occur at two different periods of that disease. It is noted as one of the early symptoms, and later as the result of the general cachexia, or in localized patches as the result of ulceration and destruction of the skin. The alo-pecia appearing as a secondary symptom of the disease may be slight or complete baldness may take place, but in either case the loss is rarely permanent if the patient is under proper treatment. As a rule, in the course of a few months the hair is reproduced. The alopecia resulting from ulcerative lesions is permanent.

The treatment of the various varieties of alopecia named depends, as will be readily inferred, upon the etiological causes. Senile alopecia is rarely amenable to treatment. Idiopathic premature alopecia may fre-quently be benefited by therapeutic measures. The general health is to be looked after. In these cases arsenic in moderate doses long continued may prove of some value. The external treatment has in view the pro-motion of the nutrition of the skin, which is attained by the use of stim-ulating applications for the purpose of increasing the vascular supply. The treatment of symptomatic premature alopecia is that of the primary disease. The external remedies and formulæ which are employed in cases of alopecia for their stimulating effects will be found in detail under the head of alopecia areata.

Alopecia Areata.

Alopecia areata (syn. area celsi, alopecia circumscripta, porrigo decalvans, tinea decalvans) is an atrophic disease of the hairy system, characterized by the more or less sudden appearance of one or more circumscribed, variously sized and shaped, whitish bald patches. The scalp is the region most frequently the seat of the disease, but other hairy parts, especially the face in the male, are often invaded, and even the whole surface may be involved. Occurring upon the scalp, one or several patches may be present, which are usually rounded and circumscribed. The hair may fall out suddenly without any previous signs of weakening, the individual awaking in the morning to discover an area of partial or complete baldness on the scalp; or, as is usually the case, the loss of hair takes place insidiously or more gradually, several days or weeks elapsing before the bald patch is of sufficient size to attract observation. The parietal region is perhaps most frequently involved. In most cases but a single patch appears at first, but this usually is followed by others. The areas incline to grow larger and larger, and, as a rule, finally coalesce, eventually the whole scalp, with possibly the exception of a tuft or patch here and there, being bald. In most cases, however, the patches, after reaching a certain size, remain stationary.

The skin of the affected areas has a smooth, whitish, polished, atrophied appearance, and is usually entirely devoid of hair or with a few straggling long or short hairs scattered over it. The orifices of the follicles become less appreciable, and the skin is thin, and resembles that seen in the baldness of advanced years. The hairs surrounding the affected area are usually found to be firmly seated in their follicles, but if the patch has not ceased enlarging they may be loose and readily extracted. In some cases about the border are noted a few short atrophied hairs, resembling the short, broken-off hairs of tinea tonsurans. At first the skin may be slightly puffed, but usually it is on a level with the surrounding parts; later, it may be somewhat depressed, as though atrophied. It is neither scaly nor inflamed. Slight anæsthesia may be present. There are, as a rule, no subjective symptoms. Involving the regions of the moustache and eyebrows, the clinical phenomena are essentially the same as when affecting the scalp. In those cases in which universal loss of hair results, the process usually begins in the same way, first appearing as well-marked areas, which rapidly increase in size; new patches are added, coalescence results, and eventually the entire surface is involved. After the disease has come to a standstill it may so remain indefinitely, or lanugo hairs may appear from time to time, reach an inch or a fraction thereof in length, may become slightly darkened, and then fall out. Finally, in favorable cases, instead of falling out, their growth continues; they become dark, and recovery takes place. In these latter cases the disease may have existed several months before signs of a permanent regrowth show themselves; on the other hand, several years may have elapsed.

The disease is met with in both sexes, in children and adults, and among the wealthy and the poor. It is not a rare disease, nor is it common. Impaired nutrition as the result of functional nerve-disturbance is probably the important etiological factor, leading to the view that the affection is a trophoneurosis. It is often seen to follow neuralgias, nervous shock, and debility. Morphœa and vitiligo, both diseases of a neurotic character, are occasionally seen in association with it. In the greater number of cases no appreciable cause is discoverable. It is not parasitic, nor is it contagious. Microscopic examinations have given negative results, the skin remaining normal and the glandular structures unchanged. Atrophy of the hair shafts and bulbs, and occasionally breaking and bulging of the hairs, are usually noted. The atrophic condition of the bulbs is similar to that seen in hairs which have reached the end of their normal life.

The disease with which alopecia areata may, by the inexperienced, be sometimes confounded is tinea tonsurans, and yet the incomplete baldness, the short, stumpy, split, gnawed-off-looking hairs, the scaliness, the increased prominence of the follicular openings, and the history and course which characterize ringworm, are entirely different from the clinical signs of alopecia areata. Where there is doubt the microscope is to be employed. It is to be remembered, also, that ringworm of the scalp is not seen in individuals past the age of puberty. The peculiar clinical features of the disease will distinguish it from other forms of baldness.

TREATMENT.—The uncertainty of the duration and ultimate termination of the disease is to be kept in view in expressing an opinion. It may be stated, with a degree of positiveness, however, that in young individuals the eventual result is, as a rule, good ; but occurring in persons past adult age, the prognosis as to a regrowth is not so favorable, and becomes less so as age increases. The length of time elapsing in favorable cases before the hair reappears, as already mentioned, is uncertain it may be several months, or on the other hand, as many years. On both points proper and persevering treatment has sometimes a material influence.

Local and general measures are called for. Of the two, the general treatment is the more important, and among remedies employed arsenic stands prominent. It should be continued for months. In addition, such tonics as iron, quinine, cod-liver oil are to be advised as the case demands. In some instances potassium iodide in moderate doses is of service.

External treatment is of value, and is in most cases to be advised. The object in view is a stimulation of the vascular supply, and through this an improvement in the nutrition of the papillæ and hairs. The same remedies in various combinations are employed as in the treatment of other forms of alopecia. Rubefacients and irritants, such as alcohol, the essential oils, sulphur, tar, cantharides, corrosive sublimate and other salts of mercury, carbolic acid, iodine, turpentine, ammonia, chrysarobin, and spiritus saponatus kalinus, are variously used. They are, as a rule, employed either in alcoholic or ethereal fluids or in the form of oils or ointments. It is to be borne in mind that the scalp tolerates strong remedies. The applications are to be made once or twice daily, according to the demands of the case, and with considerable friction, employing for the application a flannel rag or mop. Such remedies as iodine, corrosive sublimate, are usually to be painted or dabbed on.

Sulphur, two to four drachms to the ounce; corrosive sublimate, one to four grains to the ounce of alcohol; tar, ol. cadini, or ol. rusci, one to four drachms to the ounce of alcohol or ointment,—are all serviceable remedies. Cantharides and capsicum are stimulating, and may be prescribed as in the following formula:

> ℞. Tinct. cantharidis,
> Tinct. capsici, *āā.* f ℥iss;
> Olei ricini, f ℨij;
> Alcoholis, f ℨvj;
> Spts. rosmarini, f ℨij. **M.**

The following, containing the oil of mace, is also serviceable:

> ℞. Olei myristicæ exp., f ℨij;
> Alcoholis,
> Spiritus lavandulæ, *āā.* f ℥ij. **M.**

Carbolic acid may be used as follows:

> ℞. Acidi carbolici cryst., ℨij;
> Alcoholis, f ℥iij;
> Olei ricini, f ℨiv;
> Spts. rosmarini, f ℨiv. **M.**

Aqua ammoniæ may sometimes be employed with benefit, as in the formula recommended by Wilson:

> ℞. Olei amygdalæ dulc.,
> Aquæ ammoniæ fort., *āā.* f ℥ss;
> Spiritus rosmarini, f ℥ij;
> Olei limonis, f ℨss. **M.**

Blistering the affected areas by means of a cantharidal vesicating fluid, frequently repeated, sometimes proves of advantage. Friction with oil of turpentine once or twice daily may in some cases be practised with benefit; when the skin becomes sensitive it should be discontinued for a few days. Chrysarobin in ointment, 5 to 15 per cent. strength, is an active irritant which may be cautiously employed. Oleate of mercury, 10 to 30 per cent. strength, rubbed in once or twice daily, is useful in some cases, and the same may be said of the other mercurial ointments, such as citrine and white precipitate ointments. Electricity sometimes proves of service, and may be tried in obstinate cases.

Atrophia Pilorum Propria.

Atrophia pilorum propria, or atrophy of the hair, may be either symptomatic or idiopathic. As a symptomatic affection it is seen as a result of such diseases of the scalp as seborrhœa and the parasitic affections, and also following various constitutional diseases, such as syphilis and fevers, in consequence of impaired nutrition. The hairs become dry, brittle, atrophied, and exhibit a marked disposition to split up. Idiopathic atrophy of the hair is characterized in one of its forms (fragilitas crinium) by a brittle state of the hair-shaft, an irregular and uneven formation of its structure, and a tendency to separate into its filaments. It is seen about the scalp and beard, and may be slight or markedly developed. A somewhat similar condition of the hair of the beard has been described (Duhring), in which the bulb is atrophied and the shaft split up, fission taking place within the follicles, causing irritation of the skin. Another form (trichorexis nodosa) of the idiopathic affection is characterized by shining, semi-transparent, rounded swellings of the hair-shaft, seen usually upon the beard and moustache. At first sight they look not unlike the ova of pediculi; one or several may be present upon a single hair. Upon close inspection they are seen to be localized swellings of the hair-structure. At these points the hairs readily break off, leaving a brush-like end; if many of these are present, which is usually the case, they give the impression that the hair has been singed. The medullary as well as the cortical substance, as determined by microscopical examination, is swollen, and in consequence of the swelling of the medullary portion the cortex is burst and split into filaments. In regard to the cause of idiopathic atrophy of the hair nothing is known, and but little can be done in the way of treatment. Shaving and cutting the hair have exceptionally been followed by a normal growth.

Atrophia Unguis.

Atrophy of the nail is commonly an acquired affection. It is characterized by deficient development or growth of the nail-substance, as shown by a thin, brittle, soft, crumbly or worm-eaten condition. The nail may be pale, opaque or dark in color. It may occur in consequence of injury or disease of the nerves of the part, or as a result of some general disease, as syphilis, or from general debility. Eczema, psoriasis, and allied diseases, which may be productive of hypertrophy of the nails, may also cause atrophic changes. Treatment of atrophy of the nail depends upon the cause. In simple atrophy, and also in that due to eczema and psoriasis, arsenic is of value.

Atrophia Cutis.

Atrophy of the skin, or atrophia cutis propria, in its various forms is not infrequently encountered. It may occur as an idiopathic affection, or as a symptom in connection with other well-known diseases. Thus, as an example of the former condition the well-known striæ atrophicæ may be cited, while lupus, syphilis, and tinea favosa are sometimes followed by symptomatic atrophy. Injuries to nerves are also at times followed by more or less cutaneous atrophy, usually in connection with wasting of the subcutaneous structures, the skin becoming thin, dry, shrivelled, and yellowish or brownish in color. Atrophy of the skin may be general, as in the senile form, or localized, as in morphœa. Where degenerative atrophy exists the skin is usually somewhat hardened, yellowish or whitish in color, and has a waxy, fatty appearance. In the condition known as glossy skin, generally seen upon the fingers, the skin is reddish, smooth, and shining as though varnished, the affection resembling chilblains. The hairs are usually shed, and excoriations or fissures often exist. It is accompanied with pain of a burning character.

Cases of general idiopathic atrophy of the skin have from time to time been reported, the disease in almost all instances being more marked in some localities than in others, occurring in the form of more or less extensive patches. The disease originally described by Hebra and Kaposi with the name xeroderma, or parchment-skin disease, may here be referred to. The lesions consist of numerous disseminated pigment-spots, resembling freckles; telangiectases, or minute congeries of blood-vessels; atrophic macules of variable size; with more or less shrinking and contraction of skin, followed in most cases by epitheliomatous tumors and ulceration. The disease almost invariably begins in early years, is prone to show itself in several children of the same family, and lasts during life. The advanced stages of scleroderma and morphœa likewise show marked atrophic changes, which, however, will be considered in speaking of those diseases.

Senile Atrophy.—This form of atrophy, taking place as the result of old age, may be simple or degenerative, both usually occurring together. The integument becomes thin and wasted, the surface being dry, wrinkled and more or less discolored by pigmentation, with loss of hair. In degenerative atrophy the connective tissue of the corium becomes changed into a fine or coarse granular matter or into a homogeneous vitreous mass. Fatty metamorphosis and marked pigmentary deposits are also common.

Maculæ et Striæ Atrophicæ.—Atrophic streaks and spots may occur idiopathically or symptomatically. The idiopathic form is that most frequently encountered, and occurs without known cause, generally making its appearance insidiously. It is characterized by lines or streaks constituting the so-called linear atrophy, striæ atrophicæ; or by spots, maculæ atrophicæ. The streaks are more frequently met with, and consist of irregular curved or tortuous lesions, usually about a line in width and of variable length, running parallel with one another. The macules are rounded or ovalish, varying in size from a pinhead to a finger-nail. Both are smooth and glistening, and the skin is thinned and scar-like. They are slightly depressed or grooved, and possess a pinkish, whitish, or bluish-gray color. They may appear upon any region, but the abdomen, buttocks, and thighs are the favorite localities. They pursue a slow course over a period of years or a lifetime, occasioning no inconvenience. The first stage of either variety of the disease is characterized by erythema, the lesion being reddish, hyperamic, and slightly raised or puffed. This sooner or later disappears, followed by depression and atrophy.

The symptomatic form of the affection is usually noted to take place as the result of extreme distension of the cutaneous structures. It occurs sometimes in obese subjects, and in the latter stages of pregnancy upon the abdomen and mammæ, and over large abdominal and other tumors where the skin is greatly stretched, constituting the so-called lineæ albicantes.

CLASS VI.—NEW GROWTHS.[1]

Keloid.

KELOID is a connective-tissue new growth, characterized by one or more irregularly-shaped, variously-sized, elevated, smooth, firm, somewhat elastic, pale-reddish, cicatriform lesions. It ordinarily begins as a nodule or tubercle, pea- or bean-sized, which slowly, usually in the course of years, increases in dimension. When fully developed, the growth appears as an ovalish, elongated, cylindrical, fungoid or crab-shaped patch, occupying usually an area of one or several inches, distinctly elevated, sharply defined, and firmly implanted in the skin. In some cases the lesion does not exceed the size of a pea or a bean. The color is usually pinkish-white. The surface is smooth, shining, and commonly devoid of hair, with no tendency to scaliness or ulceration, and generally marked by ramifying vessels. It is firm and elastic to the touch. The disease sometimes appears in the form of streaks or lines. It is seen most frequently upon the sternum, although other regions, as the neck, mamma, ear, sides of the trunk, or back are often invaded. It is more common in the colored race. The lesion is usually single, though several may coexist. Itching to a slight degree is sometimes present, and more or less pain, especially on pressure, may also exist. Depending upon the origin of the growth, whether arising spontaneously or upon the site of various injuries of the skin, keloid is termed, respectively, spontaneous, or true, and cicatricial, or false. Clinically and pathologically, both varieties are the same.

It is often met with as the result of burns, cuts, flogging, and all ulcerative affections. Not infrequently it takes its origin in the scars of acne and variola; occasionally it is seen to develop on the lobe of the ear, taking its start at the point where the ear has been pierced. Pathologically, the lesion is a connective-tissue new growth, made up of a dense, fibrous mass of tissue, whitish in color, having its seat in the corium. The clinical features of keloid are so characteristic that no difficulty is experienced in recognizing it. The course of the disease is chronic, usually lasting throughout life; in exceptional instances spontaneous involution has been noted.

Treatment is usually negative. Removal by excision or caustics is, as a rule, followed by a return of the growth, and sometimes in an aggravated form. If its destruction or extirpation is decided upon, it should not be done while the growth is still progressive. Improvement has been reported by Vidal from multiple linear scarification. If the formation is painful, various anodyne applications may be made. Iodine, mercurial, and lead plasters may be tried with the object of promoting absorption. Painting the growth with a solution composed of potassium iodide one drachm, and an ounce each of soft soap and alcohol, followed by the application of lead plaster spread on a piece of soft leather, has been advised by Wilson. The use of lead plaster alone, applied continuously as a plaster, is sometimes followed by softening and diminution in size.

[1] Lepra (leprosy), an important disease of this class, appears, in Vol. I. p. 785, as a separate article by J. C. White.

Fibroma.

Fibroma (molluscum fibrosum, fibroma molluscum) is a connective-tissue new growth, characterized by sessile or pedunculated, soft or firm, rounded, painless tumors, varying in size from a pea to an egg or larger, seated beneath and in the skin. A single growth may occur, or, as is more commonly the case, they are present in large numbers, and usually scattered over the greater portion of the body, having a preference for the softer tissues,—for example, the trunk. They may be of various shapes, rounded and sunken in the skin itself or in the subcutaneous tissue, or club- or pear-shaped and pedunculated. They usually begin as soft masses in the skin. If but one tumor exists, it is apt to be pedunculated or pendulous, and to attain considerable dimensions, in some cases weighing several pounds. In these instances surface-ulceration is occasionally noted as the result of mere weight or pressure. As commonly met with, however, the growths are numerous, several hundreds existing, varying from a pea to a cherry in size, with larger ones scattered here and there. The overlying skin is normal, pinkish or reddish, or may be loose or stretched, hypertrophied or atrophied. They are unattended with pain. They may make their appearance at any age, often in childhood, and grow as a rule slowly. After reaching a certain size they are apt to remain stationary; in rare instance spontaneous involution of some of the growths has been noted to take place. The affection is not common. It is often inherited, and may show itself in several members of the same family. Those in whom it is observed are usually noted to be stunted in their physical and mental development. The general health is not involved. Opinions are divided as to whether the growths take their origin in the connective-tissue framework of the fatty tissue, in the connective tissue of the corium, or in that of the walls of the hair-sac. The developed tumors consist of a connective-tissue capsule enclosing a whitish fibrous mass, with the central portion more or less soft and pulpy, out of which may be squeezed a small quantity of yellowish fluid. Small, recent tumors are composed of gelatinous, newly-formed connective tissue, while old growths consist entirely of a dense, firmly-packed fibrous tissue.

They are to be distinguished from the tumors of molluscum epitheliale by the absence of an aperture or depression upon their summits. They can scarcely be confounded with multiple neuromata or with lipomata, as the accompanying pain of the former and the lobulated structure and soft feel of the latter are sufficiently distinctive. Their removal, if desired, may be effected by the knife, or in the case of the large and pedunculated growth by the ligature or by the galvano-cautery.

Neuroma.

Neuroma cutis, or neuroma of the skin, is characterized by the formation of variously-sized fibrous tubercles, containing new nerve-elements, having their seat primarily in the corium, and accompanied in their development by violent paroxysmal pain. It is exceedingly rare, there being but few cases recorded. It appears on the shoulders, arms, thighs or buttocks in the form of numerous, disseminated, pinhead to hazelnut in size, round or ovalish tubercles or nodules, which at the outset may be either painful or painless; in the later stages, however, pain, both spon_taneous and upon pressure, is a constant symptom. The growths are firm, immovable, and elastic, and are seated in the corium, extending into the deeper structures. They may be covered scantily with fine, lamina_ted, glistening scales, as in the case reported by one of us. Anatomically, the tumors are composed of nerve-fibres, yellow elastic tissue, blood_vessels, and lymphoid cells. Excision of a portion of the nerve-trunk leading to the affected area has been practised in one case (Kosinski's) reported, with permanent relief; in another (Duhring's) the relief was merely temporary.

Xanthoma.

Xanthoma (also called vitiligoidea and xanthelasma) is a connective-tissue new growth, characterized by the formation of yellowish, circum-scribed, irregularly-shaped, variously-sized, non-indurated, flat or raised patches or tubercles. Two varieties are met with. The macular, or flat form (xanthoma planum) is commonly seen upon the eyelids, looking not unlike pieces of chamois-skin inserted in the lids. This form may also be encountered occasionally on other parts of the face, as well as upon the body. The patches are smooth, opaque, usually sharply defined, and to the touch soft and apparently normal in texture; they are on a level with the surrounding integument or slightly raised, and of a creamy or yel-lowish color. They vary in size and shape, and may coalesce, forming a band extending across the eyelids, especially the upper lids. The tuber-cular form (xanthoma tuberosum) is usually met with upon the neck, trunk, and extremities, the eyelids seldom being invaded. It occurs as small, isolated nodules, or in patches slightly raised above the level of the skin, consisting of aggregations of tubercles of the size of a milletseed or larger. Both forms of the disease not infrequently occur in the same indi-vidual. After reaching a certain development it is apt to remain stationary throughout life, and with no involvement of the general health. As a rule, the lesions are few in numbers; on the other hand, rarely they may be numerous (xanthoma multiplex). The affection is usually encountered in middle and advanced life, although it is occasionally met with in the young. It is more common in women than in men. Jaundice has been frequently noticed as preceding or accompanying it, especially the tuber-cular variety. Pathologically, it is a connective-tissue new growth with fatty degeneration. Excision, where practicable, constitutes the sole method of treatment.

Myoma.

Myoma cutis, or dermato-myoma (known also as liomyoma cutis), is a rare affection, consisting of tumors of the skin composed of muscular fibres. They occur either as single or multiple tumors, varying in size from a lentil to an egg, localized in a special region, as the nipple, scrotum, labia majora, thigh, hand, or foot; or, more rarely, numerous, and scattered over the greater portion of the whole body. They are either flat or pedunculated, rounded or oval in form, pale-red in color, with a smooth surface; although generally painless, they are sometimes tender upon pressure. The growth consists essentially of a new formation of unstriped muscular fibres. At times it is composed largely of connective tissue (fibromyoma), or it may contain an abundance of blood-vessels, giving rise to cavernous erectile tumors (myoma telangiectodes). The disease is benign.

Angioma.

Angioma, or nævus vasculosus, is a congenital formation composed chiefly of blood-vessels and having its seat in the skin and subcutaneous tissue. Several forms of the affection are met with, all of which, however, may be grouped under two heads—non-elevated and prominent. The former (nævus flammeus, nævus simplex, angioma simplex) is illustrated by the so-called port-wine mark, or claret-stain, known in German as feuermal, and in French as tache de feu. The prominent variety (angioma cavernosum, nævus tuberosus) may be turgescent, erectile, pulsating, tumor-like, circumscribed growths, with an uneven or rugous surface. In shape nævi are usually roundish, but may be irregular; in color, bright or dark red, violaceous, or bluish; and in size as large as a pea or a bean, or in some cases involving areas several inches in diameter. As a rule, they are single formations. They may occur on any part of the body, but are most frequently seen about the face. Their course varies. In many instances, after attaining a certain size, they remain stationary, or in some cases may retrograde or undergo spontaneous involution, this remark applying more particularly to the flat variety in early life. Ordinarily, they are permanent deformities. They become pale under pressure, and the more prominent growths are markedly compressible. Anatomically, the growth consists of a dilatation and hypertrophy of the arterial and venous blood-vessels of the corium and subcutaneous tissues, and in some instances there is increase in connective tissue. In some cases the connective-tissue hypertrophy is made up mainly from the adipose layer (angioma lipomatodes). Occasionally there may be more or less pigmentation.

In the treatment, the extent, form, and region involved are to be considered. Various methods have been advised for their removal. For pinhead-sized nævi puncturing with a red-hot needle, or with a needle charged with nitric or chromic acid, may be employed. Those of pea size may be treated by caustic applications. Sodium ethylate, as recommended by Richardson, is an efficient caustic for the more superficial forms: it should be pure and applied with a glass rod; a dry dressing is to be employed and the crust permitted to loosen itself. Painting a nævus with liquor plumbi subacetatis will, if repeated daily for several weeks or months, sometimes succeed. Caustic potash in solution, from one to two drachms in the ounce, and nitric acid, may both be cautiously used. An ointment of a drachm of adhesive plaster and nine grains of tartar emetic applied to small nævi will, according to Neumann, cause free suppuration and healing. A solution of eight grains of corrosive sublimate in a drachm of collodion is sometimes effective. Injections of astringent and irritating liquids, such as the tincture of the chloride of iron and cantharidine, as formerly practised, possess no advantage over safer methods. Linear and punctate scarifications—in the latter the needles being charged with a 50 per cent. solution of carbolic acid or a 25 per cent. solution of chromic acid—have been recommended. In small formations vaccinating the nævus is often successful. The galvano-cautery and the actual cautery are both serviceable in treating the smaller nævi. Electrolysis constitutes a valuable plan of treatment. A current of from six to twelve cells is usually required. One or more platinum needles are attached to the negative pole and a single needle or charcoal point to the positive pole. Slight frothing at the points of insertion indicates that the action has been sufficient. Suppuration and sloughing should not occur if proper care is exercised. If the nævus is extensive, only a small portion is to be treated at the one sitting. In the port-wine mark this method promises the best results; the color is made much lighter, and exceptionally is made to disappear entirely. In prominent, and especially in pedunculated, tumors a ligature may be employed.

Lymphangioma.

Lymphangioma (also described as lymphangioma tuberosum multiplex) is a rare disease, characterized by numerous, scattered, pea- or bean-sized, ovalish or rounded, brownish-red, glistening, smooth, slightly-elevated tubercles, having a somewhat translucent look, occurring for the most part about the trunk. They are firm and elastic to the touch; are situated in the cutis, but are not sharply defined; they can be readily made to sink below the level of the surrounding integument, owing to their marked compressibility. At times they have a lilac or bluish tinge. The growths bear some resemblance to the large papular syphiloderm. They are generally congenital or appear in childhood. Anatomically, they consist of immensely dilated and hypertrophied lymphatic vessels. The course of the disease is slow, and evinces no disposition to malignancy. The general health is not involved.

Lupus Erythematosus.

Lupus erythematosus (also known as lupus erythematodes, seborrhœa congestiva, and lupus sebaceus) is a small-celled new growth, characterized by one or more circumscribed, variously sized and shaped, reddish patches, more or less covered with adherent grayish or yellowish scales. The affection usually begins as a rounded, circumscribed, pinhead- to pea-sized, slightly elevated lesion, which increases in size by peripheral extension until considerable surface is involved; or, as is often the case, the disease starts with several such spots, which grow and generally coalesce, sooner or later involving considerable surface. The spots are at first erythematous and slightly scaly, with but little elevation, later becoming thickened, with a more or less raised border sharply defined against the healthy skin, covered with small, firmly adherent yellowish or grayish scales, with enlarged and plugged or patulous follicles, the centre of the patch being somewhat depressed. The color is pinkish, reddish, or violaceous. In the beginning the disease often closely resembles seborrhœa, —so much so that it was originally described by Hebra as seborrhœa congestiva. The scaling is usually scanty, but in exceptional instances may be abundant. At times the lesions show little tendency to peripheral growth, the large areas of disease resulting from the continuous appearance of new patches in proximity which run together. Occasionally the patches are small, discrete, and numerous, when the disease is apt to be disseminated over considerable surface.

Lupus erythematosus is seen most frequently about the face, one or several patches, varying in size from a pea to a silver dollar, ordinarily being present. The nose and the checks are favorite localities, and, seated here, the disease is apt to be symmetrical, extending from one cheek across the nose to the other cheek, in shape representing rudely the outline of a bat or butterfly with outstretched wings. The lips, ears, scalp, and other parts of the body are often affected. The progress of the disease is variable; the patches, as a rule, reach a certain size, and then remain stationary or retrogress, or, as generally happens, the central portion becomes depressed and more or less atrophied. The resulting scar is whitish, usually soft, punctate, and superficial. As old patches disappear it is not uncommon to see new patches appearing close by. It is essentially a chronic disease: the individual lesions may be acute in their course, and when such is noted, as a rule new areas of disease continue to appear in rapid succession. Ordinarily, however, the individual patches themselves are chronic in their course. The disease is not attended with ulceration. The subjective symptoms of itching and burning are usually mild in character, and sometimes are entirely wanting.

The condition of the general health is, as a rule, good. The disease is seen more frequently in women than in men, and is rarely observed before puberty, being chiefly encountered in early adult and middle age. The causes are not known. It frequently begins as a seborrhœa, but it may occur (although rarely) upon the palms of the hands, where sebaceous glands are not to be found. It is a notable fact, however, that the disease is most commonly encountered in those who are subject to disorder of these glands. It is observed more often in persons of light complexion. It is comparatively rare. The condition of the general health apparently exercises no causative influence.

Pathologically, the process is essentially a chronic inflammation of the cutis, superinducing degenerative and atrophic changes. In the majority of cases the disease originates in the sebaceous glands, but later all parts of the skin become affected. It is even authoritatively stated that it may in some instances take its start in the subcutaneous connective tissue. In some respects it has the character of a new growth, which until late years it has been considered. In the light of recent investigations, however, it seems possible that it may be a chronic inflammation leading to degenerative changes. The process never ends in the formation of pus. There is small-celled infiltration about the follicles and glands, the blood-vessels are dilated, the surrounding tissue is infiltrated with embryonic corpuscles, and the sebaceous glands are enlarged and their walls infiltrated with small cells. The whole affected area is, in fact, infiltrated with a small-celled inflammatory new growth. If retrograde changes occur, the infiltration may disappear by absorption without leaving a trace. On the other hand, and as is usually the case, degenerative metamorphosis, resulting in absorption and atrophy, takes place.

There is very little difficulty in recognizing a fully-developed patch of lupus erythematosus, as its features are usually characteristic. The sharply circumscribed outline, the reddish or violaceous patch with elevated border, the tendency to central depression and atrophy, the plugged-up or patulous sebaceous ducts, the adherent grayish or yellowish scales, together with the region attacked (generally the nose and cheeks), are characters which, when taken together, are common to no other disease. Lupus vulgaris may be excluded by the absence of papules, tubercles, and ulceration. The sebaceous involvement and the peculiar atrophy and superficial scarring are, moreover, not seen in lupus vulgaris. Erythematous lupus begins, as a rule, during adult life; lupus vulgaris usually in childhood. In psoriasis the course and symptoms peculiar to that disease will distinguish it from lupus erythematosus. It is scarcely possible to confound the disease with eczema or syphilis. In some cases in the beginning of the affection it may resemble seborrhœa; in fact, it often has its starting-point in that disease. The inflammation, infiltration, sharply-defined characters, atrophy, and scarring are absent in seborrhœa.

TREATMENT.—The prognosis of lupus erythematosus, as regards the general health and welfare of the patient, is good, but respecting the disappearance and cure of the disease an opinion should always be guarded. Occasionally the patches yield readily, but, on the other hand, cases are frequently met with that prove exceedingly rebellious, responding only after long-continued treatment. Constitutional remedies are in most cases of but little value. Occasionally arsenic and cod-liver oil, used continuously for a long period, prove serviceable. Iodized starch, in the dose of one or two teaspoonfuls three times daily, has been recommended, and in some cases potassium iodide has a favorable influence.

It is to the external treatment, however, we look for positive effects. In the selection of remedial applications it is to be remembered that the patches of disease sometimes disappear spontaneously, occasionally with little or no scarring, and therefore treatment that would have as an effect marked scarring or disfigurement is to be avoided. The simplest remedy, at times useful, is soft soap, the sapo viridis of the shops. This may be used as such or in solution in alcohol, two parts of the soap to one of alcohol, constituting the well-known spiritus saponatus kalinus. It is to be energetically rubbed into the diseased parts once or twice daily. The application of the sapo viridis as a plaster is a more energetic method. After several days the soap is to be discontinued and a soothing ointment applied. In addition to its therapeutic properties, sapo viridis—or, better, its alcoholic solution—may be advantageously employed to cleanse the parts preparatory to other remedial applications. Mercurial plaster constantly applied to the patches will in some cases effect a cure. A 10 to 25 per cent. oleate-of-mercury ointment, rubbed on the parts once or twice daily, is sometimes of value.

In almost every case where the inflammatory symptoms are marked the following lotion will prove palliative, and in some cases of the mild and superficial form of the disease it has in time effected a cure:

℞. Zinci sulphatis,
  Potassii sulphidi,   āā. ʒij ;
  Aquæ,   f ℥iij ;
  Alcoholis,   f ℥j.

The salts are to be dissolved separately in the water, and then mixed, and after reaction the alcohol is to be added. Properly made, the resulting lotion is without odor, contains a whitish sediment, which when agitated gives the lotion a milky appearance. It is to be shaken, and the parts dabbed with it for from fifteen to thirty minutes twice daily, allowing it to dry on. Sulphur ointment and alcoholic sulphur lotion, such as are used in the treatment of acne, are also sometimes serviceable. Tincture of iodine, either alone or with an equal part of glycerin, painted over the parts once or twice daily until a coating forms, in some cases proves useful. The same may be said of the following formula:

℞. Iodinii,
  Potassii iodidi,   āā. ʒiv;
  Glycerinæ,   ʒj.

M.—Sig. Paint over the part until a coating is produced. Painting pure carbolic acid over the patches is sometimes followed by good results. A mixture that is serviceable as a stimulant is the following:

℞. Olei cadini,
  Alcoholis,
  Saponis viridis,   āā. ʒiij.

M.—Sig. Rub into the patches night and morning.

Stronger applications are often necessary if the disease fails to yield to the simpler remedies. Pyrogallic acid in ointment, from forty to ninety grains to the ounce, and chrysarobin in the same strength, are serviceable. The latter is a dangerous remedy to use about the face, occasioning at times a violent conjuctivitis with œdema. Pyrogallic acid is safer, and sometimes proves more satisfactory when applied in flexible collodion or liquor gutta-perchæ than in ointment form, as in the following formula:

℞. Acidi pyrogallici,   ʒj ;
  Liquor. gutta-perchæ, f ℥iv.

M.—S. Apply with a brush. This is to be painted over the patches several times daily until considerable reaction takes place or a crust forms, then discontinued, and as soon as the crust is removed or falls off the the application is to be repeated. If there is much scaling, thirty grains of salicylic acid may be added to the above formula. In most cases it is advisable as soon as the crust forms to remove it, and immediately to resume the pyrogallic-acid painting. Cantharidal blistering fluid, repeatedly applied, has been recommended. Nitrate of silver, either in stick or strong solution, is a comparatively safe caustic, and is at times useful. Treatment by linear scarifications, especially in obstinate, sluggish, and infiltrated patches, is often valuable. The scar left is, as a rule, insignificant. Erasion with the curette is a method that sometimes proves of advantage in the severer and deeper-seated forms of the disease. Although in almost all instances stimulating or active treatment is demanded and well borne, there are cases occasionally met with in which, on account of the inflammation and pain, soothing applications must, for a time at least, be employed. These cases, it will be found, are aggravated by stimulating remedies.

Lupus Vulgaris.

Lupus vulgaris (known also as lupus exedens, lupus vorax) is a cellular new growth, characterized by variously-sized, soft, reddish-brown patches, consisting of papules, tubercles, and flat infiltrations, eventually terminating in ulceration and cicatrization. The disease appears differently as seen in the several forms and stages of its development. All the varieties usually begin in one and the same way.

The primary lesions are pinhead- to small pea-sized, deep-seated, brownish-red or yellowish papules, having their seat in the deeper part of the corium. They are softer and looser in texture than normal tissue, and as the disease progresses form variously sized and shaped patches. They may be so closely aggregated as to form flat infiltrations. The patches tend to be round, serpiginous, or ill defined. As the papules increase in size they may be distinctly recognized both by the eye and by passing the finger over the surface; later even reaching the size of small peas. The lesions having attained a certain size or development and being covered with imperfectly-formed epidermis, may so remain for a time, or retrogressive changes may immediately occur. They may disappear by absorption, fatty degeneration taking place, leaving a desquamating, atrophic or cicatricial tissue—lupus exfoliativus—or disintegration and destruction of the diseased skin may occur, resulting in ulceration—lupus exedens, or exulcerans. This latter is the usual course of the disease. The ulcerations are rounded, shallow excavations with soft and reddish borders. If the ulcerations are the seat of exuberant granulations, the condition is known as lupus hypertrophicus. Papillary outgrowths may occur in the healing ulcers, and a rough, verrucous condition results—lupus verrucosus.

The lesions of lupus are seldom painful. The ulcers secrete a slight or moderate amount of pus which forms crusts. Soft or firm cicatricial tissue finally results. In almost all cases of long standing the several stages of the disease may be recognized, each lesion, whether the first or the last, going through a similar course, either of absorption and exfoliation or ulceration and cicatrization. The deeper parts may be involved in the process, subcutaneous connective tissue, cartilage, and mucous membrane being liable to invasion. The mucous membrane of the mouth, gums, velum and larynx may even be primarily the seat of the lupus infiltration, considerable destruction eventually resulting. The face, especially the nose, is the most common site of the disease. Occurring about the eye, the process may eventually destroy that organ. The ears are likewise frequently attacked. Not infrequently the extremities, and occasionally the trunk, are invaded. The disease begins, as a rule, in childhood. It is always a destructive process, usually resulting in disfiguring cicatrices.

The causes of the disease are obscure. Although it usually appears in early life, it is never congenital. Heredity has little if any influence. It is comparatively rare in this country, less so in England and Ireland, but is more common in Austria, Germany and France. It is most generally observed among the strumous and debilitated, but is also frequently seen in those who enjoy all the advantages of life and who are otherwise in average health. It is entirely distinct and independent of syphilis. The French consider it a scrofuloderm (scrofulide), and yet in many cases there is clinically a considerable difference. On the other hand, cases are met with in which its close relationship, if not identity, with the scrofuloder-mata is not to be questioned. The view that it is a tuberculosis of the skin due to the same cause as at present advanced for tuberculosis of the lungs—the bacillus—has lately been suggested. The disease attacks both sexes, but is somewhat more common in women than in men.

Anatomically, the process is a chronic inflammation, consisting essen-tially of small-cell infiltration, affecting primarily the corium, eventually spreading to other parts. The epithelial structures are usually involved in the first stages of the disease. Recent lesions are rich in vessels, the vascularity when retrogressive changes take place rapidly decreasing, beginning at the centre of the nodule. The cutaneous tissues undergo cicatricial contraction, a part, however, being organized into coarse con-nective tissue. In addition to the formation of the nodular mass, the cell-infiltration is found to spread along the vessels of the corium and papillæ, and also into the deeper portions of the skin. The papules may be so close and the cell-infiltration so extensive that a large area of disease results and undergoes the same changes as an individual lesion. The sweat and sebaceous glands are involved. Sometimes epithelial hyperplasia takes place, the epithelial outgrowth from the rete dipping down and joining similar outgrowths from the cells of the sweat-glands and hair root-sheaths, forming an epithelial network which may become a histological basis for the development of epithelioma. The occurrence of this latter disease in lupus tissue, in association or as a sequela, has been noted by several observers. According to the latest investigations the infiltration of lupus is due chiefly to cell-proliferation and outgrowth from the proto-plasmic walls and adventitia of the blood-vessels and lymphatics. The fibrous-tissue network, vessels, and a portion of the cell-infiltration are thus produced, the fixed and wandering connective-tissue cells of the inflamed stroma of the cutis being responsible for the other portion of the new growth.

DIAGNOSIS.—Ordinarily, the features of lupus vulgaris are so distinc-tive as to render a diagnosis a matter of no difficulty. The characteristic soft, small, reddish-brown subcutaneous papule—the primary efflorescence of the disease—is generally to be found, especially about the periphery of the patch, and when present is diagnostic. At times, however, it bears resemblance to syphilis, epithelioma, lupus erythematosus, and acne rosacea.

It is chiefly in the serpiginous forms of the late tubercular and ulcera-tive syphilodermata that the resemblance to lupus vulgaris is sometimes very close. There are several points of difference. Syphilis is much more rapid in its course, marked ulceration following frequently within a few weeks or months of its appearance. With lupus, on the other hand, years may elapse before the same amount of destruction results. In lupus there are usually several points of ulceration; in syphilis, one or several, which incline to coalesce. The ulcers of lupus are apt to be super-ficial, whereas those of syphilis are usually deep, with a punched-out appearance. Lupus papules are small, soft and but slightly elevated, and frequently reappear in the scars left by the disease; the papules or tubercles of syphilis are larger, more elevated, firm and harder, and are seldom seen in the scar or track of the disease. The secretion of the syphilitic ulcer is abundant, purulent and offensive, and the crusts thick, often oystershell-like, and of a greenish or blackish color; the secretion of lupus ulceration is slight, odorless, the crusts thin and scanty and of a reddish or reddish-brown color. The scar of lupus is generally hard, shrunken, yellowish, and more or less distorted, while that of syphilis is soft and, compared to the amount of ulceration, but slightly disfiguring. The bone-structures are not involved in lupus; they may be in syphilis. The two diseases have different histories: lupus generally begins in child-hood and runs a slow and chronic course; syphilis is usually seen after adolescence or adult age, and progresses more rapidly. In syphilis, more-over, other evidences of the disease may usually be found.

Lupus vulgaris differs from epithelioma in several important points. The edges of the epitheliomatous ulcer are hard, elevated, and waxy; the base is uneven, and the secretion is thin, scanty, and apt to be streaked with blood; the ulceration usually starts from a single point; it is often painful; the tissue-destruction may be considerable; and, finally, epithe-lioma is, as a rule, a disease of advanced age. Lupus vulgaris differs essentially in all these particulars.

As a rule, there is no difficulty in differentiating lupus vulgaris from lupus erythematosus. The absence of papules, tubercles and ulceration is sufficiently distinctive. Lupus erythematosus is, moreover, a super-ficial disease, pinkish or violaceous in color, showing itself in cir-cumscribed patches covered with thin adherent scales, and with usually evident involvement of the sebaceous glands. It rarely begins before adult age, whereas lupus vulgaris, as a rule, first appears in childhood. Attention to the ordinary characters of acne rosacea—the hyperæmia, the dilated vessels, comedones, acne papules and pustules, its advent at or after maturity, and the history—will prevent an error in diagnosis.

TREATMENT.—Lupus vulgaris is always a chronic disease, and one that calls for a guarded opinion as to treatment. Although it be removed, relapses are prone to occur, and new papules may show themselves even about the scar resulting from treatment. If it is localized the chances of permanent cure are more favorable. The deformity attending and fol-lowing the disease is often great,—contraction of joints, destruction of car-tilages, and sometimes partial closure of the orifices resulting. The gen-eral health is usually good. Death by tuberculosis of the lungs has been noticed in some cases.

Treatment has in the main two objects,—to limit the development or spread of the disease and to remove the morbid tissue that is already present. In accomplishing the former constitutional treatment is occa-sionally useful; although much cannot usually be attained in this way, yet from our own observations we are convinced that in some cases the disease may be favorably influenced and its spread limited. Cod-liver oil, administered in full doses and for a long period, is sometimes of decided value. Potassium iodide is another remedy which at times proves serviceable. Iodoform in half-grain doses three times daily has been recommended, as have also muriate of lime, in the dose of twenty grains three times a day, and calx sulphurata, in small doses. Hygienic measures are to be enforced, and a generous, nutritious diet advised.

External remedies are essential in every case, and constitute the only plan of treatment to be relied upon. Removal of the diseased tissues by caustics or operation is the method practised. In the earlier stages of the disease or before adopting radical measures it is advisable to make an attempt to bring about absorption by the employment of stimulating applications. Equal parts of tincture of iodine and glycerin, or one part each of iodine and potassium iodide and two parts of glycerin, may be painted over the parts daily or every other day. Mercurial plaster, renewed once or twice a day and kept constantly applied, is valuable in some cases. Corrosive sublimate in the form of a lotion or ointment, one-half to two grains to the ounce, has lately been advised. Cashew-nut oil applied with friction has been recommended for the non-ulcerative form. Tar and sulphur ointments may also be employed. Chrysarobin, either in the form of an ointment or as a solution in liquor gutta-perchæ, has also been advised.

For the radical treatment of the disease there are numerous caustics in use, but there are some which are more positive in their effect and whose action may be controlled. Nitrate of silver, pyrogallic acid, arsenic, caustic potash, the curette, scarifier, and the actual and galvano-cautery are all valuable. Nitrate of silver is best used in stick form. The lesions are forcibly pierced and bored with the stick, and thoroughly cauterized. The operation is to be repeated every three or four days. It is a safe remedy, and is especially useful about the face, as the scars left are soft and smooth. Pyrogallic acid in the form of an ointment or plaster, from 15 to 25 per cent. strength, is often of great value. It is a mild and safe caustic; it is usually painless and leaves a smooth, soft scar. The ointment should be stiff and adhesive, and kept applied constantly for several days or more, renewing twice daily. The following formula serves well:

Ŗ. Acidi pyrogallici,   ₃ij;
Emplastri plumbi,   ₃j;
Cerati resinæ comp., ₃v.

M.—Sig. Apply as a plaster. In winter the lead plaster may be omitted. The remedy may also be applied in liquor gutta-perchæ, but is not so satis-factory. The tissues become soft and blackish, and then the parts are to be poulticed and the slough removed; and if the diseased tissue is not sufficiently destroyed the dressing is to be renewed. Subsequently the ulcer is dressed with mercurial ointment or a simple salve. Healing should take place in the course of a few weeks. Iodoform is well spoken of. In deep-seated infiltration the upper epidermic layers should first be removed by a solution of caustic potassa. The iodoform is then put on and a layer of cotton is applied over it, and the dressing remains undisturbed for a week. The lupus nodules are soon destroyed. Several repetitions of the remedy may be necessary. Excepting the preliminary application of the potassa the method is painless.

A solution of caustic potash is sometimes employed for the destruction of the lupus deposit. It is thorough in its action, but is painful and must be used with great caution. The cicatrices left after the use of this caustic are apt to be large and hard. In the application, as soon as the diseased tissue has been thoroughly destroyed by the caustic, the further action may be stopped by neutralizing the alkali with diluted acetic acid. Arsenic in the form of paste is another valuable caustic. It has the advantage of sparing the healthy, and even the cicatricial, tissues. Hebra's modification of Cosme's paste is an eligible formula:

℞. Acidi arseniosi, ℈j ;
Hydrargyri sulphuret. rub., ℥j ;
Ugt. simplicis, ℥j.

M. Ft. ugt.—Sig. Spread upon a piece of kid or cloth and apply as a plaster. The paste is to be applied for two or three days consecutively, at the end of which time the parts are somewhat swollen and painful. The lupus nodules are seen as black, necrosed spots. Poultices are then applied until the slough comes away, usually in a day or two; subsequently a mild, stimulating ointment is employed. Rapid cicatrization usually takes place, and the cicatrices are, as a rule, satisfactory. The chief objection to arsenical applications is the intense pain that usually develops soon after the remedy is applied. In other respects the method has its advantages.

Acetate of zinc in crystal form, repeatedly applied to the lesions, has been advised. It is painful at the time of application, but the pain may be somewhat relieved by washing the parts with water. Red iodide of mercury in the form of a strong ointment (equal parts of the salt and a fatty base), applied upon a piece of kid or cloth, will have a speedy caustic effect. There are other caustic remedies which may be mentioned. Chloride of zinc, with an equal part of chloride of antimony and sufficient hydrochloric acid to dissolve the zinc chloride, and enough powdered licorice added to make a paste, and applied as a plaster, is an efficient caustic. It produces an eschar in twelve to twenty-four hours. The parts are then dressed with a simple ointment, and healing allowed to take place. It is a strong caustic, and is destructive to healthy as well as diseased tissue. The same may be said of Vienna paste, consisting of equal parts of lime and potassa. The latter mixture is made into a paste at the time of application by adding alcohol. It is not to be applied more than five to ten minutes, and its further effects are to be counteracted by the application of acetic acid. In the application of such powerful and destructive caustics it is advisable to protect the adjacent skin with strips of adhesive plaster. Salicylic acid has lately been recommended in the form of an ointment of the strength of one to two drachms to the ounce. It is thickly spread on linen and applied continuously. The remedy is a mild one and acts slowly. Mention may also be made of lactic acid, applications of which, it is stated, have been productive of beneficial results.

Of late years the mechanical removal of the lupus deposits has been largely practised. In small patches excision of the entire diseased area has been recommended, but as considerable healthy tissue is necessarily removed with it, and the resulting scar is deep and disfiguring, it is not to be advised. Excision followed by transplantation of healthy skin has also been advocated. An excellent method of removal is by means of the dermal curette, or scraping-spoon. It is one that answers well in many cases. The diseased tissue should be thoroughly scraped out. It is painful, and it is often necessary to operate under ether. The healthy tissues are unyielding and cannot be readily scraped away, so that only the morbid deposit is removed. As it is difficult to remove the new growth from the interstitial spaces, we are in the habit of supplementing the operation with a caustic, either cauterizing lightly with caustic potash, or, what is advisable in the greater number of cases, applying the pyrogallic-acid ointment for several days following the curetting. This method—the curetting and subsequent cauterization—has, on the whole, proved satisfactory.

Linear or punctate scarification is another method of treatment that is often valuable. It is of most service in the non-ulcerating forms. Linear scarification is the more satisfactory. The parts are thoroughly cross-tracked and a simple ointment applied. If the bleeding is marked, cold compresses may be applied. Anæmia of the parts results, the papules are disturbed, and the new growth rapidly undergoes retrogressive changes. If the area to be operated upon is large, the patient should be anæsthetized. Charging the knife, or if punctiform scarifications are practised the pointed instrument, with iodized glycerin (one part iodine to twenty of glycerin) has been advised, as rendering a successful result the more certain. The scar following the curette and linear and punctate scarification is usually soft and white, much less disfiguring, as a rule, than that following the action of the stronger caustics. Destruction of the new growth by means of the galvano-cautery or by the actual cautery has from time to time had its advocates. Piercing the individual lesions with a platinum needle-point heated to dull red by means of the battery has been strongly advised; comparative absence of pain, rapidity, and good results are claimed for it.

Scrofuloderma.

Scrofuloderma is a term employed to designate certain morbid conditions of the skin which are dependent upon that state of the system known as scrofula, or struma. The most common form of the cutaneous manifestation is that which has its beginning in one or more of the lymphatic glands. The gland slowly increases in size, without any of the ordinary signs of inflammation, and after reaching the dimensions of an almond may so remain or undergo fatty or cheesy degeneration. As a rule, however, sooner or later the gland grows much larger, the new-cell growth breaks down, the superjacent skin becomes hyperæmic, thin, sensitive, and of a violaceous or purplish color. Finally, the tumor breaks, and a thick, cheesy pus mixed with blood is discharged; sinuses are apt to form, the skin ulcerates, and the process may so continue for months, partial cicatrization taking place, and then again breaking down. The resulting ulcers are irregular or ovalish in shape, with undermined edges, and the surrounding thin and chronically inflamed skin of a violaceous color. Their bases are uneven and covered with pale, unhealthy-looking granulations. If there is crust-formation, it is seen to be thin, grayish or brownish. The process is slow and chronic. The scars are irregular, knotty, contracted, and often hypertrophic. The affection is seen most frequently about the neck, especially under the lower jaw. Other evidences of scrofula are usually present.

A less frequent cutaneous manifestation consists of one or several large, rounded, ovalish or irregularly-shaped, flat pustules upon an inflamed or violaceous base. The crust forms slowly, is thin and flat, and of a brownish color. The ulceration beneath has the peculiar scrofulous characters. The scars which follow are soft, flat, and superficial.

A scrofuloderm occasionally met with consists of one or several papillary or fungoid growths of a bright or dull violaceous red color, with an ulcerated and discharging surface. They occur perhaps most frequently about the hands, are chronic, and often lead to deep-seated ulceration, which may involve the bones and give rise to deformity. The disease resembles the verrucous and hypertrophic varieties of lupus vulgaris.

Another variety of disease, seen usually in scrofulous subjects, described by one of us (Duhring), manifests itself as small pinhead- to pea-sized, disseminated, yellowish, flat papulo-pustules upon a red or violaceous base, which slowly dry to crusts, and leave punched-out-looking scars resembling those of variola. The lesions are irregularly distributed, occurring for the most part about the face and extremities. The process may continue for years. The lesions resemble those of the small pustular syphiloderm.

The manifestations of scrofula are at the present time supposed to be due to the specific infecting agent, the bacillus. Other conditions which have been considered influential, and which are unquestionably important predisposing causes, are heredity, blood-marriages, insufficient and unwholesome food, continued exposure to wet and cold and impure air. It generally develops in childhood, often after measles, scarlatina, and similar diseases. Negroes are especially predisposed to it. The scrofulodermata are, as a rule, readily distinguished by their peculiar clinical characters. Other symptoms of scrofula are, moreover, usually present and aid in the diagnosis. It is to be differentiated from the gummatous ulcerations of syphilis by its history, course, locality, the absence of the specific infiltration at the borders of the ulceration, and the violaceous tint.

The constitutional treatment is the same as employed in other scrofulous affections—cod-liver oil, syrup of the iodide of iron, sulphide or muriate of lime, phosphorus, and iodine preparations being the most reliable remedies. The diet should be liberal, consisting of a large proportion of animal food. Hygienic measures are active adjuvants. The external treatment of scrofulous ulcerations consists in the use of stimulating applications. Mercurial ointments, corrosive sublimate in alcohol, one-fourth to one grain to the ounce, and yellow wash, are serviceable applications. Iodoform, in powder or ointment, is often of benefit. A 1 or 2 per cent. nitrate-of-silver-ointment may also be mentioned. Curetting, as in lupus vulgaris, is one of the most valuable methods of treatment, especially useful in the fungoid variety. Milton has had good results with calomel or gray powder, taken at night two or three times weekly for a few weeks, and a saline every morning in sufficient dose to produce a daily evacuation. The mercurial is then intermitted for two or three weeks. Bitters and mineral acids are given if the appetite fails. A simple ointment is used locally.

Syphilis Cutanea.

Syphilis (syphiloderma, dermatosyphilis, syphilis of the skin) manifests itself in various forms upon the integument. Preceding or ushering in the early eruptions there is sometimes considerable systemic disturbance, such as slight fever, loss of appetite, muscular pains, and headache. In the greater number of cases, however, general symptoms are wanting. Along with the cutaneous manifestations there are usually other signs of the disease. In the early eruptions the lymphatic glands are enlarged, and sore throat and mucous patches may exist. Sometimes there is loss of hair. In the later syphilodermata pains in the bones, bone lesions, and other symptoms may be observed. The early eruptions are generalized; the later manifestations are usually limited in extent, and have a tendency to appear in circular, semicircular or crescentic forms. There are rarely any subjective symptoms. The color of established syphilitic lesions is usually a dull brownish-red or yellowish-red.

Syphilis may show itself as a macular, papular, vesicular, pustular, bullous, tubercular or gummatous form of disease. In many instances, although a particular efflorescence may predominate, lesions of other varieties may be found intermingled.

SYPHILODERMA ERYTHEMATOSUM (syn., exanthematous syphilide, syphilis cutanea maculosa, roseola syphilitica, macular syphiloderm) is a general eruption, showing itself usually six to eight weeks after the appearance of the chancre. The appearance of the eruption is retarded by treatment. It consists of macules of various sizes and shapes, for the most part the size of a pea or small bean and rounded, on a level with the surrounding skin cr slightly raised, giving the skin a mottled or marbled look. At first the spots disappear under pressure, but later, owing to the presence of more or less pigmentation, they persist. Their outline, which is ill defined, is usually brought out more distinctly on exposure. They vary in color from a pale pink to a dull violaceous red, depending upon their duration and also upon the natural complexion of the individual, and as they fade away become yellowish or coppery. As a rule, they exist in profusion, so much so as to cover not infrequently almost the entire surface, appearing without order of distribution; exceptionally they exist sparsely and faintly, in which case the eruption may be overlooked. The face, backs of the hands, and feet frequently escape. Subjective symptoms are wanting. The efflorescence may appear with or without systemic disturbance, but malaise and slight fever frequently precede it. The chancre or its scar, enlarged inguinal and cervical glands, erythema of the fauces, rheumatic pains, and more or less falling of the hair usually accompany its development. It may manifest itself slowly and insidiously, a week or two elapsing before its height is reached, or the invasion may be sudden, taking place in the course of twenty-four or forty-eight hours. This syphiloderm probably occurs in the majority of cases of syphilis, but in many instances is so faint as to escape observation. As a rule, it responds rapidly to treatment.

It is to be distinguished from measles, rötheln, urticaria, simple erythema, tinea versicolor, and certain medicinal eruptions. The catarrhal symptoms, the fever, form, and situation of the eruption of measles; the rapid formation and disappearance of the patches of simple erythema; the wheals and intense itchiness of urticaria; the slight scaliness, peripheral growth, and distribution of tinea versicolor; the small roundish, confluent pinkish or reddish patches, precursory pyrexic symptoms, the epidemic nature, short duration of rötheln; and the history, fever, form, and duration of the medicinal rashes,—are points of difference which serve to distinguish these diseases from the syphiloderm.

So-called Syphiloderma Pigmentosum, or pigmentary syphilide, may here be referred to. It is a rare manifestation, and is characterized by rounded, ovalish or irregularly-shaped, variously-sized, discrete or confluent, pale grayish, yellowish, or brownish, usually ill-defined faint macules. It occurs most frequently about the neck, is seen almost exclu‑ sively in women, and is encountered during the latter half of the first and in the second year of the disease. It develops slowly, and may con‑ tinue one ⁕or two months or as many years, and is uninfluenced by anti‑ syphilitic treatment. It is a simple pigmentary affection, similar, appa‑ rently, to chloasma, from which and tinea versicolor it is to be differen‑ tiated.

SYPHILODERMA PAPULOSUM (syn., syphilis cutanea papulosa, papular syphilide, papular syphiloderm) is characterized by the formation of vari‑ ously-sized papules. The lesions are small or large, and in some cases undergo various modifications.

The Small Papular Syphiloderm (syn., miliary papular syphilo‑ derm, lichen syphiliticus) consists in an eruption of disseminated or grouped, more or less confluent, firm, small or minute, rounded or acu‑ minated papules, the size of a pinhead or milletseed. Their summits may be smooth or covered with fine scales, or may show pointed pustula‑ tion ; this last symptom occurring especially in those through which a hair protrudes. Miliary pustules, scattered here and there over the sur‑ face, may also be present. At first the eruption is bright- or dull-red, but later it generally assumes a violaceous or brownish tint. In some cases the lesions are numerous and grouped, forming patches. The eruption is seen most frequently about the trunk and upon the limbs. It may appear during the third or fourth month or later. Large flat papules or moist papules may exist simultaneously. It has a chronic course, with a tend‑ ency to relapse, and is usually rebellious to treatment. It is to be dis‑ tinguished from keratosis pilaris, lichen scrofulosus, psoriasis punctata, papular eczema, and lichen ruber. The extent of the eruption, the color, grouping, with usually the presence of pustules and large papules and other concomitant symptoms of syphilis, are points of differentiation.

The Large Papular Syphiloderm (syn., lenticular syphiloderm) is cha‑ racterized by the formation of large, flat, circular or ovalish, firmly-seated, more or less raised pale- or dull-red papules, varying in size from a small split pea to a dime. In their early stage they are usually smooth, but they subsequently become covered with exfoliating epidermis. The forehead, region of the mouth, neck, back, flexor surfaces of the extremities, scrotum, labia, perineum, and margin of the anus are all favorite localities. The lesions, as a rule, develop slowly, and, having attained various sizes, remain for weeks or months. It is one of the commonest forms of cutaneous syphilis ; it may be an early or late erup‑ tion, and shows a disposition to relapse. As a rule, it yields readily to treatment. The lesions may undergo more or less modification, due either to the locality in which they exist or to other influences. Ordinarily, they persist as typical papules, and gradually pass away by absorption. At times they become soft and spongy, while occasionally they become excoriated, with slight moisture and crusting. This latter condition is usually observed about the junctures of the mucous membrane and the skin.

A common change is into the Moist Papule (syn., mucous papule, mucous patch, broad, or flat, condyloma ; *Fr.* plaques muquese). This takes place upon those regions where opposing surfaces and natural folds of skin are subjected to more or less contact, as about the nates, umbilieus, axillæ, beneath the mammæ, etc. The lesions are more or less moist, covered with a grayish, sticky, mucoid secretion consisting of macerated epidermis. They are usually flat, and may coalesce, and so form large patches. They may become hypertrophic, warty, and papillary, constituting the vegetating syphiloderm (syphilis cutanea vegetans). In this form the lesions become elevated, more or less circumscribed, and may assume a warty character, resembling the cauliflower formation, with a contagious secretion which dries to yellowish-brown crusts. Heat, moisture, friction, and uncleanliness favor their development. They usually disappear rapidly under local treatment.

Another modification which the papule frequently undergoes is into the squamous papule, forming the Papulo-squamous Syphiloderm (syn. squamous syphiloderm, syphilis cutanea squamosa, psoriasis syphilitica). The papules become somewhat flattened, and are covered with dry, grayish, adherent scales. The scaling may be slight or relatively abundant, but is rarely as luxuriant as in psoriasis. On removing the scales the papular character of the lesion may readily be detected. As a rule, the eruption is not extensive ; it may show itself on any part, and is exceedingly persistent. It is most frequently encountered on the palms and soles, where, on account of the peculiarities in the structure of the skin, the lesions are somewhat modified. Occurring on these parts, it is known as the palmar or plantar syphiloderm. The lesions partake more of the nature of macules than papules; they are slightly raised and are irregular in outline, and, as a rule, ill defined, varying in size from a pea to a finger-nail. They may coalesce and form roundish serpiginous or crescentic patches covered with dry, scanty, semi-detached, grayish flakes of epidermis, which are most abundant about the edges ; at times the exfoliation is marked, and then the patches are distinctly squamous, as in psoriasis. It is, as a rule, symmetrical, and is frequently observed in the centre of the palms or soles and upon the ball of the thumb and about the volar surfaces of the fingers. It is rebellious to treatment. It may be an early or late manifestation, but is usually the latter.

The papulo-squamous form of the syphiloderm may resemble eczema and psoriasis. In eczema heat, itching, and sometimes discharge, together with the history and course, will be sufficient points of distinction. Psoriasis upon the palms rarely occurs except as a part of a general eruption ; the character and abundance of the scales. their lamellar arrangement, the red rete beneath, and the absence of infiltration are diagnostic. The differential diagnosis of the papulo-squamous syphiloderm and psoriasis when occurring on the other parts of the body are fully given in treating of the latter disease.

SYPHILODERMA VESICULOSUM (syn., vesicular syphilide, syphilis cutanea vesiculosa) is an exceedingly rare form of cutaneous syphilis, and in the majority of cases may be more properly classed under the head of the pustular variety. The lesions vary in size from a pin-head to a split pea. If small, they are more or less acuminated, dis-seminated, or grouped, usually involving the hair-follicles; if large, semiglobular or flat, with or without a tendency to umbilication. The vesicles, as a rule, pass into pustules. It is an early eruption, occurring usually within the first six or eight months; is rarely extensive, pursues a rapid course, and is generally associated with other symptoms of the disease.

SYPHILODERMA PUSTULOSUM (syn., pustular syphilide, syphilis cutanea pustulosa) is an important manifestation, although not so common as the macular and papular varieties. The lesions assume one of several forms, although not infrequently they are found intermingled.

The Small Acuminated Pustular Syphiloderm (syn., miliary pustular syphiloderm) is characterized by the formation of milletseed-sized acuminated pustules, usually seated upon minute reddish papular elevations. The puriform contents dry to crusts, which fall off and are followed by a slight fringe-like exfoliation around the base, constituting a grayish ring or collar. The lesions commonly involve the hair-follicles, are present in great numbers and scattered over the whole surface, and may be either disseminated or in groups; in relapses the eruption is usually localized. Variously-sized larger papules are sometimes seen scattered sparsely over the surface. It may be an early or a late secondary eruption. Minute pinpoint atrophic depressions and stains are left, which gradually become less distinct. Other symptoms of syphilis are usually present. The diagnosis is rarely difficult.

The Large Acuminated Pustular Syphiloderm (syn., acne-form syphiloderm, acne syphilitica, variola-form syphiloderm) consists of small or large split-pea-sized pustules, more or less acuminated, resembling the lesions of simple acne or variola. The resulting crusts are yellowish or brownish, usually thick and bulky, and are seated upon ulcerated bases. The lesions may develop slowly or rapidly, with or without malaise or febrile symptoms, are disseminated or grouped, at first looking more or less papular. In the subacute or relapsing cases the eruption is apt to be localized. It pursues a rapid and usually a benign course, and is to be distinguished from acne, from the potassium-iodide eruption, and from variola. The usual limitation of acne lesions to the face and shoulders, their rapid formation, and the chronic character of the disease, together with the absence of the concomitant symptoms of syphilis, are points which may be utilized in the diagnosis. Variola differs in the intensity of the general symptoms, the umbilicated pustules, and the definite duration of the disease. The acute character, bright color, course, and history of the potassium-iodide eruption are generally sufficiently characteristic.

The Small Flat Pustular Syphiloderm (syn., impetigo-form syphiloderm, impetigo syphilitica) shows itself in the form of pea-sized, flat or raised, discrete, irregularly-grouped, or confluent pustules. The crusts, which form rapidly, are a yellow, greenish-yellow, or brownish-yellow color, more or less adherent, thick, bulky, uneven, with a tendency to become granular and to crumble. Where the lesions are confluent there results a continuous sheet of crust. Beneath the crusts there may be superficial or deep ulceration. The eruption is most frequently observed about the nose, mouth, and hairy parts of the face, on the scalp, and also about the genitalia. When upon the scalp it is apt to resemble pustular eczema; the erosion or ulceration beneath, however, will serve to differentiate it.

The Large Flat Pustular Syphiloderm (syn., ecthyma-form syphiloderm, ecthyma syphiliticum) appears in the form of large pea- or dime-sized, flat pustules, with a deep red base. Crusting usually follows immediately. There are two forms of the lesion—a superficial and a deep. In the superficial variety the crust is flat, rounded, or ovalish, yellowish-brown or dark brown, and seated upon a superficial erosion or ulcer, having a grayish or yellowish secretion. It may occur upon any region, but is most common on the back, shoulders, and extremities; the lesions are sometimes numerous. It appears, as a rule, within the first year and runs a benign course. In the deep variety the crust is raised and more bulky, dark-greenish or blackish, inclining to become conical and stratified, like an oyster-shell, constituting what is designated rupia. A crust of the same character occurs in the bullous syphiloderm. If the crust is removed, an excavated ulcer is seen, having a defined or irregular outline and a greenish-yellow, puriform secretion. It is a late and a malignant manifestation, and is not infrequently met with in hospital and dispensary practice.

Syphiloderma Tuberculosum (syn., tubercular syphilide, syphilis cutanea tuberculosa) is characterized by one or more firm, circumscribed, rounded, acuminated, or semiglobular, deeply-seated, smooth, glistening or slightly scaly elevations, yellowish-red, brownish-red, or coppery in color, varying in size from a split pea to a hazelnut. They rarely occur in great numbers, and are, as a rule, confined to certain regions, and show a decided tendency to occur in groups, often forming segments of circles. When several such groups coalesce, the result is a serpiginous tract, the so-called serpiginous tubercular syphiloderm. The face, back, and extremities are favorite localities. The lesions develop slowly, are unaccompanied by subjective symptoms, and usually occur as a late manifestation, at times appearing many years after the initial lesion. A history of earlier symptoms of the disease is usually obtainable.

The eruption terminates or disappears either by absorption or by ulceration. If the former, a pigment-stain, which is usually persistent, and in some cases slight atrophy, mark the site of the lesions, and there may be also a slight amount of exfoliation. If ulceration results, it may be superficial or deep, more frequently the latter. It begins on the summit or in the interior, and the result is a deep, punched-out, more or less crescentic ulcer with a gummy, grayish-yellow deposit or covered with a crust. If the ulcerative process takes place in a patch of grouped tubercles, an extensive excavated ulcer may result. Sometimes the ulceration occurs in a crescentic or serpiginous course. In some instances from the ulcerating surface spring up papillary, wart-like, or cauliflower exorescences, with a yellowish, offensive, puriform secretion, the so-called syphilis cutanea papillomatosa. This condition is most frequently encountered upon the scalp.

Tubercular syphiloderm is to be differentiated from lupus vulgaris, leprosy, and cancer—especially the first, to which it at times bears a close resemblance. In syphilis the lesions are firmer and deeper, and form more rapidly, than in lupus; moreover, the disease is usually one of adult life and middle age, whereas lupus appears, as a rule, first in childhood.

SYPHILODERMA GUMMATOSUM (syn., gummatous syphilide, syphilis cutanea gummatosa) consists in the formation of a rounded or flat, slightly raised, moderately firm, more or less circumscribed tumor, hav_ ing its seat in the subcutaneous tissue, which later shows a tendency to break down. As a rule, only one or two tumors are present. The growth is variously known· as a gumma, gummy tumor, and syphiloma. The lesion, which is usually a late manifestation, begins as a small, pea-sized deposit beneath the skin, which gradually increases in size; the overlying skin, which is at first of a natural color, becoming pinkish or reddish. It may eventually attain the size of a walnut or may be even larger. It is firm or soft and doughy to the touch, is usually painless, and tends to break down, disappearing by absorption or ulceration, the ulcer being usually deep with perpendicular edges. It is to be distinguished from furuncle, abscess, and fatty and fibrous tumors. In most cases other symptoms of syphilis are present.

SYPHILODERMA BULLOSUM (syn., bullous syphilide, syphilis cutanea bullosa, pemphigus syphiliticus) appears in the form of discrete, disseminated, rounded or ovalish blebs, varying in size from a pea to a walnut, and containing a serous fluid which rapidly becomes cloudy or thick. In some cases the process is distinctly pustular from the beginning. The blebs, which are, as a rule, partially or fully distended, after a vari- ble time dry to crusts of a yellowish-brown or dark-greenish color, which may be thick and raised or conical and stratified, the latter constituting rupia, as in the case of the large, flat pustular syphiloderm. They are easily removed, and cover erosions or ulcers which secrete a greenish- yellow fluid. It is a rare manifestation, occurring late, is variable in its course, and is seen usually in broken-down individuals. It is not infre- quent in hereditary syphilis in the new-born.[1]

ANATOMY.—Anatomically, the syphilitic deposit consists of a round- cell infiltration. It is most typically shown in the papule and tubercle ; in the macule there is hyperæmia, with beginning tissue-cell proliferation, but the specific cell-infiltration is not distinguishable. The process usually involves the mucous layer of the epidermis, the corium, and, in the deep lesions, the subcutaneous connective tissue. The extent and depth of the infiltration depend upon the size and form of the growth.

TREATMENT.—Cutaneous syphilis, as in the case of all other manifes- tations of this disease, requires constitutional treatment, and generally local medication also. In order that relapses may in a great measure be obviated, prolonged treatment by appropriate remedies is essential. Even with such management and under the .best circumstances relapses will frequently occur. The advantage of temperate and regular living and hygienic influences in promoting a disappearance of the manifestations and keeping the disease in abeyance cannot be too strongly urged. In syphilitic subjects anæmia, dyspepsia, malaria, or any similar condition is apt to render the syphilis more violent, and, if present, should receive appropriate treatment. Ill health from any cause predisposes to a relapse.

[1] For the cutaneous manifestations of hereditary syphilis see article by J. William White on that subject in Vol. II. p. 254.

The remedies which, in a sense, may be considered to exert a specific action in syphilis are mercury and potassium iodide. They are indispensable in the treatment of the disease. Both are important, although the former is the more valuable. As a rule, mercury is the remedy to be given in the first stages of the disease, and the cases are exceptional in which its use is not permissible. In such instances potassium iodide is to be prescribed. As the later stages of the disease approach the iodide of potassium becomes relatively more important. Even in the late syphilodermata, however, mercury in small doses holds a prominent place in the treatment, as it seems to possess a greater influence in preventing relapses. In the administration of mercury salivation is to be carefully guarded against, as its occurrence is detrimental to the health of the patient, and indirectly as well as directly it exerts an unfavorable influence on the course of the disease. Beyond slight tenderness of the gums its action should never be pushed.

There are several methods of administering mercury, but that by the mouth is for many reasons the best. For this purpose various preparations, such as blue mass, calomel, corrosive sublimate, the protiodide and biniodide, as well as other mercurials, are used. In the average case the protiodide is one of the best, and is probably in most general use. It is given in pill form in the dose of one-fourth or one-half a grain three times daily. If gastric or intestinal disturbance, such as pain and diarrhœa, is produced by its use, as is occasionally the case with this and all other preparations of mercury, a small proportion of opium may be added to each pill. Blue mass is an important mercurial in the early syphilodermata, and is given in doses of two or three grains three times daily. For bringing the system rapidly under the influence of the mineral, an important consideration in some cases, calomel in doses of one or two grains combined with opium, three or four times a day, is the most active. Corrosive sublimate is slow in its action, but is usually well borne and shows but slight disposition to salivate. The dose is one-twenty-fourth to one-eighth of a grain in pill or solution three times daily. It is rarely employed in early syphilis, but is a useful mercurial for long-continued administration, and also in the later stages of the disease.

Inunction is another method of introducing mercury into the system, and is especially useful in treating the disease in the infant. For this purpose two preparations are used—blue ointment and oleate of mercury. The latter, 5 to 20 per cent. strength, has lately been somewhat extensively employed, but it is not comparable in value for this purpose to the blue ointment. The sole advantage of the oleate is its light color. The blue ointment may always be prescribed with confidence as to its effect; the same cannot be said of the oleate. Various regions are selected for the inunctions—the arms, axillæ, thighs, abdomen, chest, and back being taken in turn, so as to obviate as far as possible local irritation. About a drachm of the blue ointment suffices for an inunction. For infants the preparation should be weakened. By means of inunctions the system may rapidly be brought under the influence of the remedy.

Another method of introducing mercury is by hypodermic injections. Corrosive sublimate is the preparation commonly employed; about one-tenth of a grain, with about the same same quantity of morphia, dissolved in fifteen minims of water, constitutes the average amount for an injection, one being made daily. The back, especially the lateral regions, is the part usually selected. The method has the advantage of rapidity of action, twenty to thirty injections sufficing, as a rule, to remove the lesions. At the same time potassium iodide, if indicated, may be given by the mouth. The method, however, is objectionable, the injections producing pain, inflammatory swelling, and induration, and not infrequently abscesses. Ptyalism, a possible accident also, is to be guarded against.

The mercurial vapor bath is in many cases of value. Calomel or the black oxide of mercury is commonly used, about thirty grains of either to the bath. A vaporizing apparatus, containing the mineral and water required, is placed beneath the stool or chair, and the patient enveloped in a sleeveless flannel gown and covered over with a rubber blanket, the bath lasting about thirty minutes. The patient remains covered until cooled off, and then goes to bed in the flannel gown. The plan has cleanliness and simplicity as well as effectiveness to commend it. The corrosive-sublimate water bath is another method that is useful, especially for infants—ten to thirty grains to the bath for an infant, and two to four drachms for an adult. From fifteen minutes to half an hour should be passed in the bath.

Potassium iodide is, as already stated, indispensable in the treatment of late manifestations. The average dose is ten to twenty grains three times daily, but in many obstinate cases much larger doses may be necessary. It is usually given after meals, but it may be taken largely diluted half an hour before eating to greater advantage. Mercury should be, for reasons already stated, prescribed with it, the two remedies constituting the so-called mixed treatment. Another remedy frequently of use in the treatment of syphilis, especially in obstinate cases of ulceration, is opium in the dose of one or two grains three times daily, which in some cases possesses the power of arresting the activity of the process.

Local treatment remains to be considered. In the macular and small papular eruptions it is rarely called for, but in the more severe syphilodermata their disappearance may be hastened by external applications. The mercurial vapor and water baths already mentioned are serviceable; also an ointment of ammoniated mercury, a drachm to the ounce, a 5 to 20 per cent. oleate-of-mercury ointment, and citrine ointment with two to four parts of lard, constitute excellent local remedies. Mercurial plaster is frequently of value, especially in reducing infiltrations. In the palmar and plantar syphilides strong ointments are necessary, and should be well worked into the skin. Moist papules always require treatment; cleanliness is of great importance. Applications of solutions of chlorinated soda, corrosive-sublimate lotion, and a lotion of carbolic acid, followed by a dusting-powder of calomel, oxide of zinc, or starch, may be advised. The ulcerative lesions, after the removal of crusts by means of hot water or oily applications, are to be treated with the ointments or lotions named above.

Epithelioma.

There are three varieties of epithelioma or skin cancer—superficial, deep-seated, and papillomatous. The superficial, or flat, form begins as a minute, firm, reddish or yellowish prominence, or it may begin as an aggregation of such lesions. The process may remain in this stage for months or years; sooner or later, however, the summit of the growth becomes slightly scaly and shows a softened or excoriated centre. From this central point a small quantity of fluid oozes, which forms a yellowish or brownish crust. This scale or crust becomes detached from time to time, either intentionally or by accident, and is followed by another similar in character, but possibly larger than that which had preceded. At the same time the underlying nodule or nodules slowly increase in size.

In this condition it may remain for months or years, but sooner or later the process becomes more active. New nodules form about the edges of the patch, and in a variable period go through the same steps as those forming the original lesions. The excoriation or ulcer becomes more marked, being as large as a pea or a dime, irregular in outline, more or less crusted. It is defined against the surrounding healthy skin by a flat or slightly elevated, more or less hardened, infiltrated border. The ulcer, which has usually an uneven surface, secretes a scanty, thin, viscid fluid, which dries to a firm, adherent crust. At points there may be a disposition to spontaneous involution, the epithelial growth being cast off by suppuration, depressed scar-tissue taking its place. The ulcerative process, however, generally progresses until often a sore of considerable size may form. The general health remains unaffected. The superficial variety may form as described, and may so continue its course, or it may at any stage pass into the more malignant, deep-seated variety.

This latter variety may begin as a tubercle or nodule in the normal skin, or it may, as already stated, start from the superficial or other variety. Where it develops typically a pea-sized, reddish, shining tubercle or nodule, or an area of infiltration, forms in the skin, or even in the subcutaneous connective tissue, which grows slowly or rapidly, usually from six months to a year or more elapsing before exciting solicitude. Sooner or later, depending on the virulence of the process, ulceration takes place, superficial or deep-seated in character, depending upon the amount of infiltration. The surface of the ulcer is granular and reddish and secretes an ichorous discharge, and the edges are indurated and, as a rule, everted. As the infiltration spreads the ulcer enlarges peripherally, and at the same time involves the deeper parts, muscle, cartilage, and bone often becoming implicated. The glands also become involved, burning or neuralgic pains are felt, and the strength gradually declines, until from septicæmia, marasmus, or implication of vital parts death results.

The third variety, the papillomatous, may arise in the form of a papillary or warty growth, or it may develop, as is more commonly the case, from either the superficial or the deep-seated variety. At an advanced period its surface is papillomatous or warty, is ulcerated and fissured, bleeds easily, and discharges an ichorous fluid, which dries and forms a brownish crust.

Epithelioma is most frequently encountered about the face; the nose, eyelids, and cheek all being favorite localities. The neck, the hands, and the genitalia also suffer frequently. If seated about the genitals, its course is apt to be more rapid and destructive. The predisposing causes are not well understood. The disease rarely shows itself before middle life, and is much more common in men than in women. It is not, as a rule, inherited. The exciting causes are frequently to be found in long-continued alterations in the epithelial structures, such as, for example, occur in warts. Any locally irritated tissue may be the starting-point of the disease. The process consists in the proliferation of epithelial cells from the mucous layer. The cell-growth takes place downward in the form of finger-like prolongations or columns, or it may spread out laterally, so as to form rounded masses, the centres of which usually undergo horny transformation, resulting in onion-like bodies, the so-called cell-nests or globes. The rapid cell-growth requires increased nutriment, and hence the blood-vessels become enlarged; moreover, the pressure of the cell-masses gives rise to irritation and inflammation, with corresponding serous and round-cell infiltration.

Epithelioma is to be differentiated from syphilis, wart, and lupus. Occurring about the genitals, it may be confounded with chancre, but the history, duration, character of the base and edges will serve to differentiate the diseases. The syphilitic lesion, wherever occurring, runs a much more rapid course than epithelioma. In tubercular syphilis several points of ulceration are usually seen; in epithelioma usually only one. The secretion from syphilitic ulcerations is generally abundant and of a yellowish, creamy character; in cancer it is scanty, viscid, stringy, and streaked with blood. The ulcer of syphilis rarely has the elevated, infiltrated border usually seen in epithelioma. Warts or warty growths must be distinguished by attention to their history and course; observation extending over months may at times be necessary before a positive opinion as to the existence of epithelial degeneration is warrantable. In lupus vulgaris the deposits are peculiar and are multiple, while in epithelioma the lesion is usually a single formation. The former generally begins in early life; the latter is a disease of the middle-aged and old. It remains to be stated that occasionally cancer and lupus occur combined, the former usually following the latter.

TREATMENT.—The variety, extent, and rapidity of the process are always to be duly considered in the prognosis. The superficial form may exist for many years without causing alarm. The deep-seated variety is always to be viewed as a serious disease, and is often fatal. Relapses after operation, even where this has been well performed, are frequent. The treatment is in most cases—for the time, at all events—successful. If the diseased tissue is thoroughly removed, the relief may be permanent or may at the least extend over several years. If, however, cauterization or operation is not thorough, the parts are scarcely healed before symptoms of a recurrence manifest themselves. Internal treatment does not seem to exert any beneficial effect upon the disease. In regard to local treatment, whatever operation or remedy is capable of removing or destroying the growth may be employed, caustics, the curette, and the knife all being available for this purpose.

Among the caustic agents, potassa in stick or in solution is one of the most valuable. Chloride of zinc in paste or stick form may also be mentioned as being of service, but it is a painful caustic. Arsenical pastes are efficient, and have the advantage of sparing the healthy tissues; one consisting of equal parts of powdered acacia and arsenic, to which a small proportion of morphia may be added, will be found serviceable;

it should kept applied in the form of a plaster for from six to twenty-four hours, or until the pain, which is apt to be severe, becomes unbearable, and then poultices applied. Pyrogallic acid, from one to four drachms to the ounce of resin cerate, is a very valuable remedy. Its action is slow; it should be renewed twice daily, and its application continued for a week or longer. As a rule, it is painless.

One of the best plans of treatment is that with the dermal curette. The diseased tissue is thoroughly scraped away, the wound dressed with some simple ointment, and healing allowed to take place. Sometimes after the use of the curette it is advisable to cauterize lightly with caustic potash or to apply an ointment of pyrogallic acid for a few days to ensure complete destruction of the disease. There are other cases in which excision constitutes the most useful method of treatment. In cases in which there is much loss of tissue a plastic operation may be performed, being preceded by a thorough removal of the diseased tissues. The galvano-cautery is another method which may be resorted to.

Sarcoma.

Sarcoma cutis, or sarcoma of the skin, is a rare affection, consisting of shot-, pea-, hazelnut-, or larger-sized, variously-shaped, discrete, non-pigmented or pigmented tubercles or tumors. They are smooth, firm, and elastic, are not markedly painful upon pressure, and show a tendency to reach the surface and ulcerate. The overlying skin is at first normal and somewhat movable, but as the lesions approach the surface it becomes reddened and adherent, or if of the pigmented variety the skin acquires a bluish-black color. The multiple pigmented sarcoma (melano-sarcoma) appears, as a rule, first on the soles and dorsal surfaces of the feet, and later on the hands, the lesions manifesting a disposition to bleed.

The disease described by Geber and one of us (Duhring) under the name of inflammatory fungoid neoplasm is doubtless a form of, or closely allied to, sarcoma. It manifests itself by the formation of several distinct kinds of lesions, the more important consisting of flat or slightly-raised coin- to palm-sized, rounded or ovalish, superficial or deep-seated, smooth, scaly, or crusted patches of a pale-pinkish or deep-reddish color; and prominent, rounded, or ovalish, soft, firm, or solid, furrowed or lobulated, tubercular or fungoid tumors, varying in size from a pea to an egg, somewhat depressed in the centre, and pale-red, deep raspberry-red, or violaceous in color. The flat patches with involution assume a mottled or streaked purplish, yellowish, or salmon color. The tumors may appear suddenly within a few hours or a day, or gradually in the course of weeks or months. After reaching a certain size they tend to soften, diminish in size, and undergo spontaneous involution or ulcerate. Itching and burning are usually complained of, but are variable. All regions may be attacked. It is rare. The so-called lymphadenoma, lymphadénie cutanée, and mycosis fungoïde of the French may also, doubtless, be properly classified as a variety of sarcoma.

The disease is to be distinguished from the papular, tubercular, and gummative syphilodermata, lupus, leprosy, and carcinoma. As a rule, sooner or later, a fatal termination takes place. Treatment is palliative. Surgical interference may be of service in particular situations. Hypodermic injections of Fowler's solution in increasing doses have, it is stated, influenced the disease favorably.

CLASS VII.—NEUROSES.

Dermatalgia.

DERMATALGIA, or neuralgia of the skin, is characterized by pain having its seat solely in the skin, unattended by structural change, and associated usually with a morbidly sensitive condition of the part. The symptoms are purely subjective, as in pruritus. The skin shows no alteration. It is usually a local disorder, confined to a small area, and is met with, as a rule, in adult age. It consists in a highly-sensitive state of the integument, with a feeling of positive pain having its seat in the superficial layers of the skin, which is remarkably sensitive to external impressions; the touch, contact of the clothing, and even the air, exciting more or less pain. In character the sensation is burning, pricking or darting, or like electric shocks. It is generally worse at night. The affection may exist idiopathically or symptomatically, the latter being the more common and accompanying lesions of the nervous centres. Its frequent connection with rheumatism has been pointed out by Beau and other writers, from which fact it is sometimes called rheumatism of the skin; but in other cases it occurs in persons apparently in good health. Hysteria has also been noted as a cause. The general treatment depends upon the exciting cause, but local measures may be demanded to relieve the disagreeable or painful sensations, among which the galvanic current, applications containing belladonna, aconite, or iodine and blistering may be tried.

Pruritus.

Pruritus is a functional disease of the skin, characterized solely by the sensation of itching, without the existence of structural change. The affection must be clearly separated from the many other cutaneous diseases accompanied by itching. In pruritus the single symptom is itching, varying in kind and degree. There are no primary structural lesions, but secondary lesions, resulting from scratching and local irritation, are not infrequently present. The sensation is variously described by the sufferers, being often likened to the crawling of small insects over the surface. The desire to rub or scratch is irresistible. In other cases the sensation is a tingling, or as though some irritating substance, as flannel, was in contact with the surface. It exists in all degrees of severity, and frequently proves a source of great distress. It may occur at any age, but is most often met with in middle life and in old age, constituting so-called pruritus senilis. The itching may be constant or intermittent, but is usually the latter, occurring in most cases paroxysmally, and being almost invariably worse at night.

The disease may be local or general, but it seldom invades large portions of the surface at one time. In most cases it is a local disorder, the common regions being the genitalia and anus. The trunk, especially in elderly persons, is also not infrequently invaded. Occurring about the female genital organs, it constitutes the pruritus vulvæ of writers, having its seat in the labia or in the vagina. It is a very distressing form of disease, and is met with, as a rule, in middle life and old age. In the male the anus and the scrotum are the regions generally attacked, the perineum sometimes also being involved simultaneously. The anus in either sex is liable to invasion, the disease occurring here in children as well as in adults. All of these local varieties, as stated, are worse at night, and sometimes prove so harassing as to interfere greatly with sleep.

The causes which give rise to the affection are varied. Thus it is sometimes called forth by gestation and by the various disorders of menstruation, and in other instances, in either sex, by organic diseases of the genito-urinary tract. Diseases of the kidney and of the liver, especially jaundice, are frequently accompanied by pruritus. The nervous system is not infrequently at fault. Gastro-intestinal derangement, the ingestion of certain medicines (as opium), intestinal parasites, and hemorrhoids, are all well-known causes. The disease is strictly functional in nature, and is due to reflex nervous action.

The diagnosis rests with the subjective symptoms as given by the sufferer. There are no primary lesions; the secondary lesions, however, are sometimes so extensive as to suggest other diseases, especially prurigo and eczema, but there should be no difficulty in differentiating these diseases if their clinical features are kept in mind. Prurigo—a disease, practically speaking, unknown in this country—it will be remembered, is characterized by well-defined papules, and moreover shows predilection for the lower extremities. The subjective symptoms of pruritus often simulate those due to the presence of lice. In all cases these parasites, whether of the head, body, or pubes, should be carefully excluded in the diagnosis, for it sometimes happens that pediculosis is looked upon and treated as pruritus, the true nature of the affection being unsuspected. Pediculosis, it must not be forgotten, is occasionally met with in the upper walks of life, where it is at times extremely difficult to account for the source of contagion. Inspection of the skin and of the underclothing should be made in all suspected cases.

The treatment naturally varies with the determined or probable cause. The local origin of the affection should, in the first place, be inquired into. The internal remedies are to be selected with the view of meeting the requirements of the case. The various functions of the body should receive due attention, the bowels, in all cases tending to constipation, being kept open by laxatives, preferably saline preparations. The diet should be directed, all stimulating or injurious food and drink being interdicted. Quinine, arsenic, belladonna, strychnine, carbolic acid, tincture of gelsemium, and pilocarpine are remedies which may be tried in obstinate cases. In all cases the cause should be diligently sought for, for until this is discovered and removed there can be but little hope of complete recovery. External remedies, though extremely grateful to the patient, and of course very useful, as a rule are only palliative. There are cases, however, in which they prove curative. Water in the form of very hot or cold douches, and alkaline and sulphur lotions and baths, are sometimes serviceable, employed either alone or in connection with other remedies. In the local varieties of the disease antipruritic and stimulating lotions are especially serviceable. One of the most valuable remedies is carbolic acid, in the strength of from fifteen to forty grains to the ounce, to which may be added small quantities of glycerin and alcohol. A strong lotion consists of carbolic acid, one drachm and a half; potassa, twenty grains; water, eight ounces. The tarry preparations considered in eczema, especially liquor carbonis detergens and liquor picis alkalinus, are useful, as are likewise thymol, a few grains to the ounce of glycerin and alcohol, and oil of peppermint. The latter remedy, pure or mixed with glycerin, may be applied with a brush. Sometimes a simple chloral lotion is efficacious. In like manner lotions of acetate of lead, ten to thirty grains to the ounce; dilute hydrocyanic acid, a few drachms to the pint; hyposulphite of sodium; chloroform; chloroform and alcohol; diluted acetic acid; diluted ammonia-water; diluted nitric-acid; and corrosive sublimate,—may be tried. R. W. Taylor recommends the following:

> ℞. Fol. belladonnæ,
> Fol. hyoscyami, āā. ʒij;
> Fol. aconiti, ʒss;
> Acidi acetici, fʒj. M.

This may be diluted with water a drachm to the ounce, or may be used with equal parts of glycerin, painted on the skin or in the form of an ointment, a drachm or two to the ounce. Tobacco, used as an infusion, two or three drachms to the pint, is often efficacious, especially in pruritus vulvæ. The fluid extract of conium, applied with a brush, and iodoform in ethereal solution, applied as a spray, may likewise be resorted to where the disease involves this region. Camphor and borax may be mentioned as being sometimes of service, as in the following formula:

> ℞. Sodii boratis, ʒij;
> Glycerinæ, fʒiv;
> Spts. camphoræ, fʒss;
> Aquæ rosæ, ʒv. M.

Another lotion, containing borax and morphia, may be given:

> ℞. Sodii boratis, ʒiv;
> Morphiæ sulph., gr. xv;
> Glycerinæ, fʒss;
> Aquæ, q. s. ad fʒviij. M.

In some cases ointments prove more acceptable than lotions. Tar, carbolic acid, thymol, and the mercurials are all valuable used in this form, varying in strength with the locality and amount of surface to be treated. The smaller the area, as a rule, the stronger the remedy. Chloroform, chloral, and camphor also may be used in the form of ointments. About one drachm each of chloral and camphor to the ounce constitutes a good antipruritic remedy; the active ingredients are to be rubbed together and then added to the ointment.

In pruritus of the anus one of the most valuable and neatest remedies is carbolic acid with glycerin or olive oil, in the strength of from fifteen to forty grains to the ounce. Very hot water applied with a soft linen compress or sponge will usually afford temporary ease, and may be employed from time to time in connection with other more active rem-

edies. In some cases we have had rapid and good results from an ointment of balsam of Peru, a drachm and a half to the ounce. Equal parts
of belladonna ointment and mercurial ointment, and a solution of corrosive sublimate, about a quarter of a grain to the ounce, may also be
mentioned; and where there are fissures occasional pencilling with a
solution of nitrate of silver will afford relief, the latter application,
made with a piece of sponge fastened on a stick, being also useful in
pruritus vulvæ.

A long list of formulæ have been vaunted for the relief of pruritus of
the female genitalia, a few of which may be given. In addition to the
remedies already mentioned the following formulæ will sometimes prove
valuable. The fluid preparations may be used as vaginal injections or
may be applied by means of a brush, tampon or cloth, according to their
nature. Hyposulphite of sodium, a drachm to the ounce; sulphurous
acid, sufficiently diluted; alum, sulphate of zinc, tannic acid, acetic acid,
borax, and boric acid, may all be made use of in the form of injections.
In this variety of the disease, as well as in pruritus of the anus, a 6 per
cent. solution of cocaine, applied with a brush, or the oleate used as an
ointment in the same strength, may be prescribed.

The prognosis should in all cases be guarded, the ability to relieve the
disorder depending mainly upon the nature of the cause. The majority
of cases, due to no evident cause, prove obstinate. But in all instances
the patient should be encouraged to persevere in the treatment, and the
hope of an ultimate cure extended to him.

PRURITUS HIEMALIS.—This is a peculiar form of pruritus, characterized by a somewhat harsh and dry state of the skin, accompanied with
smarting and burning, unattended primarily by structural change,
dependent upon atmospheric influences, and occurring chiefly in winter.
It makes its appearance usually in the late autumn, becoming worse with
the colder weather, and disappearing in the spring. The disease manifests predilection for certain regions, notably the extremities, especially
the inner surfaces of the thighs, the popliteal spaces, and the calves;
but in a less degree it may also invade other localities. In its milder
form it is a common affection in cold climates. At times the itching is
severe, leading to scratching and excoriations, while in other cases it
merely amounts to an annoyance. It possesses the peculiarity of manifesting itself chiefly at night, coming on during the evening or shortly
after bed is entered. The symptoms usually vary with the weather, being
better and worse as the temperature is mild or cold. The affection in
most instances repeats itself each year, and may thus continue indefinitely
or it may partly or wholly disappear. As stated, the disorder is due to
atmospheric influences, but is aggravated by irritating underwear and
scratching. It occurs in both sexes, at all ages after puberty, and in
those who bathe freely as well as in those who make sparing use of
water. It does not seem to be influenced by the state of the general
health, nor does internal treatment affect it favorably. Among the
various external remedies, preparations containing glycerin, the petroleum ointment, carbolic acid and tar in the form of ointments and lotions,
as in eczema, and alkaline lotions and baths,—may be mentioned as being
most useful. The simple vapor bath is also in some cases beneficial.

CLASS VIII.—PARASITES.

Tinea Favosa.

TINEA FAVOSA, or favus, is a contagious, vegetable parasitic disease, due to the achorion Schönleinii, characterized by discrete or confluent pea-sized, circular, pale-yellow, friable, cup-shaped crusts, usually perforated by hairs. It is seen commonly upon the scalp, and at times on other hairy regions, involving the hairs and hair-follicles (tinea favosa pilaris), or the non-hairy portions of the integument may be attacked (tinea favosa epidermidis), and cases are occasionally met with in which the nails are the seat of the disease (tinea favosa unguium). The scalp is the usual seat. It begins as a more or less circumscribed, superficial inflammation, with slight scaling, followed by the appearance of one or more yellowish points underneath the superficial epidermis and surrounding hair-shafts. They increase in size, and reach the dimensions of small peas, constituting the so-called favus cups, favi, or favus scutula. They are sulphur-colored, friable, circumscribed, round or oval, with depressed centres, and each pierced with a hair. In their early stage they are bound down to the skin by a layer of epidermis, which surrounds and envelops their periphery. The crusts are elevated from a half to several lines above the surrounding skin, distinctly umbilicated, and if detached an excavated, reddened, atrophied or suppurating surface is disclosed.

The crusts are composed of closely-packed, concentrically-arranged layers, and although they are at first discrete, sooner or later, from increase in number and size, they coalesce, and then their peculiar features are scarcely, if at all, distinguishable, irregular masses of thick, yellowish-white, mortar-like crusts taking their place. If removed, the surface is usually found atrophied, dry or inflamed and moist, and hairless. The hair-shafts are soon involved, the nutrition of these structures impaired, and in consequence the hairs become dry, lustreless, brittle, break off or fall out, and eventually the papillæ are entirely destroyed. Pustules and suppuration are in some instances noted about the borders and beneath the crusts. The pressure of the growing fungus gives rise to atrophy of the skin, which may be seen as depressed, firm, shining, cicatricial-looking areas. The general surface may also be attacked, either together with the scalp or alone. On non-hairy regions, however, the disease is rarely persistent. If the nails are invaded, they become thickened, yellowish, opaque, and brittle. Favus is usually attended with itching, especially when occurring upon the scalp. The odor of the crusts is peculiar, and may be likened to that of mice or stale straw. Upon the scalp the disease is always chronic, if untreated lasting indefinitely.

It is more common in children than in adults, and is seen almost exclusively among the poor. It is comparatively rare in this country. It is contagious. The disease is also encountered in the lower animals, from which doubtless it is not infrequently contracted. The affection is due solely to the growth in the upper layers of the skin of the achorion Schönleinii. This vegetable parasite grows luxuriantly, and constitutes almost entirely the whole mass of the crusts. It can be readily seen by subjecting a small portion of the crust, moistened with diluted liquor potassæ, to microscopical examination, a power of three to five hundred diameters sufficing. It consists of both spores and mycelium. The mycelium is composed of pale-grayish or pale-greenish narrow, flat threads or tubes branching and anastomosing in all directions. The spores are small, variable as to size, round, oval, flask- or dumb-bell-shaped, and are to be seen in abundance in the meshes of the mycelium. Intermediate forms between the spores and mycelium are always present. The hair-follicles and hair-shafts are found to be more or less invaded. If the nails are attacked, the fungus can be easily detected in a section or in scrapings, the mycelium predominating.

As a rule, favus is easily recognized. The small, pale, yellow, friable cup- or saucer-shaped crusts and the peculiar odor are sufficiently characteristic. In some chronic cases, where the crusts are merged into a mass, perhaps mixed with dirt and pus, it resembles pustular eczema; but the condition of the hair, the atrophic patches, and the odor will serve as distinguishing points. Tinea tonsurans can scarcely be confounded with this disease, as it is wanting in the peculiar crust-formation and the tendency to scarring. In doubtful cases the microscope is to be employed.

Favus of the scalp is not only a chronic disease, but is also rebellious to treatment. In neglected cases permanent baldness, atrophy, and searring sooner or later occur. On the non-hairy portions of the body it is rarely obstinate; involving the nails, it is slow to yield. The first step in the treatment of a case of favus of the scalp, the common seat of the disease, is a removal of the crusts. This is readily accomplished by saturating the parts with simple or carbolized oil, and subsequently washing with soap and hot water. The hair on and around the patches is to be clipped as a preliminary measure; keeping the hair of the entire scalp cut short facilitates treatment, but is not essential. The hairs in the diseased areas are then to be carefully extracted by means of the broad-bladed forceps. This part of the treatment, epilation or extraction of the hairs, is indispensable if the eventual result is to be successful and permanent. Before epilating, the surface to be operated upon is to be anointed with a simple oil. After the operation a parasiticide is to be thoroughly applied, so that it may penetrate the hair-follicles. The whole surface involved is thus treated. Another plan of epilation is that in which the hair is drawn with some force between the thumb and an ordinary tongue-spatula, those that are diseased and loose coming out, while those that are sound remain. In this method the hair is not clipped. The plan is more simple and less tedious than forceps epilation, but is not so satisfactory, as the hairs are more likely to break off, and, moreover, many that are diseased are left unextracted.

Whatever parasiticide is used should be well and thoroughly applied to the affected areas. Those that have the greatest penetrating power are to be selected. Corrosive sublimate, three or four grains to the ounce of alcohol or ether; a 25 per cent. oleate-of-mercury ointment; carbolic acid and glycerin, one part of the former to three or more of the latter,—may be mentioned as among the most useful. Tar, sulphur, and ammoniated mercury and citrine ointments, of officinal strength or weakened; sulphurous acid; a solution of hyposulphite of sodium, a drachm to the ounce, —are also efficient parasiticides. Chrysarobin, in ointment or in chloroform, a drachm to the ounce, has been well spoken of, but must be used cautiously. After several weeks' treatment applications may be suspended for a week or more, so that the condition may again be determined. In ordinary well-developed cases from three to six months' active treatment is required for a removal of the disease.

Favus of the non-hairy portions of the surface requires, after a removal of the crusts, the application of a mild parasiticide, the disease, as a rule, readily yielding. In favus of the nail as much as possible of the affected portion is to be pared or cut away, and a simple parasiticide applied once or twice daily. In those who are debilitated and ill-nourished favus may possibly be rendered less obstinate by suitable internal treatment, with proper nourishment and pure air.

Tinea Trichophytina.

Tinea trichophytina, or ringworm, is a contagious vegetable parasitic disease, due to the trichophyton, its clinical characters varying according to the part invaded. It is a common disease, more frequent in children than in adults, and is met with to a varying extent in all countries. It is contagious, but individuals vary as regards susceptibility. The fungus (the trichophyton) consists of spores and mycelium. The latter consists of long, slender, delicate, sharply-contoured, pale-grayish, straight or crooked, branching, ribbon-like threads, containing spores and granules. They are remarkable for their length. The spores are round, small, highly refractive, grayish or pale-greenish bodies, and are either single or arranged in rows, which may be isolated or joined to mycelium. The appearances of the disease, and to a certain extent its treatment, are so different when affecting the general surface, the scalp or the bearded region that separate descriptions are called for. When seated upon the general surface the disease is commonly known as tinea circinata (tinea trichophytina corporis); on the scalp, tinea tonsurans (tinea trichophytina capitis); on the bearded region, tinea sycosis (tinea trichophytina barbæ).

TINEA CIRCINATA, or ringworm of the body, is characterized by one or more circular or irregularly-shaped, variously-sized, inflammatory, slightly vesicular or squamous patches. It usually begins by the formation of one or more roundish, slightly-elevated, sharply-limited, somewhat scaly, hyperæmic spots, which in some cases show minute papules or vesicles, especially about the periphery. As the process advances, usually in the course of a few days, the inflammation is more marked and the scaliness increased. The patches assume, as a rule, a distinctly annular character, and as they grow by extending peripherally, their centres clear up, so that when fully developed they are usually about an inch in diamete', and consist of a more or-less normal central area, then an intermediate pale-reddish scaly portion, and the red, elevated, and scaly or papulo-vesicular or vesicular border defined against the healthy skin. In rare instances vesico-pustules may form. There may be one, several, or many patches present, but as a rule they are not numerous. After attaining a certain size they may remain stationary for a short time or may begin to disappear spontaneously. Where two or more are in close proximity, they may increase in size, gradually coalesce, and form gyrate or irregularly-shaped lesions. At times, instead of the typical annular patches, the disease may appear in the form of disseminated, small, reddish, slightly scaly, ill-defined spots, which may appear and disappear rapidly, the patient rarely being free of lesions. Although any portion of the general surface may be invaded, there are certain regions of predilection, as the face, neck, and backs of the hands. It is commoner in children than in adults.

Involving surfaces that are in close contact, as the axillæ, between the buttocks, and the inner surfaces of the thighs, it tends to spread extensively, is more inflammatory, and often proves rebellious to treatment. Invading these parts, the condition, under the impression that it was an eczema, was described by Hebra as eczema marginatum. It is most common, however, about the thighs, and seated here is termed tinea circinata cruris. It begins usually in the same manner as ringworm on other regions, but on account of the heat, moisture, and friction of the parts its characters become changed. The patch becomes inflamed, slightly elevated, coalescing with similar patches, until the greater part of the inner surface of the thighs and buttocks may be involved. The groins and mons veneris may also be invaded. When fully developed it is characterized by extensive, irregularly-shaped, inflammatory patches, with at times a slightly moist surface, and is usually well defined against the surrounding healthy skin by a more or less raised border, which may show papules or vesicles. Sometimes beyond the general area involved may be seen more or less typical ringworm patches. As met with in this country, it is usually mild in character. In Southern Europe it is encountered more frequently, is of a severer type, and is often intractable. It is met with usually in adults. Relapses are not uncommon.

The course of ringworm of the general surface may be acute or chronic. It may disappear in a few weeks, or, on the other hand, may continue indefinitely. As commonly met with in this country, it is, as a rule, readily responsive to treatment. It is frequently seen in association with ringworm of the scalp. Itching in variable degree is usually present. Invading the nails, the affection is designated tinea trichophytina unguium. These structures become dry, opaque, dirty white or yellowish, thickened, of irregular shape, bent, soft, or brittle and laminated, the changes taking place especially about the free border. The nails of the toes are seldom affected. As a rule, not more than two or three of the finger-nails are attacked. It is commonly associated with chronic ringworm on other parts of the body.

The fungus (trichophyton) in tinea circinata has its seat in the epidermis, especially in the corneous layer. The first effect of its invasion is hyperæmia, subsequently inflammation, usually mild in character, with more or less scaling. A microscopical examination, with a power of two to five hundred diameters, of scales from the periphery of a patch, moistened with liquor potassæ, will show both mycelium and spores, the latter comparatively few in number. In fact, the fungus in ringworm of the body is rarely to be found in abundance. In tinea trichophytina unguium the substance of the nail is invaded, scrapings of which will show the fungus, usually the mycelium, generally but few spores being present.

The affection is to be recognized by its peculiar clinical features, and, if necessary, by means of the microscope. This instrument should always be employed in cases of doubt. At times it bears resemblance to eczema and seborrhœa, and to psoriasis. From eczema it may be distinguished by its circular or annular form, its sharply-defined margins, its tendency to clear up in the centre, its slight desquamation, and its history and course; the itching is usually less marked than in eczema. Seborrhœa, when occurring on the chest and back, often consists of circular patches similar in general features to ringworm, but the scales are greasy, and are seated upon non-inflamed skin; the scaliness of ringworm is the result of inflammation, while that of seborrhœa consists of dried sebaceous matter. Moreover, in the latter affection the sebaceous follicular openings are perceptibly enlarged, and are indicative of the nature of the disease. In psoriasis at times the patches clear up in the centre, and in such instances a mistake in diagnosis might occur. The scaliness of psoriasis, however, is always a marked feature; it is usually insignificant in ringworm. Moreover, the characters of the scales are different. Occasionally the circinate tubercular syphiloderm has been confounded with ringworm, but the nature of the patch in the former disease, consisting of an irregular and incomplete ring of elevated tubercles or infiltrations, with, at times, ulceration, is so entirely different from the latter affection that an error should not occur. It can scarcely be confounded with favus if the peculiar yellowish, cup-shaped crusts of that disease are kept in mind; the clinical features of the two affections are also in other respects dissimilar.

The treatment consists in the application of the milder parasiticides, the disease rarely proving obstinate. In exceptional cases, where the affection is persistent, it will sometimes be found that the general nutrition is below the standard; and in such instances constitutional remedies of a tonic nature, as cod-liver oil, iron, quinine, and arsenic, are serviceable. In children the skin is delicate and strong remedies are not well borne; nor are they, as a rule, necessary. The parts should be first washed with soap and water, and then the remedial applications made; the lotion or ointment should be applied two or three times daily. If a lotion, it should be dabbed on thoroughly; if an ointment, it should be thoroughly rubbed into the patches. The sulphite or hyposulphite of sodium, in lotion or ointment form, a drachm to the ounce; sulphurous acid, full strength or diluted; ammoniated mercury, thirty to sixty grains to the ounce of lard or vaseline; corrosive sublimate, two to four grains to an ounce of alcohol or water; an ointment of sulphur, a drachm or two to the ounce; tar ointment, a drachm or two to the ounce; carbolic acid, ten to thirty grains to the ounce of water or lard,—are all parasiticides of value which may be employed in this disease. In obstinate cases chrysarobin, five to thirty grains to the ounce of lard, may be cautiously used, or it may be applied in collodion or gutta-percha solution, 5 to 10 per cent. strength. In tinea circinata cruris applications such as the above, but stronger, are serviceable. R. W. Taylor speaks well of a solution of corrosive sublimate in tincture of benzoin, two to four grains to the ounce, painted over the parts. The chrysarobin ointment or solution already mentioned may also be especially referred to. Hebra's modification of Wilkinson's ointment (see Scabies for formula) is useful in these cases. In tinea trichophytina unguium the nail should be pared or scraped, and one of the parasiticides applied.

TINEA TONSURANS.—Tinea tonsurans, or ringworm of the scalp, is characterized by circular or irregularly-shaped, variously-sized, scaly, more or less bald patches, showing the hair to be diseased and usually broken off close to the scalp. It is met with in children, especially in those under the age of twelve years; it is rarely seen after puberty. It begins as one or more small, round, erythematous, scaly spots, which may be minutely papulo-vesicular or vesicular about the periphery. Soon by peripheral growth typical circular patches of various sizes are formed, averaging about an inch in diameter. More or less itching is usually complained of. A typical patch is circumscribed, slightly elevated, reddish, grayish or slate-colored, with more or less scaling, usually thin or bran-like in character, with the hairs broken off close to the scalp. The color varies with the complexion of the individual; in marked blondes it has usually an inflammatory tint, while in those of dark hair and skin it is bluish-gray or the color of slate. The hairs on the affected areas are involved early in the disease, becoming lustreless, dry, brittle, twisted, breaking off close to the skin, with their free extremities ragged and uneven, having a gnawed or nibbled look. They are easily extracted, or often break off within the follicles, appearing then as blackish dots. A variable degree of baldness occurs, which, however, is rarely permanent. In some instances the patch is non-inflammatory and free of scales, the loss of hair, which is more or less complete, taking place rapidly, such cases bearing resemblance to alopecia areata. As a rule, several patches varying in duration and size are present. They may remain discrete, or coalesce and form irregular areas. The vertex and parietal regions are favorite localities, although any region of the scalp may be invaded. It is not uncommon to see patches of the disease on the non-hairy portions of the body at the same time.

In some cases, especially in those ill nourished and scrofulous, the inflammation may be of a higher grade, resulting in the production of discrete or grouped pustules, terminating in crusting; or the disease may assume the condition known as tinea kerion. This latter is seen most commonly in scrofulous subjects. Beginning ordinarily as a simple patch of ringworm, the affected area soon becomes inflamed, swollen, œdematous, elevated, red, shining and boggy, covered with a mucoid secretion which is poured out from the openings of the hair-follicles. The stubby hairs soon fall out, leaving the patch more or less bald. The surface is uneven and studded with the foramina, or small cavities, containing the mucoid or sero-purulent secretion, corresponding to the dilated hair-follicles. It bears resemblance to abscess and carbuncle. An analogous condition is not uncommon in tinea sycosis. It may occur with the usual form of tinea tonsurans or alone. Occasionally the disease cures itself in this way. It may, however, be chronic. Its causes are not understood: it may be due to the presence of the fungus in the deeper portions of the hair-follicles, or at times to over-treatment. It is a rare manifestation.

Other unusual forms of the disease are occasionally noted. The spots may in the early stages be merely scaly, with or without inflammatory symptoms, and the hairs long and firmly seated, resembling eczema or seborrhœa. Later, however, the hairs break and the characteristic stumps are the result. As ringworm becomes chronic (its usual course) the clinical features become different. The disease exists in irregular areas—as a rule, non-inflammatory and more or less scaly, especially about the follicles. The hairs are short, stubby, and broken off near the skin or in the apertures of the follicles; in the latter case the skin has a punctate or dotted appearance. This condition is noted especially in brunettes; in blondes the hairs are somewhat longer and apt to drop out insidiously. Or, the disease may be disseminated, involving here and there over the scalp small groups of follicles, the hairs being short, the follicles slightly enlarged, with a tendency to scaliness; in these cases the disease may be easily overlooked.

Ringworm of the scalp is a common affection, and is observed among the rich as well as the poor, but is most frequent in those suffering from malnutrition. It may be communicated by means of caps, combs, brushes, and the like. It is frequently seen in schools and children's asylums, sometimes affecting a large proportion of the inmates. The fungus (trich-ophyton) invades the epidermis, hair-follicle, bulb, and shaft. The fol-licle becomes distended and raised; the hairs are permeated with the fun-gus (spores markedly predominating), are disintegrated, and destroyed. The perifollicular tissue may, in severe cases, be invaded. The spores are present in great abundance, the mycelium existing scantily.

As a rule, there is no difficulty in recognizing the disease. The pres-ence of stumps of hair having a gnawed or nibbled look, the prominent follicles, more or less baldness, and slight or decided scaliness, together with the history and course, constitute a clinical picture that is scarcely mistakable. If necessary, microscopical examination of the hair will give positive information. For this purpose one or two of the short, stubby hairs should be selected, placed upon a slide, a drop of liquor potassæ added, allowed to stand a few minutes, and then examined with a power of two to five hundred diameters; the hairs will be found full of spores, the shafts being completely disintegrated. If a few drops of chloroform are poured upon a patch of ringworm of the scalp and allowed to evaporate, the hairs and follicular openings affected become whitish or light-yellow, which, according to Duckworth, is pathogno-monic. It is to be differentiated from squamous eczema, seborrhœa, psoriasis, and alopecia areata. The history of eczema is different: it rarely begins as circular spots, spreading peripherally; the margins are always more or less irregular; the hairs are not involved, but remain seated firmly in the follicles; the itching is marked, whereas in ring-worm it is usually slight. Seborrhœa is non-inflammatory; the scales are greasy; the hairs are not broken off; and the margins of the patch are ill defined. In psoriasis the scaling is a marked feature; the hairs are not involved; and the disease is usually to be found typically expressed on other parts of the body. From alopecia areata ringworm may be differ-entiated by its clinical features; in the former disease the baldness is usually complete, the skin devoid of scales, non-inflamed, smooth, shin-ing, and the follicles, as a rule, less prominent than normal; the absence of the characteristic stumps of ringworm may also be noted. In obscure cases the microscope is to be employed.

An opinion regarding the length of time required to cure ringworm of the scalp should always be guarded; while some cases respond in several weeks, in others several months or more may be required. Relapses are liable to occur. External remedies are, as a rule, alone required. In chronic cases, however, where a condition of malnutrition exists, proper food, fresh air, and suitable internal remedies, as cod-liver oil, iron, and arsenic, are to be advised ; cleanliness is of importance.   The patches should be washed frequently with warm water and castile soap or sapo viridis, the frequency depending upon the scaling and the amount of disease, and also somewhat upon the remedies employed.   Occasional washing of the entire scalp is also to be advised.   Remedial applications should be, as a rule, made twice daily.   In acute or recent cases, in which the fungus has not penetrated deeply into the hair-follicles, it often yields to the ordinary parasiticides, without the necessity of epilation.   In cases commonly encountered, however, the disease has already lasted some length of time, and epilation becomes essential.   The main difficulty in the treatment of tinea tonsurans is to bring the remedy in contact with the fungus; otherwise the affection would be as easily curable as that occurring on the general surface.   To a great extent epilation aids in overcoming this difficulty, as the parasiticide is then able to permeate the emptied follicle ; and in addition to this advantage the extracted hairs take with them the fungus contained within their structures.   The hair within and around the affected areas should be clipped short, or, if the patches are numerous, the hair of the entire scalp should be cut, or, what is preferable in many cases, shaved.   If the scalp is shaved, a few days elapse before epilation is possible.   On a shaved head there is no chance for any diseased area, however small, to escape observation ; in the treatment of the disease as met with in institutions this procedure is almost essential.   In epilation the loose hairs on the patches and about the borders should first receive attention.   For this purpose a small, broad-bladed, short forceps may be employed, a few hairs at a time being seized.   A portion of the diseased area should be carefully gone over each day until all are removed.   After each epilation the parasiticide is to be applied.

Corrosive sublimate, two to four grains to the ounce of alcohol or water, is a reliable remedy ; also oleate of mercury, in the form preferably of a 25 per cent. ointment.   An ointment such as the following is serviceable in many cases :

> ℞. Ugt. picis liquidæ,
> Ugt. hydrarg. nitrat., āā. ʒij ;
> Ugt. sulphuris,   ʒiv.
> M. Ft. ugt.

Or, in place of the tar ointment in the formula, carbolic acid in the same or less quantity may be substituted.   The officinal tar, sulphur, and ammoniated mercury ointments may also be referred to as useful.   In small disseminated patches carbolic acid in glycerin, one to three drachms of the former with enough of the latter to make an ounce, will often prove serviceable.   Thymol sometimes proves of value, and may be prescribed as advised by Malcolm Morris :

> ℞. Thymolis,   ʒss ;
> Chloroformis, ʒij ;
> Olei olivæ,   ʒvj.   M.

Coster's paste is also serviceable :

> ℞. Iodinii,   ʒij ;
> Olei picis, ʒj.   M.

This is painted on the patch, and permitted to remain on until the crust comes off, then is reapplied : a few applications are sometimes sufficient. In tinea kerion the hairs are extracted and a mild parasiticide applied : sulphurous acid, a weak solution of corrosive sublimate, carbolic acid, ten to twenty grains to the ounce of water, or a weak ointment of the oleate of mercury or of white precipitate, may be employed.

If the disease proves obstinate, resisting the above treatment, it may be necessary to adopt stronger applications with a view of producing an acute inflammation in the part. To be efficacious the inflammatory action should be marked. For this purpose croton oil is used. It should never be employed when the disease is extensive ; or if used in such cases a small area only, not exceeding that of a quarter dollar, should be treated at one time. Although valuable, the remedy is severe, and must be used cautiously. It may be applied pure or weakened with two or three parts of olive oil. An application requires but a small quantity, as it is apt to involve the skin beyond the area of application. In some cases a single application is sufficient ; in others several or more are necessary before the requisite amount of follicular inflammation and suppuration results. The applications should be made by the physician, as it is not a safe remedy to entrust to attendants. After the application the part should be poulticed, and subsequently epilation practised and mild parasiticides employed. Instead of using croton oil, the patches may be painted with glacial acetic acid or cantharidal collodion once a week, and mild parasiticides, as sulphurous acid, carbolic-acid lotion, or sulphur ointment, applied in the interval. From time to time in the treatment of the disease, usually at intervals of from three to four weeks, applications should be discontinued a few days, and a microscopic examination of the scales and hairs made : if fungus is found, treatment is to be resumed.

TINEA SYCOSIS.—Tinea sycosis, or parasitic sycosis, is a disease confined to the hairy portions of the face and neck in the adult male, involving the hair and hair-follicles, with inflammation of the skin and subcutaneous connective tissue, and the formation of tubercles and pustules. It is popularly known under the name of barber's itch. It usually begins as one or more small, red, scaly spots, similar, in fact, to ringworm on the non-hairy portions of the surface. The redness and scabness increase, and swelling and induration are noticed. In a short time the hairs are involved, become dry, brittle, inclined to break, and begin to fall out, the same changes occurring as noted in ringworm of the scalp. The fungus passes to the hair-follicles ; perifollicular inflammation is set up, and results in the formation of deep-seated tubercles, varying in size from a pea to that of a cherry, giving the part a distinct nodular appearance. These coalesce and give rise to lumpy patches. The surface is of a deep reddish or purplish color ; pustulation is noted about the openings of the hair-follicles. More or less crusting may take place ; if removed, the hairs may come away with it. The amount of suppuration depends upon the grade of inflammation. Sometimes the hair-follicles are destroyed and permanent alopecia results.

The disease may involve a small area, appearing as a sharply-circumscribed, prominently-raised, deep-seated, nodular, coin-sized patch, with or without a purulent discharge from the emptied hair-follicles or with crusting; or the whole bearded region of the neck and chin may be invaded. It is not common on the upper lip or the upper bearded portion of the cheeks. Burning and itching are usually present, but are variable as to degree. The disease tends to chronicity. It is not uncommon at the same time to see patches .of ringworm on other portions of the body. It is markedly contagious, although individuals differ as to susceptibility. It is often contracted at the hands of a barber. The fungus (trichophyton) which gives rise to the disease invades the same parts as when seated upon the scalp—the epidermis and the hair and hair-follicles; the latter are usually found permeated with spores, the mycelium being scanty.

The affection is not common, its frequency varying in different countries. It is to be distinguished from simple (non-parasitic) sycosis, pustular eczema, and the vegetating syphiloderm. In simple sycosis the process is comparatively superficial and confined to the hair-follicles; the hairs are not involved, and in the beginning, at least, are seated firmly in the follicles. In tinea sycosis the skin and subcutaneous connective tissue are extensively involved, resulting in the formation of nodular masses—a condition that is characteristic; the hairs are affected, are loose, and often fall out. In doubtful cases the microscope will determine. From pustular eczema it may be differentiated by its history and course : its clinical features are entirely dissimilar. Eczema is never attended with the nodular and tubercular formation peculiar to this disease, nor are the hairs affected. The absence of ulceration will distinguish the disease from the vegetating syphiloderm. Tinea sycosis when occurring as a circumscribed patch may sometimes resemble carbuncle.

. In the treatment epilation with the use of parasiticides is employed ; as a rule, the disease yields readily to treatment. Crusts, if present, are to be removed by means of oily applications and washings with castile soap (or if necessary sapo viridis) and warm water. The parts should be clipped or shaved, preferably the latter. Although this operation is painful at first, later it may be accomplished without much discomfort ; shaving every second or third day is frequent enough. In the interval epilation is to be practised. The milder parasiticides, as sulphite or hyposulphite of sodium, a drachm to the ounce of water or ointment; sulphurous acid, full strength or diluted ; citrine ointment, two or three drachms to the ounce of vaseline or lard ; and a weak sulphur ointment,—are all useful. A 10 to 30 per cent. ointment of oleate of mercury is a valuable remedy ; the same may be said of a solution of corrosive sublimate, two to four grains to the ounce of water or alcohol. In addition, the other parasiticides mentioned in the treatment of ringworm of the body or scalp may be referred to. The applications should be made twice daily ; together with epilation they should be continued until microscopical examinations of the hairs give negative results.

Tinea Versicolor.

- Tinea versicolor is a vegetable parasitic disease due to the microsporon furfur, characterized by variously-sized, irregularly-shaped, dry, slightly furfuraceous, yellowish, macular patches, occurring for the most part upon the trunk and in adults. The affection may be slight, consisting of sev. eral small patches on the upper part of the chest, or so extensive as to involve the greater part of the trunk, neck, axillæ, flexures of the elbows, groins, and in very rare instances the face. It never occurs on the scalp, hands, or feet. As commonly met with, it is a disease of the trunk, especially the anterior portion of the thorax. It begins as small yellowish or brownish, fawn-colored, furfuraceous spots scattered over the region affected. These gradually increase in size, new spots may appear, and considerable surface may be invaded. In size they vary from a pea to large irregular patches, and are scarcely, if at all, elevated. The larger patches are irregular, and usually formed by coalescence of several smaller spots. Rarely patches may clear up in the centre and assume an annular form.

The number of patches varies; as a rule, a half dozen or more are present; in other cases they may be numerous. They show more or less furfuraceous scaling, varying with the amount of perspiration and the frequency with which the parts are washed. The scaling, even when it is insignificant or when the patches are apparently smooth, may be easily detected by scratching or scraping the surface. Slight itching is ordinarily present, especially when the parts are unusually warm; it is rarely marked. The color is usually a pale or brownish yellow. In sensitive skins at times the affection causes more or less hyperæmia, and the spots have a reddish hue. The course of the disease is variable, sometimes spreading rapidly, while in most cases its progress is slow. It is, as a rule, persistent, existing years. Relapses are not uncommon.

The cause of the disease is the vegetable fungus, the microsporon furfur. It invades the superficial portion of the epidermis. The affection is but slightly contagious. Those between the ages of twenty and forty, of either sex indifferently, are most frequently the subjects of the disease; it rarely if ever occurs in children or in elderly people. It is commonly observed in those whose nutrition is below the standard, especially in persons having pulmonary phthisis. It is a common affection, and occurs, in varying proportions, in all parts of the world. Scrapings or scales moistened with liquor potassæ may be examined with a power of three to five hundred diameters, and the peculiar features of the fungus well brought out, as the fungus exists in abundance. It consists of mycelium and spores, the former appearing as short, slender, variously-sized, straight or curved, twisted, wavy, or angular threads, crossing one another in all directions. In appearance they are homogeneous or granular, and often contain spores, especially about the joints. The spores are ovalish or round, sharply contoured, small in size, with a nucleus and slightly granular plasma. They show a marked tendency to aggregate and form groups—an arrangement which is characteristic of this fungus. The growth is found in every stage of development from mycelium to spores.

There should be no difficulty in recognizing the disease if its characters and distribution are kept in mind. In doubtful cases the microscope will prevent error. It is at times confounded with chloasma, vitiligo, and the macular syphilide. In chloasma, in which there is merely an increase of pigment in the rete, there is no scaling, the outlines are ill defined, and it is usually seen about the face—a region that is practically exempt in tinea versicolor. Moreover, the coloration in the parasitic disease is due to the fungus, which has its seat in the superficial epidermis and can be readily scraped off. With ordinary care it is impossible to mistake vitiligo for the disease in question. The macular syphiloderm is to be distinguished by attention to the distribution, character, and size of the lesions. Tinea versicolor is practically a disease of the trunk; the macular syphiloderm is usually distributed over the whole surface; and if it is the latter disease concomitant symptoms of syphilis are almost invariably present.

The disease is readily curable; any simple parasiticide properly and thoroughly applied will soon effect its removal. Lotions, as a rule, are to be preferred, inasmuch as they are more cleanly and more satisfactory. Washing the parts involved frequently with green soap (sapo viridis) and warm water is to be advised as an adjuvant, and will in some cases suffice to remove the disease. Alkaline baths, three or four ounces of carbonate of sodium or potassium to thirty gallons of water, are also useful. Various parasiticides are employed. Sulphite or hyposulphite of sodium, a drachm to the ounce; corrosive sublimate, two or four grains to the ounce of alcohol and water; sulphurous acid, pure or diluted; a saturated solution of boric acid; Vleminckx's solution, diluted with three to six parts of water,—are among the most useful. Sulphur and ammoniated mercury ointments, carbolic acid, ten to twenty grains to the ounce of lard, may be mentioned as serviceable. The frequency of application depends upon the extent and obstinacy of the disease, once or twice daily usually sufficing. After the disease is apparently cured treatment should be continued, although less actively, for a few weeks or a month, in order that a relapse may be avoided.

Scabies.

Scabies, or itch, is a contagious animal parasitic disease, due to the Sarcoptes scabiei, characterized by the formation of cuniculi, papules, vesicles, and pustules, followed by excoriations, crusts, and general cutaneous inflammation, and accompanied with itching. The amount of disturbance depends upon the duration of the disease and the sensitiveness of the skin. The itch mite (Acarus scabiei, Sarcoptes scabiei, or Sarcoptes hominis) through contagion finds its way upon the skin, and begins to burrow its way through the upper layers of the epidermis. The female only is found within the epidermis, the male, as generally supposed, never penetrating the skin. As the female burrows she lays a varying number of eggs, a dozen or more; by this time the burrow, or cuniculus, has usually attained its full length of several lines. It is to be seen as a narrow whitish or yellowish linear epidermic elevation, as a rule irregular and tortuous, and with a dotted or speckled look. It contains the female, its excrement, and a variable number of eggs. In a short time the ova are hatched, and the mites are rapidly multiplied. New burrows appear and are to be seen in all stages of development, and thus the disease progresses.

According to the sensitiveness of the skin will the lesions produced in consequence of the irritation of the mite vary. Usually, inflammatory points, papules, vesicles, pustules, and excoriations are to be seen scattered over the regions involved. The hands, especially the sides of the fingers, are almost invariably the parts first attacked, the mite gradually invad. ing other parts of the body, as the anterior surfaces of the wrists, fore. arms, elbows, and arms, the axillary folds, about the mammæ in females, between the buttocks, about the penis, the inner sides of the thighs. The face and scalp are never invaded, except in infants. Itching is a marked symptom, usually worse at night. In well-advanced cases the secondary symptoms, such as papular elevations, vesicles, impetiginous and ccthy. matous pustules, which are often torn by the scratching invoked, the crusts and excoriations of various characters, and a variable amount of cutaneous inflammation, with infiltration and pigmentation, taken together with the presence of burrows, constitute a clinical picture of the disease. In many cases the cuniculi are in a great measure obliterated by the scratching; their remains, however, may usually be detected. In persons with eczematous skin true eczema may be developed.

The disease is due solely to the presence of the itch mite. It is met with in persons of all ages and in every station of life, but for obvious reasons is more common and its ravages more marked among the poor. It is encountered in all parts of the world, but is especially frequent in the various European countries. In the United States it is comparatively infrequent, and is seen chiefly in the seaboard cities, and many of the cases can be traced to direct importation from abroad. It is markedly contagious. The Sarcoptes scabiei is almost microscopic in size, appearing as a yellowish-white rounded body. The male is but half the size of the female, and is rarely met with, apparently having no direct part in producing the cutaneous disturbance seen in the disease. The full-grown female, as may be determined by microscopical examination, is ovoid or crab-shaped, the dorsal surface convex and the ventral surface flattened, the back being studded with a varying number of short, thick spines and several long spike-shaped processes, all with their points directed backward. The head is small, rounded, or oval, without eyes, and closely set in the body, and is provided with palpi and mandibles. There are eight legs, four situated close to the head and four posteriorly. The entire parasite scarcely exceeds a fifth of a line in length. The female mite is to be looked for at the blind end of a burrow or at the roof of a vesicle.

Scabies when fully developed may usually be recognized without difficulty. The pathognomonic symptom is the presence of the parasites or the burrows. In the early stage cuniculi are not yet fully formed, but often the mite may be extracted from a recent vesicle. Burrows are usually most typically seen upon the sides of the fingers. The distribution of the eruption, however, is, in most cases, a sufficient basis for a diagnosis, the fingers, hands, flexor surface of the wrists, elbows, axillæ, buttocks, penis, mammæ in females, being especially invaded. It may be remembered also that the face and scalp, except in infants, are not involved. The multiform nature of the eruption is one of its prominent characteristics. It is a progressive disease. A history of contagion is often obtainable. It is to be distinguished from vesicular and pustular eczema and pediculosis. The more or less discrete vesicles and pustules of scabies, the localities affected, its progressive course, and the presence of burrows and a history of contagion will serve to differentiate from eczema. Pediculosis corporis involves the covered portions of the surface only, and the regions usually involved are different from those invaded in scabies. In scabies the hands are almost invariably the parts first and most markedly involved. The characters of the lesions are also different.

The disease yields rapidly to proper treatment. Various remedies are employed for the destruction of the parasite and its ova. The most common, and one that is thoroughly efficient, is sulphur. It is usually prescribed in ointment, one to four drachms to the ounce. In irritable skins, or where the secondary dermatitis is marked, the weaker proportions are advisable. A proportion of two drachms to the ounce is the average strength, and will be found suitable for the majority of cases. For children a drachm to the ounce is sufficiently strong; in these cases a half drachm of balsam of Peru may be added. This latter remedy is of itself a parasiticide. A compound sulphur ointment, known as Hebra's modification of Wilkinson's ointment, frequently employed abroad, is made up as follows:

> ℞. Sulphuris sublimatis,
>   Olei cadini,   āā. ʒij ;
>   Cretæ præparatæ,   ʒiiss ;
>   Saponis viridis,
>   Adipis,   āā. ʒj.

Styrax is another balsam that is destructive to the itch mite, used in the proportion of one part to two of lard. Naphthol, a drachm to the ounce of ointment, is, according to Kaposi and others, an especially reliable remedy, possessing the advantages of being without color or odor, and also favorably influencing the dermatitis. Usually, especially in sensitive skins, it may be prescribed in rose-water ointment; in others the following formula, which has been well spoken of by Kaposi, may be employed : ℞. Naphthol, 15 parts; pulv. cretæ alb., 10 parts; saponis viridis, 50 parts; adipis, 100 parts.

Before beginning the remedial applications the patient is to take a soap-and-warm-water bath. The ointment is then rubbed into every portion of the body with the exception, in adults, of the head. The localities favored by the parasite should receive special attention. About an ounce of ointment is required for an application. It is to be so applied twice daily for three days, and then a soap-and-water-bath is to be taken. The itching becomes less marked after the first application, but may persist in a mild degree for several days after the ointment has been discontinued. The secondary dermatitis produced by the parasite and the scratching usually subsides soon after the removal of the cause; if slow, it is to be treated with mild and soothing applications, such as are employed in the treatment of eczema.

Pediculosis.

Pediculosis, phtheiriasis, or lousiness, is a contagious animal affection, characterized by the presence of pediculi and the lesions which they produce, together with scratch-marks and excoriations. Three varieties of pediculi, or lice, infest the human body, differing both in their male and female forms, and each variety inhabiting a different portion of the body. The three varieties are—pediculus capitis, pediculus corporis, and pediculus pubis. They obtain nourishment by a process of suction, in so doing giving rise to a minute wound, in consequence of which a small amount of blood and serum exudes; more or less hyperæmia and infiltration may occur, giving rise to marked itching, and the scratching induced results in excoriations. The varieties of pediculosis are designated according to the names of the species of pediculi.

PEDICULOSIS CAPITIS.—This is a condition due to the presence of the pediculus capitis, or head louse. This pediculus is seen, as a rule, upon the scalp only; in feeble and bedridden individuals it is, at times, seen upon other parts of the body. It is an insect of a grayish color, and varies in length from one and a half to three millimeters, the female being larger than the male. It is oval in shape, consisting of head, thorax, and abdomen, the last named occupying more than half its length and made up of seven clearly-defined segments, marked off from one another by deep notches. The thorax is broad, and from its sides project six legs, each one hairy and provided with a crab-like hook at its extremity. The head is somewhat triangular, with a pair of short, five-jointed antennæ and two black, prominent eyes, and furnished with a sucking apparatus. They are extremely prolific, the progeny of a single louse numbering several thousands in about eight weeks. The eggs, or nits, are deposited upon the hairs near the roots; several may often be found on a single shaft. If seen on the hair some distance from the scalp, it is due to the fact of the hairs having grown since the nits were deposited. They are pyriform, whitish bodies, about one-fourth of a line in length, securely glued to the hairs, hatching out in five or six days. The young become capable of reproduction in three weeks. According to the duration of the affection and the habits of the individual, they are to be seen in small or large numbers. They may be found upon the scalp or crawling over the hair, the occipital region being especially favored. Pediculosis capitis is commonly seen in children, and it is also not infrequent in women; it is met with usually among the poorer classes. The irritation from the attacks of the pediculi upon the scalp gives rise to scratching, resulting in serous and purulent oozing, which, mixed with blood and dirt, mats the hair and forms crusts. In marked cases the hair soon acquires a disgusting odor. An eczematous condition is soon brought about. Excoriations, vesicles, and pustules may often be seen beyond the limits of the scalp, upon the back of the neck and shoulders, and upon the forehead. From the constant irritation, intolerable itching, loss of sleep, etc. the general health may finally suffer. Pediculosis capitis may be recognized without difficulty. The ova, or nits, may be seen even at a distance, and the parasites themselves may always be detected if a search is made. An eczematous eruption of the occipital region in children and women, especially of the poorer classes, should always give rise to suspicion and an examination. This condition is often a result of pediculosis, but it is to be remembered also that an eczema of the scalp may have at first existed, furnishing a favorable habitat for the parasites.

Treatment is satisfactory; with ordinary care the condition may soon be removed. Cutting the hair, though facilitating treatment, is not necessary. The main object is the removal or destruction of the parasites and their ova; this accomplished, the irritation and excoriations will soon disappear or yield to simple treatment. The best plan is with ordinary petroleum. The parts should be saturated with it and then bandaged, care being taken to prevent the oil from running down the neck or on to the face. The dressing is to be allowed to remain on about twelve hours, usually over night, and the scalp washed with soap and water in the morning. One or two applications, if thoroughly made, are sufficient. An oily solution of naphthol, 5 per cent. strength, has been well spoken of. Tincture of cocculus Indicus is also a reliable application. Ointments may be employed in place of lotions, but are not so cleanly or, as a rule, so satisfactory. In some cases, however, where an eczematous condition exists, especially if the hair is short, they may be employed with good results. An ointment of staphisagria, or one of white precipitate, twenty to sixty grains to the ounce, may be referred to. Oleate of mercury, in solution or ointment, 20 to 30 per cent. strength, is also serviceable. The parasites and nits are usually destroyed by any of these applications; the latter, however, remain clinging to the hair. Their removal may soon be brought about by applications of alcoholic lotions, diluted acetic acid or vinegar, alkaline lotions, and the use of a fine comb.

PEDICULOSIS CORPORIS.—Pediculosis corporis is due to the presence of the pediculus corporis, or body louse (more properly pediculus vestimenti, or clothes louse), resembling in its shape and anatomical structure the head louse, but is larger, measuring from one to four millimeters: the female is also larger than the male. Its period of growth and reproductive powers are also as great. In color, when devoid of blood, it is dirty white or grayish. The eggs are similar to, but larger than, those of the pediculus capitis. It dwells in the clothing, trespassing upon the integument only to obtain nourishment, where it may, when existing in numbers, often be surprised in the act of drawing blood or crawling over the surface. The ova are deposited in the folds and seams of the clothing, in which localities also the parasites are usually found. The excoriations, therefore, are to be seen especially about those portions of the body which are closest to these parts of the clothing, as, for example, about the neck and shoulders, the waist, hips, thighs, etc. The primary lesions consist of minute reddish puncta with slight areolæ, the points at which the pediculi have drawn blood. Not infrequently, instead of simple hemorrhagic points, a wheal marks the site of attack; at times also papules, pustules, and even furuncles, result. Intense itching is set up, and as a consequence excoriations, scratch-marks of various kinds, and blood-crusts are to be seen. Eventually, from the long-continued irritation and hyperæmia, a brownish or blackish pigmentation results. The affection is met with chiefly among the poorer classes, in the middle-aged and elderly; children are seldom attacked. It is not common in this country. The presence of the ova or the pediculi in the seams and folds, the characteristic reddish puncta, and the multiform lesions and excoriations upon the regions above named are sufficiently diagnostic. It is not to be confounded with pruritus and scabies, in which diseases the distribution and causes of the lesions are altogether different.

As the pediculi live in the clothing, treatment consists in their destruction, by baking or boiling of the wearing apparel, and in ordinary attention to cleanliness. Repeated examinations should be made, so that no pediculi or ova are permitted to remain. Alkaline baths, three to four ounces of sodium bicarbonate to the bath, and lotions similar to those employed in the treatment of pruritus, will allay the itching and aid in the removal of the secondary lesions. In those cases where the patient cannot immediately subject the clothes to the above treatment an ointment of staphisagria, made by digesting two drachms of the powder in an ounce of hot lard and straining, may be applied to the skin.

PEDICULOSIS PUBIS.—Pediculosis pubis is a condition due to the presence of the pediculus pubis, or crab louse. It is the smallest of the three varieties, measuring from one to two millimeters. It has a short, rounded, flat body, and an oval head, which is furnished with two long, five-jointed antennæ and a pair of inconspicuous eyes. The thorax, which is small and imperceptibly merged into the abdomen, is provided with six jointed, hairy legs with hooked claws. The margins of the abdomen are slightly indented, and from it projects eight stubby, prehensile feet armed with bristles. It is more or less translucent, and of a yellowish-gray color. As in the other varieties, the female is larger than the male. It is liable to escape detection on account of its translucency, and the fact that it is apt to remain seated near the roots of the hairs, clutching the hair with its head downward and buried deep in the follicles. The ova are similar in construction, but smaller than those of the other varieties; they may be readily seen attached to the hairs in the same manner. The excrement, minute reddish particles, may be detected lying around the bases of the hairs. It infests adults chiefly, being usually contracted through sexual intercourse. Although its favorite habitat is the region of the pubes, it may also infest the axillæ, the sternal region of the male, the beard, eyebrows, and even eyelashes. The amount of irritation varies—at times insignificant, while in other cases it is severe. Pediculosis pubis may be mistaken for pruritus or eczema, but an examination will disclose the ova, and if carefully sought for the pediculi may always be found, usually near the roots of the hair, looking not unlike dirt-specks or freckles; the excrement may also be detected. For their removal any of the lotions or ointments mentioned in the treatment of the other varieties may be employed. A lotion of corrosive sublimate, two to four grains to the ounce of alcohol or water; infusion of tobacco; 10 to 20 per cent. ointment of oleate of mercury; ammoniated mercury ointment; a 5 to 10 per cent. oily solution or ointment of naphthol,—are all efficient. The parts should be washed with soap and water twice daily, and the remedy applied after each washing. In order to ensure complete destruction of the ova the applications should be continued for some days after the pediculi have been destroyed.

LEPTUS.—Two species of leptus are met with as attacking man: Leptus Americanus (American harvest mite) and Leptus irritans (irritating harvest mite, harvest bug, mower's mite). The former is a minute, brick-red colored, elongate, pyriform creature with six legs, barely visible to the naked eye. Its favorite sites of attack are the scalp and axillæ, partly burying itself in the skin, giving rise to a small inflammatory papule. The latter species is more common, differing from the former merely in having a roundish oval form. It buries itself in the skin, giving rise to inflammatory papules, vesicles, and pustules. Its sites of predilection are the ankles and legs. The minute red mite met with especially about blackberry-bushes in the low grounds of Pennsylvania, New Jersey, and Delaware is probably the same species. Both varieties are common, during the summer, in our South-western States. For treatment a weak sulphur ointment or ointments of the other mild parasiticides may be employed.

PULEX PENETRANS, OR RHINOCHOPRION PENETRANS.—This creature —the sand-flea, known also as chigoe, chigger, and jigger—is almost microscopic in size, closely similar to the common flea, but has a proboscis as long as its body. It is common in tropical countries, and also met with in our Southern States. It (the impregnated female) burrows into the skin, depositing the ova, resulting in inflammatory swelling, large vesicles or pustules, and even ulceration. The toes, especially beneath and alongside of the nail, and other parts of the feet are the regions attacked. The treatment consists in extraction; it usually comes away in the form of a sac about the size of a small pea, its size due to the distension of the abdomen with ova. As a preventive the essential oils are used about the feet.

FILARIA MEDINENSIS.—This parasite, the guinea-worm, known also as dracunculus, is only encountered in tropical countries. The young bore into the skin and subcutaneous tissue, in which their growth takes place; sooner or later marked inflammation is produced, resulting in painful furuncular tumors, which finally break, showing the presence of the worms. The lower extremities, especially the feet, are the favorite regions of attack. The worm varies from several inches to three feet in length, according to its age, and is one-half or three-fourths of a line in thickness. The treatment consists in extracting the worm inch by inch, from day to day, as soon as discovered, care being exercised not to break it. Poultices may be applied.

CYSTICERCUS CELLULOSÆ.—This affection is characterized by rounded or ovalish, smooth, elastic, firm or hard, movable, pea- to hazelnut-sized tumors, more or less numerous, usually seated just beneath the skin, new tumors showing themselves from time to time. After reaching a certain size they may remain stationary. Although not painful upon pressure, spontaneous pains may be complained of. Microscopical examination reveals the cysticerci.

ŒSTRUS.—This parasite (known also as breeze, gad-fly, and bot-fly) is met with in Central and South America, and also in other countries. The neck, back, and extremities especially are liable to be attacked. The ova are deposited in the skin, and there result inflammatory, boil-like tumors or swellings with a central opening, from which issues a sanious fluid; or the lesion may assume a linear, tortuous, or serpiginous form. Sooner or later the grub is detected, and may be easily squeezed out or extracted.

DEMODEX FOLLICULORUM.—This microscopic parasite (also known as steatozoon, entozoon, acarus, and Simonea, folliculorum) is to be found in the sebaceous follicles. It is harmless, giving rise to no disturbance. It is worm-like in form, made up of a head, thorax, and a long abdomen.

It is more apt to be found in those with thick, greasy skins. Several of them often exist in a single follicle.

CIMEX LECTULARIUS, OR ACANTHIA LECTULARIA.—This insect (the common bed-bug) and its various residing-places are well known. It gives rise to a cutaneous lesion of the nature of an urticarial wheal, with a central hemorrhagic point which remains after the swelling has subsided. As a result of the scratching to which the irritation and itching give rise excoriations are often observed. A larger species (Conorhinus sanguisuga), known as the blood-sucking cone-nose and big bed-bug, has been met with in Southern Illinois and Ohio; its bite is said to produce severe inflammation of the skin. For the relief of bed-bug bites lotions containing alcohol, vinegar, lead-water, ammonia-water, and similar remedies may be sponged upon the parts. Pyrethrum powder and corrosive sublimate are the best preventives against bugs in beds.

PULEX IRRITANS.—This, the common flea, is found universally, especially in hot and warm climates. As a result of its bite erythematous spots with minute central hemorrhagic points are seen. The presence of the areola distinguishes the lesions from those of simple purpura, which at times they may resemble. The cutaneous disturbance is usually slight, but in some individuals, and especially in tropical countries, the discomfort to which these creatures give rise is often considerable.

CULEX.—Gnats, or mosquitoes, are often productive of considerable cutaneous irritation, the typical lesion being a wheal-like elevation. The itching is best relieved with ammonia-water.

IXODES.—There are several species of wood-ticks met with in our woods which are liable to attach themselves to the human skin. Inserting their proboscis and head deeply into the tissues, they suck blood until often they swell up several times their natural size. They should be induced to relinquish their firm hold by dropping olive oil or one of the essential oils upon the skin; they should never be extracted with violence.

MEDICAL OPHTHALMOLOGY.

MEDICAL OPHTHALMOLOGY.

By WM. F. NORRIS, M. D.

INTRODUCTION.—The object of the following essay is to give, as far as practicable in the limits of an encyclopædic article, an account of the eye symptoms which may be seen in the course of diseases of the general system and in connection with the pathological conditions of the various organs of the body. The eye has always been looked on as a valuable indicator of general systemic disturbance. Its expression has been noted as showing the general vigor or feebleness of the patient, as well as his varying mental moods, while paralysis of its external and internal muscles has in all times been regarded as a sign of disturbed intracranial action or disease. In order to judge of the state of the circulation the physician habitually looks at the lips, the tongue, and the nails, where the capillaries are covered by translucent material, to appreciate the state of the circulation. How much better are we enabled to do this when, by the use of the ophthalmoscope, we look at the interior of the eye and see the blood-columns in the veins and arteries of the head of the optic nerve and the retina laid bare to our view without any opaque covering whatever! Such an examination, besides showing the state of the circulation, will frequently reveal a neuritis which may be due to some intracranial disease, or show a degeneration of the optic nerve which may point to impaired power and tissue-change in the spinal cord or the brain; or there may be characteristic retinal changes associated, as, for instance, with disease of the kidneys, or extravasation of blood which may be dependent on general or local causes; these frequently serving as important indices of the state of the nerves and vascular tissues in other organs in the body.

In so vast a field, and in one so new as regards ophthalmoscopic appearances, there remains still much to be accomplished. Useful knowledge has accumulated slowly, but numerous enigmatical appearances have been referred to their true causes, while many which at first sight seemed important have been proved to be either anomalies of formation or to have no pathological import. A complete and accurate description of all the eye symptoms in all diseases is an herculean task, because it presupposes the careful study of vast numbers of cases in every department of medicine : it is therefore out of the question for any one man to complete such a description from his individual efforts, and he must either remain content with a mere sketch or collate the combined experiences of many observers in different fields in order that it may be in any way reasonably perfect. To keep such an article within any moderate limits it has been necessary to condense much, and to consider only those points which the combined testimony of many observers shows to be important and of frequent occurrence. For similar reasons the writer has abstained from giving a complete list of all authorities treating of the subjects herein discussed, and has referred only to those which appeared to him to be some of the most important. Those readers who wish a more complete bibliography can readily obtain it by referring to the various monographs hereinafter quoted, and also by consulting the well-known essays of Foerster,[1] Robin,[2] and of Mauthner,[3] or the treatises of Albutt[4] and of Gowers.[5]

Such an article is necessarily a chapter on symptomatology, giving the eye symptoms in various diseases and pathological conditions, and the reader will therefore look in vain in it for any directions as to the treatment of such maladies, or for formulæ showing advantageous modes of administering medicines. The writer has intended, by describing and grouping eye symptoms, to enable the practitioner more readily to diagnosticate the various pathological conditions of other parts of the economy. The reader should look for a description of treatment in the various articles of this work which are devoted to the discussion of such diseases and morbid states. Local diseases of the eye, except so far as they are manifestly related to or caused by general disease, have been avoided in this paper, these topics being appropriate to a treatise on the diseases of the eye.

Changes in the Eye-ground and its Appendages due to Diseases of the Circulatory Apparatus—Heart, Blood-vessels, and Blood.

The ophthalmoscope has laid bare to our view a living nerve of special sense, the highly-developed end-organ in which it terminates, and the blood-columns circulating in them. In no other part of the body has Nature vouchsafed to us so clear an insight into her mysteries. In a state of health the index of refraction of the walls of the retinal blood-vessels is so nearly coincident with that of the surrounding media that they either entirely escape our observation or are only slightly indicated, thus allowing us to see only the blood-columns which circulate within them. Owing to the distance from the heart and to the restraining influence of the intraocular pressure, as well as to the minute size of the vessels in question, the pulse-wave has so far died out as to be ordinarily invisible, even by the aid of the eye-lenses which Nature has so kindly placed as magnifying-glasses to assist us in the study of intraocular phenomena. Even where we avail ourselves of the upright image in examining the normal eye-ground, by which an amplifying power of seven to fifteen

---

[1] " Beziehungen der Allgemein-Leiden und Organ-Erkrankungen zu Veränderungen und Krankheiten des Sehorgans," in *Graefe und Saemisch's Handbuch der Augenheilkunde,* Bd. vii., 1877.

[2] *Des Troubles oculaires dans les Maladies de l'Encephale,* Paris, 1880.

[3] *Lehrbuch der Ophthalmoscopie,* Vienna, 1868, and *Gehirn und Auge,* Wiesbaden, 1881

[4] *On the Use of the Ophthalmoscope,* London, 1871.

[5] *Medical Ophthalmoscopy,* London, 1879.

diameters is obtained, we cannot usually detect any pulsation in the ves_ sels, although exceptionally we may observe pulsation which is always venous and confined to the larger twigs of the venæ centrales as they pass over the disc and dip into the nerve-substance. By slight pressure on the eyeball with the finger venous pulse can always be produced. This phenomenon consists of an emptying of the vein from the optic pylorus toward the periphery, followed by a rush of return blood in an opposite direction, which takes place in eyes where the intravenous and intraocular pressures are nearly balanced. Under these circumstances the injection of a fresh quantity of arterial blood into the eye causes a tem_ porary increase of intraocular pressure, which is transmitted through the vitreous to the main trunks of the veins, compressing them at the point nearest the heart (where the intravenous pressure is least) before the column of entering blood which has been hindered by the capillary resist_ ance has had time to flow around to re-establish the current. Stronger pressure on the eye will produce an arterial pulsation by causing the intraocular pressure to become so high that the blood enters only during the systole of the heart and diastole of the arteries. This is not infrequently seen in glaucoma, where there is an augmentation of the intraocular pressure, but is never visible in the normal eye of a healthy individual. It should be kept in mind that the venous pulse often produces a slight change in the adjacent arteries which ought not be mistaken for arterial pulsation.[1] Wadsworth and Putnam[2] describe an intermittent variation in the size of the retinal veins independent of the pulsation produced by the heart's action, and having a period of about five respirations, analogous to the variation of arterial tension found in animals. Besides the arterial pulse already alluded to, pro_ duced by augmented intraocular tension, where the normal force of the circulation is not sufficient to drive the blood in a continuous stream into the tense eyeball, we have an analogous condition where the intraocular tension may be normal, but the arterial tension is diminished, and a full stream of blood can enter only during the diastole of the arteries or max_ imum of intravascular pressure. We may notice examples of this in *insufficiency of the aortic valves,* and in some very rare cases described by Quincke[3] and Becker,[4] who found it accompanied by an alternate flushing and pallor of the optic disc analogous to the capillary pulse which may at times be observed in the finger-nail under similar condi_ tions of the general circulation. The arterial pulse may also accompany any cause which permanently or temporarily reduces the blood-pressure in the arterial system, such as pressure of a tumor on the ophthalmic artery or of a swollen nerve on the central retinal artery (as in neuritis) : or, again, by feeble impulse of the heart, as in cases of fainting or in degeneration and dilatation of the walls of the blood-vessels.[5] Becker relates[6] a case of arterial pulsation in a left eye, supposed to be due to aneurism of the aorta at a point where the left carotid is given off, whilst

[1] For a minute study of the phenomenon, vide Jaeger, *Med. Zeitschrift,* 1854. See also his *Ergebnisse des Untersuchung mit dem Augenspiegel, etc.,* 1876, pp 60, 61. See also Becker, *Arch. f. Oph.,* vol. xviii., part 1, p. 270.
[2] Vide *Trans. of the Amer. Oph. Society,* 1878, pp. 435–439.
[3] H. Quincke, *Berl. klin. Wochenschrift,* No. 34, 1868.
[4] O. Becker, *Arch. f. Ophth.,* vol. xviii., 1, pp. 207–296.
[5] Wordsworth, *R. L. O. H. Rep.,* vol. iv. p. 111.   [5] *Loc. cit.,* pp. 253–256.

the other eye presented the usual appearance of healthy retinal circulation : an aneurism at the origin of the innominate might reverse this and
give arterial pulsation in the right eye. Usually, the pulse-phenomena
in the retina are confined to the vessels on the optic disc and its immediate vicinity, but both Jaeger[1] and Becker[2] give cases where it was visible over the entire eye-ground. In cases of *congenital malformation of
the heart* with cyanosis, such as defective closure of the foramen ovale or
stenosis of the pulmonary artery, the retinal vessels show markedly the
general distension of the veins and the change of color of the blood.
Liebreich[3] gives a striking picture of such a case, and Leber[4] remarks
that in two cases observed by him the dilatation affected the arteries as
well as the veins. Knapp[5] describes a case of swelling of the discs, with
a vast number of thickened arteries and veins which radiated from them,
many twigs reaching the fovea centralis. The autopsy showed general
enlargement and hypertrophy of the whole vascular system without disease of the heart. Arcus senilis is often an accompaniment of fatty heart
and an indication of extensive fatty degeneration of other tissues of the
body, such as the small arteries of the brain and the recti muscles of the
eye.[6]

Since 1859, when Graefe[7] by means of the ophthalmoscope first diagnosticated this condition of the retina (which Schweigger[8] a year and a
half later substantiated by anatomical proof, demonstrating a closure of
the central artery by an embolus in it just behind the lamina cribrosa),
embolism of the central artery of the retina has been a favorite explanation of all cases of sudden one-sided blindness. Since that date Sichel,[9]
Nettleship,[10] Priestly Smith,[11] and Schmidt[12] have all published careful
clinical studies of similar cases with autopsies. Embolism is less frequent in this situation than in many other parts of the body, and this,
as has been pointed out by Foerster, is probably due to the fact that the
ophthalmic artery is given off from the external carotid nearly at a right
angle, and while it in turn again sends off its smallest branch—the central retinal artery—at nearly the same angle ; consequently, emboli are
more readily carried past their orifices into some other vascular area supplied by the main stem. Mauthner has suggested that the transitory but
complete blindness which sometimes precedes embolism of the central
artery may be due to the stoppage of the orifice of the artery (where it
comes off from the ophthalmic artery) by a previous embolus which has
been too large to enter the artery, and which, owing to the favorable
position of the orifice, has been washed beyond into some of the other
branches. In the majority of such cases the ophthalmoscope shows that
the retinal arteries are diminished in size and partially filled with blood,
while a white opacity of the fibre-layer of the retina extends centrifugally
from the disc and between it and the macula lutea. When the opacity surrounds the latter, the fovea centralis (where the fibre-layer dies out) shows

[1] *Ophth. Hand Atlas*, p. 75, Fig. 52.   [2] *Loc. cit.*, pp. 220, 221.
[3] *Liebreich's Atlas*, Tab ix. Fig. 3.   [4] *Graefe und Saemisch*, vol. v. pp. 524–526.
[5] *Trans. Amer. Ophth. Soc.*, 1870, p. 120.   [6] Canton, *The Arcus Senilis*, London, 1863.
[7] *A. f. O.*, v. 1, S. 136.   [8] *Vorlesungen über den Gebrauch des Augenspiegels*, S. 140.
[9] A. Sichel, *Archiv der Phys. Norm. et Path.*, No. 1, pp. 83–89 and pp. 207–213 (quoted
by Leber).
[10] *R. L. O. H. Rep.*, vol. viii., pp. 9–20.   [11] *Brit. Med. Journ.*, 1874, April, p. 452.
[12] H. Schmidt, *A. f. O.*, **xx.**, 2, pp. 287–307.

by contrast as a reddish or at times a cherry-red spot. The state of the disc itself appears to differ in different cases : some authors have described it as unusually pallid, whilst others claim that it still retains more or less of its natural pinkish hue. In cases reported,[1] where the disc is said to be of normal color, this circumstance is probably due to collateral circulation which has been established with the ciliary vessels at the optic entrance. Where the obstruction of the artery is complete the blindness is permanent, and the disc and retina become atrophic. Embolism also occurs in the branches of the central retinal artery, and in such instances there is loss of a corresponding part of the field of vision. In some cases there is hemorrhagic infarction.[2] It is never present in embolism of the main stem of the central retinal artery. Inasmuch as this latter vessel is an end-artery, the absence of infarction and subsequent sphacelus is interesting. The intraocular pressure probably prevents the back current of venous blood into the obstructed area, while the nearness of the vessels of the chorio-capillaris allows the retina to obtain sufficient nutriment to prevent death without allowing it to carry on its functions. In the case of embolism of a branch, all the retinal blood being under the intraocular pressure, there would be no hindrance to the entrance of venous blood from the areas of the retina supplied by other arterial branches, although, as above mentioned, the infarction is not present in all such cases. *Thrombosis of the central retinal vein* is also a rare affection, only recognized and diagnosticated of late years. Michel[3] reports 7 cases, with plates of the ophthalmoscopic appearances in 4 of them. The patients were all between fifty-one and eighty-one years of age, and all had rigidity of the peripheral arteries. The suddenness of the attack recalls the symptoms of embolism, but in thrombosis the blindness is said never to be absolute. The ophthalmoscopic appearances are described as consisting of a diffuse and intense reddish haze of the fibre-layer of the retina, hiding the outlines of the disc and usually extending one and a half disc-diameters from it. This area of haze shows numerous small hemorrhages, mostly linear, in the direction of the retinal fibres, and beyond it the arteries and veins of the retina again become visible. The veins are dilated, excessively tortuous, and carry dark blackish blood. In the periphery of the retina the hemorrhages are rounded and splotchy, whilst a dark rounded hemorrhage occupies the fovea centralis. There is no swelling or prominence of the disc. When the thrombosis has been complete, atrophy of the intraocular end of the optic nerve follows. Zehender[4] makes two classes of cases—the marasmic in old people, and the phlebitic in young—reporting an interesting case in a patient twenty-six years old. Leber[5] details a case of hemorrhagic retinitis with thrombosis of some of the venous trunks in the retina, which were swollen to two or three times their usual calibre, and filled with very dark, almost blackish, blood : as they approached the disc they rapidly diminished in size, and were almost thread-like as they dipped into it. Galezowski[6]

[1] Vide case by Schmidt, *Archiv f. Ophthalm.*, xx., 2, p. 288.
[2] Knapp, *Archives of Ophthalmology and Otology*, vol. i. p. 84 (with plates), and Landesberg, in same journal, vol. iv. pp. 39, 40, have each given cases of embolism of a branch of the retinal artery, with infarction.
[3] *A. f. O.*, xxiv., 2, pp. 37-70.
[4] In clinical lecture reported by Angelucci, *Klin. Monatsblätter f. Augenheilkunde*, 1880, p. 23. [5] *Graefe und Saemisch*, vol. v. p. 531. [6] *Gaz. méd. de Paris*, 1879, p. 217.

cites two instances—one in a case of injury to the ciliary region, and one after injury to the eye by steam. In the latter, the thrombosis affected the artery, and the subject was forty-nine years of age.

Retinal hemorrhage is of frequent occurrence. It is often associated with inflammation in cachectic conditions of the system, as in the various forms of symptomatic retinitis, but is also found where there is not any demonstrable constitutional disease. Here, as in the other tissues of the body, apoplexies are favored by disease of the coats of the vessels, by alteration in the state of the blood, and by increased intravascular pressure. Anatomical examination has shown in the most common form of disease in the retinal vessels fatty degeneration of their walls, with calcareous deposits in them, and a condition (denominated sclerosis) in which the coats become thickened, homogeneous, and of a higher index of refraction. In this hardened tissue there is a condition similar to amyloid degeneration, but no reaction is to be obtained from iodine (Leber). No ruptures can be seen with the ophthalmoscope, but the vessels appear to pass on in contact with the hemorrhage without change of course or calibre. These circumstances have led Leber[1] to suppose that most retinal hemorrhages are due to diapedesis, and not to rhexis. When the blood escapes into the fibre-layer of the retina, it frequently diffuses itself along the course of the fibres and between them, and gives rise to linear and striated hemorrhages, while in the deeper layers its progress is barred by the connective-tissue elements—notably by the radiating fibres of Müller—and forms irregular masses which appear as more or less rounded clumps when looked at by the ophthalmoscope. Such extravasations of blood are frequently absorbed, or, again, they may leave black spots of pigment as the only marks of their presence. At other times they produce yellowish-white masses which disappear slowly, and often leave connective-tissue cicatrices behind them, dragging upon and displacing the retinal elements. When the hemorrhage is considerable, it may cause primary distortion of the images and impairment of vision by pressure on the rods and cones. At times it breaks through the limitans interna into the vitreous, giving rise to floating opacities, more rarely spreading itself out in a layer between the vitreous and the retina. The writer well remembers such an instance in the case of an apparently healthy woman about forty years of age, who, while sitting quietly in church, noticed that objects looked red and that a dense cloud came before the eye. Examination with the ophthalmoscope showed a large hemorrhage which covered the entire region of the macula and extended far beyond it, overlapping the temporal edge of the disc. This hemorrhage was slowly absorbed, and four years later the patient had a vision of $\frac{20}{xx}$, and no trace of hemorrhage was visible in the entire eyeground. Liebreich[2] gives a good illustration of a similar case in a woman of forty-five years of age who, after suppression of the menses, had a similar state of affairs. Leber[3] has seen several such cases, in one of which the hemorrhage was changed into a brilliant white mass. This was entirely absorbed, leaving only a small pigmented stripe at its lower border as the sole trace of the previous large extravasation of blood. Occasionally retinal hemorrhage

[1] *Graefe und Saemisch*, vol. v. p. 554.   [2] *Atlas*, Table viii. Fig. 2 (1863 ed.).
[3] *Graefe und Saemisch*, v. p. 553.

ushers in glaucoma. Retinal apoplexies, like extravasations of blood in the conjunctiva of the eyeball, often come without apparent cause. In many cases they are finger-posts pointing to grave disease of the vessels in other parts of the body. The writer recalls a patient of seventy years of age who believed himself in perfect health until alarmed by a retinal hemorrhage, which a few months later was followed by a cerebral apoplexy which caused his death.

Aneurism of the central retinal artery is of excessively rare occurrence. Sous of Bordeaux quotes[1] the elder Graefe and Scultetus as having anatomically demonstrated the existence of the lesion, and Mackenzie refers[2] to a pathological specimen in the collection of Schmidler of Friburg where there was an aneurism of the central artery of each retina. Sous was the first who recognized it with the ophthalmoscope, and describes it as a red egg-shaped, pulsating dilatation of one of the main branches near the disc. Vision was so far destroyed that the patient was unable to recognize the largest letters. Martin describes[3] a similar case, while Magnus records what he supposed to be an arterio-venous aneurism following severe contusion of the eyeball, and Mannhardt a case of rupture of the choroid with a gray pulsating mass in the disc, which was also supposed to be aneurismal in nature. Schirmer has recorded[4] a case of widely-spread congenital telangiectasis of the face with a similar condition of the retinal veins of one eye. Liebreich[5] has pictured curious bead-like dilatations of the veins in a glaucomatous eye. Jacobi[6] gives three woodcuts of varix-like tortuosities of the retinal veins. Offsets extending from the retinal vessels forward into the vitreous have been observed during life and described by Coccius,[7] Becker,[8] Jaeger,[9] Samelsohn,[10] Jacobi,[11] and Norris.[12] They probably occur to some extent in many severe inflammations of the eye, and have been not unfrequently found and described in anatomical examinations of that organ; but their development is usually attended with so much cloudiness of the media as to prevent accurate ophthalmoscopic examination.

When carefully examining eyes with the ophthalmoscope, it is not a very unusual circumstance to see a small grayish tag arising from the lymph-sheath of the central retinal vessels and extending a short distance forward into the vitreous. These tags usually present slow, sinuous movements, following motions of the eyeball. It is, however, rare to have such obliterated vessels extend through the vitreous and show their previous distribution in the posterior capsule of the lens, as in the instances reported by Zehender,[13] Liebreich,[14] and Becker;[15] in Zehender's case the artery was patulous and blood-bearing. Little[16] has also depicted a case where the hyaloid artery was filled with blood. The central canal of the vitreous, which is occupied in the fœtal eye by the artery in question, is readily demonstrated in pigs' eyes by allowing colored fluid to

---

[1] *Annales d'Oculistique*, 1865, pp. 241–243.
[2] *Practical Treatise on the Diseases of the Eye*, London, 1854, 4th ed., p. 1042.
[3] *Atlas d'Ophthalmoscopie.* [4] *A. f. O.*, vii., 1, pp. 119–121.
[5] *Atlas*, Plate xi. Fig. 1. [6] *Klin. Monatsblätter*, 1874, pp. 253–260.
[7] *Glaucom.*, 1859, p. 47. [8] *Bericht der Wiener Augenklinik*, 1866, pp. 65–74.
[9] *Ophth. Hand-Atlas*, Table xv. p. 72. [10] *Klin. Monatsblätter*, 1873, pp. 216–218.
[11] *Klin. Monatsblätter*, 1874, pp. 252–260. [12] *Trans. Amer. Oph. Soc.*, 1879, p. 548.
[13] *Klin. Monatsblät. f. Augenheilkunde*, 1863, pp. 260–349. [14] *Ibid*, p 350.
[16] *Annales d'Oculistique*, 1865, p. 350. [16] *Trans. Amer. Ophth. Soc.*, 1881, pp. 211–213.

flow into it from its central end. According to H. Müller,[1] atrophied remnants of the artery are always present in the eyes of oxen. Manz[2] gives an anatomical description and plate of a continuance of the lymph-sheath of the central artery through the vitreous forward to the capsule of the lens, the remnants of the artery being found only in its proximal portion : observation had been impossible during life on account of corneal opacities. The same writer describes a convolution of vessels as penetrating the posterior part of the vitreous from the retina in the eyes of some Australian reptiles (Trachyeaurus and Lygosoma), and regards it as a similar formation to the pecten of the bird's eye. According to Ammon, some forms of congenital cataract are connected with the too early obliteration of the hyaloid artery, which is so important in furnishing nutriment to the growing lens.

Von Graefe remarks, however, that this very unusual yet incomplete development of the retinal vessels is common in congenital amaurosis. He reports[3] an instance in a blind eye of a boy ten years of age, who also exhibited a convergent squint and nystagmus. Mooren[4] also gives a case of entire absence of the retinal blood-vessels in a child seven months old. Pathological conditions of the blood often give rise to visible changes in the eye-ground.

LEUCÆMIC RETINITIS.—Liebreich[5] was first to call attention to a retinitis which is due to leucæmia. In his *Atlas* he gives an interesting picture of it, and states that he had then already had an opportunity of seeing six cases in the splenic variety of the disease. His plate shows a diffuse retinitis with scanty hemorrhages, with marked change in the color of the eye-ground and of the blood in the retinal veins and arteries. The blood-columns, especially in the veins, have acquired a slight rose tint, and have become less intense in color, whilst the hemorrhages appear slightly redder. He also describes white splotches like those of the retinitis of Bright's disease, differing from the latter only in the more peripheral situation. In one case these splotches were examined by Recklinghausen, and found to consist of patches of sclerotic degeneration of the nerve-fibres. Becker has pictured[6] two interesting cases, where, besides the diffuse retinitis with scanty hemorrhages, the main characteristics were the yellow color of the eye-ground and large white plaques with a red hemorrhagic border in the periphery. In the few cases, which the writer has had an opportunity of studying in the wards of his colleagues, the most striking change has been that of the color of the eye-ground and of the blood. In none of these were there either the white patches with red border or any extensive hemorrhage. We probably must not expect them in all cases and at all stages. In one of the patients, a negress, who was examined at the time of her admittance to the hospital, before any diagnosis had been made, the change in the color of the blood and fundus was so marked that he was able to call attention to it, as a probable case of leucæmia, and had the satisfaction of having the diagnosis confirmed by subsequent careful examination. Leber[7] states that the disease sometimes assumes the form of hemorrhagic

---

[1] *Gessamm. Schriften*, p. 365. [2] *Graefe und Saemisch*, vol. ii. pp. 97–99.
[3] *Arch. f. Ophth.*, vol. i., part 1, pp. 403, 404.
[4] *Ophthalmiatrische Beobachtungen*, 1867, p. 260. [5] *Atlas*, Plate x., 1863.
[6] *Archives of Ophthalmology* (Knapp and Moos), vol. i., 1869, pp. 341–358, Tab. B. and C.
[7] *Graefe und Saemisch*, vol. v. p. 599

retinitis, such as is often seen in cases of disease of the heart and blood-vessels. Gowers[1] thinks that there is a much greater tendency to hemorrhage in leucocythæmia than in simple anæmia, and that the effused blood is of a pale chocolate color, while white or yellowish splotches, often edged by a halo of blood-extravasations, are commonly present. Immermann has seen the retinal affection occurring in mylogenic leucæmia, but in most of the instances above cited they accompanied the splenic form of the disease. In one of Becker's cases, in which Stricker examined the blood, the bulk of the white corpuscles exceeded that of the red ones, whilst some individual white corpuscles were so much increased in size that one white one might readily contain fifty red ones. Leber[2] describes a leucæmic tumor of the lids with exophthalmos, and marked leucæmic retinitis with hemorrhages, which affected both eyes of a patient who had enlargement of the liver and spleen. He quotes Chauvel as having recorded a somewhat similar case. In both of Leber's and Chauvel's patients there was also disease of the kidneys, as evidenced by the presence of albumen and casts in the urine. Another leucocythæmic tumor of the orbit has been described by Osterwald.[3]

PERNICIOUS ANÆMIA.—Biermer (1871) was the first to call attention to the retinal changes in this grave and rare disease. Since that date Horner[4] and Quincke[5] have given us the results of the careful study of a considerable number of cases. The former had seen 30 cases, and remarks that the color of the blood, the distension and tortuosity of the veins, and the numerous hemorrhages recall the cases of leucæmic retinitis : in all of his cases the discs were entirely white. The latter, in his latest paper on the subject, records 17 cases, and gives a careful chromo-lithographic picture of one of them. He describes the affection as an œdema of the retina with numerous hemorrhages, many of which have white or grayish centres, whilst others envelop the blood-vessels, and by irregularly distending their lymph-sheaths cause them to appear varicose. The œdematous condition of the retina produces an appearance as if a thin bluish-white film had been spread over the fundus oculi. The writer has had an opportunity of observing three cases of this rare affection : in each there was a diffuse retinitis, the veins were distended, the blood pallid, and the disc was dirty white with a faint greenish tint, whilst the eye-ground was decidedly yellow in hue. In one of them there were no other pathological appearances ; in the second, only a few small hemorrhages into the lymph-sheath of some of the vessels near the macula ; in the third, numerous irregularly round or ovoid hemorrhages with yellowish-white centres. It is evident, however, from the reports of Quincke, that any one case might in its various stages present all these phases. Horner considers[6] the colorless centre of the hemorrhages to be due to a commencing absorption of the blood, while Manz[7] holds that these yellowish-white spots are the dilated extremities of retinal capillaries.

HEMORRHAGE.—Loss of blood may be the cause of impaired vision from transient anæmia of the retina or of the cerebral centres, but not un-

[1] *Medical Ophthalmoscopy*, 1879, p. 192.   [2] *Arch. f. Ophth.*, xxiv. 1, pp. 295–312.
[3] *Ibid.*, xxvii., 3, pp. 202–224.
[4] *Klinische Monatsblätter für Augenheilkunde*, 1874, pp. 458, 459.
[5] *Deutsches Archiv f. klinische Medizin*, 1877, pp. 1–31 (with plate).
[6] Quoted by Quincke, *loc. cit.*, p. 23.   [7] *Med. Centralblatt*, 1875, pp. 675–677.

frequently, in some manner which we are not yet able satisfactorily to account for, it gives rise to permanent blindness. This failure of sight may come on immediately after the hemorrhage, but it is usually noticed at periods varying from two to fourteen days after the loss of blood. Fries[1] has written an admirable monograph on the subject, and gives 26 cases collected from various authors. According to his tables, 35¼ per cent. of the cases are due to hemorrhage from the stomach or intestines; 25 per cent. to uterine hemorrhage; 25 per cent. to abstraction of blood; 7.3 per cent. to epistaxis; 52 per cent. to bleeding from wounds; and 1 per cent. each to hæmoptysis and urethral hemorrhage. Many of these cases are preopthalmoscopic, and consequently the exact pathological changes in the retina and optic nerve are necessarily matters of conjecture. Jaeger has given us two most interesting cases of blue degeneration of the optic nerve, with comparatively little change in the calibre of the main vessels of the disc and retina.[2] In both, the loss of blood occurred during labor; in the first, two births happened without accident; at the third and fourth labor there was severe hemorrhage, each followed by considerable and lasting impairment of vision, leaving ability to read Jaeg. No. iii. for a short time, and only by close approximation. In the other case there were four confinements, all accompanied by hemorrhage, each leaving the vision more and more impaired, until after the fourth labor there was no light-perception. At this time the ophthalmoscope showed only blue discoloration of the nerve, followed six years subsequently (after recurrent headaches from taking cold) by a more complete atrophy of the disc and retina, the former appearing of a dirty-green color and having acquired a saucer-like excavation, whilst the retinal vessels had undergone great diminution in their calibre. In most recorded cases no examination of the fundus has been made until long after failure of sight, and then there has generally been found some stage of atrophy; but when the ophthalmoscope has been used early in the case the eye-ground seems to have presented various appearances. Thus, Jaeger[3] says that soon after the hemorrhage the eye-ground presents a diminution in the calibre of the veins and arteries, with a light-blue discoloration of the optic disc, without any other demonstrable tissue-change. Graefe[4] saw slight diminution of the calibre of the retinal arteries and an increased pallor of the disc in a case where blood was vomited and passed by stool fourteen days after the occurrence of the blindness. On the other hand, Schweigger[5] (in two cases), Nagel,[6] Hirschberg,[7] Nägeli,[8] Horner,[9] and Landesberg[10] have all noted the occurrence of neuritis.

PROGNOSIS.—The prognosis is very unfavorable, and but few cases are recorded where there has been any improvement of sight.

PATHOLOGY.—The pathology of the affection is not well made out. Samelsohn,[11] who has reported a number of interesting cases, supposes

[1] Sigmund Fries, "Diss. Inaug." in Klin. Monatsblätter f. Augenheilkunde, 1878.
[2] Ergebnisse der Untersuchung mit dem Augenspiegel, 1876, p. 87.
[3] Loc. cit., 1876, p. 87.   [4] Arch. f. Ophth., vol. vii., part 2, p. 146.
[5] Handbuch der Augenheilkunde, 1875 (3d ed.), p. 522.
[6] Behandlung der Amaurose und Amblyopie mit Strychnine, 1871, p. 51.
[7] Bericht über die zehnte Vorsammlung der Ophth. Gessellschaft Heidelberg, 1871, pp. 53-60.
[8] Jahrbuch f. Ophthalmologie Literatur, 1879, p. 253.
[9] Klin. Monatsblätter f. Augenheilkunde, 1877 (supplement), pp. 53-60.
[10] Ibid., 1875, pp. 98, 99.   [11] A. f. O., xviii., 2, pp. 225-235.

that where there is a great loss of blood the brain becomes anæmic and occupies less room in the skull, and serum exudes from the blood-vessels to fill the vacuum. As the patient regains strength and blood is re-formed, the increased intracranial pressure drives the fluid into the subvaginal space of the optic nerves and causes neuritis. In other cases a hemorrhage into the sheath of the nerve is assumed as the cause. For those very exceptional cases where, after slight loss of blood, there is sudden and complete blindness without marked changes in the optic nerves and retinæ (and prompt reaction of the pupils to light), we are obliged to assume some lesion of the optic centres. Samelsohn[1] attempts to explain it by comparison with the observations of Lussana, Brown-Séquard, Ebstein, and Schiff, who found that wounds of the brain involving the anterior prominences of the corpora quadrigemina and the thalamus opticus may cause hemorrhage into the mucous membrane of the stomach; consequently, he assumes a central lesion which produces simultaneously the blindness and the hemorrhage. All this is, however, but ingenious speculation, and the true pathology is still to be made out by careful autopsies.

The study of the eye-ground after death is difficult; for, apart from any hindrances due to the position of the body or to social customs, Nature soon interposes an efficient barrier to such examination by the rapidity with which cloudiness of the corneal epithelium and of the lens substance sets in. These optical hindrances advance sufficiently soon to make it impossible to focus accurately any object in the eye-ground. Poncet[2] asserts that this may be remedied to a certain extent by dropping water into the conjunctival sac, which will render the cloudy epithelium sufficiently transparent to permit examination from two to five hours after death. Most observers agree that in the human eye there is an immediate blanching of the disc and choroid, causing the latter to assume a pale-yellowish hue with a faint tint of rose, and that the arteries (by promptly emptying themselves) escape observation, while the veins retain for a time a considerable amount of their contents, the blood-columns often being discontinuous and broken. Later, these changes are followed by a gradually increasing haze of the retina, which gives the appearance of a bluish-white veil spread over the fundus. Schreiber[3] gives an instructive picture of the eye of a patient dying of phthisis, and another of the same eye five minutes after death. Gayat, who had the opportunity of studying this subject in the eyes of five individuals recently decapitated by the guillotine, describes the formation of a small red spot at the fovea centralis similar to that seen in embolism of the central artery.[4] On the other hand, Becker[5] thinks that the emptying of the vessels after death is rather the exception than the rule, basing his observations not on ophthalmoscopic examinations, but on the fact that in opening freshly enucleated glaucomatous eyes, and in the eyes of those who had been hung, he had observed all the vessels, arteries as well as veins, full of

[1] *A. f. O.*, xxi., 1, pp. 150-178.
[2] *Archives générales de Médecine*, Série 6, t. xv., 1870, pp. 408-424.
[3] Separat Abdruck aus dem *Deutschen Arch. f. klin. Med.*, Bd. xxi. pp. 100, 101, Plates vii. and viii.
[4] *Annales d' Oculistique*, 1875, pp. 1-14.
[5] "Sitzungsbericht der Ophth. Gesellschaft," in *Klin. Monatsblätter f. Augenheilk.*, 1871, p. 385.

blood. Weber1 also, while admitting that the vessels both in men and animals usually empty themselves soon after death, describes as an exception a case in which there was no visible change in the blood-columns of the retinæ of the eyes of a patient with brain tumor, and a consequent optic neuritis, who was gradually dying of paralysis of the organs of respiration. This circumstance, in the opinion of the narrator, was very probably due to the obstruction to the escape of blood from the eye which would naturally be caused by the swollen and prominent optic neive. Landolt and Nuel[2] assert that there is an increase in the refraction in rabbits' eyes after death, causing any existing hypermetropia to approach emmetropia. They call attention to the difficulty of such determinations, owing to rapidly-forming haze on the corneal epithelium and to more or less complete emptiness of the retinal vessels.

Diseases of the Organs of Respiration.

Diseases of the organs of respiration appear to have little direct influence upon the nutrition of the eye, except in so far as they cause venous stasis by obstruction of the circulation through the lungs. Jaeger was the first to call attention to this fact in cases of pneumonia and pleurisy. The stasis manifests itself by an increase in the calibre of the veins, with a broadening of the light-reflex from them and a marked change in the color of the blood, causing the venous columns to become dark bluish-red. The writer has often seen this condition well marked in cases where there was not sufficient interference with the oxidation of the blood to cause an appreciable cyanosis of the skin. A higher degree of impeded circulation in the lung doubtless gives rise to the retinal hemorrhages, which, according to Foerster, are not infrequent in emphysema. Schreiber[3] mentions that in the hectic fever of phthisis the dilatation of the retinal vessels causes a congested appearance of the eye-ground, in marked contrast with the anæmic pallor of the skin of the patients. In 1871, Horner[4] published 31 cases of herpes corneæ occurring either during the course of severe catarrhal affections of the respiratory organs or immediately following such attacks. The eruption, which first appeared upon the lips, and then upon the eyeball, usually took place after the culmination of the febrile symptoms. The progress of the affection is slow, the ulcers left by the bursting of the vesicles healing in a period varying from two to six weeks. The herpes was monolateral, except in one case of double pneumonia in a drunkard, where the eruption occupied the entire central area of both corneæ. In preophthalmoscopic times Sichel called attention to blindness after pneumonia and bronchial catarrh, which he thought was due to cerebral congestions occurring in the height of these diseases.[5] He considered these congestions harmless so long as the patients remained quiet under antiphlogistic treatment, but deemed them noxious in their influence upon the eye as soon as freedom was allowed. Seidel[6] relates

[1] *Klin. Monats. f. Augenheilk.*, pp. 383–385. [2] *A. f. O.*, xix. 3, pp. 303, 304.
[3] *Veränderungen des Augenhinter-grundes bei Internen Erkrankungen*, 1878, p. 87.
[4] "Bericht der Ophth. Gesellschaft," in *Klin. Monatsblätt.*, 1871, pp. 326–328.
[5] Zehender, *Handbuch der Augenheilkunde*, vol. ii. pp. 188, 189.
[6] "Sehstörungen bei der Pneumonie," *Deutsches Klinik*, 1862, No. 27.

cases of amblyopia with contracted pupils and eyeballs which were painful on the slightest pressure. He says that coincident with croupous pneumonia on the fifth day there was color-blindness, followed two days later by a disappearance of the amplyopia, with a return of the pupils to their normal size.

Affections of the Eye caused by Diseases of the Digestive Organs.

TEETH.—Ophthalmic literature furnishes many instances of diseases of the eye said to be caused by affections of the teeth. These vary in severity from slight conjunctivitis and photophobia, or temporary failure of accommodation, to absolute amaurosis. It is natural to suppose that affections of the dental division of the trigeminus might readily give rise to reflex disorders in parts supplied by branches of the same main trunk. Although the writer has been on the lookout for such affections, he has seen very few cases of eye disease which could be logically attributed to disease of the teeth, and has known at least two sound teeth which were uselessly sacrificed to mistaken theories of pathology. Perhaps the most noteworthy effort to assign dental neuralgia as a cause of amaurosis is the well-known paper of Jonathan Hutchinson in the *Royal London Ophthalmic Hospital Reports* for 1865. An attentive study of the interesting cases there recorded shows that but few of them can be considered as affording convincing evidence of the point which he desires to prove, and few are probably more keenly aware of this fact than the distinguished surgeon himself when he writes: "I am quite alive to some of the sources of mistake which attend the attempt to prove the occurrence of paralysis from reflex irritation consequent on a peripheral cause: chief among them we have, of course, the possibility that the neuralgia itself may have been due to central disease, and that the extension of the latter may have complicated other nerves."[1] That amaurosis does, however, sometimes follow dental irritation is proved by Hutchinson's first case in the above-quoted paper, where neuralgia of the eyeball with great intolerance of light was cured by extraction of a carious molar tooth. Perhaps the most striking case on record is that of Galezowski,[2] where a small fragment of wood which had entered the cavity of a carious tooth (probably from picking the teeth with a wooden toothpick), lodged at the extremity of one of the fangs, is said to have caused absolute blindness of the eye, with dilatation of the pupil on the same side. After a blindness of eleven months the tooth with the foreign body was extracted, causing the evacuation of a few drops of thin pus from the antrum; after which the patient improved and vision gradually returned, so that on the ninth day after the operation he could see with the affected eye as well as with the other. Schmidt, after an examination of 96 patients with carious teeth, formulates the following conclusions: "1. That we may have a more or less considerable limitation of the accommodation

---

[1] "A Group of Cases illustrating the Occasional Connection between Neuralgia of the Dental Nerves and Amaurosis," by Jonathan Hutchinson, F. R. C. S., *R. L. O. H. Rep.*, vol. iv. pp. 381–388.

[2] *Archives générales de Médecine*, t. xxiii. pp. 261–264.

in consequence of pathological irritation of the dental branches of the trigeminus. 2. This may occur on both sides. Where the affection is one-sided, it is always on the side of the affected tooth. 3. It is usually an affection of the young, very seldom or never occurring in old age. 4. That the diminution of the power of accommodation is due to increased intraocular pressure caused by reflected irritation of the vaso-motor nerves of the eye." These conclusions are interesting, but cannot be considered absolutely correct, in consequence of the fact that there are no recorded tests for astigmatism or insufficiency, and that accurate examination of the state of refraction was impossible through want of a mydriatic, which may in measure have accounted for the existent diminution of accommodation. More extended and minute investigations of the subject are desirable.

STOMACH, INTESTINES, AND LIVER.—Amblyopia and amaurosis with severe gastric symptoms are not very uncommon, but, although such cases are made much worse by the ingestion of indigestible substances, constipation, etc., it has nevertheless always appeared to the writer that the primary lesion lay in the nervous system. Galezowski, however, lays stress on this subject, and discriminates between a true and false locomotor ataxia; the latter being, according to this author, symptomatic of stomachic and intestinal lesions. Many of the older writers relate cases of amaurosis from worms in the intestines. Thus Laurence[1] gives an instance of sluggishness and partial dilatation of the pupils with dim vision which promptly disappeared after the evacuation of seat-worms consequent on an enema of turpentine. Hays calls attention[2] to a case recorded by Welsh of Massachusetts where complete amaurosis in a child instantly ceased on a worm being puked up. Many similar instances might be adduced which in modern books are either passed over in silence or looked at with a shrug of incredulity. Although the writer has had no personal experience with such cases, he can readily understand that in children the irritation of worms might easily give rise to enough reflex disorder of the spinal cord and brain as to cause impairment of the accommodation and partial dilatation of the pupils. (The effects of hæmatemesis and hemorrhage from the bowels have been already discussed.)

That jaundice shows readily in the conjunctiva is well known to all practitioners, and yellow vision is described as an occasional symptom of severe icterus. Jaeger calls attention to a light-yellow color of the eyeground and retinal vessels under these circumstances. Junge,[3] Stricker,[4] and Buchwald[5] have all recorded cases of retinal hemorrhage in cases of grave disease of the liver. Litten[6] says that for ten years he has examined every case of liver disease under his charge with the ophthalmoscope, and found retinal hemorrhages only in fifteen cases. These occur only when icterus is present, but are not due, as Traube assumes, to the action of the biliary acids on the blood-corpuscles. If they were so, we should have blood-stained lymphatic sheaths instead of corpuscular diapedesis and massing of the exuded blood. Of these 15 cases, 4 were cases of congestive jaundice, 4 of carcinoma, 1 each of acute fatty degen-

[1] Amer. ed. by Hays, 1847, p. 554.   [2] *Ibid.*, 1847, p. 555.
[3] *Heinrich Müller's Gesammelte Schriften*, pp. 331–335.   [4] *Berliner klin. Wochenschrift.*
[5] Foerster, *loc. cit.*   [6] *Deutsche med. Wochenschrift*, 25 März, 1882, pp. 179–182.

ᴇration and phosphorus-poisoning, 1 of abscess, 2 of cirrhosis, 1 of hydrops cystides filleæ. The hemorrhages were usually in the nuclear layers, and seldom presented white centres, as in leucocythæmia. In the case of phosphorus-poisoning there were large white plaques with marginal inflammation. Litten considers that the pigment-spots reported in the retina in cases of liver disease (his own cases and Landolt's) are due not to cirrhosis hepatis, but to a congenital or acquired disposition to connec_ tive-tissue hyperplasia [syphilis?]. Foerster[1] has called attention to a group of cases which he ascribes to hyperæmia of the liver and plethora abdominalis, where we find discomfort in the use of the eyes from the accompanying retinal hyperæmia and diminution of the range of accom_ modation, and where the ophthalmoscope frequently shows premature senile degeneration of the lens, manifested by striæ occurring in the extreme periphery. Every careful observer will doubtless agree to the accuracy of this description, and to the advantages of proper hygiene, exercise, and the alterative mineral waters (Karlsbad, Saratoga) in such cases.

SPLEEN.—The effect of disease of the spleen in causing disease of the eye has already been alluded to in the discussion of leucæmic retinitis.

Xanthopsia appears to be a very infrequent complication of liver disease. Moxon,[2] who records seven cases of fatal obstructive jaundice, has never seen it. He remarks that in these cases the vitreous and lens remained perfectly clear, while the blood-serum was saffron-yellow and the sclerotic deeply stained (yellow or olive-green). Rose[3] gives the only case with which the writer is familiar, in which it was carefully studied and demonstrated with the spectroscope. Here the violet end of the spectrum was shortened as in poisoning by santonin, and the blue blindness was so marked that a few days before his admission to the hospital the patient had excited the astonishment of his fellow-workmen by mistaking the color of a door which had been freshly painted blue. The autopsy showed here also that the vitreous and aqueous were colorless, but the cornea was clearly yellow. This Rose thinks insufficient to have caused the xanthopsia, and therefore attributes it to the effect of the jaundice in the nerve-centres.

HEMERALOPIA.—The curious affection hemeralopia, which we well know to be a constant accompaniment of some forms of congenital nerve-atrophy (retinitis pigmentosa), and also to affect, at times, considerable numbers of persons exposed to the glare, overwork, and exposure of an active campaign, is probably always due to some form of malnutrition or disorder of the digestive apparatus, and in many cases it is associated with jaundice and disease of the liver. That glare of light is not necessary to its production is shown by its development in convalescent hospitals. Reymond of Turin reports it as developing in an individual affected by pellagra on whom he had operated for cataract, and who during the four weeks subsequent had never been out of his room. Cornillon[4] reports 5 cases of hemeralopia during jaundice, and of these 4 came under his observation

---

[1] *G. u. S.*, vol. vii. p. 74.
[2] "Clinical Remarks on Xanthopsia and the Distribution of Bile-Pigment in Jaundice," *Lancet*, Jan. 25, 1873, p. 130.
[3] "Die Gesichtslauschungen im Icterus," *Virchow's Archiv*, vol. xxx. pp. 442–447.
[4] *Le Progrès médicale*, No. 9, Fèvrier 26, 1881, pp. 157–159.

in a single winter in the hospital in Vichy. It never appeared early in the congestion of the liver, but always after jaundice had existed for some time, and disappeared without special treatment—often to recur when the disease of the liver became more marked. Parinaud[1] has reported 4 such cases in all, with jaundice, the conjunctiva being yellow, but the media not tinged. There were no ophthalmoscopic changes. One of these cases was malarial hepatitis, the other three probably cirrhosis. A curious change in the ocular conjunctiva has been noted in many of these cases of hemeralopia, and attention was first called to it by Bitot.[2] He observed 29 cases at the Hospice des Enfants Assistés at Bordeaux. The bulbar conjunctiva in the palpebral fissure, usually at the outside of the cornea, becomes dry and anæsthetic (epithelial xerosis), and a number of minute points form in it, and the little patch becomes like mother-of-pearl, iridescent and silvery. They become paler before they disappear, and come and go with the advent and cessation of the hemeralopia. Pressing on the conjunctiva over the spot by rubbing the lids over it often causes little fragments of the dry patch to crumble off. The adjoining conjunctiva is dry and less pliant, more like parchment. The extensive occurrence of hemeralopia during the severe Easter fasts of the Greek Church has been noted by Blessig. There is frequently diarrhœa associated with this condition. Teuscher also speaks of conjunctival xerosis and hypopyon keratitis in the young slave-children in the Brazilian coffee-plantations, associated with gastric catarrh and diarrhœa.

Diseases of the Kidneys and Skin.

DISEASES OF THE KIDNEYS.—As has been abundantly proved by careful autopsies, inflammation of the retina may be developed during any form of *Bright's disease*, either with the enlarged mottled kidney of acute parenchymatous nephritis, the large white kidney, the amyloid kidney, or the cirrhotic kidney of chronic disease. In the vast majority of cases the retinal inflammation appears during the later stages of the last-named form of disease, and seems to be in some way dependent upon blood-poisoning, which has been caused by the degenerating kidney.

The retinitis presents various aspects, not only in different cases, but also in the different stages of its development in the same case, and distinguishes itself mainly from other forms of inflammation of the retina by its marked tendency to fatty degeneration. As seen at an eye hospital the disease usually presents a type quite different to that which predominates in the wards of a general hospital. In the former class of cases the blood-poisoning seems to fall with peculiar intensity on the nervous system, and the patients come complaining of headache, dizziness, and dim vision, these being the only marked symptoms of the malady, while the anæmia, dropsy, and other symptoms are either absent or present in so slight a degree that the patients have not supposed themselves to be suffering from any constitutional malady or to need any medical advice. In the walking cases the retinal changes are usually very extensive (and those in the cerebrum would possibly be found equally developed if we

[1] *Archives générales de Médecine*, April, 1881, pp. 403–414.
[2] *Gaz. méd. de Paris*, No. 27, 4 Juillet, 1863.

had only as accurate a method of investigating them), whilst among hos-pital inmates we often see only a few white splotches in the retina, either with or without hemorrhages, and occasionally only a slight atrophy of the optic disc due to a previous retinitis. In the wards of a general hos-pital we have a much better opportunity to study the early development of the retinitis, and ,it is there most frequently encountered among those suffering from dropsy and dyspnœa—patients whose waxy skin and general appearance indicate at a glance how seriously their nutrition has been impaired by the ravages of the disease. When the individual lives and is not markedly relieved by the rest and treatment adopted, we fre-quently have an opportunity of seeing the development to a greater or less degree of the typical form of the affection.

In typical cases the retinal changes commence with slight œdema of the disc and surrounding retina, associated with a few irregular white splotches and striated hemorrhages in the fibre-layer. These white patches multiply and extend, but are usually confined within an area of two or three disc-diameters from the optic entrance. In high grades of the affection they coalesce and form a broad zone around the disc, which is itself swollen and prominent, its outlines being hidden by the opaque nerve-fibres which diverge from it. From time to time fresh hemorrhages occur, which are striated when in the fibre-layer, and of irregularly round-ed outline when they invade the deeper portions of the retina. These were formerly supposed to be absolutely characteristic of the disease, but it is now asserted by several good observers that similar appearances have been seen in the neuro-retinitis caused by brain tumor or by basilar meningitis where there was no accompanying disease of the kidney. Graefe,[1] Schmidt and Wegner,[2] Magnus,[3] Leber,[4] Carter,[5] and Eales[6] have each reported such cases. The hemorrhages are usually either entirely absorbed or leave behind them a fatty clot, which adds an additional white patch to the splotches already existing in the retina. In many cases occur-ring in the last stages of the disease, a remarkably yellowish tint of the fundus is observed, together with decided alteration in the color of the blood-columns in the retinal blood-vessels, the blood in the arteries being too yellow, and that in the veins presenting too little of its usually pro-nounced red-purple tint. In short, there is a state of affairs approxi-mating in some degree to that which we find in cases of pernicious anæmia.

Exceptional forms of albuminuric retinitis have been recorded where the only change seen in the fundus oculi was a pronounced choking of the disc similar to that with which we are familiar in cases of brain tumor. The writer has seen cases which at the start could not be diagnosticated by the ophthalmoscope from cases of retinal hemorrhage due to other causes. Magnus has published similar cases.

In the course of Bright's disease uræmic amaurosis is much more rarely encountered than albuminuric retinitis. It is, however, occasionally developed in cases in which albuminuric retinitis already exists. It is rapid in its development, and in its subsidence is without retinal changes, the blindness being evidently due to some transient affection of the cerebral centres.

[1] *A. f. O.,* xii. 2.   [2] *Ibid.,* xv. 3.   [3] *Ophth. Atlas,* Taf. vi. Fig. 2.
[4] *Graefe und Saemisch,* Bd. v. p. 581.   [5] *Diseases of the Eye* (Am. ed.), p. 382.
[6] H. Eales, *Birmingham Med. Review,* Jan., 1880. p 47.

DISEASES OF THE SKIN.—The *eczema* of the lower lid, nose, angle of the mouth, and external meatus of the ear which so frequently accompanies the phlyctenular conjunctivitis of scrofulous children is probably the most common example of coincident skin and eye disease. Lepra is a frequent cause of severe affections of the eye in localities where it is endemic. Bull and Hansen[1] assert that the cornea is frequently attacked. They divide the manifestations of the disease upon this membrane into two varieties—the one in which there is a diffuse infiltration of the tissue, and the other where there is a formation of tubers. The first variety is a gray opacity limited to the border of the cornea, not separated from its circumference by any such clear area as is found in arcus senilis. This opacity becomes vascularized, and may remain quiet for years till another attack of hyperæmia occurs, which, also in time receding, leaves the tissue more opaque than before. In the second there are nodes which appear to start at the margin of the cornea and to accompany either its superficial or its deep layer of vessel-loops : this latter form is more dangerous to vision. The paralysis of the orbicularis muscle which is a frequent attendant upon the smooth form of the disease allows an exposure of the membrane to irritants which often produce a third form of inflammation. The iris also exhibits the smooth and the tuberous forms of the disease. Iritis occurring in lepra is, however, by no means pathognomonic; 50 per cent. of all cases exhibiting synechiæ are the result of extensions of corneal inflammations due to orbicular paralysis. The superciliæ and the eyelashes are said to be frequent seats of leprous tubercules. In the lids the first symptom is the falling of the eyelashes, which is dependent upon the formation of the tubers before they become manifest to sight and touch. Mooren[2] maintains that chronic skin eruptions favor the development of cataract by causing creeping inflammatory processes which alter the character of the exudations into the vitreous humor, and moreover claims that when such skin eruptions have their seat in the scalp they favor the occurrence of retinitis by maintaining a constant hyperæmia of the meninges. He further cites a case where he observed a decrease in the acuity of vision corresponding with the breaking out of a skin eruption, and an increase in the power of vision coincident with the disappearance of the eruption. Foerster[3] agrees with Mooren in the statement that cataract may be formed in cases where chronic skin affections favor the development of marasmus. Rothmund[4] reports a noteworthy curiosity to the effect that cataract followed a peculiar degeneration of the skin in three families living in separate villages in the Urarlberg. The skin of these patients showed a fatty degeneration of the rete Malpighii and of the papillæ, with consecutive thinning and atrophy of the epidermis : this was most marked on the cheeks, chin, and the outer surfaces of the arms and legs. In the individuals thus affected the skin disease commenced between the third and sixth months of life, whilst the cataract appeared in both eyes between the third and sixth years. Rothmund thinks that the same congenital predisposition to disease exists in both organs, because the lens is developed out of an unfolding of the external skin.

[1] *The Leprous Diseases of the Eye,* Christiania, 1873.
[2] *Ophthalmologische Mittheilungen,* 1874, p. 93.
[3] *Graefe und Saemisch's Handb.,* vol. vii. p. 152.   [4] *A. f. O.,* xiv., 1, p. 159.

Disturbances of Vision caused by Disease of the Sexual Organs.

The eyes and their appendages frequently exhibit the effects of perverted function or diseased conditions of the sexual organs. As might be expected, these ocular effects are most marked in the female, whose generative apparatus is so much more complex and extensive. While it is true that there are thousands of women with grave disease or derangement of these organs who are free from any uncomfortable eye symptoms, still, clinical experience shows that there are crowds of others who present eye lesions due entirely to such causes. Still more frequently do we see some slight optical defect (previously scarcely noticed) become so unbearable that the patient is unfitted for any useful employment. In fact, at most eye hospitals, and still more markedly in private practice, we find an excess of female over male patients. This excess becomes more palpable when we throw out of consideration the large number of male patients who are under treatment for injuries of all sorts the result of mechanical occupations not pursued by females, and the inflammations due to direct exposure to storm, cold, and intense heat.

MENSTRUATION.—When menstruation is profuse its effects are with difficulty distinguished from those of anæmia and loss of blood, but where it is retarded, irregular, or scanty the effects are more readily traced. All surgeons of experience are agreed that it is undesirable to perform operations for cataract or to make iridectomy at the menstrual period, and it is well known that eyes which have been progressing favorably after operations become congested and irritable during the monthly period. In trachomatous eyes retardation of the catamenia often causes the eruption of a fresh crop of granules, while in cases of phlyctenular and interstitial keratitis there are still more frequently relapse and exacerbation of the disease. Vaso-motor disturbances connected with the period of puberty and with that of cessation of the menses are of daily occurrence: we constantly see cases at these epochs where some slight astigmatism or hypermetropia, which has previously given no practical annoyance to the patient, becomes absolutely unbearable. The eyes become watery and sensitive to light; there is marked congestion of the retina with tortuosity of its veins, together with serous infiltration and swelling often sufficient to obscure the margins of the disc. These symptoms frequently entirely disappear when the menses have either become established or have permanently ceased. In some rare cases the symptoms are anomalous and striking: thus the writer has seen vicarious menstruation from the lachrymal caruncle, and a case of pemphigus of the upper lid occurring regularly at each menstrual period for some months. In another patient menstruation came on during the thirteenth year with intense headache, epistaxis, and photophobia, and for a long time afterward there was utter inability to use the eyes for school-work even during the catamenial interval. At almost every menstrual epoch during a period of eight years there has been a recurrence of these symptoms, although they subside sufficiently in the interval to allow the patient to use her eyes for a very limited amount of near work. At the first examination the ophthalmoscope showed that the retinal fibres were swollen and œdematous, hiding the outlines of the discs, while the lymph-sheaths of the retinal vessels at their point of emergence from the disc presented an almost snow-white appearance. The discs and the retinæ have never quite resumed a normal appearance.

Disturbances in the circulation of the eye and its appendages are frequently associated with the menopause. The writer recalls a case where for years there was headache with intense congestion of the palpebral and bulbar conjunctiva, with a fulness and pressure on the orbits at each menstrual period, all these symptoms disappearing with the cessation of the menses. The most striking examples of the influence of the menses on the eyesight are those where the flow has been suddenly checked. Rejecting examples from the older authors, where the want of exact helps to diagnosis might leave room for a different interpretation of the symptoms, we will content ourselves with two examples where the testing of the eyesight and the ophthalmoscopic examination were made by skilled observers. Thus, Mooren—to whom we are indebted for a careful discussion of the relations between uterine disease and disturbances of sight —recites[1] the case of a peasant-woman aged twenty-three years who had complete stoppage of the menstrual flow from exposure to wet during the catamenial period : this was accompanied by high fever and delirium, with pain in the region of the right ovary. When these symptoms subsided, she noticed that there was absolute loss of sight in the right eye, and so great a diminution of it on the left that she could only distinguish movements of the hand. The ophthalmoscope showed on the right side a multiple detachment of the retina, and on the left an intense neuroretinitis. Rest in bed, inunctions of mercurial ointment, and cataplasms over the region of the ovaries, with leeches to the septum of the nose and the neck of the uterus, gradually brought about amelioration of the symptoms, with restoration of the eyesight in the left eye. As might be expected, the retinal detachment and consequent loss of vision in the right eye remained permanent. In confirmation of this case, but in contrast with it as regards the retinal symptoms, is the one related by Samelsohn.[2] The patient (a peasant-girl) by standing in a cold running brook while at work had her menses suddenly stopped. There was no marked uterine or abdominal pain. The patient complained of a feeling of pressure on the orbits, and experienced a gradual failure of sight with contraction of the field of vision. In five days there was absolute amaurosis of both eyes (no sensation of light and no phosphenes to be obtained by pressure). The sight gradually returned in each eye, this being preceded by a copious flow of tears, so that in sixteen days the patient could read small print fluently. In seven weeks the menses returned. There were no ophthalmoscopic symptoms : each eye, both during the attack and subsequent to it, showed only striation of the retina and tortuosity of its veins, the calibre of the retinal arteries being unchanged. Unfortunately, any pupillary changes that might have been recognized were annihilated by previous instillation of atropine into the eye. In the first case there was every probability in favor of a serous effusion into the subarachnoidal and the intravaginal spaces. The latter case is more difficult to explain : if it were due to orbital or intracranial neuritis, why should there not have been some ophthalmoscopic changes during the

[1] Arch. f. Augenheilkunde, Bd. x., 1881.
[2] Berliner klin. Wochenschrift, Jan., 1878, pp. 27–30.

time that the patient was under observation? If to effusion within the cranium or to local circulatory disturbances in either the corpora quad-rigemina or the occipital lobes, why were there not other symptoms of intracranial disturbance?

In further illustration of the effects of a stoppage of menstruation, Mooren[1] cites the case of a peasant-woman aged thirty-one who had complete suppression of the menses after the birth of her fourth child, and where subsequently an almost continuous headache, dimness of vision, and eventually epileptiform attacks, followed. The ophthalmoscope showed a double neuritis so intense as to lead to the supposition of a possible cerebral tumor. Mercurial inunctions with seton to the back of the neck were resorted to without result. Emmenagogues also failed to give relief. An examination of the uterus was now made, which showed great enlargement and hyperplasia, especially of its mouth and neck, for which scarifications and sitz-baths were employed with good result. The headache and epileptoid attacks disappeared, and the vision improved so far that the patient (who when admitted to the hospital could only decipher Jaeger No. xviii.) could read fluently Jaeger No. iii.

DISPLACEMENTS OF THE UTERUS.—Anteflexion and retroversion of the uterus are frequent causes of retinal hyperæsthesia. In this connection we may quote from the same author two cases, as showing how slight mechanical irritations of the uterus may cause eye disturbance—one where a patient had an episcleritis and a chronic metritis with malposition of the uterus, in whom there was an exacerbation of the ciliary neuralgia and of the local eye inflammation every time that the ulcerated os uteri was cauterized or a pessary introduced; and a second with an adhesive kolpitis, in whom the introduction of a pessary caused unpleasant feelings about the head and oppression in the cardiac region, accompanied on two separate occasions by capillary hemorrhages into the retina, all of these symptoms diappearing rapidly after the removal of the pessary. Mooren[2] has also seen a double neuro-retinitis caused by retroversion of the uterus. The sight was so much impaired that the patient could with difficulty decipher Jr. No. xx.; but it was entirely regained within a few months after the uterus had been replaced in its proper position. No other treatment was employed.

PELVIC CELLULITIS.—Still more frequently are the reflex eye disturb-anecs caused by parametritis and the various forms of pelvic cellulitis. Every practitioner has had abundant opportunity of studying the easy fatigue of the eye, the burning and stinging conjunctival sensations, the orbital and periorbital pains, the retinal hyperæsthesia and sensitiveness to artificial light, which characterize the early stages of the affection, accompanied later on by symptoms of retinal anæsthesia. Inasmuch as the cause of these symptoms is irremediable, we find in the majority of cases that it is impossible to relieve the sufferings of the patient; this cause consisting in the cicatricial shrinking of the parametrium and the pelvic connective tissue. Sleep gives relief only so long as it lasts, and the patients upon awakening, instead of feeling rested, often experience their greatest pain and discomfort. Foerster[3] and Freund, who were the first to demonstrate this

---

[1] *Loc. cit.,* p. 551. [2] *Ophthalmologische Mittheilungen,* 1878, p. 97.
[3] "Allgemein-Leiden und Veränderungen des Sehorgans," in *Graefe und Saemisch,* vol. vii. pp. 88–96.

form of parametritis, call special attention to the fact that the patients have their good and bad days entirely independent of any use of the eyes. In many of the milder cases, however, we find that the sufferings of the patients are enhanced and aggravated by the presence of some defect, such as astigmatism, hypermetropia, or insufficiency. Although the careful correction of such defects will give considerable relief and enable the patients to use their eyes for near work for a much longer period, never-theless the pain and discomfort are out of all proportion to the amount of error. Of course, we are very far from having converted such eyes into useful instruments for every-day work or for long-continued labor, but we have removed an appreciable source of irritation from an over-sensitive nervous system, and done much to relieve the tœdium vitæ in cases which perhaps for months previously have been unable to amuse or occupy themselves by the use of their eyes in either reading, writing, or sewing.

MASTURBATION is also an occasional cause of reflex eye disturbances. Mooren[1] relates two aggravated cases in women who for years had been excessively addicted to the vice. In both of these there were accommo-dative asthenopia and tenderness in the ciliary region, dread even of moderate illumination, which increased from year to year. In both cases there were attacks of dyspnœa and other disturbance of innervation of the pneumogastric nerve. Cohn has also published a number of cases of eye disease in the male sex due to the same cause. The main symptoms were a feeling of pressure on the eyes, bright dots moving before them, and a sensation as if the air between the patient and the object looked at was wavy and trembling. In some of the individuals a discontinuance of onanism and a moderate indulgence in sexual intercourse effected a complete cure. Travers[2] gives a case of loss of sight from excessive venery, and another from masturbation. Mackenzie[3] quotes Dupuytren as relating the case of a man who lost his sight on the day after his wed-ding, but where it was promptly restored by the use of a cold bath with stimulants and the application of counter-irritation to the skin of the lum-bar region. Foerster[4] has recorded a case of kopiopia hysterica in a man where, from the eye symptoms alone, he diagnosticated disease of the genital organs, and where it was afterward proved that there was inabil-ity to copulate, the patient having extremely small testicles and there being a thin whey-like discharge from the urethra.

CONGESTION AND INFLAMMATION OF THE OVARIES.—Disease of the ovaries is frequently associated with retinal œdema and hyperæs-thesia. In women complaining of weak and painful eyes pressure in the ovarian region often causes pain. Where only one ovary is tender to the touch, we often notice that the patient complains more of the cor-responding eye, although there may be no difference or abnormality in the ophthalmoscopic appearance of the two eyes. Under this head may be appropriately mentioned the eye symptoms of patients affected with hystero-epilepsy, a disease which is always associated with ovarian trouble, of which Charcot has given us so graphic a picture. He says that previous to the attack the patient experiences an aura which starts from the abdomen. The convulsion is ushered in by a loud cry, which

[1] *Loc. cit.*
[2] *Synopsis of Diseases of the Eye*, 1820, p. 145.
[3] *Diseases of the Eye*, 1854, p. 1075.
[4] *G. u. S. Handb.*, vol vii. p. 95.

is accompanied by pallor of the face and loss of consciousness. These symptoms are succeeded by twitching and rigidity of the face-muscles, with foaming at the mouth, followed by contortions of the muscles of the trunk, abdomen, and lower limbs, the paroxysm terminating with sob-bing, weeping, and laughing. Landolt has given us a careful description of the eye symptoms in such cases, and groups them into four stages. In the first, the outer and inner tunics of the eye appear healthy and the acuity of vision is normal, but there is a contraction of the form- and color-folds, always more marked on the affected side. In the second group the acuity of vision begins to fail, and the symptoms become more marked on the hitherto sound side. In the third with the more affected eye fingers can scarcely be counted, while the field of vision is limited to a few degrees from the fixation point; at this stage the ophthalmoscope shows a serous swelling of the retina, with fulness and tortuosity of its veins. In the fourth stage there is a partial atrophy of the optic nerve on both sides.

PREGNANCY.—Cases of amaurosis occurring during pregnancy, in which the vision was impaired after delivery, are recorded by Beer, Ramsbotham,[1] and other writers of the preophthalmoscopic period. Some of them, at least, may probably be accounted for by the occurrence of albuminuric retinitis in the puerperal state, but no such interpretation can be put on the more recent cases reported by Lawson[2] and Eastlake,[3] which in their main features strongly recall the amaurosis after loss of blood, although there is no history of any similar hemorrhages. In Lawson's case, we have an amaurosis which commenced during the gestation of the eighth child, and recurred during the ninth and tenth pregnancies. After the eighth labor the patient recovered sufficient sight to be able to sew; the amount of vision being gradually lessened after each gestation until finally complete atrophy of the optic nerve ensued. In Eastlake's case, the patient (æt. thirty-four) had borne nine children at full time. The labors were normal in character, and the amount of blood lost was not excessive. On the second or third days after the second and each subsequent delivery, sudden loss of vision occurred, and the woman became insensible. On recover-ing her consciousness, her sight did not at once return, the amaurosis remaining from three to five weeks. After the last labor there was com-plete and permanent loss of sight in both eyes: Z. Laurence examined this case with the ophthalmoscope, and reports only a slight contraction of the retinal arteries, without other positive lesion. Zehender,[4] in treat-ing of the subject, remarks that "almost every busy eye-surgeon has encountered similar sad cases."

PUERPERAL PHLEBITIC OPHTHALMITIS.—According to Mackenzie, this dread malady, which, as a rule, causes the death of the patient, may develop at any time from the third to the thirtieth day after delivery. It fre-quently attacks both eyes, and in those cases which do not terminate fatally eyesight is usually lost. Hall and Higginsbottom,[5] Mackenzie,[6] Fischer,[7]

[1] *Med. Times and Gazette*, March 7, 1834.   [2] *R. L. O. Hos. Rep.*, vol. iv. pp. 65, 66.
[3] *Obstet. Trans.*, vol. v. p. 79 (1864).   [4] *Handbuch der Augenheilkunde*, vol. ii. p. 180.
[5] *Medico-Chirurgical Transactions*, 1829, vol. xv. p. 120.
[6] *Treatise on Diseases of the Eye*, London, 1854.
[7] *Lehrbuch der Entzündungen und Organischen Krankheiten des Menschlichen Auges*, 1866,
p. 285.

Arlt,[1] and Hirschberg[2] have all given good clinical descriptions of the disease, with careful autopsies. As in other forms of metastasis, it is ushered in with a chill. Soon after, transient darting pains are felt in the eye, which are sometimes associated with photopsies and followed by serous infiltration of the conjunctiva bulbi. Later, owing to effusion in the capsule of Tenon and to the swelling of the orbital tissues, the eye projects forward and its motility is impaired, these symptoms being accompanied by a clouding of the cornea and the formation of pus in the anterior chamber. If the patient lives, we may have either discharge of pus through the cornea or sclera, or its gradual absorption : in either case, the eyeball shrinks to a small stump. Anatomical examination shows that the starting-point of these symptoms is a septic embolism of either the choroidal or central retinal blood-vessels. According to Hirschberg, " In other pyæmic affections in which the eye is attacked with septic embolism life is dangerously threatened, but there is a larger percentage of recovery with permanent blindness (single or double) than in the puerperal form."

Influence of Lactation.—The asthenopia, feeble accommodation, photophobia, and obstinate phlyctenular inflammations of the conjunctiva and cornea which occur during prolonged lactation are subjects of daily observation to every ophthalmic surgeon. They unfrequently fail to yield to appropriate remedies so long as the patients continue to nurse their children. Besides these symptoms, Critchett[3] has called attention to the sudden unilateral affection of sight which occurs during lactation, and is due to hemorrhage situated either in or behind the retina. This author has frequently seen such cases coming on without pain.

PATHOLOGY.—As regards the pathology of these affections we are still very much in the dark. Mooren in his elaborate paper (previously quoted) considers that the reflex disturbances of the retina and optic nerve may either be transmitted directly, or may cause primarily a spinal myelitis, which in its turn affects the eyes. He points out that the subperitoneal connective tissue of the pelvis and the uterus is so rich in blood-vessels, lymphatics, and nerves that Rouget has likened it to cavernous tissue. He asserts that the uterine and pelvic nerves re-enter the lumbar cord, while the veins anastomose freely with the veins of the spinal column ; and quotes Röhrig to show that electric stimulation of the ovary causes a rise in the general blood-pressure and a diminution of the heart's action— effects which he attributes to irritation of the vagus. He further maintains that any long-standing or often-repeated congestion of the visual centres, of the optic nerve, or of the retina would cause increase of connective tissue and a subsequent tendency to contraction, while the lymph which is poured out, acting on the cylinder axis of the nerves, causes them first to swell, and finally to absorb (Rumpf,[4] Kuhnt[5]).

[1] *Die Krankheiten des Auges*, 1863, Bd. ii. pp. 167, 269.
[2] *Archives of Ophthalmology*, 1880, vol. ix. p. 177.
[3] *Medical Times and Gazette*, 1858, p. 118.
[4] *Untersuchungen am d. Physiol. Institut. d. Univ. Heidelberg*, Bd. ii. Heft 2.
[5] *Ueber Erkrankung der Sehnerven bei Gehirnleiden*, 1879.

Febrile and Post-febrile Ophthalmitis.

VARIOLA.—Various affections of the eye which at times impair its functions, and at others destroy vision, frequently arise during the course as well as during the subsidence of smallpox. When pocks form in the skin of the eyelids, they cause the lids to swell to such an extent as to completely close the eye : many patients so affected relate how, after being blind for a week or ten days, they again recovered their eyesight. The cicatricial processes which ensue often produce falling of the eyelashes with incurvation of the tarsus, which changes the direction of the ciliæ and causes the lashes to rub against the eyeball. During the first stage of the disease there is always flushing and congestion of the conjunctiva, frequently associated with increased flow of tears and sensitiveness to strong light. In some cases we find small elevated yellowish spots, often in groups of two or three, surmounted by an area of vascularization on the edges of the lids and in the tarsal conjunctiva. Similar efflorescences are at times seen in the conjunctiva bulbi and on the limbus corneæ. These coincide in the time of their appearance with the eruption on the skin, and are probably of the same nature, although from the difference in the anatomical structures they do not present the same appearance as the pocks in the skin. Hebra, who has observed and analyzed twelve thousand cases, says that 1 per cent. of the total number presented efflorescences in the conjunctiva. Neumann, Knecht, Schely, Buck, and other German authorities describe them ; and Adler in his able monograph (*On Eye Diseases during and after Variola*) gives an accurate account of them. In opposition to the above statement it should be mentioned that Gregory maintains that no mucous membranes except those of the fauces, larynx, and trachea are capable of taking on variolous inflammation. Marson [1] also, who from his position at the London Smallpox Hospital had unusual opportunities for witnessing the disease, maintains " that pustules never form on the conjunctiva ;" Coccius [2] is also of the same opinion. These authors call attention to the fact that the well-known abscesses of the cornea which occur during the drying and desquamation of the eruption, and which have frequently been described as pocks by the older authors, cannot in any sense be considered as pocks. Beer, however, while calling these formations pocks, distinctly states [3] that they occur during the suppurative or drying stage. There seems to be no good reason why the above-described conjunctival efflorescences, which come on simultaneously with the skin, should not be considered as analogous in their natures, although from the absence of the corium in the conjunctiva they cannot assume the well-known form of the skin eruption. At times the conjunctivitis becomes catarrhal, and even purulent, leaving in some cases an acute dacryo-cystitis (Adler), and more frequently a low grade of blenorrhœa of the lachrymal duct. Beer states that " those authorities may be right who suppose that there is a real eruption of pocks in the mucous membrane of the tear-sac, because no other sort of inflammation of it is so apt to cause complete closure in its entire length." [4] The cornea may present either diffuse or interstitial keratitis. Malacia or abscesses are more fre-

[1] *London Med. Gazette*, 1838–39, pp. 204–207.
[2] *De Morbis Oculi humani que e Variolis exedi*, etc., Leipzig, 1871.
[3] *Lehre von den Augenkrankheiten*, vol. i. p. 527.
[4] *Op. cit.*, p. 525.

quent in the severe cases, where there are evidences of metastases to other organs. They usually form in the outer quadrant of the cornea, and are accompanied by marked ciliary injection, the patients complaining of stitches in the ball with frontal and temporal neuralgia. Prolapse of the iris and often the formation of a staphyloma are produced by the perforation of resultant ulcers; sometimes the entire cornea is swept away. Marson declares that he has seen this last condition occur within forty-eight hours from the time of the commencement of the corneal affection. Iritis is a less frequent complication. It is of the seroplastic variety, and, according to Adler, comes on only after the twelfth day and in cases where the progress of the disease is slow and insidious. It is always accompanied by some degree of cyclitis and by vitreous opacities. Four cases of glaucoma are on record as occurring during variola; and one (that of Adler) is noteworthy from the fact that the prodroma of glaucoma coincided with those of the smallpox. It was successfully operated on, notwithstanding the fact that the incision was made difficult by the necessity of avoiding a pock on the limbus of the cornea. Fortunately, the present generation has rarely an opportunity of seeing great numbers of eye affections from smallpox, and when they do occur, the partial protection from previous vaccination often modifies their severity. In these days of antivaccination societies, it is interesting to turn back to the accounts of the disease given by those who were in active practice at the time of Jenner's great discovery, and to see how serious the matter appeared when viewed through their spectacles. Thus, Andreæ says, "No disease is so dangerous to the eyesight as the smallpox, and before the introduction of vaccination it caused as much blindness as all other eye inflammations put together."[1] Benedict[2] also bears testimony to the great diminution in the intensity of variolous ophthalmia after the introduction of vaccination.

Writing later, Himly[3] says: "Smallpox, formerly a rich source of all eye diseases by which the doctor was most busied, is at present only feebly represented by the varioloids (*i. e.* smallpox modified by cowpox)." Mackenzie[4] states that "in former times smallpox proved but too often the cause of serious injury to the eyes, and even of entire loss of sight. It was by far the most frequent cause of partial and total staphyloma." Dumont in his work on blindness, the result of his own observations at the Hospice des Quinze-Vingts at Paris, and from its extensive statistics in previous years, records that out of a total of 2056 blind, 262 were blind from variola (or 12.64 per cent.); and, further, that the old records of the hospice showed 17.9 per cent., whilst at present (1856) it was 12 per cent. amongst the older inmates, and but 7 per cent. amongst the more recently admitted. He quotes Carron du Villars as giving the ratio before Jenner at 35 per cent. From immunity we become careless, so that when an epidemic breaks out (as that in Mayence in 1871) we have a state of suffering which forcibly brings back our remembrance of old times. Thus, Manz asserts that "the pestilences of the last (Franco-German) war have revived the remembrance of a disease which in the

[1] August Andreæ, *Grundriss der Gesammten Augenheilkunde*, vol. ii. p. 260.
[2] P. W. G. Benedict, *De Morbis Oculi humani inflammatorii*, lib. iii. p. 367.
[3] *Krankheiten u. Missbildungen des Auges*, Berlin, 1843, p. 481.
[4] *Diseases of the Eye*, p. 500.

beginning of this century was a terror to humanity, but which in the last decade was so rare that many now living physicians know it only by the writings of the older authors: the late epidemics, however, have enlarged their experience, and added a new contingent to the almost extinct army of the smallpox-scarred blind."[1]

RUBEOLA.—Preceding the outbreak of the skin eruption, or coincident with it, every case of measles presents a greater or less degree of catarrhal conjunctivitis, often accompanied by lachrymation, itching, and burning of the lids, slight pain, and photophobia. In from two to three weeks the catarrh usually disappears of itself, but in many cases leaves behind it an asthenopia and sensitiveness to light which often lasts for months. In some fortunately rare cases the catarrh increases, and we have a severe muco-purulent inflammation of the eyes, causing partial or total sloughing of the cornea, and thus leading either to the formation of a staphyloma or to the total loss of the eye. Moreover, we often have the development of phlyctenular keratitis as one of the sequelæ, especially among the weak and badly nourished. Some authors (Rilliet and Barthez, Mason, Schmidt-Rempler, De Schweinitz, etc.) relate cases where diphtheritic conjunctivitis, with all of its well-known symptoms—yellow, ropy-like secretion, great bulbar chemosis, and hard board-like infiltration of the lids—set in during the course of the disease. Keratomalacia (a rapid sloughing of the cornea with marked anæsthesia of the ball, without swelling of the lids) was probably first observed as a consequence of measles by Fischer.[2] He had seen three cases, each accompanied by suppression of the skin eruption, severe fever, and delirium. The corneæ were entirely destroyed in twenty-four to forty-eight hours, and the children died soon after the development of the eye affection. Beger and Begold (Leber) have each reported similar cases. Sometimes in the course of this disease, amaurosis, either permanent or transient, is doubtful. Graefe[3] gives a case where failure of sight came on during convalescence, and where for a week there was absolute loss of perception of light, without any other ophthalmoscopic appearances than a slight neuritis, the patient gradually recovering his eyesight. In an epidemic of measles with severe cerebral symptoms, Nagel[4] records a case of a child where on the third day sopor, convulsions, opisthotonos, and dilatation of the pupils set in. The patient remained soporose for ten days, and then, on regaining consciousness, was found to be entirely blind. On the twenty-fifth day from the setting in of the convulsions, perception of light was dubious, and the pupils, which remained insensitive to the reflection from the ophthalmoscopic mirror, contracted slightly on exposure to the full glare of daylight. There was eventually complete recovery both of health and eyesight, the return of the latter being apparently hastened by the use of strychnia. The same author relates two other cases, in one of which the ophthalmoscope showed neuritis. One of them was fatal, the other terminated in recovery, and in neither was there any return of eyesight. In some cases of measles where Bright's disease of the kidneys is pre-existent or sets in during the

[1] *Jahresbericht f. Ophth.*, 1873, pp. 178–183.
[2] J. N. Fischer, *Lehrbuch der Entzündungen und Organischen Krankheiten des Menschlichen Auges*, Prag, 1846, p. 275.
[3] *A. f. O.*, xii., 2, p. 138.   [4] *Behandlung der Amaurosen*, pp. 24–30.

attack, there may be the development of the characteristic form of reti‧
nitis albuminuria.

SCARLATINA.—In scarlatina we have usually a hyperæmia of the conjunctiva coincident with the skin eruption.   Inflammatory affections of
this membrane and of the cornea are much less frequent than in measles.
Martini[1] remarks that only in one case in twenty is there any inflammation of the eye.   Beer[2] informs us that the tears are more irritating than
in morbillous ophthalmia, and that the photophobia is more persistent.
When ichorous ulcers form, they attack not only the cornea, but also
the white of the eye, and spread much more rapidly in this situation
than in the conjunctival leaflet of the cornea.   Kerato-malacia occurs
more frequently than in rubeola.   Bonman[3] relates that in a severe epidemic of scarlet fever five boys in one family were taken sick, and
that two of them lost their sight from sloughing of the cornea within a
week of their seizure.   Of these, one died, and the other was brought to
him with a shrunken globe and without light-perception.   The eyes of
the other three children were not affected.   Arlt in the first volume of
his work on diseases of the eye[4] has given us a clinical description of this
form of kerato-malacia.   The patient, a boy of four and a half years,
was first seen by him on the eighth day of the disease.   The child was
very pallid, with a burning-hot skin, hoarse voice, slight diarrhœa, and
flat abdomen.   The right cornea was evenly clouded throughout, swollen,
and softened, while the left had lost its brilliancy and was slightly clouded,
presenting the appearance of an eye thirty-six hours after death.   The
conjunctivæ of both eyes were white, with a few vessels and ecchymotic
spots in their lower parts.   On the tenth day, the right cornea was converted into a mass as soft as schmeer-käse, and was beginning to be
thrown off on the centre, where there was a hernia of the hitherto unaffected membrane of Descemet.   Both eyes eventually had the cornea completely destroyed, and the patient died on the seventeenth day.   Iritis is
more frequent than after measles.

Considering the frequency of acute nephritis in this disease, the retinal
lesions are comparatively rare.   Schreiber[5] gives two interesting plates
of chorio-retinitis after scarlatina.   Ebert[6] at a meeting of the Berlin
Medical Society in 1867 called attention to some cases of transient blindness in the course of scarlatina without ophthalmoscopic changes; and
Graefe, who presided at the meeting, remarked that in all these cases of
absolute blindness there was still reaction of the pupil to the light, and
that therefore there could be no neuritis or decided lesion between the
corpora quadrigemina.   He considered the prognosis favorable so long
as there was pupillary reaction, and not necessarily bad where it was
wanting.   Although this is the rule, the prognosis is certainly more favorable when the pupil reacts promptly and to moderate light.   Hirschberg[7]
has recorded a case of blindness following meningitis, where light-perception failed to return, although the pupillary reaction lasted several
weeks.

[1] *Von dem Einflusse des Secretions Flussigkeiten,* vol. ii. pp. 267, 268.
[2] *Lehre von dem Augenkrankheiten,* Bd. i. pp. 536, 537.
[3] *Lectures on the Parts concerned in the Operations in the Eye,* London, 1870, p. 110.
[4] *Krankheiten des Auges,* vol. i. pp. 211--213.
[5] *Veränderungen des Augenhinter-grundes,* Plates iii. and iv , Figs. 7 and 8.
[6] *Berliner klin. Wochenschrift,* Jan. 15, 1868, pp. 21-23.   [7] *Ibid.,* 1869, p. 387.

Relapsing typhus fever is frequently followed by amblyopia and inflammation of one or both eyes. Considerable variety in the intensity and in the symptoms of the disease has been manifested in different epidemics, and the ratio of the percentage of eye cases has greatly varied. In most outbreaks of relapsing typhus fever amblyopia is followed by inflammation. This was the sequence of the symptoms in the epidemic in Dublin in 1826, in Glasgow in 1845, and in Finland in 1865, although in the last-mentioned the inflammatory symptoms were less prominent and severe than in the first two. The eye symptoms rarely develop during the first attack of the fever, but usually occur after a second or third attack or during convalescence. The earliest careful study of the eye symptoms in a severe epidemic is that of Wallace,[1] who tells us that "there is often that haggard and worn aspect, that sickly, mottled, pallid hue of skin, that sleepy, exhausted, and oppressed appearance of the eye, which is more easily observed than described. The patient only half opens the lids of the affected organ. They are of a purplish-red color and humid. Their subcutaneous vessels are preternaturally enlarged. The vascularity of the sclerotic and conjunctiva is greatly increased. The vessels of the former describe a reticulated zone round the cornea, and those of the latter run in a direction more or less straight to the edge of this membrane, and sometimes appear to pass on the edge. The hue of the redness is peculiar; it is a dark brick-red. The pupil is generally much contracted, and its edge thickened and irregular. The iris is altered in color, generally greenish, and incapable of motion. There exists dimness of the cornea, which may be compared to the appearance glass assumes when it has been breathed upon. There is often a turbidness of the aqueous humor, and a pearly appearance of the parts behind the iris may be observed by looking through the pupil. There is great intolerance of light, and a copious, hot lachrymal discharge. The vision will be found for the most part so extremely imperfect that the patient can merely distinguish light from darkness, and he is often tormented by flashes of light which shoot across his eye, and these occur more particularly in dark places; or he is troubled by brilliant spectres or by the constant presence of muscæ volitantes. There is very considerable pain, which returns in paroxysms, and these are almost always more severe at night. The pain is sometimes referred to the ball of the eye, sometimes to one of the lids, sometimes to the temple or to the circumference of the orbit." Mackenzie agrees in the main with the foregoing description: his cases were also accompanied by severe inflammation, with hypopyon and copious precipitates in the membrane of Descemet and on the anterior capsule of the lens. He also called attention to the diminution of the intraocular tension and the consequent flabbiness of the eyeball, and states that out of 1877 cases of fever admitted to the Glasgow Infirmary during the epidemic of 1843, 261 (one-seventh) were attacked by the disease of the eye. Anderson,[2] who describes the same epidemic later in the course, takes exception to Wallace's statement that there is always an amaurotic stage at the outset of the disease. He computes these cases at two-thirds of the entire number, and tabulates five cases of inflammation without

---

[1] "An Essay on a Peculiar Inflammatory Disease of the Eye, and its Mode of Treatment." *Trans. Med.-Chir. Soc. of London* (read Dec. 11, 1827).
[2] "Post-febrile Ophthalmitis," *Monthly Journ. Med. Sci.* 1845, pp. 723-729.

amaurosis. He also describes and gives plates which show opacities of the vitreous, posterior synechia, pigment on the anterior capsule, posterior polar cataract, and other forms of lenticular degeneration; these conditions ensuing not only in this disease, but in all other affections where the circulation in the ciliary body and the constitution of the vitreous are profoundly involved. Schweigger, in describing an epidemic in Berlin, says that in one-third of the cases of ophthalmia there was simple unilateral iritis, and that in a second third there was diffuse punctiform or flocculent vitreous opacities without any trace of iritis or external symptoms of disease; while in the remaining third there was iritis with vitreous opacities in common: when it ensues in its usual form the effects of annular synechiæ or detachment of the retina; rarely from suppuration of the corneæ. Although of late years the Russian writers have materially added to our knowledge of the affection, nevertheless in most essentials their observations agree with those above quoted. Thus, Blessig[1] gives an account of an epidemic in St. Petersburg, while Logetschnikow[2] describes an epidemic in Moscow in which he encountered over 700 cases of this form of ophthalmia. Larionow[3] relates the history of a mild epidemic in the Russian army of the Caucasus, and tabulates 767 cases of the fever, in which are also included a number of cases of exanthematic typhus and a few cases of typhoid fever. Exclusive of the ischæmia of the retina and feebleness of the accommodation which were present in every case during convalescence, there were 3 cases of serous retinitis, 2 of hemeralopia, and only 3 of iritis; while in 10 per cent. of these there were vitreous opacities. He did not see a single case of genuine irido-choroiditis in the entire number. Estlander[4] has given a masterly description of two epidemics which he observed at Helsingfors in Finland, both of which occurred after a failure of the crops and consequent famine. In the first of these epidemics, which was of a mild type, only 3 out of 222 patients died, and the concomitant eye affections were few in number; while in the latter, 18 out of 242 patients died, and extensive vitreous opacities with severe inflammation of the eyes were frequent. He agrees with Mackenzie that the fever attacks few children under ten years of age, and says that although the disease is much more liable to attack people between twenty and thirty years of age, here it is less frequent than it is in patients between ten and twenty years of age, where it exists in one half of the cases. Arlt[5] agrees with this, and says that it is due to the fact that hunger and malnutrition are in general much worse borne by adolescents than by adults. As regards the period of the disease at which the eye symptoms come on, Estlander says that out of 28 carefully observed cases it developed 6 times during the fever or a week after its cessation, 11 times between the second and fourth week, 5 times in the second month, and 6 times from the third to the fifth month. These figures agree well with those given by Mackenzie, and show that there is both a feeble state of constitution and a prolonged convalescence from

[1] *Congrès internationale d'Ophthalmologie*, Paris, 1868, pp. 114–117. .

[2] "Entzündung der Vorderen Abschnitten der Choroidea als Nachkrankheit der Febris Recurrens," *A. f. O.*, Bd. xvi., 1, S. 352–363.

[3] *Klinische Monatsblätter f. Augenheilkunde*, 1878, pp. 487–497.

[4] *A. f. O.*, xv. 2, pp. 108–143.

[5] *Klin. Darstellung der Krankheiten des Auges*, 1881, pp. 289–291.

this severe fever. Pepper,[1] in a previous volume of this work, has given an interesting account of an epidemic in this city in which he states that eye affections were of rare occurrence.

Exanthematous typhus fever is occasionally followed by the same train of symptoms as pointed out in discussing Larionow's statistics, who gives vitreous opacities as the most frequent forms of the eye affection. Out of a total of 57 fever patients with typhus exanthematicus, he found 1 case each of iritis, keratitis, and neuro-retinitis, 2 cases of contraction of the field of vision, 5 of subconjunctival ecchymosis, and 2 of conjunctival catarrh.

Abdominal Typhoid Fever.—Severe eye complications are less frequent in this disease than in either of the foregoing affections. During convalescence from this, as from all other exhausting diseases, there is usually feebleness of the accommodation, and occasionally the development of vitreous opacities, with or without the formation of cataract. The most common eye affections show as an optic neuritis or paralysis of some of the muscles supplied by the third pair of nerves, and are due to a complicating meningitis.

Yellow Fever.—In this disease most writers have called attention to the accompanying ocular symptoms—flushing and injection of the conjunctiva with increase of lachrymation, followed later by a change of the color of this membrane to a yellow hue, which precedes a similar change of the color of the skin of the face and other parts of the body. The first epidemic of the disease in Philadelphia occurred in 1762. Redman,[2] in describing it, says: "The patients were generally seized with a sudden and severe pain in the head and eyeballs, which were, I think, often, though not always, a little inflamed or had a reddish cast." Another severe epidemic of the disease visited the city in 1793, of which Rush[3] has given us a valuable account. Among the premonitory signs he enumerated "a dull-watery-brilliant, yellow or red eye, dim and imperfect vision;" and he defines his meaning by saying that the dull eye was found among the severe cases, and the brilliant one where the poison was less intense. Later in the disease there was "preternatural dilatation of the pupil," and in one case "a squinting which marks a high degree of morbid affection of the brain." There were hemorrhages, chiefly from the nose and uterus, and in but one case "a dropping of blood from the inner canthus." A dimness of sight was very common in the beginning of the disease, and many were affected with temporary blindness. In some there was a loss of sight in consequence of gutta serena or a total destruction of the substance of the eye. The eyes seldom escaped the yellow tinge. There were a number of cases of uncommon malignity without this symptom, but sometimes the yellow color appeared on the neck and breast before it invaded the eyes. Wood,[4] who witnessed a later epidemic (also in Philadelphia), says that even in the earliest period of the disease the white of the eye is often reddened and turbid, and in bad cases appears sometimes as if bloodshot. As before stated, in the course of the disease

[1] Vol. I. P. 399.
[2] "An Account of the Yellow Fever of 1762," by John Redman, M. D. (read before the College of Physicians of Philadelphia, Sept. 7, 1793).
[3] *An Account of the Bilious Remitting Yellow Fever as it appeared in the City of Philadelphia in the Year 1793*, by Benjamin Rush, M. D., Philada., 1794.
[4] G. B. Wood, *Treatise on the Practice of Medicine*, vol. i. p. 321, 1858.

this redness yields to a yellow or orange color. Féraud,[1] in speaking of the symptoms of the second stage, lays great stress on the brilliancy of the eyes, their lachrymose condition, the fulness and nicety of the conjunctival injection, the dilatation of the pupil, and the presence of photophobia; adding that this congestion is diminished during the remission of the fever if the attack is not severe, but that if the conjunctiva darkens and assumes an icteric aspect, which becomes more and more intense, the case is undoubtedly severe. He adds that ocular hemorrhages occur in some grave cases during the second stage, producing subconjunctival suffusion and a flow of blood from the neighborhood of the commissure of the lids. Such "hemorrhages have frequently caused conjunctivitis, keratitis, and even such an accident as phlegmon." Fernandez[2] gives three cases of delirium, suppression of urine, and loss of vision. One of these cases was examined with the ophthalmoscope, but no changes were found in the eye-ground. One case recovered, having entirely regained his eyesight; the other two died.

Intermittent Fever.—Intermittent ophthalmia is but rarely encountered in countries where only a mild form of intermittent fever is present; in fact, it was so rare in Scotland that Mackenzie in the earlier editions of his work denied its existence, but a larger experience enabled him (in 1854) to give three cases. In 1828 and 1829 it was so infrequent in Marburg that Hueter devoted two papers to its study—one of a case of the quotidian type, and the second of the septan form of the ophthalmia. In countries where the malarial poison exists in more intense form, we have quite a different state of affairs; thus Levrier[3] describes it as of common occurrence in the district of Landes in France, and says that its most frequent form is a periorbital and ocular neuralgia, accompanied by intense congestion of the conjunctiva, with increased flow of tears and a greater or less degree of photophobia, occurring in those who have had frequent attacks of intermittent fever. Wehle, whose observations were made in Hungary, describes an erysipelatous swelling of the lids with small hemorrhages in the palpebral conjunctiva, redness and swelling of the bulbar conjunctiva with intense photophobia, and occasional clouding of the cornea. Arlt[4] relates eight cases of chronic interstitial keratitis, all occurring in emaciated patients who had had severe malarial fevers, in Slavonia and Hungary. Only three of these stayed for prolonged treatment, which consisted of the use of Karlsbad water, followed by the preparations of quinine and iron; all of these recovered, and their eyes cleared, leaving only the faintest trace of corneal opacity. Galezowski[5] gives a case of malarial keratitis, and Griesinger,[6] after describing the usual symptoms of the disease (similar to that noted by Levrier), speaks of cases of long duration accompanied by clouding of the cornea and atrophy of the eyeball. He has also encountered an intermittent form of iritis. Mackenzie describes a case of it (one of those above referred to) which eventually ended in amaurosis. While affections of the retina and optic

[1] Béranger-Féraud, "La Fièvre jaune à la Martinique," quoted by Juan Santos Fernandez, Archiv. of Ophthalmology, x., 4, 1881, pp. 440–445.
[2] Loc. cit.
[3] J. F. Levrier, Thèse de Paris, 1879, "Des Accidents oculaires dans les Fièvres intermittentes," p. 56.
[4] Klinische Darstellung der Krankheiten des Auges, 1881, pp. 121, 122.
[5] Quoted by Levrier, loc. cit., p. 39.   [6] Traité des Maladies infectueuses.

nerve from malarial fever would seem to be rare in temperate latitudes, Guéneau de Mussy,[1] however, relates a case of optic perineuritis with retinal apoplexies. Macnamara, observing in India, says the serous retinitis is not uncommon in malarial fever, and that in severe cases of this disease amaurosis is not infrequent. Galezowski and Kohn each reports a case of atrophy of the optic nerves after a severe attack of inter. mittent fever, but it is not quite evident from the clinical history whether the blindness might not be attributed to the large doses of sulphate of quinia which had been administered.

ERYSIPELAS.—Erysipelas of the face and head frequently causes swell. ing of the lids and chemosis of the bulbar conjunctiva, and occasionally gives rise to an orbital cellulitis which by its effects on the optic nerve impairs or destroys sight. Beer[2] speaks of an idiopathic erysipelatous conjunctivitis which may not be accompanied by swelling of the lids. The conjunctiva is of a pale, somewhat livid-red hue, in which no distinct vessels are vis. ible, there being numerous bright-red ecchymotic spots in the subconjunc. tival tissue. Vesicular prominences form around the cornea, and become so large as to project between the lids. The folds and interstices of this swollen membrane are covered with thin mucus, which often adheres so closely to the cornea as to make it look hazy, but which can be washed off, leaving the corneal surface as brilliant as in its normal state. The conjunctival swelling finally subsides, and the membrane again adheres to the selerotic. Even after there is apparent absorption of the ecchy- moses, the places where there were extravasations of blood are slow in adhering to the sclera, and often roll into folds with every motion of the eye. Mackenzie describes the conjunctiva as of a pale yellowish-red color: it rises in soft vesicles around the cornea, and these change in shape with every motion of the eye. There is slight photophobia and a pricking sensation, with a large quantity of white mucus, which is secreted by the conjunctiva and the Meibomian glands. Where a low grade of orbital cellulitis ensues we may have only slight prominence of the eye and some interference with its motions, in which a complete subsi- dence of the symptoms without any failure of eyesight may take place. We may encounter more severe cases, where the intense swelling and inflammation of the orbital tissues so impair the functions of the optic nerve and retina as to permanently destroy the eyesight, and at times destroy life by the extension of the inflammation to the meninges. The cellulitis may attack one or both orbits. Poland[3] has recorded a case of protrusion of both eyes where, after death, the ophthalmic veins and the cavernous sinuses were found full of pus; while Cohn[4] has reported another fatal case of double erysipelatous cellulitis, in which post-mortem showed purulent phlebitis of the orbit and brain with embolic infarcta in the lungs. All cases of double exophthalmos from erysipelas do not end as fatally: Jaeger has recorded two cases of recovery, where in each one eye remained permanently blind, while the other was restored to sight. He has given us accurate and beautiful ophthalmoscopic plates of the

[1] *Journal d'Ophthalmologie,* p. 1, 1872.
[2] J. J. Beer, *Lehre von den Augenkrankheiten,* vol. i. 398, 399. (He also gives a colored plate of the appearance, Taf. 1, p. 3.)
[3] *R. L. O. H. Rep.,* vol. i., pp. 26–31, 1857.
[4] *Klinik der Embolischen Gefässkrankheiten,* 1860, p. 196.

lesions in the blind eyes, these plates showing atrophy of the optic nerve, with great thickening of walls of the retinal vessels, which in some places totally hide their contents, while in others the blood-columns are still faintly visible. In one case the inflammation of the lids had been so severe that they had grown together in the middle of the palpebral fissure and had also formed an attachment to the eyeball. These cicatricial bands were divided with the knife, only to find a blind eye with dilated pupil. In one of Jaeger's cases there were pigment-masses in the choroid. Coggin[1] describes a case of double exophthalmos with blindness where the corneæ were so denuded of epithelium that no ophthalmoseopic examination was practicable. Three weeks later the media were clear and the discs atrophic, the vessels being visible as empty white cords. These effects be attributed to thrombosis. Knapp[2] has recorded a most interesting case of erysipelas where there was severe fever with high temperature (104.8°) and marked protrusion of both eyes, in which he had an opportunity of observing the eye-grounds in all stages of the disease. On the ninth day ophthalmoscopic examination showed that the yellow spot and disc were both invisible, and that their localities could only be determined by the radiation of the tortuous veins, which were gorged with blood so dark as almost to be black, the retinal arteries being invisible. The posterier portion of the eye-ground was milky white, while the anterior was reddish white: numerous hemorrhages were scattered through the retina, more or less linear in shape in the posterior part and irregularly rounded in the anterior portion. Two days later the orbital swelling was less, and the arteries were visible, though much reduced in size, and the eye-ground was beginning to resume its normal color. About a month after seizure the patient was convalescent and he could go out. At this time the disc was atrophic, and there was a whitish cloud in the region of the yellow spot, with numerous hemorrhages: both arteries and veins presented isolated areas of perivasculitis, accompanied by snow-white patches of greater or less extent, which were of the same calibre as the adjacent dark-red blood-columns in each of them. Two months later, the disc was still atrophic, the hemorrhages had been absorbed, the blood-vessels were mostly visible as white cords—one of them presenting the usual appearance, while two showed blood-contents for a short distance surrounded by dense white walls. The white intercalary portions of the vessels seen in the examination two months after the onset of the disease are considered by Knapp to be thrombi. Arlt, Jr., reports a case of gangrenous erysipelas of the lids with loss of the eye, and mentions that his father had seen several similar cases.

[1] D. Coggin, *Trans. Amer. Oph. Soc.*, vol. ii. pp. 570–572 (session 1878).
[2] *Trans. Amer. Oph. Soc.*, 1883, and *Arch. of Ophthalmology*, 1884 (with plates and lithographs).

DISEASES OF THE NERVOUS SYSTEM.[1]

SYMPTOMS of impaired function in the eyes and their appendages have always been regarded as valuable indices of disease of the nervous system; and when it is considered that six of the twelve pairs of cranial nerves send branches to these organs, and that the second, third, fourth, and sixth pairs are distributed exclusively to them, and that they are further supplied with twigs from the cervical and cerebral sympathetic nerves, it can be readily appreciated that a vast variety of nerve lesions, interfering with some of these connections either at their origins or in their course, may produce either impaired vision in the eye or loss of power in some of its appendages. Moreover, the retina and optic nerve originate as sprouts from the anterior cerebral vesicle, and retain respectively the structure of a ganglion and of a cerebral commissure. From these circumstances, as well as from the close connection of their blood and lymph circulations with those of the cerebrum, they frequently become delicate exponents of intracranial changes.

Affections of the Second Pair (Nervi Optici).

NEURITIS.—Five years after the discovery of the ophthalmoscope Graefe called attention to the fact that in many cases of intracranial disease the intraocular ends of the optic nerve presented marked changes. He had already discovered that when these changes were inflammatory in character they presented two main varieties—the one in which there was intense swelling of the intraocular end of the nerve (designated by him stasis papilla); and the other, in which there was a dull-red suffusion of the disc. In the first variety, which he attributed to increased intracranial pressure from tumor or other cause, the disc projected into the eye and formed a small tumor, often prominent to an extent equal to its own diameter, the oedematous and opaque nerve-fibre being permeated by tortuous, enlarged, and often newly-formed capillary vessels, which hide the arteries and allow only the projecting branches or lips of the tortuous and dilated retinal veins to be perceived as they slope down in the swollen papilla to regain their normal level in the retina; the other, which he thought was due to meningitis spreading along the nerve, was characterized by a slightly swollen disc of a dull-red color, with opacity of its nerve-fibre sufficient to completely hide its normal boundaries, associated with tortuous veins and arteries that were often diminished in size. Since that time volumes have been written on the subject, and it has given rise to most extended and searching discussion, causing researches to be instituted which have added much to the knowledge of the anatomy and pathology of the central connections, circulation, and lymph-supply of the optic nerves. To-day the first variety is usually designated

[1] In the foregoing sections the relationship between definite diseases and their concomitant eye symptoms have been dealt with; whereas in this division of the subject this has been found so impracticable that it had to be discarded in favor of an anatomical basis upon which to place the various affections. This change has necessitated the disuse of the representative headings of names of disease, and the substitution of absolute physical conditions with their hypothetical causes.

as choked disc or papillitis, and the second as interstitial or descending neuritis. When typical cases are seen at the height of the disease, it is easy to make a distinction between the two varieties, but
usually they shade off so imperceptibly, the one into the other, and
the consecutive atrophies present so absolutely the same appearance, that
no experienced observer would at all times claim an ability to distinguish
between them. In the choked disc the intense swelling is limited to
the intraocular end of the nerve, and therefore vision is little interfered
with until the swelling becomes so great, or the contraction of the subsequent cicatrization so decided, that by pressure on the nerve-fibre they
become atrophic and incapable of reporting the retinal image to the
brain-centres, while in interstitial neuritis, owing to the primary interference with conduction, vision is impaired from the beginning. The
choked disc usually develops slowly, requiring a period varying from a
few days to two, three, or four weeks to attain its maximum, and it may
exist unchanged for a long time before atrophy sets in. The writer once
had an opportunity of observing a case in which the choking was produced by a cerebral gumma, and where for nearly a year the discs
remained swollen and vision was still $\frac{6}{6}$; and another of intense swelling,
where the discs projected at least from one and a half dioptrics (one mil-
limeter), in which for a period of three months vision was $\frac{6}{6}$ and the
field almost normal. Mauthner,[1] Blessig, and Schiess-Gemuseus[2] each
record cases of marked choking of the discs lasting for some time, where
the patients retained perfect central vision to the day of their death.
Double choked discs are almost always a symptom of grave intracranial
disease when all local causes in the eyes or orbits have been excluded.
Even in the very exceptional cases where they form part of the symptoms of Bright's disease they are probably indicative of intracranial effusion. The lower grades of inflammation of the optic nerve are apt to be
accompanied by marked proliferation of the connective tissue between the
nerve-bundles. There are many cases of congestive atrophic change of
the optic nerve where at first central vision is but little affected. In
judging of the appearance of neuritis the observer should be sufficiently
familiar with the changes in the eye-grounds of healthy individuals
which occur from local causes not to allow himself to be led astray by
the often very decided neuro-retinitis constantly encountered in hard-
worked eyes with uncorrected astigmatism and slight degrees of ametro-
pia; and not to mistake these changes, which are simply an expression
of that local congestion which leads ultimately to softening and elongation of the eyeballs, for changes due to incipient cerebral disease, although
each is accompanied by neuralgia. While, after careful study of the
various forms of neuritis optici during the last few years, it is acknowledged that increased intracranial pressure is apt to cause choking of the
disc, and that basilar meningitis frequently gives rise to interstitial neuritis, we are still far from having such a clear comprehension of the subject as to render the profession unanimous as regards its pathology; some
observers claiming that choked disc is essentially a vaso-motor paralysis
of the affected part, while others maintain that it is caused by infiltration
of the disc and optic nerve with abnormal fluids which have been secreted
within the cranium, and by increased intracranial pressure have been

[1] *Ophthalmoscopie*, p. 293, 1868.   [2] *Klinische Monatsblätter f. Augenheilkunde*, 1870, p. 100.

forced between the sheaths of the optic nerve and between it and its pial envelope. The ingenious explanation proposed by Graefe, tha: stasis papilla is produced by the damming up of the return blood in the cerebral sinuses, thus causing impeded circulation with increased blood-pressure in the ophthalmic vein and its branch (the central retinal vein), has generally been abandoned since the investigations of Sesemann and Merkel have demonstrated the free anastomosis between the facial and the orbital veins in whatever method the primary congestion may be brought about. The latter part of his explanation, in which he compared the rigid tissue of the lamina cribrosa to a multiplier, by its construction tending to augment any existing plethora in the head of the nerve, is still worthy of consideration. While the theory of vaso-motor paralysis is a most enticing one, it is, however, difficult to understand why paralysis of any of the fibres of the sympathetic should always be accompanied by such a limited local congestion without affecting the retinal tissue in their peripheral parts or without any branch leading to the iris, ciliary body, or choroid. Granting that there is some special filament of the carotid plexus distributed to this region of the nerve, it is hard to comprehend how it can be acted upon by tumors of almost any size or consistence situated in the most varied parts of the brain, and also why pressure on the various portions of the intracranial nerve, chiasm, and optic tracts (which so frequently cause hemianopia and partial atrophies) should not be associated with choking of the disc.

THE LYMPH-SPACE THEORY—Since the anatomical researches of Schwalbe and of Retzius have given us a clear understanding of the lymphatic circulation in the eye, the effusions into the sheaths of the optic nerve that have been found in many cases of choked disc that have been examined post-mortem have been shown to be due to the effects of blocking up of the lymph-channels and of the effusion of cerebral fluids (lymph-pus and blood) in the intervaginal space of the nerve or between it and its pital sheath. In support of this, Manz in 1870 showed that injection of fluid into the cranial cavity of rabbits would produce a marked neuritis which was readily demonstrable by the ophthalmoscope; while Schmidt proved that the spaces of the lamina cribrosa of the optic nerves of the calf could be distended by fluid thus injected. In experiments on the human cadaver the writer has repeatedly seen that colored fluids could be readily driven between the sheaths of the optic nerve by injections from the subarachnoid and subdural spaces, and also that when high pressure was used and the injection made directly into the intravaginal space of the nerve, the fluid found its way from the subdural into the perichoroidal space. He once obtained traces of the colored fluid in the lamina cribrosa of the nerve. Since this mode of communication between the cavity of the cranium and the eye has been duly appreciated, a large number of autopsies have shown that choking of the disc has been accompanied by dilatation of the outer sheath of the nerve by lymph-pus or blood which has found its way down from the cranial cavity. It has also been demonstrated that proliferation of the intravaginal (arachnoid) tissue, and the formation of tumors (psammoma and tubercle) at the distal end of the nerve, will produce choking of the disc by causing local accumulations of fluid. On the other hand, there are cases where this distension of the sheaths has been

774 MEDICAL OPHTHALMOLOGY.

carefully looked for and not found ; and those who hold the *vaso-motor theory* consider that it is in any case an accompanying accident, and not the cause, of the choking of the disc. The experiments of Rumpf and Kuhnt, however, add to its probability, by which the deleterious influence of lymph on the axis-cylinder of nerves adds to the probability of the above theory ; moreover, even if it is granted that this accumulation of lymph or other fluid within the sheaths of the optic nerve is the cause of choking of the disc, it seems very unreasonable to the writer to expect to find it in all stages of the complaint. It is everywhere admitted that a cerebral tumor may exist for a long time without causing papillitis, and also that inflammation of the discs may exist for months or years, until they have become entirely atrophic, before the brain disease shall have caused death. Choking of the disc is essentially a temporary symptom. Although severe cerebral irritation may cause a great transient increase of cerebro-spinal fluids, which in their turn may produce the most intense inflammation of the intraocular end of the nerve, yet when the atrophied nerve comes to be examined months or years later they leave no traces sufficiently lasting to positively prove their previous existence. Whatever theory may be adopted as to the mode of production of optic neuritis, its clinical importance is admitted by all. Where it exists on both sides, and is accompanied by other cerebral symptoms, it usually points to increased intracranial pressure.

Since the earliest times, impaired vision and other ocular symptoms have been recognized as accompaniments of diseases of the brain. In more recent, but still preophthalmoscopic, times the statistics showing the percentage of blindness in brain tumor are most interesting: thus, Abercrombie noted failure of vision in 17 ($38\frac{5}{10}$ per cent.) out of 44 cases, while Ladame, in a study of 331 cases, estimated that there is disturbance of vision in about 50 per cent. This percentage represents the cases of atrophy consequent upon neuritis only. It must be remembered, however, that many die of the brain disease while the disc is still choked, and that this state of the eye-nerve may exist for a long time without any appreciable failure of vision, making it evident that should we look for choked disc with the ophthalmoscope while there are as yet no symptoms of failing sight, the above percentages would still be higher. In support of this we find that there is a rise of double optic neuritis to 93 per cent in a series of 88 cases of brain tumor, 43 of which have been recorded by Annuske[1] and 45 by Reich,[2] these being here adduced because in all of them there was a careful ophthalmoscopic examination. Gowers thinks that this is an over-estimate, but admits that optic neuritis occurs in four-fifths (or 80 per cent.) of all cases of cerebral tumor. In considering this question we cannot too carefully keep in view the facts so well stated by Hughlings-Jackson,[3] that optic neuritis is essentially a transient symptom, and that, although it often occurs early in the disease, it may in some cases be developed only in the latter stages of the complaint. Jackson states that he frequently examined a case with the ophthalmoscope in which there was no appearance of choked disc till six weeks before the patient's death, when marked papillitis developed, the

[1] *A. f. O.*, xix., 3, pp. 165, 300.
[2] *Klin. Monatsblätter f. Augenheilkunde.* 1874, pp. 274, 275.
[3] *Med. Times and Gazette*, Sept. 4, 1875.

autopsy showing a tumor in the left cerebral hemisphere. In fact, where the tumor does not occupy the cortical sight-centres, the intercalary gan_glia, or press on the tractus opticus or chiasm, it may exist a long time without producing any affection of the optic nerve or deterioration of vision. No neuritis will take place by increase of intracranial pressure so long as the growth of the tumor is slow and there is a corresponding absorption of brain-substance; but should the growth of the tumor be rapid, or any other cause exist by which increased pressure, with consequent irritation and effusion, would take place, infiltration of the nerve and its sheaths with lymph or inflammatory products would ensue, and give rise to swelling and increased growth of connective tissue. In cases of cerebral tumor, however, and where the growth presses on the intracranial portion of the optic nerves, or where the chiasm is compressed and atrophied by the protuberant and bulging floor of the third ventricle, as in the two cases recorded by Foerster,[1] optic atrophy may be produced without the occurrence of previous choked disc.

HEMIANOPIA (HEMIOPIA, HEMIANOPSIA).—We may, however, have serious affections of the sense of sight without any marked alteration in the retina or optic nerve. Careful study of the various forms of hemianopia and other symmetrical defects in the field of vision will often surprise us by the extent of the defect which it reveals, and sometimes serve as a guide to the localization of the cerebral lesion which produces the defect. Hemianopia (or the not-seeing of half an object) is usually of the homonymous lateral variety, in which, if the centre of any object be fixed by the macula lutea of each eye, then either all parts of the object lying to the right-hand side of the points of fixation or else all parts lying to the left of that point become invisible. There may also be temporal hemianopia (hemianopia heteronymous lateralis),[2] in which the nasal side of each retina is blind, and the temporal field of each eye consequently abolished. In such case the right eye sees nothing to the right of the fixation-point, and the left eye nothing to the left of it. The external half of each retina may be blind, in which case there is loss of the nasal field of each eye and of the entire binocular field of vision. In all of these cases the dividing-line between the blind and seeing parts of the retina is a more or less vertical one, but there are also cases where the dividing-line is horizontal, and we thus have an upper or lower hemianopia. From a clinical standpoint the first-named variety (homonymous lateral hemianopia) is markedly distinguished from the others by its usual more rapid development, and by the absolutely sharp dividing-line which runs vertically through the retina at the macula; this field of vision retaining its form without subsequent development of zigzags or other irregularities. All other varieties of hemianopia develop more slowly, and their boundaries—which are usually not perfectly vertical or horizontal, and do not generally extend to the fixation-point—may vary from time to time. The homonymous lateral variety is of far more frequent occurrence than the other forms: out of 30 cases carefully observed by Foerster, where perimetric measurements

[1] *G. u. S.*, vol. vii. p. 141.
[2] If we retain the word hemiopia (half-seeing), then this variety is termed medial hemiopia, because the lateral halves of the retina are still intact and vision is practicable in the median or nasal field of each eye.

of the fields were taken, 23 were of this variety, while the remaining 7 presented the heteronymous temporal form. The subject of homonymous lateral hemianopia is so important clinically, and so interesting as regards the probable course of the fibres in the optic nerves, chiasm, and cerebral centres, that it appears desirable to state briefly a few of the most decisive facts in regard to it which have been substantiated by careful autopsies.

1. In 1875, Hirschberg[1] published a case of right-sided homonymous hemianopia with perfect central vision. At first there was no paralysis of sensation or motion, but subsequently aphasia and right hemiplegia set in. The autopsy showed a large sarcomatous tumor which had caused atrophy of the left tractus opticus.

2. Hughlings-Jackson and Gowers[2] (1875) relate a case of left homonymous hemianopia with hemianæsthesia and hemiplegia of the same side. The autopsy showed softening of the posterior part of the right thalamus opticus without other lesion.

3. Curschmann[3] (1879) gives the case of a patient who drank sulphuric acid, which corroded the œsophagus and affected the aorta, causing embolus of the right brachial artery. On the day following there was complete left hemianopia. The autopsy showed a large area of cerebral softening in the right occipital lobe without other lesions. In the discussion of this case at the session of the Berlin Society of Psychiatry and Nerve Diseases, Westphal[4] related a case of unilateral convulsions without loss of consciousness where there was homonymous hemianopia, and in which the autopsy showed a large area of softening in the white substance of the occipital lobe in the side opposite to the defect in the field of vision.

These cases might be multiplied, but the writer has selected them because they were made by careful and competent observers, and the lesions were so marked and limited in character as not to allow of any other intepretation than that given. If we admit the validity of the evidence, we have proved conclusively that, from a clinical and a pathological standpoint, binocular homonymous lateral hemianopia may be produced by lesions of the optic tract, of the posterior part of the thalamus opticus, and of the occipital lobe of the brain of the side opposite to the defect in the field of vision; and that, therefore, there must be a partial, and not a total, crossing of the fibres of the optic tracts at the chiasm. Moreover, as Foerster has most pertinently remarked, such a state of affairs does not violate the physiological law of the total crossing of other nerves, because in the binocular field of vision the partial crossing causes all objects to the right of the point of fixation to be seen by the left hemisphere, while those to the left of it are seen with the right hemisphere. While this problem appears sufficiently plain, and the view above advocated is adopted by the majority of writers of the present day, it is by no means equally satisfactory when looked at from a purely anatomical or physiological standpoint. Newton[5] in 1704 had already appreciated the importance and difficulty of the subject, and in

[1] *Virch. Arch.*, Bd. lxv.   [2] *R. L. O. H. Rep.*, vol. viii. p. 330.
[3] *Centralblatt f. Augenheilkunde*, 1879, p. 256.   [4] *Loc. cit.*, p. 181.
[5] *Optiks*, London, 1704, p. 136.

the hope that others might further investigate it asked the question whether the fibres from the right sides of both retinæ do not so unite at the chiasm as to go together to the right side of the brain, those from the left side of each retina pursuing a similar course to the left hemisphere. He further remarks that "if he is correctly informed that the optic nerves of such animals as have a binocular field of vision join at the chiasm, while those of the animals who have no binocular vision, such as the chameleon and some fishes, do not so join."[1] Since his day the majority of authors have adhered to this view, until Biesiadecki,[2] by careful anatomical studies and lectures, attempted to prove that in both men and lower animals there is a total crossing of the fibres at the chiasm. Twelve years later Mandelstamm,[3] by clinical observations of nasal hemiopia and dissections of the chiasm, maintained the same view. In the same year Michel[4] supported the same doctrine, and since then Schwalbe[5] and Scheel[6] have each advanced the same view. However, Von Gudden,[7] also basing his opinions upon dissections, takes the opposite ground, and has since endeavored by a series of experiments, in which he enucleated one eye of young rabbits and dogs, to prove[8] that if the animals were allowed to live until central atrophy set in there is a partial atrophy of both optic tracts, more marked on the side opposite to that of the enucleated eye, because the crossed bundle is by far larger than the direct.

From similar experiments on rabbits, Mandelstamm[9] maintains that there is a total crossing at the chiasm, and Michel,[10] who repeated Von Gudden's experiments, arrived at the same conclusion. Brown-Séquard[11] asserted that a medial cut of the chiasm in rabbits produces amaurosis of both eyes, which would indicate that there is total crossing, while Nicati[12] a year later showed that a median section of the chiasma in young cats did not produce blindness of each eye, the animal following with the eye and the head the movements of a light held at a considerable distance from the eyes.[13] The condition of the optic nerve and brain obtained from the human subject, where by accident or by disease one of the eyes has been destroyed long before death, seems in the main to speak for partial decussation. Thus, Biesiadecki, while maintaining total decussation, could only conclude from such specimens of degenerated nerves and tracts that the greater part of the fibres of the atrophic nerve went to the tract of the opposite side. Woinow[14] demonstrated preparations to the Ophthalmic Society at Heidelberg where the left eye had been blind for forty years, and the atrophy, which had travelled up the left nerve, was plainly visible in both optic tracts. Schmidt-Rimpler[15] also showed atrophy of both tracts

---

[1] *Loc. cit.*
[2] "Chiasma Nervorum Opticorum der Menschen und der Thiere," *Sitzungsberichte der Wiener Akadamie.*
[3] *A. f. O.*, xix., 2, pp. 39-58.　　　　　　　　　　[4] *Ibid.*, xix., 2, pp. 59-84.
[5] *G. u. S*, vol. ii. p. 324.
[6] *Klin. Monatsblätter f. Augenheilkunde* (extra number 2), 1874.
[7] *Arch. f. Psychiatrie,* vol. ii. p. 21.
[8] *A. f. O.*, xx., 2, p. 226, and also *Ibid.*, xxv., 1, p. 1, 1879.
[9] *Ibid.*, xix., 2, p. 47.　　　　　　　　　　[10] *Ibid.*, xxiii., 2, p. 227.
[11] *Archiv de Physiologie*, 1872, p. 261, and 1877, p. 656.　　[12] *Ibid.*, 1878, p. 658.
[13] Cats have a larger binocular field of vision, and are better subjects for experiments than rabbits.
[14] *Klin. Monatsblätter f. Augenheilkunde*, 1875, p. 425.
[15] *Ibid.*, 1877, "Bericht der Ophth. Gesellschaft," pp. 44-48.

more marked in that of the opposite side, and Manz[1] found atrophy of both tracts after atrophy of the nerve of one side; Plink[2] reports a similar state of affairs; while Popp[3] and Michel[4] from analogous specimens draw conclusions favorable to the total crossing.

The above cases are amongst the most decisive which have been reported, and are quite sufficient to show how great the conflict of opinions is among good observers. The observations and experiments on the subject of sight-centres in the cortex cerebri are also conflicting: thus, while Ferrier places the cortical sight-centre in the angular gyrus, and maintains that its destruction will produce blindness, Luciani and Tamburini agree as to the locality of the sight-centre, but maintain that its destruction produces hemianopia; while Munk places the sight-centre in the occipital lobe, and asserts that its loss causes hemianopia and not contra-lateral blindness. In the case of hemianopia reported by Keen and Thomson,[5] where a bullet wound of the left occipital lobe produced right hemianopia without other apparent lesion, the writer has had an opportunity of personally examining it and of confirming their conclusions. The conclusions which he arrived at, associated with the knowledge which he obtained in Stricker's laboratory by witnessing experiments upon dogs and apes, where portions of the occipital lobes were destroyed, have convinced him that cortical lesions of the occipital lobes produce hemianopia. On the other hand, chiefly on clinical grounds and from the study of hystero-epilepsy, Charcot concludes that the band of uncrossed fibres in the chiasm bends again somewhere in the region of the geniculate bodies to join the crossed bundle once more in the cortical centre. According to this theory, destruction of the cortical centre should produce total amaurosis of the opposite eye, and lesions between the chiasm and geniculate bodies would produce homonymous hemianopia, while pressure in the crossing-point of those fibres (which in the chiasma are uncovered and run from the geniculate bodies to the opposite cortical centre) would give paralysis of the temporal halves of both retinæ.

As regards pure crossed amblyopia, the scheme of Charcot is scarcely borne out by his clinical facts. The latest theories of those cases which were investigated by Landolt and himself showed, as they reported, marked amblyopia on the opposite side from the lesion, but associated with contraction of the field of vision in the eye of the same side. The question, however, is so vast, and so much remains to be learned concerning the brain-centres and their communications with the optic tracts, that it can scarcely be considered sufficiently ripe for an exhaustive discussion in a paper like the present.

According to Foerster, temporal hemianopia always develops slowly without any concomitant paralytic symptoms: it does not have constant boundaries, and is now progressive and again retrogressive. He cites cases which he has observed for years where at first small negative scotoma appeared just outside of the fixation-point, and increased till there was a total loss of the temporal fields. The line of division between the blind and seeing sides of the field of vision is not sharply defined and

[1] Klin. Monatsblätter f. Augenheilkunde, 1877, "Bericht der Gesellschaft," pp. 49, 50.
[2] Arch. f. Augenh. und Ohrenheilkunde, vol. v.
[3] Inaug. Diss., Embolie der Art. Centralis, Regensberg, 1875, p. 20.
[4] A. f. O., xxiii. 2, p. 243.   [5] Trans. A. O. Soc., 1871.

not accurately vertical. In some cases there is a gradual invasion of the sound side. Although it is usually assumed that some pressure in the anterior or in the posterior angle of the chiasm is the cause, yet the writer does not know of any post-mortem examination of a case. Mauthner[1] gives short histories of 23 cases of temporal hemianopia, besides 11 cases relating to nasal hemianopia (or, according to his classification, hemianopia heteronyma medialis) from various authors, in most of which the ophthalmoscope showed either the presence of a neuritis or an atrophy of the nerve. There were two autopsies in the cases of nasal hemianopia related by Mauthner—those of Schule and Knapp—one of which showed an enlargement of the third ventricle and infundibulum, with atrophy of the nerves, and the other a high degree of ætheromatous degeneration of arteries at the base of the brain. Any cause which would produce simul-taucons pressure on the outer angles of the commissure would give rise to nasal hemianopia. Little is known regarding hemianopia above or below the horizontal line : both Mackenzie and Graefe mention its occurrence, and Knapp, Schoen, and Mauthner give interesting cases. The writer has seen a case in a woman of fifty-five years otherwise apparently in good health. The upper part of each field was wanting, and the line of division ran slightly above the fixation-point, it being nearly horizontal. The optic nerves did not present any marked departure from their normal appearance, and central vision was fair $(\frac{20}{xl})$. The only autopsy of a case of superior hemianopia with which the writer is familiar is that reported by Russell,[2] in which there was a tumor involving the bones of the base of the cranium. The patient had upper hemianopia, confined to the right eye, followed by total blindness, coming on first in the right and then in the left eye. Genuine binocular hemianopia of the superior or inferior variety is probably produced by some symmetrical affection of the optic nerves between the chiasm and the eyes.

In apparently healthy individuals transient hemianopia is not an unfrequent occurrence, and may either develop with or without other cerebral symptoms. It is usually followed or accompanied by headache, or more rarely by vertigo, tinnitus aurium, difficulty of speech, etc. Even in intelligent patients, who have not been drilled by their medical adviser to carefully analyze their symptoms, it is not recognized as half-vision, but here, as in the permanent variety of the affection, it is described as a dimness or blindness of the eye on the side in which the field of vision is defective. Some cases of transient hemianopia are accompanied by peculiar zigzag flickerings of light in the defective portions of the field of vision, which have given it the name of scotoma scintillans. We are fortunate in having an accurate description of this form of the affection by so competent an observer as Foerster, who has frequently experienced it in his own person. In his case the phenomena last from fifteen to twenty-five minutes, and commence with the appearance of dimness in both eyes, which gradually increases to a defect of the field of vision lying to one side of the fixation-point. This is soon followed by a flickering which commences in a zone around the scotoma, and increases centrifugally until it assumes the form of an arc with the convexity outward,

---

[1] *Gehirn und Auge,* 1881, pp. 373–381.
[2] *Med. Times and Gazette,* No. 47, 1873 (rep. *Nagel's Jahresbericht,* 1873, p. 361).

the flickering rarely extending beyond the vertical line which separates the two halves of the field of vision. When it has reached the outer limits of the field, it generally diminishes and fades away. From a consideration of the celebrated case of Wollaston, it is probable that transient hemianopia may be caused by some temporary congestion of a brain tumor, but in the majority of instances it is certainly allied to functional disorders like migraine. Transient hemianopia has been observed in several members of the family of one of the writer's patients, all of whom are subjects of consecutive neuralgic headaches. Leber has observed the same thing. Brewster and Quaglino have attributed it to a retinal anæmia, but a careful ophthalmoscopic examination in two well-marked cases (that of Foerster and one related by Mauthner) failed to show any retinal changes. In some cases the well-marked hemianopic character of the attack speaks for its intracranial origin, which may be temporary derangement of the circulation, possibly in the optic tracts. Dianoux tells us that in his case the attack could be cut short by keeping the head down between the legs. In some of the cases which the writer has seen it may be cut short by a liberal dose of whiskey.

Affections of the Third Pair.

While a few words on the pathology of the third and sixth nerves tend to throw light on our knowledge of cerebral localization, they will also spare a good deal of needless repetition in the detailed discussion of the eye symptoms which accompany many well-marked diseases. Complete paralysis of the third nerve may be caused by pressure on its filaments at the base of the brain without other symptoms. Where it occurs with hemiplegia of the opposite side of the body and other cerebral symptoms, it is usually due to pressure on the nerve where it runs beneath the cerebral peduncle: according to Nothnagel,[1] this localization of the disease is still more certain when paralysis of the facial and hypoglossal nerves exists on the same side as the hemiplegia (that is, on the side opposite to the third-pair paralysis). Hughlings-Jackson[2] remarks that the symptoms are only positively diagnostic of a lesion in the neighborhood of the peduncle when they appear simultaneously, but when they are concentric to each other they may be due to an affection of the cranium. Ollivier and Little[3] have each related a case where this group of symptoms has not originated in any lesion in the peduncle, but has been caused by an abscess of the middle and posterior lobes, which secondarily involved these parts.

DOUBLE THIRD-PAIR PARALYSIS.—Double third-pair paralysis is rare, but might be produced by any cause acting on both peduncles. Kohts gives a case where such paralysis was caused by a tumor of the size of a cherrystone limited exactly to the posterior tubercles of the quadrigeminal body. Nothnagel remarks that paralysis of corresponding branches of the third pair point to the corpora quadrigemina as the seat of lesion. On the other hand, Panas[4] relates a case of absolute immo-

---

[1] *Topische Diagnostik der Gehirnkrankheiten,* p. 198, 1879.
[2] In Russell Reynolds's *System of Medicine,* vol. ii., 1872.
[3] Robin, *Des Troubles oculaires dans les Maladies de l'Encephale,* p. 95.
[4] Cited by Robin, *loc. cit.,* p. 74.

bility of the eyes where the only demonstrable lesion at the autopsy was a meningo-encephalitis in the lower part of the cerebellum. Robin describes a case of double third-pair paralysis where there were ptosis and dilatation of the pupils, with a loss of all power to move the eyes except downward and outward. The diagnosis was that of an interpeduncular syphilitic gumma : there was complete recovery. In the above case it is interesting to note that while the paralysis of the left eye occurred previous to that of the right, the eye last attacked was the first to regain its motions.

PTOSIS.—Paralysis of the branch of the third pair which supplies the levator palpebræ, when it exists without any lesion of the other branches or where it is coincident with hemiplegia of the opposite side, is frequently held to indicate a cerebral lesion, which may be either cortical or have its seat in the nucleus of the nerve. According to Grasset,[1] when the lesion is cortical it is situated in the parietal lobe in advance of the angular gyrus. The localization is by no means well made out. Coignt[2] has shown that it is not always crossed, for in 5 out of 20 cases mentioned by him it existed on the same side as the paralysis. Steffen[3] gives a case of double ptosis with sluggish pupils where there was complete control over the muscles moving the globe, the autopsy showing a tubercle in the tubercular quadrigemina which had entirely effaced their normal structure.

OPHTHALMOPLEGIA INTERNA.—In those cases where affection of the orbital ophthalmic ganglia can be excluded, paralysis of the pupillary and ciliary branches of the third pair is, according to Jonathan Hutchinson, due to an affection of the twig which runs through the lenticular nucleus in the striated body. It is frequently associated with paralysis of the internal rectus, and may be accompanied by paralysis of the ciliary muscle. After diphtheritis there is often paralysis of the ciliary muscle, with prompt reaction of the iris. The writer is not aware of any recorded instance of apoplexy or other sudden onset of disease which would enable us to localize exactly the centre for pupillary contraction. According to Hughlings-Jackson, we may have in apoplexy the most varied states of the pupil (normal, dilated, or contracted) independent of the seat of lesion : he further states that upon calling loudly to the patient there will sometimes be a transient pupillary dilatation. When we look at the state of the pupils as part of general symptomatology, we find a most perplexing confusion and contradiction : in fact, notwithstanding the quantity of material both in ancient and modern literature, we are far from having any satisfactory account of the subject. This is partly due to our imperfect knowledge of the anatomy of the brain and to the great difficulty of estimating exactly pupillary changes, and partly carelessness and want of a proper system of observation. The data have for the most part been hastily compiled, without a minute statement of concomitant symptoms or the stage of the disease in which they are developed. Usually, they have been made without any proper means for illuminating the pupil or apparatus for correctly magnifying and observing its motions. In most cases the want of knowledge of the more common sources of error, such as a difference in the size of the pupils owing to difference in the refraction of

[1] Robin, p. 104.   [2] *Thèse de Paris.*
[3] *Berliner klin. Wochenschrift,* No. 20, 1884.

the eyes, posterior synechiæ, or other intraocular changes, has invalidated the results.

ASSOCIATED MOVEMENTS OF THE HEAD AND EYES.—In many central lesions, associated movements of the head and eyes are present, and, although the exact channels through which they are propagated are for the most part unknown, yet certain groups of these clinical symptoms are of so frequent occurrence as to be recognized and admitted by almost all observers. Vulpian and Prévost were the first to enter into a minute study of these movements. Vulpian in his lessons on the physiology of the nervous system (1866) states that "in cases of unilateral cerebral lesion, whether it be situated in the cerebral hemispheres, the striated bodies, the thalami optici, the cerebellum, or in the different parts of the isthmus cerebri, whether the lesion be softening or hemorrhage, there is often, immediately after the attack, a deviation of the eyes at the time of development of the hemiplegia. The deviation is in general transient, and may last either a few minutes or hours or several days. The eyes are usually turned in a direction opposed to that of the hemiplegia; thus, if the right side is paralyzed, both eyes are turned toward the left. On regaining consciousness the patient, if he tries to turn his eyes to the right, may either be entirely unable to move them, or, what is more usual, may succeed in bringing them to the middle of the palpebral aperture without being able to turn them farther in that direction. Does this phenomenon depend on a paralysis of the muscles which cause conjugate motion of the eyes, or on a spasmodic contraction of their opponents, over which they are unable to triumph?" He further states: "I incline strongly to the latter view, as it is in accordance with what we observe in animals. The analogy of the phenomena goes still farther: often the head of the patient has made a more or less marked movement of rotation on the neck—a movement as the result of which the face is turned toward the non-paralyzed shoulder, and in the cases where we cannot observe a deviation by turning back the head into its normal position, an action which can often be only brought about by considerable effort."

Prévost[1] has since formulated the following laws for cases of hemiplegia: "I. When the hemiplegic looks toward his lesion and away from his paralyzed side, the lesion is hemispherical. II. If he looks toward his paralyzed side, the latter is situated in the mesencephalon." This statement coincides with the facts reported by Hughlings-Jackson, Charcot, and many other observers. Nothnagel[2] admits that this is the rule, but quotes as an exception to it a case of his own where, with right hemiplegia and head turned to the right, the eyes were turned to the left, the autopsy showing an extensive patch of softening in the left hemisphere which involved the frontal convolutions, the central convolution, and the adjacent white substance. In addition, he cites Bernhardt as giving other exceptional cases which, in his own judgment, "considerably diminishes the diagnostic value of the phenomenon." Landouzy and Coignt[3] have attempted to define still more clearly the diagnostic value of the associated movements of the head and eyes, and, while they admit the correctness of these laws of hemiplegic paralysis, they add that in convulsive

[1] *Thèse de Paris.*   [2] *Topische Diagnostik der Gehirnkrankheiten,* p. 580, 1879.
[3] *Thèse de Paris,* 1878.

cases in which there are symptoms of irritative lesions the above rules are reversed. To explain such cases they lay down the following rules : first, that if the patient looks toward his convulsed side the lesion is situated in the hemisphere of the opposite side ; and second, if he looks away from his convulsed side (or toward the lesion) there is an irritant lesion of the mesencephalon.

NYSTAGMUS.—This is a term applied to a periodic type of involuntary oscillatory or rotatory movements of the eyeballs. The oscillatory are due to rapid alternate contraction of the straight muscles, while the rotatory indicate either similar actions of the oblique muscles alone or in conjunction with the straight. The oscillatory motions are usually horizontal, but instances of vertical nystagmus occur, as in the case recorded by Soelberg Wells.[1] Nystagmus may be either congenital or acquired, the latter variety being much the more frequent form of the affection. Congenital nystagmus is usually associated either with cataract or imperfect development of the optic nerve and retina. It is a very frequent accompaniment of albinism and pigmentary retinitis. We often see the acquired form arise during the first few months of life, when the child in its effort to see is hindered by corneal or lenticular opacities resulting from ophthalmia neonatorum. One of the most interesting of the acquired forms is that which occurs amongst coal-miners, rendering a considerable number of those thus affected unfit for work. At first the symptoms are that the lights in the mines and the objects on which the patients endeavor to fix their attention begin to dance, this being accompanied by a sensation of dizziness and discomfort. In the first part of the attack they disappear when work is stopped, and the miners come up into the daylight ; but if work be persisted in they become permanent and exaggerated. When the nystagmic motions have ceased, they may often be called into activity by placing the patient in a dark room and getting him to direct his eyes to a candle held above the horizontal line of the field of vision. The motions are usually lateral, or in some cases the centre of the cornea describes an ellipse or circle which causes the patient to see a ring of light. It has been observed to occur much more frequently in those working in shafts where there is a good deal of fire-damp ; which has caused some writers to assert that the nystagmus has been dependent upon the action of the gas. This view would seem to receive some support from an instance reported by Bright of nystagmus, in a case of suffocation from the fumes of burning coals, which he attributed to cerebral pressure. In these cases it is more probably due to fatigue of the eye and its nerve-centres in the endeavor to see in the dim light and strained position which the miner is often obliged to maintain, which is intensified by the enfeeblement of the nerve-centres due to the action of the gas : these, associated with the diminution of the light caused by the wire gauze of the safety-lamp, would further increase the strain in those obliged to work in the shafts pervaded with fire-damp. The statements of Dransart,[2] founded on the examination of a large number of miners, probably give a correct idea as to the frequency of the affection. He states that among 12,000 workmen employed by one company, there were 30 under treatment for nystagmus, which would give about two and a half patients per thousand. In any form of nystagmus the motions of

---

[1] *Lancet,* 1871, p. 662.   [2] *Annales d' Oculistique,* 7, 82, p. 177.

the eyes usually become more rapid when they are used for near work. According to Nagel,[1] excessive convergence will at times cause a temporary cessation of all nystagmic motion; and he further proved this by putting extra strain on the interni by means of prisms with their base out. The true pathology of the various forms of nystagmus is still imperfectly known. Arlt[2] supposes that there is a rapid repetition of reflex movements in the endeavor to attain distinct vision in those forms which develop on account of corneal and lenticular opacities. He explains this by the supposition that the retinal impression is strengthened by the same retinal areas being rapidly and repeatedly subjected to the action of the rays of light from the same object, while a longer period of fixation would cause retinal fatigue and blur; showing the same principle by reminding us that our perceptive powers for a test object, upon first being brought into view at the periphery of the field of vision, are much stronger when the object is shaken than when it is brought quietly toward the fixation-point. Some forms of the affection, however, are manifestly due to fatigue of the nerve-centres, and have been by some authors placed in the same category as writers' cramp. For its causation we would naturally look for the anatomical changes either in the cortical centres for the eye-muscles or in the nuclei of the third and sixth pairs. Vulpian[3] states that wounds of the medulla in dogs cause nystagmus, and Schiff asserts that wounds of the white substance of the cerebellum near the peduncles give rise to the same phenomenon; while Ferrier has produced it by the influence of electricity on the cerebellum of apes. Cohn[4] records a case of gunshot wound of the right parietal bone (near the angular gyrus) which produced nystagmus. Merkel's case, occurring in a patient with embolism of the artery of the fissure of Sylvius, would also point to lesion near the angular gyrus. Stintzing[5] gives a case where there was thrombosis of the basilar and Sylvian arteries. Oglesby[6] relates two cases where nystagmus came on suddenly with dilatation of the pupils, the autopsies showing a clot which pressed on the medulla. Fienzal[7] also gives a case where there was a tumor in the left peduncle of the brain. It is often seen during epileptic convulsions. According to Raehlmann,[8] the motions of both eyes are under the control of psychic centres which regulate them according to the necessities of vision: for Willbrand[9] it is a sign of weakness of the voluntary cortical centres which fail to regulate the reflex activity of the middle brain and cerebellum. The latter author shows that the extent of the field of vision is increased in the direction of the oscillations in those cases where direct vision is not much impaired, while there is marked contraction of the field in cases where the direct visual acuity is much diminished. He also states that there is contraction of the field in the nystagmus of miners, which is greater during the intervals of the paroxysm than during their occurrence, and, further, that the contraction is greater where the case is one of long standing.

[1] Graefe u. Saemisch, vol. vi. p. 226.   [2] Krankheiten des Auges, Bd. iii. p. 335.
[3] Comptes Rendus de la Société de Biologie, 1861 (quoted by Robin, p. 157).
[4] Schussverletzungen des Auges, p. 19.   [5] Jahresbericht f. Ophth., vol. xiv. p. 306.
[6] Brain, vol. iii., 1880.   [7] Trans. Internat. Congress, at Milan, 1881, p. 126.
[8] "Nystagmus und seine Aetiologie," A. f. O., xxiv., 4, p. 237 (1878).
[9] Klin. Monatsblätter f. Augenheilkunde, vol. xvii., 1879, pp. 419-438 and 461-480.

In some rare cases nystagmus may be produced at will. Raehlmann[1] Lawson,[2] Benson,[3] all report cases of the voluntary type. In one of those given by Lawson the patient (a gentleman in good health) " first made his eyes steady, and then set both into rapid lateral motion—so rapid that the outline of the cornea was completely lost to view." Zehen_ der[4] observed it in a case of a twelve-year-old boy, where he was able to produce it by the instillation of a strong solution of eserine. Charcot states that ordinary nystagmus is a valuable symptom of disseminate sclerosis, and that it is present in about half of these cases, while it is exceptional in locomotor ataxy. " In some patients the look is vague until the eyes are made to fix some object, when the nystagmus develops."

According to Hammond, in disseminate sclerosis, nystagmus may be the only symptom for the period of a year before other symptoms develop. Moos[5] speaks of oscillatory movements of the eyes in Menière's disease, and Schwalbach[6] describes them in a case of purulent catarrh of the middle ear where they could be produced either by syringing or by pressure on the mastoid process.

Affections of the Fifth Pair.

HERPES FACIALIS.—Herpes facialis frequently appears on the lips and angles of the mouth, and occasionally in the eye and its appendages. When upon the conjunctiva or cornea, it commences as clear watery vesicles, usually in groups, which soon burst and leave open ulcers looking very much like abrasions or scratches of this membrane. They usually occur in successive crops after fevers, especially pneumonia, although at times they may appear without any assignable cause. They are also slow to heal, but are not dangerous to the eyesight, except where they give rise to purulent infiltration leading to hypopyon.

HERPES ZOSTER OPHTHALMICUS.—Herpes zoster ophthalmicus is a far more formidable affection. The eruption, as is well known, follows the distribution of the divisions of the ophthalmic branch of the trigeminus, and when the eyeball is affected the sight is always threatened. Clear watery blisters form on the cornea, which soon burst, the exposed tissue taking on purulent infiltration, while pus is not infrequently deposited in the anterior chamber. These ulcers are slow to heal under the most careful treatment, which, as a rule, consists in washing with disinfecting solutions and applying a bandage, etc. There is almost always iritis, as evidenced by the sluggish pupil and at times by marked synechiæ.

The burning and pricking pain at the seat of eruption is marked, and there is severe neuralgia in the temple, forehead, and side of the nose. The intensity of the iritis varies considerably in different cases, and, although some terminate favorably, having had but few and slight symptoms, yet the one case reported by Noyes, where it led to cyclitis, followed by shrinking of the eyeball, which ultimately gave rise to

---

[1] *Loc. cit.*   [2] *R. L. O. H. Reports,* vol. x. p. 203.
[3] *Ibid.,* vol. v. p. 343.
[4] *Klin. Monatsblättar f. Augenheilkunde,* vol. xviii., 1879, p. 127 (note).
[5] *Arch. f. Augenheilkunde und Ohrenheilkunde,* vii. 2, p. 508.
[6] *Deutsches Zeitschrift f. prakt. Med.,* No. 2, 1878.

sympathetic irritation of the fellow-eye, shows how serious its couse-
quences may be.   Permanent opacities of the cornea are not infrequent.
The disease is, fortunately, a rare one.   It usually comes on either in
middle or declining life, although Wadsworth has reported a case in a
child four years old.   The cornea becomes anæsthetic, both in the ulcers
and over the rest of its surface, a long time often elapsing before any of
its sensibility is regained.   Horner[1] was the first to demonstrate that the
corneal ulcers originated in vesicles, and the very great diminution of
intraocular pressure in the affected eyeball, and also to show the marked
difference in the temperature of the skin of the two sides.   The temperature on the affected side is usually one and a half to two degrees higher
than on the other side, while the cutaneous sensibility is markedly diminished ; as, for instance, the æsthesiometer might give twelve lines on the
healthy forehead as against twenty-two lines on the diseased side, and the
superciliary ridges and the upper eyelid on the normal side might give
respectively nine and five lines as against seventeen and seven lines on
the affected side.   In the cases which the writer has had an opportunity
of studying he has found similar variations in intraocular tension, temperature, and sensibility.   Hutchinson[2] thinks that the affection of the
nasal branch is always accompanied by inflammation of the eyeball, and
says : "Thus far, I have never seen inflammation of the whole side of
the nose without witnessing inflammation of the eye ;" while Bowman[3]
says that he has "not found affections of the eyeball to occur. especially
in those cases of ophthalmic zoster in which the eruption followed the
course of the nasal branch."   Wadsworth[4] gives a case where the entire
side of the nose was involved, the eyeball and conjunctivæ not being
affected.   He suggests that possibly the explanation in these cases is an
anomaly of distribution described by Turner, where the side of the nose
is supplied by a long, slender infratrochlear branch.   Bowman,[5] although
realizing that peripheral excitement of sensory nerves may originate in a
central or reflected source, and induce tenderness and redness in the parts
supplied by them, yet nevertheless holds that ophthalmic zoster is a peripheral disease, having its primary seat in the branches of common sensation, the nerves probably becoming inflamed in the more superficial portions
of their trunks, as the eruption succeeding as an extension of vascular
excitement to the cutaneous tissue : he thus explains the tenderness of the
skin before it reddens and the often lasting alteration of sensibility.   In
reference to whether the neuritis causing the eruption is an ascending or
descending one, the only two careful autopsies that give answer with
which the writer is familiar are those of Wyss and of Weidner, where
both show extensive changes in the nerve-centres.   The latter, made
five years after the attack, showed cicatricial shrinking of the ganglion
of Gasser and of the root of the nerve between it and the medulla;
while that of Wyss, made within two weeks of the outbreak of the
affection, showed that the entire ophthalmic branch of the trigeminus was thickened, reddened, softened, and surrounded by extravasation
of blood from the entrance of the orbit up to the ganglion of Gasser ;
while the other branches of the trigeminus were normal in size and

[1] *Klinische Monatsblätter f. Augenheilkunde*, 1871, p. 321.
[2] *R. L. O. H. Rep.*, 1866, pp. 191–215.   [3] *Ibid.*, 1867.
[4] *Trans. of Amer. Oph. Soc.*, 1874.   [5] *Loc. cit.*

appearance. The Gasserian ganglion itself was enlarged and bright red, while that of the other side of the head was yellowish-white. · As is well known, zoster in other parts of the body not infrequently affects the two sides simultaneously; and there are recorded cases where it has twice attacked the same locality, but the writer is not familiar with any such facts as regards ophthalmic zoster.

NEURO-PARALYTIC OPHTHALMIA.—In 1822, Herbert Mayo[1] showed that section of the fifth nerve within the cranium produces insensibility of the eye; and Charles Bell[2] in 1830, while recognizing this fact, maintained that "when that sensibility is destroyed, although the motions of the eyelids remain, they are not made to close the eye, to wash and clear it, and consequently inflammation and destruction of that organ follow." Since that time the subject has been a favorite theme with both clinicians and physiologists, but opinions as to its cause have been a good deal divided. While, perhaps, a majority, with Bell,[3] Snellen,[4] Kondracki,[5] Gudden,[6] Senftleben,[7] and others, hold that the inflammation of the cornea is of traumatic origin, many writers—amongst whom may be mentioned Longet,[8] Graefe,[9] Meissner,[10] Schiff,[11] and Eckhard[12]—assert that it is caused by the impaired action of the trophic fibres of the nerve; and again others, such as Ferrier,[13] Balogh,[14] and Buchmann,[15] maintain that the inflammation is peripheral, consequent upon the drying of parts of the cornea. Clinically, soon after the occurrence of complete palsy of the trigeminus, there is an interstitial punctate keratitis, which makes the cornea so cloudy that the motions of the iris are with difficulty observed, this being accompanied by conjunctival and ciliary injection. The symptoms, especially where the paralysis is incomplete, are often much alleviated by maintenance of careful closure of the lids and repeated washing of the eye, which protects the enfeebled tissue from the action of foreign bodies. Success is not, however, always obtainable, for occasionally, even with the most complete protection of the eye, eventual sloughing of the cornea cannot be prevented. This is not a usually-accepted doctrine, but the writer is convinced[16] of its truth by a case seen within a week of the commencement of the disease, in which the cornea was not yet ulcerated, where the most sedulous care in cleansing the eye and protecting it from external irritants did not prevent the necrosis and perforation of the central part of the cornea. Since then other cases of similar import have been published. Quaglino[17] gives an instance where complete ptosis shielded the eye from all gross insults, but where, nevertheless, a central slough of the cornea formed. Laqueur[18] also found

[1] *Anat. and Physiol. Commentaries*, London, 1822, No· 2. p. 5.
[2] *Nervous System of the Human Body*, London, 1830, p. 207.
[3] *Loc. cit.*   [4] *Virchow's Archiv*, Bd. xiii. S. 107, 1850.   [²] *Idem.*
[5] *Nagel's Jahresbericht* (Lit. 1873), p. 266.
[7] *Virchow's Archiv*, Bd. lxv. Heft. 1, pp. 69-99.
[8] *Anatomie et Physiologie du Système nerveux*, t. ii. p. 161, Paris, 1842.
[9] *Arch. f. Ophthalmologie*, Bd. i. Abth. i. S. 306-315.
[10] *Henle und Pfeuffer's Zeitschrift* (3), xxix. p. 96 (quoted by Soelberg Wells).
[11] *Ibid.*, p 217 (also quoted by Wells).
[12] *Centralblatt f. Med. Wiss.* (cited by Nagel, Literature 1873).
[13] *Nagel's Jahresbericht*, (Lit., 1876), p. 51.   [14] *Ibid.*   [15] *Ibid.*, 1883, p. 153.
[16] Norris, "Case of Paralysis of the Trigeminus, followed by Sloughing of the Cornea," *Trans. Amer. Ophth. Soc.*, 1871, pp. 138-141.
[17] *Nagel's Jahresbericht* (Lit. 1874), p. 26.
[18] *Klinische Monatsblätter f. Augenheilkunde*, 1877, p. 228.

that the cornea sloughed in spite of the most careful protection. In all other cases where the cornea is exposed to air and external irritants, as in lagophthalmos or excessive exophthalmos, the case is quite different, the consequent inflammation being much better borne. While this is a fact more or less familiar to all clinicians, it is nowhere better shown than in the case of Horner,[1] where there was caries of the petrous portion of the temporal bone and complete paralysis of the facial nerve. Two years later the trigeminus was attacked, and then for the first time ulceration occurred in the hitherto sound cornea. Hirschberg[2] describes neuro-paralytic keratitis and panophthalmitis consequent upon a neurectomy of the infraorbital nerve, and quotes Langenbeck as relating a similar case after section of the supraorbital nerve.

INJURIES OF THE FIFTH PAIR.—Although daily clinical experience shows us how promptly irritation of the sensitive branches of the trigeminus are followed by symptoms of reflex action in the eye—as, for instance, a cinder in the conjunctiva will cause contraction of the pupil, or a sharp pinch of the temple will at times cause pupillary dilatation—nevertheless, instances of impairment of the eyesight due to injury of the branches of the infraorbital or supraorbital nerves, and to this alone, are of rare occurrence. Sympathetic ophthalmia is the exception in which we too frequently see inflammation of one eye cause severe and often irreparable damage to its fellow. Scattered through ancient and modern surgical works there are many interesting and well-attested cases of impaired vision, some of which should be excluded on account of the want of proper evidence, which is now obtained from testing of the acuity and field of vision and ophthalmoscopic examination. Erichsen[3] cites cases from Hippocrates, Fabricius Hildanus, and La Motte where amaurosis was produced by a wound of the brow. Chelius[4] gives a case from similar injury, while Wardrop[5] narrates three instances—one of wound of forehead, one from a blow on it with a ramrod, and one from an injury by a fragment of shell. The same author calls attention to the fact that amaurosis is more readily caused by wounds and injuries of the supraorbital and infraorbital nerves than from complete division of them. The various neurotomies and neurectomies performed upon the supraorbital branch since his day bear witness to the accuracy of his deduction. The same author quotes Morgagni as saying that Valsalva has seen amaurosis follow a wound of the lower lid which has been inflicted by the spur of a cock. Morgagni relates a similar case where the injury was inflicted by the broken glass from the windows of an upset carriage; and Beer reports a similar case of amaurosis from wound of the cheek. Guthrie[6] remarks that "when the eye becomes amaurotic from a lesion of the first branch of the fifth pair of nerves, the pupil does not become dilated; the iris retains its usual action, although the retina may be insensible and the vision destroyed." More recently, Rondeau[7]

[1] *Nagel's Jahresbericht* (Lit. 1873), p. 267.
[2] *Berliner klinische Wochenschrift,* 1880, S. 169; *Sitzung der Gesell. f. Psych. und Nerven-krankheiten,* 10 März, 1879.
[3] *Loc. cit.,* pp. 233–261.
[4] South's translation of Chelius's *System of Surgery,* vol. i. p. 430.
[5] *Morbid Anatomy of the Human Eye,* vol. ii. pp. 180, 181, London, 1818.
[6] Quoted by White-Cooper, *Injuries of the Eyes,* London, 1859, p. 92.
[7] *Des Affections oculaires Réflexes,* Paris, 1866, pp. 53, 54.

gives two cases, one of which caused lachrymation, photophobia, and eventual atrophy of the eye on the affected side, followed, fifteen years later, by loss of the fellow-eye from sympathetic ophthalmia, which had been produced by degenerative changes taking place in the shrunken bulb, and a second, in which a wound of the left brow became painful eight days after the receipt of the injury, and where pains became more severe as the wound cicatrized: in this latter case the left eye became foggy in three weeks, and soon sight was entirely lost, whilst six weeks after the accident there was dull pain in the right eye, with a sensation of cloudiness and a gradual development of photophobia in it. By local bloodletting, which caused the photophobia to rapidly yield, and a derivative and alterant treatment, the patient's right eye was so far improved that fifteen days later he could find his way about with the left eye, and could see to read with the right. Ophthalmoscopic examination showed in the left eye a serous swelling of the retina which entirely obscured the margin of the discs and gave the whole fundus a grayish tint, the veins being much enlarged and very tortuous. The right eye showed similar changes, though less developed.

Affections of the Sixth Pair.

The extremely limited distribution of the sixth pair of cranial nerves renders the clinical study of their pathology comparatively simple. The eye supplied by the paralyzed muscle turns inward to an extent corresponding to the degree of loss of power in the paretic muscle plus the energy of its opponent rectus internus. The image of the object fixed by it falls, therefore, to the inner side of the macula lutea, and, being projected outward, causes a double vision, in which the image of the deviated eye appears to be in the temporal field of the affected eye (homonymous diplopia). When the healthy eye is covered and the patient endeavors to fix any near object with the paralyzed eye, it will be found that (as in all other cases of peripheral paralysis affecting any of the extra-ocular muscles) the secondary deviation of the sound eye is considerably greater than the primary deviation of the affected one; this being accounted for by the fact that the amount of consentaneous innervation which is sufficient to cause a small motion in the paretic muscle will produce a marked effect in the sound one.

Paralysis of the external rectus is quite common, and is either transient or permanent. The former variety is often put down as rheumatic, when it is really a symptom of tabes dorsalis. The permanent paralysis is frequently an accompaniment of the affections of the base of the brain: when these are located in the middle fossa of the skull it is often associated with paralysis of the facial. If hemiplegia be present, the lesion is usually situated farther back toward the exit of the nerve from the pons. Graux[1] and Ferréol have called attention to a form of paresis which results from disease of the nucleus of the sixth pair. In this form, owing to the affection of the filament which the nucleus of the sixth nerve gives to the nucleus of the third nerve, which is distributed to the internal rectus of the other side, the amount of the secondary deviation is much

[1] *Thèse de Paris.*

diminished, and there is more or less the appearance of an ordinary con-comitant convergent squint (where, as is well known, the excursions of the two eyes are nearly equal). In one case, where the autopsy showed that a small tubercle had been developed at the junction of the medulla and pons, just beneath the surface of the fourth ventricle, there was no other symptom than this conjugate deviation of the eyes. In another case, in which there was hemiplegia (hemiplégie alterne), a tubercle was found higher up in the pons, bulging into the fourth ventricle. In addi-tion to the conjugate deviation of the eyes already mentioned, Graux and Ferréol believe that this central form of paralysis is distinguished by its gradual access, slow development, and persistence. They say that in pure cases of lesion of the nucleus it is characterized by the absence of all other symptoms, and still further assert that in those cases in which it is but partially involved the accompanying symptoms are either complete facial paralysis or alternate hemiplegia.

Affections of the Seventh Pair.

Loss of power in the orbicularis palpebrarum, and consequent lagoph-thalmos, is frequently encountered as part of paralysis of the facial nerve. Where the paralysis is complete, it prevents closure of the eyelids. Variation in the size of the palpebral fissure is, however, by no means abolished, for, owing to relaxation of the levator palpebrarum, the fissure diminishes when the patient looks down, but is increased by the activity of this muscle when he looks up.

BLEPHAROSPASM.—Spasmodic closure of the lids is frequent in phlyc-tenular conjunctivitis and in many corneal and conjunctival affections. It is evidently reflex in its origin, and often entirely out of proportion to the amount of conjunctival or corneal disease. A foreign body under the lids will frequently give rise to a similar state of reflex spasm. We also encounter a greater or less degree of twitching of the lids as part of general or local chorea.

Affections of the Twelfth Pair.

BULBAR PARALYSIS, LABIO-GLOSSAL LARYNGEAL PARALYSIS.—Affections of the eye and its appendages are rather exceptional in this form of disease. In one case Galezowski describes unilateral atrophy of the optic nerve, and Dianoux[1] bilateral atrophy in another. In the latter the atrophy came on after partial paralysis of the lips and of the muscles of deglutition, it being preceded by paralysis of the right external rectus. Hallopeau[2] quotes a case from Wachsmuth where there was partial paralysis of the facial which rendered the face immobile and effaced its wrinkles, allowing the lower lid to fall. He cites also a case of Hérard in which there was amblyopia and partial ptosis. He justly remarks that such phenomena indicate an extension of the lesion from the nucleus of the twelfth pair to other parts of the central nervous system.

[1] Quoted by Robin, *Troubles oculaires dans les Maladies de l'Encephale*, p. 335.
[2] *Des Paralysies bulbaires*, Paris, 1875, p. 41.

The pupils are sometimes described as contracted, more rarely as dilated. Leeser quotes Leubel to the effect that " paralytic myosis, when it occurs in bulbar paralysis, is generally a sign that it is complicated either by progressive muscular atrophy or with sclerosis of the brain and spinal cord."

Mental Affections.

It is admitted by all observers that affections of the pupillary branch of the third pair, such as mydriasis, myosis, and inequality of the pupils, are of comparatively frequent occurrence among all classes of the insane. There is the widest difference of opinion as to the percentage of cases in which it occurs : thus, Nasse out of 229 cases found 146 (64 per cent.) with difference in the size of the pupils, while Wernicke found 24 per cent. in the Leubus Asylum, and only 13 per cent. in the Breslau Institute. The latter author has attempted to classify the pupillary lesions into three groups :

I. Mydriasis, with loss of accommodation, where the pupil does not react to light nor with increased convergence of the eyes.

II. Where the pupillary difference is slight and the irides less prompt than normal in reaction to light, all difference of the pupils disappearing upon convergence of the eyes.

III. In which the irregularity is still less, the narrower pupil being absolutely insensitive to light, but prompt in responding to convergence, while the more dilated pupil acts promptly in obedience to both light and convergence.

In the first group there is some lesion in the course of the third pair; in the second, some lesion of the sympathetic either in the cilio-spinal centre or in its unknown intracranial distribution ; whilst in the third, which is not so readily explained, there is possibly an affection of those fibres which pass from the third pair to the optic nerve. Foerster[2] states that he has frequently seen cases where at different times the same pupil under similar circumstances showed different diameters; also asserting that variation in the relative sizes of the two pupils sometimes occurred within a few days or weeks. He also maintains that in many cases the occurrence of inequality in the pupils precedes and presages the occurrence of insanity ; and as a marked example of it he quotes the case of a friend and colleague who observed this phenomenon in himself. This person was well aware of the theories on the subject, and while yet of sound mind jokingly remarked that on account of this inequality of pupils having set in, he thought of taking up his quarters in an insane hospital. A few years later he actually died insane in the Leubus Asylum. Myosis is said to be frequent in states of mental exaltation. Seifert asserts that when it is accompanied by acute mania general paralysis will sooner or later ensue. Griesinger asserts that the same thing occurs in chronic mania. As regards the changes in the optic discs in the insane, we find usually recorded either a low grade of neuritis or of atrophy : according to Leber[3] this atrophy is histologically similar to that occurring in gray degeneration of the nerves. The outer strands are

[1] *Deutsches Archiv f. klin. Med.*, Bd. viii. pp. 1–19, quoted by Leeser, p. 94.
[2] *G. u. S.*, vol. vii. p. 227. [3] *A. f O.*, xiv., 2, p. 203.

usually those most affected. Indeed, as far as these obscure diseases are at present understood, there is no good reason why any changes should be found in the optic nerves except the congestion which accompanies acute or subacute mental disease and the nerve-degeneration of various grades which might be expected to be found in all worn-out lunatics. Illusions and hallucinations referable to the sense of sight are not uncommon in the insane, and are perhaps due to degenerative changes in the visual centres. In classifying such cases for study of the intraocular changes most writers place them under the following heads—viz.: general paralysis, dementia, mania, and melancholia,[1] the account of the changes in the eye-ground and the proportion of cases in which they occur being found to vary greatly.

GENERAL PARALYSIS.—Almost all agree that in this form of the disease we frequently have gray degeneration of the optic nerve, with pupillary symptoms which strongly resemble those found in tabes dorsalis, in some instances the autopsy showing the same location of spinal changes which characterizes the changes seen in locomotor ataxia.

DEMENTIA.—In chronic dementia Albutt found either hyperæmic or atrophic changes in the disc in 23 out of 38 cases. Noyes[2] found hyperæmia in 18 cases, and infiltration of the optic nerve and retina in 12. Jehn and Klein were unable to find changes in the discs of any of the cases which they examined.

MANIA.—Albutt found the discs hyperæmic except in one case examined during a paroxysm, in which they were pale. Out of 20 cases of acute mania, Noyes[3] found 14 which showed hyperæmia of the discs; the discs of the remaining 6 were either anæmic or normal, these latter cases all being of short duration (less than three months); the 6 cases of chronic mania had eye-grounds which showed no lesion, while the other 3 exhibited hyperæmic or inflammatory changes.

MELANCHOLIA.—In Noyes's examination 4 out of 5 cases had healthy eye-ground, and 1 moderate hyperæmia and striation. Jehn found hyperæmia in every one of 40 cases examined, 2 of these having decided neuritis, which he supposed to be due to meningeal change.

Spinal Cord.

INJURIES TO THE SPINE.—Physiologists have frequently shown that pupillary and other eye-symptoms may be produced by experimental injury to the spinal cord of animals, which would lead us to naturally expect analogous results in man in cases of spinal fracture and injury. This subject has received great attention in England, where spinal injury from railway accidents appears unusually frequent. Albutt[4] tells us that it is tolerably certain that disturbance of the optic nerve and its neighborhood is seen to follow disturbance of the spine with sufficient frequency and uniformity to establish the probability of a causal relation between the two events. Erichsen,[5] who has collected his large clinical experience

---

[1] Noyes, "Ophthalmoscopic Examination of Sixty Insane Patients in the State Asylum at Utica," pp. 6 (extra copy from *Amer. Journ. of Insanity*, Jan., 1872).
[2] *Idem.* [3] *Loc. cit.* [4] *Use of the Opthalmoscope*, London, 1871.
[5] *Concussion of the Spine*, by John Eric Erichsen, London, 1875.

into a book on *Concussion of the Spine*, after citing Plutarch to show how Alexander the Great was in danger of losing his eyesight from the blow of a heavy stone on the back of the neck, gives 53 cases (not tabulated with this view by the author), of which 49 were apparently undoubted cases of spinal injuries : of these, 13 (36 per cent.) showed decided eye-symptoms. Erichsen says : "My experience accords fully with that of Albutt. I found that in the vast majority of cases of spinal concussion unattended by fracture or dislocation of the vertebral column there occurred within a few weeks distinct evidence of impairment of vision." As enumerated by this author, these symptoms consist of difficulty of seeing in dim light, blurring and running together of the letters, and at times (in the early stages) slight diplopia. Later, there is photophobia, with contraction of the brow, which gives a peculiar frown, and at times an injection of the conjunctiva; these symptoms often being accompanied by muscæ volitantes and photopsia. He agrees with Albutt in attributing these to an ascending meningitis, while Wharton Jones considers that the eye symptoms are better accounted for by the action of the cilio-spinal centre and the sympathetic filaments springing from the dorsal and cervical cord. Wharton Jones[1] lays stress upon the undue retention of after-images and upon the small amount of comfort which a positive (convex) glass gives the patients, and "to the pain extending from the bottom of the orbit to the occiput, which is always a symptom belonging to deep-seated disturbance in the circulation of the optic apparatus." Rondeau[2] gives an interesting example of severe affection of the eyesight from apparently slight injury to the spine. The patient, seventeen years old, fell on the staircase, striking the neck and shoulders. There was complete loss of sight. Light-perception returned in a month, and four years after he could distinguish large objects in front of him, but vision remained stationary at that point. Albutt informs us that the percentage of visual affections is greater in proportion to the height of the seat of the injury in the spine.

TABES DORSALIS.—That affections of the eye are common in this grave malady is admitted by all writers, but as to their frequency and nature at the different stages of the disease, there is wide diversity of opinion : this is probably in part due to the fact that from the chronic nature of the disease, which extends usually over a period of several years, it is rare that the case remains from beginning to end under care of the same observer. The symptoms are of three varieties—viz. firstly, transient paralyses of the external muscles of the eye ; secondly, changes in the iris and ciliary body ; and, thirdly, affections of the optic nerve. The first-named symptoms are frequent in the early stages of the disease. Sometimes they affect the external muscles supplied by the third pair, and at others the rectus externus. Their transient character and frequency, while admitted by all observers, have as yet received no adequate explanation, it being indeed difficult to see why transient affections of the motor nerves should be so common in a disease which has its seat in the posterior sensory columns of the spinal cord, and which presents such formidable and irreparable lesions. The pupillary symptoms are, as a rule, those of myosis, sometimes mydriasis, and at times the so-called Argyll-Robertson

[1] *Failure of Sight after Railway and Other Injuries of the Spine and Head*, London, 1869.
[2] *Affections oculaires Reflexes*, Paris, 1866.

symptom (viz. a moderate myosis, with diminished reaction to light, but prompt response to convergence and accommodation). The last symptom is by no means present in all cases and at all stages of the complaint; but where it exists there is a remarkable resistance to the action of mydriatics. Trousseau was probably the first to call attention to this state of affairs. The writer has repeatedly seen cases where a strong solution of sulphate of atropia failed to produce any more than one-third of the usual dilatation produced by the same amount of the drug. Trousseau and Duchenne have both observed that during attacks of violent pain the pupils of ataxic patients will sometimes undergo temporary dilatation. Atrophy of the optic nerve (either partial or complete) is a frequent, and often an early, symptom of tabes dorsalis, and even may precede by many years the development of spinal symptoms. Foerster relates a case where complete optic atrophy preceded the development of all other symptoms by a period of three years, he having seen a number of other instances when atrophy preceded the other symptoms for a less period. Charcot records a case where the interval was ten years, and states that sooner or later locomotor ataxia develops in the majority of cases of optic atrophy in his wards in the Salpêtrière. Gowers gives two interesting cases, in one of which blindness came on fifteen years before the development of the other symptoms, the interval in the second being twenty years. Buzzard[1] also has recorded an observation where blindness and lightning pains manifested themselves fifteen years before the development of the other ataxic symptoms. If we were to estimate the frequency of optic atrophy as a symptom of early development of tabes dorsalis by the cases seen at ophthalmic hospitals, we should probably much overrate its proportion, inasmuch as those cases in which atrophy is a more marked and early symptom alone resort to such places. Leber found that 13 (26 per cent.) out of 87 cases at his clinic had spinal symptoms, while Gowers gives 20 per cent. as a relation existing between degeneration of the optic nerves and tabes. The latter author thinks that the ratio should really be stated as 15 per cent., because 5 per cent. was due to cases which had been sent to him for examination by his colleagues. Nettleship classifies 76 cases of optic atrophy as follows: 38 as presenting undoubted symptoms of locomotor ataxia; 11 as showing mixed spinal and cerebral symptoms (as in general paralysis of the insane); 9 with other forms of spinal degeneration without brain lesions, these associated with reflex iridoplegia without other symptoms of spinal or cerebral disease; and 15 only in which there was no manifest disorder of other parts of the nervous system. In the earlier stages of degeneration of the optic nerve in tabes dorsalis the discs are usually of a dull reddish-gray tint, and, while they are still capillary superficially, their deeper layers next to the lamina cribrosa have a decidedly diminished blood-circulation, and appear of a marked and more neutral gray color. The surface of the discs often looks more or less fluffy, there being enough haze of the retinal fibres to veil, and at times to hide, the scleral ring. Later, the superficial capillarity disappears and the discs assume a pallid, filled-in aspect, being surrounded by a scleral ring which is everywhere too broad: at this stage the main stems of the retinal arteries and veins exhibit no marked change in calibre, but later on we find them

[1] *Brain*, ii. 1878, p. 168.

shrinking, and the surface of the disc becomes excavated, the nerve itself often assuming a greenish tint. The earlier stages of such degenerations often exist for a long time, and are demonstrable by the ophthalmoscope before the sight is sufficiently impaired to prevent the patient from executing any ordinary work; this being dependent upon the facts that at first there is only a concentric diminution of the field for form and colors, while central vision remains for a long time unaffected. According to Foerster, this contraction of the field commences at the outer part. In advanced cases there are often irregular sector-like defects. This state of affairs makes it probable that while the number of cases in which total blindness precedes the development of tabetic symptoms is probably rated much too high, from the natural gathering of such cases at ophthalmic hospitals, yet, nevertheless, the frequency of incomplete gray degeneration of the optic nerves in the early stages of the complaint is probably, as a rule, much underrated.

Foerster has most justly called attention to the remarkable mental cheerfulness of persons laboring under this malady, and states that he has frequently seen cases where the patients would insist that they were improving, while examination of the acuity and of the field of vision showed steady failure of the eyesight. The writer's personal experience has on several occasions substantiated this statement. According to Cyon,[1] tabes presents three varieties: First, tabes dorsalis. This variety commences with paralyses of the eye-muscles and amblyopia. The pupils are not contracted. The amblyopia progresses. Cramp-like disturbances of innervation are always present, with a want of co-ordination of movements and anæsthesia of the upper extremities, while mental disturbances are often demonstrable. Second, tabes cervicalis. Myosis, with intense boring pains in the extremities and impotence, are its chief characteristics. Ataxia is rare, and disturbances of vision develop only late in the course of the disease. Third, a class which he considers the true form of tabes dorsalis, in which there are marked anæsthesia, formication, bladder and rectal symptoms, associated with motor disturbances which often end in paralysis. In such cases there are no eye symptoms except occasional dilatation of the pupil. The same writer has collected 203 cases reported by various authors, and gives the following tables as showing the relative frequency of eye symptoms:

Amblyopia	33 times.
Paralysis of eye-muscles	30 "
Mydriasis	3 "
Myosis	9
	75

Amaurosis with affections of eye-muscles	16 times.
Amaurosis with mydriasis	8 "
" " myosis	1 "
Affections of the eye-muscles with mydriasis	4
Amaurosis with mydriasis and affection of the eye-muscles,	2 "

He remarks[2] that the number of reported cases of mydriasis is probably excessive, and says that dilatation has been improperly noted, as, for instance, where one pupil is normal and the other contracted. As regards the frequency of the Argyll-Robertson symptoms, Vincent[3] found it

---

[1] *Tabes Dorsalis*, Berlin, 1866, p. 43.　　　　　　[2] *Loc. cit.*, p. 71.
[3] *Thèse de Paris*, cited by Robin, p. 20.

present in 40 cases out of 51, in which there were 7 cases of amaurosis with immobile pupils, 5 being marked exceptions to the rule. Out of 51 cases of tabes, the same author found myosis in 27. The statements of Vincent (as will be seen) differ materially from those of Cyon. Erb[1] found that in 56 cases, there were only 7 in which the optic nerves were affected ($12\frac{1}{2}$ per cent.), while in 17 there were affections of the eye-muscles ($30\frac{3}{10}$ per cent.). He considers myosis a frequent symptom, but thinks that the stage at which it develops is not yet determined. The anatomical cause of the want of sensitiveness of the pupils to light, while they retain their movements of convergence and accommodation, has not been well made out. Vincent[2] attributes it to a paralysis of the excito-motor filaments which supply the iris, and which he locates at the upper portion of the spine; while Wernicke thinks it due to degeneration of the filaments which go from the third pair to the optic nerve. Hugh-lings-Jackson[3] tells us that the pupils which fail to react to light often act but slightly with convergence, and in a note gives two cases of abso-lutely immobile pupils where the accommodation was nearly normal for the age. In fact, much remains to be accomplished in the study of the innervation of the iris and ciliary muscle in tabes. The proportion of cases in which cycloplegia occurs, and what relation it bears in point of time and frequency to the presence of iridoplegia, are far from being well made out. Jackson also insists that tabes does not necessarily follow in all cases of long-standing optic atrophy. On a basis of 72 cases Gowers says that some formal ophthalmoplegia interna was present in 92 per cent. He groups these cases into three stages: No. 1, where there is loss of knee-jerks, lightning pains, difficulty of standing with toes out and heels together, there being a want of ataxic gait; 2, where there is an ataxic gait, but the patient can still walk by the aid of a stick; 3, where the patient cannot walk without the assistance of another person. In 23 of his cases in the first stage (84 per cent.) symptoms of palsy of some of the intraocular muscles were found; in the second stage, 29 cases (93 per cent.); in the third stage, 18 cases (100 per cent.). Erb has called attention to the fact that reflex dilatation of the pupil from sharp stimulation of the skin of the temple is usually absent where we have the Argyll-Robertson pupil. Gowers admits that this is the rule, but has seen several cases where, although there was no attempt at myo-sis on exposure to light, yet there was marked dilatation on stimulating the skin.

Unclassified Nerve Diseases.

DIABETES.[4]

DIABETES MELLITUS.—This disease, which affects so profoundly all tissues of the body, necessarily manifests its influence on the tissues of the eyes. It frequently impairs the nutrition of the vitreous and causes the formation of cataract. The presence of grape-sugar is readily de-tected in such lenses by chemical examination. Mitchell and other

[1] *Nagel's Jahresbericht der Ophthalmologie*, 1872, p. 150.   [2] *Thèse de Paris.*
[3] *Transactions of the Ophthalmological Society of the United Kingdom*, vol. i. pp. 139-154.
[4] This affection has been placed here for convenience of classification, and because there is a form of the disease which is of neurotic origin.

experimenters have produced cataract in frogs by placing them in a solution of sugar. In such instances the lens tissue is said to become transparent when the animal is removed from its sugar bath and placed for a time in water; therefore, it is probable that the cataract has been developed by the simple abstraction of water. Diabetic cataracts are often extracted successfully, and the wound usually heals well; but we occasionally have intraocular hemorrhage during the course of healing. At times the nutrition of the patients is so impaired that a slight accident is dangerous, such as happened in a patient of the writer, where the striking of the hand against an iron bedstead caused gangrene and death. Nettleship[1] has recorded an analogous case, where accidental injury during convalescence caused death from gangrene. At times marked retinitis and hemorrhages with clear media have been encountered; thus, Jaeger in 1855 gave us an admirable picture of such a case, in which there was retinal swelling so great as to hide the outlines of the nerve, it being accompanied by numerous hemorrhages and yellow splotches. In his description of the case he also states that there was a marked central scotoma (a denser inside of a lighter one) in the field, while the periphery of the retina was so little affected that the patient could still decipher large letters (No. 18 of Jaeger's test-types). We might perhaps think that the scotomata are accidental and due to the location of the retinal changes in the given case, but later researches seem to show that we may have them in diabetes without retinal changes, Nettleship and Edmunds describing two such cases. In one of these cases there seems to be some doubt whether it was not a tobacco amblyopia which had been developed in a diabetic subject; but in the other case there was no such complication. The retinal changes which have been recorded in some cases have much resembled those due to albuminaria, but these alterations in the eye-ground have been seen in a number of cases where no albumen in the urine could be obtained.

Diabetes also may, by impairing the nutrition, diminish the power of accommodation in the young and cause a rapid increase of presbyopia in old persons (Graefe, Nagel, Foerster). Horner[2] proved that a hypermetropia of $\frac{1}{14}$ in a patient of fifty-five years of age rapidly diminished to $H. = \frac{1}{48}$, and the amount of presbyopia remained unaltered, while the general health had improved and the quantity of sugar had diminished. He attributes this rapid increase and subsequent diminution of the hypermetropia to a change in the amount of the fluid contents of the eye. Were this reporter any less careful an observer, one might be inclined to suspect swelling of the lens; but he specially mentions that there was no trace of cataract formation.

EPILEPSY.

IDIOPATHIC EPILEPSY.—In idiopathic epilepsy—that is, in those cases where no gross changes in the brain can be demonstrated by autopsy —the eye symptoms are numerous and interesting. Wecker[3] tells us that at the commencement of the spasm there is contraction of the pupils. Usually, soon after the tonic spasm sets in or coincident with it, we have marked dilatation of the pupil and an abolition of the eye-reflexes, this

[1] *Transactions of the Ophthalmological Society of the United Kingdom.*
[2] *Klin. Monatsbl. f. Augenheilkunde*, 1873, p. 490.   [3] *G. u. S.,* Bd. iv. p. 565.

being shown by the want of contraction of the orbicularis or of the pupil when the conjunctiva is touched. Reynolds, Echeverria, Clouston, and Hammond have called attention to a development of hippus (an alternate contraction and dilatation of the pupil) at the end of the convulsive paroxysms; but this is exceptional. The last author considers a state of alternate contraction and dilatation of the pupils, or a contraction of one pupil with dilatation of its fellow, to be characteristic of the convulsive stage. When the convulsions are unilateral the head and eyes are often turned toward the convulsed side. Although ophthalmoscopic examination is favored by dilatation of the pupil, yet the convulsions make it so difficult that we have quite conflicting accounts of the state of the disc and retina during the paroxysm. Six cases have been accurately examined by Albutt during the convulsion, in three of which there was congestion of the disc, and pallor in the remainder. Jackson also reports cases of pallor during the convulsion. More lately, Schreiber[1] has examined three cases in which he found pallor in the convulsive stage, this being very marked in one case, where the convulsion was violent. Gowers, on the other hand, maintains that in convulsions which commence locally without initial pallor of the face he was unable to perceive any alteration of the calibre of an artery which he kept continuously in view during the convulsion. The same author tells us that during the stage of cyanosis the veins of the retina become distended and dark, and that once in the status epilepticus he has seen a congestion of the discs with œdema, which subsequently disappeared. He does not consider that there is any abnormal appearance of the discs in the intervals between the attacks, while both Albutt and Bouchut hold that they are congested. In several of the chronic cases which the writer has had an opportunity of examining there has been a low grade of atrophy of the discs with concentric limitation of the field of vision. That this, at least, is common in advanced cases is well shown by the observations of Michel,[2] who in 1867 published careful examination of the eye-ground, acuity, and field of vision of 58 epileptics. In 15 of these cases there were no visible changes; in 10, hyperæmia; in 1, hyperæmia with œdema; 1 of hyperæmia passing into atrophy; 10 of unilateral atrophy (9 of the right nerve and 1 of the left); 13 cases of atrophy of both optic nerves; the remaining cases showing changes in the eye-ground which were probably attributable to other causes. Auræ which affect the special senses have been recorded, and have been usually described as flashes of light or balls of fire. Maisonneuve (quoted by Robin) gives an instance where the auræ consisted in convulsions of the eyelids. Gowers gives 119 cases of auræ which affected the special senses, 84 of these being of the sense of sight. He divides the latter into five classes: I. Sensation in the eyeball; II. Diplopia; III. Apparent increase or diminution in the size of objects; IV. Loss of eyesight; V. Distinct visual sensations, consisting sometimes of flashes of light, colored spectra, and rarely some more specialized sensation, such as an apparition. The only one of these cases in which there was an autopsy appears to have been one of symptomatic rather than idiopathic character, as there was found a tumor of the occipital lobe which had extended as far forward as the angular gyrus.

[1] *Ueber Vorändenungen des Augenhintergrundes, etc.*, 1878 (S. 42).
[2] *Inaug. Diss.*, von Dr. Julius Michel, Würzburg, 1867.

HYSTERO-EPILEPSY.—The remarkable co-ordinated convulsions which are associated with hemianæsthesia, and which have been so minutely described by Charcot as characteristic of this disease, are constantly accompanied by subjective or objective disorders of the visual apparatus. Visions of animals, such as rats, vipers, crows, cats, etc., frequently pre_ cede the convulsive seizure, followed by a transient loss of sight; a return of the illusions (sometimes pleasant and gay, at others erotic in their nature, or again sad or terror-striking) coming on in a later stage. It is said that processions of animals are often seen, which usually come and go on the hemianæsthetic side as the attack passes off and the patient becomes quiet. The objective symptoms have been carefully studied by Landolt in Charcot's wards. They were found by him to consist in a diminution of the acuity of vision and a concentric limitation of the field for form and color. All these symptoms are bilateral, and much more marked on the anæsthetic side, they occurring before any ophthalmo_ scopic changes are visible. These are followed later by alterations in the eye-ground, which consist at first of slight congestion and œdema of the discs, followed by partial atrophy. The difference in the affection of the two eyes was so marked that Charcot at first described it as a crossed amblyopia, but he admits that the lesion is bilateral, as above described.[1]

EXOPHTHALMIC GOITRE.

GRAVES'S DISEASE; BASEDOW'S DISEASE.—The most prominent cha- racteristics of this affection are an irritability of the heart with increased fre- quency of the pulse, and enlargement of the thyroid gland and a swelling of the tissues of the orbit, which cause the eyeballs to become prominent. The size of the goitre and the amount of protrusion of the eyeball vary very much in different cases. Frequently there is a symptom to which Graefe was the first to call attention—namely, a disturbance of the usual consensual movements of the eyeball and upper eyelid. When the patient looks downward below the horizontal line, the lid no longer accompanies the eyeball in its motion, but halts in its course. This derangement in the action of the lid is supposed to depend upon some defect in the innervation of the orbicularis, as it is not present in cases of equal prominence of the eyeball from other causes. The amount of secretion from the tear-glands and from the conjunctival surface is also at times much diminished. Owing to the prominence of the eyes and the relaxation of the orbicularis, the fissure of the lids is wider open than usual, and the eye has a peculiar stare. At times, when the prominence of the eyes is very great, the lids fail to cover the balls during sleep, and the cornea becomes inflamed and ulcerated from exposure to air and dust. The disease rarely develops till after puberty, and is more frequent in females than in males: in the former it often develops after childbirth. It is so frequently accompanied by disease of the reproductive organs that Foerster, in his paper on the "Relation of Eye Diseases to General Dis- ease,"[2] places it in the section devoted to eye symptoms from diseases of the sexual organs. Ophthalmoscopic examination usually shows a slight thickening of the fibre-layer of the retina in and around the disc, with dilatation and tortuosity of the veins—a state of affairs which may often

[1] *Leçons sur les Localisations dans les Mal. du Cerveau*, vol. i. p. 119 (foot-note), Paris, 1876.
[2] *Graefe und Saemisch*, vol. vii. p. 97.

be fairly attributed to venous stasis caused by the swelling tissues. In addition to these symptoms there is sometimes, as Becker has pointed out, a dilatation of the arteries, which may almost equal the veins in calibre. At times there is an arterial pulse. As found by autopsies, the anatomical changes are usually enlargement and dilatation of the heart, hypertrophy and various degenerative changes in the thyroid glands, and a state of hyperæmia at times associated with hypertrophy of the fat tissue of both orbits.

Affections of the General System.

CHOLERA.—In this disease the eyelids are said to show an early development of cyanosis, which .becomes more marked as this symptom develops in other parts of the body. The contents of the orbits shrink and the eyes are drawn back in their sockets, there being an imperfect closure of the lids, which leads at times to necrosis of the exposed lower part of the cornea. There is a marked diminution in the secretion of tears, and often a dilatation of the veins of the exposed part of the conjunctiva bulbi, which are turgid with the black blood, this state being at times accompanied by subconjunctival hemorrhages. The pupils are usually contracted. The retinal arteries are much diminished in size, and the veins although not dilated, are filled with blackish blood. Owing to the great feebleness of the circulation, the slightest pressure with the finger on the eyeball produces arterial pulse; Graefe[1] in some cases describes a pulsating movement of interrupted blood-columns in the veins, such as is sometimes seen in incomplete embolism of the arteria centralis.

RHEUMATISM AND GOUT.—In the older books on diseases of the eye we constantly meet references to rheumatic and arthritic forms of inflammation of that organ. In the later works on the subject the list has been greatly reduced, partly because an anatomical classification has been attempted, and partly because many such affections have been attributed to other causes, such as syphilis, etc. Catarrho-rheumatic ophthalmia, rheumatic iritis, rheumatic paralysis of the eye-muscles, etc. have been so classified, not on account of their occurrence in the course of attacks of acute rheumatism, but because the writers have been unable to attribute them to any other source than that designated as having taken cold. That recurrent attacks of iritis are frequent in some individuals who have recurrent attacks of chronic inflammation of the joints is a fact familiar to many practitioners, amply attested by the cases published by Hutchinson[2] and by Foerster.[3] As regards gout, the direct proofs of its relations to eye disease are still less manifest, and most cases supposed to be attributed to this cause by both the older and more modern writers are to be classed as primary or secondary glaucoma.

SYPHILIS.—All the tissues of the eyeball and eyelids may at times manifest the signs of this dread and searching dyscrasia, although it is

---

[1] *A. f. O.*, xii. 2, p. 210.

[2] "A Report on the Forms of Eye Disease which occur in connection with Rheumatism and Gout," by Jonathan Hutchinson (*R. L. O. H. Reps.*, vol. vii. pp. 287–332; also vol. viii. pp. 191–216).

[3] "Beziehungen der Allgemein-Leiden, etc., zu Veränderungen des Sehorgans," *Graefe u. Saemisch*, vol. vii. pp. 155–160.

rarely so marked in its character as to be distinguished with certainty from other forms of eye disease by its appearance alone. Primary syphilis of the lid is rare, but when it occurs it is liable to be mistaken for epithelioma, where there is absence of a distinct history of infection. In the eyeball itself the uveal tract (iris, ciliary body, and choroid) is the favorite seat of disease. Iritis is said by Fournier[1] to be developed in from 3 to 4 per cent. of all cases of syphilis, and, according to Coccius, $11\frac{6}{10}$ per cent. out of 7898 cases of eye disease in Leipzig were due to this cause. Syphilitic iritis certainly constitutes a large proportion of the cases of inflammation of the iris seen in hospital practice: Coccius places the percentage at $46\frac{6}{10}$ per cent., while Wecker puts it at 50 to 60 per cent. It usually develops during the subsidence of the secondary skin affections, and is often to be distinguished by its insidious course and the amount of plastic exudation which accompanies it. There is ciliary injection and sluggishness of the pupil, with the formation of synechiæ, before there is any very decided pain or photophobia, this latter being usually strongly developed at a later period. The formation of gummata in the iris, which are generally seen in the smaller circle, is much rarer, generally developing in the tertiary stage of the disease; occasionally they are developed in the ciliary body. In the former situation they usually disappear under active treatment, leaving fair vision in the eye, but when situated in the latter place they usually lead to shrinking and atrophy of the eyeball, even under the most vigorous treatment. When iritis occurs in infants it is generally specific in origin. When they are born with posterior synechiæ and complicate cataract, similar occurrences during intra-uterine life may be suspected. Syphilitic choroiditis is frequent, but its frequency is probably overrated on account of a disposition to assume syphilis as a cause of cases of choroiditis in which the pathology is not evident. Foerster has very properly pointed out that a majority of the cases of disseminate choroiditis are not due to this cause, and that the changes are developed slowly, and remain stable for a long time even when not treated; while the usual form of specific choroiditis shows rapid progress, with failure of the sight, photopsies, vitreous opacities, hemeralopia, and zonular defects in the field of vision. Opinion, however, is divided on this point: Wecker thinks that two-thirds of the cases of disseminate choroiditis are due to syphilis. In many of the chronic cases of syphilitic choroiditis there is a wandering of the pigment out of the cells of the choroidal epithelium, and a distribution of it into the lymph-sheaths of the retinal vessels and capillaries, these changes producing ophthalmoscopic appearances which closely resemble those of typical pigmentary degeneration of the retina. Affections of the head of the optic nerve and superficial layers of the retina, such as are represented by Liebreich,[2] are much more rare, but the writer has repeatedly seen them both at Liebreich's Paris clinic and in our own hospitals. They are characteristic, and usually accompany the tertiary symptoms. There is a dense haze which seems to lie partly in front of the retina, and to extend around the disc for a space of one and a half to two disc-diameters, generally including the macula lutea, and rapidly diminishing as it approaches the equator. Vision is usually much reduced, and even under persistent

[1] Quoted by Foerster, *Graefe und Saemisch,* vol. vii. p. 189.
[2] Plate 10, Fig. 2, ed. 1863.

antisyphilitic treatment it is slow to clear up.   Hereditary syphilis frequently manifests itself in an interstitial keratitis, which begins with small irregularly-rounded dots near the centre of the cornea.   They gradually become more numerous, and coalesce, until the membrane appears as if a thin layer of ground glass had been imbedded in its tissue, leaving the epithelium clear and bright.   Although there is no ulceration, yet there is a great tendency to the formation of new blood-vessels, which often goes on until the entire cornea is permeated by them and becomes of a dull venous blood-like red color.   These vessels are continuous with superficial and deeper shoots which pass in from the two layers, normally forming loops in the corneal periphery.   This form of keratitis is usually accompanied by marked photophobia, pain, ciliary injection, and low grades of iritis.   The pathological processes which take place in the cornea during the disease generally leave it more or less clouded, and often much misshapen by softening and alteration of its curvature.

TUBERCULOSIS.—Except in children, the eyeball is rarely the seat of a deposit of tubercles, and even then it is much more likely to give evidence of their seat in the membranes of the brain by its secondary affection than to be itself directly affected by them.   When they form in the eye, they may affect the choroid, the intraocular end of the optic nerve, the retina, or the iris.   Jaeger was the first to call attention to their ophthalmoscopic appearances.   Their favorite seat, as is well shown in one of Jaeger's plates, is the macular region and its vicinity.   They develop in the stroma of the choroid, and appear as whitish-yellow spots varying from one-eighth the diameter of the optic disc to the size of the disc itself, and by aggregation may form even larger masses.   They are usually seen in cases of well-marked acute miliary tuberculosis, although doubtless they are often overlooked, on account of not giving rise to any symptoms; besides, thorough ophthalmoscopic examination of such sick and restless children is difficult, and the general diagnosis is usually well made out from other symptoms.   They may, however, precede all other symptoms, as in the cases reported by Steffen[1] and Fraenkel.[2]   Development of tubercular masses in the intraocular end of the opticus has been described by Chiari,[3] Michel,[4] and Gowers.[5]   In the case cited by the last author the growth extended from the disc to the ora serrata, which during life gave rise to the peculiar reflection from the eye so often seen in intraocular tumor.   According to Cohnheim,[6] tubercle is to be found in the choroid in all cases of acute miliary tuberculosis.   Other observers, however, have not been able to support him in this assertion: Albutt,[7] who repeatedly searched for them both in living and dead subjects, failed to find them; Garlick[8] during two years' experience at a children's hospital found them but once; Heinzel[9] in ten cases of general tuberculosis in children was at the autopsies unable to find any tubercles of the choroid.   According to Stricker, they may at times develop very rapidly, coming on in from twelve to twenty-four hours.   Tubercles have been

[1] Jahresbericht f. Kinderheilkunde, 1870 (Gowers).
[2] Berliner klinisches Wochenschrift, 1872, pp. 4–6 (Foerster).
[3] Wien. Med. Jahrbücher, 1877, p. 559.   [4] Archiv der Heilkunde, 1873.
[5] Medical Ophthalmoscopy, 1879, p. 250.
[6] Virch. Arch., 1867, Bd. xxxix. p. 49 (Foerster).
[7] Quoted by Gowers, p. 203.   [8] Quoted by Gowers, Med. Ophth., p. 200.
[9] Quoted by Foerster, p. 99, Jahrbuch der Kinderheilkunde, Neue Folge, viii., 3, p. 331.

found in the retina in the cases of papillary tuberculosis already referred to, and also with cases of tubercle in the iris (Perls, Manfredi). At times, tubercles in the iris occur in scrofulous and feeble children, appearing as growths in all respects closely resembling syphilitic gummata. As in the latter case, they are accompanied by severe iritis, and at times with hypopyon. Tuberculosis of the conjunctiva is a very rare affection. It is described as commencing with swelling of the lids, and when these are everted exuberant granulations of the conjunctiva are seen which are most frequently situated in the retrotarsal folds. These granulations are at first of a grayish-red color, but when they have existed for some time, superficial erosion of their surface occurs, and uneven yellowish-red ulcers are formed. The disease usually occurs in young people, and generally affects but one eye. Haab[1] has given a description of six cases of it, with reference to a few instances described by other authors.

Toxic Amblyopiæ.

TOBACCO AND ALCOHOL.—These two lesions strongly resemble each other, and it is impossible to differentiate them when we find them in persons who are addicted to the abuse of both of these drugs; consequently, for a time, in Germany, there was a disposition to underrate the potent destructive agency of the latter drug, but every practitioner of experience in eye disease must have seen cases of tobacco amblyopia in which there has been no abuse of alcohol. The best proof of the deleterious influences of tobacco on the eyesight is the improvement which results by simple abstinence from its use where the vision has been seriously affected by its influence. In the earlier stages of both forms of amblyopia there is a contracted pupil and a slight dimness of vision, the patients claiming that they see better in feeble light and twilight. The ophthalmoscope shows a slight œdema of the disc with tortuosity of the veins, the rest of the eye-ground appearing normal. Later, the usual appearances of blue-gray atrophy set in. In the earlier stage there are often color scotomata, which are usually ovoid in form and lie between the disc and the macula lutea. Unless carefully looked for with color squares of one to two millimeters in diameter, they are apt to be overlooked. Later, there is a marked reduction of central vision. When the atrophy has progressed farther, there is decided contraction of the field.

LEAD-POISONING.—The deleterious effects of lead on the eyesight are undoubted, although rare in proportion to the cases of colic and wrist-drop produced by this metal. When amaurosis develops, it is usually either in acute lead-poisoning or after a gradual saturation of the system, as is shown by repeated attacks of lead colic. In either case the amaurosis is usually accompanied by dilatation of the pupils, delirium, and convulsions. The amaurosis generally passes off, and the pupils contract with the return of vision, although it may remain permanent, and leaves the patient with atrophic nerves, as in a case observed by Trousseau, where the patient was subsequently transferred to the Salpêtrière. The only two cases which the writer has had an opportunity of witnessing showed

[1] "Die Tuberculose des Auges," *A. f. O.*, xxv., 4, p. 163.

marked choking of the discs and severe cerebral symptoms.   One of these cases died and one recovered: both were results of the use of white lead as a cosmetic.   Rognetta[1] quotes Vater as reporting a case of hemianopia produced by lead-poisoning, which recovered when the lead colic was cured.   Trousseau[2] quotes Andral as giving a case of diplopia due to the same cause, and disappearing as the patient recovered.

QUININE.—Over-doses of quinine seriously impair the eyesight, and in some cases have produced temporary but absolute blindness.   The usual symptoms are a deterioration of central vision and a contraction of the field.   The ophthalmoscopic examination reveals a pallid disc with marked diminution in the size of the retinal arteries and veins.   In many of the reported cases it is difficult to decide positively how much of the amaurosis is due to the quinine and how much to the disease for which the patient is under treatment.   This is especially true where the patient has been suffering from severe intermittent fever or from exhausting hemorrhages complicating uterine disease, which are well known frequently to produce more or less complete atrophy, with shrinking of the vessels.   There are, however, a sufficient number of well-observed cases on record to satisfactorily establish the lesion.   One of the most striking is a case of poisoning recorded by Giacomini, where the patient took at one dose three drachms of sulphate of quinia by mistake for cream of tartar.   This was followed by severe headache, pain in the stomach, dizziness, unconsciousness, with slow and scarcely perceptible pulse and infrequent respiration.   The pupils were widely dilated.   On regaining consciousness the patient found that he was almost blind, the weakness of sight lasting a long time.   As the poisoning occurred in the preophthalmoscopic era, there is of course no description of the eye-ground.   In all recorded cases, while central vision has been either partially or entirely regained, the field of vision has remained permanently contracted.

SANTONIN.—In very large doses santonin produces dilatation of the pupil, amblyopia, and complete color-blindness.   Smaller doses produce a shortening of the violet end of the spectrum and cause yellow vision.   The disturbance of vision usually lasts only a few hours.   The poison seems to be eliminated by the urine, as the sight is said to become normal while traces of the drug can still be seen in the secretion of the kidneys.   Rose has given us a most careful study of this subject in his papers entitled " Color-Blindness from Santonin "[3] and " Hallucinations in Santonin Intoxication."[4]

SALICYLATE OF SODIUM.—Gatti[5] reports a case of transient amblyopia, due to the ingestion of one hundred and twenty grains of salicylate of sodium, in a sixteen-year-old peasant-girl who had acute articular rheumatism.   There were no changes in the eye-ground except a fulness of the veins, which persisted after the eyesight had returned.   There was mydriasis.   No phosphenes could be produced.   As the urine did not present any traces of salicylate of sodium, it would seem to show that it was not eliminated by the usual emunctories.

[1] *Recherches sur la Cause et la Siège d'Amaurose.*   [2] *Thèse de Concours.*
[3] *Virch. Arch.*, Bd. xx., 1860 (Separat Abdruck, S. 48).
[4] *Ibid.*, Bd. xxviii., 1863 (Separat Abdruck, S. 12).
[5] *Gaz. d. Ospital Milano*, p. 129, 1880; *Nagel's Jahresbericht*, 1882 (Lit. 1880), p. 245.

MEDICAL OTOLOGY.

MEDICAL OTOLOGY.

By GEORGE STRAWBRIDGE, M.D.

In this article on Medical Otology it is proposed to include those dis_
eases of the ear that are frequently seen by the general practitioner, and
especially those that exist as sequelæ to some general disease, and where
the ear complication would be treated in connection with the general
disorder.

Examination of a Patient.

As nearly all ear patients are afflicted with varying degrees of deafness,
one of the first points of inquiry will be as to their hearing power. There
are three tests commonly employed for this purpose: the ticking of a
watch, the human voice, and the tuning-fork.

1st. The Watch.—By this method of examination the patient is placed
with closed eyelids, so as to exclude the visual power as a factor in the
examination, as it is a curious fact that many people are apparently
unable to distinguish between seeing a watch and hearing its tick, and
therefore so long as they can see the watch they will imagine that they
can hear it ticking. Bring the watch (held by the physician) from a
distance toward the patient until the tick is heard, and note the distance
in inches. The plan of holding the watch close to the ear, and then
slowly removing it until the extreme limit of hearing is attained, gives
an incorrect result as regards the distance that the watch can be heard,
due to the fact that the impressions produced on the terminal endings of
the auditory nerve by the watch-tick continue a sensible time after the
watch-tick has passed out of the nerve-limit, and therefore the watch-tick
can still be noted. Prout has prepared a convenient method for recording
the hearing power. Note the number of inches that the watch-tick can
be heard by a normal ear, and let this serve as a denominator of a fraction, the numerator of which is the number of inches that the same
watch-tick can be heard by the ear of the person under examination.
For instance: a normal ear can distinguish my watch-tick at a distance
of twenty inches; if, now, the patient's ear can perceive the same sound
at only five inches, the hearing power would be noted as $\frac{5}{20}$. By this
it is not meant that the hearing power is one-fourth of normal hearing,
as it would be only one-sixteenth of normal hearing, as the volume of
sound is inversely in proportion to the square of the distance.

2d. The human voice tells more about the hearing power for practical
purposes than does the watch. There are many persons who can readily

hear the watch-tick at several inches, and yet who hear very imperfectly ordinary conversation, and also many who hear very well the human voice and very badly the watch-tick. The method of examination is to speak ordinary words in a tone that can be heard by the average ear a given number of feet, and to note the distance in feet that the ear under observation can detect the words that are spoken. In this way can be noted the hearing power of the human voice, the numerator of the fraction being the distance that the word can be heard by the observed ear, the denominator being the distance that the word can be distinguished by the normal ear.

The patient should always be examined with closed eyelids, as deaf people quickly learn by watching the movements of the lips of the speaker to know the words that are being spoken. Another precaution is to have the ear to be tested directly opposite the mouth of the observer, the other ear being firmly closed.

3d. The Tuning-Fork.—Bone-conduction of sound is used by this method. The great use of the tuning-fork is in determining diseased conditions of the auditory nerve and internal ear, and it enables one to make a differential diagnosis as to whether deafness is due to a diseased condition of the sound-conducting apparatus or whether the nerve portion of the ear is at fault. For instance: a patient complains of deafness. This may be due to some obstruction in the external auditory canal, such as impacted cerumen, or it may be due to a diseased middle ear, with thickening of its membranes, or it may be due to a diseased internal ear. The watch and human voice would only show the ear to be defective in its hearing power, and it may be from any of the above-mentioned causes. The tuning-fork, in vibration, placed on an incisor tooth or on the frontal bone, would bring out the fact that if the deafness was due to a diseased middle ear or obstruction in the external auditory canal, the tuning-fork would be heard best by the defective ear; but if due to a disease of the internal ear, it would be heard the least distinctly by the defective-hearing ear. Mack explains this by the supposition that the sound-waves are prevented from freely escaping through the sound-conducting apparatus, and are reflected back on the auditory nerve-elements, and thus make a double impression. Tuning-forks having the note C are best adapted for this examination.

EXAMINATION OF THE EXTERNAL CANAL AND TYMPANIC MEMBRANE.—This can be done by direct or by reflected light, better by the latter. A mirror and speculum are needed. The mirror should be concave, with a focal distance of from 5″–7″ and a diameter of 2½″–3″, with a ball-and-socket-joint and head-band, so as to allow of the two hands being free, the head holding the mirror in the required position. The mirror should have a central perforation of 2‴–3‴, with a brass back, rendering it less liable to break. As a light-source can be used the light from an argand burner, but preferably sunlight reflected from a cloud or white wall.

The Ear Speculum.—The Wilde or Gruber speculum answers equally well. The Wilde speculum is cone-shaped, and best of German silver: it is easily cleansed and has four sizes. The Gruber speculum has a larger mouth and gives a large visual field. It has a parabolic curve, for the purpose of admitting more light; there are also four sizes. The speculum should be warm when in use, and is to be held in position in the canal by the thumb and forefinger of the left hand. Often in the examination of an external canal an angular-toothed forceps is needed to remove foreign substances.

The cotton-holder is a most important instrument, furnishing a means of thoroughly drying the external canal of any fluid with the least pos- sible amount of irritation—much less than that caused by the use of the ear-syringe. It is a slender steel rod 6″ long, having a number of serra- tions at one end to more easily allow cotton to be wrapped around it ; the other end has a convenient handle. In using this instrument a small tuft of well-cleansed cotton is wrapped around the holder, so that one half of the length of the cotton tuft projects beyond the end of the instru- ment. By slight adaptation with the fingers the cotton roll can be made soft or quite firm, and large or small in proportion to the amount of cotton used. The cotton-holder should always be used under the light from the head-mirror.

The curette is of the same length as the cotton-holder, but is made of heavier steel, and terminates at one end in a small ring of a diameter of from 2–3 mm. It is useful in removing scabs, etc. from the external canal, also in loosening impacted cerumen.

Probes are also needful. A good middle-ear probe is made of a single piece of silver, of the same length as the cotton-holder, and tapering down to a slender shank with a small knob-like ending.

The ear syringe, a most excellent instrument, is now made of rubber, holding two ounces of fluid, and has a bulbar extremity, so as to avoid injuring the external canal or tympanic membrane. The syringe has a finger-rest, with the piston ending in a ring, so as to admit of its use with one hand. In using a syringe warm water should be always employed, and at a temperature that the finger would indicate as being quite warm. Also at first force the water very gently into the meatus, so that the patient shall not be startled ; also it is well to bear in mind that many patients become very giddy under its use, necessitating either very gentle use or its being abandoned for the time.

EXAMINATION OF THE EUSTACHIAN TUBE.—The main point is as to whether the tube permits the free passage of air up to the middle ear. This can be ascertained by three methods: 1. Valsalva's method; 2. Politzer's method; 3. Catheterization of the tube.

Valsalva's method consists in forcing air through the tube by a forced expiration, the mouth and nasal passages being at the same time firmly closed. The patient can distinctly feel the air pressing against the tym- panic membrane, causing it to bulge outwardly, provided the tube is open. This proceeding has certain disadvantages, sometimes causing head congestions and giddiness.

Politzer's Method.—In this proceeding a gum air-bag is used as the means of forcing air into the tube. In the act of swallowing the soft palate is drawn against the posterior wall of the pharynx, and at the same time the pharyngeal mouth of the tube is well opened, so that air forced through the nasal passages at such a moment, being prevented from passing downward by the up-drawn palate, is forced up through the Eustachian tube into the middle ear. The success of this procedure depends entirely upon the inflation being made at the same moment that the soft palate is drawn up against the pharyngeal wall; otherwise the air would naturally pass by the widest passage, in this case downward into the stomach. The usual plan of inflating at the moment that the patient is told to swallow fails, from the fact that patients differ so materially in the quickness with which they respond to an order. Many in their anxiety will swallow before the word is given, others will allow an appreciable time to pass before swallowing, so that the inflation will fail. For this reason I have adopted the following plan : It is well known that in the act of swallowing the larynx is drawn forcibly upward, and also that the moment of the extreme elevation is nearly coincident with the moment that the soft palate is drawn against the wall of the pharynx. The prominence of the thyroid cartilage (the so-called pomus Adami) enables one to easily watch until the maximum elevation of the larynx is reached, and then quickly, by a forcible contraction of the air-bag, to thoroughly inflate the middle ear. The Politzer method so thoroughly accomplishes the object, and with the least possible irritation, that the use of the catheter in the majority of cases is no longer indicated. The method of Politzer is as follows: The patient takes some water in the mouth ; the air-bag has attached to it a short piece of gum tubing ending in a nose-piece in shape like an olive, or sometimes a small gum catheter is attached to it. This is placed in the lower nasal passage and the nose held firmly closed over it with one hand, the second hand grasping the air-bag. The patient is then told to swallow, so as to cause elevation of the soft palate (this can also be accomplished by the patient speaking quickly some word like *hoc*), and the air-bag is forcibly pressed. In this way the air is quickly driven, viâ the nasal passage and Eustachian tube, into the middle ear. In little children it is sufficient to quickly inflate, as the crying of the child elevates the soft palate to a certain degree, and so cuts off the downward passage into the stomach.

External Ear Diseases of the Auricle.

ECZEMA.—This disease occurs very frequently in infants during dentition, where irritation of the dental branches of the fifth pair of nerves causes irritation in other branches of the same nerve, including those distributed to the skin of the face and auricle, causing acute attacks of the disease. It is also frequently observed that successive teeth penetrating the periosteum will cause fresh attacks of this skin irritation, so that as long as the teething process continues, so long is the eczema apt to continue, and treatment will probably prove only palliative. Eczema occurs also in both the male and female approaching the period of adolescence, a time when other forms of skin disease are especially common.

The aged do not escape this annoying malady, where it is apt to occur in the chronic form, and is due to want of nerve-force in the skin branches of the nerves distributed to this part—a wise provision of nature allowing nerve-power to fail first in the nerves distributed to parts where the harm done is a minimum one, rather than in the nerve-centres, where disease fatal to life would result. The treatment in this class of cases would be radically different from the preceding divisions, where nerve-irritation is the cause.

DIAGNOSIS.—The acute form shows the same diagnostic appearance as does eczema occurring elsewhere—the same redness and swelling of skin, followed by the vesicular eruption with serous oozing and loss of epi_ thelium. In the chronic variety there is marked thickening of the skin, and the auricle is often covered with crusts, but here and there a deep fissure in the skin, from some one of which pus will exude.

Marked itching and burning and a sensation of fulness occur, both in the acute and chronic forms.

COURSE.—The acute variety may last only a few days, but as a rule tends to recur at frequent intervals. The chronic variety can last almost any length of time, and will often prove to be most obstinate.

TREATMENT.—Acute Variety.—The first indication is to relieve the burning and itching. This is often best done by the use of some mild anodyne powder which protects the part from the air and tends to relieve the existing skin irritation. Finely-powdered starch dusted over the part is a good remedy. One of the best anodyne powders is that of McCall Anderson :

> ℞. Pulv. camphoræ,   ʒiss ;
> Pulv. zinci oxid.   ʒss ;
> Pulv. amyli,   ʒj.

To be dusted over the inflamed surface.

Often there will be difficulty in preventing the powder from falling off. When this is the case a very thin coating of the skin with the oxide- of-zinc ointment furnishes an excellent ground for the powder to adhere to. The oxide-of-zinc ointment alone is also an excellent application.

In the chronic variety a more stimulating application is needful, and some preparation of tar will prove valuable, such as—

> ℞. Ungt. picis liquidæ,   ʒj-ʒiij ;
> Ungt. zinci oxid.   ʒj.

The crusts that collect on the auricle are best removed by a poultice of bread and milk, or a cotton pad moistened with olive oil can be bound over it for a few hours, and will serve to cleanse the part. In the very chronic cases, where points of suppuration are found, a caustic application like nitrate of silver is needed. Careful regulation of the diet and habits of the patient is indicated ; an outdoor life, abstinence from alcohol and tobacco, nutritious food, will greatly aid. Iron, quinine, cod-liver oil can be used frequently with good results, while in teething children incising of the gums will sometimes give temporary relief.

Diseases of the External Auditory Canal.

IMPACTED CERUMEN.—This disease occurs very frequently, and, as a rule, is considered a matter of very little moment by the profession at large, whereas, in fact, it is often a symptom of grave disorders of the middle ear. Roosa mentions that in 1448 cases observed by him in private practice, only 101 were cases of inspissated cerumen alone, the great majority showing in addition serious disorders of other parts of the organ of hearing. The ceruminous glands are found chiefly in the car- tilaginous portion of the external canal, and, according to Kessel, resemble the sweat-glands not only in the time and manner of their development, but also in their external form and minute histology. This is also true of the contents of the ceruminous glands, as far as the microscope allows us to judge, the only difference being that in cerumen masses of very fine corpuscles of coloring matter are found.[1] The ceruminous glands secrete but slowly, and the cerumen tends to harden and become dark in color as it grows older. The removal of the secretion is probably effected by several factors. Numerous experiments prove that the epithelial lining of the external canal has a constant motion from within outward; necessarily any substance resting on it will move with it. Cerumen could in this way be constantly extruded from the external canal; and the cerumen, becoming dry and hard by exposure to the air, would tend to separate from the skin by curling itself into small rolls, and so drop out from the external meatus. The question naturally arises, Why does the cerumen form such impacted masses as are met with? We submit the following explanation:

In many of these cases the secretion is largely above the normal, and catarrh of the naso-pharynx is found associated with it. Pomeroy first noticed this connection, and suggested the probability that the ceruminous function is greatly affected in catarrhal disease, on the theory that the earlier stages of catarrh would result in hyperæmia, and consequently augmented function, of the ceruminous glands, which if continued may result in atrophy with abolition of function, precisely as results in inflammation of the mucous membrane lining the fauces.[2]

The pneumogastric nerve by its pharyngeal branch is connected with the pharynx, and by its auricular branch with the external auditory canal, so that irritation of the pharyngeal branches of the nerve, as would occur in pharyngeal catarrh, could readily excite reflex irritation in the auricular branch, with increase of function of the parts to which it is distributed, causing increase of the ceruminous secretion. Conversely, atrophy of the nerve would be followed by atrophy of function of correlated parts. The external canal often presents a sharp angle in its course near the meatus, and this also would tend to cause an accumulation of cerumen.

It is a well-established clinical fact that the great majority of cases of impacted cerumen are found to be associated with serious diseased conditions of the middle ear especially, and probably the diseased middle ear is often an important factor in causing impaction to take place; so that it frequently happens that the patient will experience no increase of hearing after removal of such an impacted mass, owing to the diseased middle ear that may be present. I remember one case where the hearing was absolutely lessened after removal of a ceruminous plug; doubtless in this case the solid conduction through such a mass was better than through an air-filled auditory canal.

SYMPTOMS.—Sudden loss of hearing: this is due to the fact that the mass grows slowly from the periphery toward the centre, and as long as a small central opening remains the hearing power will remain good. Some sudden jolt or misstep, or some quick-acting force, will cause occlusion of this narrow passage, with consequent sudden loss of hearing. The tuning-fork, placed on the incisor teeth, will be best heard on the affected side by reason of vibrations being impeded by the mass in their passage through the external canal.

[1] Vide Stricher, *Textbook*, p. 951.	[2] *American Otological Soc. Trans.*, 1872.

Tinnitus aurium and vertigo are often present, both being due to the mass pressing inward the tympanic membrane, with consequent increase of pressure on the labyrinthine fluid by the chain of small bones pressing on the membrane of the foramen ovale. These symptoms are sometimes alarming to the patient, as in his judgment indicative of serious brain lesion.

DIAGNOSIS.—Examination of the external canal with the speculum and reflected light reveals a dark amber-colored mass lying in the external canal, which can be very hard, the result of exposure to the air for a length of time, as well as the union with it of epithelial débris of the skin of the canal; or it may be soft, like syrup, in its consistence.

The PROGNOSIS is to be guarded until the condition of the middle ear is known.

TREATMENT.—If the mass is hard in its character, its removal is best effected by the forceps or curette or blunt hook, it being understood that the external canal is well illuminated, so that the course of the instrument can be carefully watched. The curette or blunt hook will loosen the attachments of the mass to the sides of the canal, and then it can be readily removed by the forceps, care being taken not to injure the tympanic membrane. In such a way a hard plug can be removed at one sitting that otherwise would require repeated efforts to accomplish the same purpose.

If these instruments are not at hand, the next best method is to effect the removal with the syringe and warm water. A caution is to be given in the use of the syringe. There are a great number of people who are not able to have the external ear syringed, even though gently, without becoming giddy, and if the syringing is then continued the vertigo will end in a fainting attack. My rule is to caution the patient of the above fact, and always promptly stop at the first symptom of vertigo. Sometimes a short rest will allow the operator to proceed, but often it is necessary to postpone any further attempt at removal until a succeeding day. Always use quite warm water. If in a fair trial with the syringe it is found that the mass does not soften and break up, it is better to make an application of olive oil to it, and at a subsequent time repeat the attempt at removal. Soft masses of cerumen are best removed by the use of warm water and the syringe.

In some few cases inflammation of the external auditory canal will complicate the treatment, and the question will come up as to whether it is best under such circumstances to attempt the removal of the impacted mass. As a rule, the removal of the mass is the best means of combating such an inflammation, and therefore an attempt at removal should be made unless the inflammation is very acute, when treatment of this complication would be in order, and the removal of the plug deferred for the moment. In all cases the condition of the middle ear and hard pharynx should be noted after the removal of the impacted mass, and these parts often will need treatment.

Furuncle of External Auditory Canal (Acute Circumscribed Inflammation).

ETIOLOGY AND PATHOLOGY.—In a great number of cases furuncle is to be regarded as an evidence of general bodily debility. For example, in the richer classes it is often a result of over-dissipation, while in the poorer classes insufficient food, bad clothing, and such like are important factors. Local irritations of the external canal may cause the disease, such as rubbing the canal with a hairpin or toothpick to relieve itching. The use of alum and nitrate-of-silver washes in the canal will cause a furuncle in some cases. Furuncle occurs in the outer third of the canal as a rule, and often develops around a ceruminous gland, and will generally be followed by a number of others.

SYMPTOMS.—Pain is the most marked one—in the beginning of the attack of an intermittent character, with a tendency to increase toward and in the night; but as the attack advances pain becomes more marked, and may extend over the entire temporal region well down into the neck. The jaw movement also becomes very painful. The furuncle will rupture at any time, from the third day up to the tenth day, according to its location. The more deeply seated it is, the slower will be its progress toward maturity. The pain quickly disappears after the rupture, and then a short interval of rest is followed too often by the recurrence of the same disease. A varying degree of deafness is usually present, due to partial closure of the canal by the swollen soft tissues, and also it may be in rare cases through involvement of the tympanic cavity in the inflammation. Fever is often present. The great objective symptom will be the circumscribed swelling found in the cartilaginous portion of the canal and often along its anterior wall, and will show great increase of pain by but slight pressure. The swelling as it matures becomes more circumscribed, and will end in a pus collection and subsequent rupture.

DIAGNOSIS.—The disease most likely to be confounded with it would be an acute middle-ear inflammation, with involvement of the periosteum of the osseous part of the canal; but the history of the case would clear up this point.

The PROGNOSIS is favorable as to hearing, but with great probability of successive crops of the same disease.

TREATMENT.—The local application of heat and moisture is a remedy of great value, and a good method of application is to bend the head into a horizontal position, as by resting the side of the head on a table, and then fill up the external canal with water as warm as the ear will allow without causing pain; then quickly place over the auricle towels that have been dipped in very warm water and wrung dry by being twisted in a second towel, and over this a large pad of warm flannel or some similar covering. The heat and moisture will be retained for quite a time, and then the procedure can be repeated until relief from pain is obtained. In the interval the auricle is to be covered with a pad of cotton. A steam atomizer furnishes a convenient way of applying heat and moisture. Dry heat is sometimes preferred: a flannel bag filled with bran or hops and well warmed in a hot oven would carry out this indication; also a hop pillow moistened by hot whiskey is a good application.

An application of leeches affords great relief from pain. The best point to place a leech (which should be a Swedish leech) is just in front of the tragus. Two or three leeches can be applied at this place, and by encouraging the after-bleeding by warm applications any desired amount of blood can be taken. The after-bleeding can be readily controlled by the use of styptic cotton.

Incision of the Furuncle.—It is a mooted question as to whether an incision is capable of giving relief, and when it should be done. My own experience has been that the application of a leech has given greater relief than the use of a knife in those cases when the furuncle has been deep seated. Later on, when the swelling has become circumscribed and shows evidence of pus, the incision is clearly indicated.

General treatment is to be of a tonic character, and during the acute stage, when the pain is severe, anodynes are indicated.

Foreign Bodies in the External Auditory Canal.

1. VEGETABLE PARASITES.—Aspergillus flavescens and Aspergillus nigricans are found on the inner part of the canal and over the external surface of the tympanic membrane. This growth largely depends for its development upon a diseased condition of the epithelial layer of the skin lining the external canal, such as is found in cases of chronic middle-ear suppuration and in eczema of the skin of the external canal, by furnishing a moist nidus for its development.

SYMPTOMS.—Intense itching in the external canal, with a sense of fulness; also sometimes pain, with tinnitus and difficulty of hearing. The growth is found in the inner part of the canal, or over the surface of the tympanic membrane in the form of yellow or black flakes according to the variety. It may be found in spots or may form a complete covering to the canal-walls, so that when removed it forms a mould of the canal, leaving a raw skin surface, on which the growth rapidly reproduces itself. The disease is found in an acute and a chronic form, and in a few days can attain full development; also there exists a marked tendency to relapse as long as any portion remains undestroyed.

PROGNOSIS.—Favorable.

TREATMENT.—The main point is to thoroughly remove the parasite. This is best effected by the use of warm water and the syringe, carefully picking off any small portion that may remain by the forceps or curette. My practice is then to fill up the external canal with alcohol, allowing it to remain a few moments, and then to carefully dry the canal by the aid of styptic cotton. This procedure may have to be repeated every second day for a number of times until the growth is entirely destroyed. Wreden recommends the use of the hypochlorate of lime in the strength of one or two grains to the ounce of water, the salt to be freshly dissolved in water at each application. The condition of the middle ear and the integument of the external canal is to be considered after the removal of this growth, and treated as indicated by the state of the case.

2. INSECTS IN THE EXTERNAL AUDITORY CANAL.—Cases of this character occur frequently during the summer season to persons who by lying on the ground give insects an opportunity to crawl into the external canal. The common house-fly also affects an entrance into the canal quite often; also during the summer it is not uncommon to find grubs or larvæ in the canals of patients suffering from suppurative inflammation of the middle ear resulting from the deposit by insects of their eggs in the moist coverings of the canal. The movements of insects in the sensitive exter-

nal ear cause great pain to the patient, and their removal is sometimes difficult. For instance, the grub is provided with two hooks, by means of which it adheres tenaciously to the skin, so that it may be necessary to remove each one separately with the forceps. The quickest method of removal, as a rule, is to wash out the insect by the use of warm water and a syringe; and if this is not at hand the insect can be drowned by filling the canal with water, olive oil, or some demulcent liquid.

OTHER VARIETIES OF FOREIGN BODIES, such as grains of corn, beans, peas, cherry-stones, beads, buttons, pieces of slate-pencil, are found in the external canal, and the symptoms that are present arise partly from the presence of the body, but more frequently from the irritation produced by attempts at removal.

SUBJECTIVE SYMPTOMS.—Difficulty of hearing, often due to the foreign body filling up the external canal and thus excluding all sound-vibrations. Tinnitus aurium and vertigo are often present, and caused by pressure of the body on the tympanic membrane with resulting abnormal labyrinthine pressure; also a variety of reflex conditions are noted as a result of the presence of a foreign body in the external canal, such as coughing and vomiting, partial paralysis, etc.

OBJECTIVE SYMPTOMS.—The appearance of the external canal will depend greatly upon the amount of pressure that the foreign body has exerted. For instance, a body loosely lying in the canal will irritate but little; on the contrary, a hard body like a cherry-stone firmly impacted in the canal will quickly cause a severe inflammation.

DIAGNOSIS.—As a rule, the foreign body, can be readily seen with the aid of the mirror and speculum, unless the canal has become swollen to such an extent as to hide the body from sight. Probing and such-like procedures are not advisable.

TREATMENT.—The question comes up if it is good practice to make an attempt at immediate removal of a foreign body if the external canal is in a condition of acute inflammation. Unless grave head symptoms are present it is often good practice to delay, and reduce the inflammation by proper treatment, and then remove the foreign body. In other words, there is more risk by a forcible removal during a stage of acute inflammation than to permit the foreign body to remain until the inflammatory stage is past. Numbers of cases are on record where foreign bodies have remained for years in the external canal without causing serious sequelæ. Also, be sure a foreign body really exists in the canal, as it is not uncommon for patients to come with the statement that such is the case, and yet no foreign body has been discovered.

The majority of foreign bodies can be removed by the use of the syringe and warm water. The impacted bodies—and particularly those having a hard, smooth surface—present the greatest difficulties. A good plan is to try first the syringe and warm water, and if not successful try with a toothed angular forceps to grasp the body. If, as is often the case, it is found that the forceps slips off the body, then the curved blunt hook is to be used. This can be passed by the body and then turned on its axis, so that the hook is firmly placed behind it, and then a slow upward movement will often dislodge the body. On some occasions I have used two hooks, holding the body between them, and thus dragging it out. It is also better to desist after a fair trial until a succeeding day, rather than make excessive efforts at removal, which will often cause violent inflammation to follow. After the body is dislodged examine the condi_ tion of the tympanic membrane, as this is often found to be perforated by the foreign body.

Diseases of the Middle Ear.

ANATOMY.—The cavity of the middle ear is of small dimensions: antero-posterior diameter, 13 mm.; vertical diameter at the anterior part, 5.8 mm.; vertical diameter at the posterior part, 15 mm.; trans_ verse diameter at the anterior part, 3–4.5 mm.; transverse diameter at the opposite drumhead, 2 mm. (Von Tröltsch). It is situated in the petrous portion of the temporal bone and surrounded by bony walls, with the exception of the opening covered by tympanic membrane and the opening of the Eustachian tube, having a mucous periosteal covering, very thin, transparent, and colorless. This membrane covers not only the tympanic cavity, but is reflected over the chain of small bones and tendons of the tensor tympani and stapedius muscles. It is essentially a mucous membrane, and may be considered a continuation of the naso-pharyngeal mucous membrane reflected through the Eustachian tube to the middle-ear cavity; also subject to the same pathological changes as other mucous membranes.

The tympanic cavity normally is an air-filled cavity, and allows of free vibration of the tympanic membrane and its ossicles, as well as the membrane covering the oval and round foramina; and it is readily understood that any interference with the vibration of this sound-conducting apparatus will at once affect the hearing.

Its arterial blood is supplied from the middle meningeal, stylo-mastoid, ascendant pharyngeal, posterior auricular, tympanic, and internal carotid arteries. These freely anastomose with each other. The veins pass internally through minute openings of the petrosal squamous fissure to the veins of the dura mater, and thence into the superior petrosal sinus, and also externally into the venous ring surrounding the tympanic membrane, and also to the veins of the meatus (Schwartze). This is important to bear in mind, as furnishing an easy passage for the extension of middle-ear inflammation to the brain membranes.

The nerves forming the tympanic plexus are as follows : The mucous membrane is supplied by the tympanic plexus, formed from the tympanic branch of the petrous ganglion of the glosso-pharyngeal nerve—from the branch of the superficial petrosal and branches of the sympathetic nerve. The otic ganglion receives fibres from the inferior maxillary nerve, from the auriculo-temporal nerve, and from the sympathetic plexus, and it is distributed to the tensor tympani and tensor palati muscles.

The mastoid cells lead directly from the tympanum. They consist of one large opening, the antrum, and the lower mastoid cells. These cells consist of a large number of varying-sized cavities, and are enclosed by a dense layer of bone. The mucous membrane lining these cells is a direct extension of the tympanic membrane, and liable to the same pathological conditions as that mucous membrane.

The Eustachian tube connects the cavity of the tympanum with that of the naso-pharynx, and is mainly intended for the introduction of air into the tympanic cavity. It has a length of 35 mm., partly bone (11 mm. in length), partly cartilaginous (24 mm. in length). The pharyngeal opening is 8 mm. high and 5 mm. wide; the tympanic orifice, 5 mm. high and 3 mm. wide (Schwartze). The mucous membrane lining this canal is a continuation of that of the naso-pharynx, and affords an easy way for the transmission of disease from the naso-pharynx to the middle ear. The Eustachian tube at rest is probably closed, although this is a matter still discussed; but it is essential for normal hearing that the air-pressure exerted on the tympanic membrane through the external auditory canal should be equalized by that exerted through the Eustachian tube. This necessitates the opening of the tube from time to time for free admission of air into the tympanic cavity. This is accomplished by the action of the musculus dilator tubæ, the tensor veli palatini, and the salpino-pharyngeus muscle. In the act of swallowing the tube opens; also, if the nostrils are closed and the act of swallowing is performed, air will be pumped out of the middle ear; on the contrary, if the nostrils are open air will be forced into the middle ear.

Diseases of the middle ear can involve the superficial layers of the middle-ear mucous membrane only, and may be of a catarrhal character. Hyperæmia and swelling of the epithelial cells, with increased mucous secretion, will be found. Later on, if the inflammation assumes a higher degree, a serous fluid will be profusely poured out, with lessening of the mucous secretion. When the deeper epithelial cells are involved, then pus-cells often appear, and a suppurative process becomes established, with frequent destruction of the soft tissues of the middle ear.

These different grades of inflammation are seldom found distinct, but run one into another. A case can start as a pure catarrhal inflammation; this, after attaining its acme, may end in recovery or degenerate into a chronic catarrh; or, on the contrary, it may advance into an acute puru-lent inflammation with a subsequent chronic stage.

CAUSES OF INFLAMMATION OF THE MIDDLE EAR.—Change of tem-perature, causing a sudden cooling of the body, is a frequent cause of this disease; for instance, exposure to wind from a partly-open window, a sudden rush of cold water into the external canal, as in surf-bathing, etc. Irritating foreign bodies in the external auditory canal may also cause this disease.

But inflammation of the middle ear occurs most frequently as a sequela of diseases affecting the general body. Among these may be mentioned, in order of their relative importance—

1. Scarlet Fever.—This disease is apt to cause the purulent form of middle-ear inflammation, and often of a very grave character. The ear complication can occur during the existence of the rash or immediately after its cessation (Thomas), and may run a rapid course, causing destruc-tion of the tympanic membrane and middle-ear ossicles. Destruction of the facial nerve in its passage through its bony canal is not infrequent. Wendt has noticed in severe cases that the periosteum of the mastoid process, also that of the squamous and petrous portions, may participate in the purulent process, and end in subsequent caries of the bone. The severity of the ear complication will largely depend upon the condition

of the naso-pharyngeal mucous membrane. Light attacks of scarlet fever with slight throat symptoms would most probably cause slight irritation of the middle-ear mucous membrane, while the anginose variety would cause most violent inflammatory sequelæ.

2. Measles is apt to cause the catarrhal variety of middle-ear inflam_ mation rather than the purulent form. It occurs during and immediately after this eruption, and is a direct continuation of the naso-pharyngeal inflammation viâ the Eustachian tube. Hearing, as a rule, is diminished, due to the swollen mucous membrane of the Eustachian tube and middle ear, and also to fluid accumulations that often exist in the middle ear. Wendt[1] draws attention to the fact that chronic affections of the auditory apparatus, such as formation of adhesions between the ossicles or between the tympanic membrane and wall of the tympanum, may arise while the soft parts are in a swollen condition, and often chronic catarrhal sequelæ may be traced to this cause.

3. Tuberculosis is often associated with the catarrhal and purulent varieties of middle-ear inflammation, having, as a rule, a subacute course, the patient's attention sometimes only being drawn to his ear by the escape of pus from the middle ear into the external canal, the medium of communication being the mucous membrane of the pharynx viâ the Eustachian tube. Wendt[2] states that as yet the presence of tubercles has not been authenticated, although the clinical observations of rapid destruction, especially of the tympanic membrane, would seem to indicate it.

4. Retro-nasal catarrh is a frequent cause of middle-ear inflammation, the disease being communicated along the mucous membrane of the Eustachian tube. All degrees of inflammation are found, the catarrhal variety being the most frequent, while acute nasal catarrh is a cause of a large number of ear complications. Chronic retro-nasal catarrh is apt to cause a chronic middle-ear catarrh, that progresses insidiously, and almost unnoticed by the patient until the deafness begins to interfere with the ordinary affairs of life.

5. Scrofulosis causes most frequently the catarrhal form of middle-ear inflammation; and this is a direct continuation of the catarrhal affections of the naso-pharyngeal mucous membrane viâ the Eustachian tube. Birch-Hirschfeld[3] asserts that scrofulosis is the cause of the largest number of those cases in which weakening or destruction of the function of hearing has occurred during childhood; also, that the large number of scrofulous individuals found in deaf-and-dumb asylums is explained in this way; and that after the scrofulosis is cured the deafness remains as a result of permanent pathological middle-ear changes produced by the former disease.

6. Smallpox may cause several varieties of middle-ear hyperæmia, and frequently also a hemorrhagic catarrhal process is met with. Not seldom is found a suppurative inflammation, with extensive destruction of the soft tissues and ossicles, with permanent subsequent deafness. There is probably no reason to doubt that a pustule itself can develop in the middle-ear mucous membrane, just as is found in the cornea, and cause an acute inflammatory process; but, as a rule, the middle-ear mucous membrane is secondarily involved as a consequence of inflammatory process existing in the naso-pharyngeal mucous membrane.

[1] *Ziemssen*, ii. 112. [2] *Ibid.*, vii. 77. [3] *Ibid.*, xvi. 794.

7. Diphtheria is a cause of middle-ear inflammation. Wendt[1] states that in a fifth of the entire number of cases of croup and diphtheria; and in two-fifths of those cases in which the naso-pharyngeal space participated, but in no case without immediate connection with the corresponding affections of this space, he found an extension of the specific process into the middle ear. In some cases the tubal prominences were covered with membrane terminating at their orifices; in other cases a membranous cast of the cartilaginous portion of the tube was found. As a rule, the pathological changes noted were hyperæmia of the mucous membrane of the middle ear and catarrhal and purulent inflammation.

8. Syphilis causes most frequently the catarrhal variety of middle-ear inflammation; the purulent variety is also met with, but much less frequently, the disease of the naso-pharyngeal mucous membrane determining largely the grade of inflammation. Hereditary syphilis may cause this complication, as well as the primary disease, but not so frequently. Hutchinson has observed some cases of deafness in which the disease was situated either in the labyrinth or auditory nerve, the middle ear being healthy. Also, deafness may be caused by syphilitic affections of the external auditory canal, causing obstructions to sound-vibrations passing through it.

9. Typhoid fever may cause either the catarrhal or purulent form of middle-ear inflammation. For instance, Hoffmann[2] found fourteen cases of deep-seated disturbance of the faucial mucous membrane; he also met with perforation of the tympanic membrane four times—twice in connection with caries of the mastoid process.

It is easy to understand why middle-ear complications should complicate such a disease as typhoid fever, where the mucous membranes generally are the favorite seat of inflammation. Disease of the internal ear and auditory nerve are not uncommon after typhoid fever.

10. Bright's disease is a cause of hemorrhage into the middle ear. Schwartze reports in the year 1869 the case[3] of a young man who suffered from albuminuria with retinal hemorrhages; also, enlargement of the liver and spleen existed. He suddenly complained of pain in the right ear. The tympanic membrane was of a red color and devoid of concavity. Three days later an abundant serous discharge existed, with a small blood-coagulum, the patient dying a few days later of the kidney disease. Examination showed a hemorrhagic inflammation of the mucous membrane of the right tympanic cavity, which was also found filled with a bloody purulent fluid. The left tympanic cavity also was found filled with a similar fluid. A number of other similar cases are reported.

11. Whooping cough has been noted in several cases to have caused hemorrhage into the middle ear, with perforation of the tympanic membrane, with subsequent partial deafness.

The two principal types of acute middle-ear inflammation are the catarrhal and purulent; and these up to a certain stage have similar symptoms, but when pus has formed it gives rise to conditions that must be described as peculiar to purulent inflammation alone.

[1] *Ziemssen*, vii. 71.   [2] *Ibid.*, i. p. 159.
[3] *Archiv für Ohren Heilkunde*, Bd. iv. p. 12.

Acute Catarrh of the Middle Ear.

This may be described as acute catarrh of the mucous membrane lining the middle-ear cavity. The prominent symptoms are as follows :

1. Pain—This is, as a rule, of the most violent character. It is described as a boring or tearing pain situated in the ear itself, and often extending over the entire temporal region : any muscular exertion like swallowing or sneezing causes increase of it. The external ear becomes swollen, and so exquisitely tender to the touch that the least pressure over the tragus causes the patient to flinch very markedly. The pain tends to increase during the night up to the early morning hours, and to lessen during the day. The immediate effect of a middle-ear inflam_mation is to render the entire region of that side of the face tender, so that any movement of the jaws or neck becomes painful. It is also not uncommon to find the sympathetic glands of the neck becoming enlarged and tender, and they may go on to suppuration. The adult will complain most vigorously of the pain, so that there will be no difficulty in locating it; but in the infant or young child the greatest difficulty may be experienced in determining its precise seat, owing to its inability to express in language its suffering. Two points may be mentioned as aids in the diagnosis: (*a*) the cry of a young child suffering from an acute inflammation of the middle ear has a peculiar shrill, continuous character, an intermission sufficient only to inspire being noticed ; (*b*) pressure over the tragus of an inflamed middle ear will cause a quick shrinking away of the little sufferer, thus showing the seat of the disease.

2. Loss of Hearing Power.—This depends partly on a lessening of the vibratory power of the conducting apparatus, partly due to a thickened tympanic membrane, and also to the fact that the mucous membrane covering the middle ear and chain of small bones becomes swollen, and so clogs their movements. Again, the tympanum may be filled with a mucous or muco-serous fluid, instead of being an air-chamber, as in the normal condition, so that vibrations of the conducting apparatus may cease entirely, while at the same time increase of intra-labyrinthine pressure takes place. A tuning-fork placed on the incisor teeth or on the forehead is heard more distinctly on the deaf side, due to the sound-vibrations being retarded in their outward passage through the diseased middle ear ; also, the voice of the patient is heard by himself with increased resonance, due to the same cause (retarded sound-vibrations), and the patient unconsciously lowers the voice below its normal tone.

3. Giddiness is not uncommon, due partly to increase of labyrinthine pressure, and in some cases to a sympathetic irritation and congestion of the vessels of the basilar brain membrane. Fever is always to be looked for in acute middle-ear disease.

4. Noises in the ear (tinnitus aurium), resembling the noise produced by the escape of steam or the singing of crickets, etc., are common, and are due to a variety of causes. For instance, a large number of these noises (according to Theobold's theory) depend upon muscle and blood-vessel movements, causing vibrations that in a normal condition pass out through the external auditory canal without being noticed ; but if their outward passage is impeded by obstructions existing in the middle ear, like thickened tissue or the existence of fluids, as mucus or pus, or by

obstructions in the external auditory canal itself, such as impacted cerumen, etc., then these vibrations are thrown back and impress for a second time the auditory nerve-endings, and thus become noticeable sounds. (A familiar example is to shut the external auditory canal by closing the meatus: a tidal noise is at once noticed.) A crackling noise is often caused by air entering the middle ear and bubbling up through the confined fluids.

OBJECTIVE SYMPTOMS.—The tympanic membrane is at first slightly injected, particularly along the manubrium and the anterior and posterior folds; but as the inflammation advances the entire membrane becomes intensely injected and red. The cone of light is either very small or may be entirely absent, due to the membrane having lost its high reflective power. At this stage exudations into the middle ear frequently show themselves, and if of sufficient quantity may cause an outward bulging of the membrane: frequently the tympanic membrane at its lower third becomes less transparent, and in some cases fluid collections show a dark border-line stretching across the tympanic membrane, and movable by change of position of the head.

DIAGNOSIS.—This disease can be hardly mistaken: the only difficulty that can arise is whether the case is one of simple acute catarrh or is one of commencing purulent inflammation, as the symptoms are identical in each up to the formation and escape of pus, when no doubt can arise.

TREATMENT.—This must be directed against the acute inflammation that exists, then as quickly as possible to restore the mucous membrane to its normal condition and return to the sound-conducting apparatus its normal vibrating power.

Local bleeding is to be considered among the most important remedies, and therefore is taken first. This is best done by the use of the Swedish leech, applied to the tragus, as at this point the blood is most easily drawn from the tympanic cavity, in number from one to three; and if the taking of a larger quantity of blood is desired, this can be accomplished by encouraging the after-bleeding by hot fomentations. When great pain exists, when the auricle is tender and pressure on the tragus produces marked increase of pain, the application of a leech is indicated. In children it is best to refrain from the use of leeches.

The use of heat and moisture is most valuable. An effective method of application is as follows: Place the head of the patient in a horizontal position, with the affected ear turned upward, and fill the external auditory canal with water at the temperature, say, of 100° Fahr. Place quickly over the auricle towels that have been dipped in very hot water and wrung out as dry as possible, and over these a large flannel pad. This makes an excellent dressing, and one retaining the heat and moisture for a length of time. When it cools repeat the same proceeding until relief is obtained, when a large dry cotton pad can take the place of the previous dressing. Patients suffering from acute catarrh of the middle ear should be confined to the house, and, still better, to bed. All physical exercise aggravates this disease, and a suitable anodyne may be given to procure sleep if it be found necessary. Paracentesis of the tympanic membrane is sometimes indicated in those cases where the membrane shows distinct bulging and perforation is clearly close at hand; also in some cases where, notwithstanding previous treatment, the pain still continues with great severity. This operation is best done by incising the posterior half of the membrane by means of a broad paracentesis needle. The incision should be made at a point midway between the periphery of the membrane and the handle of the hammer, and on the dividing-line of the upper and lower posterior quadrants, the cut to be made downward. Paracentesis of the membrane is to be done while the head of the patient is well supported and the membrane illuminated by means of a light reflected from the head-mirror. Immediately after the operation wet hot flannels should be applied to the ear to relieve the pain.

The condition of the pharyngeal and nasal mucous membrane should be thoroughly attended to, as from this source a large number of cases of acute middle-ear catarrh have their origin. Nitrate-of-silver solutions are often of great service as a local application to the naso-pharynx. Tannic acid makes a good astringent gargle, and is more particularly adapted to those cases where a pure astringent effect is needed. Chlorate of potash is an excellent gargle, and often proves of great service. It may not be out of place to state that the use of alcohol and tobacco tends to keep up an irritated condition of the naso-pharyngeal mucous membrane, and they should be dispensed with. As part of the treatment inflations of the middle ear are used to aid in the removal of abnormal secretions from the tympanic cavity and to restore the sound-conducting apparatus to its normal condition. This can be thoroughly carried out by the Politzer proceeding. This consists in forcing air (by compressing a rubber hand-bag, Politzer's air-bag, so called) through the lower nasal passage up the Eustachian tube, and so into the middle ear. The patient holds a small quantity of water in the mouth. The nasal end of the tubing connected with the air-bag is placed in one of the lower nasal passages, and the nose tightly closed over it. The patient is then told to swallow, and at the same moment the air-bag is forcibly compressed, and the air is thus compelled to travel along the nasal passage and up the Eustachian tube into the middle ear. The act of swallowing causes the soft palate to be forcibly pressed up against the posterior pharyngeal wall, and at the same time causes the Eustachian tube orifice to open widely. A column of air thus used will expel large accumulations of mucus from the Eustachian tube, and to some extent from the middle-ear cavity, and at the same time the thorough distension of this cavity throws into motion the tympanic membrane and chain of small bones—a most desirable proceeding. In acute conditions the inflation should be made only after all pain has ceased, and then at first very gently; but in a short time a thorough inflation two or three times repeated, say every two or three days, is most beneficial. The inflation of the middle ear by the use of the Eustachian catheter is a more irritating procedure, and does not accomplish the purpose any more completely than the Politzer method. Therefore the latter is to be preferred in adults, while in children it is the only available method that can be used.

Chronic Catarrh of the Middle Ear.

Various classifications of this disease have been made by different authors: I prefer the division that Buck has used in his textbook. The following summary will give an idea of it:

Chronic catarrh is a name that has been given to a class of cases where deafness and tinnitus are prominent symptoms, and where no suppurative action in the middle ear has existed at any previous time, and where the internal ear is supposed to be in a healthy condition. In some of these cases there will be found a marked hypertrophy of the mucous membrane, and sometimes of the submucous connective tissue, accompanied with excess of secretion, with the same condition existing in the nasopharyngeal membrane. The tympanic membrane often becomes sunken, and therefore strongly concave outwardly. The short process of the malleus is very prominent, and the handle of the malleus, by being drawn forcibly backward, becomes apparently shortened (foreshortening of the malleus handle, so called).

The membrane loses its vibratory power to some extent, and the cone of light is either very small or is entirely absent. The color of the membrane changes to a more or less opaque white, with often a line of vascularity along the manubrium, or it may assume the color of ground glass; white calcareous deposits are not seldom met with; marked evidences of catarrhal inflammation exist in the naso-pharynx, such as increase of mucoid secretion, with enlargements of the tonsils, and often granular pharyngitis may be found. The mucous membrane of the Eustachian tube is often involved in the process: marked swelling of its mucoid tissue, with the tube filled with secretions, prevents free entrance of air into the middle-ear cavity. In the nasal mucous membrane, beyond the ordinary catarrhal conditions, polypoid formations are common; also thickening of the mucoid and submucoid tissues prevents the free passage of air.

In another class of cases coming under the head of chronic catarrh of the middle ear a very different set of symptoms from the class first described are noticeable. In these cases perhaps catarrhal symptoms have at one time existed, but have completely passed away, and the mucous membrane not only of the tympanic cavity, but also of the pharynx and Eustachian tube, has undergone a fibroid degeneration, causing destruction of the glandular elements and ending in an atrophied mucous membrane (the so-called proliferous degeneration of some authors). The tympanic membrane in these cases is abnormally thin and very transparent, sometimes much sunken, no doubt due to connective-tissue adhesions in the middle-ear cavity. The external auditory canal is devoid of cerumen and hair; also the same change in the mucous membrane of the nasopharynx and Eustachian tube gives a smooth, transparent appearance to their surface. In this class of cases in post-mortem examinations there have been found the stapes firmly ankylosed to the margin of the fenestra ovalis; the chain of small bones firmly ankylosed; fibroid adhesions in the mastoid cells; and adhesions between the tympanic membrane and the labyrinthine wall.

CAUSES.—A percentage of cases result from a previous acute middle-ear catarrh. Others apparently originate as a chronic condition and slowly advance. Beyond all doubt, a large percentage are inherited, as the same disease can be traced back through several generations, where signs of the disease were noted in early youth, with slow advance as years go on. It is also a matter of interest to note that these cases are apt to show sensible advance in women at the birth of a child.

PROGNOSIS, as a rule, bad, both as to the possibility of preventing increase of deafness and of doing away with tinnitus—a most annoying factor.

TREATMENT is successful in proportion to the catarrhal symptoms that exist, and which are to be treated on the general plan laid down for catarrhal inflammation. A great number of these cases call for a tonic plan of treatment, such as iron tonics, cod-liver oil, etc.

Local treatment consists in inflations of the middle ear by the Politzer method. In those cases where a thin, sunken membrane exists care should be observed not to use undue pressure, lest a rupture of the membrane result. In those cases where tinnitus aurium is a prominent factor a few drops of ether placed in the Politzer bag cause a more stimulating effect from the inflation than the use of pure air, and is sometimes of service in lessening this annoyance. It is an important part of the treatment that the general health should be in the most vigorous possible condition.

Acute Purulent Inflammation of the Middle Ear.

The disease proceeds very frequently from some inflammation in the naso-pharyngeal cavity, the mucous membrane of the Eustachian tube furnishing a ready way of communication between the pharynx and middle ear.

The exanthematous diseases furnish a large proportion of these cases. Scarlet fever stands first on the list, as causing the largest number of these cases, and also those of the most serious character. Measles, smallpox, diphtheria, the different forms of fever, such as typhus and typhoid, cerebro-spinal meningitis, pneumonia, bronchitis, etc., are complicated by this form of inflammation, and the ear disease represents simply a continuation of the naso-pharyngeal inflammation which occurs so frequently in the above-mentioned diseases. Another set of causes come under the head of change of temperature, such as exposure to draughts of air and sea-bathing, where the cold water entering the external auditory canal acts directly upon the tympanic membrane. Some few cases occur as the result of injury, such as blows upon the ear or direct injuries to the tympanic membrane.

COURSE.—The same pathological conditions are to be noted here as in the acute catarrhal attack, with the difference that the inflammation goes on to a higher grade—namely, pus-formation. In this form of disease there exists marked hyperæmia and swelling, not only of the superficial but also of the deep-seated tissue, with pus-formation, and generally perforation of the tympanic membrane, with occasional ulceration and destruction of other parts of the middle ear. The neighboring cavities of the antrum and mastoid cells participate more or less, while blood-vessels penetrating the superior wall of the middle ear furnish a ready means of communication between the inflamed middle-ear tissues and the brain-membrane, so that the wonder is not that brain complications result, but that they occur so seldom.

The changes in the tympanic membrane in the first stage are marked hyperæmia and swelling of the tissue, so that it often assumes a uniform red appearance, without a trace of the malleus or cone of light. Pus-formation in the middle ear is quickly followed by bulging of the tympanic membrane, due to increase of middle-ear pressure; and this in the great majority of cases is followed by perforation of the tympanic membrane, due not only to increase of pressure, but also to a destructive ulcerative process in the membrane itself. The latter process is seen in those cases of great destruction of the tympanic membrane that occurs in scarlet fever, where almost entire destruction of the membrane is often found. Perforation may occur at any part of the membrane.

SYMPTOMS AND COURSE.—These are very much the same, up to a certain point, pus-formation, as have been described under the head of Acute Catarrh—namely, the great pain, deafness, tinnitus, headache, tenderness on pressure over the tragus, increase of pain by movement of the jaw, followed often by quick relief by perforation of the membrane and escape of pus through the external auditory canal, with a subsequent, subsidence of inflammation and restoration of the tympanic membrane. A moderate attack may run a course of from two to six weeks, and end in entire recovery, or it may end in a chronic suppuration with its sequelæ.

DIAGNOSIS.—It often will be difficult at the outset to know if the case is one of acute catarrh or whether it will advance to a purulent inflammation; but as the disease goes on to pus-development and subsequent drum-perforation, no doubt can exist as to its true character. The perforation can often be seen, and air may be forced through it with a whistling sound by a forcible expiration of the patient. In regard to whether complications exist, such as mastoid or brain involvement, several points can be given as aids in the diagnosis. When mastoid involvement exists, the soft tissues over it become swollen, very tender on pressure, with pain in that part of the bone; also, often swelling of the posterior upper wall of the external auditory canal, a part adjacent to the mastoid process.

In those cases where the inflammation tends toward the cranial cavity, the pain spreads over the entire side of the head, and often becomes marked in the occipital and frontal regions, and is of a peculiar lancinating character. Vertigo is also present, even if the head is in a quiet horizontal position, but greatly increased by movement of the head. The body-temperature in acute purulent inflammation in adults is not altered as a rule, but in children it is raised.

PROGNOSIS.—An uncomplicated case if properly treated will generally result in a good recovery, and often with but slight impairment of the hearing power. If allowed to run its course, it may cause serious and permanent changes in the middle ear destructive to hearing, and may end either in a chronic purulent inflammation with bone destruction or in involvement of brain membranes or brain tissue proper.

TREATMENT.—In the early stages absolutely the same treatment as recommended for acute catarrh is indicated—the use of leeches, hot-water applications, rest in bed, anodynes, etc. When pus has formed and the tympanic membrane is bulging, paracentesis is indicated (method of operation, vide p. 917), to be quickly followed by the use of hot water to relieve the pain of the operation; the gentle use of the syringe and warm water will keep the canal free of pus during the suppurative process; also the external ear is to be kept covered by a cotton pad or some other like application as long as pain and tenderness exist.

In young children suffering from scarlet fever it is of the utmost importance to cleanse frequently the pharynx of its muco-purulent secretions. This can be done by means of a probang or cotton wrapped on a curved end of whalebone, and afterward some detergent wash can be used, such as a strong decoction of green tea containing alum or a solution of common salt. The muriated tincture of iron, one part to five parts of water, is an excellent local application to be applied with a camel's-hair brush. Chlorate of potash makes a valuable gargle. In young children Meigs suggests the use of a powder containing one part of chlorate of potash to six parts of sugar, and a pinch of this placed on the tongue and allowed to dissolve.

By such a plan of treatment an acute purulent case will be best carried over the acute stage, and in many instances will end in entire recovery without the necessity of local treatment; but in some cases the purulent discharge from the middle ear will continue, and it remains to consider the best local remedies for checking this discharge and when they are to be used. It is with me an absolute rule that no remedy is to be used with a view of checking a purulent discharge until absolutely all pain has passed away and no pain is caused by pressure on the tragus or over the mastoid. During the interval the local treatment will consist of cleansing the external canal from the contained pus by the use of the syringe and warm water, the canal being afterward dried by cotton on a cotton-holder. If the discharge is small in quantity, the use of cotton on a cotton-holder will be sufficient to cleanse the canal, and causes less irritation than the syringe and warm water. The frequency with which the ear is to be cleansed will depend upon the amount of the discharge, as it should be done as little as is consistent with keeping the external canal free from pus. It is also useful for the patient by the Valsalva method of self-inflation to cleanse the middle ear from the therein-contained pus just before the time of using the syringe. If this is not feasible, the Politzer method of inflation answers the same purpose. When all pain has passed away, and if the discharge still continues, it will be proper to make a local application. My favorite one is insufflation of a small quantity of finely-powdered boracic acid (a convenient rubber blower is made for this purpose). This application answers well also in chronic purulent middle-ear affections. In applying this powder a very small portion only is to be used, so that there can be no danger of blocking the discharge by the powder obstructing its passage through the middle-ear cavity. A small portion is to be placed in an insufflator and blown in, the application to be repeated every few days. I would also mention the great importance of keeping the external canal closed by a wad of absorbent cotton, which not only absorbs the pus as it slowly escapes, but also prevents the immediate contact of air with the middle-ear cavity—a most desirable aid in the cure.

Chronic Purulent Inflammation of the Middle Ear.

Urbantschitsch[1] calls attention to two distinct pathological conditions that are to be noted in this disease—the one a swelling and hypertrophy,

[1] Vide *Textbook*, p. 351.

the other a thinning, of the mucous and submucous tissues. The thickening consists in an infiltration, with subsequent connective-tissue development, either in the submucous or over the free surface of the mucous membrane, causing in the first case a diffuse tissue hypertrophy; in the latter case forming a circumscribed connective-tissue formation, papillary excrescences, and nodes. The condition accompanied with thinning of the tissue is to be considered a higher grade of purulent inflammation, by which it results that a portion of the normally existing tissue disappears, and is not again reproduced, while the newly-developed inflammatory products do not advance to organization, but are thrown off in the purulent discharge. In this way can be explained why at one time, by examination through the external canal and perforated tympanic membrane, there is found a swollen connective tissue, while at another time the bone can be seen through the thinned membrane.

CAUSES.—As a rule, it is a sequela of a previous acute attack. And it is also safe to say that a large number of chronic purulent cases are the result of bad treatment or non-treatment of the acute attack. To mention the causes of chronic suppuration is to repeat those causing the acute variety, such as diseases of the naso-pharynx resulting from scarlatina, variola, measles, typhus, tuberculosis, bronchitis, syphilis, etc.; also the external irritating causes, effect of change of temperature, as by draughts of air, cold water entering the external auditory canal, etc.

SUBJECTIVE SYMPTOMS.—Difficulty of hearing is always present. This is often caused by masses of granulations or collections of pus, filling up largely the tympanic cavity. These with a hypertrophied mucous membrane could sensibly interrupt sound-vibrations; and it will not be out of place to remark that the recovery of hearing will depend largely on what amount of change can be effected in these different conditions. Tinnitus aurium is not a constant factor; a few patients suffer from discomfort caused by pus passing down the pharynx, causing nausea.

OBJECTIVE SYMPTOMS.—More or less swelling of the external canal, while the constant passage of purulent fluids over the skin results in exfoliation of its epithelial layer and a subsequent weeping from the skin tissue. The secretion varies from an abundant discharge to a minimum of a few drops per day. It may be watery or muco-purulent, or of a thick, creamy, tenacious consistence. Odor is common, and if the bone is involved of a most disagreeable character. The perforation in the tympanic membrane may vary in size from that of a pin-head to a loss of the greater part of the entire membrane; also, the membrane is found thickened, with an occasional calcareous deposit in its fibrous layer. Granulations and polypoid growths are found in the external canal and middle-ear cavity. The mucous membrane of the naso-pharynx will show the various changes that are found associated with the different diseases that cause this complication.

DIAGNOSIS.—This is without difficulty as a rule. The discharge, the perforation that often can be seen, the whistling caused by the air being forced through the middle ear and the perforation in the tympanic membrane by the Valsalva or Politzer method of inflation, are very significant of middle-ear suppuration. The pulsation often noticed at the bottom of the external auditory canal, and which has been considered indicative of perforation, is caused by a thin surface of fluid in contact with a

pulsating blood-vessel, and therefore is not necessarily a sign of perfora_
tion of the tympanic membrane, as fluids are found in the external
auditory canal from inflammation of its coats, and in such a case pulsa_
tion might occur; but this is but seldom the case, and the removal of the
fluid would remove any doubt as to whether the fluid was a result of
external-ear inflammation or caused by purulent middle-ear disease.

The course of a chronic purulent inflammation is very variable. In
many cases under proper treatment healing and restoration of tissue go
on rapidly. The secretion grows daily less and of a thicker consistence,
and the mucous membrane of the middle ear rapidly returns to a normal
condition. The perforation in the tympanic membrane becomes smaller,
and often entirely closes, so that in a young person the restoration may
be so complete that it is difficult to know where the seat of perforation
has been. In one case in my practice in a child of ten years, where the
membrane had been destroyed to at least three-fourths of its extent, a
full restoration took place. In another class of cases the course is not
so favorable. The tympanic membrane is largely destroyed, and is not
regenerated. The chain of small bones may be either partly or entirely
lost. Granulations form in the mucous membrane of the middle ear, and
the bony walls of the tympanum undergo partial necrosis, the pus appearing as an acrid, irritating fluid with more or less odor. The graver complications of purulent inflammation are apt to occur in those cases of
chronic purulent inflammation where there has been a stoppage of the
free discharge of pus from the middle ear, causing it to collect in the
antrum and mastoid cells.

TREATMENT.—The first indication is to cleanse as thoroughly as possible the middle-ear cavity of the muco-purulent fluid that may have collected. This is best accomplished by forcing air up the Eustachian tube
and through the middle ear by either the Politzer or Valsalva method
of inflation. The fluids thus forced out into the external canal can be
removed by the use either of warm water and the syringe if large in
amount, or by cotton on a cotton-holder if small in quantity : the latter
plan is less irritating, and also completely dries the external canal. No
local application ought to be made as long as any pain exists.

The local applications that my experience has shown to give the best
results consist of boracic acid and iodoform. (The latter is objectionable
on account of its odor.) The powder-insufflator furnishes a convenient
method of applying these powders, and only small quantities should be
used, so that no possible plugging of the middle ear can take place.
Some authorities prefer fluid applications instead of powder. Weak solutions of sulphate of zinc, from one to four grains to the ounce, are frequently used : a few drops, warmed, are poured into the external canal
and allowed to remain a short time, and then removed by a twisted tuft
of cotton on a cotton-holder. Nitrate-of-silver solutions are to be used
on a cotton-holder ; and if a very strong solution is used it should be
neutralized with salt and water.

The frequency of application of any remedy will depend upon the amount
of discharge; but as the discharge lessens, so should the remedy be less
frequently applied. The same rule applies to the cleansing of the ear, as
I have no doubt that excessive use of the syringe often tends to re-establish and increase the discharge. In some cases, where the discharge has

become very small in quantity, a thick scab will form over the tympanic perforation, and· restoration of the tympanic membrane will rapidly advance under such a covéring, showing that it is good practice not to remove such a scab, provided pus is not thereby prevented from escaping. A cotton plug should always be worn in the external canal of a purulent ear, as it acts as an absorbent of the purulent secretions, as well as protects the middle ear from the irritating contact of the air.

The naso-pharyngeal cavities are to be considered and appropriately treated ; also, a general tonic treatment is often indicated.

SEQUELÆ OF PURULENT INFLAMMATION.—I. Brain involvement, either of the meninges or its substance proper: *a*, purulent meningitis ; *b*, abscess of the brain ; *c*, phlebitis with thrombosis of the sinuses. II. Mastoid disease.

I. Brain Involvement.

It will be proper for a clear understanding of the subject to briefly consider the anatomy of the middle-ear cavity with reference to this complication. The middle-ear cavity is practically surrounded by bony walls, with the exception of the foramen closed by the tympanic membrane and the opening of the Eustachian tube. The roof of the middle ear is of varying thickness, and is perforated by a number of canals for the passage of blood-vessels, forming a direct communication between the circulation of the middle ear and the meninges of the brain; also, the petro-squamous suture in the earlier years of life before complete ossification has set in provides a way for spreading of the inflammatory process from the tympanum to the brain tissue ; also, cases are recorded where caries has formed actual openings in this bony roof, through which pus has entered into the brain cavity. The floor of the tympanic cavity is very thin, and forms a fossa in which lies the jugular vein, so that involvement of this vein in the inflammatory process could occur by the close apposition of these parts. The anterior wall is formed in part by the carotid canal, and cases are noted where defects in this bony wall are found. Under such circumstances the coats of the artery would lie in direct contact with the middle-ear membranes. Also, it is to be noted that small twigs from the carotid artery pass through its bony canal and anastomose with vessels of the middle ear, furnishing a way for the spread of inflammation from the middle ear to the carotid artery that may result in thickening of its walls.

The superior and posterior surfaces of the petrous bone are in direct contact with the brain membranes. The posterior wall contains the passage into the mastoid cells by way of the antrum, through which middle-ear inflammations spread and involve the mastoid cell cavities, and may result in some cases in thrombosis of the transverse sinus.

The inner wall presents two weak points—the one the round foramen, covered with membrane ; the other, the oval foramen, covered with the stirrup and the annular ligament. Inflammation can cause destruction of these coverings and give free access of pus through their foramina into the labyrinth, and thence through the internal auditory canal into the brain cavity. It is not difficult, therefore, with so many ways of communication between the middle ear and brain cavity to have easy spread of inflammation between these two regions.

. (*a*) PURULENT MENINGITIS may arise from continuance of the inflamma tion along the veins which penetrate the roof of the tympanic cavity in their passage from the middle ear to anastomose with the blood-vessels of the meninges, or may in rare instances be caused by pus entering the brain cavity by way of the internal ear, or it can result from caries of the petrous portion of the temporal bone.

SYMPTOMS.—Fever will be present; distressing headache; vertigo, a most significant symptom, and often present even when the head is quiet and in a horizontal position, but greatly increased by the vertical posi- tion and motion; pain of a lancinating character, shooting over the entire affected side and even down the neck; the occiput and vertex are favorite points for pain to locate. Nausea and hiccough are present. Abdomen depressed; pupils reacting to light but feebly; slow pulse; and in some cases paralytic symptoms are prominent. Post-mortem appearance: men inges congested, and lymph and pus often found at various points. Dura mater over the diseased petrous bone will be found thick, congested, and pus may be found between it and the bone. Caries of the petrous bone also is found in some cases.

(*b*) ABSCESS OF THE BRAIN.—With the exception of wounds and injuries, chronic purulent middle-ear inflammation is the most frequent cause of brain abscess. Meyer, in a collection of 89 cases of brain abscess tabulates the causes as follows: Typhus, 1; intercranial tumor, 2; disease of nasal mucous membrane, 3; disease of the blood-vessels, 5; inflamma tion of neighboring parts of the brain, 5; unknown causes, 11; suppura tion of distant organs, especially the lungs, 19; caries of the petrous bone, 20; injuries, 21. Lebert collected 80 cases of brain abscess, and found that one-fourth were caused by purulent middle-ear inflammation, caries of the petrous bone being frequently present; in one-seventh of the cases the brain abscess appeared before puberty, in the remaining cases mostly between the sixteenth and thirtieth years; also, that in some cases the abscess developed in the part of the brain lying over the bony roof of the middle ear; in other cases it was found in a distant part of the brain or the cerebellum, probably developing as a metastatic abscess. Toynbee considered the retention of purulent products in the middle ear or mastoid cells as the chief cause of brain complications from ear sources: he also endeavored to show that an inflammation of the external auditory canal will tend to implicate the cerebellum and lateral sinus—that inflam - mation of the middle-ear cavity would extend to the cerebrum, and that of the labyrinth to the medulla oblongata. But, practically, such a rule will not hold good, and Gull has modified Toynbee's law as follows: The cerebellum and lateral sinus may suffer from mastoid disease, while the cerebrum is threatened by caries of the roof of the tympanic cavity.

Brain abscess is generally located in the medullary substance, very rarely in the cortex. The middle portion of the brain hemisphere is the most frequent seat of abscess, and very often in that part adjacent to the diseased ear. The abscess may be located directly over the diseased bone, so that the dura mater forms its covering on one side and the brain tissue on the other, or it may be located in the brain parenchyma with perfectly healthy brain tissue between it and the diseased bone. Meyer traces the origin of a brain abscess from ear disease in this manner: A chronic catarrh of the middle-ear mucous membrane results in an hypertrophy of the mucosa on one side and a chronic inflammation of the neighboring bone on the other side. Caries of the petrous bone, so caused, produces inflammation and adhesion of the dura mater, and from here as a starting-point the inflammation spreads into the brain tissue. In rare cases the brain abscess has been found connected by a fistulous tract with the diseased bone.

SYMPTOMS.—Headache is generally present in varying degree, often of a lancinating character. Vertigo frequently present. Fever generally present, with or without chill. Convulsions frequent, with loss of consciousness and unsteadiness of gait, and often paralysis of different parts of the body. The pupils are often contracted, and not unfrequently this disease may closely resemble typhus fever. Lebert noticed in his cases that failure of the intellect was not the rule, but paralysis of sensibility occurred in two-thirds of them. It is also to be noted that cases occur where all these symptoms are absent. This disease can run an acute or chronic course. In the acute condition a fatal termination is caused by the great destruction of brain tissue involved in the suppurative process. In the chronic cases the abscess becomes encapsulated, but finally terminates by rupture of the abscess and escape of pus into the ventricles or over the surface of the brain. In Lebert's cases the fatal termination occurred in half of them during the first month, in one-third of the remainder toward the end of the second month, and in the remaining cases in a varying time between the third and eighth months.

(c) PHLEBITIS WITH THROMBOSIS.—This sequela of middle-ear suppuration is not infrequent. Von Dusch in 32 cases of phlebitis with thrombosis found that purulent middle-ear disease was the cause of 20 of them. It is frequently found in the venous sinuses in proximity to the petrous portion of the temporal bone, especially in the lateral and petrosal sinuses, and often caused by caries of the petrous bone.

Phlebitis with thrombosis of the lateral sinus is characterized by a swelling of the mastoid region which extends downward into the neck, due to an extension of the phlebitis from the lateral sinus along the veins leading from that sinus through the mastoid process to the exterior of the skull. Giddiness and unsteady gait are often present. If the inflammation involves also the superior longitudinal sinus, it will cause symptoms such as epileptic convulsions and violent hemorrhage from the nose. Wreden considers that the epileptic seizure is due to a capillary hemorrhage in the cortical substance of the posterior cerebral lobes, caused by obstruction of the veins passing over the brain substance. The nose-bleeding is due to the fact that a part of the blood circulating through the veins of the nasal passages, and then through the superior longitudinal sinus, is hindered by the sinus obstruction and accumulates in the veins of the nasal passages, and finally causes a rupture in some part.

Phlebitis with Thrombosis of the Cavernous Sinus.—Urbantschitsch gives the following summary of this complication:[1] A thrombosis of the cavernous sinus can be caused by a thrombus in the internal jugular or facial veins or by a clot passing from the superior petrosal sinus into the

[1] Vide *Textbook*, p. 367.

cavernous sinus, or, finally, by inflammation and thrombosis in the venous circulation of the carotid canals.

PROMINENT SYMPTOMS.—Retro-bulbar œdema and exophthalmos, caused by stoppage of the blood from passing from the orbit into the cavernous sinus. This may result in a mechanical compression of the retinal vessels and temporary blindness; also, occasionally swellings appear about the eyelids and nose. Compression of the oculo-motor and abducens nerves as they pass along the outer wall of this sinus may cause paralysis of these nerves, and consequent inward turning of the eye, with ptosis of the eyelids; also, pressure on a branch of the fifth pair of nerves as it passes along the outer wall of the sinus may cause neuralgia in the parts supplied by the branch, or neuralgia in the supraorbital region.

Phlebitis with thrombosis of the internal jugular vein is marked by a well-defined swelling extending from the angle of the jaw downward along the line of the sterno-cleido-mastoid muscle, painful on pressure, with marked distension of the veins of the face and neck, especially the external jugular vein. Later on, when the collateral circulation is established, the superficial veins are apt to return to their former calibre. If the inflammation extends downward, it can involve the vena cava; and if upward, the facial veins, causing a swelling of the cheeks and eyelids. The process can also extend from the facial to the orbital veins, and thence into the cavernous sinus. Pressure of the thromboid mass on the internal jugular vein, on the glosso-pharyngeal hypoglossus and pneumo-gastric nerves at the opening of the jugular foramen, will cause nervous symptoms corresponding to the nerve involved.

PROGNOSIS of a phlebitis with thrombosis, as a rule, is unfavorable. Chronic middle-ear suppuration can also form a starting-point of meta-static abscess, also of tubercular formations in the lungs and other organs of the body. I have also been much impressed with the frequent occur-rence of kidney complications, such as granular nephritis, in this disease. A gradual absorption of pus will develop a general bodily weakness, and it is a fairly well established fact that, as a rule, patients suffering from chronic middle-ear suppuration are not apt to be long lived: many life insurance companies now order that this disease will prevent the case from being considered a first-class risk.

II. Mastoid Disease.

The mastoid process of the temporal bone presents an outer convex with an inner concave surface. On the upper and posterior borders of the bone are found several canals, through which the external vessels form a union with those of the dura mater; also, by which the outer cranial veins form a union with the transverse sinus. There is also an important suture—the petro-squamous suture, which admits of the pas-sage of blood- and lymph-vessels. These vessels furnish a channel for the spread of inflammation from the antrum outwardly, involving the tissues of the neck, and inwardly to the brain membranes and brain tissue proper; phlebitis with thrombosis of the lateral sinus can also occur. The interior of the mastoid process contains one large opening, the antrum, with numerous communicating air-cells, and all lined with an extension of the tympanic mucous membrane. Inflammation of the mastoid process, as a rule, is an extension of inflammation from the middle ear. The cause will be found in an obstruction to the free escape of the purulent products from the antrum out through the middle ear. It is also found that in a great number of cases of purulent middle-ear inflammation the air-cells are closed by a process of sclerosis. There are two forms of mastoid disease—1, periostitis of the bone; 2, inflammation of the mucous membrane of the mastoid cells.

1. Periostitis of the Mastoid Bone is caused either by external injuries, or more frequently by inflammation extending from the mastoid cells outwardly to the periosteum.

SYMPTOMS.—Pain, severe in character, also fever. Redness over the mastoid and great sensibility to the touch, followed by marked swelling, which may extend far down the neck, involving the lymphatic glands. Later, pus will be found between the periosteum and bone, and in a few cases caries of the bone.

2. Inflammation of the Mucous Membrane of the Mastoid Cells is caused generally by extension of inflammation from the middle-ear cavity, either of a catarrhal or purulent character, causing the cell-cavities to quickly fill up with the inflammatory products which escape through the antrum and middle-ear cavity into the external canal. If this way is closed, the fluids accumulate in the mastoid cells and form conditions favorable to involvement of the internal organs.

SYMPTOMS.—Severe pain, tenderness, and redness of skin over mastoid, but not the marked swelling that is found in periostitis. During such an inflammation facial paralysis may develop, showing that the inflammation has extended into the bone itself. Delirium is occasionally met with, probably due to a more or less circumscribed meningitis; coma is also occasionally noted, caused by effusion into the lateral ventricles. In many cases of antrum inflammation there is a marked swelling of the upper and posterior cutaneous covering of the osseous part of the external canal, making it a valuable symptom in determining the degree of the inflammatory action.

Caries and necrosis of the mastoid bone are resultants of the above-described conditions, and are especially found in early childhood, and generally caused by retention of pus in the mastoid cells and breaking down of their walls. This process can be limited to the cell portion of the bone or can also involve the cortex, with formation of an external fistulous opening.

TREATMENT.—Use of heat and moisture, either by hot-water fomentations or warm poultices, like flaxseed, over the entire temporal region of the head on which the diseased mastoid is located. The flaxseed poultice is to be covered with oil silk and changed as often as needful to keep it warm. The use of leeches to the mastoid is indicated by tenderness of the part to the touch, with heat and swelling of the tissue covering the bone. Two or three foreign leeches can be used, and if the abstraction of more blood is desired the after-bleeding is to be encouraged by warm moist applications. If the disease advances notwithstanding this treatment, an opening down to the bone is indicated. The incision is usually described as the Wilde incision. The length of the cut is to be from a half to one inch, down to the bone, the point of the knife entering the skin on a level with the upper wall of the auditory canal, about half an inch behind the auricle. Occasionally the posterior auricular artery is cut, but hemorrhage is readily controlled by pressure over the artery. During the entire treatment the external auditory canal is to be cleansed from time to time of the purulent secretions, so as to facilitate the dis_ charge of pent-up fluids from the middle ear and antrum. Also the condition of the pharynx is to be noted, and treated if needful. Finally, if all these measures fail to relieve, and the patient shows signs of meningeal or brain involvement, together with marked redness, tenderness, and swelling over the mastoid bone, showing that pus is being retained in the mastoid cells, there only remains the making of an opening into the mastoid process and antrum by means of a bone-drill or gouge. This is best done by a free vertical incision through the skin and periosteum covering the mastoid process. Examine then the bone, and a fistulous opening may be found which can be enlarged by a probe, and so allow the free escape of pus. If such does not exist, apply a drill to the bone at a point·a quarter of an inch posterior to the external canal and just below a horizontal line drawn tangent to its upper wall. The instrument is to have a direction inward, upward, and slightly forward. The depth to which it should penetrate varies : usually cell-structure is reached at a slight depth, when the drill should be withdrawn. If sclerosis of bone exists, it will be necessary to go deeper, but never more than three_ quarters of an inch, or about 20 millimeters. This is Buck's rule. Schwarze says, never go deeper than 25 millimeters, otherwise there is risk of plunging the drill into the labyrinth. Also, during the drilling process Buck recommends keeping the fore finger of the operating hand constantly pressed against the neighboring bone, so as by counter-pressure to reduce to a minimum the risk of wounding the lateral sinus if it should lie in an abnormal position in the path of the drill. After-treatment consists in keeping the canal open by gentle washing. The use of a bone- gouge is preferred by some to the drill, as being a less dangerous instrument.

Diseases of the Internal Ear.

ANATOMY.—The internal ear consists of a central cavity, from one end of which arise the semicircular canals, and from the other the cochlea. The interior of these contains the membranous portion and fluids of the internal ear. The cochlea contains the most important part—namely, the terminal endings of the auditory nerve. Sound-vibrations pass through the external canal and strike against the tympanic membrane, throwing it into vibration. The vibrations of this membrane are carried across the middle ear by the chain of small bones to the membrane closing the foramen ovale of the internal ear, throwing this and the labyrinthine fluid also into vibration, and these latter vibrations, impinging on the terminal endings of the auditory nerve in a way as yet unknown, produce sound.

Vessels of the Labyrinth.—The labyrinth obtains its blood partly from the arteria auditiva interna, a branch from the basilar artery which comes from the vertebral, and partly through vessels communicating with the middle ear viâ the round and oval windows, and through others passing through the long walls themselves. The arteria auditiva interna divides in the internal meatus into a vestibular and cochlear branch. The former is distributed to the soft structures of the vestibule and semicircular canals. The cochlear branch is distributed to the modiolus and layers of the lamina spiralis. The venæ auditivæ internæ empty into the inferior petrosal sinus or the lateral sinus; other branches empty into the superior petrosal sinus.

The auditory nerve or portio mollis of the seventh nerve arises by two roots in the medulla oblongata. One ganglionic nucleus of origin is in the floor of the fourth ventricle, the other is in the crus cerebelli ad medullam (Stieda). The nerve winds around the restiform body, and passes into the meatus auditorius internus, and finally divides into a vestibular and cochlear branch. The vestibular branch divides into three branches: the superior is distributed to the utricle and ampullæ of the superior vertical and horizontal semicircular canals; the middle to the sacculis, and the inferior to the ampulla of the inferior vertical semicircular canal. The cochlear branch enters the modiolus and breaks up into smaller branches, which radiate fan-shaped into the lamina spiralis, and are then distributed between the two plates of the lamina spiralis through all its turns.

TINNITUS AURIUM.—It may be assumed that the normal ear is filled with continuous sound. The blood flowing through the large arteries and veins in close proximity to it (such as the carotid arteries and jugular vein), as well as the blood flowing through the vessels of the internal ear, will give rise to sound by throwing into vibration the soft tissues surrounding them, including also the walls of the vessels themselves. This motion is sufficient to excite the auditory nerve-elements by causing vibrations of the intra-labyrinthine fluids, and so produce sound; which, being a normal condition, and one to which the ear is accustomed, will remain unnoticed.[1]

The arterial system of the body throws the neighboring tissue into vibration, but this is not recognized unless our attention is particularly directed to it; or, in other words, the entire body is filled with movement as a normal condition, and therefore attracts no attention. But let this movement be increased—for instance, by violent muscular exertion, increasing the arterial action—or lessened, as in syncope, and at once an abnormal condition draws our attention to it.

In the same way the ear is filled with continuous sound as a normal condition, and therefore it is not perceived, these sound-vibrations escaping out through the middle ear and external canal. This can be readily proved. Let the external auditory canal be obstructed artificially, either by the finger or by a cork. At once a tidal tinnitus, so called, is produced, this being caused by the normal sound-vibrations being impeded in their outward passage and being thrown back again to impress the nerve-elements for a second time. This, being an abnormal condition, is at once recognized.

Different Varieties of Tinnitus Aurium.—I. Tinnitus caused by obstruction of the normal sound-vibrations in their outward passage through the middle ear and external canal; tidal tinnitus, so called from a resemblance to the noise of the ocean. Such obstructions may exist in the middle-ear

---

[1] To Theobald we are indebted for the vascular theory of sound.

cavity, as thickening of the soft tissues of the middle ear, exudations and adhesions, as found in chronic catarrh, or in the external canal, as impacted cerumen, a swollen canal, etc. The effect of such obstruction would be to interrupt the normal sound-vibrations and cause them to be reflected back again to impress for a second time the auditory nerve-elements, causing an abnormal and therefore recognized condition. This is the most frequent variety of tinnitus, and for the reason that it is produced by the more ordinary ear diseases.

II. Tinnitus caused by abnormal sound-vibrations produced either by increase or by decrease of intra-labyrinthine pressure. In a normal condition the auditory nerve-elements are subjected to a given intra-labyrinthine pressure; now, if this pressure be altered (either by being increased or diminished) an abnormal condition ensues, and is noted as such.

a. Tinnitus produced by increased intra-labyrinthine pressure may be caused by increase of the intra-labyrinthine fluids (by effusions, hemorrhages, etc., as in Menière's disease), or can be caused by increase in the amount of blood flowing through the arteries and veins of the internal ear. In either case there will result an increase of pressure that is exerted on the auditory nerve-elements. Also, another result of such increase of pressure on the arteries of the labyrinth would be to throw them into more active pulsation, and so cause greater movement on the intra-labyrinthine fluids. These abnormal vibrations impinging on the auditory nerve-endings would be noticed as such, and give rise to tinnitus of a pulsating character corresponding to the movements of the pulsating vessels. Such a condition is noticed in an eyeball afflicted by glaucoma, or can be artificially produced by finger-pressure on a normal eye. The veins of the retina will be first thrown into movement, and as the pressure increases the arteries will show marked pulsation. Why should not a similar set of conditions in the internal ear produce similar results?

b. Tinnitus produced by a lessened intra-labyrinthine pressure may be caused either by loss of intra-labyrinthine fluid or by a lessened blood-supply to the internal ear. The latter cause being the most frequent, a familiar example of this would be the tinnitus experienced by a fainting person, a common sensation being a swimming head accompanied with strange whizzing noises in the ears. The tinnitus of anæmia is of this class, and frequently of the pulsating variety. Another explanation might be given: an anæmic heart murmur might be conveyed along the blood-vessels as through a speaking-tube, and in that way impress the auditory nerve. In this variety of tinnitus it is supposed that the sound-conducting apparatus of the middle and external ear is normal; if any obstruction exists, it would cause increase of tinnitus of this variety.

III. Tinnitus caused by a diseased condition of the auditory nerve, either in the part lying between the internal ear and brain or in the brain-centre itself — pure subjective tinnitus. Here we enter upon a subject obscure from the fact that so little pathological research has been made in this direction; but, reasoning from analogy, why cannot the auditory nerve be subject to as many diseased conditions as the optic nerve, where the ophthalmoscope has clearly shown the existence of neuritis, atrophy, and many other pathological changes, caused, it may be, by disease of the retina, or it may exist as an inflammation of the nerve itself exterior to the eyeball, or it may be due to a brain tumor pressing on the optic nerve or optic tracts, also basilar meningitis? Gummata, osseous growths, etc. have in turn caused optic neuritis; finally, lesions at the optic nerve-endings in the brain itself have caused well-defined pathological changes in the optic nerve, which by the aid of the ophthalmoscope are recognized. Now, if these changes exist in the optic nerve, why may not the same conditions be present in connection with the auditory nerve, although from its anatomical location they are not capable of demonstration, as in the case of the optic nerve? And, as in the latter phosphene symptoms are common, due to nerve-irritation, so in irritation of the auditory nerve tinnitus would be developed, but of a subjective character. (In this connection it is not out of place to remark that in obscure internal ear disease examination of the optic nerve will often give valuable information toward clearing up the ear complication.) This variety of tinnitus may in some cases be due to a reflex nerve-irritation.

Finally, tinnitus may be noticed in cases of inflammation of the middle ear where fluid has collected, and is caused by the bursting of air-bubbles in their passage through this fluid, the air gaining access to the middle ear by way of the Eustachian tube. Tinnitus so produced resembles a bubbling or crackling sound. Hinton draws attention to certain cases where the tympanic membrane has lost its normal elasticity and become stiff, any movement of such a membrane causing a crackling sound. Also, there are some cases of tinnitus produced by foreign bodies being deposited on the tympanic membrane, such as cerumen, pieces of hair, etc., making a rustling or rasping noise.

Tinnitus produced by abnormal contractions of the tensor tympani or stapedius muscles has been thought to exist. Tinnitus may be intermittent or continuous. It also has an endless variety of sound, from one almost unrecognizable to a roar so loud as to render the patient nearly distracted.

Location of the Tinnitus.—Those varieties due to a diseased external or middle ear locate the sound, as a rule, in the ear itself. Subjective tinnitus is often located in the frontal and occipital regions; often also in the ear itself. It is also to be noted that marked tinnitus may be associated with a low degree of deafness, and the converse is true: slight tinnitus may be associated with a high degree of deafness.

PROGNOSIS.—The removal of tinnitus depends entirely upon the cause of it and the possibility of its removal. Continuous tinnitus is always to be regarded as a more pronounced symptom than the intermittent form.

The TREATMENT will be directed to the removal of the cause. If the disease is located in the external canal or middle ear, or in a diseased condition of the naso-pharynx, these irritating causes should be removed by treatment already laid down in previous pages. The treatment of subjective tinnitus will be guided by the same principles. Determine the cause and seek for its removal. As to whether any particular drugs exist peculiarly adapted to the removal of tinnitus, I would say that in tinnitus of a subjective character or due to nerve-irritation the bromides are indicated in appropriate doses. Inflation of the middle ear with air impregnated with ether (a few drops of ether dropped into a Politzer air-bag and the inflation made by the Pollitzer method), at intervals of three or four days, in some cases proves of benefit.

Deafness after Cerebro-Spinal Meningitis, Scarlet Fever, Mumps, etc.

This opens up a chapter in which our knowledge derived from post-mortem examination is very limited. In a given number of such cases the inflammation probably extends from the brain to the labyrinth; in others the changes that are found exist chiefly in the middle ear, so that it must be supposed that the inflammation in such cases has originated in the middle ear, and has secondarily invaded the labyrinth. In some cases, such as deafness after mumps, Toynbee is of the opinion that the peculiar poison of that disease affects the nervous apparatus of the ear, as the deafness comes on suddenly, and is usually complete, without evidence of disease in any other part of the ear. In this class of cases the prominent symptoms are deafness—which is total—and staggering gait, with vertigo. This symptom may last many weeks, and then cease. As a rule, examination of the tympanic membrane is negative, and the seat of disease is to be sought for in the labyrinth, whether it may be an inflammation of the soft structures or an effusion, causing increased intra-labyrinthine pressure. In many cases the suddenness of the attack would point to an effusion as the more probable cause.

Brunner in a comparison of five cases of deafness after mumps[1] gives the following symptoms and course of the disease: 1. The nervous deafness after mumps can be one-sided or double-sided, the former being more frequent. 2. It is complete, and, according to past experience, incurable. 3. It develops rapidly, with vertigo and subjective noises, the later symptom lasting a long time. 4. There is little or no fever. 5. Pain is never or very seldom present. 6. Consciousness is not lost; excessive vertigo a prominent symptom. 7. It happens both in children and adults.

Menière's Disease.

A. Guye of Amsterdam has published a very full summary of the history of this disease.[2] The following is extracted from it: Under the head of Menière's disease is included those cases of inflammatory processes in the semicircular canals or in the middle ear producing vertigo, which is either continuous, or caused by normal movements of the head, or appearing only at intervals of weeks or months; also, that this disease is of a secondary nature, and is due to inflammatory processes in the tympanum or antrum. In typical cases the vertigo is accompanied by sensations of rotation: first a sense of rotation about a vertical axis and toward the affected side; this is followed by a sensation of rotation about a transverse axis forward and backward. The vertigo then becomes complete, and is followed by fainting, with or without loss of consciousness and vomiting. The attack in some cases may last for a few minutes to a half hour; in others every movement will tend to produce vertigo for

[1] *Archiv Otology*, vol. xi., No. 2, p. 103. [2] *Ibid.*, vol. ix., No. 3.

several days. In chronic cases the feeling of vertigo to a slight degree persists between the attacks. Guye considers the causes of middle-ear catarrh as the factors most likely to cause Menière's disease. Syphilis is also noted in some cases.

TREATMENT.—In some cases an alterative treatment is most serviceable, such as iodide of potassium, also the bromide of potassium; quinine is also by some recommended. The use of alcohol and tobacco is to be forbidden.

The disease known as boiler-makers' deafness, because generally found among men laboring in machine-shops, where they are subjected to loud noises connected with the work they are engaged on, is thought to be due to a paralysis of the terminal endings of the auditory nerve due to concussion. The middle ear sometimes shows some thickening of the tympanic membrane. Treatment is without avail.

In internal-ear diseases a few common symptoms can be noted. All cases show deafness, and in most of them of an absolute degree. And here is where the tuning-fork proves a valuable aid in diagnosis of deafness due to middle-ear disease, in which cases the tuning-fork is heard best on the deaf side, and to deafness due to internal-ear disease, where the tuning-fork is heard the least on the deaf side. Vertigo and a staggering gait are quite common symptoms, probably due to irritation of the semicircular canals. Prognosis as a rule is bad, as far as recovery is concerned, and an alterative treatment is often indicated. Electricity, I would state, in my experience has not proved to be of any avail.

Deaf-Mutism

may be either congenital or acquired. Two-thirds of all cases will come under the first class, and often depend upon a mal-development of some part of the central nervous system or the ear itself, or may be due to intra-uterine disease of the ear. There is a strong tendency for this disease to be inherited, and particularly in children where there exists a blood-relationship between the parents. The acquired cases may arise from defects in the central nervous system or in the internal ear, or may be due to diseases affecting the middle ear, such as purulent inflammation; and this latter cause is to be noted, as no doubt proper treatment of the middle-ear disease in many cases would have prevented such a result.

All deaf cases become mute, unless the disease has occurred in adult life, when the patient has already acquired the power of language. A deaf-mute does not speak, because he cannot hear, and therefore speech is an unknown quantity.

The TREATMENT would consist in treating any middle-ear disease that might exist, such as the sequelæ of purulent inflammation, and the instruction of the patient in acquiring the power of intercommunication either by the methods long employed of finger-reading, or, much better, by the lip method, so called, where the power of speech is given to the patient. Such cases should attend schools where such instruction is given, commencing at five years of age, and many cases now attest the value of the latter method of instruction.

DIFFERENT METHODS OF DETECTING FEIGNED DEAFNESS.—The

Moos Method.—Stop the external canal of the sound ear with a cork; place a vibrating tuning-fork on the head. If the person under examination declares that he does not hear the fork with either ear, he is feigning deafness, as it would be heard well by the sound ear.

The Urbantschitsch method makes use of the human voice. First determine that good hearing power exists in the sound ear; then shut the external canal of this ear with a cork and address the individual with a few loudly-spoken words. If he denies hearing at all, he is feigning, as a good hearing ear, by simple closure of the external canal, will be still able to hear loudly-spoken words.

Another method is to determine the distance at which the person can hear certain words and repeat them correctly. Then have the patient close the eyes and let the examiner try by lengthening and shortening the distance, and note the result. Often he will hear and repeat words spoken at long distances, and apparently not be able to repeat words spoken at short distances.

Müller's Method.—Speak into the sound ear through a tube or paper roll different words as softly and quickly as the examined person can repeat; then let a second examiner repeat the same in the deaf ear. Of course nothing will be heard by the person feigning. Then let the first examiner repeat his performance; the feigner will quickly repeat after him. Suddenly begins the second examiner to softly and quickly speak in the deaf ear, but choosing different words from the first examiner. A really one-sided deaf person will repeat the words spoken into the sound ear only, while the feigner will be in doubt, and will not be able to separate the words heard by both ears, so as only to repeat the words heard by the sound ear.

INDEX TO VOLUME IV.

END OF VOLUME IV.

Lightning Source UK Ltd.
Milton Keynes UK
UKHW012138180219
337529UK00012B/1351/P